CRAIG E. GREENE, DVM, MS

Professor, Department of Small Animal Medicine
College of Veterinary Medicine
University of Georgia
Athens, Georgia

INFECTIOUS DISEASES OF THE DOG AND CAT

W.B. SAUNDERS COMPANY
A Division of Harcourt Brace & Company

Philadelphia   London   Toronto   Montreal   Sydney   Tokyo

W.B. SAUNDERS COMPANY
A Division of
Harcourt Brace & Company

The Curtis Center
Independence Square West
Philadelphia, Pennsylvania 19106

Library of Congress Cataloging-in-Publication Data

Greene, Craig E.

Infectious Diseases of the Dog and Cat / Craig E. Greene.

p. cm.

ISBN 0–7216–2339–5

1. Dogs—Infections.   2. Cats—Infections.   I. Title.

SF991.G743   1990
636.7′089′69—dc20   89–10834

Editor: Linda E. Mills
Designer: W. B. Saunders Staff
Production Manager: Bill Preston
Manuscript Editors: Lorraine Zawodny and Mary Prescott
Illustration Coordinator: Walt Verbitski

Infectious Diseases of the Dog and Cat   ISBN 0–7216–2339–5

Printed in the United States of America.

Last digit is the print number: 9   8   7   6   5   4

This book is dedicated

to Jeanne and Casey, who made a
personal sacrifice while it was
being written;

to the contributors, whose time
and effort made it possible;

and to people whose research
and publications have advanced
our understanding of canine and
feline infections.

CONTRIBUTORS

Lawrence W. Anson, DVM, Diplomate, ACVS
Assistant Professor, Department of Veterinary Clinical Sciences, College of Veterinary Medicine, The Ohio State University, Columbus, OH
MUSCULOSKELETAL INFECTIONS

Max J. Appel, DVM, PhD
Professor of Virology, New York State College of Veterinary Medicine, Cornell University, Ithaca, NY
CANINE DISTEMPER

Jeffrey E. Barlough, DVM, PhD, Diplomate, ACVM
Assistant Professor, Department of Medicine, School of Veterinary Medicine, University of California, Davis, Davis, CA
FELINE CORONAVIRAL INFECTIONS

Stephen C. Barr, BVSc, MVS, MACVSc, PhD, Diplomate, ACVIM
Assistant Professor of Medicine, New York State College of Veterinary Medicine, Department of Clinical Sciences, Cornell University; Internist, Veterinary Teaching Hospital, New York State College of Veterinary Medicine, Cornell University, Ithaca, NY
AMERICAN TRYPANOSOMIASIS

Jeanne A. Barsanti, DVM, MS, Diplomate, ACVIM
Professor, Department of Small Animal Medicine, College of Veterinary Medicine, University of Georgia; Internist, University of Georgia Veterinary Small Animal Teaching Hospital, College of Veterinary Medicine, University of Georgia, Athens, GA
GENITOURINARY INFECTIONS; BOTULISM; CRYPTOCOCCOSIS; COCCIDIOIDOMYCOSIS

Rudy W. Bauer, DVM
Athens Veterinary Diagnostic Laboratory, Department of Veterinary Pathology, College of Veterinary Medicine, University of Georgia, Athens, GA
ACANTHAMEBIASIS

Derrick Baxby, PhD, MRC Path.
Senior Lecturer, Department of Medical Microbiology, University of Liverpool, Liverpool, UK
FELINE COWPOX VIRUS INFECTION

Malcolm Bennett, BVSc, PhD, MRCVS
Research Fellow, Departments of Veterinary Clinical Science and Veterinary Pathology, University of Liverpool Veterinary Field Station, "Leahurst," Neston, Wirral, UK
FELINE COWPOX VIRUS INFECTION

Ernst L. Biberstein, DVM, PhD, Diplomate, ACVM
Professor of Microbiology, School of Veterinary Medicine, Microbiology Service, Veterinary Medical Teaching Hospital, University of California, Davis, Davis, CA
LABORATORY DIAGNOSIS OF FUNGAL AND ALGAL INFECTIONS

Patricia Carey Blanchard, BS, DVM, PhD, Diplomate, ACVP
Assistant Adjunct Professor, Department of Veterinary Pathology, University of California, Davis, Davis, CA; Pathologist, California Veterinary Diagnostic Laboratory System, Tulare Branch, Tulare, CA
STREPTOCOCCAL AND OTHER GRAM-POSITIVE BACTERIAL INFECTIONS

Edward B. Breitschwerdt, DVM, Diplomate, ACVIM
Professor of Medicine, Department of Companion Animal and Special Species Medicine; Internist, Veterinary Teaching Hospital, North Carolina State University, Raleigh, NC
ROCKY MOUNTAIN SPOTTED FEVER AND Q FEVER; RHINOSPORIDIOSIS; BABESIOSIS

Janet P. Calpin, BS
AALAS Technologist, Animal Resources, College of Veterinary Medicine, University of Georgia, Athens, GA
LABORATORY DIAGNOSIS OF PROTOZOAL INFECTIONS

Clay A. Calvert, DVM, Diplomate, ACVIM
Associate Professor, Department of Small Animal Medicine, University of Georgia, Athens, GA
CARDIOVASCULAR INFECTIONS; CANINE VIRAL PAPILLOMATOSIS

Leland E. Carmichael, DVM, PhD, Diplomate, ACVM
John M. Olin Professor of Virology, Baker Institute, New York State College of Veterinary Medicine, Cornell University, Ithaca, NY
CANINE HERPESVIRUS INFECTIONS; CANINE BRUCELLOSIS; CANINE VIRAL ENTERITIS

Sharon A. Center, DVM, Diplomate, ACVIM
Associate Professor, New York State College of Veterinary Medicine, Cornell University, Ithaca, NY
HEPATOBILIARY INFECTIONS

Francis W. Chandler, DVM, PhD, Diplomate, ACVP
Professor of Pathology, Department of Pathology, Medical College of Georgia; Director, Barton Immunopathology Laboratory, Medical College of Georgia Hospital and Clinics
CANDIDIASIS; TRICHOSPOROSIS; PNEUMOCYSTOSIS

Susan M. Cotter, DVM, Diplomate, ACVIM (and Oncology)
Associate Professor of Medicine, School of Veterinary Medicine, Tufts University, North Grafton, MA
FELINE VIRAL NEOPLASIA

Hollis Utah Cox, DVM, PhD, Diplomate, ACVM
Professor of Veterinary Bacteriology, Department of Veterinary Microbiology and Parasitology, School of Veterinary Medicine; Chief, Diagnostic Microbiology and Parasitology, Veterinary Teaching Hospital and Clinics, School of Veterinary Medicine, Louisiana State University, Baton Rouge, LA
STAPHYLOCOCCAL INFECTIONS

Thomas M. Craig, DVM, PhD
Professor, Department of Veterinary Microbiology and Parasitology, College of Veterinary Medicine; Clinical Parasitologist, Veterinary Teaching Hospital, Texas A&M University, College Station, TX
HEPATOZOONOSIS

Michael J. Day, BSc, BVMS (Hons), PhD, MRCVS, MASM
Postdoctoral Research Fellow, MRC Cellular Immunology Unit, Sir William Dunn School of Pathology, University of Oxford, Oxford, UK
RHINOSPORIDIOSIS; ASPERGILLOSIS AND PENICILLIOSIS

Steven W. Dow, Diplomate, ACVIM
NIH Fellow, Feline Retrovirus Laboratory, Department of Pathology, Colorado State University, Fort Collins, CO
ANAEROBIC INFECTIONS; CARDIOVASCULAR INFECTIONS

David W. Dreesen, DVM, MPVM, Diplomate, ACVPM
Associate Professor of Medical Microbiology, College of Veterinary Medicine, University of Georgia, Athens, GA
RABIES

J.P. Dubey, MVSc, PhD
Zoonotic Diseases Laboratory, Livestock & Poultry Sciences Institute, United States Department of Agriculture, Beltsville, MD
TOXOPLASMOSIS AND NEOSPOROSIS; ENTERIC COCCIDIOSIS

Robert W. Dunstan, DVM, MS, Diplomate, ACVP
Associate Professor, Department of Pathology, College of Veterinary Medicine, Michigan State University, East Lansing, MI
SPOROTRICHOSIS

Charles K. English, MS; Lt., MSc, USN
Department of Pathology, Georgetown University Schools of Medicine and Dentistry, Washington, DC
CAT SCRATCH DISEASE

James F. Evermann, MS, PhD
Professor, Clinical Virology, College of Veterinary Medicine, Washington State University, Pullman, WA
LABORATORY DIAGNOSIS OF VIRAL AND RICKETTSIAL INFECTIONS

William R. Fenner, DVM, Diplomate, ACVIM (Neurology)
Associate Professor, Department of Veterinary Clinical Sciences, College of Veterinary Medicine, The Ohio State University; Staff Neurologist, Veterinary Teaching Hospital, College of Veterinary Medicine, The Ohio State University, Columbus, OH
BACTERIAL INFECTIONS OF THE CENTRAL NERVOUS SYSTEM

Duncan C. Ferguson, VMD, PhD, Diplomate, ACVIM
Associate Professor of Physiology and Pharmacology and of Small Animal Medicine, College of Veterinary Medicine, University of Georgia, Athens, GA
ANTIBACTERIAL CHEMOTHERAPY

Carol S. Foil, MS, DVM, Diplomate, ACVD
Associate Professor, School of Veterinary Medicine, Department of Veterinary Clinical Sciences, Louisiana State University; Dermatologist, Veterinary Teaching Hospital and Clinics, Louisiana State University, Baton Rouge, LA
DERMATOPHYTOSIS; MISCELLANEOUS FUNGAL INFECTIONS

Richard B. Ford, DVM, MS, Diplomate, ACVIM
Associate Professor of Medicine, College of Veterinary Medicine, North Carolina State University, Raleigh, NC
CANINE INFECTIOUS TRACHEOBRONCHITIS

William J. Foreyt, PhD
Associate Professor, College of Veterinary Medicine, Washington State University, Pullman, WA
SALMON POISONING DISEASE

S. Dru Forrester, DVM, MS
Lecturer, Department of Small Animal Medicine and Surgery, Texas A&M University, College of Veterinary Medicine; Veterinary Clinical Associate, Veterinary Teaching Hospital, College of Veterinary Medicine, Texas A&M University, College Station, TX
CANINE EHRLICHIOSIS

James G. Fox, DVM, MS
Professor and Director, Division of Comparative Medicine, Massachusetts Institute of Technology, Cambridge, MA; Adjunct Professor of Comparative Medicine, Tufts University School of Veterinary Medicine, North Grafton, MA
ENTERIC AND OTHER BACTERIAL INFECTIONS

Rosalind M. Gaskell, BVSc, PhD, MRCVS
Senior Research Fellow, Department of Veterinary Pathology, University of Liverpool Veterinary Field Station, "Leahurst," Neston, Wirral, UK
FELINE COWPOX VIRUS INFECTION

Peter W. Gasper, DVM, PhD
Assistant Professor of Hematopathology, College of Veterinary Medicine and Biomedical Sciences, Colorado State University, Fort Collins, CO
PLAGUE

Ellie J. C. Goldstein, MD
Clinical Professor of Medicine, University of California, Los Angeles, School of Medicine, Los Angeles, CA; Director, R. M. Alden Research Laboratory, Santa Monica Hospital Medical Center, Santa Monica, CA
BITE AND SCRATCH INFECTIONS

John R. Gorham, DVM, PhD, Diplomate, ACVM, ACLAM
Research Leader, Animal Disease Research Unit, College of Veterinary Medicine, Washington State University, Pullman, WA
SALMON POISONING DISEASE

Russell T. Greene, DVM, PhD, Diplomate, ACVIM, ACVM
Instructor, Clinical Microbiology, College of Veterinary Medicine, North Carolina State University, Raleigh, NC
LYME BORRELIOSIS

Craig E. Griffin, DVM, Diplomate, ACVD
Clinical Instructor, School of Medicine, University of California, Irvine, Irvine, CA; Director, Animal Dermatology Clinics, Garden Grove and San Diego, CA
INTEGUMENTARY INFECTIONS

David A. Harbour, BSc, PhD
Lecturer in Veterinary Virology, University of Bristol Veterinary School, Bristol, UK
FELINE ASTROVIRAL INFECTIONS

Elizabeth M. Hardie, DVM, PhD, Diplomate, ACVS
Assistant Professor of Surgery, College of Veterinary Medicine, North Carolina State University, Raleigh, NC
ENDOTOXEMIA; ACTINOMYCOSIS AND NOCARDIOSIS

Lenn R. Harrison, VMD, Diplomate, ACVP
Veterinary Pathologist, Veterinary Diagnostic and Investigational Laboratory, University of Georgia, Tifton, GA
ACANTHAMEBIASIS

John W. Harvey, DVM, PhD, Diplomate, ACVP
Professor, Department of Physiological Sciences, College of Veterinary Medicine, University of Florida; Chief, Clinical Pathology Service, Veterinary Medical Teaching Hospital, College of Veterinary Medicine, University of Florida, Gainesville, FL
CANINE EHRLICHIOSIS; HAEMOBARTONELLOSIS

Johnny D. Hoskins, DVM, PhD, Diplomate, ACVIM
Professor, Department of Veterinary Clinical Sciences, School of Veterinary Medicine, Louisiana State University; Veterinary Internist, Veterinary Teaching Hospital and Clinics, Louisiana State University, Baton Rouge, LA
STAPHYLOCOCCAL INFECTIONS

Peter J. Ihrke, VMD, Diplomate, ACVD
Professor of Dermatology, Department of Medicine, School of Veterinary Medicine, University of California, Davis; Chief of Service, Dermatology, Veterinary Medical Teaching Hospital, School of Veterinary Medicine, University of California, Davis, Davis, CA
INTEGUMENTARY INFECTIONS

Spencer S. Jang, BA
Clinical Laboratory Technologist Supervisor, Microbiology Service, Veterinary Medical Teaching Hospital, University of California, Davis, CA
LABORATORY DIAGNOSIS OF FUNGAL AND ALGAL INFECTIONS

Kenneth L. Jeffery, DVM
Mesa Veterinary Hospital, Ltd., Mesa, AZ
COCCIDIOIDOMYCOSIS

Cheri A. Johnson, DVM, MS, Diplomate, ACVIM (Internal Medicine)
Associate Professor, Small Animal Clinical Sciences, College of Veterinary Medicine, Michigan State University; Chief of Medicine, Veterinary Teaching Hospital, Michigan State University, East Lansing, MI
GENITOURINARY INFECTIONS

Boyd R. Jones
Reader, Small Animal Medicine, Massey University; Head, Small Animal Clinic and Hospital, Massey University, Palmerston North, New Zealand
ENTERIC AND OTHER BACTERIAL INFECTIONS

Robert L. Jones, DVM, PhD, Diplomate, ACVM
Associate Professor, Department of Microbiology, College of Veterinary Medicine and Biomedical Sciences, Colorado State University; Head, Bacteriology Section, Diagnostic Laboratory, Colorado State University, Fort Collins, CO
LABORATORY DIAGNOSIS OF BACTERIAL INFECTIONS

Arnold F. Kaufmann, DVM, MS
Chief, Bacterial Zoonoses Activity, Division of Bacterial Diseases, Center for Infectious Diseases, Centers for Disease Control, Atlanta, GA
TULAREMIA

Ann B. Kier, DVM, PhD, Diplomate, ACLAM
Associate Professor, Departments of Pathology and Laboratory Animal Medicine, University of Cincinnati Medical Center, Cincinnati, OH
CYTAUXZOONOSIS

Carl E. Kirkpatrick, DVM, PhD*
Formerly, Assistant Professor, Department of Pathobiology, College of Veterinary Medicine, University of Illinois, Urbana, IL
ENTERIC PROTOZOAL INFECTIONS

Joe N. Kornegay, DVM, PhD, Diplomate, ACVIM
Professor of Neurology, College of Veterinary Medicine; North Carolina State University; Staff Neurologist and Neurosurgeon, Veterinary Teaching Hospital, College of Veterinary Medicine, North Carolina State University, Raleigh, NC
MUSCULOSKELETAL INFECTIONS

Gail A. Kunkle, DVM, Diplomate, ACVD
Associate Professor, College of Veterinary Medicine, University of Florida; Dermatology Service Chief, University of Florida Veterinary Medical Teaching Hospital, Gainesville, FL
MYCOBACTERIAL INFECTIONS

Michael R. Lappin, DVM, PhD, Diplomate, ACVIM
Assistant Professor, Department of Clinical Sciences, College of Veterinary Medicine and Biomedical Sciences, Colorado State University, Fort Collins, CO
TOXOPLASMOSIS AND NEOSPOROSIS; LABORATORY DIAGNOSIS OF PROTOZOAL INFECTIONS

*Deceased

Alfred M. Legendre, DVM, MS, Diplomate, ACVIM
Professor of Medicine, College of Veterinary Medicine, University of Tennessee; Internist, Veterinary Teaching Hospital, University of Tennessee, Knoxville, TN
BLASTOMYCOSIS

Randall Lockwood, PhD
Humane Society of the United States, Washington, DC
BITE AND SCRATCH INFECTIONS

Dennis W. Macy, DVM, Diplomate, ACVIM
Associate Professor of Medicine, College of Veterinary Medicine and Biomedical Sciences, Colorado State University, Fort Collins, CO
PLAGUE

Andrew M. Margileth, MD
Professor, Pediatrics, Department of Pediatrics, Uniformed Services University of the Health Sciences, F. Edward Hebert School of Medicine; Consultant, Department of Pediatrics, Walter Reed Army Medical Center, Bethesda Naval Hospital, Washington, DC
CAT SCRATCH DISEASE

Charles L. Martin, BS, DVM, MS, Diplomate, ACVO
Professor, Department of Small Animal Medicine, College of Veterinary Medicine, University of Georgia; Director, Veterinary Teaching Hospital, University of Georgia, Athens, GA
OCULAR INFECTIONS

Linda Medleau, DVM, MS, Diplomate, ACVD
Associate Professor, Department of Small Animal Medicine, College of Veterinary Medicine, University of Georgia; Dermatologist, Veterinary Medical Teaching Hospital, College of Veterinary Medicine, University of Georgia, Athens, GA
CRYPTOCOCCOSIS

V. Pang, DVM, PhD
Pig Research Institute of Taiwan, Miaoli, Taiwan, Republic of China
ENCEPHALITOZOONOSIS

Roy V.H. Pollock, DVM, PhD
Director of Veterinary Support and Affairs, Norden Laboratories, Lincoln, NE
CANINE VIRAL ENTERITIS

R. Charles Povey, BVSc, PhD, FRCVS
President, Langford, Inc., Guelph, Ontario, Canada
FELINE RESPIRATORY DISEASES

Annie K. Prestwood, DVM, PhD
Professor, Department of Parasitology, College of Veterinary Medicine, University of Georgia, Athens, GA
LABORATORY DIAGNOSIS OF PROTOZOAL INFECTIONS; CRYPTOSPORIDIOSIS

Hugh W. Reid, BVM and S, PhD, MRCVS, Diplomate, TVM
Principal Veterinary Research Officer, Moredun Research Institute, Edinburgh, UK
ARBOVIRAL INFECTIONS

S. Rosendal, DVM, PhD
Professor, Department of Veterinary Microbiology and Immunology, Ontario Veterinary College, University of Guelph; Associate Supervisor of the Clinical Microbiology Laboratory of the Veterinary Teaching Hospital of the Ontario Veterinary College, University of Guelph, Guelph, Ontario, Canada
MYCOPLASMAL INFECTIONS

Edmund J. Rosser, Jr., DVM, Diplomate, ACVD
Assistant Professor of Dermatology, Department of Small Animal Clinical Sciences, Veterinary Clinical Center, College of Veterinary Medicine, Michigan State University, East Lansing, MI
SPOROTRICHOSIS

Philip Roudebush, DVM, Diplomate, ACVIM
Associate Professor and Chairman, Department of Clinical Sciences, College of Veterinary Medicine, Mississippi State University, Mississippi State, MS
BACTERIAL INFECTIONS OF THE RESPIRATORY SYSTEM

Fredric W. Scott, DVM, PhD
Professor of Virology, College of Veterinary Medicine, Cornell University, Ithaca, NY
FELINE PANLEUKOPENIA

J. A. Shadduck, DVM, PhD, Diplomate, ACVP
Texas A&M University College of Veterinary Medicine, College Station, TX
ENCEPHALITOZOONOSIS

N. J. H. Sharp, BVM, MVM, MRCVS, Diplomate, ACVS
Research Assistant, College of Veterinary Medicine, North Carolina State University, Raleigh, NC
ASPERGILLOSIS AND PENICILLIOSIS

Emmett B. Shotts, Jr., PhD
Professor of Medical Microbiology, College of Veterinary Medicine, University of Georgia, Athens, GA
LEPTOSPIROSIS

Robbert J. Slappendel, DVM, PhD
Associate Professor of Internal Medicine, Department of Small Animal Medicine, Faculty of Veterinary Medicine, State University of Utrecht; Clinical Hematologist and Head of Intensive Care, University Clinic for Companion Animals, Utrecht, The Netherlands
LEISHMANIASIS

E. Elizabeth Sparger, DVM, Diplomate, ACVIM
NIH Research Fellow, Department of Medicine, School of Veterinary Medicine, University of California, Davis, Davis, CA
FELINE VIRAL NEOPLASIA

Cheryl A. Stoddart, MS, PhD
Postdoctoral Fellow, Department of Microbiology and Immunology, Stanford University School of Medicine, Stanford, CA
FELINE CORONAVIRAL INFECTIONS

J. R. Szabo, DVM, PhD, Diplomate, ACVP
Health and Environmental Sciences, Texas, Lake Jackson Research Center, The Dow Chemical Company, Freeport, TX
ENCEPHALITOZOONOSIS

Gregory C. Troy, DVM, MS, Diplomate, ACVIM
Professor, Department of Small Animal Clinical Sciences, Virginia Polytechnic Institute and State University; Hospital Director, Veterinary Teaching Hospital, Virginia-Maryland Regional College of Veterinary Medicine, Virginia Polytechnic Institute and State University, Blacksburg, VA
CANINE EHRLICHIOSIS

David E. Tyler, DVM, PhD, Diplomate, ACVP
Professor of Pathology, College of Veterinary Medicine, University of Georgia, Athens, GA
PROTOTHECOSIS

Shelly L. Vaden, DVM, Diplomate, ACVIM
Graduate Student, College of Veterinary Medicine, North Carolina State University, Raleigh, NC
CANINE INFECTIOUS TRACHEOBRONCHITIS

Marc Vandevelde, DVM, Dr. Habil
Professor and Director, Institute of Animal Neurology, School of Veterinary Medicine, University of Bern, Bern, Switzerland
PSEUDORABIES; NEUROLOGIC DISEASES OF SUSPECTED INFECTIOUS ORIGIN

Douglas J. Wear, MS, MD, Col., Marine Corps, USA
Chairman, Department of Infectious and Parasitic Diseases and Pathology, Armed Forces Institute of Pathology, Washington, DC
CAT SCRATCH DISEASE

Dennis W. Wilson, BS, MS, DVM, PhD, Diplomate, ACVP
Assistant Professor, Department of Veterinary Pathology, University of California, Davis; Pathologist, Veterinary Medical Teaching Hospital, University of California, Davis, Davis, CA
STREPTOCOCCAL AND OTHER GRAM-POSITIVE BACTERIAL INFECTIONS

Alice M. Wolf, DVM, Diplomate, ACVIM
Associate Professor, Texas A&M University College of Veterinary Medicine; Internist, Texas Veterinary Medical Center, Texas A&M University, College Station, TX
HISTOPLASMOSIS

PREFACE

This book is a sequel to the text *Clinical Microbiology and Infectious Diseases of the Dog and Cat*, which I edited in 1984. The most obvious change in this book over its predecessor is the choice of a new title instead of a second edition. This name change reflects my decision and that of the publisher to focus the book as a clinical reference tool. Our aim was to provide a complete source of information on the principles and practice of treating infectious diseases in dogs and cats for veterinary students during their clinical training and for practicing veterinarians. Institutional and research workers in animal health fields may find it similarly valuable. The basic microbiology and immunology sections from the previous book have been eliminated. These subjects have been covered elsewhere in texts devoted solely to their content. Exclusion of this material was also intended to keep the book affordable for veterinary students. Zoonotic diseases of dogs and cats are discussed in applicable chapters under the heading Public Health Considerations rather than in a tabular chapter as in the previous text. Clinical signs of the respective zoonoses in people are described so that veterinarians can be knowledgeable in alerting their clients to potential diseases they may contract from association with their dogs or cats. Human health physicians may also find this information of value.

The subject of infectious diseases is a rapidly advancing area of discovery. Despite my attempt to make the preceding text of 1984 complete and comprehensive at the time of publication, it was soon out of date. In the last six years, many new infections of dogs and cats have been recognized. Either new agents have been discovered, or known existing pathogens have now been recognized as causing disease in dogs and cats.

Diseases caused by newly discovered agents include transmissible acidophil cell hepatitis (Chapter 17), feline astroviral infection (Chapter 25), feline immunodeficiency virus infection (Chapter 26), neosporosis (Chapter 86), cutaneous coccidiosis (suspected caryosporosis), and intrahepatic biliary coccidiosis (all in Chapter 87).

Previously recognized infections that have now been established to occur in dogs or cats include Q fever (Chapter 38), Lyme borreliosis (Chapter 46), L-form infections (Chapter 50), trichosporosis (Chapter 73), öomycosis (Chapter 74), and acanthamebiasis (Chapter 85).

Diseases that were given brief mention before but now have been given expanded coverage under individual section headings include otitis externa (Chapter 5); infectious myocarditis (Chapter 6); infectious pericardial effusion (Chapter 7); pleural infections and eugonic fermenter-4 infection (Chapter 8); canine parvovirus-1 infection and canine rotaviral enteritis (Chapter 21); melioidosis and glanders (Chapter 50); groups A, B, C, G and other streptococcal infections, *Rhodococcus equi* infection of cats, listeriosis, and anthrax (Chapter 56); nasal and disseminated aspergillosis (Chapter 71); miscellaneous fungal infections (Chapter 74); pug dog encephalitis and feline poliomyelitis (Chapter 90).

Diseases that now have chapter status are feline syncytial virus infection (Chapter 28), feline paramyxoviral encephalitis (Chapter 29), feline cowpox infection (Chapter 30), enterovirus infections (Chapter 33), mumps (Chapter 34), arboviral infections (Chapter 35), chlamydiosis (Chapter 40), mycoplasmosis (Chapter 41), endotoxemia (Chapter 44), anaerobic infections (Chapter 49), dermatophilosis (Chapter 54), feline abscesses (Chapter 55), staphylococcal infections (Chapter 57), bite and scratch infections (Chapter 58), plague (Chapter 59), tularemia (Chapter 60), cat scratch disease (Chapter 61), candidiasis (Chapter 72), and cryptosporidiosis (Chapter 88).

This book has been redesigned to facilitate finding information for diagnosis and treatment of infections. Section I discusses clinical problems with infectious diseases, such as environmental control of infections, immunodeficiency disorders, and immunization. Principles of diagnosis and therapy of infections in various organ systems are described with an emphasis on infections caused by commensal or saprophytic bacteria. Each of the four remaining sections, II through V, includes current information on diseases caused by viruses, rickettsiae, and mycoplasmas; bacteria; fungi and algae; and protozoa, respectively. Each of these major sections is introduced by a chapter discussing routine diagnostic testing for the type of microorganisms covered in that section. The aim of these diagnostic chapters is to help the clinician determine indications and methods for sample collection and submission to the laboratory, interpretation of results, and when applicable, performance of in-office diagnostic procedures. The chapter following the diagnostic chapter covers the indications and pharmacologic considerations of antimicrobials used to treat the particular classes of organisms discussed in the section.

Many modifications have also been made to improve the readability of the book. The typeface has been changed for easier reading. Drug dosage tables have been furnished to give complete and consistent prescribing information in each chapter. Within all disease chapters, greater emphasis is placed on clinical findings, diagnosis, therapy, prevention, and public health considerations. The references have been cited numerically rather than in parentheses to reduce distraction to the reader. References primarily include those published since the 1984 text or those that concern diseases not discussed there. Consequently, those interested in a complete bibliographic listing for each disease should consult both this and the preceding text. Taken together, bibliographic information in both texts should provide the reader with a relatively extensive listing of veterinary literature on a given subject.

All appendices in the preceding text have been updated and expanded. Newer features in selected appendices include immunization recommendations and biologics available in the United States, Canada, Great Britain, Australia, and New Zealand (Appendices 1 to 5). The Compendium of Animal Rabies Vaccines, 1990, is included (Appendix 6). Interstate and international regulations for shipment of dogs and cats with respect to infectious disease evaluation and vaccination are listed in Appendix 7. In Appendix 14, antimicrobial drug dosages are cross-referenced with tabular listings throughout the text.

CRAIG E. GREENE

ACKNOWLEDGMENTS

One person can ultimately be held responsible for coordinating and editing a textbook, but the work cannot be completed without the assistance of many others. My contributors were unselfish in their commitment to add yet another task to their already busy schedules. I certainly could not have done the work or provided the needed expertise without their assistance.

I definitely would not have considered committing myself to another textbook without the faithful assistance of Janet Calpin, a technician in Animal Resources at the University of Georgia. As in *Clinical Microbiology and Infectious Diseases of the Dog and Cat*, she was my "right hand" in all phases of this book from the start to the finishing touches. Her commitment to excellence and consistency helped to see the book to completion. Anyone who benefits from this book should appreciate her dedication, because it would not have been written without her. Lucy M. Rowland, Medical Resources Librarian, was extremely helpful on numerous occasions in locating bibliographic information and keeping me abreast of the latest publications. Nancy Wolski compiled information on vaccines for the appendices and produced computer graphic images for some of the illustrations. The secretaries of the Department of Small Animal Medicine, Diane Embrick, Mamie Watson, and Randi Gilbert, helped with the mailing and receipt of all the manuscripts. Many people in the Educational Resource Center, headed by Dr. Lari Cowgill, helped me throughout the production of this book. Susan Burer, Administrative Secretary, was extremely courteous and saw to it that my requests for work were handled without delay. Vivian Freeman and Linda Tumlin similarly handled my duplicating requirements. Photographic needs were managed by Jeanne Ann Davidson and Susan Snyder. The successful art work of medical illustrator Kip Carter and the illustrations of Dan Beisel were used again. Cynthia Krauss added several new line drawings to the list. Many new graphic and carto-graphic illustrations were done by Betsy Furbish, and some of those done by Harsh Jain were used again. I greatly appreciate the lending of photographic material by many persons. They are acknowledged in the respective figure legends.

Many people helped me with their expertise in reviewing particular sections of the book. Dr. Willy Burgdorfer and Dr. Tom Schwan of Rocky Mountain Laboratories, Hamilton, MT, reviewed the information and illustrative materials on tickborne diseases. Dr. Dan Fishbein, Centers for Disease Control, Atlanta, GA, and Dr. Cynthia Holland, University of Illinois, Urbana, IL, reviewed the sections on ehrlichiosis. Dr. Ernst Biberstein, University of California, Davis, CA, evaluated material on streptococcal infections. Dr. Leland Carmichael, Cornell University, Ithaca, NY, reviewed the section on infectious canine hepatitis.

Dr. David Watson, University of Sydney, Sydney, Australia, and Dr. Elizabeth Lee, Massey University, Palmerston North, New Zealand, provided me with information concerning the biologics marketed in their respective countries.

I am indebted to those who have provided me research and clinical support on infectious diseases over the years. Drs. Mike Lappin, Andre Jaggy, and Abigail Kaufman are three graduate students who have worked with me on infectious disease research problems involving toxoplasmosis, distemper, and Lyme borreliosis. Mandy Marks, Nancy Wolski, and Lynn Reece have been invaluable research technicians. Richard and Joanne Moyer of Crozet, VA have provided financial support through the memorial fund of Edward Gunst, Richmond, VA.

I would also like to thank Dean David Anderson; Dr. John Oliver, head of the Department of Small Animal Medicine; and the faculty, staff, and students of the University of Georgia College of Veterinary Medicine for making it a respected veterinary institution as well as an enjoyable place to work.

The people at W. B. Saunders have done an exceptional job in their efforts with this book. When Darlene Pedersen, who was my initial editor, was promoted, I was placed in the very capable and understanding hands of Linda Mills. Linda saw to it that all the loose ends were met at Saunders and coordinated all phases of preparation of the manuscript. She also provided me with moral support when several setbacks appeared to doom the final accomplishment of our task. Lorraine Zawodny was responsible for the copy editing. She was always available and willing to help. Her impeccable editing and medical knowledge gave the book a consistent format and readability while helping to rectify errors in grammatic or scientific terminology. This book will be current at the time it is published. Al Beringer and his staff typeset the text entirely from electronic copy. There was only a few weeks' delay from the time the author-updated and copy-edited manuscript was supplied until the galleys were available. Only six months elapsed from the time the final version of the chapters was delivered until publication.

Many other people on the staff at W. B. Saunders deserve acknowledgment. Bill Preston was helpful in the final production phases from the galleys. Maureen Sweeney provided the cover design, and the administrative efforts of Peter Clifford and Connie Vrato were greatly appreciated.

CRAIG E. GREENE

CONTENTS

SECTION IV
FUNGAL AND ALGAL INFECTIONS

APPENDICES

CLINICAL PROBLEMS

SECTION I

1 ENVIRONMENTAL FACTORS IN INFECTIOUS DISEASE

Craig E. Greene

Means of Transmission

The **reservoir** of an infectious disease is the natural habitat of its causative agent. Organisms such as clostridia and salmonellae can survive and multiply in inanimate reservoirs such as soil and water. Animate reservoirs, known as **carriers**, can be clinically or subclinically infected with and shed microorganisms that cause disease. Reservoirs and carriers are distinguished from the **source** of infection, which can be any vertebrate, invertebrate, inanimate object, or substance that enables the infectious agent to come into immediate contact with a susceptible individual. In many cases, the source is the reservoir.

A pathogenic organism must evolve a mechanism that enables it to spread from the reservoir or carrier to other animals in order to perpetuate the cycle of infection. Generalized spread of the infection to many body tissues results in contamination of many body secretions. Acute localized respiratory or gastrointestinal (GI) infections usually result in heavily contaminated secretions or excretions, such as aerosols produced during coughing and sneezing or diarrhea and vomitus, respectively. Genitourinary infections are transmitted in urine, uterine or vaginal discharges, and semen. Occasionally, infectious organisms may be shed from open, draining wounds.

Clinical illness is not always encountered in animals that are shedding. Many subclinical carriers exist; they are usually in the chronic or convalescent stage of disease. Latent carriers may shed organisms intermittently, in association with reactivation of infection. Infection potential, however, generally varies inversely with the length of time over which a disease is communicable. Acute, severe illnesses usually are associated with highly contagious secretions because transmission occurs over a short time.

The **transmissibility** or **communicability** of an infection refers to its ability to spread from infected to susceptible hosts. "Contagion" and "transmissibility" have been used interchangeably; however, the former implies spread following intimate contact. Transmission can occur between members of the same population (horizontal) or succeeding generations through the genetic material (vertical). Spread of infection to offspring by the placenta or in the milk is actually horizontal transmission. Not all infectious diseases are transmissible: e.g., systemic mycotic infections originate from soil rather than spreading between individuals.

Direct contact transmission is probably the most frequent and important means of spread of infection. This involves direct physical contact or close approximation between the reservoir host and the susceptible individual. Venereal transmission of *Brucella canis* between dogs or bite transfer of feline immunodeficiency virus between cats are examples of direct physical contact transmission. Aerosol droplets from respiratory, fecal, or genitourinary secretions of dogs and cats generally do not travel farther than 4 or 5 feet; therefore, droplet spread can be considered a form of direct transmission. The spread of infection under such circumstances usually can be limited, as long as fomite transmission is prevented, by ensuring that there is adequate distance between affected and susceptible animals.

Vehicle, or indirect, transmission involves the transfer of infectious organisms from the reservoir to a susceptible host by animate or inanimate intermediates known as **vehicles** or **fomites.** Indirect transmission is dependent on the ability of the infectious agent to temporarily survive adverse environmental influences. The most common animate fomites involved in indirect transmission in veterinary practice are human hands. Inanimate fomites can include anything by which an agent indirectly passes from infected to susceptible individuals, such as food dishes, cages, and surgical instruments. Canine and feline parvoviruses are often spread in this manner owing to the short shedding period in infected animals and the relatively long period of environmental persistence of these viruses.

Common-source transmission involves the simultaneous exposure of a number of individuals within a population to a vehicle contaminated by an infectious agent. The vehicles of common-source infections usually are blood products, drugs, food, and water. Food-source outbreaks of *Salmonella* gastroenteritis have been observed in small animal practice.

Airborne spread of infection depends upon the ability of resistant microorganisms to travel for relatively long distances or to survive in the environment for extended periods until they encounter susceptible hosts. Freshly aerosolized particles containing microbes rarely remain airborne for more than 1 meter unless they are smaller than 5 μm in diameter. **Droplet nuclei**, which are desiccated aerosolized particles containing resistant microbes, may also be carried alone or on dust particles by air currents for extended periods and distances. Resistant respiratory pathogens such as *Mycobacterium*

tuberculosis and *Histoplasma capsulatum* are commonly spread by this means.

Vector-borne disease may be considered a specialized form of vehicular or indirect contact spread in which invertebrate animals transmit infectious agents. Vectors are generally arthropods that transmit infection from the infected host or its excreta to a susceptible individual, to its food and water, or to another source of immediate contact. Vectors such as flies may transfer organisms externally, or **mechanically**, on their feet or internally within their intestinal tracts. The ability of organisms to survive in the vector without further propagation has been demonstrated with *Shigella* and *Salmonella* infections. **Propagative transmission** means that the infectious agent multiplies in or upon the vector prior to transfer. Transmission of the plague bacillus, *Yersinia pestis*, by fleas occurs in this manner. **Transovarial** transmission results when the vector transfers the organism to its progeny, as in the case of ticks transmitting *Rickettsia rickettsii*, the agent of Rocky Mountain spotted fever. **Transstadial** transmission, the transfer of infection only between molting stages in the life cycle of the vector, occurs in canine ehrlichiosis. True biologic (**developmental** or **cyclopropagative**) transmission by arthropod vectors involves an obligate developmental stage in the life cycle of the vector. Some of the protozoal pathogens of the dog and cat (e.g., *Hepatozoon*, *Trypanosoma*, *Leishmania*) have a developmental life cycle in the vector.

Environmental Control of Microbes

The health of both humans and domestic animals depends upon the ability to control microorganisms that cause or have the potential to cause disease. Destruction of the organisms occurs when the microenvironment is changed adversely by physical or chemical means. Several levels of microbial disinfection are recognized. Good decontamination always requires cleaning to remove organic residues and debris. With prior cleaning, most of the organisms are removed and disinfectants are more effective.[1]

Sterilization is the process by which microorganisms are completely destroyed by chemical or physical means. All life forms, including heat-resistant spores, are killed. Sterility is an absolute condition; there is no partial sterilization process.

Disinfection is the destruction of most pathogenic microorganisms, especially the vegetative forms, but not necessarily bacterial spores. Although disinfection may be brought about by physical as well as chemical agents, a disinfectant is usually a chemical means of control used on inanimate objects. **Antisepsis**, a special category of disinfection, is the inhibition or destruction of pathogenic microbes on the skin and mucous membranes. It is assumed that all pathogenic vegetative microbes are destroyed; however, resident flora may still persist. It is important that the antiseptic not be toxic to animal tissues. To reduce tissue toxicity, chemicals must be either more dilute or applied for a shorter period than would be necessary to produce sterility.

Sanitation is the reduction of the number of bacterial contaminants to a safe level. A sanitizer is not concentrated enough, nor is it in contact with the organisms long enough, to effect disinfection.

In practice, in the absence of bacterial spores, sterilization and disinfection produce identical results. However, when spores are present, only the harshest of measures can ensure sterility. Unless the item to be treated can withstand sterilization procedures via autoclave or ethylene oxide (EO), either physical or chemical disinfection must be relied upon to reduce the number of microorganisms to a safe level.

PHYSICAL AGENTS

Heat

Use of either **moist** or **dry** heat is one of the oldest physical controls of microorganisms. Of the two, moist heat, especially under pressure, is more efficient, requiring shorter exposure at lower temperature than is needed for disinfection by dry heat. When used correctly, steam under pressure is the most efficient means of achieving sterility. The recommended temperature-pressure-exposure time to produce sterilization with an autoclave is 121°C at 15 lb/in^2 for 15 minutes or 126°C at 20 lb/in^2 for 10 minutes. Steam heat is also most effective for the elimination of resistant protozoal cysts, such as *Toxoplasma* and coccidia. Hot-air ovens are the most common dry heat sterilizers, but to be effective, they must provide a consistent heat source. Dry heat sterilization can be assumed if objects are maintained at 160 ± 10°C for a minimum of 1 hour, preferably 2 hours. Microwave oven sterilization times of dry materials are similar to those of dry ovens once the sterilization temperature is reached.[2] The only advantage of microwave use is the shorter time it takes to achieve these temperatures. Dry heat is recommended for sterilizing cutting instruments and glassware or items that might be damaged by moisture, such as glass syringes and reusable needles.

Radiation

Ionizing or high-energy radiation can be produced by radioactive elements, which are sources of γ-rays, or by a cathode-ray tube that produces x-rays. γ-rays and x-radiations induce ionization of the vital cell components, especially nuclear DNA. Owing to the cost and dangers of this equipment, this type of microbial control has found practical application chiefly in the industrial field. Pharmaceuticals, plastic disposables, and suture materials generally are sterilized by the manufacturer by means of ionizing radiation. Nonionizing, or low-energy, radiation, in the form of ultraviolet (UV) light, has found practical application in the destruction of airborne organisms. Because low-energy rays do not penetrate well, they are used primarily as surface-active agents. The bactericidal range of UV light is 2400 to 2800 angstroms (Å). UV lamps usually produce radiation in the range of 2537 Å and work at maximum efficiency at temperatures of 27° to 40°C. They depend upon air convection currents to circulate airborne organisms. Germicidal lamps must be positioned above eye level to prevent retinal burns. For best efficiency, the lamps can also be placed in air conditioning or heating ducts.

CHEMICAL AGENTS

The antimicrobial properties of various chemical disinfectants are summarized in Table 1–1 and Appendix 10.

Alcohols

Ethyl and isopropyl alcohol are rapidly bactericidal against vegetative bacteria but have little effect against spores. Alcohols can be virucidal, provided there is adequate exposure time. Ethyl alcohol is more effective against the nonenveloped viruses than isopropyl alcohol, whereas the reverse is true for the enveloped viruses. Ethyl alcohol is

Table 1–1. Antimicrobial Properties of Common Classes of Chemical Disinfectants

| CLASS OF DISINFECTANT | BACTERIA | | | | FUNGI | VIRUSES | |
	Gram Positives	Gram Negatives	Acid Fast	Spores		Enveloped	Nonenveloped
Alcohols							
Ethyl	+	+	+	−	−	+	+
Isopropyl	+	+	+	−	−	+	−
Halogens							
Chlorine (hypochlorite)	+	+	+	+	+	+	+
Iodine	+	+	+	±	+	+	±
Aldehydes							
Formaldehyde	+	+	+	+	+	+	+
Glutaraldehyde	+	+	+	+	+	+	+
Phenolics	+	+	+	−	+	+	±
Surface-Active Compounds							
QUATs (cationic)	+	±	−	−	+	±	−
Amphoterics (anionic)	+	±	+	−	+	±	−
Biguanides	+	+	−	−	−	?	?
Ethylene Oxide	+	+	+	+	+	+	+

+ = effective; ± = somewhat effective; − = not effective; ? = effectiveness not known; QUATs = quaternary ammonium compounds.
See Appendices 9 and 10 for specific recommendations.

effective against *Proteus* and *Pseudomonas*. Alcohol is effective only as long as it remains in contact with the item to be disinfected. Because it evaporates readily, repeated applications may be needed to ensure adequate effect. Alcohol is used primarily on viable tissues as an antiseptic agent. Because water is essential for the antimicrobial action, absolute (100%) alcohol has no disinfecting qualities. Concentrations found to be most bactericidal are between 50% and 95% by volume. The two most widely used concentrations are 70% and 85%. The alcohols are inactivated by organic soil, and they are ineffective if diluted to less than 50%. Alcohols dissolve lens-mounting cement, blanch asphalt tiles, and harden plastics on long-term exposure.

Halogens

These compounds are ineffective or unstable in the presence of organic material, soaps, or hard water. They are active against a wide variety of viruses and resistant bacteria, such as *Proteus* and *Pseudomonas*.

Household bleach, a 5.25% sodium hypochlorite solution diluted up to a maximum of 1:30 (v/v), is a common form of chlorine used for disinfection. The germicidal activity of chlorine compounds is dependent upon an acid pH of the solution. Increasing the temperature of the solution decreases the exposure time needed. Other than aldehydes, this is one of the few chemicals that will inactivate parvoviruses. Solutions of bleach are deactivated by light. They should be kept in opaque containers and be diluted fresh daily.

Iodine is only slightly soluble in water; therefore, disinfectant solutions are made by dissolving it in alcohol or combining it with organic compounds. Iodine is sporicidal, fungicidal, and somewhat virucidal, depending on exposure time and concentration. Unlike chlorine, iodine exerts its effect over a wide range of pH.

Iodophors are iodine solutions complexed with a detergent; the latter helps to increase the contact of the iodine with the surface to be disinfected. The advantages of iodophors over iodine are that they are nonstaining and produce minimal tissue damage. Organic matter may reduce their activity, especially with dilute solutions, but the effect is less marked than with hypochlorites. Povidone iodine is a complex of polyvinylpyrrolidone and iodine (Betadine Solution, The Purdue Frederick Co, Norwalls, CT). Solutions of 10% (undiluted) to 1% (1:9) povidone iodine have been used for skin and wound disinfection. A 1:50 dilution of povidone-iodine is recommended as an ocular surface disinfectant for use in presurgical situations.[3] Polyhydroxydine is a potent iodine-containing wound and skin antiseptic (Xenodine, Squibb Animal Health Division, Princeton, NJ). It has been effective in treating canine wounds when used undiluted (100%) or as a 1:9 dilution (10%).[3a] As long as the iodophor solution maintains its color, it is effective.

Aldehydes

These have been employed as gaseous sterilants as well as chemical disinfectants. The exposure time needed for *formaldehyde* to effect sterilization is long, because the gas does not penetrate well, and has been replaced by more efficient gases. A 100% formalin solution is approximately 40% formaldehyde in water. A 20% formalin solution (8% formaldehyde) is a high-level disinfectant, and its biocidal activity can be increased by addition of 70% alcohol, but the solution is irritating to tissues and mucous membranes. *Glutaraldehyde* is chemically related to formaldehyde but is more reactive, even in the presence of organic materials, soaps, and hard water. A 2% aqueous alkaline solution is equivalent to 20% formalin in alcohol in biocidal activity. The alkaline solution is much more biocidal but less stable. Stability is maintained for about 2 weeks at pH 7.5 to 8.5. At the dilution at which it is used, glutaraldehyde is slightly irritating to the skin and mucous membranes and very irritating to the eyes. Both glutaraldehyde and formalin are used as high-level disinfectants for instruments, including lensed instruments, such as endoscopes, and plastic tubing and catheters. Following disinfection, items should be rinsed thoroughly with sterile distilled water. A glutaraldehyde-phenate complex (Sporicidin, Sporicidin International, Washington, DC) has been shown to be as effective at 1:16 dilution as undiluted glutaraldehyde and as stable and less irritating.

Phenolics

These are good housekeeping disinfectants because they remain stable when heated and after prolonged drying, will redissolve upon contact with water. They remain active in the presence of organic soil, soaps, and hard water and usually are the disinfectant of choice in treating fecal contamination, such as with *Salmonella*. They must be thoroughly rinsed from areas contacted by cats because of greater toxicity in this species, and they are irritating to the skin and mucous membranes. *Hexachlorophene*, a phenolic derivative commonly formulated with hand soap, is used as a degerming agent for the skin and mucous membranes because it causes little tissue irritation. Used only once, hexachlorophene is not more effective than soap in eliminating microorganisms. Its activity is reduced by organic material. Hexachlorophene is also neurotoxic when absorbed from the skin, and its use should be avoided over extensive areas and in neonates and animals with severely abraded skin.

Surface-Active Agents

These are chemicals that alter the surface tension of the organism and are classified as cationic or anionic. The *quaternary ammonium compounds* (QUATs) are cationic detergents that have been used for disinfection and antiseptic purposes, although their activity as disinfectants may have been overrated. They are inactivated by organic material, soaps, and hard water. They should not be used in preparation of skin for surgery because they are inactivated by detergents used in surgical scrubs. QUATs are algicidal, fungicidal, bactericidal, and virucidal (against enveloped viruses) at medium concentrations. When properly used, QUATs are effective bactericides against both gram-positive and gram-negative bacteria; however, they display greater activity against gram-positive organisms. They have an unusual ability to kill *Giardia* cysts at refrigerated and room temperatures (see Prevention, Chapter 84).[4] They are ineffective against tubercle bacilli, *Proteus*, *Pseudomonas*, bacterial spores, and the nonenveloped viruses even at high concentrations. When the temperature is increased from 20°C to 37°C, the concentration of the solution can be reduced by half.

QUATs also have been used in medicine as antiseptics and in flushing infected wounds. They are thought to form a film over the skin with the inactive part of the compound directed toward the skin, possibly trapping bacteria but not killing them.

The germicidal part is directed toward the environment, preventing further contamination. Degerming the skin with a more effective antiseptic before applying a QUAT may overcome the problem. Care must be taken not to allow undiluted QUATs to contact exposed tissues. Chemical burns occurred after using undiluted (17%) benzalkonium chloride on skin surfaces of dogs and cats.[4a] Cats also developed oral and esophageal ulcerations after licking treated skin areas.

Anionic surfactants or *amphoterics*, organic acids that have the detergency of anionic compounds, are effective against both gram-negative and gram-positive bacteria and are reported to be fungicidal but not sporicidal. Unlike QUATs, they are effective against *Proteus* and *Pseudomonas*. Amphoterics are effective in one application and are not inactivated by serum or hard water, although soaps and detergents affect them adversely. Like QUATs, they leave a film on the skin that will block the transfer of organisms from unwashed to washed hands. Amphoterics are nontoxic to tissues and noncorrosive to moist surfaces, and they have a deodorizing ability. They can greatly reduce the total number of bacteria on hospital floors.

Biguanides

Chlorhexidine, the most commonly used disinfectant of this class, has gained popularity as a wound antiseptic because of its low tissue toxicity. It is effective against *Proteus* and *Pseudomonas*. It has no residual activity following a single application. It has been shown to be an effective and nonirritating antiseptic for irrigation of canine wounds.[5] Concentrations of chlorhexidine of 0.5% in water or alcohol have been shown to reduce bacterial contamination when

used in canine wounds or as a surgical antiseptic, but they retard granulation tissue formation and epithelization.[3a] Lower concentrations of chlorhexidine (0.1%) were less antiseptic but did not inhibit wound repair. These compounds retain some activity in the presence of organic material and hard water but are inactivated by soaps.

Ethylene Oxide (EO)

When properly used, this gas is the most effective chemical sterilant. Like other chemical disinfectants, EO is subject to limitations imposed by temperature, moisture content, concentration, and exposure time. It has been recommended that routine sterilization be performed at 30°C to 55°C. If the temperature is not properly maintained, the gas may condense, or if the exposure time is too short, sterility failures can occur. Most EO sterilizers used in hospitals are designed to produce 50% to 60% relative humidity; it must not fall below 30%, or sterility failure will occur.

EO sterilization is not recommended for some plastics and pharmaceuticals or for animal feeds and beddings. The gas reacts with or is absorbed by these items. Solutions in sealed glass containers cannot be sterilized because the gas cannot penetrate glass. Instruments and other items should be clean, dry, and as free of contamination as possible prior to EO sterilization. Items are placed in semipermeable plastic wraps. Following the sterilization process, articles must be aerated to allow the residual gas to dissipate, because the absorbed gas is irritating to skin and mucous membranes. Recommended routine aeration procedures are as follows: at room temperature, 48 to 168 hours, depending upon the items sterilized and their use; with forced-air cabinets, 8 to 12 hours, depending upon the cabinet temperature.

Nosocomial Infections

Nosocomial (hospital-acquired) infections can arise endogenously from the spread of indigenous microflora or exogenously from contact with organisms on external sources. Exogenous sources of infection commonly include other animals and fomites such as

human hands, rodents, arthropods, food dishes, catheters, and hospital cages. Transmission can occur by airborne, contact, or vehicle routes. Many nosocomial infections result from opportunistic spread of the normal microflora rather than newly acquired agents. The prevalence rate of nosocomial infections in human and probably veterinary hospitals is 5% to 10% of hospitalized patients.

Not all infections that develop in the hospital environment are nosocomial in origin. Infections that are present or incubating at the time of admission are excluded. Moreover, nosocomial infections may not become clinically evident until after the patient has been discharged from the hospital. Hospitalized animals are more prone to infection because of increased exposure to pathogens, concurrent immunosuppressive illness, and, in recent years, increased stress imposed by technologic advances in medical practice (Tables 1–2 and 1–3). Excessive use of antimicrobial therapy may increase the risk of colonization with antimicrobial-resistant pathogens.

DEVELOPMENT OF ANTIBACTERIAL RESISTANCE

Microorganisms have evolved means of overcoming the effects of antimicrobial drugs. Most resistance mechanisms are under genetic control. Spontaneous chromosomal mutations are relatively rare in bacterial populations; extrachromosomal transfer of genetic material or plasmids is more important. Plasmid transfer occurs

Table 1–3. Factors Predisposing the Hospitalized Patient to Nosocomial Infection

MECHANISM	EXAMPLES
Decreased external defense mechanisms	Burns, decubital sores, smoke inhalation, IV and urinary catheters, surgery, trauma
Impaired humoral antibody defense	Congenital deficiency, failure to obtain colostrum, splenectomy, dysproteinemias
Impaired phagocytic and cellular immune mechanisms	Glucocorticoid therapy, antineoplastic drugs, congenital immune defect, diabetes mellitus, congestive heart failure, malignant neoplasia, malnutrition, neutropenia, gangrene
Alteration in microbial flora	Antimicrobial therapy, environmental reservoirs, contaminated equipment, improper isolation procedures, contaminated food or water

Table 1–2. Organisms Commonly Implicated as Opportunists in Compromised Hosts

VIRUSES	Feline leukemia virus Feline herpesvirus Feline calicivirus Canine distemper virus
BACTERIA	Citrobacter Escherichia coli Enterobacter Klebsiella pneumoniae Mycobacterium Nocardia asteroides Proteus Pseudomonas aeruginosa Serratia marcescens Staphylococcus aureus Staphylococcus epidermidis
FUNGI	Aspergillus Candida Cryptococcus Histoplasma Mucor
PROTOZOA	Pneumocystis carinii Toxoplasma gondii

most frequently during bacterial conjugation, although alterations in bacterial nucleic acid may also occur through bacteriophages (via transduction) or acquisition from naked nucleic acid (via transformation), or through exchange between bacterial and host DNA (via translocation). Plasmid transfer also commonly occurs between bacteria of different genera.

Genetic acquisition of bacterial resistance to antimicrobials may manifest in a variety of ways, including changes in permeability to the drug, in receptors for the drug, or in metabolic pathways. Plasmid resistance is frequently associated with cross-resistance among a number of structurally related antimicrobials.

The prevalence of antibiotic resistance commonly increases in proportion to the frequency of use. Resistance very often develops with streptococci, staphylococci, Escherichia coli, Salmonella, Proteus, and Klebsiella.[6, 7] Suppression of normal enteric flora and proliferation of antimicrobial-resistant strains occur with partially absorbed antimicrobials or those that are excreted in the bowel in active form, such as tetracyclines, chloramphenicol, ampicillin, metronidazole, furazolidone, amoxicillin, and cloxacillin.[8] Antibiotic resistance in fecal coliform bacteria has been documented in domestic pets in association with the increased use of antibacterial drugs in such animals.[9] Heightened antibacterial resistance among pets in rural environments was correlated with the increased use of antibiotics in livestock feeds. These findings should caution veterinarians against indiscriminate use of antimicrobials; moreover, similar resistance patterns have been identified in human contacts of both types of animals.

Antimicrobial resistance in human medicine has been shown to be more of a problem in hospitalized patients, in whom antibiotic usage is widespread, than among patients in general. Similar findings probably exist in veterinary practices. The development of new antibacterial drugs has just barely kept ahead of evolving resistance patterns. Widespread or indiscriminate usage of gentamicin and trimethoprim-sulfonamide by veterinarians may threaten the efficacy of these relatively new antibiotics in the near future. The availability of a large number of antibacterial drugs should not give the veterinarian a sense of security because many drugs have become obsolete as a result of evolving bacterial resistance.

Development of bacterial resistance can be prevented by certain adjustments during antimicrobial therapy.[6] Measures include restriction of prophylactic drug therapy, use of fully effective doses at adequate intervals, use of narrow-spectrum antibacterials specific for the isolated organisms, isolation of animals receiving long-term antibacterial therapy, selection of antibacterials against which the isolated organisms are not prone to develop resistance, changing of antibacterials after an effective treatment period, restriction of indiscriminate use of antibacterial drugs, and use of topical or local rather than systemic therapy whenever possible.

CONDITIONS ASSOCIATED WITH NOSOCOMIAL INFECTIONS

Urinary Catheterization

This procedure is probably the most common cause of nosocomial infection in veterinary practice. Fluid washout from urine flow is a primary defense mechanism of the urinary tract. Catheters upset this barrier by permitting entry of organisms at the urethral meatus and catheter junction. The distal urethra and prepuce or vagina are normally inhabited by commensal organisms. When catheters are left in place, these bacteria can

migrate in retrograde fashion and infect the rest of the urinary tract, which is normally sterile. Transient bacteremia also may occur following manipulation of urinary catheters in infected patients. To prevent infection, the external genitalia must be thoroughly cleansed, after which catheterization must be performed under strict aseptic conditions. Short-term, repeated, nontraumatic catheterization is preferable to placement of long-term indwelling catheters. Prophylactic topical or systemic antimicrobial therapy does not reduce the prevalence of infection unless the catheter is left in place less than 4 days (see Indwelling Catheters, Chapter 11).[10] Antimicrobial therapy should not begin until the catheter is removed. At this time the urine can be cultured, the sediment examined, and the animal started on therapy, which should be modified when the culture results are received. Antimicrobial therapy instituted while the catheter is in place merely selects for resistant infections.[10, 10a, 11] Periodic instillation of a disinfectant such as hydrogen peroxide into closed urinary drainage systems has not been effective in preventing catheter-associated bacteriuria in people.[12]

Intravenous Catheterization

Intravenous (IV) infusions are both essential and life-saving in veterinary practice. Since the development of flexible plastics, IV catheters are maintained in the patient for longer periods; however, the possibility that the infusion system can become contaminated is greater. The improper use of indwelling catheters has resulted in a high prevalence of nosocomial bacteremias. IV catheter–related infections are more common than realized in veterinary practice.[10a, 13] Infusion bottles, bags, or administration sets can become contaminated from hairline cracks produced during manufacture. Organisms may enter infusion systems when the administration set is inserted into the bottle, allowing the influx of room air, when the vacuum is released, or when medicaments are added. Organisms can also be introduced at the connection of the infusion set with the IV catheter.

Bacteria can also enter the IV infusion system at the site of penetration by the catheter tip by migrating between the catheter and skin surfaces. The prevalence of local infection is greatly increased when IV cutdown sites are used and catheters are in place for longer than 24 to 48 hours. Organisms producing localized infection at the catheter site may be infused systemically during the administration of fluid or during flushing of clogged catheters. Bacteria can also migrate in retrograde fashion, even against gravity flow, from the contaminated catheter to the infusion bottle.

Organisms of the family Enterobacteriaceae, such as *Klebsiella*, *Enterobacter*, *Serratia*, as well as *Citrobacter* and *Pseudomonas* proliferate readily at room temperature in 5% dextrose and can reach concentrations of 10^5 and 10^6 organisms/ml without producing obvious clouding of the solution. *Serratia* has been incriminated as the most common cause of IV catheter infection in small animal practice.[14-16] Benzalkonium chloride solutions should not be used for skin preparation because these antiseptic solutions can support the growth of *S. marcescens* and other microorganisms. Many other common contaminants, such as *Staphylococcus*, *Pseudomonas*, *E. coli*, and *Proteus*, do not survive or proliferate in 5% dextrose, although *Candida* can grow very slowly.

Lactated Ringer's, normal saline, and other isotonic fluids have been less commonly incriminated as the cause of nosocomial bacteremia than have dextrose solutions; however, they can support the growth of a variety of organisms. Parenteral hyperalimentation fluids and other hypertonic solutions readily support the growth of *Candida*. Blood products, even when stored at refrigerated temperatures, can become contaminated and support the growth of cold-growing microorganisms such as *Pseudomonas* and some coliforms.

Clinical signs of catheter-associated infection include localized swelling and warmth at the insertion site and venous cording. The systemic spread of infection is characterized by fever, hypotension, tachycardia, and GI and central nervous system (CNS) signs. Overwhelming infections associated with endotoxemia are more likely to occur when gram-negative organisms are involved and in immunosuppressed patients. Clinical signs in such cases are shock, collapse, coma, and death.

Diagnosis of IV infusion–associated infection is frequently made when the clinical signs improve suddenly following termination of fluid therapy. However, because bacteremia may seed many organs, clinical signs can persist after the infusion is discontinued. Culture or Gram staining of catheter tips has been recommended[10a, 17, 18] and is a more rapid and practical means of determining presence of infection. However, this alone may not always confirm the presence of bacteremia. When blood cultures are performed, organisms should correspond to those found at the catheter site. It is also possible for pseudobacteremia to occur when the infected catheter site locally seeds the venous effluent being sampled. Therefore, at least two to three blood samples should be taken from different sites at intervals of at least 10 minutes once the catheter has been removed. Adequate skin preparation and antisepsis at the collection sites are essential.

IV catheter–associated infections can be prevented with adequate precautions. Hands should be washed prior to catheter placement. The hair at the catheter site should be carefully shaved to avoid microabrasions of the skin. Gentle mechanical cleansing of the skin with an iodophor or with soap and water for 2 to 5 minutes should be followed by alternate disinfection using 70% alcohol and 1% to 2% tincture of iodine or iodophor solutions. Iodine-containing antiseptics are effective against most bacteria and fungi, with the exception of spores. Tincture of iodine preparations, superior to iodophors for the final application, are frequently too irritating for repeated usage.

To restrict movement, catheters should be firmly stabilized with adhesive tape. A small amount of a broad-spectrum antimicrobial ointment, such as one containing organic iodine or neomycin-bacitracin-polymyxin, should be applied at the point of skin penetration, and the site should be covered with a sterile occlusive dressing, or if only tape is to be used, then it must be sterile. The date and time of catheter insertion should be recorded. No catheter should be left in place longer than 72 hours. If the catheter must remain in place for longer periods, the IV site should be inspected and dressed with a new sterile dressing at 48- to 72-hour intervals. Concurrent administration of antibiotics does little to prevent IV catheter–associated infection, but causes the development of an antimicrobial-resistant infection.

When a small volume or slow infusion

rate is required, use of multiple small infusion bottles is preferred to that of one large bottle. The rationale for this is that should the system become contaminated, the time for microorganism multiplication is minimized. Infusion bottles should be checked for turbidity and vacuum, and infusion bags should be squeezed prior to use to detect leaks. Infusion filters 0.22 μm in diameter are available to restrict the flow of microorganisms through the fluid line into the patient; however, they will not prevent passage of endotoxins and pyrogenic factors. Drugs should be added to infusion fluid containers in uncontaminated surroundings following proper disinfection of the site of addition to the infusion fluid.

Respiratory Infections

The upper respiratory passages have anatomic defense mechanisms that prevent most inhaled particles from reaching the lower airways. However, invasive procedures such as tracheostomy, fiberoptic endoscopy, transtracheal catheterization, nebulization, and endotracheal intubation bypass these defense mechanisms and expose the respiratory tract to increased numbers of organisms, especially gram-negative organisms. The occurrence of nosocomial pneumonias was much higher in endotracheally intubated human patients receiving histamine type 2 blockers.[19] Retrograde contamination of the oropharynx with gram-negative bacteria from the stomach was thought to be responsible.

Decreased respiratory clearance function has also been associated with an increased risk of nosocomial respiratory infections. Decreased clearance activity can occur with CNS depression, neuromuscular paralysis, chronic obstructive lung disease, and impairment of pulmonary alveolar macrophage function. Inhalation anesthesia, nebulization, humidification, and ventilatory support increase the risk of nosocomial infection due to cross-contamination. Appropriate disinfection protocols for the equipment used in these procedures is discussed later in the chapter (see Prevention of Nosocomial Infections).

Wound Infections

Nonsurgical defects or breaks in the skin are associated with an increased risk of con-

tamination and subsequent infection. Establishment of infection depends upon the type and depth of the injury, damage to vascular supply, devitalization of tissue, and delay in presentation for treatment. Wounds involving intestinal perforation and burns are always contaminated and therefore require immediate attention. Deep-sample culturing of infected wounds must be performed with surgical entry or needle penetration because surface contaminants are commonly present. Material thus obtained should be sealed in an airtight container and submitted to a laboratory as soon as possible, in an attempt to culture anaerobic agents that often are present.

Extensive debridement or surgical drainage of wounds may be required to prevent wound infections and to reduce extensive swelling or abscess formation. Wounds should be covered to prevent extensive drying of devitalized tissues, and drainage should be encouraged by incomplete closure or drain placement. Occlusive dressings containing adequate absorbent material should be changed whenever drainage is present. To encourage formation of sufficient granulation tissue, limbs should be immobilized or supported. Chronic nonhealing scar tissue should be resected from the wound. Prolonged hospitalization and the indiscriminate use of topical or systemic antibiotics favor the overgrowth of resistant bacteria.

GI Infections

Enteric pathogens, such as parvoviruses, coronaviruses, *Salmonella*, and *Giardia*, may spread among dogs or cats in a veterinary hospital or animal-holding facility. Outbreaks are usually the result of poor sanitation, inadequate disinfection, and crowding of animals. Wards, treatment areas, waiting rooms, cages, exercise runs, and feeding utensils are all sources of infection. All outbreaks of gastroenteritis among recently hospitalized patients should be investigated as to the cause and possible source of infection. Fecal examinations and cultures for protozoa and parvovirus should be performed when economically feasible.

Prevention of GI infections requires intensive cleaning and disinfection procedures. All feces within the hospital should be removed as soon as possible, and the contaminated site should be thoroughly disinfected with a diluted (1:32) chlorine bleach solution. Use of smooth, impervious floor and cage surfaces will facilitate disinfection and cleaning. Crowding of animals in the waiting room and in hospital wards should be avoided. Hospitalized animals should not be moved from cage to cage, but each should be assigned to one cage. Those having episodes of acute vomiting or diarrhea either before or after being admitted to the hospital should be isolated.

Decubital Ulcers

These are the most common nosocomial skin infections to develop in incapacitated animals maintained in immobile or recumbent positions on unpadded surfaces. Abrasion and continuous pressure over bony surfaces cause devitalization of skin and secondary bacterial invasion. Immunosuppressed animals may develop septicemia as a result of decubital sores. *Pseudomonas* commonly contaminates these wounds. Identification of the invading microorganism and antibacterial therapy usually are of little benefit unless the primary cause is eliminated. Prevention is easier than cure; it involves frequent turning of recumbent patients and the use of padding in their cages.

PREVENTION OF NOSOCOMIAL INFECTIONS

Most nosocomial pathogens, whether acquired endogenously or exogenously, do not produce disease by themselves. The risk of nosocomial infections is greatest for immunocompromised or surgery patients and for newborns. Prevention of these infections can be achieved only by strict monitoring of the known predisposing causes. Attempts should be made to reduce the contact of high-risk patients with potential pathogens by segregating them from the general hospital population or minimizing their hospital stay. Additional measures include using indwelling catheters only when necessary, minimizing surgical procedures, and practicing routine disinfection. Chemical disinfection procedures in veterinary hospitals are reviewed in the following section and summarized in Table 1–4.

Antimicrobial Prophylaxis

Prophylactic use of antimicrobial drugs is a controversial subject. The unnecessary use of antibiotics has caused justifiable concern because of the increased prevalence of resistant microorganisms. Antibiotics alter the patient's microflora and allow infection by resistant bacteria. It has long been thought that microflora were responsible for bacterial superinfections following prophylactic administration of antimicrobial drugs; however, invasion by exogenous, resistant organisms is more likely. Prolonged use of antibiotics may not lessen an animal's susceptibility to infection but may merely alter the microbial flora that cause the problem.

There are certain justifications for instituting treatment with antimicrobial drugs prior to documenting that an infectious process exists. Immunosuppressed hosts that have been exposed to disease may require antimicrobial therapy; however, most clinicians would argue that close monitoring of the patient should be followed by IV administration of antimicrobials only if fever or other signs of infection appear. High-risk conditions associated with immunosuppression and secondary infection include diabetes mellitus, persistent neutropenia, Cushing's disease, immunosuppressive or cancer chemotherapy, and chronic bronchopulmonary disease. Traumatic or contaminated wounds and burns may require topical or systemic chemotherapy.

Preoperative and intraoperative administration of antimicrobials has been shown to reduce the prevalence of postoperative infection in surgery of the bowel, respiratory and biliary tracts, and oropharyngeal region.[19a] Organisms that contaminate relatively avascular subcutaneous tissue, bone fragments, or serosal surfaces are often commensals of skin and mucosal surfaces. There are surgical situations in which antimicrobial therapy administered prior to the procedure for anticipated infection may be beneficial. These include surgical procedures performed on contaminated wounds following trauma, procedures performed at infected sites, procedures in which contamination is expected, such as in the immunosuppressed patient, and procedures involving prolonged exposure (> 4 hrs) of healthy tissue (Table 1–5).[20] Short-term, clean surgical procedures in dogs and cats have no difference in infection rates when

Table 1–4. Treatment Time Required for Chemical Disinfection of Hospital Equipment

	TYPE OF DISINFECTION[a]	DISINFECTANT[b]	EXPOSURE TIME[c]
Objects with smooth hard surfaces	H	17	3–12
	H	8–10	15–18
	H	11	5
	I	1–3, 6, 8–10, 12	30
	L	1, 4, 7, 13, 14–16	10
	L	8–10	5
Rubber tubing (completely filled) and catheters	H	17	3–12
	I	6, 10, 12	30
	L	7, 13, 14–16	10
Polyethylene tubing (completely filled) and catheters	H	17	3–12
	H	8–10	15–18
	I	1, 2, 6, 10, 12	30
	L	1, 7, 13–16	10
Thermometers (wiped thoroughly clean)	H	8–10	10–12
	I	2, 5, 10	30
	L	6	10
Lensed instruments	H	9–11	10–12
	I	9, 10	30
	L	7, 13–16	10
Hinged instruments (free of organic material)	H	9, 10	10–12
	I	2, 8–10	20
	I	6, 12	30
	L	8–10	10
	L	1, 7, 13–16	20
Inhalation, anesthetic, and endoscopic equipment	H	9, 11	10
	H	17	3–12
	I	2, 10	20
	L	1, 14–16	20
	L	10, 11	5
Housekeeping (floors, furnishings, and walls)	I	3, 6, 12	20
	L	4, 7, 13–16	10

[a]H = high-level disinfection (free of all microorganisms; equivalent to sterilization); I = intermediate-level disinfection (free of all vegetative bacteria and fungi, tubercle bacilli, and most viruses); L = low-level disinfection (free of vegetative bacteria and fungi and most enveloped viruses).

[b]1 = 70–90% ethyl or isopropyl alcohol; 2 = 70–90% ethyl alcohol; 3 = hypochlorite (1000 ppm); 4 = hypochlorite (100 ppm); 5 = 0.2% iodine + alcohol; 6 = iodophors (500 ppm); 7 = iodophors (100 ppm); 8 = 20% formalin + alcohol; 9 = 20% formalin aqueous; 10 = 2% activated glutaraldehyde aqueous; 11 = 0.13% activated glutaraldehyde + phenate complex; 12 = 2% phenolic aqueous; 13 = 1% phenolic aqueous; 14 = quaternary ammonium compounds; 15 = amphoterics; 16 = chlorhexidine; 17 = ethylene oxide.

[c]For H time in hours; for I and L time in minutes.

antimicrobial prophylaxis is compared with placebo treatment.[21] Antimicrobials should be administered to an animal before and during surgery when the genitourinary tract is infected and prior to routine dental procedures. Prophylactic antimicrobial therapy is also desirable in conjunction with surgical drainage of abscesses.

The success of prophylactic antimicrobial therapy before surgery involves timing administration of the drug so as to achieve maximum concentrations during the operative procedure. With delays of up to 4 hours after the procedure, animals respond as if treatment had not been given.[22, 23] Oral therapy is given 1 hour, IM injections one-half hour, and IV therapy immediately before the beginning of the operation and continued for no longer than 12 hours thereafter.[24] Antimicrobials penetrate formed tissue exudates and blood clots poorly but will be readily incorporated in the latter if they are present in the plasma during clot formation.

Measures should be taken to reduce the risk of infection following antimicrobial prophylaxis since infection with resistant organism is more likely. Hospitalization, stress, and invasive procedures should be avoided in immunosuppressed patients. If antibiotics are used, they should be bactericidal drugs whose effectiveness is limited as much as possible to the suspected contami-

Table 1–5. Classification of Surgical Wounds and Indications for Prophylaxis[a]

CLEAN	CONTAMINATED
1. Elective surgery	1. Fresh traumatic wound
2. No entry into mucosal surface	2. Spillage from mucosal surface
3. No break in asepsis	3. Acute inflammation encountered
4. No inflammation or drainage encountered	4. Dental prophylaxis[b]

CLEAN CONTAMINATED	DIRTY
1. Entry into GI, GU, RT mucosae	1. Abscessed material present
2. No unusual contamination	2. Viscus perforated
3. Minor break in asepsis	3. Older (>4 hr) traumatic wound
	4. Suppuration encountered

[a]Data from National Research Council. *Ann Surg* 160:1–192, 1964.
[b]For dental prophylaxis, see Gingivitis, Chapter 9
GI = gastrointestinal tract, GU = genitourinary tract, RT = respiratory tract.

nant (Table 1–6). A full course of antibiotics at the proper dosage should be used, because anything less is often ineffective in the absence of an adequate immune system.[25] If results of susceptibility testing are conflicting or indicate that organisms are not susceptible to the drug being used, antibiotics should not be changed if the patient appears to be responding.

There are several disadvantages of antimicrobial chemoprophylaxis, some so serious that the risk of therapy may outweigh the benefits. Bacterial resistance or drug toxicities may occur. Prophylaxis with antimicrobials may suppress normal microflora and increase the risk of infection with resistant microorganisms (superinfection).

Isolation Precautions

Restricting animal movement and contact within a veterinary hospital are important means of controlling spread of nosocomial infections. As a general rule, animals entering the hospital should be currently vaccinated (see Chapter 2) or should be vaccinated if their status is uncertain. Any animal infested with ectoparasites should be dipped on admission if its condition permits. Immunosuppressed patients should not be housed in the hospital or if admitted, should be moved to a separate area. In the event that infection is identified in an animal, four categories are proposed for which isolation precautions are indicated (Table 1–7).

Class 1 infections have very little chance of spread between individuals, and the zoonotic potential is low. Systemic mycotic and algal infections are primarily contracted by environmental exposure. Systemic herpesvirus infection is a threat only to neonates, and dogs showing only neurologic signs with canine distemper are unlikely to spread disease. No additional precautions are needed, and routine cage cleaning, hand washing, and disinfection of hospital equipment are all that is necessary.

Class 2 infections are of greater risk of transmission than class 1. Close contact is required between animals with papillomatosis or feline leukemia virus infections or

Table 1–6. Indications and Drugs for Antimicrobial Prophylaxis

			RECOMMENDED DRUG	
INDICATIONS	EXAMPLES	MICROORGANISM	First Choice	Alternative
Clean contaminated[a] surgery	Bowel or genital surgery	Aerobic	Gentamicin	Spectinomycin or trimethoprim-sulfonamide
		Anaerobic	Metronidazole	Clindamycin
	Bite wounds	Aerobic	Ampicillin	Cephalosporins
		Anaerobic	Clindamycin	Penicillins
Complicated clean surgery	Prolonged surgery[b]	Staphylococci, streptococci	Cephalosporins	Clavulanic-amoxicillin
	Orthopedic prosthesis	*E. coli*	Cephalosporins	Penicillinase-resistant penicillins
Neutropenia	Cancer chemotherapy, ehrlichiosis, and estrogen intoxication	Gram-negative	Trimethoprim-sulfonamide	Cephalosporins, aminoglycoside
		Gram-positive	Cephalosporins	Penicillinase-resistant penicillin
		Anaerobic	Clindamycin	Metronidazole

[a]No gross contamination in field but historic complications.
[b]Longer than 3 hours.

Table 1–7. Classification of Infectious Diseases Based on Zoonotic and Nosocomial Potential

CLASS 1[a]	**CLASS 3**[d]
Systemic herpesvirus infection (puppies)	Drug-resistant bacterial infections *(Klebsiella, Pseudomonas)*[c]
Canine distemper (neurologic form)	Canine brucellosis[c]
Histoplasmosis	Leptospirosis[c]
Cryptococcosis	Giardiasis[c]
Coccidioidomycosis	Cryptosporidiosis[c]
Prototheosis	Toxoplasmosis (feline enteroepithelial)[c]
	Campylobacteriosis[c]
	Dermatophytosis[c]
	Sporotrichosis[c]
CLASS 2[b]	**CLASS 4**[e]
Drug-susceptible bacterial infections	Canine parvoviral diarrhea
Feline leukemia and other viral neoplasias	Other enteric infections
Feline immunodeficiency virus infection	Feline panleukopenia
	Infectious canine hepatitis
Canine viral papillomatosis	Canine distemper (multisystemic form)
Feline infectious peritonitis	Canine viral respiratory diseases
Haemobartonellosis	Feline viral respiratory diseases
Canine ehrlichiosis	Feline chlamydiosis[c]
Babesiosis	Rabies
Pneumocystosis	Salmonellosis[c]
American trypanosomiasis	Shigellosis[c]
Leishmaniasis	*Mycobacterium tuberculosis* infections[c]
Rocky Mountain spotted fever[c]	Plague
Lyme disease (canine borreliosis)	
Atypical mycobacterial infections	
Blastomycosis	

[a]Acquired from the environment or limited shedding or susceptibility period.

[b]Close contact or vector transmission required or environmentally nonresistant organisms.

[c]Zoonotic potential with direct transmission to people.

[d]Transmission by infected body secretions with organism of moderate environmental resistance and zoonotic potential.

[e]Serious zoonotic pathogens or high level of transmission.

feline infectious peritonitis. Many of these infections can be spread by contact with infected body fluids. Most other infections in this group are vector-transmitted, so that proper arthropod control will minimize the risk of spread from infected individuals. Most of the organisms cannot survive outside the host and are susceptible to routine disinfectants.

Class 3 infections are spread by close or direct contact with infected individuals or their excreta, but the risk of transmission via body fluids and excreta can be minimized by sanitary measures. These animals can be admitted to the general hospital population, but they should remain in their cages so as to restrict the contact of their urine and feces with other animals. Their cages should be identified as to the particular illness. Hand washing and cage cleaning must be critically practiced between animals, and feces or diarrhea, urine, and vomitus should be removed immediately. Dilute (1:30) bleach for viruses and phenolic compounds for bacteria should be used for disinfection. *Toxoplasma* and *Cryptosporidium* oocysts are inactivated by 10% ammonia solutions or by boiling water or steam cleaning. *Giardia* cysts are most susceptible to some dilute (1:100 or greater) QUAT disinfectants.[4]

Class 4 animals should be strictly isolated in a separate ward and should not be admitted to the general animal population. Animals with upper respiratory infections are preferably not admitted to the hospital and should be treated as outpatients. These highly contagious diseases are spread by air or contact. Body exudates or secretions are highly infectious, or the organisms are resistant to most methods of control. Persons handling these animals should wear protective outer garments, shoe covers, and rubber gloves. Contaminated wastes from these areas should be double-bagged in plastic and disposed of separately. Cages should be thoroughly disinfected once the animal is discharged. If the patient had *Salmonella*, the cage surface should have negative culture results before being used again.

Hands

These are the most common reservoirs or fomites for microorganisms associated with nosocomial infection, and handwashing is probably the *single most important* and immediate way of reducing hospital-acquired infections. Hands should be washed routinely with water and mild, noncaustic soap or detergent after handling or examining patients and especially after contact with blood, secretions, and excretions. The mechanical effect of soap and water cleansing is most important in reducing the numbers of transient bacteria on the skin surface. Frequent use of antiseptics should be avoided because they can burn or dry the skin. Preexisting dermatitis will result in the persistent carriage of large numbers of microorganisms, which negates the effect of handwashing. Bar soaps, allowed to dry between uses, appear to have a lower prevalence of contamination than liquid soaps. Liquid soap canisters can become contaminated and must routinely be emptied, cleaned, and disinfected before being refilled. Iodine-containing soaps are superior as scrubbing agents for use prior to surgery; however, they may produce dermatitis in sensitive individuals. A comparison of the available handwashing soaps and antiseptics appears in Table 1–8. Handwashing sinks and bathing tubs in all areas of a veterinary hospital can be disinfected with chlorine bleach to reduce contamination with organisms such as *Pseudomonas*. Rubber gloves may be used as an adjunctive means of reducing spread of infection when handwashing must be done so frequently as to prove impractical or irritating to the skin.

Airborne Contaminants

These can be reduced by having impervious floor coverings and using wet mops or filtered vacuums throughout the hospital. Air conditioning systems should be electronically filtered if possible and should be designed to reduce turbulent airflow. The best ventilation systems have air inlets near the ceiling and air outlets near the floor, allowing air to travel downward toward the heavily contaminated floor region. Air exchange rates of 6 to 10 times per hour have been shown to efficiently reduce the number of airborne microorganisms in animal holding facilities while producing minimal air turbulence.[26]

Surgery

Nosocomial infections have increased owing to the more invasive and prolonged surgical procedures and the use of synthetic implants. The major source of bacteria contaminating surgical wounds is the patient's endogenous microflora. Such nosocomial infections can also arise from inadequate sterilization of surgical equipment, from operating room air, or transfer from the veterinary staff or hospital environment. Microbes indigenous to the hospital environment are most problematic because they are often antimicrobial-resistant. A classification of human surgical wound contamination that can be applied to veterinary practice is summarized in Table 1–5.[27]

Many factors contribute to the likelihood of postoperative infection. Preparation of the surgical site is critical. Skin trauma produced during surgical preparation greatly increases the local bacterial population. Delayed wound healing caused by excessive numbers of sutures, foreign implants, or devascularized tissue serve as foci for infection following contamination. Although surgically placed drains allow for removal of blood or pus in dead-space areas, they may delay closure or allow for entry of organisms into wounds. The risk of tissue infection is directly proportional to the increased amount of tissue handling and trauma. Vascular compromise to tissue and bleeding into tissue spaces are major contributory factors. The duration of surgery has a major influence on the overall risk of wound infection. Drying of tissues and airborne contamination are also major causes. Infection rates may double for every hour of operative time. Nosocomial infections develop in 1% of pa-

Table 1–8. Comparison of Commonly Used Topical Soaps and Antiseptics

AGENT	ADVANTAGES	DISADVANTAGES
Hand soap	Noncaustic, inexpensive	Liquids and moist bars support bacterial growth
Hexachlorophene (phenolic)	Good for *Staphylococcus*	Must use daily, CNS toxicity with absorption, minimal effect on gram-negative bacteria and fungi
Benzalkonium chloride (QUAT)	Inexpensive	Ineffective, harbors opportunistic bacteria (e.g., *Serratia*)
Alcohol	Relatively inexpensive, need 70% aqueous, ethanol superior	Volatile, flammable, drying, bacterial resistance common
Iodine (halogen)	Good for viruses, fungi, and vegetative and sporulated bacteria; most effective as tincture; sustained germicidal action	Irritating, hypersensitivity, stains skin, drying
Iodophors (halogen)	Water soluble, low irritation, less staining	Reduced potency compared with iodine, drying

tients after surgeries that last less than 30 minutes and in 14% after operations lasting longer than 3.5 hours.

Host factors are equally important in the defense against surgical infections. Localized infections at distant sites can spread to operative wounds by hematogenous routes. Host immunosuppression by concurrent disease or an inherent immunodeficiency disorder may increase the risk. Prolonged hospitalization increases the risk from infection with antimicrobial-resistant bacteria. Wet dressings reduce the fibrin seal formation on a wound and may allow for the maceration of tissue and proliferation of bacteria at the incision site. Prophylactic antibiotics should not be used indiscriminately in surgical procedures but only when contamination of tissues is expected (see Antimicrobial Prophylaxis).

Surgical Equipment

This should be appropriately sterilized with steam autoclaves or EO, rather than by cold disinfection, and should be stored in dust-free enclosed cabinets. Cold disinfection should be avoided when possible as it may be associated with the increased risk of infections from soil saprophytes such as *Clostridium tetani*. All surfaces in operating rooms that do not contact the patient should be routinely disinfected with phenolic compounds. Floors can be washed with disinfectants and wet-mopped or polished. Wet mops or vacuums with filtered exhaust elements can pick up excess disinfectant and loosening debris.[28] Built-up disinfectant films can be removed with a solution of 0.12 liters (one-half cup) of vinegar in 3.8 liters (1 gallon) of water. Dry mops and brooms should never be used to clean hospital floors because they disseminate microorganisms in dust. Personnel should wear face masks to minimize aerosol contamination in surgery areas. Handwashing and gloving for surgery is superior to handwashing alone in minimizing the spread of skin microflora to the patient. Antisepsis of the skin at the incision site is similar to that used in preparing IV catheter sites, but there is a final application of tincture of iodine or iodophor solution just before the animal is draped.

Anesthesia and Nebulizer Equipment

This should be washed with water and detergents. This equipment may be heat sensitive, so it may need to be sterilized with EO gas or soaked in 2% glutaraldehyde for 30 minutes, followed by aeration or sterile water rinse, respectively. All equipment should be completely dry before it is used. Solid rubber face masks that can withstand heat disinfection may be flash autoclaved at 56°C for 3 minutes.

Rubber anesthesia circuits can be disinfected by immersion in 80°C water for 15 minutes. Soda lime canisters should be completely emptied and disinfected by similar means when needed.

Nebulizers and humidifiers can be disinfected by flushing hydrogen peroxide (20% by volume in water) through the system. Acetic acid at a concentration of at least 2% has been used, but it is somewhat ineffective against the more resistant gram-negative bacteria. Chlorhexidine (0.02%) is better for this purpose, especially when it is used at a temperature of 50°C. Temperature-controlled nebulizers that can be maintained at 45°C during use have the lowest prevalence of contamination. Periodic disinfection of nebulizer chambers with chlorine bleach or sterilization with EO gas is also recommended.

Endoscopic Equipment

This should be cleaned with soap and water as soon as possible after each use to remove gross soil, rinsed thoroughly with clean water, then rinsed with a disinfectant solution. Iodophors and bleach are corrosive to metal parts. Flexible endoscopes should be effectively disinfected or sterilized between uses whenever possible, particularly if they are used to examine normally sterile areas such as the respiratory and genitourinary tracts. Flexible endoscopes can be sterilized by soaking in alkaline glutaraldehyde for 10 minutes, then rinsing with sterile water. Sterilization can be achieved with EO gas, but many endoscopes cannot withstand the 63°C aeration temperature that is commonly used and require more prolonged aeration at lower temperatures. Unlike rigid metal endoscopes, most flexible endoscopes

Table 1–9. Susceptibility of Bacteria to Heat Disinfection

PROCEDURE	ORGANISMS KILLED	TEMPERATURE		TIME	COMMENTS
		°C	°F		
Dishwashing					
Automatic wash	Most vegetative	60	140	20 sec	Add degergent
Sterilization	All vegetative, most spores	82	180	10 sec	Add detergent
Manual wash	Some vegetative	43–49	110–120	10–20 sec	Add detergent
	All but spores	76.5	170	30 sec	Add disinfectant
Cage Cleaning	Gram-negative rods, gram-positive cocci	49	120	2–4 min	Steam or hot water
	Gram-negative rods	48–60	120–140	Instantaneous	Steam or hot water
	Gram-positive cocci	71	160	2–4 min	Steam or hot water
	All but *Bacillus* spores	82	180	Instantaneous	Steam or hot water
	Bacillus spores	82	180	> 1 min	Steam or hot water
Anesthetic Tube Cleaning					
Mild disinfection	Most vegetative	55	132	3 min	Hot water
Pasteurization	All but spores	80	176	15 min	Hot water
Clothes Washing (Automatic)	All spores	>71	>160	25 min	Add detergent, add bleach to increase cidal activity

cannot tolerate sterilization by steam autoclaving.

Cages

Animal-holding facilities must receive adequate disinfection. Mere cleansing of cages with liquid disinfectants between uses is insufficient. Steam cleaning on a monthly basis is the most effective means of ward and cage sanitation. Transient washing at 82°C is considered optimal for cage disinfection except against spores of *Bacillus*, which can be killed if the washing is prolonged for a minute or more. Lower temperatures may be effective in destroying vegetative bacteria (Table 1–9).

Clothes and Dishes

Disinfection of these articles requires higher temperatures that can be achieved with automatic clothes washers; because dishwashers use water at higher temperatures, they disinfect better than manual dishwashing (see Table 1–9). At these high temperatures, most organisms will be killed; bacterial spores are the exception. Low-temperature (22°C) washing using laundry chemicals and bleach followed by drying is

as effective as high temperature (71°C) washing to eliminate pathogenic bacteria.[29]

References

1. Russell AD, Yarnych VS, Koulikovskii AV: *Guidelines on Disinfection in Animal Husbandry for Prevention and Control of Zoonotic Diseases.* Geneva, World Health Organization, 1984, 62 pp.
2. Jeng DK, Kaczmarek KA, Woodsworth AG, et al: Mechanism of microwave sterilization in a dry state. *Appl Environ Microbiol* 53:2133–2137, 1987.
3. Roberts SM, Severin GA, Lavach JD: Antibacterial activity of dilute povidone-iodine solutions used for ocular surface disinfection in dogs. *Am J Vet Res* 47:1207–1210, 1986.
3a. Lee AH, Swaim SF, McGuire JA: Effects of chlorhexidine diacetate, povidone iodine, and polyhydroxydine on wound healing in dogs. *J Am Anim Hosp Assoc* 24:77–84, 1988.
4. Zimmer JF, Miller JJ, Lindmark DG: Evaluation of the efficacy of selected commercial disinfectants in inactivating *Giardia muris* cysts. *J Am Anim Hosp Assoc* 24:379–385, 1988.
4a. Bilbrey SA, Dulisch ML, Stallings B: Chemical burns caused by benzalkonium chloride in eight surgical cases. *J Am Anim Hosp Assoc* 25:31–34, 1989.
5. Amber EI, Henderson RA, Swaim SF, et al: A comparison of antimicrobial efficacy and tissue reaction of four antiseptics on canine wounds. *Vet Surg* 12:63–68, 1983.
6. Powers TE: General principles underlying the clinical use of antimicrobials. *Coll Vet Med Rev (Mississippi State Univ)* 2:7–21, 1982.
7. Kaufmann J: Nosocomial infections: *Klebsiella. Compend Cont Educ Pract Vet* 4:303–311, 1984.
8. Jones RL: Control of nosocomial infections. In Kirk

RW (ed): *Current Veterinary Therapy IX.* Philadelphia, WB Saunders Co, 1985, pp 19–24.

9. Monaghan C, Tierney V, Colleran E: Antibiotic resistance and R-factors in the fecal coliform flora of urban and rural dogs. *Antimicrob Agents Chemother* 19:266–270, 1981.

10. Barsanti JA, Blue J, Edmonds J: Urinary tract infection due to indwelling bladder catheter in dogs and cats. *J Am Vet Med Assoc* 187:384–388, 1985.

10a. Lippert AC, Fulton RB, Parr AM: Nosocomial infection surveillance in a small animal intensive care unit. *J Am Anim Hosp Assoc* 24:627–636, 1988.

11. Breitenbucher RB: Bacterial changes in the urine samples of patients with long-term indwelling catheters. *Arch Intern Med* 144:1585–1588, 1984.

12. Thompson RL, Haley CE, Searcy MA, et al: Catheter associated bacteriuria. Failure to reduce attack rates using periodic instillations of a disinfectant into urinary drainage systems. *JAMA* 251:747–751, 1984.

13. Burrows CF: Inadequate skin preparation as a cause of intravenous catheter–related infection in the dog. *J Am Vet Med Assoc* 180:747–749, 1982.

14. Wilkins RJ: *Serratia marcescens* septicaemia in the dog. *J Small Anim Pract* 14:205–215, 1973.

15. Fox JG, Beaucage CM, Folta CA, et al: Nosocomial transmission of *Serratia marcescens* in a veterinary hospital due to contamination by benzalkonium chloride. *J Clin Microbiol* 14:157–160, 1981.

16. Armstrong PJ: Systemic *Serratia marcescens* infections in a dog and a cat. *J Am Vet Med Assoc* 184:1154–1158, 1984.

17. Cooper GL, Hopkins CC: Rapid diagnosis of intravascular catheter–associated infection by direct Gram staining of catheter segments. *N Engl J Med* 312:1142–1147, 1985.

18. Collignon P, Chan R, Munro R, et al: Rapid diagnosis of intravascular catheter related sepsis. *Arch Intern Med* 147:1609–1612, 1987.

19. Driks MR, Craven DE, Celli BR, et al: Nosocomial pneumonia in intubated patients given sucralfate as compared with antacids or histamine type 2 blockers. *N Engl J Med* 317:1376–1382, 1987.

19a. Romatowski J: Prevention and control of surgical wound infection. *J Am Vet Med Assoc* 194:107–114, 1989.

20. National Research Council, Division of Medical Sciences. Ad hoc committee of the Committee on Trauma: Postoperative wound infections. The influence of ultraviolet irradiation of the operating room and other factors. *Ann Surg* 160:1–192, 1964.

21. Vasseur PB, Paul HB, Enos LR, et al: Infection rates in clean surgical procedures: a comparison of ampicillin prophylaxis versus a placebo. *J Am Vet Med Assoc* 187:825–827, 1985.

22. van den Bogaard AEJM, Weidema WF: Antimicrobial prophylaxis in canine surgery. *J Small Anim Pract* 26:257–266, 1985.

23. Oates JA, Wood AJJ: Antimicrobial prophylaxis in surgery. *N Engl J Med* 315:1129–1138, 1986.

24. Mercer HW: Calculation of dosage regimens of antimicrobial drugs for surgical prophylaxis. *J Am Vet Med Assoc* 185:1083–1087, 1984.

25. Hawthorn JW, Rubin M, Pizzo PA: Empirical antibiotic therapy in the febrile neutropenic cancer patient: clinical efficacy and impact of monotherapy. *Antimicrob Agents Chemother* 31:971–977, 1987.

26. Smith CW, Schiller AG, Smith AR: Monitoring the cleanliness of your surgery room floor. *J Am Anim Hosp Assoc* 16:531–532, 1980.

27. White WJ: Energy savings in the animal facility: opportunities and limitations. *Lab Anim* 11:28–35, 1982.

28. Smeak DD, Olmstead ML: Infections in clean wounds: the roles of the surgeon, environment and host. *Compend Cont Educ Pract Vet* 6:629–634, 1984.

29. Blaser MJ, Smith PF, Cody HJ, et al: Killing of fabric-associated bacteria in hospital laundry by low-temperature washing. *J Infect Dis* 149:48–57, 1984.

2 IMMUNOPROPHYLAXIS AND IMMUNOTHERAPY

Craig E. Greene

Immunoprophylaxis

Immunoprophylaxis involves enhancement of a specific immune response in an animal in an attempt to protect it against infectious disease. This response can be **actively** induced through the use of vaccines containing microorganisms, their components, or metabolic products. Immunity can also be **passively** transferred by the administration of humoral or cellular factors obtained from a previously sensitized donor. Immunoprophylaxis also implies preexposure immunopotentiation and should be differentiated from **immunotherapy**, which is the attempt to increase nonspecifically the immune response in an already infected animal. Immunoprophylaxis is more commonly used in the prevention of viral and bacterial diseases because of the relatively few antigens responsible for immunologic control of such infectious agents. Fungal, protozoal, and metazoan pathogens and neoplasms, all containing more complex antigenic determinants, are presently best controlled immunologically with nonspecific immunotherapy.

PASSIVE IMMUNIZATION

Artificial (passive) transfer of specific antibodies or other immunocompetent substances has been used classically to treat a variety of infectious diseases in humans and animals. The use of passive immunization has been decreasing in recent years; currently, it is used in small animal veterinary practice only in a few special instances (Table 2–1). Passive administration of serum or immune globulin has a beneficial role in protecting colostrum-deprived neonates (< 2 days old) against certain diseases. Active immunization must be avoided because of the risk of inducing disease with modified live vaccines and the poor response to inactivated vaccines at this age. Antisera, given to older (<8-weeks-old) kittens that become inadvertently exposed to feline panleukopenia virus, will provide protection much sooner than that produced following vaccination. Passive immunization may also temporarily benefit severely immunosuppressed dogs and cats receiving cancer chemotherapy that may become exposed to infectious agents during a course of hospitalization. Immune sera may also be of prophylactic or therapeutic benefit in treating litters of puppies that are clinically affected with neonatal herpesvirus infections (see Treatment, Chapter 18). Serum, in such cases, should be prepared from recovered bitches that have previously had affected litters. Hyperimmune serum was beneficial in treating parvoviral-infected dogs within 4 days PI (first days of clinical illness).[1] A commercial multivalent homologous hyperimmune immunoglobulin preparation (Stagloban P, Hoechst Veterinr Gmb, Munich, West Germany) is available in West Germany for this purpose. Passive immunization with antitoxin is used in the initial treatment of dogs and cats with tetanus (see Chapter 48). Monoclonal antibodies have been used as

Table 2–1. Comparison of Passive and Active Immunoprophylaxis

	PASSIVE	ACTIVE
Advantages	Immediate protection Works for agents that are poor immunogens	Stronger protection Longer protection Anamnestic response
Disadvantages	Allergic reactions Immune reactions Delays ability to vaccinate Short-lived protection Transfer of disease more likely	Delayed response
Indications	Exposed susceptible neonates Colostrum-deprived neonates Exposed immunosuppressed animals Replaces immunocompetent tissues	Unexposed susceptible neonates Booster vaccinations Routine immunization

specific passive immunotherapy for infectious agents, but because they are usually produced in rodents, species tolerance is low to systemically administered foreign immunoglobulins.

The efficacy of passive immunization depends upon many factors, including the antibody titer to the specific agent involved, the relative importance of serum antibody in controlling the particular infection involved, and the timing of administration of antibody compared with exposure. Owing to the large amounts of foreign protein that are administered, allergic reactions are more likely with passive immunization. Transfer of infectious agents is more likely with administration of serum when noncommercially prepared products are used. Unfortunately, the administration of immunoglobulins also delays the ability to stimulate active immunity in the host by vaccination. Large amounts of exogenously administered antibody may negate endogenous antibody production by tying up exogenous antigens or by direct feedback mechanisms that are not clearly understood. The duration of protection received from passively administered antisera is short lived. The amount received is finite and like all exogenous proteins, undergoes accelerated elimination from the body, especially if it originates from a different species.

Although not readily available commercially, canine and feline immune sera can be prepared in veterinary practices by sterilely harvesting serum. Immune serum is derived from healthy individuals or from groups of animals that have recovered from the disease in question, whereas hyperimmune serum comes from animals that have been repeatedly vaccinated against specified infectious agents. Veterinarians who prepare their own serum must carefully screen donors for insidious blood-borne infectious diseases such as feline leukemia or immunodeficiency virus infections or canine brucellosis or ehrlichiosis.

Oral administration of sera, either alone or in the milk substitute, is probably the most effective means of treating colostrum-deprived neonates in their first hours of life. Immunoglobulins, rapidly absorbed by neonates for up to 72 hours, also provide some local protection from intestinal pathogens. This local protection is only temporary because unstable serum antibodies are destroyed by proteolytic enzymes once the neonate develops improved digestive function. Other routes used are intramuscular (IM), subcutaneous (SC), intramedullary, and intraperitoneal. The dose of 2 to 4 ml/kg varies, depending on the titer of the preparation. Immune sera is not usually administered IV to small puppies or kittens because of the tendency to produce immunologic reactions in the recipient and because of the difficulty in cannulating a vein.

MATERNAL IMMUNITY AND VACCINATION

Newborn dogs and cats have the inherent capacity to respond immunologically to numerous antigens at birth, but this response is slower and inferior compared with that of

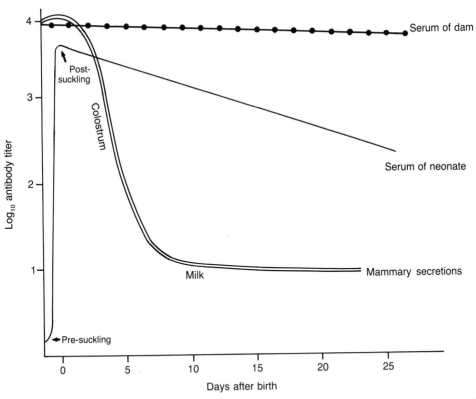

Figure 2–1. Correlation between antibody in serum and mammary secretions of dam and serum of neonatal puppy or kitten following birth.

the older animal. Under normal circumstances, protection against infection during these early weeks of life is afforded by passive transfer of immunoglobulins and small amounts of cellular material from the dam. The amount (2% to 18% of total) of antibody transferred in utero from an immune dam protects colostrum-deprived puppies or kittens but makes them refractory to immunization for several weeks. Subsequently, that immunoglobulin absorbed in colostrum gives the neonate a titer almost equal to that of the dam, and the quantity varies depending on the disease being considered (Fig. 2–1 and Tables 2–2 and 2–3). The decline of maternal antibody in neonates is similar to that for passively administered immunoglobulins, with each disease having a characteristic half-life for elimination (Table 2–4). Similarly, antibody class is important with respect to titer loss. Serum maternally-derived IgA, IgM, and IgG in neonates are lost in the order given.

The absolute titer of maternal immunoglobulin in the serum of a neonate depends upon the quantity of immunoglobulin received during nursing and the absolute titer of the dam. The amount is also inversely

proportional to the size of the litter. These values are so variable among individual animals that quantitative predictions cannot be made short of direct measurement of serum immunoglobulins of the dam or puppy. Such measurements (nomogram determinations) are usually impractical; therefore, veterinarians use multiple vaccines, given at 2- to 4-week intervals, in an attempt to break through maternal immunity before exposure to virulent virus (Figs. 2–2 and 2–3). Frequently given vaccines may also accelerate the depletion of the maternal antibody present in the neonate's circulation.

Attempts to overcome the interfering effects of maternal antibody on vaccination have included use of antigenically related vaccines, such as measles for canine distemper virus; alternate routes, such as intranasal administration for canine or feline respiratory viruses or *Bordetella*; or different vaccine strains or types that are able to overcome maternal immunity at a younger age.

ACTIVE IMMUNIZATION

Vaccination, the production of an active immune response, involves stimulating the

Table 2–2. Comparison of Maternal Immunity for Selected Canine and Feline Infectious Diseases[a]

| | SERUM TITER OF NEONATE | | | HALF-LIFE MATERNAL ANTIBODY (days) |
| | (% of Dam's Titer) | | (% of Neonate's Titer) | |
DISEASE	Pre-suckle	Post-suckle	Obtained in Utero/Colostrum	
Canine distemper[2, 3]	3	77	4/96	8.4
Infectious canine hepatitis[4, 5]	NR	92	NR/NR	8.6
Feline panleukopenia[6, 7]	<1	97	1/99	9.6
Canine parvoviral infection[8, 9]	5.7	60	10/90	9.7

[a]NR = not reported

Table 2–3. Effect of Maternal Immunity on Vaccination for Selected Canine and Feline Infectious Diseases[a]

| | MINIMUM TITER PREVENTING REPLICATION | | MINIMUM AGE (WEEKS) | | |
DISEASE	Virulent Virus (Method Determined)[b]	Vaccine Virus	To Begin Vaccinating Colostrum-Deprived	To Begin Vaccinating Colostrum Recipients	To Stop Vaccinating Colostrum Recipients
Canine distemper[2, 3]	1:20-1:30 (SN)	1:30 (SN)	2–3	6	12–14
Infectious canine hepatitis[4, 5]	NR	1:5 (SN)	2–3	6	12
Feline panleukopenia[6, 7]	1:30 (SN)	1:10 MLV (SN)	4	6	12
Canine parvoviral infection[8, 9]	1:80 (HI)	<1:10 (HI)	5	6–9	16–18

[a]HI = hemagglutination inhibition, NR = not reported, SN = serum neutralization (viral neutralization).
[b]Absolute titers will vary between laboratories.

Table 2–4. Half-Life of Maternally Derived Immunoglobulins in Neonatal Dogs and Cats

DISEASE	HALF-LIFE (days)	USUAL DURATION OF PROTECTION AGAINST DISEASE* (weeks)
Canine distemper[3]	8.4	9–12
Canine parvovirus[9, 11]	9.7	8–11
Infectious canine hepatitis[5]	8.4	9–12
Feline panleukopenia[7]	9.5	8–14
Feline leukemia[12]	15	6–8
Feline rhinotracheitis[13, 14, 15]	18.5	6–8
Feline calicivirus infection[16, 17]	15	10–14
Feline enteric coronavirus infection[18]	7	4–6

*The duration of maternal antibody protection against disease usually corresponds to the interval over which vaccines are ineffective. In some diseases, such as canine parvovirus infection, 3 to 5 weeks' additional time may be needed for maternal antibody interference with vaccination to disappear.

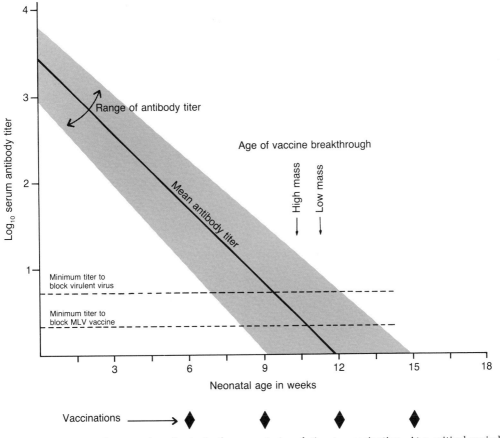

Figure 2–2. Elimination of maternal antibody in the neonate in relation to vaccination. At a critical period, the antibody titer may block an MLV vaccine but fail to protect against infection with virulent virus. Higher antigen mass or less attenuated vaccines break through this maternal antibody barrier sooner than lower antigen mass or more attenuated products.

Figure 2–3. Comparison of response to sequential (2-week interval) vaccination in neonates with *(top)* and without *(bottom)* maternal antibody protection. The presence of maternal antibody delays the neonate's ability to produce successful active immunization.

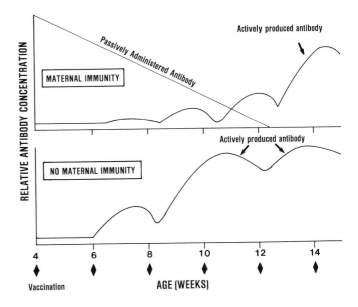

host with antigenic extracts or whole cultures of microorganisms. Clinical use of vaccination in small animals has been limited primarily to diseases caused by viruses and bacteria.

Vaccine Production

The development of tissue culture of viruses has greatly improved both the quality and the means of manufacturing veterinary vaccines. Commercial production, licensing, and marketing of biologics is rigidly controlled by the United States Department of Agriculture (USDA), the Ministry of Agriculture in the United Kingdom, the Bureau of Animal Health in Australia, and the Department of Agriculture in Canada. Vaccines are evaluated for safety as demonstrated by tests for sterility, toxicity, and the presence of adventitious agents. Efficacy of products marketed in the United States is confirmed in many cases by challenge studies that are performed *only 2 weeks* following completion of the initial vaccination series. Serologic responses are frequently followed for longer periods but unfortunately do not represent an absolute measure of protection in all types of infectious disease. Subsequently, vaccines are subjected to field testing by a limited number of practicing veterinarians before they are released for general usage.

Within the limits of testing guidelines, it is obvious that many products are initially marketed without complete knowledge of duration of immunity or adverse side effects. Reputable manufacturers are receptive to reports of complications encountered by practicing veterinarians and in turn keep the veterinary profession informed of continuing efficacy studies.

Fortunately, veterinary vaccines, unlike the human counterparts, can be more extensively tested on the species in which they are to be used, and appropriate challenge tests can be performed. The efficacy of a vaccine is determined by subsequently exposing vaccinated and unvaccinated animals to the same challenge dose and measuring the incidence and severity of clinical disease that follows. Seroconversion may be a valuable indicator to susceptibility to infection with certain diseases, such as that caused by canine parvovirus, in which experimental challenge produces minimal clinical illness.

Directions given by the manufacturers for handling of vaccines should always be followed accurately because of the labile and occasionally harmful nature of biologic products. If lyophilized products are used, vaccines should always be mixed with the diluents provided. Different products should never be mixed to produce combined vaccines unless this is permitted by the instructions. Serial numbers of vaccines should be entered in medical records to assist in tracing vaccine breaks or vaccine-induced illnesses.

The commercial production of combined vaccines in recent years has made vaccination protocols more convenient for both the veterinary profession and pet owners, increasing the likelihood that animals will be properly vaccinated. Interference testing, required for licensing, helps assure the veterinarian that antigens in combined products will produce immunity equal to individual antigens administered separately with no increased risk of complications.

Types of Vaccines

Live agents in vaccines must be modified (attenuated) so that they retain immunogenicity and ability to replicate in the intended host but do not produce illness. Attenuated vaccines produce cell-mediated and long-lived humoral immune responses as compared with noninfectious (inactivated or purified antigen) vaccines. This is because T cell stimulation is superior with attenuated products. Because they replicate in the host, initial antigenic content is of low importance; however, any factor that neutralizes or inactivates the vaccine will make it ineffective. Attenuation of agents is usually achieved by adapting them to unusual hosts or subjecting them to prolonged storage or, more recently, by serial passage in tissue culture. Vaccines also have been developed by inoculating only partially attenuated strains of organisms at sites other than those of their tissue tropism. This principle has been used to produce parenteral vaccines against respiratory pathogens. These agents undergo limited replication at the alternative sites, but unfortunately, they frequently produce a systemic rather than a local antibody response.

Quality control is an essential factor in live vaccine production to ensure that cell lines used in attenuating vaccine viruses do not contain latent pathogens, especially since veterinary vaccine production usually involves the use of primary and secondary cell cultures. Primary cell cultures are those derived from harvesting tissues taken directly from an animal. Secondary cultures originate from further cultivation of primary cell lines. Established (continuous) cell lines that are used for routine diagnostic virology are usually too anaplastic for vaccine production. Unlike human vaccines, those for animals are usually produced in cell lines of the species for which the vaccine is intended, which increases the risk of contamination with potentially pathogenic, latent, or passenger viruses. For this reason, quality control and careful screening for adventitious agents are important in live vaccine production.

Live vaccines are usually lyophilized, which increases their stability and storage lifespan. Temperature is another important factor determining storage lifespan, and vaccines should always be stored at 0°C. Commercially prepared live vaccines usually contain excess antigen, since some deterioration is expected.

Noninfectious vaccines are produced in a similar fashion to live vaccines. Inactivated products contain agents subjected to various forms of denaturation without destroying their immunogenicity. Heat and light treatments have been relatively ineffective because in many cases, they destroy immunogenicity without complete inactivation. Chemical inactivation with formalin produces slight modification in antigenic composition of the product, reduction in immunogenicity, and severe irritation to the animal at the site of injection. Ethyleneimine and β-propiolactone are inactivating agents that overcome many of these disadvantages. Subunit or genetically engineered vaccines are composed of purified immunogenic components of infectious agents in an attempt to increase the specificity and quantity of the immunogen while reducing its allergenicity.

Adjuvants, or nonspecific immunostimulatory drugs, are frequently added to noninfectious products to increase the duration and level of immunity they produce. Emulsified water-in-oil preparations have historically been used in veterinary products to facilitate antigen persistence. However, newer vaccines contain adjuvants such as mineral gels consisting of aluminum hydroxide, aluminum phosphate, and alum. Other adjuvants work by altering or stimulating lymphocyte responses to antigens.[19a] Adjuvants will be discussed further under Immunotherapy. Because noninfectious vaccines fail to replicate in the host, the antigenic mass present is a critical determinant in the efficacy of a particular product. In general, noninfectious vaccines must be given at least twice to produce an anamnestic response that equals one attenuated vaccination (Fig. 2–4).

Noninfectious vaccines usually require at least two vaccinations before an anamnestic response is produced. Despite this shortcoming, immunity that is stimulated by inactivated or subunit products is commonly sufficient for clinical protection and routine use. Following vaccination with inactivated products, many partially protected animals probably become infected upon exposure to virulent agents. They develop a mild or subclinical infection that further boosts their immunity to the disease.

For a further discussion of subunit vaccines, see Developmental or Experimental Vaccines. For a comparison of the three major vaccine types, see Table 2–5.

Evaluation of Vaccine Protection

Immunity following vaccination takes several days to develop, but it may last for years. Following first-time or primary exposure to an antigen, the initial protection is usually provided by interferon and later by an immunoglobulin response. The primary response is slower in onset than a secondary or anamnestic response and initially is predominantly composed of IgM (Fig. 2–5).[20] A secondary response that follows re-exposure to the antigen is characterized primarily by IgG.

Both humoral and cell-mediated responses are important in protection from infection. Vaccines have an important role in stimulating both mechanisms. Unfortunately, humoral immune responses have often been measured following vaccination and equated with protection of an animal from infection. The significance of an absolute antibody titer is only meaningful when standarized serologic procedures are used and when this is related to titers giving protection of animals to challenge infections. Furthermore, protection against many

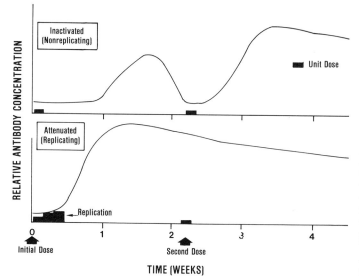

Figure 2–4. Comparison of antibody response following inoculation with inactivated *(top)* and live attenuated *(bottom)* virus vaccines. One dose of the live attenuated virus vaccine continues to drive the immune response. Two doses of inactivated vaccine are required to produce a similar effect. (Modified from Mims CA: *The Pathogenesis of Infectious Disease.* Academic Press, 1977, p 225, with permission.)

respiratory and GI infections is based on secretory rather than serum immune responses. Therefore, challenge of the animal with a virulent agent is a more reliable measure of vaccine efficacy. Cellular memory of past exposure to an antigen may persist long after serum antibody titers decline.

Vaccination Failures

The many causes of vaccination failure in dogs and cats are summarized in Table 2–6. A few of the more pertinent features are discussed in this section. Veterinarians should realize the difference between *vaccination* and *immunization*. Not all vaccines will effectively immunize those patients to which they are given because of inherent host factors, difficulties with the vaccine, or errors made in the process of administration. Vaccination in the presence of maternal antibody is the most common cause of vaccine interference in young animals and has been discussed previously.

Use of cytotoxic agents or glucocorticoids may be associated with a decreased response to vaccination, depending on the dosage and duration of treatment. When glucocorticoids are given long term, the use of alternate-day therapy is less likely to cause immunosuppression. Glucocorticoids are less likely to interfere with booster vaccinations; however, they are not recommended when initial attempts are made to induce an immune response to a particular antigen.

Moderate dosages of prednisolone were administered to previously unvaccinated 13-week-old puppies for a 3-week period prior to vaccination for canine distemper.[21] Dosages of 1 or 10 mg/kg were given every 12 hours for the first week, once daily for the second week, followed by alternate-day therapy for the last week. The dogs were challenged with virulent virus 3 days after vaccination. Although in vitro lymphocyte stimulation testing showed a depressed response compared with control dogs, all vaccinated puppies receiving glucocorticoid therapy were immune to challenge.

Antibody responses to measles and distemper virus vaccination have also been studied in dogs more severely immunosuppressed with concurrent methotrexate and antithymocyte sera.[22] Dogs immunosuppressed prior to canine distemper vaccination developed vaccine-induced systemic illness and encephalitis and died. Those that were immunosuppressed following distemper vaccination and were later challenged with virulent canine distemper virus resisted challenge but had no increase in neutralizing antibody titer.

Dexamethasone, at a daily dosage of 0.25 mg/kg, was given to dogs prior to and following their first vaccination with rabies vaccine.[23] There was no decrease in the serum antibody titer of treated compared with untreated animals.

Changes in body temperature may influ-

Table 2–5. Comparison of Different Vaccines

MODIFIED LIVE VACCINE	INACTIVATED VACCINE	SUBUNIT VACCINE
Advantages		
Rapid protection	No reversion to virulence	No postvaccinal illness
Prolonged protection	Increased activity with added	Minimal extraneous foreign protein
Lower antigen mass needed	adjuvants	Higher potency obtainable
Can administer by natural route	Stability in storage	
Stimulate secretory antibody (SIgA)		
Better able to stimulate cell-mediated immunity		
Better stimulator of interferon		
Disadvantages		
Risk of adventitious agents	Minimum of 2 doses needed for	Costly to produce
Can produce vaccine-induced illness in immunosuppressed hosts	maximum protection	Many technical difficulties in manufacture
Susceptible to inactivation	Increased risk of allergic complications	
Require more rigorous testing for potency and reversion to virulence	Shorter duration of immunity than modified live vaccines	
Require replication in host	Higher antigen mass needed	
Might revert to virulence	Restricted to parenteral use	
	Adjuvants frequently required	
Indications		
Outbreaks	Pregnant animals	Pregnant animals
For production of mucosal immunity	Debilitated or immunosuppressed animals	Debilitated or immunosuppressed animals
Routine vaccination	Colostrum-deprived neonates (passive immunization preferred)	When live vaccines produce disease but potency not required
		To reduce allergenicity of inactivated products
Diseases in Which Vaccines Are Used		
Canine: Parvoviral enteritis	Canine: Coronaviral enteritis	Canine: Leptospirosis (envelope)
Hepatitis	Parvoviral enteritis	Bordetellosis
Bordetellosis	Hepatitis	cell wall antigen
Parainfluenza	Bordetellosis	Feline: Leukemia (glycoprotein
Distemper	Leptospirosis	gp 70)
Feline: Panleukopenia	Feline: Panleukopenia	
Calicivirus	Calicivirus	
Rhinotracheitis	Rhinotracheitis	
	Leukemia	
Canine and feline: Rabies	Canine and feline: Rabies	Canine and feline: Rabies (glycoprotein G)

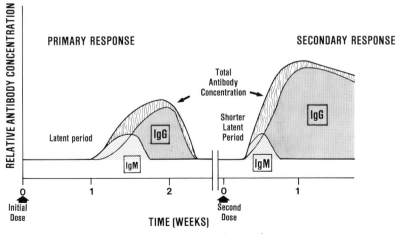

Figure 2–5. Primary and secondary humoral immune responses.

Table 2-6. Causes of Vaccination Failure

HOST FACTORS	VACCINE FACTORS	HUMAN ERROR
Immunodeficiencies	Inactivated during handling	Improper mixing of products
Maternal antibody interference	Improper storage	Exposed at time of vaccination
Age: very young or very old	Vaccines do not protect 100% of population	Concurrent use of antimicrobials
Pregnancy		Simultaneous use of antisera
Stress	Disinfectant used on needles and syringes	Too frequent administration (<2-week interval)
Pyrexia, hypothermia	Wrong strain	Disinfection of skin?[a]
Incubating disease at time of vaccination	Excessive attenuation	Wrong route of administration
Drugs: cytotoxic, glucocorticoids		
Anesthesia?[a]		
Hormonal fluctuations		
General debilitation		

[a]? = uncertain.

ence the immune response. Elevated rectal temperature, artificially induced by high environmental temperature and humidity, has been shown to inhibit the serologic response of 8- to 12-week-old puppies to canine distemper vaccination.[24] Puppies with elevated rectal temperatures ($\geq$ 39.8°C [103.6°F]) that were kept under these conditions developed clinical illness following subsequent challenge with virulent distemper virus, while those with lower rectal temperatures were protected. The serologic response following vaccination for infectious canine hepatitis was not affected by these conditions.

Hypothermia is also known to decrease the measured in vitro cell-mediated immune response of dogs, and probably cats, to vaccination.[25] Anesthesia and surgery were shown to have little influence on the serologic response of dogs to distemper vaccination although the cell-mediated immunity (CMI), as measured by in vitro lymphocyte stimulation, was depressed.[26]

Inactivation of modified live vaccine is less commonly a cause of vaccine failure because of present-day manufacture and lyophilization of vaccines, refrigerated storage, and use of heat-sterilized disposable syringes rather than chemically disinfected syringes. Most vaccines have adequate particle numbers to overcome possible reductions in antigen mass that occur during handling and storage. Even with all factors taken into consideration, no vaccine produces immunity in 100% of the population to which it is administered. This biologic variation is responsible for vaccine breaks in a low percentage of cases with all vaccines. Protection of 70% of the population may be effective in reducing the prevalence of diseases when communicability is low, such as has oc-

curred with rabies; however, it is unacceptable in preventing rapidly transmitted diseases such as canine parvoviral enteritis. Depending on the disease, the acceptable efficacy of protection allowed for most vaccines is between 65% and 95%, meaning a certain percentage of animals will be unprotected in any vaccinated population.

Veterinarians are often blamed for animals developing disease following apparently adequate vaccinations. It is possible that the animal was incubating the disease prior to vaccination. Other factors, however, are under direct control of the veterinarian. Many of these vaccine breaks may be caused by inattention to precautions that should have been taken during the vaccination procedure. Dogs and cats may contact pathogenic agents for the first time when they enter the veterinary hospital for vaccination. This may occur in the hospital waiting room or ward area because of improper traffic flow or inadequate disinfection or isolation procedures for already infected animals.

Vaccine interference can occur whenever antigens are administered at too frequent an interval. It is better to administer several attenuated vaccines simultaneously than to give them 1 to 4 days apart because of the blocking effect that the first vaccine may have on the second (Fig. 2-6). This interference may relate, in part, to the production of interferon by infected cells. Whenever possible, modified live vaccines should not be administered in the face of other infectious diseases for this reason. Postponement of vaccinations for at least 2 to 3 weeks following illness or prior to sequential vaccinations with the same or a different product has been shown to be sufficient to overcome this interference.

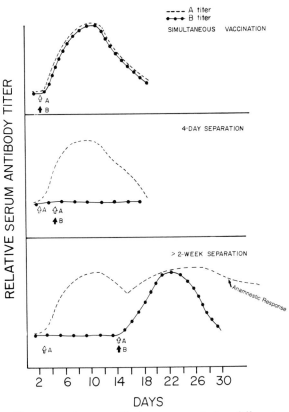

Figure 2–6. Serum antibody responses to two different antigens, homologous (A) and heterologous (B). *Top,* With simultaneous vaccination, a response to both antigens occurs. *Middle,* A 4-day interval between the first inoculation with antigen A and a repeated inoculation with antigen A and a single inoculation with antigen B prevents a response to either, presumably because of inactivation by factors such as interferons. *Bottom,* A 2-week or greater interval between the same repeated vaccinations (used in the middle example) is followed by a primary response to antigen B and an anamnestic response to antigen A.

In some circumstances, the route of vaccination is also critical in maximizing the immune response since modified live virus (MLV) rabies vaccines, feline respiratory vaccines, and measles vaccines are more effective when given IM rather than SC. For MLV rabies vaccines, this discrepancy may be explained by the fact that vaccine virus replicates better in innervated muscle as opposed to less innervated subcutaneous tissue.

VACCINATION RECOMMENDATIONS FOR SPECIFIC DISEASES

The diseases to be discussed are those for which vaccines are commercially available

to small animal practitioners. Specific chapters on each disease should be consulted for additional information. Overall recommendations for canine and feline immunization protocols are summarized in Appendices 1 and 2, respectively. Appendix 5 lists the manufacturers of veterinary biologics in English language–speaking countries.

Canine Vaccination Recommendations

See Appendices 1 and 3.

Canine Distemper. (Also see Prevention, Chapter 16.) Only modified live virus vaccines have been effective in protecting dogs against canine distemper. Distemper vaccination is presently performed in combination with other antigens at 3- to 4-week intervals, beginning at 5 to 8 weeks of age. Most presently used vaccines are able to break through maternal immunity by the time the animal is 12 weeks of age. Colostrum-deprived puppies should be vaccinated with distemper vaccine beginning at 2 to 3 weeks of age.

Measles vaccination, alone and in combination with that for distemper, has been recommended in the first vaccination given to puppies between 6 and 9 weeks of age. It is used to create a heterotypic immune response in the presence of a high concentration of maternally derived distemper antibody, at a time when vaccination with MLV distemper vaccine would fail. Measles antigen does not produce as strong an immune response as distemper antigen. Measles virus does not typically produce a strong humoral response to canine distemper virus (CDV) but rather cell-mediated immune protection. Distemper antigen has been combined with measles by some vaccine manufacturers with the assumption that it would produce a superior homotypic response in those puppies whose maternal immunity is weak. Measles vaccines should never be given to bitches older than 12 weeks of age, and its use is usually not recommended after 9 weeks of age. Maternal antibodies to measles antigen, present in bitches' colostrum if they are bred and have a litter following the first heat, will interfere with the effectiveness of measles vaccine subsequently given to the pups. Furthermore, by 12 weeks of age, maternal immunity will have waned sufficiently that distemper vaccine alone should be effective.

Immunity to distemper in a previously unvaccinated, unexposed dog lasts for 10 months when only one CDV vaccine is given or when a distemper-measles vaccine is followed by one distemper vaccine.[27] To ensure protection until a yearly booster is given, at least two vaccinations with CDV antigen should follow in the puppy vaccination series whenever measles or combined distemper-measles antigens are used as the first vaccine. At least two vaccinations with CDV vaccine should also be given, 3 to 4 weeks apart, whenever dogs over 12 weeks of age are presented for their first vaccination. Measles vaccine is more effective when given IM. CDV vaccines appear equally effective whether given IM or SC.[28] Vaccination of dogs with MLV-CDV vaccine IV may be effective in preventing disease when it is given within 3 to 4 days following initial exposure to virulent distemper virus. Dogs should be given one vaccination booster whenever such exposure occurs, regardless of their previous vaccination history.

Distemper is a disease that can develop following stress, concurrent illness, or immunosuppression of currently vaccinated dogs. Distemper vaccine virus may occasionally induce illness itself (usually 7 to 10 days postvaccination) if it is given to severely immunosuppressed dogs or with particular batches of vaccine[28a] (see Vaccination Failures and Postvaccinal Encephalomyelitis). Therefore, care must be taken not to vaccinate dogs against distemper, especially neonates < 3 months old that have a known or suspected parvoviral infection (see Prevention, Chapter 21). Measles vaccine might be used in lieu of distemper vaccine under such circumstances since it is less likely to produce vaccine-induced encephalitis (see Canine Parvoviral Infection).

Infectious Canine Hepatitis. (Also see Chapter 17.) Vaccination for infectious canine hepatitis (ICH) is usually done in combination with that for distemper and other diseases, beginning at 6 weeks of age. Modified live adenovirus vaccines are used in the United States because of their ability to produce a superior immune response. Vaccination for ICH has brought about a marked reduction in the prevalence of a disease that was once widespread. Outbreaks or isolated cases still occur when vaccination of pup-

pies is delayed or incomplete. The shedding of modified viruses and viral stability outside the host have been responsible for inadvertent immunization of many dogs. Vaccines for ICH contain either homologous canine adenovirus-1 (CAV-1) or a closely related respiratory isolate, canine adenovirus-2 (CAV-2). The former is shed in the kidneys and the latter in upper respiratory secretions; however, the amount that is shed varies between individual products. Another side effect of MLV–CAV-1 vaccine is its ability to produce anterior uveitis (blue eye) in a small percentage of dogs. The prevalence of this complication can be increased if the vaccine is inadvertently given IV. CAV-2 vaccines do not frequently cause this potential complication. Intranasal CAV-2 vaccines can protect puppies, despite maternal antibody interference, by stimulating local immune responses.[28b]

Adjuvanted inactivated CAV-1 and CAV-2 vaccines have been used in the United Kingdom.[29] Although inactivated vaccines produce a lesser serologic response, they are not shed by the host nor do they produce uveitis. A booster dose must be given annually, whereas in many cases, the MLV products produce lifelong immunity.

Canine Infectious Tracheobronchitis. (Also see Prevention, Chapter 19.) Infectious tracheobronchitis, or kennel cough, is incited by a number of respiratory pathogens with variable degrees of virulence and immunogenicity. Modified live distemper and CAV-2 viruses, both of which can cause respiratory tract infections, are included in routine parenteral vaccines. Modified live parainfluenza virus and *Bordetella bronchiseptica* bacterin may be added in parenteral combinations; however, herpesvirus- and reovirus-containing products are not available. The duration of immunity produced by respiratory vaccines against most primary respiratory pathogens, such as parainfluenza virus and *Bordetella*, has not been well established. Serum antibody titers that last for relatively long periods following parenteral vaccination with these antigens have little role in providing protection against infections of the respiratory or other mucosal surfaces. Secretory antibody and other local immune mechanisms are more important. Parenteral canine respiratory vaccines usually do not produce protection until 2 to 3 weeks following the second vaccination.

Originally, parenterally administered *Bordetella* bacterins contained lipopolysaccharide that produced fever, swelling, pain, or abscess formation at the site of injection. Newer products have modified whole-cell or purified cell wall components that obviate these side effects. Some reduction in efficacy has been associated with the purification process.

Intranasal vaccines, including both modified live parainfluenza virus and *B. bronchiseptica*, have been developed in an attempt to increase the local immune response to vaccination (see Appendix 3). Intranasal *Bordetella* vaccine has been shown to protect against clinical illness and to reduce the shedding of organisms following challenge exposure.[30] Most animals were protected against infection by 4 to 14 days following vaccination. Intranasal parainfluenza and *Bordetella* vaccines may protect within 72 hours following their use, so that they can be used to help prevent illness in an outbreak in a kennel or in pets prior to hospitalization or boarding. The clinical illness resulting from intranasally administered canine respiratory vaccine is mild or unnoticeable as compared with that seen with topically applied feline respiratory vaccines.

Use of vaccines against tracheobronchitis is recommended when an increased risk of respiratory infection is known or suspected. When anticipated, dogs initially should be vaccinated with at least two parenteral or one intranasal vaccine at least 10 to 14 days prior to possible exposure at dog shows, kennels, or veterinary hospitals. With intranasal vaccines, the animal could be vaccinated immediately prior to exposure as a less desirable but practical alternative. Puppies as young as 2 to 3 weeks of age can be given intranasal vaccine since it is not as affected by maternal antibody as parenteral products. Annual or more frequent boosters are recommended in animals that are exposed to a high prevalence of tracheobronchitis. Parenteral parainfluenza virus and *Bordetella* vaccines have minimal side effects. They are marketed in combination with distemper vaccines, so for convenience separate administration is not required.

Canine Parvoviral Enteritis. (Also see Prevention, Chapter 21.) Vaccination for canine parvoviral enteritis has become an essential part of the vaccination program in dogs. Parvovirus is as contagious as canine distemper virus, but it is much more stable in the environment. This means that over 90% to 95% of dogs in the population may have to be successfully immunized to break the chain or spread of infection. Produced from either feline origin (feline panleukopenia virus) or canine origin (canine parvovirus-2 [CPV-2]) isolates, they are available as noninfectious or MLV vaccines.

In canine parvoviral infection as with other diseases, MLV vaccines offer a longer duration of immunity (see Table 2–7). Although antibody titers may wane earlier with inactivated products, under field conditions, dogs may be partially protected and when exposed to virulent virus, may become subclinically infected, which boosts immunity. Some inactivated CPV-2 vaccines have produced resistance to challenge infection in pups 1 year after the second of two inoculations.[31] Equal protection can be provided by one MLV–CPV-2 injection. MLV products also offer relatively better protection against shedding of virulent virus following challenge than do inactivated vaccines. For this reason, older dogs that will be housed with younger susceptible animals should be vaccinated with MLV vaccines. MLV–CPV-2 products themselves are consistently shed in the feces of vaccinated dogs, albeit at a lower level than that following natural infection. The amount of fecal shedding, which decreases with attenuation, is of no clinical significance, although accidental exposure of other dogs to vaccine virus with seroconversion may occur. MLV products are not recommended in immunosuppressed or pregnant dogs or in puppies less than 5 weeks of age. Ideally, bitches should be vaccinated with MLV–CPV-2 products at least 2 weeks prior to breeding. If already pregnant with an uncertain level of antibody, the bitch can be given two doses of inactivated CPV-2 vaccine 3 to 4 weeks apart in the last trimester.

When given to puppies, none of the presently available vaccines break through maternal immunity as effectively as virulent canine parvovirus, although the MLV–CPV-2 vaccines have greater activity in this regard.[32] MLV–feline origin parvoviral vaccines have not produced as consistent an immune response as MLV–CPV-2 products in puppies that completed their vaccination series between 12 to 16 weeks.[32a] Maternal antibody interference was important, but not the sole reason for this inconsistent protec-

Table 2–7. Comparison of Vaccines Available for Canine Parvovirus Infection

	FELINE-ORIGIN VACCINES[a]		CANINE-ORIGIN VACCINES	
	Inactivated	**Modified Live**	**Inactivated**	**Modified Live**
Recommended for use in pregnancy	Yes	No	Yes	No
Shedding of vaccine virus	No	No	No	Yes
Prevent shedding of virulent virus	No	Yes	No	Yes
Relative magnitude of humoral response	Low	Intermediate	Low	High
Relative protection following challenge after 2 weeks[b]	Variable	Variable	Variable	High
Duration of humoral response	3–8 mo	6–12 mo	9–12 mo	≥20 mo
Recommended revaccination interval	6–12 mo	12 mo	12 mo	12 mo
Relative particle mass of vaccine required	High	High	High	Low
Minimum dose recommended (≥14–16 weeks of age)	2–3	2	2	1

[a]Use only higher-particle-mass vaccines adapted for dogs.
[b]Assume no interference from maternal antibody.

tion. Passively acquired serum antibody has also been effective in prolonging the incubation period, reducing viremia and subsequent clinical illness, and reducing fecal excretion of virulent CPV-2 following experimental challenge.[1] However, repeated exposure to virulent virus leads to an accelerated decline in maternal antibody titers.[33] Thus maternal antibody may fall below protective levels, requiring earlier vaccination, in areas of high environmental contamination.

Vaccination for parvoviral infection in young puppies is most commonly recommended in conjunction with the series of inoculations for canine distemper. Some commercially available MLV–CPV-2 products are claimed to break through maternal immunity as early as 6 weeks of age.[34,35] Unfortunately, some puppies may not be protected, even with MLV–CPV-2 vaccine until up to 18.5 weeks of age.[32,36] Therefore, repeated vaccination of puppies for parvoviral infection is essential. Administration of at least four vaccines in a series, prior to 18 weeks of age, was associated with more consistent seroconversion of puppies than with lower numbers of vaccinations.[36a] Oronasal vaccination has not been any more successful than parenteral vaccination in breaking through maternal antibody interference.[37] Dogs that are older than 16 to 18 weeks of age at first presentation should receive at least two vaccinations 3 to 4 weeks apart, although theoretically, if MLV–CPV-2 is used, one vaccination may be sufficient for protection against parvoviral infection.

Although virulent CDV and CPV-2 have been shown to produce immunosuppres-

sion, this has not been well documented for attenuated canine distemper or canine-origin parvoviral vaccine viruses. Although in vitro lymphocyte stimulation testing has been shown to be suppressed following vaccination with MLV–CPV-2 vaccines,[37a] no clinical evidence of immunosuppression has been documented with their use. Nevertheless, vaccines may cause problems in dogs simultaneously infected with virulent viruses. Enhanced parvoviral disease has been reported in dogs that received commercial distemper-hepatitis-leptospirosis vaccination several days before experimental infection with virulent CPV-2.[38] Postvaccinal distemper encephalitis was documented only when distemper vaccine was given to young (3-week-old) puppies incubating virulent parvoviral disease[39] but not in older (11- to 15-week-old) puppies.[40]

Although it has been suggested that combined vaccination with MLV-CDV and CPV-2 vaccines causes immunosuppression,[41] more controlled experimental studies that evaluated six commercial products have refuted these claims.[40] Despite the general fact that MLV parvoviral and distemper vaccines are safe when combined, recommendations have been made by some not to use them together for the first vaccinations given to puppies less than 9 to 10 weeks of age. These same recommendations state that parvoviral vaccine be used alone for the first immunization (6 weeks of age), to be followed by subsequent distemper vaccination 3 weeks later (9 weeks of age) or vice versa. Unfortunately, during this 3-week interval, puppies with reduced maternal immune protection will be highly susceptible to infection with either virulent distemper or parvovirus, depending on which is omitted. Another recommendation has been to give the vaccines alternatively on a weekly basis, although spacing MLV inoculations too closely may cause vaccine interference. Alternating between distemper and parvoviral vaccines in young puppies on a weekly or greater interval is therefore not recommended, unless there is a high prevalence of postvaccinal encephalitis. Measles vaccine may be substituted for distemper antigen in the first vaccination of very young puppies (< 9 weeks of age) to reduce potential distemper vaccine–induced encephalitis when pups with concurrent virulent parvoviral infection must be vaccinated.

The antigenic composition of canine parvovirus has been slightly altered since it was initially recognized in 1978.[42] Despite this fact, commercial vaccines produced from original isolates still protect dogs against subsequent challenge with more recently recovered strains.[43] Similarly, immunodiagnostic tests based upon monoclonal antibodies to original isolates are still sensitive in detecting newer strains of virus.[43a]

In general, parvoviral vaccination should be started at 6 to 8 weeks of age, along with canine distemper vaccination, because of the high prevalence of infection and the chance that vaccination at this age may protect some puppies with lower maternal antibody titers. Early vaccination (6 to 8 weeks of age) can induce protection against distemper and parvovirus in some cases. Vaccination of puppies for parvovirus should continue at 3- to 4-week intervals until dogs are at least 16 weeks and, in some cases, 18 weeks of age because of the prolonged maternal antibody interference that seems to exist with this disease.

Administration of parvoviral vaccines on a weekly basis is not routinely recommended because of the possibility of vaccine interference by closely spaced inoculations (see Fig. 2–6). A 2-week interval is the accepted minimum. A 1-week interval should only be considered when outbreaks of parvoviral enteritis develop in puppies less than 18 weeks of age, and established vaccine protocols have been unsuccessful. At such times, MLV–CPV-2 vaccine could be given in combination with some other antigens, on a weekly basis, between 6 and 12 weeks of age. After this time it could be given every 2 weeks until the pups are 18 weeks old.

Pups from breeds with a high prevalence rate for developing infection, such as Doberman pinschers, Rottweilers, or pit bull terriers, should also receive vaccines until they are 18 weeks old. Vaccination for parvovirus might seem indicated earlier than 6 to 8 weeks of age in cases where the prevalence of the disease is high or in colostrum-deprived puppies. However, only inactivated products should be used in puppies less than 5 weeks of age because of potential damage to rapidly dividing cells, such as those in the myocardium. Veterinarians should advise pet owners to ensure that puppies are isolated and not exposed to other dogs or litters during the early neonatal period and until the vaccination series for distemper and parvoviral infection are complete. They should also attempt to keep suspected parvovirus-infected dogs that may contaminate waiting rooms and hospital wards from coming into contact with susceptible puppies in their environment.

Coronaviral Infection. (Also see Prevention of Coronaviral Infections, Chapter 21.) An MLV vaccine against canine coronaviral (CCV) infection that was approved and released for use in dogs in the United States was withdrawn soon after its release because of a suspected coronaviral-induced encephalomyelitis (see Postvaccinal Encephalomyelitis). Inactivated coronaviral vaccines are available (see Appendix 3).[44,45,45a] The manufacturers recommend that two vaccines be given 2 to 3 weeks apart, beginning at 6 weeks of age. However, puppies completing their vaccination schedule when less than 12 weeks of age should be given an additional dose between 12 to 16 weeks because of the potential maternal antibody interference. Inactivated vaccines cause no adverse reactions and appear to be safe and not to cause interference when used simultaneously with other biologics.[45a,46] As with many vaccines, immunity studies of only 2-weeks' duration after the second dose are available. Serum and intestinal antibody concentrations, although potentially less conclusive measures of protection, have been evaluated for longer periods. Noninfectious vaccines for CCV do not totally prevent infection of exposed dogs but reduce the degree of viral replication throughout the intestinal tract. Secretory IgA has been increased in challenged vaccinated animals as compared to unvaccinated controls.[45,45a] Because secretory antibody titers are generally short-lived and a parenteral noninfectious product is being used, booster vaccines are recommended yearly or sooner if the need for confirmed protection arises.

CCV generally produces less morbidity and minimal mortality as compared with CPV-2 (see Canine Viral Enteritis, Chapter 21). Combined infections with CPV-2 and CCV can be more severe than with either infection alone.[47] There may be some justification in vaccinating dogs against CCV as a means of protecting them against severe CPV-2 infections.

Vaccination against CCV is recommended when clients desire all possible means of protection against viral diarrhea or in endemic areas. Previously unvaccinated animals may not respond in time to its use in an outbreak. The use of this vaccine on a routine basis depends upon the cost to the client for this additional protection and the inconvenience to the practitioner of maintaining inventories of separate preparations. Otherwise, routine use of these noninfectious CCV vaccines can help reduce the severity of infection, and adverse reactions appear few.

The CCV vaccine has been combined with distemper, adenovirus, parainfluenza virus, and parvovirus multivalent products. Combination of *Leptospira* bacterins and inactivated CCV antigen in the same product has caused some difficulties. Increased allergic reactions to the *Leptospira* fraction have been found when CCV adjuvants are present. There does not appear to be a problem with administering *Leptospira* bacterin at another site at the same time. To avoid potential interactions, CCV vaccine could be used in puppies between 6 and 9 weeks of age and then leptospiral vaccination instituted thereafter. An additional dose of CCV vaccine will still be needed at 12 weeks of age or older. When leptospiral bacterin is marketed in a combined product with CCV vaccine, both can be used simultaneously.

Leptospirosis. (Also see Prevention, Chapter 45.) *Leptospira* vaccines for dogs contain the inactivated bacterins of *L. canicola* and *L. icterohaemorrhagiae*. Vaccination with these products is not routinely recommended in animals less than 9 weeks of age because of the allergenic nature of the vaccines. Anaphylaxis may be noted within 1 hour following the second or third vaccination of puppies given the initial series (see Type 1 Immunologic Complications). A prior allergic reaction to a combination booster in any dog is probably caused by the *Leptospira* bacterin, which should be eliminated in subsequent vaccinations. Combination of this vaccine with inactivated adjuvanted vaccines, such as those for CCV disease, will increase the risk of anaphylaxis. *Leptospira* bacterin is marketed in a liquid form and is usually used to reconstitute the lyophilized components in combination vaccines.

Unfortunately, *Leptospira* bacterins do not produce as high a level or as long a duration of immunity as other agents used in canine vaccines. Certain *Leptospira* products would have to be administered two or three times over 2- to 3-week intervals to produce immunity that might last 6 months. Such protocols of vaccination are impractical under most circumstances since this vaccination is usually performed in conjunction with routine distemper and hepatitis vaccination. A few companies have products that are claimed to provide protection from challenge for up to 12 to 14 months. Unfortunately, none of the present *Leptospira* vaccines protect against the carrier state that may develop after exposure to virulent organisms; they only decrease the development of clinical illness. Newer subunit vaccines containing the immunogenic envelope of *Leptospira* are being developed to overcome the disadvantages of presently available products.

Rabies Vaccination Recommendations

(Also see Chapter 31.) Rabies vaccines have been extremely effective in reducing the prevalence of this disease in dogs. As a result, the incidence of human disease has decreased substantially, whereas the relative importance of feline rabies has increased. The first vaccines for rabies, derived from nervous tissue of infected adult animals, evoked severe autoimmune reactions in the CNS. Subsequently, more purified, extraneurally produced MLV vaccines were cultivated in avian embryo and tissue culture media. Certain MLV vaccines have produced postvaccinal rabies in dogs and cats (see

Postvaccinal Encephalomyelitis). Because of this problem, the trend has been to switch to the use of inactivated rabies vaccines. In the United States, only one MLV vaccine is presently USDA-approved for use in cats (see Appendix 6).

Some inactivated vaccines provide a similar duration and level of protection compared with MLV products. Advantages of using inactivated vaccines are the absence of postvaccinal encephalomyelitis and the ability to use one brand of vaccine for many species. The most recent Compendium of Animal Rabies Vaccines (see Appendix 6), published by the National Association of State Public Health Veterinarians, should be consulted.

To give immunity similar to that of attenuated products, inactivated rabies vaccines must contain high viral content and must contain adjuvants such as aluminum hydroxide. These modifications may be associated with a greater degree of allergic reactions, especially in cats (see Postvaccinal Complications).

All MLV rabies vaccines must be given IM at one site in the thigh. MLV vaccines require fixation to nerve endings to be effective and these are more plentiful in muscle as compared with subcutaneous tissue. Inactivated vaccines were initially required to be given IM until appropriate challenge studies in SC vaccinates could be completed.[48] In general, inactivated rabies vaccine given IM often give stronger immune responses than those given SC. Because of the significant antibody responses that occurred following SC vaccination, many of the inactivated vaccines originally certified by challenge studies for IM use were given preliminary 3-year licensing approval for SC use by the USDA. Because the serologic studies did not always predict the protection following challenge, the approval for 3-year vaccination protection for SC vaccination based on IM administration was withdrawn until challenge studies were completed.[48] Consult the Compendium (Appendix 6) for the approval recommendations for the route of administration of and duration of protection afforded by particular products.

Both dogs and cats should receive their first rabies vaccine no earlier than 3 months of age; this is frequently given on the last visit of the neonatal vaccination series (Appendices 1 and 2). Subsequent boosters in dogs are administered 1 or 3 years later,

depending on the vaccine used and local public health laws. Because of the confusion it might cause in diagnosis and management, rabies vaccination is *not* recommended for wild animals that are kept as pets; however, when needed, only inactivated products should be used.

Feline Vaccination Recommendations
(See Appendices 2 and 4.)

Feline Panleukopenia. (Also see Prevention, Chapter 23.) Both inactivated and MLV vaccines are effective in preventing this disease. In the absence of maternal antibody interference, at least two doses of inactivated vaccine are required in kittens to equal the protection afforded by one dose of MLV vaccine. Therefore, at least two MLV or three inactivated vaccine doses should be given at 3- to 4-week intervals when kittens are presented for the initial series at 8 to 9 weeks of age. The second MLV vaccine ensures that an anamnestic response will occur if the first vaccine was blocked by maternal antibody. Maternal antibody interference is usually gone by 12 weeks of age. Both are effective when used as yearly boosters, although one MLV vaccine probably provides longer-term protection. Inactivated vaccines are preferred in pregnant queens, in severely immunosuppressed or diseased cats, and in kittens less than 4 weeks of age that require vaccination. Newborn kittens are immunologically responsive to feline panleukopenia by 7 days of age; however, use of the MLV vaccine must be avoided prior to 4 weeks of age because of its potential for producing cerebellar degeneration.

In this disease, homologous immune serum can provide immediate protection to exposed unvaccinated kittens (see Passive Immunization). Subsequent vaccination should be delayed for at least 2 weeks.

Feline Respiratory Disease. (Also see Prevention, Chapter 27.) Calicivirus and rhinotracheitis virus vaccines are available as MLV and inactivated parenteral and as MLV intranasal products. Parenteral vaccination for respiratory infections produces a slower response to protection, usually requiring at least two vaccines at a minimum of 3 to 4 weeks apart (Fig. 2-7).[48a] In contrast, intranasal vaccines may provide protection within 48 hours in a susceptible cat but may

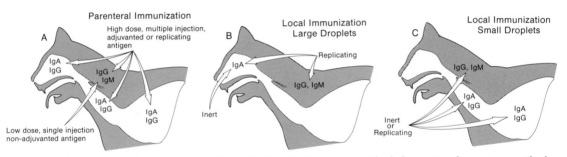

Figure 2–7. Comparison of the serum and tissue fluid antibody response *(shaded areas)* and secretory antibody production at various levels of the respiratory tract *(unshaded areas)* following parenteral vaccination *(A)* or local vaccination with large ($\geq$ 10 μm) *(B)* or small (< 10 μm) *(C)* antigen-containing droplets. (Data adapted from Wilkie BN: *J Am Vet Med Assoc* 181:1074–1079, 1982, with permission.)

typically produce a high incidence of mild contagious respiratory illness following vaccination.[48b] Despite their improved efficacy, veterinarians dislike using the intranasal and conjunctival route of vaccination because of the increased prevalence of postvaccinal disease. However, those using parenteral vaccine should also be careful to prevent accidental oronasal exposure of cats to aerosols or spilled vaccine during administration because postvaccinal respiratory disease may occur. Although it is more painful, IM vaccination reduces the chance of vaccine contamination of the skin surface or of the environment and has been shown to be more consistent in producing an immune response than the SC route. However, the protection afforded against the development of respiratory diseases is usually incomplete and temporary whether parenteral or intranasal vaccination is used. Cats that contract respiratory viruses following vaccination may have milder clinical illness than they would have had without vaccine protection.

Colostric immunity to feline respiratory viruses is thought to last for approximately 6 to 14 weeks, depending on the virus (see Table 2–3). Intranasal vaccines can break through this immunity earlier because of the reduced importance of serum antibodies to protection against infection or inactivation of vaccine virus on the respiratory mucosa.[49] Early vaccination, between 5 to 9 weeks of age, with intranasal MLV or parenteral adjuvanted inactivated vaccines may be beneficial in breaking through maternal antibody interference and in controlling feline viral rhinotracheitis in catteries when respiratory disease develops in kittens prior to the recommended initial vaccination series, between 9 and 12 weeks of age.[49]

Inactivated respiratory virus vaccines are safe for use in debilitated cats, in kittens less than 4 weeks of age that have been deprived of colostrum, and in pregnant queens, although the protection is weaker than that provided by MLV products. With these exceptions, MLV vaccines should always be used to protect cats in case of an outbreak, and then the intranasal vaccine is preferred.

Feline "pneumonitis vaccines" are available MLV products for parenteral administration. They offer some degree of protection against clinical illness caused by *Chlamydia psittaci*, but immunity is not complete. The routine use of this vaccine is not essential because of the relatively lower prevalence of infection and the milder clinical illness produced by this agent. Exposed vaccinated cats develop milder clinical illness than unvaccinated animals. Maternal antibody interference does not appear to be important with this vaccine and no teratogenic effects are known, so that kittens can be vaccinated as early as 3 weeks of age when neonatal conjunctivitis is a problem (see Chapter 27). At least one parenterally administered MLV chlamydial vaccine has been shown to protect cats against experimental challenge for as long as 1 year.[50] Feline pneumonitis vaccines are available in various combinations with the respiratory viruses and feline panleukopenia virus. Therefore, vaccination for pneumonitis, although it is probably not essential, can be accomplished without much additional expense or inconvenience to cat owners. Routine vaccination against feline respiratory disease is often necessary in cats that are stressed or congregated in catteries, research facilities, and multiple cat households.

Feline Leukemia Virus (FeLV) Infection.
(Also see Prevention of Feline Leukemia Virus Infection, Chapter 26.) Vaccination for FeLV is different from that of any other disease of cats. The disease is one that can be tested for prior to vaccination. The course of infection is invariably chronic and fatal in persistently viremic, bone marrow–infected cats. The vaccines, although potentially beneficial, do not give complete protection, and cats can be already latently infected at the time of vaccination and remain undetected by FeLV testing until a later date. Thus vaccinated cats can still develop the disease. Veterinarians must take an extra amount of time for client education and prevaccination screening for infection. Although not ideal or completely effective, existing vaccines may boost a cat's immune response against a very harmful viral infection. Clients should be advised of the incomplete protection these vaccines afford. The decision of whether or not to vaccinate cats with the presently available products rests with the practitioner.

Vaccines available in the United States are a subunit vaccine, **Leukocell 2** (Norden Laboratories, Lincoln, NE) and a whole virion vaccine, **Covenant** (Diamond Scientific, Des Moines, IA). Leukocell 2 contains soluble, unassembled and noninfectious FeLV proteins with adjuvants. Leukocell, the predecessor of Leukocell 2, was given IM or SC in a three-dose series with the first two doses spaced at 2- to 3-week intervals, and the last dose given 2 to 3 months later. Leukocell 2 is administered SC to cats that are 9 weeks of age or older in two doses, given 3 to 4 weeks apart. Covenant contains whole virus and additional gp70 (an envelope protein) antigen that is chemically inactivated and adjuvanted. It is recommended for use in clinically healthy cats 10 weeks of age or older. Cats are given two doses IM, spaced at 3- to 4-week intervals. Annual revaccination with a single dose is recommended for these vaccines.

A genetically engineered vaccine (see Developmental or Experimental Vaccines) has been developed for FeLV infection (Leucogen, Virbac Pharmaceutical, Nice, France) has been developed in Europe.[50a] A specific subcomponent (p45) of the gp70 envelope is produced in *E. coli*, purified, and adjuvanted using a saponin derivative (Quil A, see Immunostimulatory Complexes). Two vaccinations are recommended, to be given two weeks apart for adequate protection. Yearly vaccination is recommended.

Vaccination for FeLV infection is a controversial subject. Many questions have arisen about the efficacy, administration, and safety of FeLV vaccines. These will hopefully be answered below.

EFFICACY OF VACCINES. In efficacy studies for FeLV vaccines, challenge has involved glucocorticoid-induced immunosuppression prior to oronasal exposure to virulent virus so that a high proportion of unvaccinated controls become infected. Results of challenge studies are better indicators of protection than serum antibody titers; however, as with most vaccines, challenge has been done only 2 weeks after the last vaccination.

Antibody titers to gp70 and feline oncornavirus cell membrane antigen (FOCMA) have been measured to determine longer-term immunity following vaccination because of the difficulties and expense of conducting challenge studies at various intervals. These antibodies would seem to be important in protection against viremia (gp70) and tumor development (FOCMA). Not all antibodies to gp70 measured by enzyme-linked (ELISA) or fluorescent (IFA) immunoassays are virus neutralizing. Only serum-neutralizing antibodies have been directly correlated with protection against FeLV infection. Although increases in neutralizing and gp70 antibodies after vaccination have been variable, increases seen in FOCMA antibodies have been more consistent. Still, the relationship of FOCMA antibodies to protection against neoplasia is not absolute. Furthermore, although helpful as a research tool, the measurement of serum antibodies to gp70 or FOCMA is impractical and unnecessary in clinical practice.

Results of challenge studies of the vaccines, completed by their respective manufacturers in specific pathogen-free (SPF) cats, are summarized in Table 2–8.[51,52,52a] Most of the clinical and experimental data exist for the original Leukocell vaccine. Following challenge, persistent ($\geq$10 weeks) viremia was found in 20% of vaccinates and 70% of unvaccinated cats. FeLV-related neoplasia developed in 20% of vaccinates and 70% of controls when cats were subsequently followed over a 2-year period. Because these studies have been under experimental conditions and involved such a small number of cats, the extent of protection to natural exposure is still uncertain.

Table 2–8. Comparison of Response to Challenge with Virulent FeLV in Vaccinated and Nonvaccinated Glucocorticoid-Immunosuppressed Specific Pathogen–Free Cats[a]

VACCINE	ROUTE	STUDY NUMBER	VACCINATED		NONVACCINATED	
			Number of Cats	Percentage Aviremic[b] (%)	Number of Cats	Percentage Aviremic[b] (%)
Leukocell	IM[c]	1	25	80	10	30
Covenant	IM[d]	1	23	100	22[e]	46
Covenant	SC[f]	2	29	96.5	19[e]	58
Leukocell 2	SC[g]	1	11	100	10	50
Leukocell 2	SC[g]	2	26	96.2	12	66.7
Leukocell 2	SC[g]	3	25	72	10	40
VacSYN	SC[h]	1&2	44	91	20	15

[a]Challenge with virulent virus strains two weeks after the last vaccination.

[b]Aviremic (ELISA) at 10 weeks postchallenge with Leukocell and Leukocell 2 in study 1, at 3 weeks with Covenant, and at 9 weeks with Leukocell 2 in study 2. Virus isolation determination of viremia and ELISA at 12 weeks postchallenge with Leukocell 2 in study 3 and at 4 weeks postchallenge with VacSYN.

[c]Series of three vaccines given IM. Summary of trial conducted in 1985. (Norden Product Info.)

[d]Series of two vaccines given IM. Summary of three trials (#87-03, #87-33, #88-16) conducted in 1987 and 1988, Diamond Scientific, University Edition Covenant FeLV Vaccine Technical Seminar, 1988.[52]

[e]Nine cats in trial #88-16 served as controls for both the IM and SC vaccine trials.

[f]Series of two vaccines given SC. Summary of two trials (#88-06, #88-16) conducted in 1988, Diamond Scientific, University Edition Covenant FeLV Vaccine Technical Seminar, 1988.[52]

[g]Series of two vaccines given SC. Summary of trials conducted 1987–1988. (Norden Product Info.)[52a]

[h]Series of two SC vaccinations. Summary of two trials in 1988 and 1989. (Synbiotics Product Info.)

In independent studies with Leukocell,[52, 53a] thirty-seven kittens from either SPF or conventional sources and from FeLV-negative queens were divided into vaccinated (n = 23) or control (n = 14) groups. The kittens were vaccinated at 9- and 12-weeks of age and were commingled beginning at 14 weeks of age in a room containing one asymptomatic, naturally-infected, FeLV-positive challenge cat for every 5 kittens. The kittens were maintained in contact with the viremic challenge cats for 24 weeks. Serologic studies in the vaccinate and control kittens indicated high anti-gp70 titers in 2 kittens from each group prior to challenge exposure.[53b] All kittens had increased anti-gp70 and anti-FOCMA titers following vaccination. Seventy percent of vaccinates and 64% of controls were viremic 10 weeks after first exposure to the challenge cats and remained persistently viremic. Approximately 35% of the cats from each group (all FeLV-positive) died of various disorders including feline infectious peritonitis (FIP), respiratory disease, myelogenous leukemia, and myocarditis. Failure of the vaccine to protect these cats was attributed to such factors as potential prevaccination exposure to FeLV or to failure of the vaccine to protect against heterogenous naturally occurring strains of virus.[53a, 53b]

In another independent study with Leukocell in client-owned, vaccinated cats, there was a marked increase in both gp70 and FOCMA antibodies in approximately 37% of aviremic, previously seronegative cats.[53] This value was 93% in aviremic, previously seropositive cats, indicating the vaccine may be inducing an anamnestic response in cats that had already been exposed to the virus. In a third study, only a small percentage of aviremic, seronegative cats developed serum neutralizing antibodies, whereas a greater percentage developed FOCMA antibodies after vaccination.[54] These studies have questioned the reported efficacy of the original Leukocell vaccine under natural circumstances. In most of these studies, cats were given two instead of the recommended three doses, making direct comparison with the manufacturer's data difficult. A study in which three doses were used showed increased efficacy compared with the two-dose regimen.[53c]

For Covenant and Leukocell 2, only the manufacturers' efficacy data are available. With Covenant, persistent viremia was defined in cats that were viremic at 3 (instead of 9 to 12) weeks postchallenge as for Leukocell or Leukocell 2. The reported percentage of aviremic vaccinated cats postchallenge was 100% and 96.5% in two separate studies for Covenant as compared with 80% for Leukocell and 72 to 100% for three studies with Leukocell 2 (Table 2–8). However, the shorter (3 versus 12 weeks) observation period for viremia and the higher percentage of nonviremic unvaccinated cats as compared with that for Leukocell (46% and 58% versus 30%) suggest a relatively weaker challenge infection for Covenant. For Leukocell 2, the percentage of nonviremic, unvaccinated and vaccinated cats is similar to that for Covenant, suggesting a similar challenge severity. The lower percentage of aviremic vaccinated (72%) and unvaccinated (40%) in study 3 may reflect increased sensitivity of detection of viremia because virus cultivation rather than direct ELISA methods were used to identify virus in blood. All of the vaccines might show comparable efficacy if tested under equal circumstances. As suggested by independent observations on Leukocell, protection afforded by the newer vaccines under natural conditions may not be as predictable as found by these laboratory studies in SPF cats.

PROTECTION AGAINST LATENCY. Cats can harbor FeLV in their cell genome without complete viral expression (see Pathogenesis of FeLV, Chapter 26). Latency appears to be a phase in the course of elimination of infection in viremic cats. Most cats which are only transiently viremic gradually eliminate this latent virus within a 6- to 30-month period.[55,56]

In one study, Leukocell was not effective in preventing latency from developing in challenged cats;[54] however, the duration of observation was only several weeks after challenge, and only two doses of vaccine instead of the recommended three doses were given. In other studies by the manufacturer, cats previously vaccinated with three doses and subsequently challenged were shown not to be latently infected when tested by bone marrow cultivation 2 years after challenge.[57] The absence of latent infections in this later study may merely represent natural elimination of the virus, which is difficult to determine owing to the long time interval of evaluation and lack of inclusion of unvaccinated control cats in this evaluation. It has not been conclusively demonstrated that available vaccines can prevent the development of or accelerate the elimination of latent infections.

VACCINE SAFETY. Adverse reactions to FeLV vaccines have primarily been of an allergic nature. They do not cause immunosuppression in uninfected cats or any change in the course of illness of already viremic cats, nor do they appear to activate latent infections.

They are noninfectious vaccines and will not produce FeLV infection or make cats viremic. Anaphylactic reactions have been minimized by switching to SC rather than IM administration with additional purification and removal of non-essential preservatives and proteins (see Type I, Immunologic Complications).

No data exist on the prevalence of such reactions, but IM is more likely than SC administration to produce such complications because of the more rapid absorption of antigen. Precautions should be taken to limit the number of antigens given simultaneously to cats if such allergic reactions are noted. Limited safety studies have involved use of these vaccines in exotic cats.[58]

PREVACCINATION TESTING. Should only clinically healthy and FeLV-negative cats be vaccinated? There are some low-risk groups for infection such as cats from single-cat households, FeLV-negative catteries, and isolated environments. Whether these individuals should be tested is usually based on the practitioner's decision or advice given to the client and the client's reaction to the cost involved.

Although there is some expense and inconvenience to prevaccination testing of all cats, it is not always comparable to the cost to the client of the complete vaccination series. In this regard, it could be recommended that *all* cats of *all* ages be tested for FeLV viremia prior to vaccination. The ELISA test results can usually be used as the criteria for response to vaccine.[54] Vaccines do not seem to benefit ELISA-tested viremic cats; their use under such circumstances would be wasteful and misleading. On the other hand, latently infected cats that test negative on the ELISA may still be able to benefit from vaccination. Use of the IFA test for initial vaccination screening may miss some ELISA-positive immune carrier cats that may not benefit from vaccine and may later develop persistent viremia or disease.

The arguments against prevaccination testing have included high cost and inconvenience since some client costs for testing are as much or greater than that for a single injection of vaccine. Because of the possibility that FeLV test–negative cats could still be infected and because the vaccines do not protect all cats from becoming infected, a negative FeLV test result does not assure that a vaccinated cat will not become infected in the future.

Although less likely, kittens can be prenatally or neonatally infected with the virus, so that age is not a precise predictor of infection. In general, the prevalence of infections in kittens is lower than in cats over 6 months of age. Furthermore, maternal antibodies may transiently suppress viremia in an infected kitten. For these reasons, and because of the confusion surrounding interpretation of FeLV test results, some practitioners have resorted to vaccination without testing of clinically healthy cats.

In kittens, testing can often be done on the first vaccination visit which is often at 6 to 8 weeks of age. Vaccination does not begin until 9 to 10 weeks of age, by which time the results will be available. The reluctance to test such young animals results from the time commitment and technical problems related to bleeding such young cats. These problems can be overcome because of newer tests for FeLV that require smaller blood samples or can be performed on saliva or tears (see Diagnosis of FeLV, Chapter 26).

If cats are presented at 9 to 10 weeks of age or older, a prevaccination blood sample can be obtained and the animal can be given the first dose. This saves the client an additional visit. If the test is negative, the vaccination series can be continued. If the test is positive, the series must be discontinued and a second ELISA test must be performed 4 to 8 weeks later. If the test is negative, the cat may be presumed to have recovered from natural infection, and the need for vaccination is optional. If the second test is positive, an IFA test should be done. This will determine if the bone marrow is infected, since most IFA-positive cats have a poor prognosis and remain persistently viremic.

NUMBER OF VACCINES. As with other inactivated products, antigen mass and repetitive vaccination offer the best assurance of protective response.[59] Cats receiving only one dose of the initial series and not revaccinated within a 2-month period should have their vaccination series started over, although no data are available. Subsequent annual revaccination with a single dose is given 1 year from the date of the last vaccination of the initial series.

VACCINATION OF HIGH-RISK CATS. Multicat households, catteries, and research facilities allow for close contact and, therefore, the greater risk that FeLV infection will be spread. Because efficacy of vaccines is *never* 100% under *natural* circumstances, clients should be advised not to place FeLV-vaccinated cats in the same environment with viremic cats. Similarly, in established FeLV-free populations, vaccination should not be a substitute for routine FeLV testing and elimination of viremic cats. Because of the short period of residence compared with the time and expense to induce protective immunity, vaccination of all cats entering humane shelters may not be justifiable. Testing and removal of all incoming viremic cats may be of more benefit. Studies that have claimed a reduction in FeLV infections in infected populations where vaccination is instituted have been misleading.[60] The initial prevalence of infection cannot be accurately compared with subsequent incidence data since vaccination has been coupled with removal of infected cats.

Feline Infectious Peritonitis (FIP) Virus Infection. (Also see Prevention, Chapter 24.) Mutant strains of feline infectious peritonitis virus have been developed for use as vaccines.[61,61a] The only favorable results have been with intranasal administration of MLV vaccines. Protection in one study was approximately 40% when cats were challenged with virulent virus.[61] In another study,[61a] using a temperature-sensitive vaccine strain given intranasally, protection against virulent virus challenge in 20 vaccinated cats was 85%, whereas 83% (of 12) nonvaccinated control cats died.[61a] The vaccine stimulated local secretory antibody and systemic cell-mediated immune responses to FIPV. These results may be explained by restricted replication of the temperature-sensitive strain in the pharyngeal region. Fortunately, intranasal vaccination has not precipitated a more severe and accelerated disease syndrome as compared with the disease in challenged vaccinates. This has been a problem with prior FIP vaccine development.

Developmental or Experimental Vaccines

No vaccine is presently available for canine brucellosis (also see Chapter 52). As in most diseases in which facultative intracellular pathogens are present, inactivated vaccines have been relatively ineffective. Both live *Brucella ovis* and avirulent *B. canis* strains have been shown to offer some degree of protection to dogs when challenged with virulent *B. canis*. Unfortunately, with the currently available diagnostic tests, these vaccines interfere with the ability to distinguish between infected and vaccinated animals. It is unlikely that a commercial vaccine will be developed.

A vaccine developed to protect puppies against neonatal herpesvirus has been shown to provide partial protection (see Prevention, Chapter 18). Unfortunately, the low prevalence of the disease and the incomplete protection against infection that is afforded make its usefulness questionable. Proper management is more valuable in control of the disease.

For many years, improvements in the efficacy of existing vaccines were (1) to be able to give parenterally administered products locally for mucosal diseases, such as respiratory infections; (2) to develop new live vaccines for diseases where inactivated vaccines were only available; and (3) to purify products to remove nonessential, potentially allergenic proteins. Presently, the future of vaccine development will rely on producing noninfectious vaccines using genetic or immunologic methods, such as subunit fractionation, attenuation with genetic manipulation, recombinant DNA techniques, synthesis of antigenic peptides, or immunization with anti-idiotypes.[62-65]

With subunit vaccines, viral particles are split and fractionated and nucleic acid is removed or inactivated while maintaining surface components to stimulate an immune response. One of the already available FeLV vaccines comes closest to this type of product. Other subunit or purified antigenic component vaccines have been developed on a clinical basis for canine distemper, canine bordetellosis, leptospirosis, and rabies.

Attenuation of agents by genetic manipulation involves insertion of genetic code for immunizing proteins into vaccinia virus as a vector. A recombinant vaccinia virus expressing FeLV gp70 envelope protein was not successful in producing antiviral antibodies in cats.[66] Instead, inoculated cats developed neutralizing antibody against the vaccinia virus. Experimental recombinant vaccinia virus products given intradermally were capable of inducing immune responses in dogs to human influenza, herpesviruses and hepatitis viruses.[66a]

Recombinant DNA technology also allows for in vitro production of large quantities of immunogenic proteins by introducing coding into bacteria, yeasts, or continuous cell lines. Synthetic antigens can be produced by identifying the antigenic or genetic determinants using monoclonal antibodies. Once the nucleotide and amino acid sequences have been determined, the protein can be synthesized. Unfortunately, antigenically active peptides by themselves are often weak antigens and they must be adjuvanted.

Anti-idiotypic antibodies are antibodies that are produced against antigen combining sites on specific immunoglobulins directed against the infectious agent. The anti-idiotypic antibody actually resembles the antigen itself and stimulates T cells in a way similar to a vaccine. Although veterinary vaccines of this type are only in experimental stages, anti-idiotypic vaccines have the advantage of being produced by genetic manipulation and are safe because they lack the risk of infectious agents as in MLV vaccines.

Vaccination of Exotic Carnivores

Many nondomestic carnivores are vaccinated for diseases of dogs and cats, with commercially available canine and feline vaccines. Only inactivated rabies vaccines should be used. Susceptibility and recommendations for vaccinating these carnivores are summarized in Table 2–9. Because of the risk of vaccine-induced infection, there is a concern for vaccinating exotic carnivores with MLV-CDV vaccine; inactivated products are ineffective.[71] Chicken embryo–derived CDV vaccines appear to be safest in this regard for species such as the ferret.

Vaccination Requirements for Interstate Shipment of Animals

Interstate shipment of animals that are affected with or have recently been exposed to infectious diseases is prohibited within the United States. The information in Appendix 7 has been extracted from the current regulations of the United States Department of Agriculture, Animal Health and Plant Inspection Service.

POSTVACCINAL COMPLICATIONS

Many immune-mediated and nonimmune complications severe enough to restrict or

Table 2–9. Vaccination of Families of Terrestrial Carnivores and Their Susceptibility to Infectious Diseases of the Dog and Cat[a]

	SUSCEPTIBILITY/WHETHER TO VACCINATE						
	Canidae[b]	Felidae[c]	Procyonidae[d]	Ursidae[e]	Mustelidae[f]	Viverridae[g]	Hyenidae[h]
Canine distemper	+/+	−/−	+/+	+/−	+/−	?/±	+/+
Feline panleukopenia	−/−	+/+	+/+	?/−	+/+	?/±	−/−
Infectious canine hepatitis	+/+	−/−	−/−	+/−	−/−	−/−	?/±
Feline respiratory disease	−/−	+/+	−/−	−/−	−/−	−/−	−/−
Parainfluenza	+/+	+/−	?/?	?/?	?/?	?/?	?/?
Rabies	+/+	+/+	+/+	+/+	+/+	+/+	+/+
Leptospirosis[i]	+/+	+/−	+/±	+/−	+/±	+/±	+/±

[a]+ = yes, − = no, ± = optional, ? = uncertain. Data from Fowler and Theobald, 1978;[67] Appel, 1987;[68] Appel, 1988;[69] Norden, 1988.[70]

[b]Coyote, dingo, domestic dog, jackal, raccoon dog, wolf, red fox, gray fox. Only MLV chicken tissue culture vaccines or inactivated vaccines should be used on the gray fox.

[c]Cheetah, lion, jaguar, margay, ocelot.

[d]Bassariscus, coati, kinkajou, raccoon, lesser panda. Only inactivated vaccines should be used on the lesser panda.

[e]Bears.

[f]Ferret, fisher, grison, marten, mink, otter, sable, skunk, wolverine, badger. Only MLV chicken tissue culture vaccines should be used on ferrets.

[g]Binturong, fossa linsang, mongoose, civet.

[h]Hyena.

[i]Only inactivated vaccines should be used.

eliminate the use of a particular vaccine follow the use of commercial vaccines in dogs and cats. Repeated annual revaccination of veterinary patients cannot always be justified with respect to all the components included in presently available combination products. Veterinarians should be aware of potential complications caused by each vaccine component so that particular antigens can be deleted from subsequent boosters if problems arise.

Immunologic Complications

Immunologic reactions that can develop following vaccination are those relating either to hypersensitivity or to autoimmunity; they can be classified as types I, II, III, or IV pathogenesis (Table 2–10).

Type I. Type I reaction, or anaphylaxis, may occur following the use of any vaccine, although it is most commonly associated with the use of inactivated products containing large amounts of foreign protein, such as *Leptospira* bacterin. Foreign proteins, such as fetal bovine serum, used in cell culture have also contributed to this problem. With the advent of inactivated and adjuvanted viral vaccines used for rabies, feline respiratory disease, feline panleukopenia, and feline leukemia virus infection, an increasing prevalence of type I reactions has been

noted in cats.[72,72a] If anaphylaxis is a problem with some animals, it is advised to (1) modify the vaccination schedule to reduce the number of antigens given simultaneously, (2) switch to MLV instead of noninfectious adjuvanted products, and (3) use SC versus IM inoculations.

Within minutes to hours of vaccination, cats developing anaphylaxis vomit and have diarrhea. The diarrhea is usually watery but may become hemorrhagic if it is severe or persistent. Respiratory distress, manifested by dyspnea and cyanosis, is the most severe manifestation. A majority of cats will respond favorably to epinephrine and glucocorticoids, but those developing severe progressive respiratory symptoms or hemoptysis usually die. Even with recovery, diarrhea may persist in some cats for several days thereafter.

Local or systemic reactions may occur in young puppies within 1 hour after their second or third vaccination and may result in acute vomiting, diarrhea, dyspnea, collapse, or death. Puppies that survive such episodes should not be revaccinated with known allergenic components such as leptospiral antigen in combined vaccines through the remainder of their initial vaccination series. If they are revaccinated with leptospiral antigen, it should be done only after they are 16 weeks of age or older and then with cautious monitoring immediately following the injection.

Table 2–10. Postvaccinal Complications

TYPE OF PROBLEM	MECHANISM OF PRODUCTION	RESPONSIBLE VACCINES
Immunologic		
Type I	Immediate hypersensitivity: allergy, anaphylaxis	Leptospira bacterin; inactivated rabies, feline leukemia and respiratory vaccines
Type II	Cytotoxicity (hypersensitivity or autoimmunity):	
	(a) autoimmune hemolytic anemia	(a) MLV parvoviral vaccine
	(b) autoimmune thrombocytopenia	(b) MLV distemper vaccine
Type III	Immune complex (hypersensitivity):	
	(a) uveitis	(a) MLV–CAV-1 vaccine
	(b) generalized serum sickness	(b) Passive immunization
Type IV	Cell-mediated (hypersensitivity or autoimmunity):	
	(a) granuloma	(a) BCG immunotherapy
	(b) encephalitis	(b) Nervous tissue–derived rabies vaccine
	(c) polyradiculoneuritis	(c) Inactivated neonatal mouse brain rabies vaccine
Nonimmunologic		
Local reaction at injection site	Adjuvants, preservatives, inactivators	*Bordetella* and *Leptospira* bacterins; inactivated rabies vaccine
Systemic fever and malaise	Local lymphoid replication of MLV products	Any MLV vaccine
Abortion, infertility, congenital malformation	In utero or early neonatal infection	Any MLV vaccine during pregnancy; Parvoviral vaccines during neonatal period
Clinical disease in vaccinates	Incomplete attenuation or local administration of attenuated vaccines	Intranasal vaccines: feline calicivirus feline herpesvirus canine parainfluenza virus canine *Bordetella* vaccine
Postvaccinal shedding	Virus localization	Canine parvovirus—GI CAV-1 vaccine—renal CAV-2 vaccine—respiratory
Postvaccinal encephalitis	Immunosuppressed animal or relatively unattenuated virus enters the nervous system where immune defenses are poor	Canine distemper vaccine Measles vaccine Rabies vaccine CAV-1 vaccine MLV canine coronaviral vaccine

MLV = modified live virus; CAV-1 = canine adenovirus-1 (hepatitis); BCG = bacille Calmette-Guérin; GI = gastrointestinal; CAV-2 = canine adenovirus-2 (respiratory).

Inbred atopic dogs have been shown to develop enhanced antipollen IgE antibody responses when vaccinated with canine distemper, hepatitis, and leptospirosis vaccines just prior to, but not after, exposure to pollen extracts.[73] Because of this immunopotentiation, it is recommended that atopic dogs receive their booster vaccinations during winter months in the case of warmer seasonal allergies.

Type II. Type II hypersensitivity, or autoimmunity resulting in cellular injury, has been suspected or reported following the use of MLV vaccines in dogs. Autoimmune hemolytic anemia and autoimmune nonregenerative anemias (autoimmunity to erythrocyte precursors) have been suspected to occur within 1 to 2 weeks following the use of modified live canine- and feline-origin parvoviral vaccines in dogs. Affinity of the virus for erythrocytes may be explained by the hemagglutinating properties of the virus and the high antigen mass used in some of these vaccines.

Transient thrombocytopenia also was reported following the use of MLV vaccines in dogs.[74,75] Thrombocytopenia, which developed in most vaccinated dogs, was mild ($> 100,000$ and $< 200,000$ platelets/μl) and subclinical. Despite transient thrombocytopenia, no change in platelet function was detected.[55] Whether this form of thrombocytopenia is caused by autoimmune or infectious mechanisms is uncertain. Only those animals with concurrent congenital or acquired bleeding tendencies may be expected to show hemorrhagic tendencies. Veterinarians may want to delay elective surgery on animals with known bleeding tendencies for a 1-week period following vaccination.

Severe immune-mediated thrombocytopenia can also occur within 1 to 2 weeks following vaccination of dogs. These animals have overt petechiae and hemorrhagic tendencies, with platelet counts less than 50,000/μl. Glucocorticoid therapy is usually required for several weeks thereafter to increase the platelet count, and subsequent boosters must be avoided or minimized to prevent a recurrence of the problem in these dogs.

Type III. Type III hypersensitivity reactions associated with immune complex formation are involved with the anterior uveitis that occurs in some dogs receiving the MLV–CAV-1 vaccine. This local type III, or Arthus, reaction results from virus-antibody complex formation within the eye (see Pathogenesis, Chapter 17). The process resolves spontaneously unless secondary complications such as glaucoma develop.

Generalized serum sickness is the result of widespread immune-complex deposition throughout the walls of the microvasculature of certain structures, such as the renal glomeruli, joints, and uveal tract. Usually, this complication is seen only following the administration of large amounts of hyperimmune serum or globulin. Since passive immunization is used infrequently in dogs and cats, the prevalence of serum sickness is minimal. It has also developed in a dog as a complication of *Corynebacterium parvum* immunotherapy.[75a]

Glomerulonephritis and amyloidosis can result from chronic or repeated antigenic exposure. This is one reason why humans are not given booster doses on an annual basis as is the practice in veterinary medicine. Both syndromes have been experimentally produced in animals following desensitization therapy protocols using repeated injections of large quantities of foreign antigen. Neither disease has ever been correlated with the repeated administration of biologics in dogs or cats.

Type IV. Cell-mediated, or type IV, hyper-

sensitivity reactions can occur following the use of bacille-Calmette-Guérin (BCG) as an immunostimulator (see Immunotherapy). Large, exuding granulomas may develop at the site of injection. Postvaccinal encephalitis was an allergic reaction that occurred following the use of nervous tissue–derived rabies vaccines. Polyradiculoneuritis (coonhound paralysis in dogs, Guillain-Barré syndrome in humans) has been a complication of human influenza vaccination, and this phenomenon has been observed in dogs following use of suckling mouse brain inactivated rabies virus vaccines in dogs (see Postvaccinal Encephalomyelitis).

Nonimmunologic Complications
See Table 2–10.

Local Reactions. Many complications have been associated with either local irritation or production of disease by canine and feline biologics. Local reactions following vaccination include swelling, irritation, and abscess formation. These are most frequently noted with the use of inactivated products containing adjuvants or with bacterial vaccines containing large amounts of foreign protein derived from the culture media. Parenteral *Bordetella*- and *Leptospira*-adjuvanted bacterins and adjuvanted inactivated rabies, feline leukemia virus, and feline respiratory vaccines have most commonly been incriminated.

Focal cutaneous lesions developed at the site of inactivated rabies vaccine in dogs, a majority of which were poodles.[76] Hyperpigmented alopecic macules were observed. These were histologically characterized by a local nonsuppurative vasculitis with rabies virus–specific fluorescence in the wall of the blood vessels. One dog suffered from anaphylaxis when the vaccine was readministered on a subsequent booster.

Cats inoculated with combined inactivated respiratory vaccine using a water-in-oil emulsion as an adjuvant developed focal cutaneous or intramuscular swellings.[77] These were histologically chronic suppurative granulomas that appeared to be foreign body reactions to the lipid component.

Systemic Illness. Systemic illness characterized by fever and malaise may also occur as a result of self-limiting infection caused by

MLV vaccines, usually caused by replication of the vaccine virus within local lymphoid tissues without viremic spread. This commonly does not last longer than 1 to 2 days following vaccination and often explains the transient anorexia and depression noted in recently vaccinated animals.

Prenatal and Neonatal Infections. If MLV vaccines are given during pregnancy, vaccine infections can result in fetal malformation or death or infertility and abortion in the dam. Neonatal infection can also occur following the use of MLV canine or feline parvoviral vaccines in puppies or kittens less than 4 to 5 weeks of age. The general recommendation is to never use MLV vaccines in pregnant females.

Respiratory Disease. Clinical illness can develop as an expected postvaccinal event when intranasal vaccines are used for feline calicivirus and rhinotracheitis virus or canine parainfluenza virus and *Bordetella bronchiseptica* infections. The mild clinical syndrome is usually self-limiting, but the organisms may spread to other susceptible animals. The immunity to such vaccines is superior to that of parenteral vaccines; however, the clinical disease that these vaccines can produce has limited their use by many veterinarians. It should be remembered that parenteral MLV respiratory vaccines inadvertently or accidentally released into the environment can cause similar reactions.

Shedding of Vaccine Agent. Shedding of vaccine virus, which occurs with the MLV intranasal products, can also occur following administration of parenteral vaccines such as MLV canine-origin parvoviral vaccine (feces), CAV-1 vaccine (urine), and CAV-2 vaccine (respiratory secretions). This shedding may serve to vaccinate other susceptible animals that come in contact with infected secretions. Reversion to virulence has not been demonstrated with virus that is shed as a result of vaccination with the commercially available veterinary vaccines, although the potential exists.

Postvaccinal Encephalomyelitis. Neurologic disease has been the most commonly documented postvaccinal reaction described in dogs and cats. This may relate to the overt nature of neurologic illness and decreased immunocompetence of the CNS against MLV agents. Historically, complications following rabies virus vaccination have received the most attention. Allergic encephalomyelitis was a common complication following the use of the first rabies vaccines of nervous tissue origin. Myelin included in the vaccine sensitized the immune system of the animal against its own myelin. Similar problems have occurred with inactivated rabies vaccine, produced in neonatal mouse brain.[78] The CNS of the newborn mouse, normally devoid of myelin, is well adapted to the production of large quantities of rabies virus needed to produce inactivated vaccine. A few older animals were apparently inadvertently used in production of the virus, or peripheral or cranial nerve myelin was accidentally included, and this resulted in transient acute lower motor neuron paralysis 1 to 2 weeks after vaccination in a proportion of dogs. The diagnosis of acute polyradiculoneuritis was made on the basis of marked muscle atrophy, hyperesthesia, slowed nerve conduction velocities, and the return to normal function, which began after 1 to 2 weeks of paralysis. The simultaneous presence of allergic encephalomyelitis could not be excluded, since affected dogs recovered and necropsies were not performed.

Rabies infection also has been reported following vaccination with MLV vaccines. Low-passage vaccines that have caused problems in dogs are no longer licensed for use in the United States. Certain high-passage vaccines have induced postvaccinal rabies in cats, and as a result, only one is still approved for use in cats in the United States. MLV rabies vaccines should never be used in exotic carnivores because of the uncertainty that exists with respect to their susceptibility to vaccine-induced disease.

Vaccine-induced rabies in dogs and cats following MLV vaccination begins with paralysis in the inoculated limb within 7 to 21 days and progresses bilaterally and in an ascending fashion.[79–81] Affected cats have had progressive lower motor neuron paralysis with unusual extensor rigidity of the limbs.[82] Pain sensation and reflex function were decreased in an ascending fashion. Partial paresis of the forelimbs occurred. There was no chance to determine the potential recovery in cats since all were destroyed. Two dogs with postvaccinal rabies recovered within 1 to 2 months following the onset of clinical signs.[80]

Animals with vaccine-induced rabies do

not represent a health hazard because the virus is attenuated and is not shed in the saliva. Because of the difficulty in distinguishing the vaccine virus from virulent virus, expert virologists and public health officials should be contacted for recommendations concerning disposition of an affected animal (see Chapter 31).

Encephalomyelitis has been reported after combined distemper virus and CAV-1 vaccination in the dog.[83,84] Postvaccinal distemper has also been reported following immunosuppression of dogs with cytotoxic chemotherapy[85] (see Vaccination Failures, earlier) and virulent parvoviral infection (see Canine Parvoviral Enteritis, also earlier).[86] Atrophy of the Purkinje's cells in three of six pups given MLV measles vaccine at 6 weeks of age was reported.[87] Cerebellar signs were noted beginning 5 days after vaccination. MLV feline panleukopenia vaccines

and canine parvoviral vaccines should not be used in kittens or puppies less than 4 to 5 weeks of age. Cerebellar degeneration and myocarditis may develop in kittens and puppies, respectively, from vaccine virus infection. Parenteral vaccination with attenuated canine coronaviral vaccine has been associated with a disseminated vasculitis and meningitis in affected dogs.[88,89]

Influence on Drug Disposition. A potential influence of vaccines or viral infection on drug disposition exists in that they induce interferon synthesis, which in turn inhibits hepatic enzyme systems.[90] This could prolong the effects of drugs eliminated by oxidative metabolism, such as aminophylline, barbiturates, lidocaine, propranolol, chloramphenicol, tylosin, griseofulvin, and trimethoprim.

Immunotherapy

In general, immunotherapy includes any form of treatment that alters the immune system. This discussion is limited to include nonspecific means of stimulation of the immune system in an attempt to restore immunocompetence and control or treat infectious disease (Table 2–11). Nonspecific immunotherapy has been used to treat infections caused by facultative intracellular bacteria, viruses, fungal agents, or metazoan parasites for which vaccination or specific forms of chemotherapy are unavailable.

MICROORGANISMS

Microorganisms or their extracts have been used classically as nonspecific immunostimulators. Freund's *complete* adjuvant is a water-in-oil emulsion containing inactivated mycobacteria. The antigen is contained in the aqueous phase, and the mycobacteria are in the oil phase. Injection of this mixture induces cell-mediated immunity and humoral antibody formation. BCG is a nonpathogenic strain of *Mycobacterium bovis* that has been used in treating neoplasia in dogs and cats and in cats infected with feline leukemia virus. Facultative intracellular organisms such as mycobacteria that

are used as immunostimulators have a marked affinity for localizing in and stimulating mononuclear-phagocyte clearance mechanisms. An emulsion of mycobacterial cell wall (Regressin, Ragland Research Inc., Athens, GA), which has been modified to decrease toxicity and antigenicity while retaining antineoplastic activity, has been licensed for use as a cell-mediated immune stimulant for treating equine sarcoids. It has been recommended for immunotherapy for other neoplasms, such as feline leukemia, although studies demonstrating its efficacy for this purpose are not available at this time. Various other bacteria, including *Propionibacterium acnes (Corynebacterium parvum)* and certain species of *Staphylococcus* and *Salmonella*, have also been proposed as immunostimulants. Immuno-Regulin (ImmunoVet Inc., Tampa, FL) is a preparation of the bacterium *P. acnes* that acts as a nonspecific immunostimulant. Clinical studies reported by the manufacturer indicate that 20 cats positive for FeLV (only one had overt evidence of neoplastic involvement) were treated with Immuno-Regulin.[91] Twelve of the cats became negative for the virus on testing of blood in a mean time of 120 days. Larger scale controlled studies and tissue or bone marrow isolation of virus may have to be done in

Table 2–11. Nonspecific Immunotherapy

EXAMPLE OR SOURCE	MODE OF ACTION	TYPE OF IMMUNE RESPONSE	DISEASE-SPECIFIC	SPECIES-SPECIFIC
Microorganisms				
Bacteria				
BCG, Freund's complete adjuvant (muramyl dipeptide) *Salmonella, Bordetella pertussis, Propionebacterium acnes*	Cell wall components: enhances phagocytosis and intracellular killing, increases macrophage chemotaxis and T cell response	Cell-mediated Humoral: primarily IgG	No	No
Viruses				
Newcastle disease virus, Avian poxvirus	Interferon inducer	Interferon	No	Variable
Chemicals				
Macromolecules				
RNA, poly-IC, poly-AU	Interferon inducer, can enhance cellular and antibody response	Interferon Cell-mediated	No	Variable
Interferons	Antiviral, immunostimulatory	Interferon	No	No
Small chemicals				
Organic: vitamin A, fatty acids, lipids, lipopolysaccharide, Freund's incomplete adjuvant, glycosides (Quil A)	Delays antigen absorption Alters antigen presentation	Humoral	No	No
Inorganic: beryllium, alum, silica	Prolongs release of antigen	Humoral: primarily IgE	No	No
Pharmacologic agents Levamisole	Similar to thymic hormone: stimulates macrophage phagocytosis, immune killing, and chemotaxis Enhances T cell cytotoxicity, lymphokine production, and nucleic acid synthesis	Cell-mediated	No	No

[a] BCG = bacille Calmette-Guérin; poly IC = polyriboinosinic-polyribocytidylic acid; poly AU = polyadenylic-polyuridylic acid.

the future to determine the true FeLV-status of recovered cats. Limited studies have also been made in treatment of recurrent canine pyoderma.[91a]

Staphylococcal protein A (SPA) is a polypeptide of *S. aureus* Cowan 1 which has the ability to bind to the Fc (non–antigen-binding) region of certain IgG subclasses. It may combine with immune complexes and stimulate complement activation, or it may induce T cell activation, interferon-γ production, and generation of cytotoxic responses. SPA has been used in the treatment of cats with FeLV. It has been given parenterally, causing increased serum interferon concentration and cytotoxic antibody to gp70.[92] Antitumor but no antiviral effects were noted in other studies.[93] Extracorporeal immunoabsorption with SPA of plasma from FeLV-infected cats caused transient clearance of viremia and improved clinical signs associated with increased concentrations of interferon, complement, and cytoxic antibody to gp70.[94,95] The prognosis in neoplastic conditions is still poor.

INTERFERONS

Interferons (IFNs), a group of secretory glycoproteins produced by infected cells, inhibit subsequent replication of microorganisms in adjacent cells and stimulate lymphocytes for antitumor and antiviral responses via enhanced macrophage activity and lymphocyte-mediated cytotoxicity. There are three major classes of interferons, α, β, and γ. IFN-α and IFN-β are primarily responsible for antiviral effects, whereas IFN-γ is responsible for immunomodulation. Despite the broad range of effects against infections caused by many microorganisms, passive administration of preformed interferon substances is accompanied by complications. At first it was thought to be relatively host-specific, only functioning in the species in which it was produced. Now it is known that some interferons can protect a number of hosts. The major limitation to the clinical use of interferon has been the difficulty of production and purification of the large amounts that are required.

Interferon administration in small animal practice has primarily been studied in FeLV-positive cats.[96] A crude preparation produced from infected bovine cells in tissue culture was given orally to cats with nonregenerative anemia associated with feline leukemia.[97] Spontaneously and experimentally FeLV-infected cats have been given bovine IFN-β or human IFN-α or both in an attempt to stimulate their immune system. While cats remained viremic, they had dramatic clinical improvement when given 1 unit or less per day orally.[98,99] The typical interferon doses per administration for parenteral use in people are in the magnitude of 10^6 units. Although previously overlooked, oral interferon in low dosages appears to work across species lines, perhaps by stimulating oral lymphatic tissue (see also Interferons, in Antiviral Chemotherapy, Chapter 15, and Therapy of FeLV Infection, Chapter 26).

MACROMOLECULES

Several macromolecular compounds and certain viruses are known to produce antiviral and other antimicrobial activity in the host. These compounds induce interferon synthesis. Most of the substances known to induce the production of interferon have a structure similar to double-stranded RNA. Many viruses induce the formation of interferon naturally, but new synthetic nucleic acid polymers have been produced that also induce its synthesis.

The clinical use of nonpathogenic viruses to stimulate interferon production is impractical because antibodies develop to the inducing agent, inhibiting subsequent responses. Interferon production was reported in healthy female dogs with mammary tumors that were given BCG cell wall emulsion.[100]

Synthetic interferon inducers have the advantage of continuing effectiveness after successive administrations. However, since the production of interferon is transient—only lasting for about 1 week—interferon induc-

ers must be given repeatedly to be clinically useful.

Polyriboinosinic-polyribocytidylic acid (poly-IC) has been one of the most common chemical interferon inducers used in dogs and cats. Toxic side effects of poly-IC in dogs and cats are lymphopenia, lymphoid necrosis, CNS depression, hemorrhagic gastroenteritis, and incoagulability. Poly-IC was reported to be effective in protecting dogs from ICH infection, although increased concentration of interferon could not be measured.[101] Poly-IC was helpful in preventing herpesvirus infections in newborn puppies.[102]

The concentration of interferon generally peaks 8 hours following administration of the inducer and declines gradually by 24 hours. Inhibition of interferon production is pronounced if inducers are readministered at a frequency greater than every 2 weeks. Because the duration of effect of interferon is less than 2 weeks, continuous protection cannot be maintained.

Poly-IC was found to be more effective in stimulating interferon and less toxic in dogs when it was combined with poly-L-lysine and carboxymethylcellulose to form poly-ICLC.[103]

INTERLEUKIN-2

This lymphokine is produced by activated helper T cells and is responsible for stimulating specific cell-mediated cytotoxicity. It has been synthesized in large quantities through recombinant DNA technology; however, it may cause toxicity. Its potential uses include treatment of neoplastic and viral diseases.

SMALL CHEMICALS (ADJUVANTS)

Many chemical compounds have been added to inactivated biologics in an attempt to increase their effectiveness to a level comparable with that of modified live vaccines (see Table 2–10). Emulsified water-in-oil (Freund's *incomplete* adjuvant) and mineral gels such as aluminum hydroxide, aluminum phosphate, and alum have been used. They may enhance cell-mediated immunity, provide for slowed antigen degradation and release, and stimulate the function of the mononuclear phagocyte system. These products have been added to most inactivated veterinary biologics. One disadvantage of their use is that they frequently evoke local tissue reactions or abscess at the site of injection.

PHARMACOLOGIC AGENTS

Levamisole is a broad-spectrum anthelmintic that nonspecifically stimulates cell-mediated immunity in a variety of species. It potentiates mononuclear cells in the phagocytosis, chemotaxis, and intracellular destruction of bacteria. Toxicity of levamisole is relatively high; hypersalivation, vomiting, diarrhea, and CNS signs have been observed. Morphologic lesions, characterized by a perivascular, nonsuppurative, or granulomatous meningoencephalitis, were described in the CNS of treated dogs.[104,105] Potential facilitation of the cell-mediated immune system may produce the lesions in the CNS by causing the body to react against latent agents (e.g., distemper virus).

LIPOSOMES

Liposomes are synthetic microscopic structures composed of multiple concentric lipid bilayers surrounding an equal number of aqueous layers. The lipid layers are relatively impermeable to aqueous substances trapped within.

Immunologic mediators, antigenic substances, and drugs have been placed within the aqueous compartment of liposomes to facilitate delivery of these substances to selected tissues in the body. Liposomes themselves are relatively nonantigenic, nontoxic, and biodegradable because they are prepared from lipids normally found in cell membranes.

Liposomes may have potential to act as carriers of immunogens for purposes of vaccination. Immunogenicity can be increased by the addition of adjuvants within the liposomal membrane. Liposomal antigens, which normally stimulate only humoral immunity, can stimulate cell-mediated immunity if substances such as lipid A (see Chapter 1) and muramyl dipeptide are added in the membrane.

Liposomes also have been used for selective in vivo delivery of drugs to cells of the mononuclear phagocyte system, which preferentially removes these compounds from the circulation. Intracellular parasites, such as systemic fungi, mycobacteria, *Babesia canis*, *Ehrlichia canis*, *Trypanosoma cruzi*, and *Leishmania donovani*, that reside in these cells may be more susceptible to chemotherapeutic agents delivered in liposomes (see also Liposomes, in Antibacterial Chemotherapy, Chapter 43).

IMMUNOSTIMULATORY COMPLEXES

Immunostimulatory complexes (ISCOMs) are substances used to facilitate the immunologic recognition of membrane proteins of envelope viruses in subunit vaccines. The matrix of the ISCOM has often been the glycoside, Quil A (Spikoside, Isotec AB, Sweden) which in micelle form has accessible hydrophobic regions. A hydrophobic region of the membrane glycoprotein can be attached to those sites on the ISCOM matrix. ISCOM preparations from enveloped viruses are highly immunogenic and have been used to prepare feline leukemia virus vaccine (see Feline Leukemia Virus Infection).[106]

References

1. Ishibashi K, Maede Y, Ohsugi T, et al: Serotherapy for dogs infected with canine parvovirus. *Jpn J Vet Sci* 45:59–66, 1983.
2. Baker JA, Robson DS, Gillespie JH, et al: A nomograph that predicts the age to vaccinate puppies against distemper. *Cornell Vet* 49:158–167, 1959.
3. Gillespie JH, Baker JA, Burgher J, et al: The immune response of dogs to distemper virus. *Cornell Vet* 48:103–126, 1958.
4. Carmichael LE: Studies on infectious canine hepatitis. PhD diss. Ithaca, NY, Cornell University, 1959.
5. Carmichael LE, Robson DS, Barnes FD: Transfer and decline of maternal infectious canine hepatitis antibody in puppies. *Proc Soc Exp Biol Med* 109:677–681, 1962.
6. Scott FW: Feline panleukopenia. PhD diss. Ithaca, NY, Cornell University, 1968.
7. Scott FW, Csiza CK, Gillespie JH: Maternally derived immunity to feline panleukopenia. *J Am Vet Med Assoc* 156:439–453, 1970.
8. Pollock RVH: Canine parvovirus: host response and immunoprophylaxis. PhD diss. Ithaca, NY, Cornell University, 1981.
9. Pollock RVH, Carmichael LE: Maternally derived immunity to canine parvovirus infection: transfer, decline, and interference with vaccination. *J Am Vet Med Assoc* 180:37–42, 1982.

10. Mason MJ, Gillett NA, Muggenburg BA: Clinical, pathological, and epidemiological aspects of canine parvoviral enteritis in an unvaccinated closed beagle colony: 1978–1985. *J Am Anim Hosp Assoc* 23:183–192, 1987.

11. Carmichael LE, Joubert JC, Pollock RVH: A modified live canine parvovirus vaccine. II. Immune response. *Cornell Vet* 73:13–29, 1983.

12. Jarrett O, Russell PH, Stewart MF: Protection of kittens from feline leukemia virus infection by maternally derived antibody. *Vet Rec* 101:304–305, 1977.

13. Gaskell RM: Studies on feline viral rhinotracheitis virus with particular reference to the carrier state. PhD diss. Bristol, England, University of Bristol, 1975.

14. Edwards BG, Buell DJ, Acree WM: Evaluation of a new feline rhinotracheitis virus vaccine. *VM SAC* 72:205–209, 1977.

15. Povey RC: A review of feline viral rhinotracheitis (feline herpesvirus-1) infection. *Comp Immunol Microbiol Infect Dis* 2:373–387, 1979.

16. Johnson RP: Immunity to feline calicivirus in kittens. PhD diss. Guelph, Ontario, University of Guelph, 1980.

17. Johnson RP, Povey RC: Transfer and decline of maternal antibody to feline calicivirus. *Can Vet J* 24:6–9, 1983.

18. Pedersen NC, Boyle JF, Floyd K, et al: An enteric coronavirus infection of cats and its relationship to feline infectious peritonitis. *Am J Vet Res* 42:368–377, 1981.

19. Mims CA: *The Pathogenesis of Infectious Disease.* New York, Academic Press, 1977, p 225.

19a. Thein P: Adjuvants: immunomodulation and immunostimulation. *Vet Med Rev* 59:3–8, 1988.

20. Bellanti JA (ed): *Immunology II.* Philadelphia, WB Saunders Co, 1978b, p 155.

21. Nara PL, Krakowka S, Powers TE: Effects of prednisolone on the development of immune responses to canine distemper virus in beagle pups. *Am J Vet Res* 40:1742–1747, 1979.

22. Slater EA: The response to measles and distemper virus in immunosuppressed and normal dogs. *J Am Vet Med Assoc* 156:1762–1766, 1970.

23. Blancou J, Milward F, Toma B: Vaccination against rabies in carnivores treated with corticoids. *Rec Med Vet* 157:651–657, 1981.

24. Webster AC: The adverse effect of environment on the response to distemper vaccination. *Aust Vet J* 51:488–490, 1975.

25. Schultz RD: Theory and practice of immunization. In Kirk RW (ed): *Current Veterinary Therapy VII.* Philadelphia, WB Saunders Co, 1980, pp 1248–1255.

26. Kelly GE, Webster AC: The effect of surgery in dogs on the response to concomitant distemper vaccination. *Aust Vet J* 56:556–557, 1980.

27. Wilson JHG, Periboom WJ, Leemans-Dessy S: Combined distemper/measles vaccine. *Vet Rec* 98:32–33, 1976.

28. Shin DT, Gorham JR, Evermann JF, et al: Comparison of subcutaneous and intramuscular administration of a live attenuated distemper virus vaccine in ferrets. *Vet Rec* 114:42–43, 1984.

28a. Cornwell HJC, Thompson H, McCandlish IAP, et al: Encephalitis in dogs associated with a batch of canine distemper (Rockborn) vaccine. *Vet Rec* 112:54–59, 1988.

28b. Lewis DC, Dhein CR, Evermann JF: Current concepts in vaccination programs for dogs, cats and ferrets. Part 1. *Comp Anim Pract* 2:3–8, 1988.

29. Cornwell HJC, Paterson SD, McCandlish IAP, et al: Immunity to canine adenovirus respiratory disease: effect of vaccination with an inactivated vaccine. *Vet Rec* 113:509–512, 1983.

30. Cornwell HJC, Thompson H: Vaccination in the dog. *In Pract* 4:151–155, 1982.

31. Wallace BL, McMillen JK: An inactivated canine parvovirus vaccine: duration of immunity and effectiveness in presence of maternal antibody. *Canine Pract* 12:14–19, 1985.

32. Carmichael LE, Pollock RVH, Joubert JC: Response of puppies to canine-origin parvovirus vaccines. *Mod Vet Pract* 65:99–102, 1984.

32a. Thompson H, McCandlish IAP, Cornwell HJC, et al: Studies of parvovirus vaccination in the dog: the performance of live attenuated feline parvovirus vaccine. *Vet Rec* 122:378–385, 1988.

33. Macartney L, Thompson H, McCandlish IAP, et al: Canine parvovirus: interaction between passive immunity and virulent challenge. *Vet Rec* 122:573–576, 1988.

34. Gill MA, May S, Johnson T: First dose CPV takes guesswork out of vaccinating puppies against CPV infection. *Norden News* 61:4–11, 1986.

35. Churchill AE: Preliminary development of a live attenuated canine parvovirus vaccine from an isolate of British origin. *Vet Rec* 120:334–339, 1987.

36. O'Brien SE, Roth JA, Hill BL: Response of pups to modified-live canine parvovirus component in a combination vaccine. *J Am Vet Med Assoc* 188:699–701, 1986.

36a. Olson P, Klingeborn B, Hedhammar A: Serum antibody response to canine parvovirus, canine adenovirus-1 and canine distemper virus in dogs with known status of immunization: study of dogs in Sweden. *Am J Vet Res* 49:1460–1466, 1988.

37. Glickman LT, Appel MJG: A controlled field trial of an attenuated canine origin parvovirus vaccine. *Compend Cont Ed Pract Vet* 4:888–892, 1982.

37a. Mastro JM, Axthelm M, Mathes LE, et al: Repeated suppression of lymphocyte blastogenesis following vaccinations of CPV-immune dogs with modified live CPV vaccines. *Vet Microbiol* 12:201–211, 1986.

38. Potgieter LND, Jones JB, Patton CS, et al: Experimental parvovirus infection in dogs. *Can J Comp Med* 45:212–216, 1981.

39. Krakowka S, Olsen RG, Axthelm MK, et al: Canine parvovirus infection potentiates canine distemper encephalitis attributable to modified live-virus vaccine. *J Am Vet Med Assoc* 180:137–139, 1982.

40. Swango LJ: Frequently asked questions about CPV disease. *Norden News* 58:4–10, 1984.

41. Kesel ML, Neil DH: Combined MLV canine parvovirus vaccine: immunosuppression with infective shedding. *VM SAC* 78:687–691, 1983.

42. Parrish CR, Carmichael LE: Natural variation of canine parvovirus. *Science* 230:1046–1048, 1985.

43. Appel MJG, Carmichael LE: Can a commercial vaccine protect pups against a recent field isolate of parvovirus? *Vet Med* 83:1091–1093, 1988.

43a. Bartkoski MJ, Lurren M, Dees C, et al: Canine parvovirus immunodiagnosis and vaccination procedures. *Comp Anim Pract* 2:30–33, 1988.

44. Edwards BG, Fulker RH, Acree WM, et al: Evaluating a canine coronavirus vaccine through antigen extinction and challenge studies. *Vet Med* 80:28–33, 1985.

45. Gill MA, May SW, Beckenhauer WH: Immunogenicity and efficacy of an inactivated canine coronavirus vaccine. Norden Laboratories, Lincoln, NE, 1987.

45a. First Dose CV Product Information. Norden Laboratories, Lincoln, NE, 1989.

46. Fulker RH, Edwards BF, Acree WM, et al: Safety studies on a killed canine coronavirus vaccine administered simultaneously with modified-live canine viral antigen vaccines. Canine Pract 13:18–27, 1986.

47. Appel MJG: Does canine coronavirus augment the effects of subsequent parvovirus infection? Vet Med 83:360–366, 1988.

48. Most rabies vaccines must be administered intramuscularly. J Am Vet Med Assoc 186:545, 1985.

48a. Wilkie BN: Respiratory tract immune response to microbial pathogens. J Am Vet Med Assoc 181:1074–1079, 1982.

48b. Cocker FM, Newby TJ, Gaskell RM, et al: Responses of cats to nasal vaccination with a live, modified herpesvirus type 1. Res Vet Sci 41:323–330, 1986.

49. Johnson RP, Povey RC: Vaccination against feline viral rhinotracheitis in kittens with maternally derived feline viral rhinotracheitis antibodies. J Am Vet Med Assoc 186:149–152, 1985.

50. Kolar JR, Rude TA: Duration of immunity in cats inoculated with a commercial feline pneumonitis vaccine. Vet Med SAC 76:1171–1173, 1981.

51. Leukocell Product Information. Norden Laboratories, Lincoln, NE, 1985.

52. Covenant FeLV Vaccine Technical Seminar, University Edition. Diamond Scientific, Des Moines, IA, 1988.

52a. Haffer K, Derr J, Koertje W, et al: Efficacy studies of a two dose feline leukemia vaccine. Vaccine, in press, 1989.

53. Legendre AM: Feline leukemia virus vaccination. In Kirk RW (ed): Current Veterinary Therapy X. Philadelphia, WB Saunders Co, 1989, pp 1052–1056.

53a. Legendre AM: Personal communication. University of Tennessee, 1989.

53b. Fanton B: Comments on Leukocell. Contact challenge study conducted at the University of Tennessee. Norden Laboratories, Lincoln NE. Personal communication, 1989.

53c. Pollock R: Personal communication. Cornell University, 1989.

54. Pedersen NC, Johnson L, Ott RL: Evaluation of a commercial feline leukemia virus vaccine for immunogenicity and efficacy. Feline Pract 15:7–20, 1985.

55. Jones BEV: Platelet aggregation in dogs after live-virus vaccination. ACTA Vet Scand 25:504–509, 1984.

56. Pacitti AM, Jarrett O: Duration of the latent state in feline leukemia virus infections. Vet Rec 117:472–474, 1985.

57. Haffer KN, Sharpee RL, Beckenhauer WH: Feline leukaemia vaccine protection against viral latency. Vaccine 5:133–135, 1987.

58. Citino SB: Use of a subunit feline leukemia virus vaccine in exotic cats. J Am Vet Med Assoc 192:957–959, 1988.

59. Sharpee RL, Bechenhauer WH, Baumgartener LE, et al: Feline leukemia vaccine: evaluation of safety and efficacy against persistent viremia and tumor development. Compend Cont Educ Pract Vet 8:267–277, 1986.

60. Henley JP, Stewart DC, Dickerson TV: Evaluating the efficacy of feline leukemia vaccination in two high-risk colonies. Vet Med 81:470–474, 1986.

61. Scott FW: Update on FIP. 12th Annu Symp for Treatment of Small Animal Diseases, 1989, pp 43–47.

61a. Gerber JD: Protection of cats against feline infectious peritonitis (FIP) by intranasal administration of a temperature sensitive FIP virus vaccine. Norden Laboratories, Lincoln, NE, Personal communication, 1989.

62. Moennig B: Feline leukaemia prophylaxis. J Small Anim Pract 27:343–352, 1986.

63. Finberg RW, Ertl CJ: Use of T-cell specific antiidiotypes to immunize against viral infections. Immunol Rev 90:129–155, 1986.

64. Robinson AJ: The effect of molecular biology on vaccine development. N Z Vet J 34:41–42, 1986.

65. Engleberg NC, Eisentein BI: The impact of new cloning techniques on the diagnosis and treatment of infectious diseases. N Engl J Med 311:892–901, 1984.

66. Gilbert JH, Pedersen NC, Nunberg JH: Feline leukemia virus envelope protein expression encoded by a recombinant vaccinia virus: apparent lack of immunogenicity in vaccinated animals. Virus Res 7:49–67, 1987.

66a. Appel MJG, Paoeletti E: Immune response to vaccinia virus and recombinant virus products in dogs. Am J Vet Res 49:1932–1934, 1988.

67. Fowler ME, Theobald J: Immunity procedures. In Fowler ME (ed): Zoo and Wild Animal Medicine. Philadelphia, WB Saunders Co, 1978, pp 613–617.

68. Appel MJ: Virus Infections of Carnivores, vol 1. Horzenik MC (series ed): Virus Infections of Vertebrates. New York, Elsevier, 1987.

69. Appel MJ: Personal communication. Cornell University, Ithaca, NY, 1988.

70. Susceptibility of various exotic animals to canine distemper and feline distemper viruses. Norden Laboratories, Lincoln, NE, 1981.

71. Montali RJ, Bartz CR, Teare JA, et al: Clinical trials with canine distemper vaccines in exotic carnivores. J Am Vet Med Assoc 183:1163–1167,1983.

72. Karesh WB, Bottomley G: Vaccine-induced anaphylaxis in a Brazilian jaguar (Panthera onca plaustrix). J Zoo Anim Med 14:133–137, 1983.

72a. Rosenthal RC, Dworkis AS: Adverse reactions to Leukocell. J Am Anim Hosp Assoc 23:515–518, 1987.

73. Frick OL, Brooks DL: Immunoglobulin E antibodies to pollens augmented in dogs by virus vaccines. Am J Vet Res 44:440–445, 1983.

74. Straw B: Decrease in platelet count after vaccination with distemper hepatitis (DH) vaccine. VM SAC 73:725–726, 1978.

75. Dodds WJ: Bleeding diseases of small animals. Vet Ref Lab Newsl :1–4, 1984.

75a. Leifer CE, Page RL, Matus RE, et al: Proliferative glomerulonephritis and chronic active hepatitis with cirrhosis associated with Corynebacterium parvum immunotherapy in a dog. J Am Vet Med Assoc 180:78–80, 1987.

76. Wilcox BP, Yager JA: Focal cutaneous vasculitis and alopecia at the site of rabies vaccination in dogs. J Am Vet Med Assoc 188:1174–1177, 1986.

77. Stanley RG, Jabara AG: Chronic skin reaction to a combined feline rhinotracheitis virus (herpesvirus) and calicivirus vaccine. Aust Vet J 65:128–130, 1988.

78. Greene CE: Personal observations. University of Georgia, Athens, GA, 1988.

79. Barnard BJH, Geyer DHJ, DeKoker WC: Neurological symptoms in a cat following vaccination with high-egg passage Flury rabies vaccine of chicken embryo origin. *Onderstepoort J Vet Res* 44:195–196, 1977.

80. Pedersen NC, Emmons RW, Selcer R, et al: Rabies vaccine virus infection in three dogs. *J Am Vet Med Assoc* 172:1092–1096, 1978.

81. Bellinger DA, Chang J, Bunn TO, et al: Rabies induced by high-egg passage Flury strain vaccine. *J Am Vet Med Assoc* 183:997–998, 1983.

82. Esh JB, Cunningham JG, Wiktor TJ: Vaccine-induced rabies in four cats. *J Am Vet Med Assoc* 180:1336–1339, 1982.

83. Hartley WJ: A post-vaccinal inclusion body encephalitis in dogs. *Vet Pathol* 11:301–312, 1974.

84. Bestetti G, Fatzer R, Fankhauser R: Encephalitis following vaccination against distemper and infectious hepatitis in the dog. An optical and ultrastructural study. *Acta Neuropathol (Berl)* 43:69–75, 1978.

85. Slater EA: The response to measles and distemper virus in immunosuppressed and normal dogs. *J Am Vet Med Assoc* 156:1762–1766, 1970.

86. Krakowka S, Olsen RG, Axthelm MK, et al: Canine parvovirus infection potentiates canine distemper encephalitis attributable to modified live-virus vaccine. *J Am Vet Med Assoc* 180:137–139, 1982.

87. Fankhauser R, Freudiger V, Vandevelde M, et al: Purkinje cell atrophy following measles virus vaccination in dogs. *Schweiz Arch Neurol Neurochir Psychiatr* 112:353–356, 1973.

88. Wilson RB, Holladay JA, Cave JS: A neurologic syndrome associated with use of a canine coronavirus-parvovirus vaccine in dogs. *Compend Cont Educ Pract Vet* 8:117–124, 1986.

89. Martin ML: Canine coronavirus enteritis and a recent outbreak following modified live virus vaccination. *Compend Cont Educ Pract Vet* 7:1012–1016, 1985.

90. Short CR: Potential influence of viral infection and vaccination on drug disposition. *J Am Vet Med Assoc* 189:330–332, 1986.

91. Ray WF, Filliland CD, McMichael JC, et al: *ImmunoRegulin Biological Response Modifier*. Tampa, FL, ImmunoVet Inc, 1982.

91a. Becker AM, Janik TA, Smith EK, et al: *Propionibacterium acnes* immunotherapy in chronic recurrent canine pyoderma. *J Vet Intern Med* 3:26–30, 1989.

92. Liu WT, Good RA, Trang LQ, et al: Remission of leukemia and loss of feline leukemia virus in cats injected with *Staphylococcus* protein A: associa-tion with increased circulating interferon and complement-dependent cytotoxic antibody. *Proc Natl Acad Sci* 81:6471–6475, 1984.

93. Harper HD, Sjoquist J, Hardy WD, et al: Antitumor activity of protein A administered intravenously to pet cats with leukemia or lymphosarcoma. *Cancer* 55:1863–1867, 1985.

94. Snyder HW, Singhal MC, Hardy WD, et al: Clearance of feline leukemia virus from persistently infected pet cats treated by extracorporeal immunosorption is correlated with an enhanced antibody response to FeLV gp70. *J Immunol* 132:1538–1543, 1984.

95. Noorbibi KD, Engelman RW, Liu WT, et al: Remission of leukemia in cats following ex vivo immunosorption therapy using *Staphylococcus* protein A. *J Biol Response Mod* 3:278–285, 1984.

96. Weiss RC: Immunotherapy for feline leukemia, using staphylococcal protein A or heterologous interferons: immunopharmacologic actions and potential use. *J Am Vet Med Assoc* 192:681–684, 1988.

97. Tompkins MB, Cummins JM: Response of feline leukemia virus–induced nonregenerative anemia to oral administration of an interferon-containing preparation. *Feline Pract* 12:6–15, 1982.

98. Steed VP: Improved survival of four cats infected with feline leukemia virus after oral administration of interferon. *Feline Pract* 17:24–30, 1987.

99. Cummins J, Tompkins M, Olsen R, et al: The oral use of human interferon alpha in cats. *J Biol Resp Mod* 7:513–523, 1988.

100. Winters WD, Harris SC: Interferon induction in healthy and tumor-bearing dogs by cell walls of *Mycobacterium bovis* strain bacille Calmette-Guérin. *Am J Vet Res* 43:1232–1237, 1982.

101. Wooley RE, Brown J, Scott TA, et al: Effect of polyinosinic-polycytidylic acid in dogs experimentally infected with infectious canine hepatitis virus. *Am J Vet Res* 35:1217–1219, 1974.

102. Bibrack B: Aktiv interferonisierung: eine neue moglichkeit der Bekampfung des Welpensterbens. *Kleintierpraxis* 20:258–263, 1975.

103. Tsai SC, Appel MJ: Interferon induction in dogs. *Am J Vet Res* 40:256–361, 1979.

104. Vandevelde M, Boring JG, Hoff EJ: The effect of levamisole on the canine central nervous system. *J Neuropathol Exp Neurol* 37:165–173, 1978.

105. Sutton RH, Atwell RB: Nervous disorders in dogs associated with levamisole therapy. *J Small Anim Pract* 23:391–397, 1982.

106. Osterhaus A, Weijer K, Uytdehaag F, et al: Induction of protective immune response in cats by vaccination with feline leukemia virus ISOCOM. *J Immunol* 135:591–596, 1985.

3 IMMUNODEFICIENCY AND INFECTIOUS DISEASE

Craig E. Greene

Immunodeficiency diseases result whenever there is an impairment in phagocytic, humoral, or cell-mediated immune (CMI) defense mechanisms. Such defects can be hereditary, in which case they are usually noted at an early age, or acquired, as when they accompany immunosuppression caused by drug therapy or other diseases. Immunodeficiency should be suspected whenever an animal chronically does poorly or develops persistent or recurrent infections. Infections in immunodeficient animals, usually caused by opportunistic pathogens, do not respond well to antimicrobial therapy in that partial improvement or relapse is common. Paradoxically, immunodeficient states have been characterized as predisposing some animals to autoimmune disease. Presumably, this increased frequency of autoimmunity and hypersensitivity reflects an imbalance in the immune system caused by a lack of one or more immunomodulating components. It may also relate to inadequate removal of infectious agents, resulting in chronic antigenic stimulation of other components of the host's immune system.

TYPES OF IMMUNODEFICIENCY

Immunodeficient states can arise through defects in phagocytic, humoral, or CMI mechanisms (Table 3–1).

Phagocytic Defects

Phagocytic impairment is associated with an increased prevalence of pyogenic bacterial infections. A wide variety of bacteria are usually involved, most of which are normal microflora or pathogens of relatively low virulence. Recurrent infections of the skin, respiratory tract, and oral cavity are common, and recurrent bacteremia and overwhelming sepsis are also seen. Neutrophil counts may be decreased or increased, depending on whether quantitative or qualitative deficiencies are present, respectively. Qualitative defects must be detected by special techniques, including the measurement of bactericidal activity, phagocytic ability, and chemotaxis.

Humoral Defects

Humoral immune defects involving antibody production are also associated with pyogenic infections; however, capsule-forming bacteria, which resist phagocytosis, are usually involved. *Streptococcus pneumoniae* (pneumococcus), certain *Klebsiella*, and *Pseudomonas* may predominate. The site and type of infection usually depend on the immunoglobulin (Ig) deficiency that exists. Animals with specific Ig deficiencies have not been identified. Findings in humans and dogs with IgA deficiencies include increased incidence of respiratory and GI infections or allergic processes. People with IgM deficiencies have a tendency to develop overwhelming sepsis and atopy. IgE-deficient humans have less tendency to infections but are more prone to develop autoimmune disorders.

Although not always present, humoral immune defects can be suspected on the basis of a decreased globulin concentration. Serum electrophoresis can help to determine which protein class is reduced, but immunoelectrophoresis must be done to detect the type and quantity of the Ig that is deficient.

Table 3–1. Clinical Features of Various Types of Immunodeficiency Disease

	TYPE OF IMMUNODEFICIENCY		
	Phagocytic	**Humoral**	**Cell-Mediated**
Type of organism	Pyogenic bacteria (e.g., *Staphylococcus, E. coli, Klebsiella, Enterobacter, Serratia, Proteus, Actinomyces*)	Pyogenic encapsulated bacteria (e.g., *Pseudomonas,* pneumococcus)	Granuloma-producing bacteria (e.g., *Mycobacterium*), viruses, fungi, protozoa
Infectious complications	Pyoderma, pneumonia, rapid spreading cellulitis, chronic stomatitis, osteomyelitis	IgA Pneumonia, bronchitis, sinusitis IgM Overwhelming sepsis	Generalized infections
Laboratory finding	Complete blood count Neutropenia (quantitative defects) Neutrophilia (functional defects)	Total protein Hypoglobulinemia (quantitative defect) Hyperglobulinemia (functional defect) Serum electrophoresis Increased or decreased β- and/or γ- globulin	Complete blood count Lymphopenia
Additional specialized testing	Complement quantitation, phagocytic bactericidal index, neutrophil chemotaxis	Immunoelectrophoresis, lymph node biopsy, special antibody titer before and after vaccination	Lymphocyte stimulation (transformation), intradermal skin testing Skin allograft rejection

Titers against specific antigens can be measured, followed by evaluation of the antibody response to vaccination against particular agents. Biopsy of lymph nodes reveals disorganization with loss of germinal centers and normal paracortical lymphocytes. Decreases in plasma cell populations may be evident.

Cell-Mediated Deficiencies

Cellular immune deficiencies are associated with an increased risk of viral, fungal, intracellular bacterial, and protozoal infections. Animals with cellular immunodeficiencies may have smaller tonsils and peripheral lymph nodes and decreased numbers of circulating lymphocytes. More specific testing reveals decreased delayed-type hypersensitivity to skin testing with tuberculin and dinitrochlorobenzene (DNCB) and prolonged allograft rejection times. Reduced in vitro lymphocyte stimulation is also found.

HEREDITARY IMMUNODEFICIENCIES

Hereditary deficiencies in immune function are being recognized with increasing

frequency in dogs and cats. These are summarized in Table 3–2. The high degree of inbreeding that occurs within popular purebred bloodlines is likely to increase the chance that defects will be discovered.

External Defense

Primary Ciliary Dyskinesia. This defect, described in several dogs, is characterized by an absence of ciliary defense mechanisms. Typical clinical findings are those of a dog several weeks to several months of age with chronic respiratory disease, otitis media, and in some cases, transposition of viscera, all presumably related to defective microtubular formation resulting in abnormal ciliary motion.[1–3] Other abnormalities include renal fibrosis and dilation of renal tubules from impairment of renal tubular cilia; hearing loss from obstruction of the auditory tube; male infertility from spermatozoal tail dysfunction; and hydrocephalus from defective ependymal cilia. Neutrophilic movement may also be abnormal, presumably because of defective microtubules, which are important in their cytoskeleton.[1]

Phagocytic Immunodeficiencies

Canine Cyclic Hematopoiesis. This defect has been described in gray collies (gray col-

Table 3–2. Hereditary Immunodeficiencies of Dogs and Cats[a]

DISEASE	SPECIES (BREED)	MECHANISM OF DEFECT
External Defense Defect		
Ciliary dyskinesia	D (many)	Absence of ciliary motion
Phagocyte Defect		
Cyclic hematopoiesis	D (collie, Pomeranian, cocker spaniel)	Block in neutrophil release from bone marrow
Chédiak-Higashi anomaly	C (Persian)	Decreased neutrophil chemotaxis and bactericidal capacity
Granulocytopathy	D (Irish setter)	Bactericidal defect in neutrophils
	D (Doberman pinscher)	Bactericidal defect in neutrophils
	D (Weimaraner)	Neutrophil defect?
	D (Irish setter)	Reduced granulocyte adherence
Pelger-Huët anomaly	D (foxhound, basenji)	Impaired neutrophil chemotaxis (variable defect)
	C (domestic shorthaired)	
Mucopolysaccharidosis	C (Siamese)	Arylsulfatase B deficiency
Neutrophil granulation defect	C (Birman)	Eosinophilic granules in neutrophil cytoplasm
Humoral Immune Defect		
Complement deficiency	D (Brittany spaniel)	C3 absent, impairing phagocyte function
Selective IgA deficiency	D (German shepherd, beagle, shar-pei, Airedale)	Reduced serum and secretory IgA
Cell-Mediated Defect		
Thymic atrophy	D (Weimaraner)	Decreased growth hormone, decreased T cell function
Pneumocystosis	D (dachshund)	Suspected T cell defect
Thymic hypoplasia	C (Burmese)	Suspected T cell defect
Combined Immune Defect		
Combined immunodeficiency	D (Basset)	T cell defect, reduced serum IgG, IgA, with variable IgM

[a]See text for a summary of clinical findings and respective references.
 D = dog, C = cat.

lie syndrome), with isolated reports in Pomeranians and cocker spaniels.[4] Emigration of neutrophils and other cells from the bone marrow is blocked, resulting in a cyclic fluctuation in neutrophils from the bone marrow. Additional defects in lysosomal function result in decreased bactericidal capacity of neutrophils. Animals are commonly stunted and have periodic episodes of fever, anorexia, depression, and suppurative infections. Respiratory, umbilical, and septicemic infections are most common. Most animals have secondarily increased Ig concentrations and develop amyloidosis at an older age.

Chédiak-Higashi Anomaly. An autosomal recessive defect described in Persian cats and other species, Chédiak-Higashi anomaly is characterized by oculocutaneous albinism and recurrent pyogenic infections.[5] There are abnormally large melanin granules in hair shafts, and enlarged cytoplasmic granules are present in phagocytic cells. Leukocytes have decreased capacity for the intracellular killing of bacteria, which is a result

of impaired fusion of lysosomes with phagosomes, and decreased chemotaxis. Cats, unlike other species, do not experience recurrent infections, but they do show hemorrhagic tendencies as a result of defects in platelet function.

Canine Granulocytopathy. This defect in neutrophilic bactericidal capacity has been described in Irish setters as an autosomal recessive trait.[6] Dogs are homozygous for the defect and are stunted, have recurrent bacterial infections, and require constant antibiotic therapy. They develop pyoderma, gingivitis, osteomyelitis, and lymphadenopathy and have a pronounced leukocytosis that persists throughout the illness. Polyclonal hypergammaglobulinemia is a common finding in chronic recurrent infections.

Neutrophil Dysfunction in Doberman Pinscher Dogs. Chronic rhinitis and pneumonia have been reported in closely related Doberman pinschers.[7] The dogs had increased numbers of structurally normal neutrophils but with reduced bactericidal function.

Chronic sneezing, coughing, and chronic mucopurulent nasal discharge had been present since weaning in some dogs. Antibiotic treatment was temporarily effective. Some dogs, with or without respiratory signs, had poor quality of hair coat, generalized seborrhea, scaling, and a lusterless appearance. Although mortality was low, persistent nasal discharge and coughing were present in some dogs.

Recurrent Infections in Weimaraners. Young (<3 years) inbred Weimaraner dogs have suffered from a syndrome of chronic recurrent pyogenic infections.[8,9] Although neutrophils are suspected to be affected, results of neutrophil function tests in these dogs were within reference ranges. Unlike dogs with growth hormone deficiency and thymic dystrophy, these dogs have normal body size and condition (see also Cell-Mediated Immunodeficiencies). High fever, vomiting or diarrhea, lymphadenopathy, joint pain, and mucosal bleeding have been noted. Marked congestion or ulceration of mucous membranes, pyoderma, and recurrent subcutaneous swellings, and in some cases, neurologic signs have been noted. Hematologic abnormalities have included marked neutrophilia with or without a left shift and monocytosis. Urate crystalluria, presumably from excess acid breakdown from degenerating neutrophils, has been a consistent finding on urinalysis. The cause of the bleeding defect was undetermined. Culture results of blood or lesions has shown a variety of pyogenic commensal bacteria. Necropsy findings have included suppurative lymphangitis, osteomyelitis, polyarthritis, and abscesses throughout soft tissues.

Granulocyte Adherence Defect. A line-bred, cross-bred Irish setter dog had recurrent bacterial infections and persistent leukocytosis that were first noted at 2 months of age.[10] The dog's neutrophils lacked surface glycoproteins responsible for leukocyte adherence, aggregation, and chemotaxis. The dog suffered from deep skin wound infections, pododermatitis, superficial pyoderma, gingivitis, pneumonia, thrombophlebitis, and ascending osteomyelitis. Poor wound healing, persistent fever, localized cellulitis with impaired pus formation, and local lymphadenopathy were also found.

Pelger-Huët Anomaly. Decreased lobulation of granulocytic cells has been described in American foxhounds, basenjis, and domestic shorthaired cats.[11] The abnormal nuclear shape is thought to contribute to reduced cell mobility and abnormal chemotaxis. Not all affected animals appear to have chemotactic defects, and none has been shown to have increased risk of infection.

Mucopolysaccharidosis. An autosomal recessive disorder in Siamese cats, mucopolysaccharidosis is caused by an arylsulfatase B deficiency that results in bone and cartilage deformity.[12] An affected cat is small and has a flattened face, small ears, increased corneal opacity, large forepaws, and pectus excavatum. Large metachromatic granules that stain with toluidine blue are present in peripheral blood granulocytes. No increased risk of infection has yet been associated with this defect.

Neutrophil Granulation Defect. This hereditary abnormality of neutrophils has been described in Birman cats.[13] The trait is associated with autosomal recessive inheritance and causes fine eosinophilic granules in neutrophilic cytoplasm. Neutrophil function was similar to that of neutrophils from unaffected cats, and no increased susceptibility to infection was noted.

Humoral Immunodeficiencies

Defects of the Ig system have been poorly documented in dogs and cats. A hereditary C3 deficiency characterized by autosomal recessive inheritance has been described in Brittany spaniels.[14] Recurrent sepsis and localized bacterial infections similar to those seen with neutrophil defects occurred. This similarity results from the essential role of C3 in neutrophil chemotaxis and opsonization.

Selective IgA Deficiency. Low or undetectable serum or secretory IgA concentrations or both have been detected in German shepherd,[15] beagle,[16] and shar-pei[17] dogs. Chronic recurrent upper and lower respiratory infections, otitis externa, and dermatitis are the usual manifestations. Despite the selective low IgA levels in many related dogs, not all animals were symptomatic. Some affected dogs had high serum titers of rheumatoid factor.[18]

Airedale terriers with discospondylitis were found to have suppressed lymphocyte stimulation associated with serum factors, increased serum β-1 globulins and decreased serum IgA concentrations as compared with age-, sex-, and breed-matched control dogs.[19] Measurements were not made prior to infection; however, preexisting immunodeficiency may have been responsible for entry and spread of the infection to the intervertebral disc space.

Cell-Mediated Immunodeficiencies

The best-documented cell-mediated immunodeficiency in dogs has been described in Weimaraners with increased susceptibility to infection, decreased growth hormone concentration, thymic atrophy, and decreased T cell function. The deficiency can be detected in affected puppies within 1 to 3 months of birth; the signs include stunted growth, chronic wasting, and suppurative pneumonia. Dogs have a normal γ-globulin concentration but show a decreased in vitro response to lymphocyte stimulation with phytohemagglutinin. Histologic findings include reduced number of cells in the paracortical (T lymphocyte) regions of the lymph nodes and in the splenic white pulp. Dogs have shown improvement following exogenous administration of thymosin or growth hormone, indicating that a defect in the hypophysis of these dogs results in thymic abnormalities.[20]

A CMI defect has been suspected in dachshunds that have a high propensity for *Pneumocystis* pneumonia (see Chapter 89). Thymic hypoplasia and an increased susceptibility to infection in Burmese kittens have been mentioned.[21]

Combined Immunodeficiency

Basset hound dogs have been described with lymphopenia, depressed T lymphocyte function with low serum IgA and IgG and variable IgM concentrations.[22] The disease is sex-linked and dogs develop severe bacterial skin infections, stomatitis, and otitis within the first few weeks of life. Most die of systemic viral infections by 12 to 16 weeks of age. Necropsy findings include thymic, lymph node, and splenic dysplasia.

ACQUIRED IMMUNODEFICIENCIES

Immune defects secondary to many infectious diseases, metabolic disturbances, intoxications, and drug therapies have been described (Table 3–3).

Infectious Diseases

Canine Distemper. Disseminated viral infections that involve replication in and damage to lymphoid tissue, such as canine distemper, are associated with depression of CMI.[23] Persistent immunodeficiency caused by canine distemper virus usually occurs when infection develops prenatally or within the first weeks of neonatal life, when full immunocompetence has not been established. Affected dogs frequently are stunted and develop chronic infections with protozoans such as *Giardia* and rickettsiae such as *Haemobartonella*. They can also be expected to be more susceptible to viral and fungal pathogens, and they frequently have pronounced lymphopenia and hypogammaglobulinemia. Persistent suppression of CMI in neonatal puppies can be detected by decreased lymphocyte stimulation test results and a decrease in synthesis of T cell–dependent antibodies (IgG and IgA). IgM is also reduced if thymic hypoplasia results from early in utero infection. Transient depression of CMI has been reported in older neonates that are infected with virulent distemper virus. Some of this suppression has been shown to be caused by lymphocyte immunoregulatory factors in serum.[24] Depression of immunoresponsiveness following vaccination is minimal if it occurs at all.

Canine Parvovirus Infection. This virus has an affinity for replicating in rapidly dividing cells and produces severe lymphopenia and immunosuppression in neonates. An increased risk of secondary infections, including greater susceptibility to canine distemper vaccine–induced encephalitis, has been reported in 3-week-old pups (see Chapter 2). Lymphocyte transformation assay results were depressed in adult mongrel dogs shedding naturally acquired canine parvovirus in their feces.[25]

Canine Ehrlichiosis. Depression of in vitro lymphocyte stimulation and skin hypersen-

Table 3–3. Acquired Immunocompromised Conditions of Dogs and Cats

COMPONENT AFFECTED	CAUSE	COMPONENT AFFECTED	CAUSE
Damage or Penetration of External Barriers	Skin 　Burns 　Tissue necrosis 　Intravenous catheters 　Cerebrospinal fluid 　　collection Gastrointestinal tract 　Antacid usage 　Endoscopy	Complement Deficiency	Feline leukemia Immune hemolytic 　anemias Endotoxemia
	Lungs 　Heart failure 　Chronic lung disease 　Inhalation anesthesia Urinary tract 　Urinary catheters 　Cystocentesis	Humoral Deficiency	Malnutrition Dysproteinemias Cytotoxic chemotherapy Colostral deprivation
Phagocyte Defects	Quantitative 　Feline panleukopenia 　Canine ehrlichiosis 　Diphenylhydantoin 　　(dogs) 　Estrogen (dogs) 　T-2 toxin (cats) 　Methylnitrosourea 　　(cats) Qualitative 　Hypophosphatemia 　　(dogs) 　Prolonged bacteremia 　　(dogs) 　Diabetes mellitus 　Renal failure 　Systemic lupus 　　erythematosus 　Drug (aspirin, 　　glucocorticoids, 　　halothane anesthesia, 　　amphotericin B, 　　vinca alkaloids, 　　chloramphenicol, 　　tetracycline)	Cell-Mediated Deficiency	Canine distemper Canine ehrlichiosis Canine parvovirus 　infection Feline panleukopenia Feline leukemia Feline immunodeficiency 　virus infection Canine demodicosis Systemic lupus 　erythematosus Protein-calorie restriction Vitamin E and selenium 　deficiency Lymphangiectasia Newborn animals Old animals Pentobarbital anesthesia 　(dogs) Cytotoxic chemotherapy Glucocorticoid therapy

sitivity with DNCB has been reported in canine ehrlichiosis several months after initial infection, when hyperglobulinemia develops.[26] The depression does not appear to significantly alter the course of infection at this time, although certain breeds (e.g., German shepherds) have more severe illness and significantly greater depression of CMI before and after infection than other breeds. No increased susceptibility to infection has been documented in dogs with acute ehrlichiosis as yet; however, they are susceptible to pyogenic infections during the chronic neutropenic phase of the disease.

Canine Demodicosis. Dogs with generalized demodicosis have decreased in vitro lymphocyte stimulation and random neutrophil movement. Serum proteins with apparent immunoregulatory roles are responsible for the findings. No increased susceptibility to infection has been documented in vivo, although many dogs do develop severe secondary pyoderma. Secondary bacterial infection rather than the mite *Demodex canis* is responsible for the suppressive activity.[24] Neutrophilic chemotactic movement has been decreased in bacterial or staphylococcal pyoderma in dogs.[27] In some cases, with antimicrobial therapy these abnormal test results return to reference ranges accompanied by clinical improvement.[28]

Feline Panleukopenia. Feline panleukopenia virus has a predilection for rapidly dividing cells and produces permanent cell-mediated immunosuppression and thymic atrophy in kittens infected in utero. Lymphoid depletion, mild depression of in vitro lymphocyte function, and neutropenia are characteristic in neonatally infected cats, which may have a transiently increased susceptibility to infection. Overwhelming sepsis from gram-negative enteric microflora, which accompanies feline panleukopenia, may relate to the immunosuppression caused by the virus.

Feline Leukemia Virus Infection. Immunodeficiency in feline leukemia virus infection often occurs before malignant transformation of T lymphocytes.[29, 30] Feline leukemia virus directs the production of a polypeptide, p15e, that impairs in vitro lymphocyte stimulation and causes prolonged retention of cutaneous allografts. Secondary hyperglobulinemia and complement depletion have also been found. Immune complex formation may also interfere with lymphocyte function since immune complex removal has improved the clinical condition of infected cats.[31] (Also see Therapy, Chapter 26 and Immunotherapy, Chapter 2.) Infected cats that do not develop neoplasia have a high mortality rate and increased susceptibility to concurrent infection with other organisms such as commensal bacteria, pathogenic fungi, *Haemobartonella*, and feline infectious peritonitis virus. Certain forms of feline leukemia virus infection also result in severe neutropenia, which increases the risk of secondary bacterial infection.[31a, 31b] Persistent neutropenia may also develop in some cats independent of feline leukemia virus infection.[31c]

Feline Immunodeficiency Virus Infection. Cats naturally affected with this syndrome develop fever, variable neutropenia and chronic infections of the skin and mucosal surfaces.[32] Experimentally inoculated cats develop generalized peripheral lymphadenomegaly and transient neutropenia, followed by a disease-free period. In natural circumstances, other infectious agents may be needed to induce the immunosuppressive syndromes (also see Chapter 26).

Overwhelming Bacteremia. Severe endotoxemia or sepsis has been shown to impair CMI of dogs and to decrease neutrophil bactericidal function (also see Etiology, Chapter 44).

Metabolic Disturbances

Many biochemical processes that occur in noninfectious disease states interfere with normal immune mechanisms. Failure of neonates to ingest colostrum and dysproteinemia are both associated with impaired humoral antibody function. Decreased complement concentration has been noted with endotoxemia, immune-mediated hemolysis, and malnutrition. Age has a marked influence on CMI. Newborn puppies and kittens experience a hypothermic state during the first week of life that suppresses T cell function. A decline in CMI, which is also seen in older dogs and cats, may explain their increased susceptibility to infectious and neoplastic disorders. Aged animals' vaccinations should be kept current. Proper nutrition is also an important determinant of immunoresponsiveness. Protein and caloric restriction has resulted in premature thymic atrophy and decreased cell-mediated, humoral, and phagocytic responses in animals.[33] In contrast, overfed obese dogs have had an increased susceptibility to infection and severe clinical illness.

Vitamin E and selenium deficiencies in dogs have been associated with decreased in vitro lymphocyte responsiveness, decreased serologic response to vaccination, and increased susceptibility to infection with opportunistic pathogens.[34] This deficit can be accentuated by excessive intake of polyunsaturated fats (strong oxidants that counteract the effects of vitamin E).[35] Vitamin E deficiency causes the animal to produce a suppressor serum factor capable of decreasing lymphocyte responsiveness to antigenic stimulation.[35a] Increased incidence of distemper infection has been noted in a kennel in which dogs developed "brown fat" disease as a result of a vitamin E–deficient ration.[36]

Vitamin A deficiency can cause immunosuppression with opportunistic infections similar to that of vitamin E deficiency. Zinc deficiency during prenatal and neonatal periods can result in impaired cell-mediated immune responses and thymic atrophy. Immunosuppression caused by dietary deficiencies can be relieved by adequate supplementation.[36a]

Depressed phagocyte function has also been reported in humans with diabetes mellitus, systemic lupus erythematosus, and renal failure. Similarly, poorly regulated diabetic dogs had reduced neutrophil adherence as compared with controlled diabetic and nondiabetic dogs.[37] Any cause of permanent neutropenia, such as bone marrow aplasia, will significantly impair phagocyte function. Intestinal lymphangiectasia is associated with depressed CMI because of lymphocyte loss through the damaged intestinal tract.

The immune response also appears to change with aging, increasing during fetal and neonatal periods, peaking after puberty, and then declining with old age. In dogs this decline begins at 7 years of age.[38]

Iatrogenic Causes

External defense mechanisms can be impaired as a result of burns, chronic moist skin, IV and urinary catheterization, CSF collection, endoscopy, and excessive use of antacids. Leukocyte chemotaxis and phagocytosis have been shown to be impaired following administration of aspirin, glucocorticoids, tetracycline, chloramphenicol, amphotericin B, and Vinca alkaloids and with halothane anesthesia.[39] Severe hypophosphatemia produced in dogs from IV hyperalimentation has resulted in impaired phagocyte function. Splenectomy has been shown to be associated with an increased risk of septicemia in humans, apparently as a result of lost mononuclear phagocyte system function. Although splenectomy has been recommended as adjunctive therapy for autoimmune anemia and thrombocytopenia in dogs,[40] splenectomized animals have had a higher frequency of bacteremia and associated complications.[9]

Glucocorticoids cause immunosuppression through a number of mechanisms, including inhibition of macrophage phagocytosis and decreased T cell immunoresponsiveness, in addition to the decreased neutrophil function previously noted. Alternate-day glucocorticoid therapy with short-acting agents is less immunosuppressive than daily therapy or therapy using longer-acting agents.

Cytotoxic agents such as cyclophosphamide, azathioprine, and methotrexate have profound effects on both CMI and humoral immunity, as well as on phagocyte function. These effects vary according to the drug and dosage used. Care must be taken to reduce the chance of infection in dogs or cats receiving these drugs. When such animals are

hospitalized, they should be isolated in wards away from routine incoming patients. Therapy on an outpatient basis is more desirable because it minimizes the exposure to nosocomial pathogens.

Generalized anesthesia has been shown to have deleterious effects on immune function in dogs. Inhalation anesthesia with halothane has been shown to depress pulmonary macrophage function and mucociliary clearance in dogs. Pentobarbital anesthesia, halothane anesthesia with surgery, and thiamylal induction with methoxyflurane anesthesia for a keyhole renal biopsy have been shown temporarily to suppress lymphocyte stimulation in dogs.[41, 42] Responses generally returned to normal within 1 week after the procedures; however, no increased tendency to infection has been documented.

Ambient temperature appears to be important in the immune response, especially in neonatal hypothermic puppies.[43] Pups of 3 to 10 days of age in temperatures $\leq 30°C$ (86°F) had depressed cellular and humoral immune responses. They had systemic and CNS spread of CAV-1 and canine distemper vaccine viruses. Precautions must be taken to ensure that pups less than 2 weeks of age, already incapable of mature immune responses, are kept at ambient temperatures of 30°C to 37°C (86°F to 98.6°F).

References

1. Morrison WB, Frank DE, Roth JA, et al: Assessment of neutrophil function in dogs with primary ciliary dyskinesia. *J Am Vet Med Assoc* 191:425–430, 1987.
2. Edwards DF, Patton CS, Bemis DA, et al: Immotile cilia syndrome in three dogs from a litter. *J Am Vet Med Assoc* 183:667–672, 1983.
3. Afzelius BA, Carlsten J, Karlsson S: Clinical, pathologic, and ultrastructural features of situs inversus and immotile cilia syndrome in a dog. *J Am Vet Med Assoc* 184:560–563, 1984.
4. Chusid MJ, Bujak JS, Dale DC: Defective polymorphonuclear leukocyte metabolism and function in canine cyclic neutropenia. *Blood* 46:921–930, 1975.
5. Kramer JW, Davis WC, Prieur DJ: The Chediak-Higashi syndrome in cats. *Lab Invest* 36:554–562, 1977.
6. Renshaw HW, Davis WC, Renshaw SJ: Canine granulocytopathy syndrome: defective bactericidal capacity of neutrophils from a dog with recurrent infection. *Clin Immunol Immunopathol* 8:385–395, 1977.
7. Breitschwerdt EB, Brown TT, DeBuysscher EV, et al: Rhinitis, pneumonia, and defective neutrophil function in the Doberman pinscher. *Am J Vet Res* 48:1054–1062, 1987.

8. Studdert VP, Phillips WA, Studdert MJ, et al: Recurrent and persistent infections in related Weimaraner dogs. *Aust Vet J* 61:261–263, 1984.

9. Greene CE: Unpublished observations. University of Georgia, Athens, GA, 1988.

10. Giger U, Boxer LA, Simpson PJ, et al: Deficiency of leukocyte surface glycoproteins mo1,LFA-1 and Leu M5 in a dog with recurrent bacterial infections: an animal model. *Blood* 69:1622–1630, 1987.

11. Latimer KS, Rakich PM, Thompson DF: Pelger-Huët anomaly in cats. *Vet Pathol* 22:370–374, 1985.

12. Haskins ME, Patterson DF: Mucopolysaccharide storage disease in three families of cats with arylsulfatase B deficiency: leukocyte studies and carrier identification. *Pediatr Res* 13:1203–1210, 1979.

13. Hirsch VM, Cunningham TA: Hereditary anomaly of neutrophil granulation in Birman cats. *Am J Vet Res* 45:2170–2174, 1984.

14. Winkelstein JA, Cork LC, Griffin DE: Genetically determined deficiency of the third component of complement in the dog. *Science* 212:1169–1170, 1981.

15. Whitbread TJ, Batt RM, Garthwaite G: Relative deficiency of serum IgA in the German shepherd dog: a breed abnormality. *Res Vet Sci* 37:350–352, 1984.

16. Felsburg PJ, Glickman LT, Jezyk PF: Selective IgA deficiency in the dog. *Clin Immunol Immunopathol* 36:297–305, 1985.

17. Moroff SD, Hurvitz AI, Peterson ME, et al: IgA deficiency in shar-pei dogs. *Vet Immunol Immunopathol* 13:181–188, 1986.

18. Glickman LT, Shofer FS, Payton AJ, et al: Survey of serum IgA, IgG, and IgM concentrations in a large beagle population in which IgA deficiency had been identified. *Am J Vet Res* 49:1240–1245, 1988.

19. Barta O, Turnwald GH, Shaffer LM, et al: Blastogenesis-suppressing serum factors, decreased immunoglobulin A and increased β1-globulins in Airedale terriers with diskospondylitis. *Am J Vet Res* 46:1319-1322, 1985.

20. Roth JA, Kaeberle ML, Grier RL, et al: Improvement in clinical condition and thymus morphologic features associated with growth hormone treatment of immunodeficient dwarf dogs. *Am J Vet Res* 45:1151–1155, 1984.

21. Perryman LE: Primary and secondary immune deficiencies of domestic animals. *Adv Vet Sci Comp Med* 23:23–51, 1979.

22. Felsburg PJ, Jezyk PF, Haskins ME: A canine model for variable combined immunodeficiency. *Clin Res* 30:347A, 1982.

23. Stevens DR, Osburn BI: Immune deficiency in a dog with distemper. *J Am Vet Med Assoc* 168:493–498, 1976.

24. Barta O, Waltman C, Shaffer LM, et al: Effect of serum on lymphocyte blastogenesis. 1. Basic characteristics of action by diseased dog serum. *Vet Immunol Immunopathol* 3:567–583, 1982.

25. Olsen CG, Stiff MI, Olsen RG: Comparison of the blastogenic response of peripheral blood lymphocytes from canine parvovirus–positive and negative outbred dogs. *Vet Immunol Immunopathol* 6:285–290, 1984.

26. Nylindo M, Huxsoll DL, Ristic M, et al: Cell-mediated and humoral immune responses of German shepherd dogs and beagles to experimental infection with *Ehrlichia canis*. *Am J Vet Res* 41:250–254, 1980.

27. Latimer KS, Prasse KW, Mahaffey EA, et al: Neutrophil movement in selected canine skin diseases. *Am J Vet Res* 44:601–605, 1983.

28. Latimer KS, Prasse KW, Dawe DL: A transient deficit in neutrophilic chemotaxis in a dog with recurrent staphylococcal pyoderma. *Vet Pathol* 19:223–229, 1982.

29. Olsen RG, Krakowka S: Immune dysfunctions associated with viral infections. *Compend Cont Educ Pract Vet* 6:422–430, 1984.

30. Mullins JI, Chen CS, Hoover EA: Disease-specific and tissue-specific production of unintegrated feline leukemia virus variant DNA in feline AIDS. *Nature* 319:333–336, 1986.

31. Snyder H, Singhal MC, Hardy WD, et al: Clearance of feline leukemia virus from persistently infected pet cats treated by extracorporeal immunoadsorption is correlated with an enhanced antibody response to FeLV gp 70. *J Immunol* 132:1538–1543, 1984.

31a. Gabbert NH: Cyclic neutropenia in a feline leukemia-positive cat: A case report. *J Am Anim Hosp Assoc* 20:343–347, 1984.

31b. Swenson CL, Kociba GJ, O'Keefe DA, et al: Cyclic hematopoiesis associated with feline leukemia virus infection in two cats. *J Am Vet Med Assoc* 191:93–96, 1987.

31c. Swenson CL, Kociba GJ, Arnold P: Chronic idiopathic neutropenia in a cat. *J Vet Intern Med* 2:100–102, 1988.

32. Yamamoto JK, Sparger E, Ho EW, et al: Pathogenesis of experimentally induced feline immunodeficiency virus in cats. *Am J Vet Res* 49:1246–1258, 1988.

33. Law DK, Dudrick SJ, Abdou NI: The effect of dietary protein depletion on immunocompetence: the importance of nutritional repletion prior to immunologic induction. *Ann Surg* 179:168–173, 1974.

34. Langweiler M, Sheffy BE, Schultz RD: Effect of antioxidants on the proliferative response of canine lymphocytes in serum from dogs with vitamin K deficiency. *Am J Vet Res* 44:5–7, 1983.

35. Sheffy BE: Nutrition, infection and immunity. *Compend Cont Educ Pract Vet* 7:990–997, 1985.

35a. Schultz RD: Nutrition at high and deficient levels can greatly reduce immune function in dogs, cats. *DVM Magazine* 19:24–26, 1988.

36. Greene CE: Unpublished observations. University of Georgia, Athens, GA, 1982.

37. Latimer KS, Mahaffey EA: Neutrophil adherence and movement in poorly and well-controlled diabetic dogs. *Am J Vet Res* 45:1498–1500, 1984.

38. Schultz RD: The effects of aging on the immune response. *Compend Cont Educ Pract Vet* 6:1096–1105, 1984.

39. Miller EP: Glucocorticoid-induced immunosuppression. *VM SAC* 78:1199–1204, 1983.

40. Feldman BF, Handagama P, Lubberink AA: Splenectomy as adjunctive therapy for immune-mediated thrombocytopenia and hemolytic anemia in the dog. *J Am Vet Med Assoc* 187:617–619, 1985.

41. Felsburg PJ, Keyes LL, Krawiec DR, et al: The effect of general anesthesia on canine lymphocyte function. *Vet Immunol Immunopathol* 13:63–70, 1986.

42. Medleau L, Crowe DT, Dawe DL: Effect of surgery on the in vitro response of canine peripheral blood lymphocytes to phytohemagglutinin. *Am J Vet Res* 44:859-860, 1983.

43. Schultz RD: Ambient temperature affects canine immune response. *Norden News* 59:36, 1984.

4 FEVER

Craig E. Greene

ETIOLOGY AND PATHOGENESIS

Fever is a pathophysiologic elevation of body temperature that occurs in response to disease processes such as infection, metabolic disorders, and neoplasia or to pharmacologic therapy. *Fever, hyperthermia,* and *pyrexia* are usually considered synonyms for increased body temperature. However, strictly defined, fever (pyrexia) should be distinguished from hyperthermia (heat illness). *Fever* occurs when the thermoregulatory "set point" of the body is raised above the normal range of body temperature and increased endogenous heat is generated to reach this new level (Fig. 4–1A and 4–1B). *Hyperthermia* occurs when the thermoregulatory point remains unchanged but because of internal or exogenous influences, body temperature increases beyond the normal range to deleterious levels (Fig. 4–1C). Because it rarely has an infectious cause, the pathophysiology and treatment of hyperthermia will not be discussed extensively in this text. Hyperthermia should be differentiated from fever since its causes and treatment differ (Tables 4–1 and 4–2). While the need to reduce body temperature with fever is debatable, the only effective management for hyperthermia is prompt reduction of body temperature by external cooling.

Normal Temperature Regulation

Mammals are better adapted than other vertebrates to maintain body temperature within narrow limits. Dogs and cats keep their core temperatures constant within 2°C over a 24-hour period. The thermoregulatory reflex involves a complex sequence of sensory, integrating, and effector mechanisms to maintain proper energy needs.

Sensors. Peripheral neural thermoreceptors are located in the skin, whereas internal locations include the CNS (hypothalamus and spinal cord) and abdomen.

Integrator. The hypothalamus, which also contains neuronal networks that are sensitive to body temperature, receives incoming information from peripheral receptors by neural and humoral means. The thermoregulatory center is in the preoptic region of the rostral hypothalamus. This region is divided into a rostral (parasympathetic) heat loss center and a caudal (sympathetic) heat production center. The reciprocal interplay between heat loss and heat production is responsible for a final set point or accurate control of body temperature.

Effectors. Physiologic and behavioral modifications of the animal are the result of hypothalamic influences. The effector responses take advantage of heat loss and heat gain to ensure that body temperature is maintained at the set point. Body heat is lost to the environment through alterations in conduction, convection, and radiation. A major portion of heat loss occurs through the skin and can be affected by increased blood flow (vasodilation) and sweating. Respiratory heat loss through evaporation by panting is of greater importance in animals that do not sweat, such as the dog and cat.

Heat can be gained from the environment by heat transfer and also through normal metabolic processes. Increased metabolic heat production by endothermic animals primarily occurs through skeletal muscle contraction (shivering) and by catabolism of body fat.

Behavioral means of lowering body temperature include seeking shelter from sunlight and remaining inactive (Fig. 4–2A). Vasoconstriction, piloerection, and "curling up" are ways that an animal conserves body heat (Fig 4–2B).

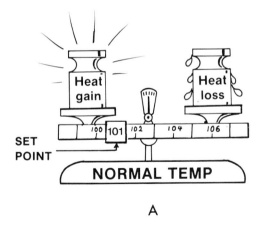

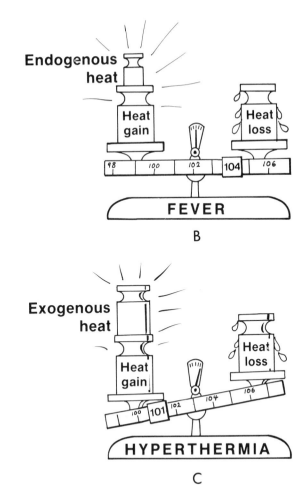

Figure 4–1. *A,* Temperature regulation in the normal animal showing a thermal set-point of 38.3°C (101°F) with balanced heat gain and heat loss mechanisms. *B,* Mechanism of fever involves a rise in set-point to 40°C (104°F), which increases endogenous heat production and conservation while maintaining a balance between heat gain and heat loss. *C,* Mechanism of hyperthermia, in contrast to that of fever, involves an increase in heat load on a normal set-point. Increased heat gain can be from exogenous (environmental) or endogenous (muscle activity) sources.

Influences on Body Temperature

Physiologic. Several physiologic influences may modify body temperature by altering the hypothalamic set point. Body temperature is not well controlled in neonates, presumably because of their ineffective hypothalamic regulation. Exercise increases body temperature as a result of increased muscular activity but never by more than several degrees. Body temperature usually rises above and then falls below normal postprandially, but the change is usually not greater than 0.5°C (1°F). Dehydration appears to be an important factor in increasing body temperature. That the temperature returns to normal after rehydration helps to differentiate the fever of dehydration from that of persistent infection. Body temperature may vary slightly throughout the estrous cycle. During the course of gestation it gradually increases, but it falls precipitously and transiently at parturition and then returns to normal.[1] Psychogenic influences on body temperature are frequently observed in excitable animals that are presented for examination in a veterinary hospital.

Pathologic. Increased body temperature is associated with disease processes that release or produce activators of fever (exoge-

Table 4–1. Causes of Hyperthermia

Increased metabolic rate
Hyperthyroidism
Increased muscle activity
Tetanus
Seizures
Hypertonic myopathies
Malignant hyperthermia
Decreased heat loss
Hot, enclosed space (car)
Occlusive cervical wraps
Laryngeal paralysis
Brachycephalic dogs and cats
Drug therapy
Phenothiazines
Anticholinergics

Table 4–2. Comparative Features of Fever and Hyperthermia

	FEVER	HYPERTHERMIA
Synonyms	Pyrexia	Heat illness, heat stroke
Mechanism	Altered hypothalamic set-point	Increased heat production, decreased heat loss, hypothalamic set-point maintained
Need of Therapy	Optional or debated	Mandatory
Therapy Used	Antiprostaglandins	External cooling

nous pyrogens), such as lipid A, a lipo-polysaccharide component (endotoxin) of the cell walls of gram-negative bacteria. These exogenous activators induce the synthesis of at least three endogenous pyrogens, interleukin 1, tumor necrosis factor (cachectin), and interferons. These cytokines are produced by immunologically active lymphocytes and bone marrow–derived cells, predominantly mononuclear phagocytes. The activated cells release pyrogens with infections (involving any type of microorganism), hypersensitivities, tissue necroses, or immune-mediated disorders.

The mechanism by which endogenous pyrogens reset the hypothalamic thermostat is uncertain because the blood-brain barrier is impermeable to them, although some evidence suggests that they selectively cross it in the region of the anterior hypothalamus

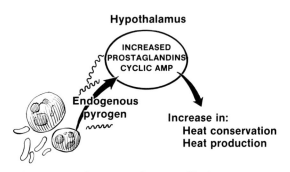

Figure 4–3. Pathogenesis of increased body temperature produced by an endogenous pyrogen.

(Fig. 4–3). Endogenous pyrogens stimulate the hypothalamus to raise the set point, making the animal feel cold. This effect induces physiologic and behavioral heat conservation and production mechanisms that raise the body temperature and maintain the febrile state (Fig. 4–4). Research suggests that endogenous pyrogen may increase the synthesis of prostaglandins, which act as intermediators between the protein pyrogen and the thermostatic set point. Injection of prostaglandins into the thermoregulatory centers in the CNS of the dog and cat can cause a rise in body temperature set point. Antipyretic drugs, such as aspirin, are also known to block prostaglandin synthesis and may reduce fever by this mechanism. Other experimental data indicate that increases in adenosine 3′,5′-monophosphate (cyclic AMP), norepinephrine, and the ratio of sodium to calcium concentration in the hypo-

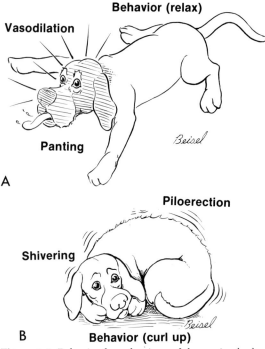

Figure 4–2. Behavioral mechanisms of decreasing body temperature *(A)* and increasing body temperature *(B).*

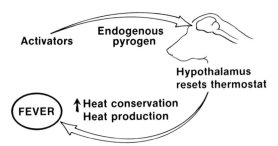

Figure 4–4. Hypothalamic regulation of body temperature in the febrile state.

thalamus can cause body temperatures to rise above physiologically normal ranges. These mechanisms are probably not involved in the pathogenesis of fever following experimental infection because in many cases, they require supraphysiologic concentrations or experimental modification.

Arginine vasopressin (AVP), a peptide synthesized in the hypothalamus, is most noted for its antidiuretic effects minimizing water loss. AVP concentrations in plasma increase during fever. AVP also stimulates lymphocyte proliferation, acts as corticotrophin-releasing factor, and acts centrally as a true antipyretic. AVP may be the substance that helps to regulate fever, preventing dangerous increases in body temperature.[2]

A number of other pathologic phenomena are associated with the febrile response. Fever is often accompanied by an elevated erythrocyte sedimentation rate because of increased synthesis of fibrinogen by the liver and globulin by plasma cells in response to inflammatory processes. The liver also makes a variety of other proteins, including haptoglobins, which bind hemoglobin; ceruloplasmin, which binds copper; and C-reactive protein. C-reactive protein binds to bacterial surfaces and fixes complement, thereby providing a rudimentary defense mechanism. Most of these proteins migrate as α-2 globulins, which can be detected on serum electrophoresis and which produce the acute phase reaction typified by an α-2 spike, often seen in acute inflammatory processes. Reduction in serum zinc and iron levels is a manipulation of the febrile response and is thought to be stimulated by the release of endogenous pyrogens by mononuclear phagocytes. Bacteria, which require iron for their survival, must compete for available iron, which decreases because of mononuclear phagocyte sequestration that occurs with the febrile state.[3]

FEVERS OF UNKNOWN ORIGIN

Fever of unknown origin (FUO) is the term used to describe the situation when the cause of a fever remains undetermined after 2 to 3 weeks of a thorough physical examination and associated laboratory tests. Infections probably account for at least 30% to 40% of the undiagnosed fevers encountered in clinical practice. Systemic infections such as tuberculosis, deep mycoses, and other chronic or latent infections may be difficult to diagnose during early stages (Table 4–3). Bacterial endocarditis or recurrent bacteremia from another localized focus may be hard to recognize. Localized abscesses or infections in various organs, such as the liver, pancreas, peritoneal and pleural cavities, lungs, meninges, joints, and genitourinary system, may be unrecognized for long periods because of the difficulty of assessing these areas with routine diagnostic methods.

Infectious disease is not the only cause of *persistent fever*. Noninfectious causes of fever include neoplastic and immune-mediated disorders (Table 4–4). Solid neoplasms may produce inflammation and necrosis of tissues with resultant fever. Hematopoietic neoplasias, such as lymphosarcoma, myeloproliferative disease, and plasma cell myeloma, are most likely to produce fever, probably as a result of their production of or induction of other cells to produce endogenous pyrogens. Diffuse metastatic neoplasia and carcinomas usually are also responsible. The most common sites of localized neoplasia that produce fever are the kidney, liver, gallbladder, bone, lungs, stomach, and lymph nodes. Neoplasms in the esophagus, jejunum, pancreas, colon, rectum, mammary glands, and genitourinary system are least likely to cause fever.

Immunologic disorders resulting in fever are most commonly the autoimmune or col-

Table 4–3. Systemic Infectious Diseases Commonly Associated with Fevers of Unknown Origin

VIRAL	Feline leukemia virus infection Feline infectious peritonitis Feline immunodeficiency virus infection
RICKETTSIAL	Rocky Mountain spotted fever Haemobartonellosis Ehrlichiosis
BACTERIAL	Bacterial endocarditis Mycobacterial infection Leptospirosis Borreliosis
FUNGAL	Histoplasmosis Coccidioidomycosis Blastomycosis
PROTOZOAL	Toxoplasmosis Babesiosis Leishmaniasis
METAZOAN	*Dirofilaria immitis* Ectopic migrations

Table 4–4. Noninfectious Diseases Commonly Associated with Undiagnosed Fever

NEOPLASIA	
Diffuse	Hematopoietic disorders (lymphoma, myeloproliferative disorders, plasma cell disorders) Metastatic disease (various types) Carcinomas (various types)
Localized	Common: kidney, liver, gallbladder, bone, lungs, stomach, lymph nodes Uncommon: brain, esophagus, jejunum, pancreas, colon, rectum, mammary gland
AUTOIMMUNE DISEASES	Collagen disorders Systemic lupus erythematosus Chronic autoimmunity: joints, glomeruli, platelets, erythrocytes, etc. Vasculitis
MISCELLANEOUS	Hepatic cirrhosis Immunodeficiency diseases Hyperlipemia Pulmonary embolism Hypersensitivity disorders Granulomatous diseases Thrombophlebitis Infarctions
CNS DISORDERS	Brain tumors Diencephalic lesions Heavy metal intoxication

lagen diseases. Fever in systemic lupus erythematosus may be due to immunosuppression or tissue necrosis and injury as a result of the disease or as a reaction to drug therapy.

Other mechanisms of fever production include increased metabolic activity that occurs in diseases such as hyperthyroidism. Intracranial lesions from trauma, neoplasia, or inflammation may alter body temperature by directly interfering with the hypothalamic thermoregulatory mechanisms. Many drugs are known to interfere with temperature regulation on a central or peripheral basis. Drug-induced fevers are usually continuous and persistent and resolve only when therapy is discontinued. Paradoxically, salicylates, which are known to interfere with the genesis of fever, may produce fever when given in high doses.

ASSOCIATED CLINICAL FINDINGS

Fever has both beneficial and adverse effects (Table 4–5). The advantages are primarily the favorable effects that higher body temperature has on the immunologic response. Body temperature elevation is deleterious to certain viruses, bacteria, and protozoa, including polioviruses, herpesviruses, pneumococci, gonococci, and *Leishmania*, and may indirectly be associated with host defense mechanisms.

Unfortunately, fever is commonly seen in combination with tachycardia, hyperpnea, and increased urine concentration. Experimentally, pyrogens initially cause increased thirst and water diuresis in dogs, resulting in polydipsia and polyuria.[4] Sustained fever is associated with a raised threshold in the thirst center in response to osmotic stimuli, with the result that affected animals stop drinking water and are frequently severely dehydrated. More severe and protracted fevers may result in vasomotor collapse with GI and neurologic disturbances.

Fever has been classified on the basis of characteristic patterns of correlation observed with certain disease syndromes in humans. Such correlation, which may be biased by the frequency of fever measurement in humans, is not well established in the dog and cat. As a rule, it is helpful to distinguish between acute self-limiting fever and chronic sustained or intermittent fever.

DIAGNOSIS

Physical Examination

A detailed history is paramount in the workup of a febrile patient. Age is an important consideration with respect to neoplastic disease. Prior clinical signs and infectious diseases, as well as vaccination

Table 4–5. Consequences of Fever

BENEFITS	ADVERSE EFFECTS
Impairs microorganism Decreased serum iron Suppresses bacterial replication	CNS toxicity Mental depression Precipitates seizures Enhances brain injury
Facilitates host defenses Lysosomes more efficient Lymphocyte stimulation accelerated Interferon production increased Phagocytes more efficient	Metabolic alterations Dehydration Hemoconcentration Increased metabolic rate Reduced appetite Stresses cardiac reserve

histories, should be determined. The home environment and travels of the patient should be ascertained. The presence of abnormal body discharges or secretions is important.

Physical examination should be thorough, since many causes of FUO may be missed because of inadequate detection of a disease process. Areas often overlooked during physical examination are the oral cavity, ocular fundi, ears, nose, posterior nasopharynx, deep neck region, thoracic and abdominal cavities, lymph nodes, muscles, and joints. Care should be taken to palpate the abdominal organs, including the liver, spleen, and lymph nodes, to determine their size. The umbilicus should be examined in young patients. Rectal examination is essential in mature breeding animals of both sexes. A neurologic examination may be indicated by a history of locomotor abnormalities.

Laboratory Testing

This becomes of utmost importance in the evaluation of unexplained fever. Routine hematologic tests, including CBC and platelet count, plus a biochemical profile and a urinalysis should be the initial noninvasive laboratory evaluations of the chronically febrile patient. A discussion of the hematologic and biochemical findings expected in particular infectious disorders appears under the heading Clinical Laboratory Findings in each chapter.

Thoracic radiography should be performed when clinical signs or physical examination indicates cardiac and pulmonary involvement. It can be argued that diagnostic radiologic techniques should be routine in the workup of a patient with FUO. Sometimes lesions not found by palpation and auscultation of the thorax may be detected radiographically. Radiography can be used to evaluate bone lesions that are difficult to assess on physical examination. Specialized radiographic contrast procedures may be required to outline the genitourinary and GI systems. Other involved procedures such as scanning and ultrasonography may be available at referral centers.

The most common cause of an FUO is an infectious process. Bacteriologic and fungal cultures may be necessary to determine the presence of infection and to identify the organism. Bacteremia or bacterial endocarditis can be confirmed only by repeated sterile blood collection. Blood culture results may be negative if anaerobic organisms are not specifically cultured or if the disease process involves the right heart valves (see Diagnosis, Chapter 7). In the absence of positive blood culture results, organisms may be isolated from sterilely collected urine, joint and cerebrospinal fluids, and bone marrow of bacteremic patients. Findings of culture of the throat, sputum, feces, and wounds will be significant only if known pathogens are isolated. Lymph node aspirates or percutaneous biopsy specimens of liver, spleen, and muscle may be cultured when organ localization of disease is suspected. Special care should be taken in the laboratory with cultures from animals with chronic febrile diseases because of the difficulty in isolating certain facultative intracellular parasites.

Serologic titers may be obtained when a specific pathogen is suspected on the basis of history or clinical signs. Each antibody determination has diagnostic limitations as outlined in subsequent chapters; false-positive results are usually more common than false-negative results. Measurement of specific antibody classes, such as IgM, or detection of antigenic components of the organism in serum has improved reliability of some serologic tests. Rising titers are usually required to confirm infection unless certain persistent intracellular pathogens such as *Brucella*, *Ehrlichia*, *Babesia*, or *Leishmania* are suspected. A rising titer (fourfold) is usually required to confirm active infection in toxoplasmosis, feline infectious peritonitis, leptospirosis, and most systemic mycoses. Testing for the presence of specific viruses, such as feline leukemia virus, may be performed by immunodiagnostic methods.

Immunologic testing may confirm the presence of underlying autoimmune or hypersensitivity disease as the cause of the persistent fever. Antinuclear antibody, rheumatoid factor, and Coombs' tests may be performed.

Biopsy should be made of any tissue in which suspicious lesions are found. Endoscopes can be used for visual inspection and collection of tissues or fluids. Exploratory laparotomy has been advocated as a last resort to determine the cause of chronic FUOs in humans. The advisability of this

Table 4–6. Commonly Used Antipyretic Drugs

SALICYLATES	Acetylsalicylic acid (aspirin)
PARA-AMINOPHENOLS	Acetophenetidin Acetaminophen
INDENES	Indomethacin
PYRAZOLINE DERIVATIVES	Phenylbutazone Dipyrone

procedure in animals in the absence of clinical or laboratory abnormalities that suggest abdominal involvement is questionable. Culture or biopsy of various tissues and organ fluids may be performed at the time of surgery. More recently, less invasive biopsy and cytologic examinations have been performed with fiberoptic endoscopic equipment. Previously unreachable sites, such as lumina of the nasopharynx, trachea, bronchi, esophagus, stomach, small and large intestines, urinary bladder, and pleural and peritoneal cavities, can now be evaluated by this relatively noninvasive procedure.

THERAPY

Appropriate treatment requires that fever (normally a beneficial response of the body) be distinguished from hyperthermia (which is usually detrimental). Unlike the procedure with hyperthermia, it is not always desirable to normalize the body temperature of the patient with fever.

Antipyretics

The indiscriminate or routine administration of antipyretic agents for the treatment of fever should be avoided because as a primary mode of management, this may interfere with the clinician's ability to follow the course or determine the cause of the underlying illness. Antipyretics should be avoided initially so that the severity of fever can be used to monitor the response of the disease to primary modes of therapy, such as antimicrobial or anti-inflammatory drugs.

The antipyretics are divided into several groups on the basis of chemical structure (Table 4–6). With appropriate use, salicylates are probably the most desirable and safest of the analgesic-antipyretic drugs. It is irrational to use them in combination with drugs such as phenylbutazone, dipyrone, and acetaminophen because of similarities in mode of action.

Although antipyretics are not indicated in the primary management of fever, they should be used if the temperature rises higher than 41.6°C (107°F) because of potential damage to the brain and other organs. Damage is more likely to be caused by exogenously induced hyperthermia (e.g., heat stroke and malignant hyperthermia), in which, unlike fever, the body thermostat is not under control. Antipyretics should be used in cases of increasing body temperature only when other means of reducing it have been ineffective.

Aspirin (acetylsalicylic acid) is probably the drug of choice for antipyretic therapy. The dosages of antipyretics for dogs and cats are listed in Table 4–7. Higher (25 mg/kg/day) dosages have been used safely in both species[5] but tend to be associated with an increased prevalence of GI irritation and ulceration. This problem can be partially overcome by dividing the daily dose into several treatments, by administering the drug with food, or by using buffered aspirin or buffering compounds. However, the last measure may interfere with absorption and efficacy. Not all aspirin compounds are equally effective. Crushable formulations of aspirin are more absorbable and more effective antiprostaglandin compounds. Other

Table 4–7. Recommended Dosages of Antipyretic Drugs[a]

DRUG	SPECIES	DOSE[b] (mg/kg)	ROUTE	INTERVAL (hours)	DURATION (days)
Aspirin	D	4	PO	8–24	prn[c]
	C	10	PO	12–48	prn[c]
Dipyrone	D	500–2500 mg total	IM, IV, SC	24	prn[c]
	C	125 mg total	IM, IV, SC	12–24	prn[c]

[a]D = dog, C = cat, PO = oral, IM = intramuscular, IV = intravenous, SC = subcutaneous, prn = as needed.
[b]Dose per administration at specified interval, expressed as mg/kg unless otherwise stated.
[c]GI ulceration with hemorrhage is a side effect. Hematocrit should be monitored every 3 to 5 days.

drugs, such as acetaminophen, have increased toxicity and can cause methemoglobinemia and Heinz's body formation (especially in cats); they are also more expensive than aspirin. Even when given parenterally, phenylbutazone has a tendency to cause significant GI ulceration in dogs and cats. Indomethacin should be avoided because of its known hepatotoxicity and propensity to cause fatal GI ulceration in some dogs.

Antibiotics

Fever should not be the sole justification for antimicrobial therapy. Antibiotics are useful only when a bacterial infection is the cause of the febrile response. Antibiotics may be given in an attempt to make a therapeutic or empirical diagnosis in a febrile patient, but they should never be given for longer than 1 to 2 weeks if a favorable response is not noted. If beneficial results occur, antibiotics may be continued for 4 weeks longer. Some experimental evidence

has indicated that for some antibiotics, a greater antibacterial effect or higher plasma or tissue concentration is noted at higher body temperatures.[6] For this reason, fevers should not be routinely lowered with concurrent antipyretic therapy when antimicrobial therapy is given.

References

1. Tsutsui T, Murata Y: Variations in body temperature in the late stage of pregnancy and parturition in bitches. *Jpn J Vet Sci* 44:571–576, 1982.
2. Kasting NW, Veale WL, Cooper KE: Vasopressin: a homeostatic effector in the febrile process. *Neurosci Biobehav Rev* 6:215–222, 1982.
3. Kluger MJ, Rothenberg BA: Fever and reduced iron: their interaction as a host defense response to bacterial infection. *Science* 203:374–376, 1979.
4. Szczepanska-Sadowska E, Sobocinska J, Kozlowski S: Thirst and renal excretion of water and electrolytes during pyrogen fever in dogs. *Arch Int Physiol Biochim* 87:673–686, 1979.
5. Yeary RA, Swanson W: Aspirin dosages for the cat. *J Am Vet Med Assoc* 163:1177–1178, 1973.
6. Riffat S, Nawaz M, Rehman ZU: Pharmacokinetics of sulphadimidine in normal and febrile dogs. *J Vet Pharmacol Ther* 5:131–135, 1982.

5 INTEGUMENTARY INFECTIONS

Bacterial Infections of the Skin

Peter J. Ihrke

Pyoderma is defined as a pyogenic or pus-producing bacterial infection of the skin. Despite this straightforward definition, misdiagnosis and therapeutic mismanagement of bacterial skin infections are common. Misdiagnosis may be linked to the diversity of clinical manifestations from animal to animal in various sites and at different times in the course of the disease. Pus is often not grossly visible. Both the primary and secondary skin lesions seen with pyodermas are also shared with many unrelated diseases. In addition, bacterial infections of the skin occur as secondary infections or coexist with other skin diseases. This diversity makes the proper diagnosis and management of pyodermas one of the consistent challenges in dermatology.[1–3]

Pyodermas are the second most common cause of skin disease in the dog. Only flea allergy dermatitis occurs more frequently.[4] In contrast, pyodermas are an uncommon cause of skin disease in people and in cats and other domestic animals. Besides subcutaneous abscesses from bite wounds, all other forms of bacterial skin disease are rare in the cat. The reasons for the increased frequency of bacterial skin disease in the dog in comparison with other mammalian species studied are unknown. *Staphylococcus intermedius,* a gram-positive, coagulase-positive coccus, is the primary canine bacterial skin pathogen.[5–7] This bacterium is a distinct species from *S. aureus,* the primary human skin pathogen.[8]

Although pyodermas are rare in the cat, bacterial abscesses and cellulitis secondary to cat bites are the most common feline skin diseases. *Pasteurella multocida,* a normal resident of the mouth of the cat, is the primary pathogen.[9] *P. multocida* is also a human pathogen and may cause cellulitis, abscesses, osteomyelitis, septic arthritis, septicemia, and meningitis. Reported cases of human *P. multocida* infection are generally associated with feline bite wounds (see Chapter 58). However, it should be kept in mind that pus from a feline abscess is an additional potential source of infection for people.

ETIOLOGY AND PATHOGENESIS

Normal Microflora of the Skin and Hair

The microbial flora of the skin is composed of both resident and transient bacteria. Resident bacteria are able to multiply on the skin surface and in hair follicles and are usually harmless. Transient bacteria presumably seed the skin from the mucous membranes and the environment and under normal circumstances cannot effectively compete with the established resident flora to secure an ecologic niche. Coagulase-negative micrococci, α-hemolytic streptococci, and occasional diphtheroids and clostridia are the major resident bacteria on canine skin.[10] Similar bacteria have been reported to reside on cat skin; however, fewer quantitative studies have been performed.[9] Coagulase-positive staphylococci such as *S. intermedius* and *S. aureus* have been identified as transients on canine and feline skin. In addition, *Pseudomonas* sp., *Proteus* sp., and *Corynebacterium* sp. have been isolated.[3] Controversy exists as to whether coagulase-positive staphylococci are part of the normal cutaneous flora of the dog.[11] This author believes that coagulase-positive staphylococci are found infrequently on normal dog skin and should thus be considered as transients. Somewhat paradoxically, coagulase-positive staphylococci are consistently present in 90% of normal canine hair coats.[12] Consequently, a ready population of potential pathogens is available for colonization of susceptible skin.

Microbial Alterations with Skin Disease

It has long been observed clinically that pyodermas are seen secondary to other skin diseases. Coagulase-positive staphylococci may be cultured in large numbers from dogs with keratinization defects.[10] The cultures taken from dermatitic skin in perilesional areas also indicate staphylococcal overgrowth.[13] These data imply that a conversion occurs in the bacterial flora in dogs with other skin disease such that pathogenic *S. intermedius* becomes the predominant organism cultured. Thus, dogs with various primary skin diseases may be at increased risk for the development of secondary pyodermas. A similar microfloral conversion occurs in people with atopic dermatitis.

Pure cultures of coagulase-positive *S. intermedius* are isolated from most pustules or draining tracts in dogs with pyoderma. Consequently, *S. intermedius* is regarded as the primary bacterial pathogen of canine skin. Almost without exception, when gram-negative bacteria such as *Proteus* sp., *Pseudomonas* sp., or *Escherichia coli* are cultured from a pyoderma, they are grown in conjunction with *S. intermedius* from an open lesion. If gram-negative bacteria are isolated from a pyoderma without concomitant isolation of *S. intermedius*, the technique used and the results obtained should be questioned. Infection with *S. intermedius* creates a tissue milieu that is conducive to secondary gram-negative bacterial invasion.

Various protein products and toxins are elaborated by strains of staphylococci and relate to the degree of pathogenicity in people. Similar data have not been elucidated for canine staphylococcal infections, underscoring the frequent inability to predict the course of bacterial skin disease in the dog. Protein A, identified in canine staphylococci,[14] is a protein that can prevent specific antibody access, prematurely trigger the complement cascade, and act as a chemoattractant for neutrophils (see also Chapter 57). Protein A is known to be responsible for much of the inflammatory response to staphylococci in people. The role of protein A in the pathogenesis of canine pyoderma is unknown. Leukocidin, hemolysins, epidermolytic toxin, and other soluble products may be important in the host response to pyoderma.[15] A hypersensitivity to staphylococcal antigens may promote the penetration of staphylococcal antigens by affecting epidermal permeability barriers.[16]

P. multocida is the most common bacterial isolate from feline abscesses and cellulitis. Occasionally, β-hemolytic streptococci, *Bacteroides* sp., and fusiform bacilli may be isolated.[9] On the rare occasions when coagulase-positive staphylococci are implicated in the pathogenesis of feline skin disease, *S. aureus* has been isolated most commonly.[6, 17]

Factors leading to the initiation of pyoderma are obscure. Preexisting diseases such as ectoparasitism, keratinization defects, allergy, and endocrinopathies (hypothyroidism and Cushing's disease) predispose to secondary pyodermas. In addition, poor grooming, pruritus, inflammation from any cause, and the injudicious use of glucocorticoids may be contributory.

Once pyoderma has been initiated, immunologic incompetence, coexisting disease, pruritus, severe inflammation, and improper initial therapy are all negative prognostic factors. Pruritus and severe inflammation are often hallmarks of frustrating recurrent pyodermas.

Classification of Pyodermas

Much has been published concerning the classification of pyodermas.[2, 3, 18, 19] The current schemes, based on depth of involvement in the skin, are most useful clinically since the deeper the level of inflammation, the more likely underlying causes will be present and the more aggressive the clinician must be, both diagnostically and therapeutically. Using depth of involvement as a criterion for classification, pyodermas may be subdivided as surface, superficial, and deep (Table 5–1). Detailed clinical descriptions of specific subgroups are available elsewhere.[2, 3, 20, 20a, 20b] Bacteria causing mycobacterial diseases and subcutaneous abscesses are discussed elsewhere (Chapters 51, 53, and 55).

Other classification schemes have been based on anatomic site of infection (pressure-point pyoderma), causative agent (staphylococcal pyoderma), or on primary versus secondary infection. As our knowledge increases, more pyodermas are viewed as secondary to other causes.

Surface Pyoderma. Although pathogenic bacteria (predominantly S. *intermedius*) can be cultured from superficial skin lesions, bacterial involvement is probably secondary. Acute, moist dermatitis and intertrigo are classified as surface pyodermas. *Acute, moist dermatitis* develops as a sequela to self-trauma and allergic disease. Flea allergy dermatitis is the most common underlying cause. *Intertrigo* is seen in conjunction with poor drainage and maceration at sites of skin folding. Surface pyodermas rarely are diagnostic or therapeutic problems and constitute a minority of the cases of skin disease classified as pyodermas.

Superficial Pyoderma. Superficial pyodermas are the most common bacterial skin diseases in dogs and are among the most common canine dermatoses. Lesions may be nonfollicular *(impetigo)* or follicular *(folliculitis)* and often are diagnostic challenges. Severe inflammation or intense pruritus indicates an inappropriate host response. The terms *bacterial hypersensitivity* and *pruritic superficial pyoderma* have been used to describe this confusing syndrome. Recurrence is common, and long-term management may be difficult.

Deep Pyoderma. Most deep pyodermas begin as a superficial folliculitis. Follicular rupture may lead to a granulomatous tissue response. Deep pyodermas are much less common than superficial pyodermas. Diagnosis may be less difficult than with superficial pyodermas, but therapy is often problematic.

CLINICAL FINDINGS

Dermatology has a singular advantage over most other specialty areas in medicine in that skin lesions are visible and available for careful inspection. Excellent lighting is essential for a proper physical examination. A lighted hand lens is beneficial. Frequently, clinical findings can be clarified by clipping the overlying hair from an affected area.

Primary Skin Lesions

An erythematous papule is the most common primary skin lesion seen in most superficial and some deep pyodermas. Papules are circumscribed solid elevations of the skin and usually are formed in groups. As infection proceeds, pus accumulates in an intraepidermal or follicular location to form a pustule. Small pustules may appear as papules to the naked eye. Intact pustules are often transient in canine skin. If pustules rupture on the surface, crusted papules are seen. In deep pyodermas, follicular rupture exacerbates inflammation in the adjacent dermis, resulting in a nodule or furuncle. Surface rupture of these deeper lesions may lead to fistulous tracts.

Table 5–1. Classification of Bacterial Infection of the Skin Based on Depth of Infection

SURFACE PYODERMA
  Acute moist dermatitis (pyotraumatic dermatitis, hot spots)
  Intertrigo (skinfold pyoderma): lipfold pyoderma, facial-fold pyoderma, vulvar fold pyoderma, tailfold pyoderma, obesity fold pyoderma

SUPERFICIAL PYODERMA
  Impetigo (puppy pyoderma)
  Superficial folliculitis
  Pruritic superficial pyoderma (bacterial hypersensitivity)

DEEP PYODERMA
  Deep folliculitis and furunculosis: muzzle folliculitis and furunculosis (canine acne), nasal pyoderma, interdigital pyoderma, pressure-point pyoderma, generalized deep pyoderma
  Cellulitis
  Mycobacterial infections: cutaneous tuberculosis, feline leprosy, cutaneous atypical mycobacteriosis

SUBCUTANEOUS ABSCESSES
  Feline abscess and cellulitis
  Actinomycosis
  Nocardiosis

DISEASES FORMERLY CLASSIFIED AS PYODERMAS
  "Juvenile pyoderma" (puppy strangles, juvenile cellulitis)
  Hidradenitis suppurativa (probably bullous pemphigoid or dermatomyositis)

Secondary Skin Lesions

Pustules can rupture spontaneously or be obliterated by self-trauma. Consequently, ruptured pustules become crusted papules. At that point, they may be indistinguishable from papules seen with other skin diseases. If crusted papules are grouped, crusts composed of dried pus, exudate, and keratin debris may form. Intense focal inflammation may foster a peripheral, expanding ring of peeling keratin termed a collarette. *Pruritic superficial pyoderma* or *bacterial hypersensitivity* are terms that have been used for this syndrome despite variable pruritus and a lack of proof of hypersensitivity. Self-traumatic excoriations may lead to the formation of erosions and ulcers.

Alopecia can be seen secondary to pyoderma. Hair fragments are shed from infected follicles. In addition, transient patchy alopecia can be secondary to localized telogen effluvium and possibly telogen arrest in a normally mosaic, asynchronous hair replacement pattern. Permanent, scarring alopecia secondary to folliculitis is uncommon, in contrast with the condition in people.

Distribution of Lesions

Acute moist dermatitis, usually secondary to flea allergy, is seen most commonly in the dorsal lumbosacral region. Intertrigo, or skinfold pyoderma, is seen at the specific site of the anatomic defect according to breed. Impetigo consists of noninflammatory nonfollicular pustules located primarily in the groin of prepubescent dogs. Superficial folliculitis is a pleomorphic subgrouping with crusted papules and pustules present in intertriginous zones such as the groin and axilla. Inflammation, alopecia, crusting, and pruritus are all variable and influence the character and the distribution of lesions. Folliculitis may be generalized on the thorax. The attendant patchy, partial alopecia with folliculitis is more distinctive in short-coated dogs. Improper use of glucocorticoids may contribute to the spread of pyoderma while paradoxically decreasing visible inflammation. Deep pyodermas often follow the distribution pattern of superficial pyodermas since they commonly occur as sequelae. A characteristic self-explanatory pattern is seen with interdigital, pressure-point, and nasal pyodermas. Since cellulitis is seen most commonly secondary to generalized demodicosis, the distribution follows that of the primary disease.

DIAGNOSIS

A discussion of the differential diagnosis of each subgrouping of pyoderma is beyond the scope of this chapter. Important differential diagnoses are listed in Table 5–2. For additional information, the reader is referred to textbooks of dermatology.[3, 19]

Certain diagnostic procedures help to document bacterial infections of the skin. The easiest and potentially most beneficial diagnostic test is an impression smear stained with a rapid stain such as Diff-Quik (Harleco, Gibbstown, NJ). Impression smears may be made of exudates from either intact pustules or draining fistulous tracts. Pres-

Table 5–2. Differential Diagnosis of Bacterial Infections of the Skin

SURFACE PYODERMA
Acute Moist Dermatitis
  Drug reactions, demodicosis, neoplasia—especially sweat gland adenocarcinoma and metastatic disease, early panniculitis, early vasculitis, candidiasis
Intertrigo
  Lipfold pyoderma: demodicosis, drug reactions, early pemphigus vulgaris, early bullous pemphigoid, "diabetic dermatopathy," candidiasis, localized pemphigus foliaceus
  Vulvar-fold pyoderma: urinary tract infection, bullous pemphigoid, drug reactions, pemphigus vulgaris, dermatomyositis

SUPERFICIAL PYODERMA
Impetigo
  Early flea allergy dermatitis, superficial folliculitis
Superficial Folliculitis
  Early flea allergy dermatitis, demodicosis, dermatophytosis, pemphigus foliaceus, seborrheic dermatitis, drug reaction, sarcoptic acariasis

DEEP PYODERMA
  Demodicosis, dermatophytosis, subcutaneous and deep mycoses, neoplasia—especially keratoacanthomas, panniculitis, vasculitis, drug reactions

MYCOBACTERIAL INFECTIONS
Cutaneous Tuberculosis
  Neoplasia, feline leprosy, other bacterial abscesses, subcutaneous and deep mycoses
Feline Leprosy
  Neoplasia, sporotrichosis, other subcutaneous and deep mycoses
Cutaneous Atypical Mycobacteriosis
  Sterile panniculitis, abscesses

SUBCUTANEOUS ABSCESSES
  Neoplasia, sterile panniculitis, pansteatitis

ence of both extracellular and intracellular cocci in the smear is supportive of a diagnosis of pyoderma. Bacterial culture and identification and antibiotic susceptibility testing have been overused in the management of superficial pyodermas and underused in deep pyodermas. In many circumstances, impression smears are sufficient, and the empirical choice of antibacterial agents is justified. Additional information on diagnostic bacteriology is available in Chapter 42.

Skin biopsy is a neglected but valuable procedure in the documentation of pyoderma.[21] The more often skin diseases are biopsied, the more frequently pyoderma is diagnosed, even when it is not suspected. Multiple representative specimens with an appropriate history should be submitted to a veterinary dermatopathologist.

There are no reliable diagnostic tests to determine immunocompetence. Gross information can be derived from a CBC and serum electrophoresis. An absolute neutrophilia with a lymphocyte count of at least 1000 to 1500 cells/μl should be seen in normal dogs with ongoing or recurrent pyoderma. A broad-based elevation in the serum electrophoretic pattern in the β and γ range should also be present. In vitro lymphocyte transformation assays and bactericidal tests are available, primarily as research tools.

THERAPY

The reader is referred to recent reviews for specific recommendations on the management of various subgroups of pyodermas.[1-3, 20] In general, systemic antibiotics are not needed in the treatment of most surface pyodermas. Correction of predisposing factors and topical therapy are usually sufficient.[20] Impetigo and muzzle folliculitis and furunculosis may require only topical therapy. Systemic antibiotic therapy is required for the successful management of most other superficial and deep pyodermas. Although choice and therapeutic regimens of antimicrobials may vary among clinicians, topical antibacterial or immunomodulatory therapy should be viewed as adjunctive.

Antibiotic Therapy

The basic principles of antibiotic therapy include the selection of an appropriate an-

tibiotic, the establishment of an optimum dosage, and the maintenance of that dosage for long enough to ensure cure rather than transient remission.[22]

Since pyodermas often require long-term therapy, narrow-spectrum antibiotics may be more appropriate theoretically, as they cause less alteration in GI flora. However, few problems are seen with the long-term use of broad-spectrum antibiotics. There is little clinical evidence that bactericidal agents are more effective than bacteriostatic agents in the management of uncomplicated superficial pyodermas. Bactericidal antibiotics are recommended in most deep pyodermas and in circumstances where immunosuppression is confirmed or suspected. An antibiotic with a known spectrum of activity directed against S. intermedius should be selected. Commonly, the elimination of S. intermedius is sufficient to achieve clinical cure since this species creates an environment favorable for the replication of other bacteria.

The choice of antibiotic may be empirical or may be based on the results of bacterial culture and susceptibility testing. Empirical therapy is justified since previous studies indicate probable efficacy.[23-26] Appropriate antibiotics are discussed in greater detail in various review articles.[3, 18, 19, 22]

Antibiotics effective in the management of pyodermas are listed in Table 5-3 and discussed below. Penicillin, ampicillin, amoxicillin, and tetracycline are poor choices owing to bacterial resistance.

Oxacillin, a β-lactamase–resistant penicillin, is an excellent antibiotic for canine pyodermas. Resistance and side effects are rare. Expense and administration three times daily are the only drawbacks. Food interferes with its absorption, so it should be given 1 hour before or after feeding. Other similar synthetic penicillins have given mixed results. Nafcillin may be similar in efficacy but cloxacillin and dicloxacillin have not been as effective as would be expected.

Erythromycin is an effective and inexpensive antibiotic for uncomplicated superficial pyodermas. However, vomiting is a common side effect. ***Lincomycin*** commonly shares cross-resistance with erythromycin. Although more expensive than erythromycin, it possesses the distinct advantages of twice daily administration and a lack of GI irritation.

Trimethoprim-sulfonamides are used ex-

Table 5–3. Antibiotics Useful in Canine Bacterial Skin Diseases[a]

DRUG	DOSE[b] (mg/kg)	ROUTE	INTERVAL (hr)	ASSESSMENT[c]
Narrow Spectrum				
Erythromycin	10–15	PO	8	Good inexpensive empirical choice; cross-resistance with lincomycin; causes vomiting
Lincomycin	22	PO	12	Good empirical choice, especially if owners away for long hours
Oxacillin	22	PO	8	Excellent choice if expense is no problem; food interferes with absorption
Broad Spectrum				
Chloramphenicol	44–66	PO	8	Bone marrow suppression, potential human toxicity; alters hepatic drug metabolism
Clavulanic acid–potentiated amoxicillin[d]	11–22	PO	8	Good choice, if expense is no problem; moisture-sensitive; in vitro efficacy not predictable in vivo
Trimethoprim-sulfonamides[e]	13	PO	12	Excellent empirical choice; watch for side effects
Cephalexin, cefadroxil	22	PO	12	Do not use empirically; save for unresponsive cases to limit bacterial resistance

[a]PO = oral.
[b]Dose per administration at specified interval, expressed as mg/kg unless otherwise stated.
[c]For additional information on these drugs, see Chapter 43.
[d]Based on amoxicillin fraction.
[e]Based on trimethoprim and sulfonamide dosage combined.

tensively for canine pyodermas. Advantages include economy and twice daily administration, facilitating owner compliance. Dosages of trimethoprim-sulfonamide in excess of 13.2 mg/kg based on combined dosages of both drugs given twice daily should be avoided since sulfonamide cystic urolithiasis may occur in as short a time as a 2-week period.[26a] Keratoconjunctivitis sicca is the most common side effect. A drug-induced immune hypersensitivity disorder affecting eyes and joints has been reported in Doberman pinschers (see Chapter 43)[27] and in other breeds. As a precaution, clinicians should instruct owners to stop the drug if signs such as lameness or ocular problems develop.

Clavulanic acid–potentiated amoxicillin is expensive but has minimal side effects and based on in vitro susceptibility testing, should be an excellent drug in the management of pyodermas. However, results have been disappointing, even at dosage levels higher than recommended by the manufacturer. Its susceptibility to inactivation by moisture necessitates dispensing the drug in foil strips.

Chloramphenicol has been used in the dog as an effective inexpensive drug despite reversible depression of liver microsomal enzymes and bone marrow suppression. Concerns about nonreversible, fatal aplastic anemias in people are warranted since limited human exposure can initiate this rare drug reaction. Consequently, chloramphenicol is no longer recommended.

Cephalexin and ***cefadroxil*** are expensive oral cephalosporin antibiotics given twice daily that have excellent activity against *S. intermedius*.[27a] However, since widespread abuse of cephalosporins has led to increased bacterial resistance, their use should be reserved for deep pyodermas or life-threatening disease. Side effects of these drugs are vomiting and diarrhea. More detailed information about each antibiotic is available in Chapter 43.

Bacterial culture and susceptibility testing should be performed when empirical therapy has been ineffective. In addition, culture is advisable if infections are deep, chronic, or caused by more than one species of bacteria. Antibiotics should be chosen based on proven efficacy as well as susceptibility testing. The same antibiotics that are good empirical choices are recommended based on culture and susceptibility testing results. If *Staphylococcus* is not isolated, reculture should be performed. In mixed infections, if all of the isolates are not susceptible to one antibiotic or if they share susceptibility only to a cephalosporin or aminoglycoside, then an antibiotic effective against staphylococci should be chosen.

Improper antibiotic dosage is a common reason for treatment failure. All dogs should be weighed accurately before dosages are computed. Dosage errors are seen most often with large dogs. Once a proper dosage has been established, antibiotics must be administered for long enough to ensure cure rather than transient remission. Most superficial pyodermas require at least 3 weeks of therapy, and therapy should be continued for 5 days beyond apparent clinical cure. For deep pyodermas, antibiotics should be continued for at least 2 weeks beyond apparent cure. Durations of therapy of 2 to 3 months are common.

Topical Therapy

Topical therapy is an important adjunct in the management of pyodermas used to aid in debridement, encourage drainage, and decrease pain and pruritus. Improvement in patient attitude and owner encouragement are additional benefits. Twice weekly antibacterial shampoos containing benzoyl peroxide or chlorhexidine are the most commonly employed topical therapy. Benzoyl peroxide shampoos may decrease recrudescence in susceptible dogs. Dogs with deep pyodermas require more aggressive topical therapy. After clipping, dogs with deep pyodermas benefit from daily antibacterial shampoos or twice daily whirlpools or soaks. Chlorhexidine or povidone-iodine is added to warm water in whirlpools or soaks. Whirlpools remain the least used but most beneficial topical therapy for deep pyodermas.

Immunomodulatory Therapy

Immunomodulatory therapy is controversial in veterinary dermatology. Since most clinicians use immunostimulatory drugs in conjunction with antibiotics and topical therapy, properly controlled blind studies are necessary to determine efficacy. Furthermore, immunodeficiency has been difficult to demonstrate in breeds, such as the Ger-

man shepherd, that are predisposed to pyoderma.[27b] Adjunctive immunomodulatory therapy may be attempted in dogs with confirmed or suspected defects of the immune system or in dogs with recurrent pyoderma.

Staphage lysate (Delmont Laboratories, Swarthmore, PA) is an immunomodulatory drug prepared for human use and consisting of bacteriophage-lysed S. aureus ultrafiltrate that is injected SC.[2, 3, 18] Staphage lysate contains potent bacterial antigens such as protein A that may stimulate cell-mediated immunity. Commonly a dose of 1 ml is injected SC weekly. One controlled study indicated efficacy when 0.5 ml was used twice weekly.[27c] Levamisole is given orally (2.5 mg/kg every other day) in the hope of altering lymphocyte and phagocyte function. Levamisole is probably less effective than Staphage lysate. Another controlled study has been performed with encouraging results using Propionobacterium acnes immunotherapy in treating dogs with chronic recurrent pyoderma.[27d]

Factors Complicating Management

Treatment failure and disease recurrence are associated with the lack of recognition of factors complicating management. Most antibiotic dosages for treatment of pyoderma are largely empirical, as little research has been done. Sequestered foci of infection impede antibiotic penetration in deep pyodermas, and keratin debris from ruptured hair follicles encourages foreign body granulomatous response. Antibiotics that require microbial replication for activity, such as penicillins, are less effective when necrotic tissue and obstructed drainage routes create conditions that are no longer favorable for bacterial multiplication. Consequently, higher dosages are warranted in the management of chronic deep pyodermas.

Concomitant problems such as demodicosis, keratinization defects, hypothyroidism, or steroid abuse may hinder successful management. Pruritus, either associated with a pyoderma or with an underlying pruritic disease, is an additional complicating factor. External factors such as owner compliance with therapeutic regimens, vomiting of drug, or drug inactivation must also be considered.

Assessment of Therapy

All dogs receiving systemic antibiotics for pyodermas should be reexamined in 7 to 10 days after therapy is initiated. If substantial improvement is not noted, the clinician should reevaluate therapy and review various factors that may be complicating management. The clinician must consider the possibility of unidentified underlying disease or misdiagnosis.

PUBLIC HEALTH CONSIDERATIONS

The documentation of S. intermedius as a separate and distinct species from S. aureus partially explains why humans with a normally functioning immune system do not seem to be at risk for becoming infected from canine skin or wound infections. Under usual circumstances, owners of dogs with staphylococcal pyodermas are not at risk of zoonotic infection. Alternatively, a dog with severe suppurating pyoderma would be of greater concern in a household with an immunosuppressed person.

However, in vitro transfer of R plasmid antibiotic resistance has been achieved between human and canine species of staphylococci.[28, 29] The antibiotic resistance transfer, which probably has occurred by a plasmid transfer via conjugation, does not persist in heterologous species of staphylococci. If the process of plasmid transfer between bacterial species occurs outside the laboratory, a potential increase in antibiotic resistance could emerge in the human and animal populations.

Otitis Externa   Craig Griffin

ETIOLOGY

Otitis externa results from any inflammation of the external ear canal. Numerous etiologic agents and predisposing factors have been associated with otitis externa in dogs and cats (Table 5-4).

Infectious agents are important contributors to otitis externa, and bacteria, yeasts, parasites, and viruses have all been incriminated.[30,31] In many cases, the actual role of the infectious organism as the primary cause of otitis externa has not been well established. Bacteria or the broad-based budding yeast Malassezia canis (previously Pityrosporon pachydermatis) may cause secondary infection in an ear canal predisposed to infection because of other underlying diseases or abnormalities.[30, 30a] Once established, the bacteria or M. canis may perpetuate otitis externa and contribute to chronic changes within the ear canal.[31] In other cases, the degree of otitis externa may be subclinical or not a significant enough problem to prompt the client to seek veterinary care until the ear becomes secondarily infected. The response to combination otic treatment may temporarily resolve the signs until another secondary infection occurs. To the clinician, the infectious agent falsely appears to be the main cause of the animal's problem.

Otic Microflora

The normal ear canal is colonized by a variety of microorganisms. Coagulase-positive S. intermedius can be isolated from up to 47.6% of normal ear canals[32, 33] but is the most common isolate in acute otitis externa. The other common organisms isolated in cases of otitis externa are Pseudomonas sp., Proteus mirabilis and β-hemolytic streptococci. These have been reported in less than 5% of normal ear canals[30, 31]; however, Pseudomonas sp. and P. mirabilis are the most common isolates from chronically diseased ears. Mixed infections usually are composed of S. intermedius in conjunction with a gram-negative rod. It is interesting to note that a greater percentage of sterile cultures are found in dogs with otitis externa than in normal dogs.[31, 32] In cats, P. multocida may also be isolated.

By combining cytologic evaluation with culture, the prevalence of the broad-based budding yeast M. canis in the normal dog ear has been reported to be 47% to 49%.[34, 35] Cytology is more sensitive and detects 15% to 22% of cases not found with culture.[36] In contrast, *M. canis* are cultured from 54% to 83% of the dogs with otitis externa.[30] Unfortunately, good quantitative studies have not yet been done to help determine the role of *M. canis* in canine otitis externa. At this time, it is probably most appropriate to consider *M. canis* a secondary invader contributing to or perpetuating inflammation in an already diseased ear canal.[30, 31] In cats, the relative importance of *M. canis* in disease is less certain than in dogs since 23% of normal cats and 19% of those with otitis externa have detectable yeasts by culture or cytology.[37]

The ear mite, *Otodectes cynotis*, is believed to be responsible for 5% to 10% of canine and 50% of feline cases of otitis externa.[30] Most animals develop a hypersensitivity reaction to the mite that causes the inflammation seen clinically[38]; however, some are asymptomatic carriers.[39, 40] In others, the inflammation may lead to a secondary bacterial or yeast infection. The secondary infection or possibly the hypersensitivity reaction can eventually result in the destruction of the mites. This means that the reported incidences of *Otodectes*-induced otitis that are based on demonstration of the mite are probably very low.

Viruses are a known cause of otitis externa in people. In dogs, otitis externa has been reported with canine distemper infections.

Predisposing Factors

Most microbial infections of the external ear canal are secondary to another disease or factor making the ear canal susceptible to normal or opportunistic microflora. In the author's experience, the most common predisposing diseases are keratinization disorders, atopy, *O. cynotis* hypersensitivity, and endocrinopathies. Other factors associated with otitis externa are listed in Table 5–4. Of special interest, any narrowing or obstruction of the canal by anatomic abnormalities or masses seen in such breeds as the shar pei dog will also predispose to otitis externa.

CLINICAL FINDINGS

Pruritus and a foul discharge or odor are the two major reasons clients present their pets with otitis externa. Pruritus of the ear

Table 5–4. Diseases and Factors Associated with Otitis Externa in the Dog and Cat

INFECTIONS
  Bacteria (*S. intermedius*, β-hemolytic streptococci, *Pseudomonas* sp. and *Proteus mirabilis*), yeasts, fungi, viruses, metazoal parasites (mites)

FOREIGN BODIES
  Foxtails, plant debris, dried exudates, microscopic secondary foreign bodies

ALLERGIC DERMATOSES
  Atopy, food or contact allergies

ENDOCRINOPATHIES
  Hypothyroidism, sex hormone imbalance

KERATINIZATION DISORDERS
  Primary seborrhea, secondary metabolic seborrhea, vitamin A–responsive dermatosis, sebaceous adenitis

CONFORMATIONAL/STRUCTURAL
  Stenotic ear canals, polyps, hairy ear canals

IMMUNE MEDIATED
  Pemphigus foliaceus, lupus erythematosus

NEOPLASIA
  Ceruminous gland tumors, squamous cell carcinoma

OTITIS MEDIA

MISCELLANEOUS
  Water maceration, juvenile cellulitis, systemic debilitating diseases

canal and pinna is manifest by head shaking, scratching, or rubbing the ears along the floor or other objects. Evidence of pruritus on the physical examination will be pinnal or caudal auricular alopecia, hair mats, broken hairs, excoriations, and occasional areas of acute moist dermatitis. In many uncomplicated cases of allergic otitis externa, the clinical findings will be limited to erythema and possibly slight increase in ear wax.

When otitis externa is complicated by secondary bacterial or yeast infections, the character and amount of discharge may become more purulent and moist and may develop a foul odor. Inflammation may be severe, and the ear canals may become painful. Some animals become head shy, others will show evidence of pain only when the canal is palpated.

DIAGNOSIS

The differential diagnosis of otitis externa is extensive (see Table 5–4). It is essential that the clinician take a complete history and perform physical and otoscopic examinations to reveal other evidence of allergy or other disorders that the client did not recognize or consider significant. A thorough examination of the ear, utilizing an otoscope, is needed to determine the presence of secondary changes and the extent of the inflammation and discharge, as well as the condition of the tympanic membrane.

Smears of ear canal contents are among the most useful diagnostic tools available to the clinician. Properly prepared smears help to determine the presence, as well as the roles, of bacteria and yeast in the disease. When secondary bacterial infections are contributing to the disease, leukocytes and phagocytized bacteria are usually present. When primarily wax and keratin are present, the bacteria that may be seen are most likely incidental but can still contribute to the odor and inflammation by their lipolytic action on the waxy debris.

The slide should be heat-fixed by carefully passing it over an open flame two or three times prior to staining. Heat fixing melts some wax and debris, which causes them to adhere better to the glass slide. Without heat fixing, much of the wax, lipid, and the associated yeasts may wash away in the staining process. Greater than ten yeasts per high power field are suggestive of yeast overgrowth.[31]

Occasionally, *O. cynotis* or *Demodex* sp. can be diagnosed by examination of a smear. It is important to remember that failure to find mites, especially if secondary infection is present, does not rule out their existence.

Bacterial culture and susceptibility testing are useful when the tympanic membrane is ruptured and the clinician feels systemic antibiotic therapy is warranted. Culture and susceptibility testing also are indicated in chronic otitis externa when primarily rods are found on a smear.

THERAPY

Effective treatment and management of otitis externa is best achieved by combining several principles. If possible, a definitive diagnosis should be made and specific therapy for that disease should be prescribed. Predisposing factors should be eliminated or prophylactically treated. Topical therapy is especially beneficial. Systemic antibacterial or antifungal therapy may be needed when otitis media is present. Ear canals should be cleaned and dried prior to initiating therapy. Cleaning the ear canals is frequently

needed just to complete the otoscopic examination and to determine the integrity of the tympanic membrane. Thorough cleansing of the ear canals will remove small secondary foreign bodies as well as degenerated inflammatory cells, free fatty acids, bacterial toxins, wax, and debris. In most cases, ceruminolytic agents, such as carbamide peroxide and dioctyl sodium sulfosuccinate, are most effective in emulsifying and facilitating the cleansing procedures. Once the ear canals are cleaned, topical medications can be properly applied. These products must be used with great caution if the tympanum is ruptured. If they are used, thorough rinsing with pure water is preferred. Other rinse solutions should not contain detergents or disinfectants, as they are ototoxic and are also contraindicated with a ruptured tympanic membrane.[41]

Rubber-bulb ear syringes are a very efficient way to flush the ear. Following the initial flushing, loops can be utilized to remove any remaining material. In other cases, especially those with a ruptured tympanum, a feeding tube attached to a 12-ml syringe may be used for the final flushing as well as cleaning out the bulla. In addition, this is a rapid, atraumatic way of removing residual water.

Once the ears are clean, topical therapy can be effectively utilized in the treatment plan. In general, most ear products contain various combinations of glucocorticoids, antibacterial, antiyeast, and parasiticidal agents in aqueous solution or oil vehicles. Oil vehicles are best when the ears are dry, as they will tend to moisturize the skin. In moist exudative ears, water-soluble vehicles are preferred because they are less occlusive. Besides selecting the most appropriate vehicle, the clinician must decide what active ingredients are most appropriate for each case. There is no single perfect topical ear product.

In general, glucocorticoids should be used when there is inflammation, and most commercial otic medications are so formulated. Recent studies have shown that otic preparations with dexamethasone and triamcinolone have systemic effects and result in iatrogenic adrenal suppression with signs of hyperadrenocorticism.[42, 43] With long-term therapy, the glucocorticoids used should be of as low a potency as possible.

Bacterial infections should be treated with topical antibiotics or disinfectants. In general, the aminoglycosides (neomycin, polymyxin, gentamicin), as well as chloramphenicol, are frequently effective. However, aminoglycosides are potentially ototoxic, especially when topical application is used and when the ear drum is ruptured (see Aminoglycosides, Chapter 43). Optimally, drugs that may later be needed for systemic therapy should not be used topically in acute cases, as resistance may develop. Disinfectants are an effective alternative to antibiotics. Iodine and chlorhexidine are good choices but again are ototoxic when put into the middle ear. Acetic acid at 2% is effective against *Pseudomonas* sp. and at 5% is cidal against most bacterial pathogens involved in otitis externa. Tris-EDTA preparations are also effective against *Pseudomonas* (see Topical Buffered EDTA Solution, Chapter 43).

When *M. canis* is present, the antiyeast agents such as nystatin and thiabendazole frequently are effective. In more difficult cases, 1% miconazole lotion will usually work. If a *Malassezia* otitis media is diagnosed, then the systemic antifungal ketoconazole given 10 mg/kg every 12 hours for 4 to 6 weeks is the preferred treatment (see Topical Antifungals, Chapter 63).

O. cynotis is relatively sensitive to most insecticides, including pyrethrins, rotenone, and thiabendazole. In addition to the ears, the whole body and other in-contact animals should be treated. Ivermectin at 250 μg/kg is effective against *Otodectes*. It also has the advantage of effectively eliminating mites from other areas as well. However, ivermectin is not approved for use in cats or dogs at this dosage. It is absolutely contraindicated in collies.

Many products are available that combine a variety of ingredients and effects. The clinician should become familiar with several products that are appropriate for each type of infectious agent. The most appropriate topical drug can then be prescribed based on the clinical findings, cytology, and diagnosis.

The prognosis is generally good in acute (<4 weeks' duration) cases of otitis externa when the tympanic membrane is intact. Early control of the disease is important to prevent secondary changes.

A guarded-to-good prognosis is indicated in chronic cases. Whenever the tympanic membrane is ruptured, otitis media will be present, and the prognosis becomes guarded with medical therapy alone. When second-ary changes have progressed to marked fibrosis with narrowing of the lumen or bulla, surgical intervention may be required. In cases that have calcified ear canals, surgery will be necessary to achieve good results.

References

1. Ihrke PJ: An overview of bacterial skin disease in the dog. *Br Vet J* 433:112–118, 1987.
2. White SD, Ihrke PJ: Pyoderma. *In* Nesbitt GH (ed): *Dermatology—Contemporary Issues in Small Animal Practice.* New York, Churchill Livingstone, 1987, pp 95–121.
3. Muller GH, Kirk RW, Scott DW: Bacterial skin diseases. *In* Muller GH, Kirk RW, Scott DW (eds): *Small Animal Dermatology.* Philadelphia, WB Saunders Co, 1983, pp 197–238.
4. Sisco WM, Ihrke PH: Unpublished data. University of California, Davis, CA, 1987.
5. Phillips WE, Kloos WE: Identification of coagulase-positive *Staphylococcus intermedius* and *Staphylococcus hyicus* subsp. *hyicus* isolates from veterinary clinical specimens. *J Clin Microbiol* 14:671–673, 1981.
6. Biberstein EL, Jang SS, Hirsh DC: Species distribution of coagulase-positive staphylococci in animals. *J Clin Microbiol* 19:610–615, 1984.
7. Berg JN, Wendell DE, Vogelweid C, et al: Identification of the major coagulase-positive *Staphylococcus* sp. of dogs as *Staphylococcus intermedius. Am J Vet Res* 45:1307–1309, 1984.
8. Live I: Differentiation of *Staphylococcus aureus* of human and of canine origins: coagulation of human and of canine plasma, fibrinolysin activity, and serologic reaction. *Am J Vet Res* 33:385–391, 1972.
9. Scott DE: The skin. *In* Holzworth J (ed): *Diseases of the Cat: Medicine and Surgery,* vol 1. Philadelphia, WB Saunders Co, 1987, pp 619–675.
10. Ihrke PJ, Schwartzman RM, McGinley K, et al: Microbiology of normal and seborrheic canine skin. *Am J Vet Res* 39:1487–1489, 1978.
11. Krogh HV, Kristensen S: A study of skin diseases in dogs and cats. II. Microflora of the normal skin of dogs and cats. *Nord Vet Med* 28:459–463, 1976.
12. White SD, Ihrke PJ, Stannard AA, et al: Occurrence of *Staphylococcus aureus* on the clinically normal canine hair coat. *Am J Vet Res* 44:332–334, 1983.
13. Kristensen S, Krogh HV: A study of skin diseases in dogs and cats. III. Microflora of the skin of dogs with chronic eczema. *Nord Vet Med* 30:223–230, 1978.
14. Fehrer-Sawyer SL: Identification and quantitation of protein A on canine *Staphylococcus intermedius. Proc Am Acad Vet Dermatol Am Col Vet Dermatol* 2:13, 1986.
15. Halliwell REW: Current therapy in recurrent pyodermas and topical treatments in dermatology. *Tijdschr Diergeneeskd* 111(Suppl 1):735–765, 1986.
16. Mason IS, Lloyd DH: The influence of allergic factors on the penetration of staphylococcal antigens through skin. *Proc Voorjarsdagen,* Amsterdam, 14, 1986.
17. Devriese LA, Nzuambe D, Godard C: Identification and characterization of staphylococci isolated from cats. *Vet Microbiol* 9:279–285, 1984.

18. Ihrke PJ: Antibacterial therapy in dermatology. *In* Kirk RW (ed): *Current Veterinary Therapy IX.* Philadelphia, WB Saunders Co, 1985, pp 566–571.

19. Nesbitt GH: Bacterial skin diseases. *In* Nesbitt GH (ed): *Canine and Feline Dermatology: A Systematic Approach.* Philadelphia, Lea and Febiger, 1983, pp 81–89.

20. Ihrke PJ: The management of pyodermas. *In* Kirk RW (ed): *Current Veterinary Therapy VIII.* Philadelphia, WB Saunders Co, 1983, pp 505–517.

20a. Fourrier P, Carlotti D, Magnol JP, et al: Les pyodermites du chien. *Pract Med Chir Anim Comp* 23:467–485, 1988.

20b. Wisselink MA: Investigations on the pathogenesis of deep pyoderma in the German shepherd dog. Diss. University of Utrecht, Drukkens Elinkwijk BV, Utrecht, 1989, pp 3–79.

21. Ihrke PJ, Gross TL: The skin biopsy: maximizing benefit. *In Proceedings. Am Anim Hosp Assoc* 1988, pp 299–301.

22. Ihrke PJ: Therapeutic strategies involving antimicrobial treatment of the skin in small animals. *J Am Vet Med Assoc* 185:1165–1168, 1984.

23. Medleau L, Long RE, Brown J, et al: Frequency and antimicrobial susceptibility of *Staphylococcus* species isolated from canine pyodermas. *Am J Vet Res* 47:229–231, 1986.

24. DeSaxe M, Lloyd DH: Antibiotic resistance and other characters of *Staphylococcus aureus* isolates from dogs. *In Proceedings. Assoc Vet Clin Pharm Therapeut* 1982, pp 50–57.

25. Cox HV, Hoskins JD, Roy AF, et al: Antimicrobial susceptibility of coagulase-positive staphylococci isolate from Louisiana dogs. *Am J Vet Res* 45:2039–2042, 1984.

26. Phillips WE, Williams BJ: Antimicrobial susceptibility patterns of canine *Staphylococcus intermedius* isolates from veterinary clinical specimens. *Am J Vet Res* 45:2376–2380, 1984.

26a. Ling GV: Personal communication. University of California, Davis, CA, 1989.

27. Werner LL, Bright JM: Drug-induced immune hypersensitivity disorders in two dogs treated with trimethoprim sulfadiazine. *J Am Anim Hosp Assoc* 19:783–790, 1983.

27a. Angarano DW, MacDonald JM: Efficacy of cefadroxil in the treatment of bacterial dermatitis in dogs. *J Am Vet Med Assoc* 194:57–59, 1989.

27b. Wisselink M, Bernadina W, Willemse A, et al: Immunologic aspects of German shepherd pyoderma. *Vet Immunol Immunopathol* 19:67–77, 1988.

27c. De Boer DJ, Moriello KA, Thomas CP, et al: The use of *Staphylococcus* phage lysate as an adjunct therapy for idiopathic recurrent pyoderma in the dog. *Proc Am Acad Vet Dermatol Am Coll Vet Dermatol* 5:27, 1989.

27d. Becker AM, Janik TA, Smith EK, et al: *Propionibacterium acnes* immunotherapy in chronic canine pyoderma. *J Vet Intern Med* 3:26–30, 1989.

28. Forbes BA, Schaberg DR: Transfer of resistance plasmids from *Staphylococcus epidermidis* to *Staphylococcus aureus*: evidence for conjugative exchange of resistance. *J Bacteriol* 153:627–634, 1983.

29. Naido J, Lloyd DH: Transmission of genes between Staphylococci on skin. *In* Woodbine M (ed): *Antimicrobials in Agriculture.* Monograph 23, London, Her Majesty's Stationery Office, 1984, pp 285–292.

30. Griffin CE: Otitis externa. *Compend Cont Educ Pract Vet* 3:741–750, 1981.

30a. Gabal MA: Preliminary studies on the mechanism of infection and characterization of *Malassezia pachydermatis* in association with canine otitis externa. *Mycopathologia* 104:93–98, 1988.

31. August JR: Diseases of the ear canal. *In* Solvay Veterinary, Inc: *The Complete Manual of Ear Care.* Philadelphia, Veterinary Learning Systems Co, 1986, pp 37–53.

32. Grono LR, Frost AJ: Otitis externa in the dog. *Aust Vet J* 45:420–422, 1969.

33. Dickson DB, Love DN: Bacteriology of the horizontal ear canal of dogs. *J Small Anim Pract* 24:413–421, 1983.

34. Baxter M: The association of *Pityrosporum pachydermatis* with the normal external ear canal of dogs and cats. *J Small Anim Pract* 17:231–234, 1976.

35. Trettien AL: The role of *Malassezia pachydermatis* in the external ear canal of normal dogs. *Proc Am Acad Vet Dermatol Am Col Vet Dermatol* 3:26–27, 1987.

36. Griffin CE, Rosenkrantz WR: Unpublished observations. Animal Dermatology Clinic, Garden Grove, CA, 1988.

37. Baxter M, Lawler DC: The incidence of otitis externa of dogs and cats in New Zealand. *NZ Vet J* 20:29–32, 1972.

38. Weisbroth SH, Powell MB, et al: Immunopathology of naturally occurring otodectic otoacariasis in the domestic cat. *J Am Vet Med Assoc* 165:1088–1093, 1974.

39. Grono LR: Studies of the ear mite, *Otodectes cynotis. Vet Rec* 85:6–8, 1969.

40. Frost RC: Canine otoacariasis. *J Small Anim Pract* 2:253–256, 1961.

41. Lane JG: Diseases of the ear canal. *In* Solvay Veterinary, Inc: *The Complete Manual of Ear Care.* Philadelphia, Veterinary Learning Systems, 1986, p 81.

42. Moriello KA, Fehrer SL, Meyer DJ, et al: *Proc Am Acad Vet Dermatol Am Col Vet Dermatol* 3:4, 1987.

43. Moriello KA, Fehrer-Sawyer SL, Meyer DJ, et al: Adrenocortical suppression associated with topical otic administration of glucocorticoids in dogs. *J Am Vet Med Assoc* 193:329–331, 1988.

6 MUSCULOSKELETAL INFECTIONS

Joe N. Kornegay
Lawrence W. Anson

The musculoskeletal system is rarely a predominant site affected by most infectious diseases of dogs and cats. This system, however, is often injured as a result of immunopathologic mechanisms induced by infectious organisms, or it may serve as a secondary nidus of infection. As such, initial clinical signs of certain infectious diseases may reflect musculoskeletal involvement. The causative agents, clinical features, and treatment of these conditions form the basis of this discussion.

Muscle Infections

INFLAMMATORY POLYMYOPATHIES

Etiology

Inflammatory muscle disease in dogs and cats may be subdivided into infectious and noninfectious categories. The infectious group includes diseases such as toxoplasmosis, leptospirosis, and clostridial infections, in which the causative agents selectively involve muscle (see Muscle Infections, Appendix 11). The noninfectious group includes diseases that are probably immune mediated, such as polymyositis and eosinophilic myositis.[1] This distinction is somewhat artificial because infectious agents may be the underlying cause of some immune-mediated conditions. For example, viruses and *Toxoplasma gondii* may incite the immunologic attack against muscle by altering its antigenicity and result in nonsuppurative or eosinophilic myositis. Chronic eosinophilic myositis may lead to atrophic myositis involving the masticatory muscles; however, a clear association between these latter two conditions often is not present. Eosinophilic myositis and atrophic myositis may be grouped under the term *masticatory muscle myositis* (MMM).[2] Selective involvement of the temporalis muscles in MMM apparently occurs because antibodies are directed against antigens that are specific for the type II muscle fibers that predominate in these muscles.

Clinical Findings

Animals with immune-mediated polymyositis usually have diffuse muscle pain, weakness, stilted gait, and pyrexia.[3] Those with MMM often have focal involvement of the muscles of mastication, resulting in atrophy of these muscles, trismus, and pain upon opening the mouth.

Evidence of additional organ system involvement may distinguish the infectious polymyopathies of toxoplasmosis and leptospirosis from immune-mediated diseases. The infectious myopathies, however, generally have clinical features that are similar to those of their noninfectious counterparts.

Diagnosis

A diagnosis of polymyositis or MMM is based on characteristic clinical signs, elevation of serum muscle enzymes such as creatine kinase, typical electromyographic abnormalities, and histologic evidence of myonecrosis and inflammation. All four criteria may be evident in some cases.

Diagnosis of leptospirosis or toxoplasmosis is dependent upon histologic demonstration of the causative organisms in the biopsy material, by culture, or by evaluating sequential serum antibody titers. Further diagnosis and treatment of these two infections are covered in Chapters 45 and 86, respectively.

Therapy

Because of their potential immune-mediated cause, polymyositis and MMM are treated with glucocorticoids on a reducing dosage regimen. Prednisone, given at 2.2 mg/kg once daily, is effective in most affected animals. In some cases, administration of this drug can be stopped after 2 weeks without recurrence of clinical signs, although other animals will require prolonged periodic treatment.

FOCAL MYOSITIS

Infectious polymyopathies must be distinguished from focal muscle infections, in which lameness or localized tissue swelling may be the only clinical sign. Analogous infections in people are termed pyomyositis and are usually caused by staphylococci. Infection usually occurs subsequent to blunt trauma or a penetrating wound and progresses to abscess formation. Although not common, focal muscle infections in dogs and cats do occur (Fig. 6–1) and usually follow trauma, bite wounds, or contamination of a surgical wound (see also Anaerobic Infections, Chapter 49). *Staphylococcus intermedius* and *Clostridium perfringens* are the pathogens most commonly isolated. Clindamycin is an effective drug for treatment of anaerobic bacterial myositis. Treatment should include surgical drainage and, based on results of culture and susceptibility, antibiotic therapy for 5 to 7 days (Tables 6–1 and 6–2).

Bone Infections

In most cases of osteomyelitis in dogs and cats, the infective organism reaches the involved bone either by direct extension from a contiguous focus of infection or through hematogenous spread. Lesions of the appendicular skeleton are almost always due to direct extension and often occur subsequent to either open fractures or surgery to repair a fracture. In contrast, vertebral osteomyelitis (discospondylitis) usually results from hematogenous spread of the causative organism from distant sites of infection and rarely

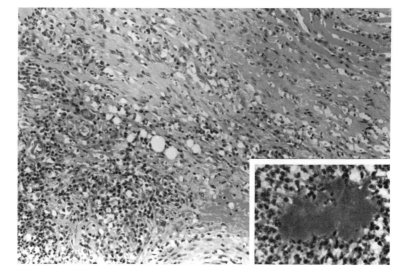

Figure 6–1. Purulent septic myositis of the temporalis muscle from a dog with acute facial swelling and hemiparesis. A section of skeletal muscle containing scattered inflammatory cells is seen in the upper right corner. This muscle is bordered by fibrous connective tissue. Numerous inflammatory cells, including many that were identified as necrotic neutrophils, are seen in the lower left corner (H and E, × 120). Inset: Aggregate of bacteria seen in another area of the lesion (H and E, × 240). *Escherichia coli* and *Corynebacterium* sp. were cultured from the temporalis muscle.

Table 6–1. Recommended Therapy for Musculoskeletal Infections in Dogs and Cats

ORGANISM	USUAL SITE[a]	SYSTEMIC ANTIBIOTICS
Staphylococcus intermedius	D, A, O	Cephradine[b] **or** cloxacillin[c] or clindamycin
Brucella canis	D	Tetracycline[d] **and** streptomycin[e]
Streptococcus sp (β-hemolytic)	D, A	Ampicillin **or** penicillin[f]
Proteus, Pseudomonas	I, O	Gentamicin **or** third generation cephalosporins **or** ticarcillin
Erysipelothrix rhusiopathiae	D, A	Penicillin[b,c]
Pasteurella multocida	I	Ampicillin **or** tetracycline
Anaerobes	M, O, I	Clindamycin **or** metronidazole **or** chloramphenicol
Mycoplasma	A	Tetracycline[d]
Borrelia	A	Ampicillin **or** tetracycline
Toxoplasma	M	Clindamycin
Aspergillus	D	Ketoconazole **or** amphotericin B
Cryptococcus	A	Ketoconazole **or** amphotericin B
Coccidioides, Blastomyces	O	Ketoconazole **or** amphotericin B

[a]D = discospondylitis, A = arthritis, M = myositis, O = osteomyelitis, I = otitis media–interna.
[b]Substitute any first generation cephalosporin.
[c]Substitute any β-lactamase–resistant penicillin.
[d]Substitute minocycline or doxycycline.
[e]Substitute gentamicin.
[f]Substitute amoxicillin, erythromycin.

follows vertebral surgery.[4] Because of these differences, appendicular and vertebral osteomyelitis are discussed separately. Otitis media is covered in a third subsection.

APPENDICULAR OSTEOMYELITIS

Etiology and Pathogenesis

The most common causes of osteomyelitis are direct implantation from penetrating wounds, spread from contiguous soft tissue infections, open fractures, or surgical repair of closed fractures.[5] Mandibular or maxillary infection can result from periodontal disease.[6] Hematogenous spread of infection to the long bones of dogs and cats is rare. The existence alone of bacteria in bone does not necessarily lead to osteomyelitis. For bacterial osteomyelitis to occur, the bone must have a compromised vascular supply, such as occurs with fractures.[7] Osteomyelitis is more common in male than female dogs, perhaps because males are more likely to be hit by a motor vehicle and therefore to sustain long bone fractures.

Staphylococcus spp. are the most common bacterial isolates.[6,7] Coliforms or mixed infections are also common. Less frequently, infections with other aerobic bacteria such

Table 6–2. Drug Dosages for Treatment of Musculoskeletal Infections[a]

DRUG	DOSE[b] (mg/kg)	ROUTE	INTERVAL (hour)	DURATION (week)
Penicillin-V	40	PO	6	4–6
Ampicillin	20	PO	8	4–6
Cloxacillin[c]	10	PO	6	4–6
Tetracycline	22	PO	8	3
Minocycline[d]	10	PO	12	4–6
Streptomycin	20	IM	12	1
Gentamicin	2	IM	12	1[e]
Cephradine[f]	20	PO	8	4–6
Clindamycin	11	PO	12	4[g]
Chloramphenicol	50	PO	8	1

[a]PO = oral, IM = intramuscular.
[b]Dose per administration at specified interval, expressed as mg/kg unless otherwise stated.
[c]Other β-lactamase–resistant penicillins can be substituted. See Penicillins, Chapter 43.
[d]Doxycycline may be substituted.
[e]Renal function should be closely monitored before continuing treatment.
[f]Other first generation cephalosporins may be substituted. See Cephalosporins, Chapter 43.
[g]Myositis therapy need only last 1–2 weeks. Osteomyelitis is treated for at least 4 weeks.

as *Erysipelothrix* have been reported.[7a] Increased sophistication in culturing techniques has led to identification of more anaerobic bacteria causing infections.[5,8] The role of anaerobes in osteomyelitis in animals with concomitant aerobic infection is unclear.

Until recently, coagulase-positive *Staphylococcus* spp. have not been differentiated, and the clinical implications of identifying the particular species have been limited. However, as *S. aureus* is a commensal organism of humans and *S. intermedius* is a commensal of dogs,[9] identification of staphylococcal species in cases of osteomyelitis is important to the subsequent identification of the source of the infection (see also Chapter 57). Specifically, *S. intermedius* may originate from the skin of the patient, whereas *S. aureus* originates from the surgeon. Accordingly, identifying the specific staphylococcal species in postsurgical osteomyelitis cases may direct the surgeon to improve preoperative skin preparation or to be more stringent in aseptic technique.

Fungal infections involving bone may be either disseminated, as with blastomycosis or coccidioidomycosis, or from extension of soft tissue lesions, as with phaeohyphomycosis (see Chapter 74).

Clinical Findings

In cases of acute osteomyelitis, inflammation, heat, swelling, and pain are often present. Infections in the immediate postoperative period are often accompanied by serous to purulent discharge from the incision. Clinical signs associated with disseminated infections may be fever, anorexia, dullness, and dyspnea, depending on the organisms and the sites of infection.[6] In the dog and cat, chronic osteomyelitis is most common.[7] Clinical signs often noted are a soft tissue swelling at the site of infection, lameness of the affected limb, and draining sinuses.

Diagnosis

History and clinical signs should direct the clinician toward a tentative diagnosis of osteomyelitis. A history of an open fracture or open reduction and internal fixation of a fracture, when accompanied by the clinical findings described above, indicates a need for further diagnostic studies. Acute osteomyelitis after open reduction of a fracture may be difficult to differentiate from a localized soft tissue or incisional infection. Leukocytosis may be present in cases of acute osteomyelitis. Bacteria isolated from blood cultures should be considered the etiologic agent in cases of suspected acute hematogenous osteomyelitis. Cytologic evaluation of aspirates or exudates may aid in the diagnosis of fungal osteomyelitis. Radiographic assessment of the infected bone may help in the diagnosis; however, radiographic changes may not be evident until 10 to 14 days after onset of the infection.[7] Radiographic evidence of soft tissue swelling in the affected area can be seen initially. With time and if the infection is not controlled, irregular periosteal reactions, cortical lysis, and increased medullary density may be seen (Fig. 6–2). Sequestra formation can occur with or without an involucrum.[6] Definitive diagnosis requires a positive culture result. Draining tracts should not be cultured; instead, fine-needle aspirates or pieces of bone and associated soft tissues obtained at surgery should be sampled.

Therapy

The axiom that it is better to prevent a disease than to treat it later certainly applies to osteomyelitis. Correct preoperative preparation, aseptic intraoperative technique, gentle tissue handling, and stable fracture fixation all aid in reducing the incidence of postsurgical osteomyelitis. For fractures, when prolonged surgical exposure is anticipated, prophylactic antibiotic therapy is indicated. Proper initial management of open fractures is important, as appropriate care may prevent complications with osteomyelitis.[10] In cases of acute osteomyelitis, hot-packing the area and creating dependent drainage may be needed. Cultures of samples from the infected site or, in some instances, blood cultures are required to identify the causative organism. Appropriate antibiotics, chosen on the basis of culture and susceptibility patterns, should be instituted as soon as possible. Gram stains of exudate or tissue may aid in the selection of an antibiotic before culture results are available. Until culture results are known, combined therapy with ampicillin and gentamicin may be in-

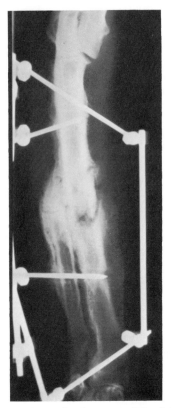

Figure 6–2. Radiograph of osteomyelitis of the radius and ulna of a 2-year-old male Great Dane 6 weeks after stabilization of an open midshaft radius and ulna fracture with a Kirschner-Ehmer apparatus. Extensive periosteal callus has bridged the ulnar fracture. The fracture site of the radius is still evident, and there is an associated sequestrum. Bone lysis is present around the tip of the pin immediately distal to the fracture site. A diagnosis of osteomyelitis was made.

stituted.[7] β-Lactamase-resistant penicillins, such as methicillin, cloxacillin, or a cephalosporin (see Tables 6–1 and 6–2) also may be effective. Clindamycin has been effective in treating experimentally induced posttraumatic staphylococcal osteomyelitis in dogs.[11] Initial parenteral therapy will aid in rapidly achieving tissue levels of the antibiotic. Antibiotic therapy should be continued for 4 to 8 weeks.

Chronic osteomyelitis requires aggressive antibiotic therapy and surgical intervention. All devascularized tissue, including bone, should be debrided. If a nonunion is present and there is inadequate stabilization, appropriate steps to provide rigid fixation are required. Without stability of the bone and associated soft tissues, the infection will not resolve. Following surgery, the surgical site may then be treated by closed or open irrigation. A cancellous bone graft can be placed

at the site after a healthy bed of granulation tissue is present.[12] Long-term antibiotic therapy, based on culture and susceptibility results, is required. Parenteral administration may be needed initially. As a high percentage of animals with chronic osteomyelitis are infected with *Staphylococcus* spp., a β-lactamase–resistant antibiotic such as cloxacillin can be used until the appropriate antibiotic is determined. Chronic osteomyelitis of the digits may perhaps be best managed by amputation.

VERTEBRAL OSTEOMYELITIS

Infections involving vertebrae are common in dogs[4, 13–16] but are rarely recognized in cats.[17] In most cases, these infections involve adjacent vertebrae and the interposed disc and are termed **discospondylitis** (Fig. 6–3). Less frequently, infections may be confined to the vertebral body, in which case the terms **spondylitis** and **vertebral osteomyelitis** may be more appropriate.

Etiology and Pathogenesis

As is true of appendicular osteomyelitis, coagulase-positive staphylococci are the or-

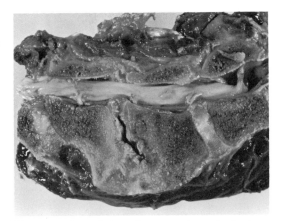

Figure 6–3. Lateral view of transected vertebral column from a 6-year-old female Great Dane with tetraparesis and depression of six weeks' duration. The C6-C7 interspace is at the center of the picture. The caudal aspect of the vertebral body of C6 and the cranial aspect of the vertebral body of C7 are irregular in appearance, suggesting that there is vertebral lysis. Fibrous tissue and new bone present dorsal to the disc space compress the spinal cord ventrally. The intervertebral disc at C6-C7 is absent. There is considerable new bone ventral to the C6-C7 disc space and sclerosis of the caudal aspect of the vertebral body of C6 and the cranial aspect of the vertebral body of C7. A diagnosis of discospondylitis was made. From Kornegay JN: *Compend Cont Educ Pract Vet* 1:931, 1979, with permission.

ganisms most commonly associated with discospondylitis. In the authors' experience, S. intermedius is isolated most frequently from dogs with discospondylitis. Streptococcus and Brucella canis are cultured less frequently. Infections of the disc space also develop in dogs with disseminated aspergillosis (see Chapter 71).

These organisms usually gain access to the vertebral column through hematogenous spread from infected sites elsewhere in the body. Urinary tract and integumentary infections, bacterial endocarditis, and orchitis have been identified as potential primary sources of infection in affected dogs. Reasons for predilection to vertebral metastasis of these infections are not clear. Presumably, the presence of subchondral vascular loops in the vertebral epiphysis slows circulation, allowing colonization of blood-borne bacteria. These bacteria then diffuse through the cartilaginous end-plate of the vertebral body to reach the disc. Infection is further disseminated to the adjacent vertebrae through freely communicating venous sinuses. In some arid geographic areas, such as the western regions of the United States and Australia, plant awn migration within the body may cause vertebral osteomyelitis. Although unproved, it is thought that after the awn is inhaled, it enters the respiratory tree, exits the lung, and follows the diaphragm to the spine.[18]

Prior trauma, spinal surgery, and immunosuppression are factors that may predispose dogs to discospondylitis of hematogenous origin. The role of immunosuppression is increasingly apparent.[16,19] Moderately suppressed stimulation test responses were noted in lymphocytes cultured in serum from four Airedales with discospondylitis.[19] That lymphocytes in these dogs responded strongly to mitogens when cultured with serum from clinically healthy dogs suggested that serum inhibitory factors may have been responsible. Increased levels of β1-globulin were present. Decreased serum concentrations of IgA found in these dogs may have impaired their resistance to infection against skin or mucosal microflora. GI sources were suspected since there was no statistical difference in the frequency of skin, vaginal, or urinary tract infections in dogs with or without discospondylitis.[14] Hypothyroidism, a predisposing factor for infections in people, was not found.

In 12 dogs with discospondylitis, normal or slightly elevated nitroblue tetrazolium re-ductase activity was found, which suggested normal neutrophil function.[16] IgG, IgM, and IgA serum concentrations were variable in all dogs. The C3 fragment of complement was increased in ten of the dogs. Lymphocyte stimulation response was depressed in six dogs; five of them had suppressed activity with fetal calf serum, suggesting the defect was inherent in the lymphocyte itself. The results of these studies suggest that immunosuppression, arising from serum factors or inherent lymphocyte defects, may be involved in the pathogenesis of discospondylitis. However, immunosuppression in these dogs may also have occurred because of the infection, rather than having an important role in initiating the infection.

Clinical Findings

Discospondylitis primarily affects large, middle-aged dogs, with males outnumbering females by approximately two to one.[4] In one study, a high percentage of dogs was less than 1 year of age.[13] Great Danes and German shepherd dogs appear to be affected disproportionately. Disc spaces in the mid-thoracic spine, C6-C7, and L7-S1 are most commonly involved, and multiple disc space involvement is relatively common. Affected dogs are usually hyperesthetic and often have evidence of systemic infection, including mental depression, pyrexia, anorexia, and weight loss. The subtlety of initial neurologic involvement delays diagnosis in most cases. If the disease remains untreated, however, proliferation of fibrous connective tissue and new bone (Fig. 6–3) causes spinal cord compression and paresis caudal to the lesion. Less frequently, vertebral instability may occur, leading to subluxation and additional or more sudden spinal cord compression.

Diagnosis

Evidence of concomitant systemic and spinal cord disease should alert the veterinarian to the possibility of discospondylitis. There are no consistent blood chemical changes, and leukocytosis is infrequently present. Pyuria, bacteriuria, or both may be identified. CSF usually is normal or has only mild elevation of protein. A definitive diagnosis usually is made with spinal radiographs, where varying degrees of vertebral lysis, sclerosis, and spondylosis are seen (Fig. 6–4). Radiographic changes may not occur until 4 to 6 weeks after the onset of infection, so dogs may have clinical signs of discospondylitis and be radiographically normal. Radioisotope bone scanning is useful in identifying early lesions in affected people and has also proved beneficial in some dogs, although this procedure is not generally available to veterinary practitioners.

When a diagnosis of discospondylitis is made or suspected despite lack of radiographic signs of disease, evaluation of *B. canis* titers and cultures of blood and urine may indirectly identify the causative organism. Bacterial blood culture results were positive in approximately 75% of dogs with discospondylitis.[20] Bacteria other than coagulase-positive staphylococci, *Streptococcus*, and *B. canis* should be viewed as contaminants unless isolated on multiple blood cultures (see Diagnosis, Chapter 7). Bacterial urine cultures and the agglutination test for *B. canis* also should be evaluated, particularly if blood culture results are negative (see Chapter 52). If treatment includes vertebral curettage, bone cultures should also be obtained. Bacteria with antibiotic susceptibilities similar if not identical to those cultured from blood usually are identified. Percutaneous aspiration of lesions, when used in conjunction with fluoroscopy, may be used to provide samples for culture.

Therapy

Treatment of discospondylitis is similar to that for appendicular osteomyelitis. How-ever, the potential for spinal cord involvement makes early diagnosis and treatment even more imperative.

Dogs with little or no neurologic dysfunction are treated with an antibiotic that is selected based on results of serology or blood cultures. Parenteral antibiotic administration for several days may be indicated in some acutely affected dogs; however, oral therapy generally is effective. Antibiotics should be continued for 4 to 6 weeks. If culture and serologic results are negative, the causative organism is assumed to be a coagulase-positive *Staphylococcus*, and β-lactamase–resistant antibiotics such as cephradine or cloxacillin are used (Tables 6–1 and 6–2). In infected humans, these two antibiotics achieve concentrations in both bone and pus that exceed the minimum inhibitory concentration (MIC) for *S. intermedius*[21] and have consistently been effective in vitro against this organism in cases of both appendicular osteomyelitis and discospondylitis in dogs (Table 6–1). Chloramphenicol, trimethoprim, ampicillin, and penicillin have not been as effective in vitro against staphylococci. Most dogs treated with an appropriate antibiotic improve almost immediately and do not relapse. Dogs that fail to respond clinically within 5 days of the onset of antibiotic therapy should be reassessed. Solitary, readily accessible lesions in dogs that do not respond should be treated surgically, at which time the lesion should be curetted and cultured. Dogs with multiple, widely separated lesions or lesions that are not readily accessible should be treated with a different antibiotic.

Although some dogs with moderate to

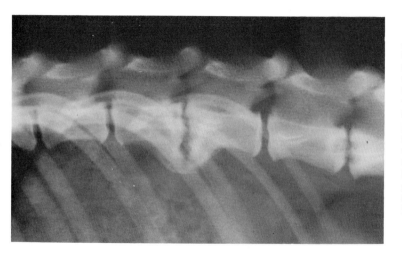

Figure 6–4. Lateral radiograph of the thoracolumbar spine from a 2-year-old female mixed-breed dog with spinal hyperesthesia and mild posterior ataxia of two weeks' duration. The T13-L1 interspace is at the center of the picture. There is lysis and associated sclerosis of the cranial end-plate of L1 and the caudal end-plate of T13. Note the new bone ventrally. Similar but less pronounced changes are evident at L2-L3. A diagnosis of multifocal discospondylitis was made.

marked (nonambulatory) neurologic dysfunction may also respond to antibiotic therapy alone, surgery may ultimately be indicated. A myelogram may be helpful in dogs requiring surgery to determine the extent and location of the compression prior to surgery. Either a hemilaminectomy or dorsal laminectomy is then done to remove the offending bone or fibrous tissue. A hemilaminectomy is preferred because the spinous processes are retained for stabilization, if needed. The lesion should also be curetted, and necrotic bone and disc material should be removed and cultured. Antibiotic therapy is instituted parenterally based on these cultures and continued orally for 4 to 6 weeks after surgery. The prognosis for these dogs must be guarded, as neurologic dysfunction may be irreversible.

A combined treatment regimen using tetracyclines and aminoglycosides should be used to treat discospondylitis due to *B. canis* (Tables 6–1 and 6–2; also see Table 52–2). Decompressive surgery may be indicated in more severely affected dogs. See Chapter 52 for a complete discussion of the treatment protocol for brucellosis.

OTITIS MEDIA–INTERNA

As is true of discospondylitis, clinical signs of otitis media–interna usually reflect neurologic rather than musculoskeletal disease. This disease is discussed here because the infection is seeded in bone of the middle ear and the bony labyrinth of the inner ear.

Normal Anatomy

Knowledge of the anatomic interrelations of the compartments of the ear (Fig. 6–5)[22] is important in understanding the pathogenesis of otitis media–interna and its treatment. Both the middle and inner ears are in the petrous temporal bone. The middle ear is separated from the horizontal portion of the external ear canal by the tympanic membrane. This membrane is composed of a loose dorsal section (pars flaccida) and a larger, more rigid ventral portion (pars tensa). The pars flaccida is pink or white and contains small branching blood vessels. The pars tensa is tough, glistening, pearly gray, and often has striations. These subsections radiate from the membranal attach-

ment of the manubrium of the malleus. Together with the incus and stapes, the malleus connects the tympanic membrane to the oval window of the inner ear. The auditory ossicles are situated in a small dorsal concavity of the middle ear, the epitympanic recess. The larger, air-filled tympanic bulla forms the remainder of the middle ear and contains the round foramen and the aural opening of the auditory tube. This latter opening is covered by the secondary tympanic membrane and communicates with the cochlea of the inner ear. The cochlea contains the peripheral sense organs of hearing. In addition to the cochlea, the inner ear consists of the semicircular canals and the utricle and saccule of the vestibule. These structures are concerned with balance.

Etiology and Pathogenesis

Otitis media–interna in dogs and cats usually is caused by extension of otitis externa. Accordingly, *S. intermedius*, *Pseudomonas aeruginosa*, *Proteus*, and *Streptococcus* are the most common bacterial pathogens, and fungi such as *Malassezia (Pityrosporon)* and *Candida* may occasionally be isolated. Because of their predilection to otitis externa, floppy-eared dogs such as cocker spaniels and poodles may be over-represented. Less frequently, otitis media–interna results from ascension of bacteria from the oral cavity through the auditory tube, which may explain the occurrence of otitis media–interna in cats, prick-eared dogs, or animals without external ear disease. Conversely, infections originating in the middle ear may reach the oral cavity through this same route.

Clinical Findings

Clinical signs of simple otitis media are similar to those of otitis externa. Aural hyperesthesia is manifested by pawing of the involved ear and discomfort upon manipulation of the animal's pinna, auditory canal, or face. In cases in which the infection has followed otitis externa, the external ear canal is inflamed and usually contains debris. On otoscopic examination, the tympanic membrane may be absent or obscured by this debris. When visible and intact, the membrane is discolored and often bulges outwards. Occasionally, a fluid line is observed,

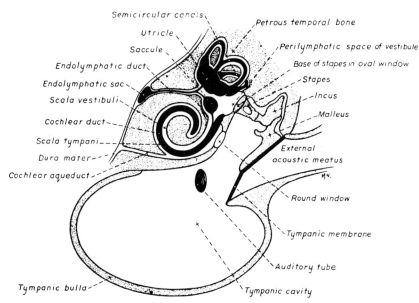

Semicircular canals
Utricle
Saccule
Endolymphatic duct
Endolymphatic sac
Scala vestibuli
Cochlear duct
Scala tympani
Dura mater
Cochlear aqueduct
Tympanic bulla
Petrous temporal bone
Perilymphatic space of vestibule
Base of stapes in oval window
Stapes
Incus
Malleus
External acoustic meatus
Round window
Tympanic membrane
Auditory tube
Tympanic cavity

Figure 6–5. Diagram of the middle and inner ear of the dog. (From Getty R et al: *Am J Vet Res* 17:364–375, 1956. Reprinted with permission.)[22]

indicating presence of serum or exudate in the middle ear. Some animals subsequently may have evidence of facial nerve paralysis or Horner's syndrome because of involvement of the facial nerve and ocular branch of the sympathetic trunk, respectively, as they pass through the middle ear.

With chronicity, there is increased likelihood that the causative organism of otitis media will spread to the inner ear. In these cases, evidence of peripheral vestibular disease occurs. Clinical signs include head tilt toward the affected side; horizontal nystagmus with the fast component in a direction opposite the involved side; and ataxia manifest variably by falling, rolling, and circling in the direction of the lesion. Most affected animals also have clinical evidence of otitis, both media and externa. When concomitant external ear disease is absent in either dogs or cats and only vestibular peripheral nerve palsy is noted, idiopathic peripheral vestibular disease should be considered. If there is evidence of central vestibular disease (postural reaction involvement, vertical or variable nystagmus, involvement of cranial nerves other than facial, and depression), extension to the brain stem or subarachnoid space may have occurred.

Nystagmus and ataxia usually resolve despite destruction of the peripheral vestibular sense organs. Reasons responsible for resolution of these signs are not clear. However, affected animals probably compensate through other sensory modalities such as vision and conscious proprioception. Head tilt may remain, but this usually is a cosmetic rather than functional handicap.

Diagnosis

Animals with clinical evidence of otitis media–interna should be anesthetized so that an otoscopic examination can be completed and radiographs can be taken. If the tympanic membrane is obscured by debris, the external ear canal should be gently flushed with a dilute (1:10) aqueous povidone-iodine solution, rinsed with sterile water or saline, suctioned, and dried. This aids in visualization of the tympanic membrane. If observed changes suggest middle ear disease, both open-mouth and lateral radiographs of the tympanic bullae should be taken. Radiographically, fluid accumulation will be reflected by increased density within the affected bulla. In advanced cases, there also may be radiographic evidence of osteomyelitis of the bulla and adjacent temporomandibular joint. If available, computed tomography offers a more definitive means of identifying these changes. Acoustic audiometry and assessment of the acoustic reflex allow for a critical evaluation of the integrity of the tympanic membrane. Although hearing can be crudely assessed clinically by observing an animal's response to noises, use of the brain stem auditory evoked response is more definitive.[23]

Therapy

Choice of treatment for otitis media–interna is dependent upon the stage of the disease. If there is not concurrent chronic otitis externa, administration for 5 to 7 days of a broad-spectrum antibiotic, such as ampicillin or chloramphenicol, may be curative (Tables 6–1 and 6–2). However, most dogs and cats with otitis media–interna usually also have chronic otitis externa and benefit from myringotomy, lateral ear resection, or both. If the tympanic membrane is intact, myringotomy should be accomplished under anesthesia at the time of otoscopic examination and radiography. Performance of this procedure is facilitated considerably by prior lateral wall resection. Either a blunted 17-gauge needle or myringotomy knife is used. Use of the needle allows simultaneous collection of fluid for culture and flushing. The needle is passed along the ventral horizontal ear canal so that it penetrates the ventral aspect of the pars tensa (Fig. 6–6).[24] Performing the procedure in this manner helps to prevent iatrogenic damage to the auditory ossicles. After fluid has been withdrawn for bacterial culture and cytologic evaluation, the middle ear is repeatedly flushed with dilute aqueous povidone-iodine solution, until the fluid recovered by suction is clear of debris and blood. The middle ear then is rinsed several times with sterile saline, and an antibiotic is instilled.

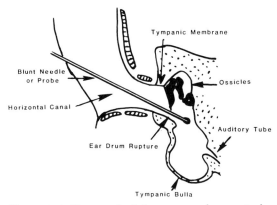

Figure 6–6. Diagram depicting proper placement of a needle for myringotomy and flushing of the tympanic bulla. (Modified from Lane G: In Pract 1:5–15, 1979. With permission.)[24]

Selection of the antibiotic is based on prior cultures of the external ear. It should be changed if follow-up cultures of middle ear fluid indicate unresponsiveness. When culture and susceptibility results are unavailable, a broad-spectrum antibiotic such as gentamicin in combination with a glucocorticoid is indicated. Aminoglycosides may have to be avoided since they affect auditory or cochlear nerve function, if these have not already been impaired when the ear drum has been damaged (see Aminoglycosides, Chapter 43). The antibiotic should be continued topically for 5 to 7 days. Animals with cytologic or cultural evidence of fungal infection should receive a topical antifungal agent for a similar period of time (see Otitis Externa, Chapter 5). Animals with nystagmus and vertigo from concurrent acute otitis interna also may benefit from antihistamines or benzodiazepines. Systemic use of antibiotics or antifungal agents is not usually indicated, unless the disease is recurrent or it is impossible to establish drainage through the external ear.

Many dogs and cats with otitis media respond to a single session of middle ear irrigation, together with daily cleaning and application of topical antibiotics. This is particularly true of animals with recent onset because the inner ear often is either unaffected or only minimally involved. Even some animals with clinical evidence of otitis interna may respond rapidly following myringotomy, suggesting their clinical signs are due to either increased pressure within the bony labyrinth or reversible inflammation of the sensory end organs. Others may require multiple sessions at 3- to 5-day intervals. Animals that fail to respond to middle ear irrigation in combination with lateral ear resection are candidates for bulla osteotomy. This procedure allows for removal of proliferative tissue and more complete drainage. Operative techniques for this procedure and lateral wall resection can be found elsewhere.[25,26]

The greatest danger of otitis media–interna is extension of the infection to the brain stem. This usually is avoided if proper treatment is initiated early. Collection and evaluation of CSF should be done when the animal is anesthetized for the myringotomy procedure if neurologic signs suggest intracranial involvement.

Joint Infections

Arthropathies of the dog can be subdivided into two broad categories, inflammatory and noninflammatory. Noninflammatory causes such as degenerative joint diseases are much more common. The inflammatory category can be further subdivided into infectious and noninfectious causes. Infectious arthropathies are the subject of this discussion.

ETIOLOGY

Bacterial joint infections may be caused by a number of different organisms; *Staphylococcus* spp., *Streptococcus* spp., and coliforms are most commonly isolated.[27] A variety of viruses, other bacteria, protozoa, and fungi have been associated with polyarthritis in dogs and cats (see Rule-Outs for Joint Infections, Appendix 11). Infectious agents may cause polyarthritis either by direct damage to the joint or indirectly through an immune-mediated pathogenesis.[28] With direct infections, the route of entry may be hematogenous, by penetrating wounds (e.g., postoperative), or by direct extension from surrounding bone and soft tissue. Polyarthritis of immune or infectious nature can be seen in animals with bacterial endocarditis[29] or other chronic infective processes elsewhere in the body.[28] The respiratory, urinary, and GI tracts are the sites most frequently involved, and immune-complex deposition is suspected.

Destruction of articular cartilage is the primary clinical concern in cases of septic arthritis. The inflammatory response and subsequent release of lysosomal enzymes degrade the cartilaginous matrix. Loss of collagenous support leads to subsequent mechanical damage during joint movement. The deposition of fibrin may also impair the normal exchange of metabolites and nutrients.

CLINICAL FINDINGS

Lameness is usually acute with both hematogenous and nonhematogenous arthritis. The affected joint(s) will usually be swollen, hot, and painful (Fig. 6–7). Nonhematogenous infections will usually be monarticular.

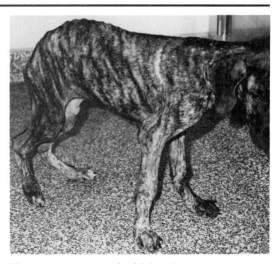

Figure 6–7. Ten-month-old female Great Dane with lameness caused by polyarthritis. Note the crouched stance and the swelling of the joints, particularly the carpi.

Animals with hematogenous infections may have evidence of both systemic and polyarticular infections.[29,30] Systemic signs include lethargy, anorexia, and fever.

DIAGNOSIS

Confirmation of a suspected case of septic arthritis requires further diagnostic studies. Early radiographic changes may include a thickened synovium, joint effusion, and widening of the joint space. As the infection becomes chronic, irregular joint surfaces and joint destruction, progressing to fibrous or bony fusion, may be noted. Analysis of synovial fluid may aid in the differentiation of infectious and noninfectious inflammatory joint disease. Synovial fluid volume and turbidity will usually be increased, with poor mucin clot formation. Viscosity will be decreased, and the total cell count, consisting predominantly of neutrophils, will be increased dramatically. Gram staining may help to identify microorganisms so that an appropriate antibiotic may be given while culture and susceptibility results are pending. Culture should be performed for both bacteria and fungi. In cases of suspected hematogenous septic arthritis, blood cultures are indicated. In people, synovial fluid cultures may be negative because of previous antibiotic therapy.[31] Synovial biopsy and culture may be needed to diagnose septic arthritis.[27] Blood cultures should be performed when systemic infection is suspected. Immune-mediated joint disease resulting from chronic persistent infections may be associated with positive antinuclear antibody or rheumatoid factor test results.

THERAPY

After diagnosis of septic arthritis, therapy must be directed at eliminating infection and salvaging the involved joint. Antibiotic therapy should be based on culture and susceptibility results of synovial fluid and intraoperative biopsies. Until results are available, a broad-spectrum β-lactamase–resistant antibiotic may be indicated (see Tables 6–1 and 6–2). Initially, antibiotics should be given parenterally, followed by oral therapy for 4 to 6 weeks. If indicated, the synovial fluid may be recultured after stopping antibiotic therapy.

Joint aspiration and irrigation may be helpful in septic joints when a diagnosis is made early in the disease course; however, in many cases, arthrotomy will be needed. Indications for arthrotomy are septic arthritis of greater than 3 days' duration, penetrating joint wounds, infections following surgery, and any infections in skeletally immature animals. All necrotic tissue should be removed, and the joint should be lavaged with copious amounts of normal saline or lactated Ringer's solution. In joints such as the stifle, medial and lateral incisions may give better postoperative drainage. In many cases, primary closure of the affected joint is not advised. Instead, treatment of the incisions as open wounds, with second intention healing, is recommended.[31]

Postoperative care will require application of sterile dressings and daily bandage changes, as healing occurs. Passive physical therapy of the affected joint may help to express exudate from the joint.[31]

The prognosis depends on the chronicity of the infection, the organism involved, and the degree of joint destruction. If diagnosed early and if appropriate, aggressive treatment is given, septic arthritis can be managed successfully. However, with increasing duration of infection and multiple joint involvement, the prognosis becomes worse. Hematogenous infection may be difficult to eradicate owing to the extent of systemic involvement. In cases in which the septic condition is cured but the degenerative changes are so severe that ambulation is affected, arthrodesis of the joint may be indicated.

References

1. Bennett D, Kelly DF: Immune-based non-erosive inflammatory joint disease of the dog. 2. Polyarthritis/polymyositis syndrome. *J Small Anim Pract* 28:891–908, 1987.
2. Shelton GD, Cardinet GH, Bandman E: Canine masticatory muscle disorders: a study of 29 cases. *Muscle Nerve* 10:753–766, 1987.
3. Kornegay JN, Gorgacz EJ, Dawe DL, et al: Polymyositis in dogs. *J Am Vet Med Assoc* 176:431–438, 1980.
4. Kornegay JN: Diskospondylitis. *In* Kirk RW (ed): *Current Veterinary Therapy IX*. Philadelphia, WB Saunders Co, 1986, pp 810–814.
5. Johnson KA, Lomas GR, Wood AKW: Osteomyelitis in dogs and cats caused by anaerobic bacteria. *Aust Vet J* 61:57–61, 1984.
6. Stead AC: Osteomyelitis in the dog and cat. *J Small Anim Pract* 25:1–13, 1984.
7. Caywood DD: Osteomyelitis. *Vet Clin North Am* 13:43–53, 1983.
7a. Houlton JEF, Jefferies AR: Infective polyarthritis and multiple discospondylitis in a dog due to *Erysipelothrix rhusiopathiae*. *J Small Anim Pract* 30:35–38, 1989.
8. Walker RD, Richardson DC, Bryant MJ, et al: Anaerobic bacteria associated with osteomyelitis in domestic animals. *J Am Vet Med Assoc* 182:814–816, 1983.
9. Berg JN, Wendell DE, Vogelweid C, et al: Identification of the major coagulase-positive *Staphylococcus* sp. of dogs as *Staphylococcus intermedius*. *Am J Vet Res* 45:1307–1309, 1984.
10. Parker RB, Waldron DR: The initial treatment of open fractures. *Vet Clin North Am* 10:707–716, 1980.
11. Braden TD, Johnson CA, Wakenell P, et al: Efficacy of clindamycin in the treatment of *Staphylococcus aureus* osteomyelitis in dogs. *J Am Vet Med Assoc* 192:1721–1729, 1988.
12. Bardet JF, Hohn RB, Basinger R: Open drainage and delayed autogenous cancellous bone grafting for treatment of chronic osteomyelitis in dogs and cats. *J Am Vet Med Assoc* 183:313–317, 1983.
13. Johnson RG, Prata RG: Intradiskal osteomyelitis: a conservative approach. *J Am Anim Hosp Assoc* 19:743–750, 1983.
14. Turnwald GH, Shires PK, Turk MAM, et al: Diskospondylitis in a kennel of dogs: clinicopathologic findings. *J Am Vet Med Assoc* 188:178–183, 1986.
15. Gilmore DR: Lumbosacral diskospondylitis in 21 dogs. *J Am Anim Hosp Assoc* 23:57–61, 1987.
16. Kornegay JN: Vertebral diseases of large breed dogs. *In* Kornegay JN (ed): *Contemporary Issues in Small Animal Practice: Neurologic Disorders*, vol 5. New York, Churchill Livingstone, 1985, pp 197–215.
17. Norsworthy GD: Discospondylitis as a cause of posterior paresis. *Feline Pract* 9:39–40, 1979.
18. Johnston DE, Summers BA: Osteomyelitis of the

lumbar vertebrae of dogs caused by grass-seed foreign bodies. *Aust Vet J* 47:289–294, 1971.

19. Barta O, Turnwald GH, Shaffer LM, et al: Blastogenesis-suppressing serum factors, decreased immunoglobulin A, and increased β1-globulins in Airedale terriers with diskospondylitis. *Am J Vet Res* 46:1319–1322, 1985.

20. Kornegay JN, Barber DL: Diskospondylitis in dogs. *J Am Vet Med Assoc* 177:337–341, 1980.

21. Hughes SPF, Nixon J, Dash CH: Cephalexin in chronic osteomyelitis. *J R Coll Surg Edinb* 26:335–339, 1981.

22. Getty R, Foust HL, Presley ET, et al: Macroscopic anatomy of the ear of the dog. *Am J Vet Res* 17:364–375, 1956.

23. Sims MH: Electrodiagnostic evaluation of auditory function in small animals. *In* Kirk RW (ed): *Current Veterinary Therapy X*. Philadelphia, WB Saunders Co. 1989, pp 805–811.

24. Lane G: Canine aural surgery. *In Pract* 1:5–15, 1979.

25. Ader PL, Boothe HW: Ventral bulla osteotomy in the cat. *J Am Anim Hosp Assoc* 15:757–762, 1979.

26. Siemering GH: Resection of the vertical ear canal for treatment of chronic otitis externa. *J Am Anim Hosp Assoc* 16:753–758, 1980.

27. Bennett D, Taylor DJ: Bacterial infective arthritis in the dog. *J Small Anim Pract* 29:207–230, 1988.

28. Bennett D: Immune-based non-erosive inflammatory joint disease of the dog. 3. Canine idiopathic polyarthritis. *J Small Anim Pract* 28:909–928, 1987.

29. Bennett D, Taylor DJ: Bacterial endocarditis and inflammatory joint disease in the dog. *J Small Anim Pract* 29:347–365, 1987.

30. Schrader SC: Septic arthritis and osteomyelitis of the hip in six mature dogs. *J Am Vet Med Assoc* 181:894–898, 1982.

31. Brown SG: Infectious arthritis and wounds of joints. *Vet Clin North Am* 8:501–510, 1978.

7 CARDIOVASCULAR INFECTIONS

Clay A. Calvert
Steven W. Dow

Bacteremia and Endocarditis

ETIOLOGY

Bacteria normally are excluded from the bloodstream by effective host defenses. On occasion, they do circumvent these barriers and gain access to the blood and cause a transient bacteremia, an event that is often unnoticed in clinically healthy individuals. In individuals with impaired immune defenses, invasion of bacteria into the bloodstream can lead to disastrous and overwhelming infection. Any heavily colonized mucous membrane surface or localized site of infection can serve as a source for direct bacterial extension into lymphatics or blood vessels, especially after tissue-manipulating procedures such as dentistry, endoscopy, proctoscopy, or rectal palpation.[1] Vascular catheters provide bacteria with direct access to the bloodstream, increasing the risk of iatrogenic bacteremia. Persistent bacteremic infections in people and animals are consistently associated with high mortality.[2-4]

Blood cultures are not routinely used for diagnosis in veterinary patients, and there have consequently been few comprehensive reviews of the epidemiology or clinical significance of bacteremia in septic and critically ill veterinary patients. The actual prevalence of bacteremia in domestic animals is probably underestimated.

EPIDEMIOLOGY

Prevalence

Aerobic bacteremia among a veterinary hospital population was found to occur in approximately 1% of the internal medicine case load and 0.3% of the general hospital accessions when blood cultures were procured because of suspected sepsis.[5] Bacteremia has been associated with various potential sources of sepsis, such as bacterial endocarditis or discospondylitis. Affected dogs have ranged in age from 1 to 11 years, which is similar to dogs with bacterial endocarditis. Although there were equal numbers of male and female dogs with bacteremia, there was almost a 2:1 male-to-female ratio of dogs with bacterial endocarditis and discospondylitis.[5]

A predisposition of large, male dogs to bacterial endocarditis has been observed.[6-8] Although chronic or subacute bacterial prostatitis has been identified in some bacteremic male dogs, a causal relationship is difficult to prove. Nonetheless, the prostate gland should be suspected as a potential source of infection in large, middle-aged, or older male dogs with bacteremia. Bacteriuria, commonly associated with bacteremia and bacterial endocarditis, may be either a cause or a consequence of bacteremia.[4]

The percentages of isolation of various organisms from dogs and cats with bacteremia and bacterial endocarditis are summarized in Table 7–1. Since the recognized prevalence of bacteremia in cats has not equaled that of dogs, most of the discussion that follows concerns the disease in dogs. Much of the information can be extrapolated for diagnosing and treating feline cardiovascular infections.

Table 7–1. Frequency of Isolation of Bacteria from Positive Blood Culture[a]

BACTERIA	CANINE ENDOCARDITIS[6,9] (n = 58)	CANINE BACTEREMIA[10,11] (n = 73)	FELINE BACTEREMIA[10] (n = 13)
Gram-Positive			
Staphylococcus intermedius	6–33	11–36	0
Streptococcus spp.	12–26	18–21	0
Enterococcus	0	4	0
Gram-Negative			
Escherichia coli	6–30	18–71	14
Klebsiella pneumoniae	0	6–28	14
Salmonella	0	13–11	29
Enterobacter cloacae	0	3–8	7
Pseudomonas aeruginosa	6	6–7	0
Proteus	0	14	0
Anaerobic			
Clostridium perfringens	0	20	0
Propionibacterium acnes	6	0	
Bacteroides spp.	0	4	14
Fusobacterium spp.	0	0	14
Pasteurella	0	3	0
Moraxella	0	2	0
Erysipelothrix rhusiopathiae	19	0	0
Corynebacterium spp.	19	3	0
Multiple	0	53	0

[a]Values are expressed as a percentage of organisms isolated. 0 = not reported.

Staphylococcus

Coagulase-positive S. intermedius (previously S. aureus, also see Etiology, Chapters 5 and 57) have been the most common bacteria isolated from blood cultures of dogs with intravascular infections and bacterial endocarditis.[4,6] Staphylococcal bacteremia is not, however, synonymous with endocarditis, especially when an obvious extravascular source for the bacteremia can be identified.[12] Common sources for bloodstream infection include abscesses and skin and wound infections. S. intermedius is normally present on canine hair and skin, and an association of cutaneous infections with staphylococcal bacteremia in dogs is to be expected. These staphylococci also may gain entry into the bloodstream of dogs from foci such as acute osteomyelitis, discospondylitis, septic arthritis, aspiration pneumonia, and genitourinary infections.[4]

Coagulase-negative staphylococcal bacteremia is usually related to IV catheter infections.[13] Permanent damage to cardiac valves often results from staphylococcal endocarditis, and antibiotic treatment must therefore be more intensive and of longer duration than is treatment of uncomplicated staphylococcal bacteremia. Sequelae to staphylococcal bacteremia, in addition to endocarditis, include metastatic abscess formation and septic shock syndromes. Dogs with staphylococcal bacteremia may develop septic embolization of the kidney, spleen, and left ventricle,[6] whereas in people metastatic abscesses also may lodge in the brain and bones. Septic pulmonary embolization occurs in people and dogs with right-sided bacterial endocarditis.[5,6,14] S. aureus bacteremia in people occasionally triggers a septic shock syndrome ("toxic shock") virtually indistinguishable from gram-negative bacillary endotoxic shock.[12]

Streptococcus

Streptococcal bacteremia is common in dogs but is somewhat less frequent than in people. Twenty-six percent of dogs with endocarditis had β-hemolytic streptococci.[6] In a larger population of bacteremic dogs with a variety of underlying illnesses, 6% of blood culture results have been positive for β-hemolytic S. canis and 5% have been positive for non–β-hemolytic S. viridans and enterococci.[3,4] Most β-hemolytic streptococci enter the bloodstream via the skin, while α-hemolytic streptococci usually enter via breaks in mucous membranes. Non–β-hemolytic streptococci are normal skin commensals and occasionally may contaminate improperly collected blood culture specimens.

Group B streptococci have been reported to cause sepsis in both dogs and cats.[15,16] In people, bacteremia caused by group D streptococci, including S. faecium and S. faecalis, usually originates from the urinary tract but also can occur following manipulation of the lower bowel.[17] Enterococcal endocarditis, which has been reported in dogs,[6,18] is especially serious because, unlike most other streptococci, enterococci are often resistant to penicillins and cephalosporins.

Gram-Positive Aerobic Bacilli

Diphtheroids, a heterogenous group of bacteria including the genus Corynebacterium, are often interpreted as contaminants when isolated from blood culture because they normally inhabit skin and mucous membrane surfaces. However, Corynebacterium has been isolated from 4% of bacteremic dogs[3] and has been associated with endocarditis in dogs.[18,19] Corynebacterium spp. have been one of the most common isolates from dogs with endocarditis of the aortic valve,[9] as has Erysipelothrix rhusiopathiae.[9,20,21] Bacillus spp. are frequent blood culture contaminants. In the immunocompromised host, however, B. cereus or B. subtilis can cause serious septicemias. Corynebacterium and Bacillus should be isolated from multiple blood cultures before bacteremia is diagnosed.

Gram-Negative Bacilli

Gram-negative bacillary bacteremia usually represents a serious opportunistic infection that has developed subsequent to significant depression of host defenses, for these bacteria are rarely considered primary invaders.[2,4,10] Gram-negative bacteremia is often associated with high mortality, and the number of such infections has increased along with the use of new antibiotics, greater use of invasive medical devices, and the trend toward more immunosuppressive therapy in the treatment of malignancies and inflammatory diseases.

Of bacteria of the family Enterobacteri-aceae, Escherichia coli is the most common bloodstream isolate from animals.[10] E. coli is abundant in the lower GI tract, which often serves as a reservoir for infection of other body sites. Urinary tract infection is the source for most gram-negative enteric bacteremias in people; the large bowel, respiratory tract, and infections of skin and wounds also serve as portals of entry to the bloodstream.

Oropharyngeal and fecal colonization with gram-negative bacilli increases progressively in seriously ill hospitalized persons as their status declines and has also been demonstrated in hospitalized dogs.[22] Other sources for bloodstream invasion by gram-negative bacilli include IV and urinary catheters, drainage tubes, contaminated IV fluids, disrupted mucosal barriers (e.g., after dental procedures or proctoscopic examination), contaminated aerosolization devices, and decubitus ulcers. In contrast to staphylococcal bacteremia, gram-negative bacteremia in dogs and cats rarely is associated with septic thrombosis and metastatic abscess formation.[10] Presumably, this may result in part because the course of gram-negative bacteremia is more progressive owing to endotoxemia (also see Chapter 44), and animals do not survive to develop embolic complications.

Although common in the environment and occasionally present on mucosal surfaces, Pseudomonas has rarely been isolated from deeper tissues of healthy patients. Because Pseudomonas is an opportunist, its rapid colonization with subsequent development of bacteremia is much more likely to occur following disruption of host defenses, especially cutaneous barriers (surgery and burns) and depletion of neutrophils, as occurs with cancer patients.[23] Extensive antibiotic use may also predispose to Pseudomonas bacteremia.

Anaerobic Bacteria

Anaerobic bacteria, particularly anaerobic gram-negative rods, are now considered serious bacteremic pathogens.[10,24] Development of anaerobic bloodstream infections may be predisposed by the presence of periodontal disease, deep abscesses, granulomas, peritonitis, osteomyelitis, septic arthritis, and septic pleural effusions (also see Chapter 49).[1] Clostridium perfringens was the most common canine isolate, whereas *Bacteroides* and *Fusobacterium* were isolated with equal frequency from cats.[3,10] A mechanically correctable lesion (abscess, perforated bowel, necrotic tissue) is often the source of anaerobic bacteremia, although impaired host defenses are not a prerequisite for infection. In people, *Bacteroides* usually enters the bloodstream via intra-abdominal sources, such as GI or genital inflammatory diseases, whereas *Fusobacterium* bacteremia often originates from infections of the respiratory tract. Characteristics of anaerobic bacteremia include high fever, thrombophlebitis, and icterus, particularly with *Bacteroides* bacteremia. Sequelae to anaerobic bacteremia include metastatic abscess formation and endocarditis. Clostridial bacteremia tends to have a relatively insidious clinical course without obvious signs of sepsis although septic shock may occur occasionally.

Polymicrobial Bacteremia

Bloodstream infection with multiple species of bacteria has been documented to occur in up to 20% of dogs[3] and 30% of cats[10] with positive blood culture results. Anaerobic bacteria, especially *Bacteroides* and *Clostridium*, are often components of polymicrobial infection in people and dogs. Clinical implications of polymicrobial compared with monomicrobial bacteremia are not clearly established. Although higher mortality rates have been reported in people with polymicrobial sepsis, no significant increase in mortality was observed in dogs or cats with polymicrobial bacteremia when compared with those with monomicrobial bacteremia.[10] Factors that predispose to polymicrobial bacteremia include neutropenia, GI and urogenital tract obstruction and infection, bowel perforation or surgery, and prostatic operations.

PATHOGENESIS

Bacteremia develops as a normal but transient phenomenon whenever bacteria-laden mucosal surfaces such as the nasopharynx and the GI and genital mucosae are traumatized.[1,2] Clinically important bacteremia may occur when the bloodstream is seeded with high numbers of bacteria via venous and lymphatic drainage from sites of infection.[1,2] Fluid accumulation, high tissue pressure, surgical or physical manipulation of abscesses, areas of cellulitis, or other infected tissues all favor lymphatic and venous spread of bacteria to the systemic circulation. In most healthy individuals, bacteria are removed from the bloodstream rapidly and effectively through phagocytosis by fixed tissue macrophages in the spleen and liver. Persistent bacteremia only ensues when bacteria multiply at a rate that exceeds the mononuclear phagocyte system's ability to remove them. Serum from healthy patients is bactericidal, largely owing to the presence of a number of humoral defense factors, including specific antibacterial antibodies of the IgM and IgG classes, as well as complement proteins, properdin, and fibronectin.[25] Bacterial capsules and other virulence factors may delay clearance of blood-borne bacteria, whereas bacteria that activate

---

Table 7–2. Factors Predisposing to Bacteremia in Dogs and Cats

SPECIFIC INFECTIOUS DISEASES	**IMMUNODEFICIENCIES**
Ehrlichiosis	Diabetes mellitus
Feline immunodeficiency virus infection	Glucocorticoids
Feline leukemia virus infection	Phagocyte defects
Canine parvoviral enteritis	Hepatic failure
Feline panleukopenia	Renal failure
	Solid tumors
SITES OF INFECTION	Hematologic malignancies
Abscesses	Splenectomy
Burns	Old age
Colitis	Shock
Stomatitis	
Pyoderma	**IATROGENIC MANIPULATIONS**
Urinary infections	Dental prophylaxis
Penetrating wounds	Endoscopic procedures
Canine and feline parvoviral infections	IV catheters
Musculoskeletal infections	Antimicrobial therapy
	Urogenital tract manipulations

complement via the alternate (antibody-independent) pathway are cleared rapidly. Glucocorticoids apparently do not affect clearance of bacteria from the bloodstream but may allow greater multiplication in extravascular tissues, thereby facilitating increased bloodstream entry.

Sources of Infection and Risk Factors

The most common sources of bacteremia include infections of the GI and genitourinary tracts, skin and wounds, respiratory tract, abdomen, and biliary tract. IV catheter–associated infections also occur. The sources of infection are not always identified.

A variety of factors, summarized in Table 7–2, have been cited as predisposing to bacteremia. When considering mortality from bacteremia and sepsis, the single most important factor influencing outcome following infection generally is the severity of the patient's underlying disease. Death from bacteremia is much less likely to occur if the animal was previously healthy.

Bacterial Endocarditis

It has been assumed that prior heart valve damage is an important predisposing factor for development of valvular bacterial endocarditis. Experimentally, it is difficult to induce bacterial endocarditis of heart valves in dogs unless the valve has been physically or chemically damaged or unless highly virulent bacteria are used. The most common congenital heart defect associated with valvular bacterial endocarditis in dogs is subaortic stenosis.[6] However, most dogs with confirmed valvular bacterial endocarditis had no history of valvular disease or congenital heart defects.[6,7]

Stress or endothelial injury leading to collagen exposure on the valve surface has been shown to result in platelet aggregation. Subsequent bacteremia may result in colonization of the platelet-fibrin thrombus. The pathogenesis of subacute bacterial endocarditis in people has been reported to involve these platelet-fibrin thrombi.[26] In addition, it is believed that prior valvular damage and a high titer of agglutinating antibody against the infective bacteria are required.[26] Certain

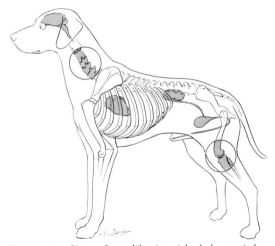

Figure 7–1. Sites of predilection (shaded areas) for bacterial embolization in bacteremia include the meninges, intervertebral disc spaces, heart valves, urinary tract, and joints.

pathogenic bacteria such as some staphylococci, streptococci, and *Pseudomonas* may produce endocarditis in the absence of predisposing factors such as the ability to adhere to normal canine heart valves or preexisting valvular damage.[27]

Time Course of Bacteremia

Relation of the time course of bacteremia to the infectious organism is not always possible. Peracute bacteremia, which develops over several hours, usually is the result of gram-negative infections, wherein endotoxemia produces severe clinical and hemodynamic abnormalities. Acute bacteremia develops over 12 to 24 hours and is most often the result of gram-negative infections but may result from staphylococcal infec-

Table 7–3. Sequelae to Bacteremia

AUTOIMMUNE DISORDERS
  Positive ANA, LE, Coombs' testing

IMMUNE-COMPLEX DISEASES
  Glomerulonephritis, polyvasculitis, polyarthritis

BACTERIAL EMBOLIZATION
  Meningitis, polyarthritis, renal microembolization

DISCOSPONDYLITIS
  Hyperesthesia, spinal cord compression

BACTERIAL ENDOCARDITIS
  Valvular insufficiency, cardiac arrhythmias

ENDOTOXEMIA
  Shock, hypotension, coagulopathy

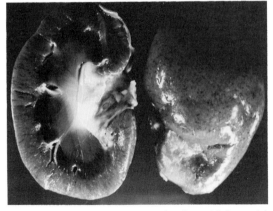

Figure 7–2. Kidney specimens of a dog with bacterial endocarditis demonstrating renal infarction due to embolization.

Table 7–4. Frequency of Various Heart Valve Involvement in 44 Dogs with Necropsy-Proved Bacterial Endocarditis

AFFECTED VALVES	DOGS AFFECTED (%)
Mitral	71
Aortic and others	34
Aortic only	23
Mitral and aortic	14
Pulmonic	2
Tricuspid	14

tion. Subacute bacteremia develops and persists for several weeks or longer and is often the result of gram-positive and sometimes anaerobic infections, although these organisms can also produce acute sepsis in the susceptible host. Chronic bacteremia of weeks' to months' duration may result from infection with microorganisms of low toxicity (e.g., *Brucella canis* or *S. intermedius*); sequestration of bacterial colonies on heart valves or in bone; abscess formation in the liver, spleen, kidneys, or muscles; or from a partial response to antibacterial therapy.

Sequelae

Secondary embolic abscesses, splenomegaly, and hematuria are more often associated with bacterial endocarditis than with bacteremia alone (Fig. 7–1; Table 7–3). Metastatic infection can result in life-threatening complications. Virtually all dogs with bacterial endocarditis of the left heart experience multiple continuous embolization and renal infarction, which may lead to renal failure (Fig. 7–2). Septic embolization of the spleen occurs in most dogs with bacterial endocarditis, although clinically apparent complications are uncommon.[6] Subacute and chronic bacteremia can result in sustained antigenic stimulation of the immune system and increased circulating immunoglobulin. Circulating immune complexes may be deposited in many tissues, leading to development of polyarthritis, myositis, vasculitis, and glomerulonephritis.

Valvular damage and dysfunction, microembolization of the myocardium, and cardiac rhythm disturbances are the principal cardiac consequences of bacteremia and bacterial endocarditis. The mitral and aortic valves are most often affected (Table 7–4; Fig. 7–3).[6, 7] Vegetations of the aortic or mitral valve lead to valvular regurgitation (insufficiency), which induces volume overload of the heart and left-sided congestive heart failure. Arrhythmias are the primary consequences of myocardial embolization. Major coronary artery occlusion and myocardial infarction are unusual in dogs with bacterial endocarditis.[6] Aortic valvular endocarditis may lead to a dissecting valvering abscess with infection of the septum or of a major component of the atrioventricular (AV) conduction system. AV heart blocks have been found in dogs with endocarditis but are uncommon.

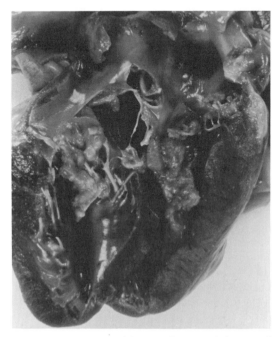

Figure 7–3. Severe proliferative lesions of the mitral valves from a dog with vegetative endocarditis.

CLINICAL MANIFESTATIONS

The clinical signs associated with bacteremia and bacterial endocarditis are similar (Table 7–5). The prevalence of lameness, sinus tachycardia, heart murmurs, cardiac rhythm disturbances, embolic complications, and immune-mediated phenomena is greater with bacterial endocarditis. Gram-negative sepsis usually manifests peracute or acute clinical signs. Bacterial endocarditis tends however to be subacute or chronic and is manifest by low-grade or episodic fever, although body temperature is sometimes normal.

Dogs with bacteremia usually display some combination of fever, lethargy, anorexia, and GI disturbances such as vomiting or diarrhea at the time of initial bacteremia. Following the initial clinical signs, dogs with gram-positive bacteremia or early bacterial endocarditis variably manifest fever, lameness, myalgia, lethargy, and anorexia. Dogs with subacute or chronic bacterial endocarditis may exhibit signs of left-sided congestive heart failure, especially if the aortic valve has been damaged. Heart failure usually develops from 2 to 4 months after the onset of clinical signs associated with bacteremia. Mitral insufficiency alone seldom results in heart failure within the first year after the diagnosis. Acute cardiogenic pulmonary edema occurring in breeds not normally affected by mitral valve endocardiosis or cardiomyopathy is often the result of bacterial endocarditis. In such cases, there is usually no history of a preexisting heart murmur, or the heart murmur may be absent at the time of presentation.

Physical examination findings from patients with bacteremia and bacterial endocarditis vary with the stage of disease and associated sequelae. In some dogs, lameness or polyarthritis may be the dominant clinical sign. However, lameness is an inconsistent finding in dogs with bacterial endocarditis.[6]

In some, heart failure or renal failure may distract the clinician's attention from an infectious disease.

Although often absent early in the disease course, systolic heart murmurs have been detected in most dogs with bacterial endocarditis.[6] The murmur usually is of recent onset or is latent in these animals. The systolic murmur of rapidly changing character, described in association with endocarditis in people, is less common in dogs. The presence of a systolic murmur whose intensity increases over a short period of time or evidence of a diastolic murmur is an ominous sign. A diastolic murmur is almost always due to aortic valve regurgitation and is strongly suggestive of vegetative endocarditis.

The presence of lameness, joint pain, muscle pain, and stiffness may suggest either immune-mediated disease or septic embolization of various tissues. In many dogs, both infective and immune-mediated arthritis simultaneously exist. Bilaterally symmetric joint involvement is more typical of the immune-based arthritis.[27a] Lumbar or abdominal pain on palpation may suggest renal or splenic inflammation secondary to septic embolization, infarction, or abscess formation.

Occasionally, erosion of an artery occurs following septic embolization, and hemorrhage occurs. Thrombophlebitis also may produce pain and edema of an extremity. Vasculitis has commonly been associated with bacteremia, and although petechiae and ecchymoses of the mucous membranes or retina are possible, such findings in spontaneous cases have been uncommon.[4–6]

DIAGNOSIS

Clinical Laboratory Findings

The leukograms of dogs with bacteremia alone and with bacterial endocarditis have

Table 7–5. *Clinical Signs in 122 Dogs with Either Bacteremia Alone or Bacterial Endocarditis*

CLINICAL SIGNS	BACTEREMIA (n = 77)	BACTERIAL ENDOCARDITIS (n = 45)
Fever (>39.4°C)	75	70
Lameness		
Total	19	34
Shifting	6	18
Vomiting	17	35
Heart murmur	6	74
Ventricular arrhythmia	5	27

been similar. A neutrophilic leukocytosis with an appropriate left shift and monocytosis have been present in most dogs with gram-positive or anaerobic bacteremia and in virtually all dogs with chronic bacterial endocarditis at some point during the course of disease. However, in one study, 19% of the dogs with bacterial endocarditis did not have a leukocytosis at any time during the course of their clinical evaluation.[6] Leukopenia and an inappropriate left shift have been more common with bacteremia alone, usually in association with peracute and acute gram-negative infections.

A normocytic, normochromic anemia commonly has been seen with subacute or chronic bacteremia and usually has been nonregenerative. A regenerative anemia occasionally has been encountered with bacterial endocarditis and probably is the result of erythrocyte destruction from physical forces associated with vegetative lesions or blood flow turbulence. Coombs' test results occasionally have been positive. Erythrocyte sedimentation rates have been faster in dogs with bacterial endocarditis.

Serum chemistry abnormalities are commonly, but not exclusively, associated with bacteremia and bacterial endocarditis. The main findings in affected dogs have been hypoalbuminemia (<2.5 mg/dl), a 2-fold or greater elevation of alkaline phosphatase (ALP), and hypoglycemia (<70 mg/dl).[5] Increased serum ALP activity was associated primarily with gram-positive infections and occasionally with gram-negative infections.[5]

Hypoalbuminemia has been a common manifestation of most types of bacteremia. Subacute and chronic bacteremia may result in transcapillary leakage due to immune-mediated or embolic vasculitis or bacterial toxins. Sepsis also has been associated with reduced hepatic synthesis of albumin, and 50% of bacteremic dogs in one study have had increased sulfobromophthalein retention, suggesting reduced hepatic function.[4] Hypocalcemia often has occurred in bacteremia and has been attributed to the hypoalbuminemia.[28]

Hypoglycemia may occur and the clinician should consider the possibility of a bacteremic episode. The mechanism of hypoglycemia is uncertain at this time; however, it may partly result from the effects of bacteria or bacterial toxins on the intermediary metabolism of glucose. In contrast,

hyperglycemia has been correlated with a higher postoperative mortality in the dog than in normoglycemic or hypoglycemic septicemic dogs and cats.[29] This may relate to the fact that hyperglycemia has been seen in early, severe septicemia, and hypoglycemia develops in more chronically affected animals.

In addition to the Coombs' test, serum tests for immune-mediated diseases, such as antinuclear antibody titer, rheumatoid factor, and lupus erythematosus (LE) cell preparation, occasionally had positive results.[6] In people, intracellular bacteria in circulating leukocytes and elevated serum teichoic acid antibodies (see Diagnosis, Chapter 57) have helped diagnose bacterial endocarditis when blood culture results were negative. Antibody to peptidoglycan was more sensitive than that to teichoic acid in determining the severity of staphylococcal bacteremia.[30]

Bacteremia may occasionally be diagnosed by direct microscopic examination of leukocytes in blood smears. Direct Gram stains of peripheral blood are usually unrewarding, because the number of microorganisms present is often much lower than the 10^5/ml necessary for detection. Wright's stains of buffy coat smears may increase the rate of detection.[31] Use of acridine orange is more sensitive than use of Gram stain, because organisms can be detected at 10^4/ml concentrations. Slides must be handled carefully to prevent inadvertent contamination.

A simple method of performing leukocyte smears involves placing one drop of fresh collected, nonclotted venous blood on a clean glass coverslip and incubating it in a moist Petri dish for 25 minutes at 37°C. The clot on the coverslip is gently washed off with normal (0.9%) saline, and the coverslip with attached leukocytes is immersed in fixative (methanol or glutaraldehyde) prior to Giemsa staining and microscopic examination.

Proteinuria, occult hematuria, and pyuria may occur in association with bacteremia or more commonly, with bacterial endocarditis in which renal infarction, glomerulonephritis, and renal microabscess formation are common sequelae. Urinary tract infections may be either a cause or an effect of bacteremia, and urine cultures should be submitted when abnormalities are found on urinalysis.

Radiographic and Electrodiagnostic Testing

Thoracic radiographs are usually of little value in the diagnosis of bacteremia and bacterial endocarditis, since left-sided congestive heart failure (e.g., left atrial enlargement, pulmonary edema, distention of the lobar veins) is only apparent in late stages in some animals. Bacterial endocarditis of the tricuspid or the pulmonic valve is uncommon, although it produces multiple embolization of the pulmonary arterial system that appears as focal areas of mixed interstitial and alveolar lung disease.

The electrocardiograms (ECGs) of dogs with bacterial endocarditis are frequently abnormal. Ventricular tachyarrhythmias, the most common arrhythmias, are in most cases not life-threatening. AV blocks, supraventricular arrhythmias, evidence of chamber enlargement, and ST segment changes are seen occasionally.

Although usually only available at referral institutions, the echocardiogram has been important in the diagnosis of bacterial endocarditis and in monitoring cardiac function in surviving dogs.[7] It has made possible the presumptive diagnosis of valvular endocarditis in the absence of positive blood culture results and diastolic heart murmurs. Two-dimensional ultrasonography has been a more accurate technique for detecting vegetative lesions.

Blood Culture

The definitive diagnosis of bacteremia requires consistent clinical signs and laboratory data and the isolation of the offending microbe from blood cultures. As primary or secondary sites of infection, urine, CSF, and joint fluid may also contain the organism. Preferably, the bacteria should be isolated from more than one blood sample. In addition, a source of infection should be sought and attempts should be made to isolate an organism from that site.

In addition to that for bacteremia, the definitive antemortem diagnosis of bacterial endocarditis requires the presence of a cardiac murmur of recent onset. The presence of echocardiographic abnormalities indicative of bacterial endocarditis is extremely useful.

When an etiologic diagnosis is established

with positive blood culture results, more appropriate and effective antibiotic therapy can be employed. Low blood culture yields are a frequent complaint but probably reflect the effects of poor patient selection, improper blood culturing techniques (e.g., timing, volume, number of specimens), and inadequate laboratory processing (e.g., failure to culture for anaerobes). By adhering to recommended guidelines for obtaining and processing blood culture specimens, the diagnostic yield from blood cultures can be improved.

Although empiric multiple antibiotic therapy often has been instituted in critically ill patients prior to obtaining culture results, the effort and expense required for blood culture has been justifiable since improper treatment may increase mortality from bacteremia.

Indications. Blood culture is indicated in acutely ill patients with fever or hypothermia; with leukocytosis, especially with a marked left shift; or with neutropenia and in patients with unexplained tachycardia, hypoglycemia, circulatory collapse, tachypnea or dyspnea, anuria or oliguria, icterus, thrombocytopenia, or DIC. Complementary cultures of urine and any other obvious sources of infection should be obtained. Blood cultures are also indicated in animals with unexplained fever, intermittent or shifting lameness, recent or changing cardiac murmur, or other signs of bacterial endocarditis.

Bacteremia in animals with endocarditis or other intravascular infections is usually continuous, and fewer blood cultures are necessary for a positive diagnosis. Generally, it is suggested that a maximum of three blood cultures obtained over a 24-hour period is usually sufficient to diagnose endocarditis.[32-34] Culturing blood during febrile episodes does not increase the frequency of positive results from patients with endocarditis. Prior antibiotic therapy rarely results in negative blood cultures and more often simply delays bacterial growth. Samples should be collected from multiple sites on the body, since multiple blood culture bottles inoculated by blood obtained from one venipuncture are regarded as one sample.

Timing of blood cultures becomes more critical when bacteremia originates from an extravascular source. Ideally, blood cultures should be drawn within the hour prior to the onset of fever, since there typically is a delay between the influx of bacteria into the bloodstream and the onset of fever.[32] As it is usually impossible to predict a fever spike, multiple blood cultures obtained over a 24-hour span are sufficient in most instances to detect intermittent bacteremia. When an infectious cause for fever of unknown origin is suspected, two blood cultures are obtained initially, followed by two additional cultures over 24 to 36 hours.[32-35] In the case of critically ill, acutely septic patients, three blood cultures should be obtained over a 30- to 60-minute period before instituting antimicrobial treatment. If possible, blood culture samples should be spaced at least 1 hour apart.

At least 5 to 10 ml of blood should be collected for each culture, because the chances of obtaining a positive culture are directly related to the volume of blood cultured.[35,36] The concentration of organisms is relatively low (5 to 10/ml) in the blood of most patients with bacteremia. A blood to culture broth ratio of 1:10 must be maintained in order to counteract the bactericidal activity of serum. Anticoagulant and antiphagocytic effects of broth additives are diminished if dilution of blood in media is less than 1:8.[5]

Technique. Prior to venipuncture, thorough skin antisepsis as for surgery is the most effective means of avoiding culture contamination. Small numbers of bacteria may persist inside hair follicles and sweat and sebaceous glands, which may be penetrated by the needle. If the vein must be palpated after skin disinfection, a sterile glove should be worn. To minimize the risk of contamination, blood samples should not be drawn through indwelling IV catheters unless venipuncture is impossible. However, in a critical situation, a recently placed indwelling IV catheter is acceptable for blood collection. Arterial blood specimens offer no advantage over venous blood specimens except that they may be helpful for detection of fungemia.[36,37] Collection of blood from separate veins is unnecessary unless a catheter-related infection or phlebitis is suspected. Finding the same organism at two different surgically prepared sites may reduce the chances of the same contaminant, especially when sampling times are close.

Blood is inoculated immediately and directly into culture media, using either a syringe and needle or a blood transfer set. A new needle should be used to introduce blood into the culture bottle after the culture bottle diaphragm has been disinfected with alcohol or iodine. Only commercial culture bottles packed under vacuum and fitted with rubber diaphragms should be used for routine blood cultures in order to minimize the risk of contamination.[38] Air must not be allowed to enter into vacuum bottles during blood injection. The blood should be dispersed in the culture medium by gently inverting the bottle two to three times. Blood culture bottles should be inoculated and can be maintained at room temperature to avoid killing temperature-sensitive bacteria[35,39]; however, incubation at 37°C is often used in the laboratory.

For suspected catheter-related sepsis, the catheter should be removed aseptically with a sterile forceps after local antisepsis of the insertion site with a 70% alcohol-soaked swab. A blood sample can be taken at the same time for culture. After removal of the catheter, the distal 5- to 6-cm catheter segment should be cut off and placed in a sterile dry tube to be sent to the laboratory. Methods for quantitating catheter-associated bacteria should be done to differentiate bacterial contamination of the catheter from clinically significant infection.[40]

Laboratory Isolation. Commercial multipurpose nutrient broth media, such as tryptic soy broth, trypticase soy broth, Columbia broth, and brain-heart infusion broth (Difco Laboratories, Detroit, MI) are all suitable for recovery of both aerobic and anaerobic bacteria. Thioglycolate and thiol broth (Difco), intended for anaerobic blood culture only, should not be relied on for multipurpose cultures because aerobic (especially *Pseudomonas*) and facultative anaerobic bacteria are not reliably isolated. Most liquid media are bottled under vacuum with CO_2 added and usually are suitable to support the growth of clinically important anaerobes. Therefore, use of special anaerobic broth is rarely necessary.

Most commercial blood culture media contain 0.05 to 0.025% sodium polyanethol sulfonate (SPS), a polyanionic anticoagulant that also inhibits complement and lysozyme activity, interferes with phagocytosis, and inactivates therapeutic serum levels of aminoglycosides. Fresh, undiluted serum is rapidly bactericidal. Dilution of blood with liquid media is essential to neutralize these serum and cellular antimicrobial properties.[38] Even at 1:10 dilutions, serum may be bactericidal to coliform bacteria, an effect that is counteracted by addition of SPS.[34] SPS is inhibitory to mycoplasmas and should not be used in media intended for their isolation. Dilution of blood in culture broth will usually lower therapeutic concentrations of antibiotics to noninhibitory levels. In situations where high levels of β-lactam antibiotics are present in blood prior to culture, β-lactamase can be added to the culture media. Para-amino benzoic acid, available in some commercial blood culture media, competitively antagonizes the actions of sulfonamides and increases blood culture yields from patients receiving sulfonamide drugs. Antibiotics can also be inactivated by mixing blood, prior to culture, in media containing adsorbent resins that nonspecifically absorb antibiotics. The advantages of such antibiotic removal bottles have not yet been clearly demonstrated, and they are expensive for routine use.[33,41]

In the laboratory, culture bottles are examined daily for evidence of microbial growth: turbidity, hemolysis, gas production, or colony formation. In aerobic culturing, the broth should appear turbid within 24 hours of inoculation. Ninety-five percent of bacteria are recovered from blood culture media within 7 days.[35] Longer incubation may be necessary for specimens from patients receiving prior antibiotic therapy or from patients with endocarditis caused by fastidious organisms. In addition to visual inspection, routine (blind) subcultures onto solid culture media usually are performed for antimicrobial susceptibility testing between 7 and 14 hours after blood collection and again after 48 hours of incubation.

Interpretation of Results. It may be difficult to determine whether a positive culture result signifies actual bacteremia or simply contamination. Contamination is best distinguished from bacteremia by culturing multiple blood specimens. Multiple isolations of the same organism imply significance because of repeatability. Knowledge of the normal canine and feline bacterial skin flora is helpful in interpreting blood culture results. Coagulase-negative staphylococci, α-hemolytic streptococci, *Micrococcus* and *Acinetobacter* are normal skin commensals on the dog. *S. intermedius* is normally present on canine hair, whereas *Micrococcus*, α-hemolytic streptococci, and *Acinetobacter* are normally present on feline skin.[42] Recovery of diphtheroids, *Bacillus* spp., and coagulase-negative staphylococci usually signifies contamination unless they are isolated from multiple specimens. Non-hemolytic streptococci and α-hemolytic streptococci from single cultures are also of uncertain significance. Clostridia in the bloodstream of dogs occasionally have been unassociated with clinical signs of sepsis, and the true significance of their presence is uncertain. The presence of bacteria of the family Enterobacteriaceae or Bacteroidaceae, *P. aeruginosa*, *S. aureus*, or *S. intermedius* and β-hemolytic streptococci or yeasts in the bloodstream is nearly always clinically significant.[39,43] In all cases, the significance of positive blood cultures should be interpreted in light of the patient's clinical status and the potential sources for bacteremia.

THERAPY

Blood cultures and bacterial antibiotic susceptibility tests are essential for the proper treatment of bacteremia and bacterial endocarditis. It is important to choose a bactericidal antibiotic that has good tissue penetration and to use high IV dosages for the first few days. Antimicrobial therapy may be continued orally at high dosages for at least 3 weeks for treatment of bacteremia and for 6 to 8 weeks for therapy of bacterial endocarditis. Blood cultures need not be repeated after antibiotics have been discontinued if endocarditis was not suspected and recovery was complete.

Despite the primary concern with the infectious agent, concomitant predisposing disorders should not be overlooked. Sources of infection should be identified and managed. Urinary and IV catheters should be removed when sepsis is suspected, and potential sites of infection should be drained, debrided, or otherwise treated.

In critically ill patients, antibiotic therapy should be started prior to the return of blood culture results, although this approach has inherent shortcomings, such as selection for microbial resistance. Subsequent therapeutic adjustments may be made on the basis of culture results. Several antibiotics may have to be given in sequence for treatment of bacterial endocarditis. Bacteriostatic anti-

Table 7–6. Choice of Antimicrobial Therapy for Bacteremia[a]

ORGANISM	SITES	FIRST CHOICE	SECOND CHOICE(S)
Staphylococcus intermedius	Pyoderma	cep, brp	amg, vanc
Escherichia coli	Bowel compromise, peritonitis	amg, tms	3rd gen cep, quin
β-Hemolytic Streptococcus	Genital, navel, and skin infections	pen, amp	1st gen cep, chlor, ery
Pseudomonas	Chronic wounds, leukopenia, burns, tracheostomy	amg[b], quin	carb, ticar
Anaerobes	Abscesses, oral cavity lesions, bowel compromise, body cavity exudates	pen, met	amp, chlor, clin

[a]cep = cephalosporins, brp = β-lactamase–resistant penicillin, amg = aminoglycoside, vanc = vancomycin, tms = trimethoprim sulfonamide, 3rd gen cep = 3rd generation cephalosporins, quin = quinolone, pen = penicillin, amp = ampicillin, 1st gen cep = 1st generation cephalosporins, chlor = chloramphenicol, ery = erythromycin, carb = carbenicillin, ticar = ticarcillin, met = metronidazole, clin = clindamycin.
[b]May combine aminoglycoside with ticarcillin or carbenicillin for maximum efficacy.

biotics, if used at all, should conclude rather than initiate this sequence.

On the basis of predisposing infections or other factors, time course of infection, known patterns of associated bacteria, and their antimicrobial susceptibility patterns, the antibiotics most likely to be effective can be predicted (Table 7–6). This knowledge is important when blood culture results are negative and in critically ill patients prior to blood culture results. Subsequently, appropriate adjustments in therapy may be necessary, based upon antibiotic susceptibility results.

In general, first generation cephalosporins and penicillins, especially β-lactamase–resistant types, are most effective in vitro for gram-positive bacteria, whereas aminoglycosides and first generation cephalosporins are most effective against gram-negative agents. Thus, a combination of an aminoglycoside, such as gentamicin, with penicillin, ampicillin, or a first generation cephalosporin is the logical choice for immediate treatment of life-threatening bacteremia in the absence of laboratory identification of an organism or its antibiotic susceptibility. The combination of first generation cephalosporins and aminoglycosides, however, is not very effective against anaerobic bacteria. When an anaerobic infection is suspected, penicillins should be used, or in some cases, clindamycin or metronidazole may be needed. Despite in vitro susceptibility testing, trimethoprim-sulfonamide is a poor choice for anaerobic infections. Penicillin formerly was the preferred drug for anaerobic bacteremia. However, those infections caused by *Bacteroides* spp. have had increasing resistance to it.[44]

Table 7–7. Antimicrobial Dosages for Bacteremia with or without Endocarditis in Dogs and Cats[a]

DRUG	SPECIES	DOSE[b] (mg/kg)	ROUTE	INTERVAL (hrs)	DURATION[c] (days)
Penicillin	B	$20–40 \times 10^3$ U/kg	IV	4–6	4–7
Ampicillin	B	20–40	IV	6	4–7
Cephalothin	B	20–40	IV	6	4–7
	B	15–25	IV	8	4–7
Gentamicin	B	2–4	IV	8	5–14[d]
Trimethoprim sulfonamide	D	15	IV	8–12	4–7
Metronidazole	B	8–15	IV, PO	8	5–7
Chloramphenicol	D	15–25	IV	6–8	4–7
	C	10–15	IV	6–8	4–7
Ciprofloxacin[e]	B	10–15	PO	12	14
Norfloxacin[e]	B	22	PO	12	14
Enrofloxacin[e]	B	5–15	PO	12	14

[a]B = dog and cat, D = dog, C = cat, IV = intravenous, PO = oral.
[b]Dose per administration at specified interval, expressed as mg/kg, unless otherwise stated.
[c]After the animal is stabilized, oral therapy should be continued when possible for periods of 3 to 6 weeks; see text.
[d]Renal function and urinalysis must be closely monitored for signs of nephrotoxicity at this dosage and frequency. Reduce dose to 1–2 mg/kg every 8 hours if renal compromise is anticipated.
[e]For dosages of other quinolones, see Chapter 43 and Appendix 14.

In order to ensure adequate serum antibiotic concentrations, the upper limit of the usual recommended dosage range of antimicrobial drugs is indicated (Table 7–7). Parenteral treatment is desirable for up to 14 to 21 days, especially for bacterial endocarditis, although this is not always practical. SC administration of ampicillin or cephalothin, or SC or IM administration of gentamicin may be substituted for the IV route when necessary or after 4 to 7 days of IV treatment. Except in animals with endocarditis, most bacteremic episodes are usually short-lived and are adequately treated by a short regimen. Ideally, oral antibiotic therapy should be instituted only after there is clinical and hematologic evidence of improvement in animals with endocarditis or uncorrected extravascular sources of infection.

Combination antibiotic therapy is often employed for gram-negative infections because they are associated with more acute progression and high mortality. Although clinical evidence supports the use of carbenicillin or ticarcillin with aminoglycosides for *Pseudomonas* and *Proteus,* these drugs must be given separately because of known in vitro incompatibilities. Amikacin, unlike tobramycin and gentamicin, is not inactivated in vitro by penicillin.[45] Continuous IV infusion of aminoglycosides has been recommended although increased nephrotoxicity has been reported as compared with intermittent pulse dosing.

Use of bactericidal rather than bacteriostatic antibiotics has been shown to result in higher concentrations of circulating endotoxin in animals with experimental gram-negative septicemia. However, clinical signs have not been more severe in animals treated with bactericidal antibiotics, and these animals have not had more suppression of bacterial replication and seeding from extravascular sites.[46]

Patients with bacteremia must be closely monitored (see also Endotoxemia, Chapter 44). Although clinical and hematologic evidence of improvement often occurs initially, relapse is common. Acquired antimicrobial resistance may develop rapidly. Clinical signs of resurging bacteremia include transient fever, deterioration of mucous membrane color, increasing capillary refill time, increasing rectal to toe-web temperature differential, decreasing blood pressure, and tachycardia. Detection of these signs of early deterioration indicates a need for intensification of therapy, including adjustments of antibiotic treatment. It also should prompt a search for a persistent focus of infection (e.g., abscess, catheter) that may be treatable.

PROGNOSIS

Several factors influence the natural course of bacteremic disorders including adequacy of therapy, severity of bacteremia, source of infection, delay before treatment, concomitant disorders, and the age and prior health status of the patient. The prognosis is better when abscesses, cellulitis, and skin and wound infections are the sources of bacteremia but is worse when gram-negative bacteria are involved because of the potentially fatal complications associated with endotoxemia. The mortality of bacteremic dogs with hypoalbuminemia and elevation of serum ALP activity and of dogs with these abnormalities plus hypoglycemia was significantly higher than that of dogs without these abnormalities.[4] Abnormalities of serum albumin concentration or serum ALP activity alone did not correlate with an increased mortality rate.[4] Late relapse and death have occurred in some dogs, usually when bacteriostatic antibiotics were chosen for treatment. The premature termination of antibiotic therapy may also result in relapse and death in bacteremic dogs, particularly those associated with bacterial endocarditis.

Although many survived the initial complications of bacteremia, aortic valvular insufficiency resulted in intractable left-sided congestive heart failure in most dogs within 2 to 3 months, and all dogs died by 9 months. Bacterial endocarditis affecting only the mitral valve is associated with a better prognosis.[6] Renal failure in a number of dogs has developed 1 to several years after having survived bacterial endocarditis. Apparently, septic embolization and infarction of the kidneys during bacteremia are the causes of renal failure.

The indiscriminate use of glucocorticoids even with antibiotics as prophylaxis is detrimental to bacteremic patients. Prophylactic antibiotic treatment usually is ineffective unless the type of bacteria and its antibiotic susceptibility are known. Bacterial resistance to frequently used antibiotics, such as ampicillin, is common. Thus, effective prophylactic antibiotic therapy usually requires the use of combinations of antibiotics, often including an aminoglycoside. Even then, the tendency to select for resistant bacteria is increased. Another common reason that glucocorticoids are administered to bacteremic dogs is the similarity in clinical manifestations of bacteremic and immune-mediated diseases. The survival rate of dogs with bacterial endocarditis given glucocorticoids was lower when compared with an overall survival rate of dogs that did not receive glucocorticoids.[6]

Infectious Myocarditis

Myocarditis (inflammation of the myocytes, interstitium, and vasculature) may result from primary or secondary causes. Both active and chronic myocardial disease may be associated with infectious diseases of dogs (Table 7–8). The respective chapters should be consulted for additional information on each. Myocarditis secondary to infectious agents may be subclinical if the inflammation is focal and limited. Severe or diffuse myocarditis results in fever, malaise, weakness, cardiac arrhythmias, and congestive heart failure. The diagnosis of myocarditis is usually made when ventricular tachyarrhythmias, with or without ST segment changes, are detected in patients with evidence of systemic disease. Specific serologic testing is available for some of the underlying diseases. Therapy is directed at the primary infectious agent, control of cardiac arrhythmia, and treatment of congestive heart failure.

Infectious Pericardial Effusion

ETIOLOGY

There are many causes of pericardial effusion in dogs and cats (Tables 7–9 and 7–10).[47–49] Pericarditis (inflammation of the fibrous and serous layers of the pericardium) due to infectious agents is the most common cause. Pericarditis may result from local (pleural or pulmonary) infections or from hematogenous spread of microorganisms. *Actinomyces* or *Nocardia* and anaerobic infections are most likely to spread from pleural infections or migrating foreign bodies.[50] Hematogenous infections of the pericardium can occur when infectious organisms embolize in the myocardial or pericardial vasculature. Bacteremias and viral infections, such as feline infectious peritonitis, can cause effusive pericarditis.

Pericarditis may be effusive or constrictive but in the dog and cat it is usually effusive. Effusions of infectious pericarditis are either modified transudates or exudates and are usually serosanguineous or bloody.

CLINICAL FINDINGS

The infectious nature of the underlying agent and the severity of pericardial effusion determine the historic findings. Weight loss, weakness, dyspnea, and mild abdominal effusion are the earliest signs. Fever is an inconsistent finding, varying with the infectious agent and time course of the disease. As the severity of the pericardial effusion worsens, dyspnea, weakness, and abdominal effusion become pronounced.

The principal physical findings reflect external cardiac compression. As the effusion becomes more extensive, the intrapericardial pressure rises to or exceeds right atrial and left ventricular diastolic pressures. Intracardiac pressure increases, ventricular diastolic filling is impaired, and stroke volume is reduced. The central venous pressure is increased, and venous return to the right atrium is impaired, resulting in right-sided heart failure. Jugular pulses and distention of the jugular veins are often present. Subsequently, increased venous pressure can

Table 7–8. Infectious Causes of Myocarditis

VIRUSES
  Canine distemper virus (neonate)
  Canine parvovirus (prenatal, neonate)
  Canine herpesvirus
PROTOZOANS
  Trypanosoma cruzi
  Toxoplasma gondii
  Hepatozoon canis
FUNGI
  Cryptococcus neoformans
  Coccidioides immitis
  Aspergillus tereus
  Paecilomyces varioti
ALGAE
  Prototheca spp.
RICKETTSIAE
  Rickettsia rickettsii
BACTERIA
  Numerous genera

Table 7–10. Causes of Pericardial Effusion in 84 Cats

CAUSE	CATS WITH SIGN (%)
Cardiac	20 (24)
Feline infectious peritonitis	16 (19)
Neoplasia	13 (15)
Infectious[a]	12 (14)
Renal failure	9 (11)
Coagulopathies	7 (8)
Miscellaneous	5 (6)
Iatrogenic	2 (2)

Data from Rush JE et al: *Proc Am Coll Vet Intern Med*, 5:922, 1987, and Harpster NK: *In* Holzworth J (ed): *Diseases of the Cat: Medicine and Surgery.* WB Saunders Co, 1987, p 820.
[a]Other than feline infectious peritonitis.

lead to pleural and abdominal effusions. The triad of increased central venous pressure, as with evident jugular pulses, weak peripheral arterial pulses, and muffled heart sounds, is strongly suggestive of pericardial effusion.

When the effusion is severe, the heart and lung sounds are not clearly audible. Mucous membrane color is often pale, and the peripheral pulses are weak because of decreased cardiac output. A reflex tachycardia is often present.

DIAGNOSIS

Thoracic radiographs will always be abnormal when pericardial effusion is severe enough to produce cardiovascular impairment. However, since the pericardial and cardiac silhouettes cannot be distinguished by simple radiographs, the size of the heart and the severity of effusion cannot be accurately determined. In some cases, pleural effusion may partially obscure the pericardial-cardiac silhouette.

Massive effusion is characterized by a

Table 7–9. Causes of Pericardial Effusion in 42 Dogs

CAUSE	DOGS WITH SIGNS (%)
Neoplasia	24 (57)
Idiopathic hemorrhagic	8 (19)
Cardiac	6 (14)
Traumatic	2 (5)
Uremic	1 (2)
Infectious	1 (2)

Data from Berg RJ, Wingfield W: *J Am Anim Hosp Assoc* 20:721–730, 1984.

greatly enlarged, round cardiac silhouette whose borders are smooth without the normal protrusions produced by the chambers. The silhouette is flattened where it contacts the thoracic walls. The parenchymal lung fields are not affected unless the lungs are involved as the primary source of infection. The lobar arteries may appear small owing to decreased right-ventricular output. Contrast radiography (positive or negative) may be performed after removal of the effusion in an attempt to identify mass lesion.

Electrocardiographic changes may be present, particularly when the degree of effusion is severe. Low-voltage complexes, electrical alternans, and ST segment changes may be present. Echocardiography is an accurate means of determining the presence and severity of effusion and of cardiac function. Two-dimensional ultrasound examination is useful in many cases in the detection of intrapericardial masses.

Pericardiocentesis is performed immediately if severe cardiovascular impairment has occurred secondary to severe effusions. Otherwise, pericardiocentesis is performed after radiographic, electrocardiographic, and echocardiographic examinations.

An area over the right thoracic wall is clipped and prepared as for surgery. Lidocaine is infiltrated into the skin and intercostal musculature between the fourth and sixth rib spaces. A 14- or 16-gauge, 15- to 20-cm over the needle, intravascular catheter (Angiocath, Deseret Co, Sandy, UT) works best for this procedure. Electrocardiographic monitoring is advised. A small incision is made in the skin with a scalpel 2 to 3 cm lateral to the sternum at the cranial border of a rib. The catheter with needle and attached syringe is inserted through the chest wall in the direction of the heart while applying negative pressure to the syringe. When the pericardium is reached, artifacts may be detected on the electrocardiogram, and pericardial fluid will be obtained. The catheter should be advanced into the pericardial sac, and the needle should be removed. A three-way stopcock and extension tubing may be used to facilitate removal of as much fluid as possible.

Cytologic analysis and microbial culture of the effusion should always be performed. Infectious pericardial effusion is either serosanguineous or (more often) bloody. The protein content is greater than 2.5 mg/dl and is often in excess of 3.5 mg/dl. Neutrophils and, to a lesser extent, erythrocytes are the predominant cell types. Macrophages and reactive mesothelial cells are usually present, especially when the effusion is chronic. Erythrophagia and hemosiderocytes may be observed. Degenerate neutrophils and infectious agents may be detected. When the latter are absent, hemorrhagic effusions due to neoplasia, idiopathic benign (hemorrhagic) pericardial effusion, and infectious pericarditis cannot be distinguished by cytology.

The presence of pyrexia, an inflammatory leukogram, or other biochemical data associated with bacteremia or sepsis is variably and inconsistently associated with infectious pericarditis.

THERAPY

If the etiology of a systemic infection is evident, aggressive antimicrobial therapy is indicated as soon as appropriate samples for culture are procured. In some cases, the infectious nature of the effusion is not appreciated until the results of cytology and culture are obtained.

Continuous drainage via an indwelling pericardial catheter or preferably surgical intervention, along with antimicrobial therapy, is recommended. Subtotal pericardectomy is recommended because surgically created pericardial fenestrations may adhere to the epicardium postoperatively, thus resealing the pericardium.

Constrictive pericarditis-epicarditis may occur and is easily recognized at the time of surgery. Although pericardectomy can be performed, extensive fibrin deposition on the epicardium is difficult to remove. Strip-

ping of the epicardium is tedious and is associated with complications, such as tearing of the myocardium and heart rhythm disturbances.

Bacterial infection, although producing fibrinous pericarditis and epicarditis, can often be treated successfully once the pericardium is removed. In the authors' experience, *Staphylococcus* and *Streptococcus* organisms are most often incriminated. Antimicrobial therapy should involve broad-spectrum, bactericidal drugs administered IV at high dosages when feasible and should always be guided by antimicrobial susceptibility results.

References

1. Black AP, Crichlow AM, Saunders JR: Bacteremia during ultrasonic teeth cleaning and extraction in the dog. *J Am Anim Hosp Assoc* 16:611–616, 1980.
2. Duma RJ: Gram-negative bacillary infections. Pathogenic and pathophysiologic correlations. *Am J Med* 78(suppl 6A):154–163, 1985.
3. Hirsh DC, Jang SS, Biberstein EL: Blood culture of the canine patient. *J Am Vet Med Assoc* 184:175–178, 1984.
4. Calvert CA, Greene CE, Hardie EM: Cardiovascular infections in dogs: epizootiology, clinical manifestations and prognosis. *J Am Vet Med Assoc* 187:612–616, 1985.
5. Calvert CA, Greene CE: Bacteremia in dogs: diagnosis, treatment, and prognosis. *Compend Cont Educ Pract Vet* 8:179–184, 1986.
6. Calvert CA: Valvular bacterial endocarditis in the dog. *J Am Vet Med Assoc* 180:1080–1084, 1982.
7. Lombard CW, Buergelt CD: Vegetative bacterial endocarditis in dogs: echocardiographic diagnosis and clinical signs. *J Small Anim Pract* 24:325–339, 1983.
8. Anderson CA, Dubielzig RR: Vegetative endocarditis in dogs. *J Am Anim Hosp Assoc* 20:149–152, 1984.
9. Sisson D, Thomas WP: Endocarditis of the aortic valve in the dog. *J Am Vet Med Assoc* 184:570–576, 1984.
10. Dow SW, Curtis CR, Jones RL, et al: Results of blood culture from critically-ill dogs and cats: 100 cases (1985–1987). *J Am Vet Med Assoc,* 195:113–118, 1989.
11. Hardie E, Rawlings CA, Calvert CA: Severe sepsis in selected small animal surgery patients. *J Am Anim Hosp Assoc* 22:33–42, 1986.
12. Sheagren JN: *Staphylococcus aureus:* the persistent pathogen. *N Engl J Med* 310:1368–1372, 1984.
13. DeLeon SP, Wenzel RP: Hospital-acquired bloodstream infections with *Staphylococcus epidermidis. Am J Med* 77:639–643, 1984.
14. Libman M, Arbeit RD: Complications associated with *Staphylococcus aureus* bacteremia. *Arch Intern Med* 144:541–545, 1984.
15. Kornblatt AN, Adams RL, Barthold AW, et al: Canine neonatal deaths associated with Group B streptococcal septicemia. *J Am Vet Med Assoc* 183:700–701, 1983.

16. Dow SW, Jones RL, Thomas T, et al: Group B streptococcal infections in two cats. *J Am Vet Med Assoc* 190:71–72, 1987.

17. Barrall DT, Kenney PR, Slotman GJ, et al: Enterococcal bacteremia in surgical patients. *Arch Surg* 120:57–63, 1985.

18. Drazner FH: Bacterial endocarditis in the dog. *Compend Cont Educ Pract Vet* 1:918–923, 1979.

19. Henik RA, Allen TA, Jones RL, et al: Case report of endocarditis in a dog due to *Corynebacterium* sp. *J Am Vet Med Assoc* 187:1458–1461, 1986.

20. Hoenig M, Gillette DM. Endocarditis caused by *Erysipelothrix rhusiopathiae* in a dog. *J Am Vet Med Assoc* 176:326–327, 1980.

21. Eriksen K, Fossum K, Gamlem H, et al: Endocarditis in two dogs caused by *Erysipelothrix rhusiopathiae. J Small Anim Pract* 28:117–123, 1987.

22. Fafoutis D: Characteristics of multiple drug-resistant bacterial strains associated with veterinary nosocomial infections. Master's thesis, Fort Collins, Colorado State University, 1980.

23. Bodey GP, Ladeja L, Elting L: Pseudomonas bacteremia: retrospective analysis of 410 episodes. *Arch Intern Med* 145:1621–1629, 1985.

24. Hirsch DC, Indiveri MC, Jang SS, et al: Changes in prevalence and susceptibility of obligate anaerobes in clinical veterinary practice. *J Am Vet Med Assoc* 186:1086–1089, 1985.

25. Sullam PM, Drake TA, Sunde MA: Pathogenesis of endocarditis. *Am J Med* 78(Suppl 6B):110–114, 1985.

26. Weinstein L: Infective endocarditis. In Braunwald E (ed): *Heart Disease: A Textbook of Cardiovascular Medicine.* Philadelphia, WB Saunders Co, 1984, pp 1166–1220.

27. Ramirez-Rhonda CH: Adherence of *Streptococcus mutans* to normal and damaged canine aortic valves. *Clin Res* 25:382A, 1977.

27a. Bennett D, Taylor DJ: Bacterial endocarditis and inflammatory joint disease in the dog. *J Small Anim Pract* 29:347–365, 1987.

28. Aderka D, Schwartz D, Dan M, et al: Bacteremic hypocalcemia. A comparison between the calcium levels of bacteremic and nonbacteremic patients with infection. *Arch Intern Med* 147:232–236, 1987.

29. Hardie EM, Rawlings CA, George JW: Plasma-glucose concentrations in dogs and cats before and after surgery: comparison of healthy animals and animals with sepsis. *Am J Vet Res* 46:1700–1704, 1985.

30. Verbrugh HA, Peters R, Gossens WHF, et al: Distinguishing complicated from uncomplicated bacteremia caused by *Staphylococcus aureus*: the value of new and old serological tests. *J Infect Dis* 153:109–115, 1986.

31. Todd JK: Nonculture techniques using blood specimens for the diagnosis of infectious disease. *Am J Med* 75:37–43, 1983.

32. Tilton RC: The laboratory approach to the detection of bacteremia. *Ann Rev Microbiol* 36:467–493, 1982.

33. Reller LB: Recent and innovative methods for detection of bacteremia and fungemia. *Am J Med* 75:26–30, 1983.

34. Washington, JA: Blood cultures. Principles and techniques. *Mayo Clin Proc* 50:91–98, 1975.

35. Isenberg HD, Washington JA, Barlows A, et al: Collection handling and processing of specimens. *In* Lannette EH, Barlows A, Hausler WJ, et al (eds): *Manual of Clinical Microbiology.* Washington DC, Am Soc for Microbiol, 1985, pp 73–98.

36. Vaisanen IT, Michelsen T, Vatonen V, et al: Comparison of arterial and venous blood samples for the diagnosis of bacteremia in critically ill patients. *Crit Care Med* 13:664–666, 1985.

37. Gleckman R, Gantz NM: Maximizing the yield from blood cultures in suspected infective endocarditis. *Crit Care Med* 11:15–22, 1983.

38. Hirsch DC, Ruehl WW: Clinical microbiology as a guide to the treatment of infectious bacterial diseases of the dog and the cat. *In* Scott FW (ed): *Infectious Diseases.* New York, Churchill Livingston, 1986, pp 1–27.

39. Washington JA: Medical microbiology. *In* Henry JB (ed): *Clinical Diagnosis and Management by Laboratory Methods.* Philadelphia, WB Saunders Co, 1984, pp 1064–1380.

40. Brun-Buisson C, Abrook F, Legrand P, et al: Diagnosis of central venous catheter–related sepsis. *Arch Intern Med* 147:873–877, 1987.

41. Hansen SL, Hetmanski J, Stewart BJ: Resin-process methods for improved isolation of organisms from blood and body fluids. *Am J Med* 75:31–36, 1983.

42. Muller GH, Kirk RW, Scott DW: *Small Animal Dermatology.* Philadelphia, WB Saunders Co, 1983, pp 197–199.

43. Calvert CA, Greene CE: Cardiovascular infections. *In* Greene CE (ed): *Clinical Microbiology and Infectious Diseases of the Dog and Cat.* Philadelphia, WB Saunders Co, 1985, pp 220–237.

44. Garvey MS, Avcoin DP: Therapeutic strategies involving antimicrobial treatment of disseminated bacterial infections in small animals. *J Am Vet Med Assoc* 185:1185–1189, 1984.

45. Holt HA, Broughall JM, McCarthy M, et al: Interaction between aminoglycoside antibiotics and carbenicillin or ticarcillin. *Infection* 4:107–109, 1976.

46. Sheneg JL, Barton RP, Morgan KA: Role of antibiotic class in the rate of liberation of endotoxin during therapy for experimental gram-negative bacterial sepsis. *J Infect Dis* 151:1012–1018, 1985.

47. Berg RJ, Wingfield W: Pericardial effusion in the dog: a review of 42 cases. *J Am Anim Hosp Assoc* 20:721–730, 1984.

48. Rush JE, Keene BW, Fox PR: Retrospective study of pericardial disease in cats. *Proc Am Coll Vet Intern Med* (abstract) 5:922, 1987.

49. Harpster NK: The cardiovascular system. *In* Holzworth J (ed): *Diseases of the Cat: Medicine and Surgery,* vol 1. Philadelphia, WB Saunders Co, 1987, p 820.

50. Lorenzana R, Richter K, Ettinger SJ, et al: Infectious pericardial effusion in a dog. *J Am Anim Hosp Assoc* 21:725–728, 1985.

8 BACTERIAL INFECTIONS OF THE RESPIRATORY SYSTEM

Philip Roudebush

From a clinical standpoint, the respiratory system is often divided into the upper and lower respiratory tracts and the pleural cavity. The upper respiratory tract consists of the nasal passages, nasopharynx, pharynx, larynx, and extrathoracic trachea. The lower respiratory tract consists of the intrathoracic trachea, bronchi, and gaseous exchange units. Specific diseases caused by viruses, fungi, protozoa, rickettsia, mycoplasma, and certain bacteria such as *Actinomyces* and *Nocardia* that primarily infect the respiratory system are covered in other chapters. This discussion focuses on bacterial infections of the respiratory system produced by invasion of normal microflora, specific bacterial pathogens, or following impairment of normal host defense mechanisms. The normal microflora of the respiratory tract are discussed because these organisms frequently become involved in both upper and lower respiratory infections.

Normal Bacterial Flora

UPPER RESPIRATORY TRACT

Surveys of the bacterial microflora of the nasal cavities, tonsils, and pharynx of clinically normal dogs have found many types of aerobic and anaerobic bacteria (Tables 8–1 and 8–2).[1-7] In a study of 92 healthy dogs, 2 or more organisms were routinely cultured from the rostral nasal cavity, whereas more than 50% of cultures surgically obtained from the caudal nasal cavity were sterile.[8] Because of marked individual variations, it is not possible to expect to find the same

Table 8–1. Bacterial Isolates from Nasal Swabs of Clinically Healthy Dogs[a, 1-3]

Staphylococcus (coagulase negative)
Streptococcus (α- and nonhemolytic)
Neisseria spp.
Bacillus spp.
Escherichia coli and Enterobacter spp.
Pasteurella multocida
Moraxella spp.
Corynebacterium spp.
Proteus spp.
Pseudomonas spp.
Staphylococcus (coagulase positive)
Streptococcus (β-hemolytic)
Clostridium spp.
Alcaligenes spp.

[a]Bacteria are listed in approximate order of frequency of isolation.

Table 8–2. Bacterial Isolates from Tonsillar and Pharyngeal Swabs of Clinically Healthy Dogs[a, 1-7]

Streptococcus (α- and nonhemolytic)
Staphylococcus (coagulase-negative)
Neisseria spp.
Escherichia coli and Enterobacter spp.
Pasteurella multocida
Bacillus spp.
Streptococcus (β-hemolytic)
Alcaligenes spp.
Klebsiella pneumoniae
Proteus spp.
Pseudomonas spp.
Corynebacterium spp.
Staphylococcus (coagulase-positive)
Clostridium spp.
Bacteroides spp.
Propionibacterium spp.
Peptostreptococcus spp.
Fusobacterium spp.

[a]Bacteria are listed in approximate order of frequency of isolation.

Table 8–3. Bacterial Isolates from Tracheal Swabs and Lungs of Clinically Healthy Dogs[6, 9]

Staphylococcus (coagulase-positive and -negative)
Streptococcus (α- and nonhemolytic)
Pasteurella multocida
Klebsiella pneumoniae
Enterobacter aerogenes
Acinetobacter spp.
Moraxella spp.
Corynebacterium spp.

organisms as nasal cavity and pharyngeal flora in each animal, but the presence of a certain range of flora can be predicted.

LOWER RESPIRATORY TRACT

The normal canine tracheobronchial tree and lung are not continuously sterile. Stud-ies using guarded culture swabs or samples of the lower trachea of clinically healthy dogs have found bacteria in 40% to 50% of samples (Table 8–3). Aerobic bacteria were isolated from 37% of lung samples, while only 10% of dogs examined had no growth from cultures of multiple samples of their lung tissue.[9] Most of the bacteria cultured from the trachea and lungs are identical to those found in the pharynx of those same dogs.

These data support the concept that oro-pharyngeal bacteria are frequently aspirated and may be present for an unknown interval in the normal tracheobronchial tree and lung. This bacterial population has the po-tential to cause or complicate clinical res-piratory infection and clouds interpretation of airway and lung cultures.

Upper Respiratory Tract Infections

BACTERIAL RHINITIS

Primary bacterial rhinitis is rare in the dog and cat. Bacterial rhinitis commonly is sec-ondary to nasal trauma or inhalation of for-eign material; reflux of liquids or food into the nose owing to pharyngeal or esophageal dysfunction; viral, fungal, or parasitic infec-tions; neoplasia; dental disease; oronasal fis-tula; or bacterial bronchopneumonia.

Clinical signs of bacterial rhinitis include sneezing, mucopurulent nasal discharge, ocular discharge secondary to nasolacrimal duct obstruction, and cough with gagging or retching. Epistaxis occurs infrequently with primary bacterial rhinitis but may be asso-ciated with underlying disease such as fun-gal rhinitis or neoplasia. Pawing at the face or nose indicates severe nasal irritation, often caused by foreign bodies or food lodged in the nasal cavity. Ulceration of the external nares and accumulation of crusted exudate occur in severe or chronic cases.

Because primary bacterial rhinitis is un-common, a thorough search for underlying problems should be performed. Diagnostic techniques include skull and nasal radio-graphs, endoscopic examination of the nasal passages, thorough oropharyngeal examina-tion, cytologic examination of exudate, bac-terial culture, and biopsy. These techniques are usually performed with the patient under general anesthesia.

The radiographic feature of chronic rhi-nitis is increased density of the nasal cavity due to excessive secretion accumulation. The turbinates are rarely destroyed, and the vomer bone is intact unless the disease is advanced. The frontal sinuses usually do not have increased density. Oblique views of the skull should be taken to evaluate the upper dental arcade.

The potential of rhinoscopy to detect sig-nificant abnormalities depends on the in-strument used and the amount of exudate or hemorrhage obscuring the field of view.[10] Rhinoscopy is invaluable in evaluating fun-gal rhinitis and a foreign body but is less helpful in nasal neoplasia. Purulent exudate and friable, hyperemic mucosa with or with-out ulceration will be viewed in bacterial rhinitis.

Cytologic specimens of lesions or exudate will be consistent with a septic, purulent exudate. Bacterial cultures are difficult to interpret because they often yield a mixed bacterial population similar to the normal nasal flora. Occasionally, a pure culture of a pathogen is helpful in choosing an appro-priate antimicrobial based on susceptibility testing. Biopsy of nasal turbinates and mucosa may be helpful in identifying nasal diseases associated with bacterial rhinitis.

Bacterial rhinitis will often resolve if the underlying problem, such as a foreign body, oronasal fistula, or dental disease, is corrected. In many patients, signs of rhinitis are temporary and may improve without treatment. Persistent or recurring signs require drug therapy for a limited period of time.

The external nares should be cleaned frequently of exudate. In the absence of specific culture results, administration of broad-spectrum antibacterials is indicated. Nebulization or vaporization will help mobilize secretions in the clogged nasal passages and soothe irritated mucous membranes. The use of sympathomimetic nasal decongestants such as phenylephrine or oxymethazoline in patients with copious serous or mucoid nasal discharge may be indicated. However, nasal decongestants are contraindicated in patients with thick, tenaceous, mucopurulent nasal discharges, because the exudate may become more viscous and difficult to expel. Glucocorticoid-responsive rhinitis associated with lymphoplasmacytic infiltrates of nasal mucosa, which may mimic bacterial rhinitis, was described.[11] The decision to institute glucocorticoid therapy is made after antibacterial therapy fails to improve clinical signs and no evidence of a primary infectious process is found during diagnostic evaluation.

CHRONIC SINUSITIS

Chronic bacterial sinusitis is uncommon in the dog, although mucus accumulation does occur when nasal diseases occlude normal drainage of the frontal sinus through the sinus osteum. Chronic sinusitis in cats occurs as a result of mucosal and bone damage secondary to feline viral respiratory infections (Chapter 27). Severe mucosal ulceration and turbinate destruction allow secondary bacterial infection of the nose and frontal sinuses. This syndrome is often called the "chronic snuffler" because the clinical signs in cats include chronic snorting and snuffling breathing, purulent nasal discharge, and sneezing. Many young cats with this syndrome are infected with feline leukemia virus (Chapter 26), which may influence their response to treatment.

Treatment is often frustrating because the underlying pathogenesis of the disease syndrome is poorly understood and many patients fail to respond to all forms of symptomatic therapy. The nasal cavity can be vigorously flushed with saline with or without antiseptic solutions to remove the exudate and inhibit bacterial growth. Drug penetration into the normal canine sinus is poor for the few antibacterials that have been evaluated and this is probably similar in cats. Drug penetration will obviously increase with inflammation, but sinusal levels are unknown. Broad-spectrum antibacterials are used for prolonged periods of time (2 to 4 months) following bacterial culture and susceptibility testing. Nasal decongestants may be helpful in individual cats, but they can exacerbate the problem by drying the exudate. Surgical turbinectomy and sinus trephination may be helpful to establish drainage of these areas and remove inspissated pockets of exudate.[12] Nasal flushing and systemic antibacterials can be used subsequent to surgical intervention. More aggressive surgical approaches have included sinus obliteration and reconstruction of apertures into the frontal sinuses.

TONSILLITIS AND PHARYNGITIS

Tonsillitis is usually bilateral but occasionally may occur as a unilateral disease when a foreign body is trapped in the tonsillar crypt. Primary tonsillitis usually occurs in young, small breed dogs that exhibit clinical signs of malaise, gagging cough with retching, fever, and inappetence. Inspection will often reveal a bright-red tonsil with an associated pharyngitis. Punctate hemorrhages on the tonsil itself and purulent exudate in the tonsillar crypt may also be visible. The tonsil will be friable and will easily bleed on manipulation. Tonsillitis is not always associated with gross enlargement of the tonsil; in fact, the benign appearance of the tonsil in some cases may be in sharp contrast with the severity of clinical signs. Specific bacteria associated with primary tonsillitis have not been studied.

Tonsillitis most commonly occurs secondarily to a preexisting disease process. Primary diseases commonly associated with a secondary tonsillitis include chronic vomiting or regurgitation, chronic gingivitis or periodontitis, tracheobronchitis, and nasopharyngeal irritation due to rhinitis.

Inflamed swollen tonsils are not an absolute indication for treatment. Elimination of preexisting problems usually results in resolution of the tonsillitis. If clinical signs are severe or persistent, then broad-spectrum antibacterial therapy for 10 to 14 days should be considered. Tonsillectomy is indicated when primary tonsillitis is a recurrent problem or hyperplastic tonsils protrude from the crypts, causing mechanical interference with breathing and swallowing.

Primary pharyngitis is uncommon but may occur concurrently with tonsillitis. Pharyngitis is usually a secondary problem as part of a widespread oral or systemic disease (see Chapter 9). Pharyngitis often accompanies viral or bacterial upper respiratory tract infections, pharyngeal foreign bodies and retropharyngeal abscesses. Treatment is aimed at underlying diseases such as removal of foreign bodies or surgical drainage of abscesses. Broad-spectrum antibacterial therapy may be used for 7 to 14 days.

LARYNGITIS

Laryngitis usually occurs as part of a widespread viral or bacterial respiratory infection such as canine tracheobronchitis or feline rhinotracheitis. Other common causes of acute noninfectious laryngitis are trauma to the larynx during endotracheal intubation and prolonged barking or dyspnea. Treatment is aimed at the coexisting infectious problem.

Lower Respiratory Tract Infections

TRACHEOBRONCHITIS

Canine infectious tracheobronchitis is a highly contagious respiratory disease of dogs and is characterized by coughing. This syndrome is associated with a wide variety of viral, mycoplasmal, and bacterial agents. Chapter 19 discusses this syndrome in detail. *Bordetella bronchiseptica* is the bacterial pathogen that has been shown to be a primary respiratory pathogen in dogs without accompanying viral or mycoplasma infection.

BACTERIAL PNEUMONIA

Etiology

Bacteria enter the lower respiratory tract primarily by the inhalation or aspiration routes or hematogenously. Whether or not a respiratory infection will develop depends on the complex interplay of many factors: size, inoculation site, and virulence of the organism and resistance of the host. Clinical conditions that predispose the animal to bacterial pneumonia include preexisting viral, mycoplasmal, or fungal respiratory infections; regurgitation, dysphagia, and vomiting; reduced levels of consciousness (stupor, coma); severe metabolic disorders (diabetes mellitus, uremia, hyperadrenocorticism); thoracic trauma or surgery; immunosuppressive therapy (anticancer chemotherapeutic agents, glucocorticoids); and functional or anatomic disorders (tracheal hypoplasia, primary ciliary dyskinesia). IV catheter–associated bacteremia is probably the most common cause of hematogenous pneumonia, especially in patients with severe underlying disease.

Bacterial pneumonia is more common in the dog than in the cat. *B. bronchiseptica* appears to be the principal primary bacterial pathogen of canine pneumonia.[13] *Streptococcus zooepidemicus* may also be a primary pathogen (see Group C Streptococcal Infections, Chapter 56).[14] Most isolates in dogs with pneumonia are thought to be opportunistic invaders, the most common of which are staphylococci, streptococci, *E. coli*, *P. multocida*, *Pseudomonas* spp. and *Klebsiella pneumoniae* (Table 8–4).[15–17] A single pathogen is isolated in the majority of cases, but mixed infections are common.[16,17] Gram-negative isolates predominate in both single and mixed infections.

Bacterial pathogens in feline pneumonia are poorly documented. *B. bronchiseptica*

Table 8–4. Most Common Isolates from the Lower Respiratory Tracts of Dogs with Suspected Bacterial Pneumonia[15–17]

MICROORGANISM	% OF DOGS
Bordetella bronchiseptica	7–22
Escherichia coli	17–29
Klebsiella spp.	10–15
Pasteurella spp.	7–34
Pseudomonas spp.	6–34
Staphylococcus spp.	9–20
Streptococcus spp.	15–27
Others	17–35

and *Pasteurella* spp. are reported most frequently.[18,19]

Clinical Findings

Historical findings and clinical signs of canine bacterial pneumonia include cough, fever, dyspnea, serous or mucopurulent nasal discharge, anorexia, depression, weight loss, and dehydration. Auscultation usually reveals abnormal breath sounds including increased intensity or bronchial breath sounds, crackles, and wheezes.[15]

Diagnosis

The diagnosis of bacterial pneumonia is confirmed by hematologic findings, thoracic radiographs, and microbiologic and cytologic examination of material from the tracheobronchial tree or lung. A neutrophilic leukocytosis with a left shift is frequently found on a CBC. Arterial blood gas values correlate well with the degree of physiologic disruption in patients with bacterial pneumonia and are a sensitive monitor of the patient's progress during treatment. Thoracic radiographs reveal an alveolar pattern characterized by increased pulmonary density in which margins are indistinct and in which air bronchograms may be seen. A patchy or lobar alveolar pattern will be present in a cranial ventral lung lobe distribution.

The definitive method of establishing a diagnosis of bacterial pneumonia is to obtain aspirates, washings, or brushings for microbiologic and cytologic examinations. Multiple procedures that bypass the oropharynx have been recommended to obtain these specimens. Blood cultures can also be helpful in identifying the etiologic agent causing bacterial pneumonia.

Transtracheal Aspiration. Because animals are unable to expectorate sputum, transtracheal washing and aspiration is a safe, simple, and clinically valuable method for obtaining tracheobronchial material for culture and cytologic examination. The technique is well tolerated by most dogs and cats, and requires only minimal restraint of the unanesthetized patient. The equipment and technique are well documented.[20]

Although complications from transtracheal washing and aspiration are uncommon, the procedure is not without risk. As with the majority of invasive diagnostic procedures, the risks are significantly decreased with experience. The procedure can be performed in cats and small dogs but is considerably more difficult. Transtracheal washing should not be attempted in the fractious or uncooperative patient without adequate chemical and manual restraint.

The most common complication associated with transtracheal washing is subcutaneous emphysema. This occurs when persistent coughing or dyspnea causes air to leak from the puncture site into the cervical subcutaneous tissues. Other complications include endotracheal hemorrhage, tracheal laceration, cardiac arrythmias, and infection at the puncture site.

Preparation of material for cytologic evaluation can be done by several methods. Visible strands of exudate may be teased onto a microscope slide, smeared, and stained. Small quantities of material can be centrifuged and smears made of the sediment. New methylene blue wet mounts and Wright-Giemsa or Gram stains of air-dried smears can be used for identification of cellular elements and bacteria. Cytologic evaluation of tracheobronchial secretions is usually consistent with a purulent exudate. Bacteria are often not demonstrable, and their absence in cytologic specimens from transtracheal aspirations does not rule out bacterial pneumonia.

An aliquot of aspirated material can be cultured directly for aerobic and anaerobic bacteria. Anaerobic culture is indicated only when aspiration pneumonia or pulmonary abscess formation is suspected. Secretions that coat the distal end of the catheter can be cultured if the amount of aspirated material is minimal. In a recent study, sensitivity of transtracheal washing and aspiration for recovery of bacteria was good, but specificity was poor.[21]

Bronchoscopy. Tracheobronchoscopy is valuable for obtaining brush catheter specimens for cytologic and microbiologic examination. The procedure requires that the patient be maintained under general anesthesia, which may be of concern in patients with bacterial pneumonia. IV anesthetic agents and a mouth speculum will allow a thorough tracheobronchial examination with a rigid bronchoscope passed through the mouth. Brush catheters and suction cannulas may be passed through the lumen of the rigid bronchoscope to obtain specimens.

The transoral approach with a flexible fiberoptic bronchoscope inserted through an endotracheal tube is preferred. The patient is anesthetized using standard procedures, is intubated, and is maintained on inhalation anesthesia. An endotracheal tube Y adapter allows oxygen and anesthetic gas to flow to the patient while the flexible endoscope passes through the endotracheal tube and into the trachea. This technique is successful in moderate- to large-sized dogs during lengthy procedures. Small dogs and cats are given an IV anesthetic, and a flexible or small diameter rigid fiberoptic endoscope is passed directly into the trachea. Brush catheters are passed through the biopsy channel of the endoscope to obtain specimens.

The advantages of tracheobronchoscopy are numerous when compared with other diagnostic techniques. Endoscopy allows the direct visualization of the tracheobronchial tree and the lesions associated with bacterial pneumonia, thereby allowing a better assessment of the patient's clinical status and prognosis. The cytologic preparations obtained by mucosal brushings through the endoscope are superior to those obtained from transtracheal washing and aspiration.

Because of contamination from the oropharynx, bacterial cultures obtained with sterile, open-end, brush-in-catheter systems passed through the endoscope have been considered unreliable in the past. A commercially available catheter (Microbiology Specimen Brush, Microvasive Inc., Milford, MA) that enhances the ability to obtain reliable cultures of lower airway secretions through a bronchoscope has been developed. This system consists of a sterile brush contained within a telescoping double catheter occluded by a polyethylene glycol plug. This system is passed through the instrumentation channel of the bronchoscope. The brush is extended into secretions to be cultured and then retracted into the inner catheter. The entire brush-in-telescope, double-catheter system is removed from the endoscope. The brush is advanced out of the catheter, where the wire is transected with sterile scissors, and the brush is placed in trypticase soy broth. The only disadvantage is the expense for a catheter system that can be used only once.

Fine-Needle Lung Aspiration. Transthoracic fine-needle aspiration can be used to procure material for microbial culture and cytologic examination directly from the lung. Fine-needle aspiration is best performed after routine diagnostic procedures such as transtracheal washing have proved negative. The technique, contraindications, and complications have been well documented in other references.[20]

A study of diagnostic procedures in a canine model of streptococcal pneumonia found that transthoracic fine-needle lung aspiration had the highest sensitivity and specificity for bacterial recovery when compared with transtracheal washing, flexible fiberoptic bronchoscopy, transbronchial lung biopsy, or blind catheter brushing.[21] Sensitivity was enhanced when "dogside" culturing was performed rather than sending the samples to the microbiology laboratory. Complications of percutaneous fine-needle aspiration are common and potentially serious. Pneumothorax is the primary complication, with a 10% to 30% incidence rate reported in one study.[21]

Blood Cultures. These have been recommended in people with bacterial pneumonia to help isolate the infectious agent. Documented bacteremia is also thought to be a poor prognostic finding. No studies in animals that document the value of blood cultures in establishing a prognosis or isolating the bacterial agent in cases of pneumonia exist. One study has confirmed that 50% of dogs with experimentally induced streptococcal pneumonia were blood culture–positive within 48 hours of onset of clinical signs.[21]

PULMONARY ABSCESS

Pulmonary abscesses, necrotic areas of lung parenchyma containing purulent material usually produced by pyogenic infection, are uncommon in dogs and cats. Most arise from aspiration of oropharyngeal or gastric contents and are termed primary lung abscess. Secondary lung abscess results from a primary underlying process such as bronchial obstruction, septic or heartworm thromboemboli, airway parasites, foreign body, bullous emphysema, tuberculous cavities, or neoplasia. Obligate anaerobic bacteria are identified more frequently than aerobes, but mixed infections are common. *Mycoplasma* spp. have also been recovered in a cat.[22]

The clinical signs in pulmonary abscess formation depend on the etiology but closely resemble those of chronic bacterial pneumonia. Clinical findings include weight loss, chronic fever, cough, and hemoptysis. Hematologic findings include leukocytosis with a left shift, anemia, and rarely hypoproteinemia. An abscess usually will appear on a thoracic radiograph as an ill-defined pulmonary nodule or mass, with or without cavitation. Abscesses are often indistinguishable from granulomas, traumatic bullae, tumors, or pneumatocysts. Cytologic examination of brushings or aspirations is consistent with a septic or nonseptic purulent exudate.

Lung abscesses are usually treated without drainage, using long-term antibacterial therapy. Choice of antibacterials should be based on culture and susceptibility findings. Clindamycin appears to be the antibiotic of choice in treatment of human anaerobic lung abscess.[23]

Eugonic Fermenter-4 (EF-4) Infection

Group EF-4 is a collection of unclassified bacterial strains designated by the Centers for Disease Control, Atlanta, Georgia. These bacteria, ecologically and culturally similar to *Pasteurella* spp., have been isolated as commensal flora from the oral cavity of dogs and cats (see Table 9–1) and from people as contaminating organisms of dog and cat bite wounds. The precise means by which EF-4 organisms produce respiratory or systemic infection is unknown, but inhalation or hematogenous dissemination from an oral site is suspected. Concurrent immunosuppression may be important for the organism to colonize other regions of the body.

Both domestic[24–26] and exotic[27, 28, 28a] cats

and domestic dogs[26, 29] have been affected. Clinical signs such as anorexia, hypersalivation, and dyspnea have been the main signs of respiratory infection in dogs and cats. Sudden death, with or without premonitory signs, has been noted in some cases. Abdominal distention from exudative peritonitis was noted in one pup.

Diagnosis has been made primarily by culture of the abscess wounds at necropsy. The organism can be cultivated on blood agar, incubated aerobically or anaerobically, and classified by its biochemical reactions.[24] In a few cases in cats, leukopenia and nonregenerative anemia have been found premortem. Multifocal nodular abscess formation is the typical pathologic finding in the lungs. The lesions are grossly indistinguishable from multifocal neoplasms or granulomas. Extrapulmonary lesions have included similar multifocal abscesses in the liver and peritoneal cavity and lymph nodes. The abscesses are histologically characterized by neutrophilic and mononuclear infiltrates surrounding sometimes visible colonies of gram-negative bacteria.

Therapy for this type of infection is unknown but can be expected to be similar to that of pasteurellosis (see Chapter 59 and Table 59–1).

THERAPY OF LOWER AIRWAY INFECTIONS

Unlike treatment of upper airway infections, that for lower tract infections must be aggressive, and systemically effective antimicrobials must be used. Drug penetration into consolidated lung tissues is more effective systemically than by topical means.

Antibiotics

Oral or parenteral antibacterials are the principal therapy for lower airway bacterial infections. It is unrealistic to expect any single antibacterial to be routinely effective against the wide variety of organisms causing bacterial pneumonia. The most important criterion for selection of an antibacterial is identification of the bacterial organism. Substantially more patients recover if antibacterial therapy is administered according to culture results and in vitro susceptibility testing than if empirically administered.[15]

Initial choices of antibacterials can be based on the shape of bacteria noted on airway or lung cytologic preparations. Cocci are usually staphylococci or streptococci. Rods are usually members of the family Enterobacteriacae, which are the most unpredictable with respect to antibacterial agents (Table 8–5).[16] Levels of antibacterials in airway secretions after oral or parenteral administration are much lower than serum levels. Therefore, systemic antibacterials should be administered in high doses for long periods of time so that maximum concentrations are reached in lung tissue and airway secretions.

Hydration

Maintenance of normal systemic hydration is an important therapeutic objective in patients with bacterial pneumonia. Dehydration hinders mucociliary clearance and secretion mobilization because normal respiratory secretions are more than 90% water.

Table 8–5. Antimicrobial Therapy for Lower Airway Bacterial Infections[a]

GRAM-POSITIVE COCCI	Amp(amox)icillin, chloramphenicol, gentamicin, trimethoprim-sulfonamide, first generation cephalosporins
GRAM-NEGATIVE RODS	Amikacin, chloramphenicol, gentamicin, trimethoprim-sulfonamide, fluoroquinolones
Bordetella	Chloramphenicol, tetracycline, gentamicin, kanamycin
ANAEROBES	Amp(amox)icillin, penicillin, second or third generation cephalosporins, clindamycin, metronidazole

[a]Consult Appendix 14 for appropriate dosages.

Aerosol

The goal of aerosol therapy is to mobilize secretions by adding water to the mucociliary blanket. A nebulizer that produces particles between 0.5 and 3.0 μm must be used to ensure that water is deposited in the lower airways. Water vaporizers or humidifiers are inadequate for this reason. The animal is placed in an enclosed chamber and a bland aerosol (normal saline) is nebulized into the chamber. The animal should be treated several times daily for 30 to 45 minutes per treatment. Since bronchoconstriction invariably develops, pretreatment with bronchodilators is recommended.

Nebulization with bland aerosols has subjectively resulted in more rapid resolution of cases of canine bronchopneumonia when used in conjunction with physiotherapy and systemic antimicrobials.[30] Physiotherapy should always be used immediately after aerosolization to enhance secretion clearance. Physiotherapy methods include mild forced exercise, increasing cough frequency by chest wall coupage or tracheal manipulation, and postural drainage.[24] Aerosol administration of nonabsorbable antimicrobials such as aminoglycosides substantially reduces the number of bacteria in airways. Routine intratracheal or aerosol administration of antibacterials is not recommended.

Supportive

Animals with severe tachypnea, dyspnea, or marked hypoxemia ($PaO_2 < 60$ torr) require oxygen therapy. The early period of highest mortality with bacterial pneumonia corresponds to the period of greatest hypoxemia. The oxygen should be humidified to prevent drying of respiratory membranes. Oxygen can be administered by oxygen cage, mechanical ventilator, intratracheal cannula, or nasal catheter.[31] Drugs such as antitussives and antihistamines that inhibit mucokinesis and exudate removal from the respiratory tract are contraindicated with bacterial pneumonia.

Pleural Infections

Purulent pleuritis, pyothorax, and thoracic empyema describe septic processes of the pleural cavity resulting in exudate accumulation.

ETIOLOGY

Pleural infections are usually polymicrobic in nature. There is a high incidence of obligate anaerobic bacteria as sole pathogens or in combination with aerobic-facultative and anaerobic bacteria. Obligate anaerobic bacteria and gram-positive filamentous organisms such as *Nocardia* and *Actinomyces* are most commonly isolated from dogs with pyothorax (see Chapter 53). Feline pyothorax is associated with a high incidence of pure obligate anaerobic bacteria and infection with *Pasteurella* spp. Other bacterial, fungal, and yeast organisms isolated from pleural exudate of the dog and cat are summarized in Table 8–6.[32–39] Sources of bacterial pleural infections are not identified in most cases but include penetrating thoracic wounds; migrating foreign bodies; esophageal perforation; hematogenous spread; lung parasites; extension from cervical, lumbar, mediastinal or pulmonary infections; and iatrogenic causes.

CLINICAL FINDINGS

Pyothorax occurs most commonly in young adult, male, nonpurebred cats and adult large-breed dogs. Clinical signs result

Table 8–6. Specific Etiologic Agents Isolated from Pleural Infections in Dogs and Cats[32–39]

MOST COMMONLY ISOLATED	LESS COMMONLY ISOLATED
Actinomyces	Aspergillus
Bacteroides	Blastomyces
Corynebacterium (aerobic	Candida albicans
and anaerobic	Clostridium
Propionibacterium)	Cryptococcus
Fusobacterium	Escherichia coli
Nocardia	Enterobacter
Pasteurella	Histoplasma
Staphylococci (aerobic	Klebsiella
and anaerobic	Proteus
Peptococcus)	Pseudomonas
Streptococci (aerobic and	
anaerobic	
Peptostreptococcus)	

from restrictive respiratory disease, including increased respiratory rate, shallow respirations, dyspnea, and orthopnea. Other signs include exercise intolerance, lethargy, anorexia, and fever. Physical examination reveals muffled heart sounds, decreased breath sounds, and hyporesonant (dull) percussion sounds, especially over the ventral portions of the thorax. Chronic or severe infections result in a dehydrated, debilitated, or hypothermic patient.

DIAGNOSIS

A diagnosis of pyothorax is confirmed by hematology, thoracic radiographs, and thoracocentesis with cytologic evaluation and culture of pleural fluid. Neutrophilic leukocytosis with or without a left shift is the most common hematologic finding. Leukogram results do not correlate with the severity of the underlying infection, however, and leukocyte counts within or lower than the reference range are found with some frequency.[40] Radiographic signs of free pleural fluid include increased hazy density of the lung fields (ventral portions of lung fields on lateral view), which obscures the cardiac silhouette; retraction of lobar borders from the chest wall; visibility of interlobar fissures; and rounding or filling of the costophrenic angles.

Cytologic evaluation of pleural fluid is usually consistent with a septic or nonseptic exudate. Cytomorphology of the neutrophil is most helpful in determining whether pleural fluid should be cultured.[41] Aerobic and anaerobic culture of pleural fluid is done whenever neutrophil degeneration is observed, regardless of whether or not bacteria are seen cytologically.

THERAPY

Treatment of pyothorax should be prompt and aggressive. Initial goals of therapy include relief of respiratory embarrassment via thoracocentesis, appropriate fluid therapy, supportive care, and systemic antibacterials. Local treatment is then initiated with pleural drainage and lavage by permanent tube thoracostomy. Advantages of closed chest drainage and lavage include avoiding frequent needle thoracocentesis, facilitating pleural fluid sampling to monitor therapeutic response, and allowing direct instillation of isotonic lavage fluid into the pleural space. Disadvantages include maintaining drain placement and patency and risking pneumothorax and chest wall infection. Mortality appears to be higher in cases treated with multiple thoracocentesis and antibacterials alone than in those treated with tube thoracostomy.[40] The average length of chest tube drainage is 3 to 7 days.

Systemic antimicrobial therapy is ineffective without lavage and drainage of the infected pleural cavity. No single antibacterial agent will inhibit the wide variety of facultative and obligate anaerobic bacteria associated with pyothorax. Penicillin or penicillin derivatives are often used because they are effective against obligate anaerobic, *Pasteurella*, and *Actinomyces* infections. Systemic antibacterial therapy should be continued for at least 4 to 6 weeks. Lack of significant improvement or the formation of lung abscesses or radiographic evidence of fluid encapsulation indicates surgical exploration or lobectomy.

References

1. Smith JE: The aerobic bacteria of the nose and tonsils of healthy dogs. *J Comp Pathol* 71:428–433, 1961.
2. Clapper WE, Meade GH: Normal flora of the nose, throat, and lower intestine of dogs. *J Bacteriol* 85:643–648, 1963.
3. Bailie WE, Stowe EC, Schmitt AM: Aerobic bacterial flora of oral and nasal fluids of canines with reference to bacteria associated with bites. *J Clin Microbiol* 7:223–231, 1978.
4. Balish E, Cleven D, Brown J, et al: Nose, throat and fecal flora of beagle dogs housed in "locked" or "open" environments. *Appl Environ Microbiol* 34:207–221, 1977.
5. Brennan PC, Simskins RC: Throat flora of a closed colony of beagles. *Proc Soc Exp Biol Med* 134:556–570, 1970.
6. McKiernan BC, Smith AR, Kissil M: Bacterial isolates from the lower trachea of clinically healthy dogs. *J Am Anim Hosp Assoc* 20:139–142, 1984.
7. Baldrias L, Frost AJ, O'Boyle D: The isolation of *Pasteurella*-like organisms from the tonsillar region of dogs and cats. *J Small Anim Pract* 29:63–68, 1988.
8. Abramson AL, Isenberg HD, McDermott LM: Microbiology of the canine nasal cavities. *Rhinology* 18:143–150, 1980.
9. Lindsey JO, Pierce AK: An examination of the microbiologic flora of normal lung of the dog. *Am Rev Resp Dis* 117:501–505, 1978.
10. Sullivan M: Rhinoscopy: a diagnostic aid? *J Small Anim Pract* 28:839–844, 1987.
11. Burgener DC, Slocombe RF, Zerbe CA: Lymphoplasmacytic rhinitis in five dogs. *J Am Anim Hosp Assoc* 23:565–568, 1987.
12. Anderson GI: The treatment of chronic sinusitis in 6 cats by ethmoid conchal curretage and autogenous fat graft sinus ablation. *Vet Surg* 16:131, 1987.
13. Bemis DA, Carmichael LE, Appel MJG: Naturally occurring respiratory disease in a kennel caused by *Bordetella bronchiseptica*. *Cornell Vet* 67:282–293, 1977.
14. Garnett NL, Eydelloth RS, Swindle MM, et al: Hemorrhagic streptococcal pneumonia in newly procured research dogs. *J Am Vet Med Assoc* 181:1371–1374, 1982.
15. Thayer GW, Robinson SK: Bacterial bronchopneumonia in the dog: a review of 42 cases. *J Am Anim Hosp Assoc* 20:731–735, 1984.
16. Hirsch DC: Bacteriology of the lower respiratory tract. In Kirk RW (ed): *Current Veterinary Therapy 9.* Philadelphia, WB Saunders, 1986, pp 247–250.
17. Jones SD, McKiernan BC: Lower respiratory tract disease in the dog: bacterial cultures and sensitivities. *J Am Anim Hosp Assoc.* In press, 1988.
18. Snyder SB, Fisk SK, Fox JG, et al: Respiratory tract disease associated with *Bordetella bronchiseptica* infection in cats. *J Am Vet Med Assoc* 103:293–294, 1973.
19. Drolet R, Kenefick KB, Hakomaki MR, et al: Isolation of group eugonic fermenter-4 bacteria from a cat with multifocal suppurative pneumonia. *J Am Vet Med Assoc* 189:311–312, 1986.
20. Roudebush P: Diagnostics for respiratory diseases. In Kirk RW (ed): *Current Veterinary Therapy 8.* Philadelphia, WB Saunders, 1983, pp 222–230.
21. Moser KM, Maurer J, Jassy L, et al: Sensitivity, specificity and risk of diagnostic procedures in a canine model of *Streptococcus pneumoniae* pneumonia. *Am Rev Resp Dis* 125:436–442, 1982.
22. Crisp MS, Birchard SJ, Lawrence AE, et al: Pulmonary abscess caused by a *Mycoplasma* sp. in a cat. *J Am Vet Med Assoc* 191:340–342, 1987.
23. Levison ME, Mangura CT, Lorber B, et al: Clindamycin compared with penicillin for the treatment of anaerobic lung abscess. *Ann Intern Med* 98:466–471, 1983.
24. Drolet R, Kenefick KB, Hakomaki MR, et al: Isolation of group eugonic fermenter-4 bacteria from a cat with multifocal suppurative pneumonia. *J Am Vet Med Assoc* 189:311–312, 1986.
25. Jang SS, Demartini JC, Henrickson RV, et al: Focal necrotizing pneumonia in cats associated with a gram-negative eugonic fermenting bacterium. *Cornell Vet* 63:446–454, 1973.
26. McParland PJ, O'Hagan J, Pearson GR, et al: Pathological changes associated with group EF-4 bacteria in the lungs of a dog and cat. *Vet Rec* 111:336–338, 1982.
27. Lloyd J, Allen JG: The isolation of group EF-4 bacteria from a case of granulomotous pneumonia in a tiger cub. *Aust Vet J* 56:399–400, 1980.
28. Fenwick BW, Jang SS, Gillespie DS: Pneumonia caused by a eugonic fermenting bacterium in an African lion. *J Am Vet Med Assoc* 183:1315–1317, 1983.
28a. Perry AW, Schlingman DW: Pneumonia associated with eugonic fermenter-4 bacteria in two Chinese leopard cats. *Can Vet J* 29:921–922, 1988.
29. Valentine BA, Porter WP: Multiple hepatic ab-

scesses and peritonitis caused by eugonic fermenter-4 bacilli in a pup. *J Am Vet Med Assoc* 183:1324–1325, 1983.

30. McKiernan BC: Respiratory therapeutics. *In Proceedings*. ACVIM Forum, Washington, DC, 1987, pp 165–172.

31. Fitzpatrick RK, Crowe DT: Nasal oxygen administration in dogs and cats: experimental and clinical investigations. *J Am Anim Hosp Assoc* 22:293–300, 1986.

32. Withrow SJ, Fenner WR, Wilkins RJ: Closed chest drainage and lavage for treatment of pyothorax in the cat. *J Am Anim Hosp Assoc* 11:90–94, 1975.

33. Sherding RJ: Pyothorax in the cat. *Compend Cont Educ Pract Vet* 1:247–252, 1979.

34. Hardie EM, Barsanti JA: Treatment of canine actinomycosis. *J Am Vet Med Assoc* 180:537–540, 1982.

35. Jonas LD: Feline pyothorax: a retrospective study of twenty cases. *J Am Anim Hosp Assoc* 19:865–871, 1983.

36. Robertson SA, Stoddent ME, Evan RJ, et al: Thoracic empyema in the dog; a report of twenty-two cases. *J Small Anim Pract* 24:103–119, 1983.

37. McCaw D, Franklin R, Fales W, et al: Pyothorax caused by *Candida albicans* in a cat. *J Am Vet Med Assoc* 185:311–312, 1984.

38. Hirsch DC, Indivieri MC, Jang SS, et al: Changes in prevalence and susceptibility of obligate anaerobes in clinical veterinary practice. *J Am Vet Med Assoc* 186:1086–1089, 1985.

39. Orton EC: Pleura and pleural space. *In* Slatter DH (ed): *Textbook of Small Animal Surgery*. Philadelphia, WB Saunders, 1985, pp 557–558.

40. Bauer T: Pyothorax. *In* Kirk RW (ed): *Current Veterinary Therapy 9*. Philadelphia, WB Saunders, 1986, pp 292–295.

41. Cantwell HD, Rebar AH, Allen AR: Pleural effusion in the dog: principles for diagnosis. *J Am Anim Hosp Assoc* 19:227–232, 1983.

9 GASTROINTESTINAL AND INTRA-ABDOMINAL INFECTIONS

Craig E. Greene

ORAL CAVITY

Normal Microflora

The normal microbial flora of the canine and feline oral cavity is composed of a wide variety of both aerobic and facultative bacteria (Table 9–1). The frequency with which individual species are isolated depends on culture methods, sampling site, and breed and individual differences. From a clinical standpoint, bacterial culture of specimens from the oropharyngeal region is meaningless because of the diversity of commensal organisms and the lack of accurate quantitative methods. Antimicrobial agents used in treating oral infections should be chosen with the composition of the resident microflora in mind (see also Chapter 58).

Gingivitis

Gingivitis or periodontitis with inflammation and recession of the perialveolar gum margins is a common finding in dogs and cats.[5b] It is usually caused by the excessive accumulation of dental plaque or tartar resulting from the deposition of by-products from the breakdown of foodstuffs and saliva by normal resident microflora (Fig. 9–1). The plaque microflora of dogs with periodontal disease has been shown to shift to increased numbers of obligative anaerobic organisms such as *Bacteroides asaccharolyticus* and reduced numbers of streptococci, enterococci, and staphylococci as compared with normal flora.[5c] Salivary microflora, which differs from plaque microflora, remains relatively constant in the presence of periodontal disease. Gingival hypertrophy and alveolar abscess formation are sequelae of tartar formation. The type of microflora present, the diet, and the animal's chewing habits may be important in the formation of tartar. Hard diets have been shown to reduce the incidence of tartar accumulation. Treatment includes the extraction of severely affected teeth, debriding necrotic or proliferative gum margins, and the scaling of tartar from less severely involved dental surfaces. Tetracycline, metronidazole, and chlorhexidine have been evaluated for treatment of periodontitis in experimentally affected dogs.[6] Tetracycline and metronidazole have been beneficial in reducing dental tartar or preventing its reformation when they have been used with or without mechanical cleansing (Table 9–2). After 1 year of tetracycline therapy, dogs with periodontal disease had less alveolar bone resorption than untreated controls.[7] Metronidazole therapy has had similar beneficial effects.[8] Flushing the dental surfaces once daily with 0.1% to 0.2% chlorhexidine[9] or alternate-day brushing[10] may delay the accumulation of tartar. Unfortunately, chlorhexidine may stain the teeth light blue, but a commercial product formulated especially for dental purposes (Nolvadent, Fort Dodge Labs, Fort Dodge, IA) does not produce staining. Numerous cleansers and brushes have been developed for daily brushing of dogs' teeth, and they warrant consideration when tartar is a problem.

125

Table 9–1. Microflora Most Commonly Isolated from the Oral Cavities of Clinically Healthy Dogs[a, 1-5]

ORGANISM	SITES
Aerobes	
Gram-Negative	
Neisseria	B
Escherichia coli	B
Pasteurella	B
Pseudomonas	B
Proteus	T
Moraxella	N
Acinetobacter	N
DF-2	N
EF-4	N
Ilj	N
Gram-Positive	
Nonhemolytic streptococci	B
β-Hemolytic streptococci	B
Staphylococcus epidermidis	B
S. aureus (intermedius)	B
Corynebacterium	N
Bacillus	B
Actinomyces	N
Anaerobes	
Bacteroides	U
Fusobacterium	U
Propionibacterium	U
Peptostreptococcus	U
Clostridium	U
Veillonella	U
Simonsiella	N
Candida	T
Mycoplasma	T

[a]B = tonsillar and nontonsillar; N = nontonsillar, supragingival scrapings; T = tonsillar; U = unspecified sites.

Bacteremia Associated with Dental Disease

Bacteremia associated with dental manipulations may be clinically nonsymptomatic, may cause acute septicemia, or subsequently may result in bacterial endocarditis or localized tissue infections. The severity of bacteremia frequently correlates with the degree of periodontitis present. Even though they are not primarily pathogenic, many anaerobes may establish themselves in tissue injured or devitalized by routine surgical procedures, sutures, or foreign implants.

Dental procedures should not be performed at the same time as other surgical procedures, because surgical wounds have been infected by bacteria released when simultaneous dentistry is performed. Whenever dentistry is performed, prophylactic administration of antimicrobial drugs is recommended (Table 9–2). Penicillin is the drug of choice for humans undergoing dental cleaning; however, IV administration of aqueous penicillin during ultrasonic dentistry in dogs did not alter the prevalence of bacteremia before or after dental manipulation.[11] On the basis of in vitro susceptibility testing, chloramphenicol, cephalosporins, erythromycin, and gentamicin have been recommended. All except erythromycin can be given parenterally while the animal is anesthetized. Gentamicin should never be used alone because it is relatively ineffective against anaerobic bacteria. For these reasons, chloramphenicol or penicillin derivatives or cephalosporins with or without gentamicin are recommended. Appendix 14 and Table 9–2 should be consulted for appropriate dosages. Therapy should begin no earlier than 4 hours prior to the dental procedure and preferably should be continued during it by IV drip. The most critical period is immediately during the procedure. Drug administration should be terminated no longer than 12 hours following the procedure because no further benefits are gained, and the risk that antibiotic-resistant bacteria will cause infections is increased.

Necrotizing Ulcerative Gingivostomatitis

In people, acute necrotizing ulcerative gingivostomatitis (ANUG), or trench mouth, is

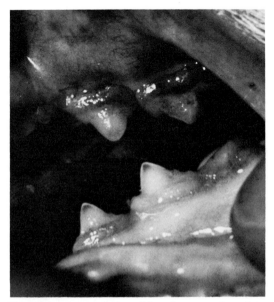

Figure 9–1. Accumulation of dental tartar and resulting perialveolar gingivitis in a cat.

Table 9–2. Systemic Therapy for Oral Infections[a]

DRUG	SPECIES	DOSE[b] (mg/kg)	ROUTE	INTERVAL (hours)	DURATION (days)
Stomatitis-Gingivitis					
Metronidazole	D	10–15	PO	12	10–28
	C	8	PO	12	7–14
	C	5–10	PO	8	7–14
Tetracycline	D	20–40	PO	12–24	prn
Clindamycin	B	5–10	PO	12	7–10
Amp(amox)icillin	B	20	PO	12	14–21
Ketoconazole	B	5–10	PO	12	7–10
Prednis(ol)one	B	0.5	PO	12	7–14
Methylprednisolone acetate	C	0.5–1	IL[c]	Once	14–28
Triamcinolone acetonide	C	0.1–0.2	IL[c]	Once	14–28
Dental Prophylaxis					
Penicillin	B	20,000 U/kg	IV	[d]	1
Chloramphenicol	B	15–25	IV	[d]	
Gentamicin	B	2	IV, SC	[d]	1
Cephapirin	B	20	IV	[d]	

[a]D = dog, C = cat, B = dog and cat, IV = intravenous, SC = subcutaneous, PO = oral, IL = intralesional, prn = as needed.

[b]Dose per administration at specified interval, expressed as mg/kg unless otherwise stated.

[c]Injection done under anesthesia as a last resort.

[d]Only given once beginning just prior to or during anesthesia for dental procedures.

a syndrome with multiple causes, characterized by oral ulcerations. Opportunistic overgrowth of oral microflora occurs in many diseases when immune defenses are impaired or oral ulcerations develop.[11a, 11b] The causes of ANUG in dogs and cats are probably equally diverse and include many acquired immunosuppressive conditions, such as diabetes mellitus, persistent neutropenia, feline leukemia virus (FeLV) and feline immunodeficiency virus (FIV, formerly FTLV) infections, and canine Cushing's disease. A virus antigenically related to feline calicivirus (FCV) was found to cause transient gingivitis and glossitis in a dog.[12] As in people, psychologic and physical stresses may be involved in some animals. Bristles of plant awns can induce a similar syndrome when they become embedded in gingival tissues.[13]

Cats subclinically infected with FCV and feline rhinotracheitis virus may relapse with overt upper respiratory infection or oral ulceration following stress or immunosuppression such as with concurrent FIV infection. Stress appears to reduce the amount of fibronectin, a receptor protein, on epithelial cells for gram-positive organisms. Thus, overgrowth with gram-negative bacteria may develop. Hard, dry cat food also appears to have a role in exacerbating palatine ulceration in cats with acute FCV infection.[14] Chronic feline ulceroproliferative stomatitis

(faucitis) has been associated with persistent FCV and FIV infections in cats.[15, 15a]

Regardless of its cause, oral ulceration presents a particular clinical syndrome characterized by reluctance to eat, hypersalivation, halitosis, and evidence of pain on opening the mouth. Hemorrhage may occur spontaneously or following oral manipulation. Although rare, systemic signs may include fever, lymphadenopathy, and depression. Ulcers may be distributed throughout the oral cavity but are usually concentrated on the dental, labial, and gingival surfaces (Fig. 9–2). Ulcers may be covered by a pseudomembranous exudate. White pseudomembranous plaques can be found in cases of candidial stomatitis. In many neutropenic cats infected with FeLV, the ulcers characteristically have minimal exudation, can progress rapidly, and may result in sloughing of large portions of the caudal oropharynx or larynx.

Faucitis is characterized by vesicular, ulcerative, and later proliferative lesions in the mucosa, usually accompanied by lymphoplasmacytic or eosinophilic infiltrations in the tissue of the caudal pharynx at the glossopharyngeal arch (fauces).[15, 16] It frequently appears among a number of cats within a household and tends to be recurrent following the initial treatment or to be unresponsive to therapy. In chronic stages, pro-

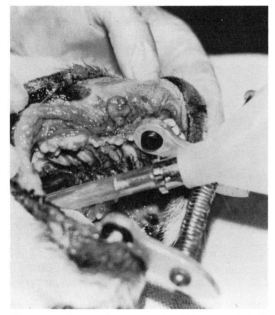

Figure 9–2. Diffuse ANUG in a dog. (Courtesy of Dr. D. W. Scott, New York State College of Veterinary Medicine, Ithaca, NY.)

liferation of granulation tissue forms large masses in the caudal pharynx (Fig. 9–3).

Animals with persistent stomatitis should first be examined for excessive accumulation of dental tartar. Systemic or underlying diseases will usually be apparent from the results of urinalysis and routine hematology, biochemistry, and FeLV and FIV testing.

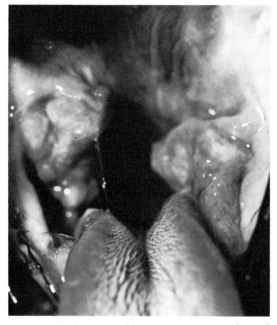

Figure 9–3. Chronic proliferative stomatitis in the oral cavity of a cat.

Neutropenia or neutrophil function defects are a common underlying cause of oral ulceration. Polyclonal hyperglobulinemia is often present in cats affected with chronic stomatitis and lymphoplasmacytic infiltrations. Results of bacterial cultures and susceptibility testing or oral cytology should be correlated with cytologic and histologic findings since most cultured organisms are merely overcolonizing already damaged tissues. Specimens for FCV isolation can be taken by rubbing sterile swabs on the gums, soft palate, and oropharynx and by placing them directly into viral transport or culture media (see Chapter 14).

Underlying disease processes and other causes of ANUG should be eliminated or treated when they are encountered. Plant awns or foreign material embedded in the gums can be scraped away with a scalpel when the gum margins are debrided. Symptomatic therapy of stomatitis includes changing the diet to soft or bland foods, both to encourage eating and to lessen the mechanical irritation of ulcers. With chronic, nonhealing ulcers, it is often beneficial to remove dental tartar and normal or diseased teeth in affected regions of the mouth. In cats, removal and biopsy of chronic proliferative lesions may be required. Some lesions that arise adjacent to and later involve the tonsillar crypt may develop into squamous cell carcinomas. Systemic therapies for stomatitis are summarized in Table 9–2. Swabbing and flushing of teeth, gums, and lesions throughout the oral cavity with 1% hydrogen peroxide can be initiated in the hospital and continued at home by the owner, although excessive use of peroxide may cause vomiting. Use of astringents such as tincture of nitromersol or thimersal, potassium permanganate, and organic iodine compounds has been advocated. Cauterization with silver nitrate or dilute acid solutions also has been recommended but may interfere with healing and epithelization. Vitamins B and C are usually administered on an empirical basis.

Topical or systemic antimicrobial therapy appears to hasten the resolution of ANUG significantly, perhaps by inhibiting the overgrowth of fusiform and spirochetal bacteria that colonize and impair healing of ulcerated lesions in the oral cavity (see Table 9–2). Candidial stomatitis is best treated by topical application of antifungal drugs, such as clotrimazole or nystatin (see also Table 63–3), or with systemic ketoconazole. Historically, tetracycline, chloramphenicol, ampicillin, or penicillin solutions have been applied topically for bacterial stomatitis, although the first two drugs frequently cause anorexia in cats. Systemic antibiotic therapy directed primarily against anaerobic bacteria appears to be more efficacious in treating stomatitis. Relapse may occur in some cases following termination of antimicrobial therapy, and a repeated course of therapy may be required.

Prednisone may be administered when antimicrobial therapy is being discontinued in an attempt to break the cycle of recurrent stomatitis. Glucocorticoid therapy may be needed if an autoimmune disease such as pemphigus is suspected; however, the immunosuppression induced by glucocorticoids can itself cause or exacerbate some cases of ANUG.

In cats with refractory stomatitis, therapy with hypoallergenic diets, levamisole, progesterones, or intralesional injection of repositol (water-insoluble) glucocorticoids under general anesthesia may be attempted as a last resort.

Tonsillitis

Chronic tonsillar inflammation is most commonly recognized in dogs and is usually accompanied by pharyngeal irritation initiated by foreign bodies, chronic coughing, persistent vomiting, and licking of infected sites, such as lesions caused by anal sacculitis. Dogs may have inappetence, hypersalivation, or sneezing and oculonasal discharge; they may scratch at their ears or repeatedly shake the head. Fever and malaise do not usually accompany tonsillitis unless it is secondary to underlying systemic infection or neoplasia.

Diagnosis is based upon a thorough oral examination, which usually requires sedation. The pharyngeal mucosa is reddened, and tonsils are enlarged and frequently protrude from the crypts as the tongue is pulled rostrally. Culture is unnecessary, and antibacterial therapy using amoxicillin, tetracycline, or trimethoprim-sulfonamide is recommended. Low, antiinflammatory dosages of glucocorticoids have shown benefit in reducing the severity of clinical signs when used in conjunction with antimicrobial therapy.[17] Surgical removal of the tonsils, followed by histologic examination, is usually the best course of action when antibacterial therapy has been ineffective or transiently curative. Chronic tonsillar enlargement, if not corrected by surgery, usually serves as a nidus for continual infection (see also Tonsillitis and Pharyngitis, Chapter 8).

ESOPHAGUS AND STOMACH

The oral cavity and ingested material are the primary sources of microorganisms that colonize the lower portions of the GI tract (Fig. 9–4). The esophagus and stomach contain a transient population of organisms after saliva or food is swallowed. Once the stomach has emptied of food, the low pH usually destroys most of the bacteria that remain. Those that persist during the fasting period are strains adapted to survival at low pH (Table 9–3). The oral cavity, esophagus, stomach, and proximal small intestine are colonized primarily by gram-positive aerobic and by anaerobic bacteria, which are usually susceptible to penicillin or its derivatives. This susceptibility is the rationale for the clinical use of such drugs in treating ulcerations and perforations and for antimicrobial prophylaxis involving surgery of these portions of the GI tract.

Material from abscesses or cellulitis that develops following perforating lesions of the oral cavity or upper GI tract should be collected with sterile syringes that are capped or sealed immediately following collection. The latter method will increase the chances of detecting anaerobic bacteria, although cultures must be instituted rapidly (see Chapter 42).

A variety of organisms including gram-positive rods and cocci, gram-negative rods and cocci, yeasts, and spirochetes have been found in the stomach of most normal dogs.[18] Nontoxigenic *Clostridium perfringens* was found in the gastric contents of normal dogs and those with acute gastric dilation. The type and prevalence of organisms in clinically healthy dogs did not differ from those found in dogs with acute gastric dilation.

SMALL INTESTINE

Intestinal Microflora

Concentrations of bacteria in the proximal small bowel are relatively low because of

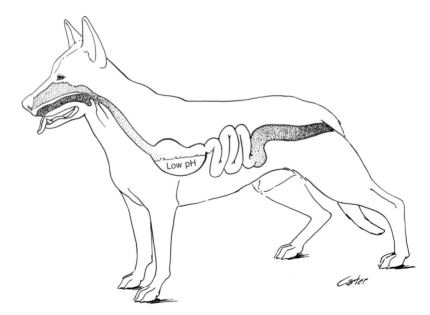

Figure 9–4. Concentration of microorganisms throughout the intestinal tract of a fasting dog. Numbers are highest in the oral cavity and colon and lowest in the midportion of the bowel.

the influence of gastric acid and bile and gradually increase toward the ileocecal region (see Table 9–3 and Fig. 9–4). Numbers of microorganisms in the distal small or large bowels are not affected by feeding, but remain relatively constant after meals. Increased numbers of organisms may be found in the stomach and upper small intestine when normal bowel defenses are impaired. Excessive use of antacids, obstruction or stasis of intestinal or bile flow, or a decrease in mucosal secretion can result in bacterial overgrowth of the small intestine.

The normal microflora of the small intes-

Table 9–3. Major Microflora of the GI Tract of Dogs and Cats

			SMALL BOWEL			
	ORAL CAVITY[c]	STOMACH[d]	Proximal[d]	Distal	CECUM/COLON	FECES
Total Counts[b]						
Fasting	10^7	10^1–10^2	10^1–10^2	10^3–10^7	10^9–10^{10}	10^{10}–10^{11}
Postprandial	10^7	10^4–10^5	10^2–10^3	10^3–10^7	10^9–10^{10}	10^{10}–10^{11}
Aerobic Organisms						
Gram-positive[e]	+	$10^{0.4}$–10^1	$10^{0.4}$–10^2	$10^{1.4}$–10^3	10^4–10^9	10^4–10^9
Gram-negative[f]	+	10^1–10^2	10^2	10^2–10^6	10^7–10^8	10^7–10^8
Anaerobic Organisms						
Gram-positive[g]	+	$10^{0.3}$–10^2	$10^{0.1}$–10^3	10^2–10^6	10^7–10^9	10^7–10^{10}
Gram-negative[h]	+	–	+	10^1	10^6–10^{10}	10^6–10^{10}
Other Organisms						
Spirochetes	+	+	+	+	+++	0
Mycoplasma	+	–	–	–	–	–
Yeasts	+	–	–	–	10^5	+

[a]+ = present but absolute quantity uncertain; +++ = present in large numbers; − = absent or data not available; 0 = normally absent. Data derived from studies in people, dogs, and cats.[2, 17a-17e]
[b]Values expressed as organisms/ml or g of intestinal contents.
[c]See Table 9–1 for information concerning frequency of isolation.
[d]All values listed are for fasting animals except where the postprandial state is indicated.
[e]*Streptococcus, Staphylococcus, Bacillus, Corynebacterium.*
[f]Enterobacteriaceae (primarily *Escherichia coli, Enterobacter, Klebsiella*), *Pseudomonas, Neisseria, Moraxella.*
[g]*Clostridium, Lactobacillus, Propionibacterium, Bifidobacterium.*
[h]*Bacteroides, Fusobacterium, Veillonella.*

tine play an important role in preventing colonization by pathogenic bacteria by competing for available nutrients, maintaining oxygen levels, and producing antibacterial substances. In addition, the normal intestinal microflora assist the body in metabolizing bile acids and drugs and have a role in synthesizing volatile fatty acids and vitamins. Puppies and kittens, lacking normal microflora at birth, derive their microflora from exposure to their dam and littermates or from the environment by 2 to 3 weeks of life.[19] Organisms that initially colonize the intestinal tract, which may vary somewhat between individuals, permanently colonize the intestinal tract and remain relatively stable in composition throughout the life of the individual. The high-meat diets ingested by most carnivores result in a predominance of streptococci and *C. perfringens* and a suppression of *Lactobacillus*. Lactose in the diet of nursing animals contributes to acidification of the colonic contents, with a resultant increase in *Enterobacter* and a decrease in *E. coli* and *Bacteroides*.

Greater knowledge of the composition of the intestinal microflora has been gained in recent years because of the development of improved techniques for culture of anaerobic bacteria. Anaerobes are now known to make up a majority of the intestinal microflora, greatly outnumbering aerobic bacteria (Table 9–3). The duodenum and upper jejunum primarily harbor gram-positive bacteria, including streptococci and lactobacilli. Anaerobes and gram-negative organisms predominate in the distal portions of the small bowel and colon. Numbers of microorganisms reach their maximum in the cecum, colon, and feces.

The composition and distribution of the normal fecal flora can be altered by disease, such as diarrhea.[19] Decreased transit time of intestinal contents and evacuation of fluid feces result in decreased numbers of lactobacilli with concomitant increases in *Bacteroides* and members of the Enterobacteriaceae. *Enterobacter*, which normally reside in the small intestine, may appear in the feces of dogs with diarrhea. The concentration of many anaerobes is reduced in the feces during diarrhea because these organisms normally require stasis and low oxygen tension for their growth.

In older veterinary literature, there are reports of spirochetes as a cause of diarrhea in dogs and cats. They are known to be a part of the normal flora throughout the GI tracts of dogs and cats and are present in greatest numbers in the oral cavity, cecum, and colon (see Table 9–3).[20] Because spirochetes are not demonstrable by routine hematoxylin and eosin staining, they had been previously overlooked by pathologists. Scanning electron microscopy and special staining procedures have shown them to be attached to the intestinal epithelium at the base of the intestinal glands. Because of their adherence to epithelial surfaces, spirochetes are not shed in the feces of normal dogs and cats, but during diarrheic episodes, they dislodge from the epithelium throughout the intestinal tract and appear in large numbers in the feces. Spirochetes should not be incriminated in diarrhea, nor should they be confused with *Campylobacter fetus* (see Chapter 50).

Pathophysiologic Mechanisms of Infectious Diarrhea

Enteropathogenic organisms, unlike resident and nonpathogenic transient microflora, have acquired means of overcoming host defense mechanisms and the inhibitory properties of the normal microflora. Adherence factors (e.g., somatic pili) that permit intestinal pathogens to establish infection allow them to attach to, multiply on, and colonize the intestinal mucosa. Some pathogenic bacteria that cause diarrhea remain on the mucosal surface and produce potent enterotoxins that disrupt fluid flux across the intestinal mucosa. Others are able to penetrate intact epithelial cells, producing inflammatory damage in the underlying mucosa. Enteric viruses damage the intestine by replicating within and destroying selected populations of epithelial cells.

Normal Function of Intestinal Villi

The normal structure and function of an intestinal villus is shown in Figure 9–5. Intestinal epithelial cells are produced by the germinal epithelium located in the intestinal crypts. Younger, undifferentiated, and primarily secretory epithelial cells, produced by the germinal epithelium of the intestinal glands (crypts), migrate up the intestinal villus as the older, differentiated, absorptive cells at the tip eventually slough

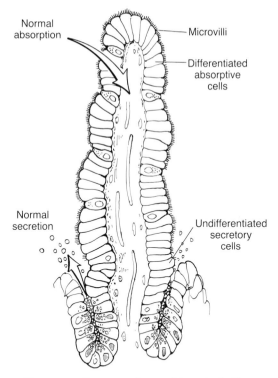

Normal
absorption

Microvilli

Differentiated
absorptive
cells

Normal
secretion

Undifferentiated
secretory
cells

Figure 9–5. Structure of normal intestinal villus.

into the intestinal lumen. Most of the absorptive process is confined to the differentiated cells at the villous tip, which also produce locally active intestinal enzymes that aid in the digestive process. The preponderance of intestinal secretion is confined to specialized goblet cells and undifferentiated cells that line the sides and depths of the crypts.

Noninvasive Enterotoxigenic Bacteria

Following attachment to the intact epithelial surface, noninvasive organisms produce a powerful heat-labile exotoxin that binds to surface receptors on the small intestinal epithelial cells. The toxin acts at a cellular level to stimulate adenyl cyclase and other unknown mechanisms to increase intracellular adenosine 3',5'-cyclic monophosphate (cyclic AMP) (Fig. 9–6A). The net effect of cyclic AMP is to increase secretion of chloride and decrease absorption of sodium by the intestinal epithelium, resulting in the loss of large quantities of water and electrolytes in the feces in the absence of morphologic injury to the intestinal mucosa.

Many bacterial species that infect dogs and cats not only produce enterotoxin-induced diarrhea following initial colonization but also cause mucosal invasion (see Table 9–4). Strains of some species, such as *E. coli*, can produce diarrhea by either mechanism. Several enterotoxin-producing strains of bacteria, such as *Staphylococcus aureus, C. perfringens,* and *E. coli,* which are common causes of food-borne diarrhea and acute gastroenteritis, are harbored in the colons of clinically normal dogs and cats. Presumably, the bacteria and toxin cause clinical illness only after being ingested or during bacterial overgrowth or intestinal stasis, when they proliferate in the small intestine. Enterotoxigenic staphylococci have been isolated from the large bowel of clinically healthy dogs.[21, 22] Enterotoxigenic *E. coli* have been recovered from dogs with acute diarrhea, but their importance alone as a cause of illness has been uncertain (see Neonatal Colibacillosis).[23, 23a] Similar isolation of enteropathogenic strains has been made from cats.[24]

Mucosa-Invading Bacteria

Following invasion of the mucosa, some bacteria produce hemorrhagic (dysenteric) stools. The two bacterial genera that produce dysentery are *Salmonella*, which usually has an affinity of the ileum, and *Shigella*, which has an affinity for the ileum and the colon. After they penetrate submucosal tissue, both produce a marked inflammatory response characterized by the influx of neutrophils. *Shigella* and many strains of *Salmonella* are phagocytized and killed, although some may persist, causing a chronic carrier state (see also Chapter 50).

Villous Atrophy

The well-differentiated apical absorptive cells of the intestinal villus are responsible for producing digestive enzymes that act locally at the intestinal brush border. Reoviruses, rotaviruses, and coronaviruses have a selective affinity for replication within and destruction of these cells, resulting in villous atrophy (see Table 9–4 and Fig. 9–6B). Impaired absorption and digestion are characteristic of this type of diarrhea. A relative increase in intestinal secretion is usually

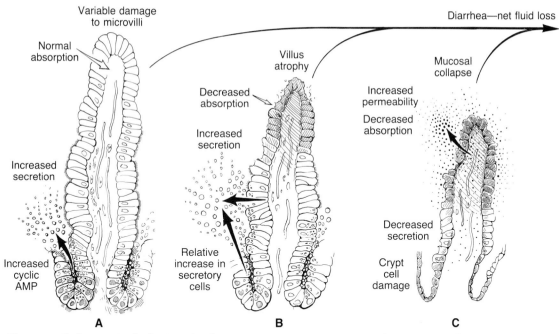

Figure 9–6. Pathogenesis of infectious diarrhea. *A,* Noninvasive enterotoxigenic bacteria (e.g., vibrios, staphylococci, and clostridia) primarily stimulate cyclic AMP. *B,* Villous atrophy results from selective infection of apical epithelial cells with certain viruses (e.g., coronaviruses and rotaviruses). *C,* Intestinal gland degeneration and mucosal collapse occur when viruses (e.g., parvoviruses) damage the germinal intestinal gland epithelium.

associated with terminal villous atrophy because of continued replication of the undifferentiated germinal crypt epithelial cells, which have more secretory than absorptive functions.

Intestinal Gland Degeneration

Because canine and feline parvoviruses require rapidly dividing cells for replication, they selectively damage the mitotically active intestinal gland epithelium so that absorptive cells at the tips of the villi are not replaced, which leads to intestinal gland degeneration and eventual mucosal collapse (Fig. 9–6C). The primary defect is in absorption; however, secretory processes are also inactivated. Damage to the mucosal barrier in most cases also results in an influx of inflammatory cells and increased vascular permeability, with the eventual exudation of serum proteins.

Diarrheal Syndromes Caused by Bacteria

See Chapter 50 for additional enteric bacterial diseases.

Neonatal colibacillosis has been described in many species, including dogs[25, 26] and cats.[24] Characteristically, puppies are affected within the first week of life and have a high mortality rate. They show acute depression, weakness, hypothermia, cyanosis, and CNS signs prior to death. Older puppies that survive for several weeks may have persistent diarrhea, abdominal discomfort, weight loss, and dehydration. Gross necropsy findings include hemorrhagic lesions on serosal surfaces of all body cavities and throughout the GI mucosa. Septicemia can be confirmed by bacterial culture from the blood or from many organs. Histologic examination reveals gram-negative bacilli in many tissues of septicemic newborns.

The cause of *E. coli* septicemia in newborn puppies may be associated with their immunologic incompetency rather than the virulence of a particular strain of organism. Enterotoxic, attaching, and effacing bacterial strains of *E. coli* exist (see Noninvasive Enterotoxigenic Bacteria). Furthermore, intestinal epithelial cells of newborn puppies are highly and nonselectively permeable to a variety of proteins (including bacteria) that are absorbed by pinocytosis. Exposure of newborns to *E. coli* prior to colostrum inges-

Table 9–4. Mechanism and Site of Action of Enteropathogenic Bacteria and Viruses

MECHANISM AND BACTERIA OR VIRUS	SITE*
Enterotoxin Production	
Vibrio cholerae	SI
Staphylococcus aureus	Stomach and SI
Clostridium perfringens, type A	SI
Bacillus cereus	SI in initial stages
Vibrio parahaemolyticus	SI
Escherichia coli	Some strains in SI
Yersinia enterocolitica	SI and colon
Klebsiella pneumoniae	SI
Campylobacter fetus	SI
Salmonella typhimurium	SI in initial stages
Mucosal Invasion	
Salmonella	Ileum in later stages
Shigella	Colon
B. cereus	SI in later stages
V. parahaemolyticus	SI in later stages
E. coli	Some strains in colon
Villous Atrophy	
Coronaviruses	SI
Reoviruses	SI
Rotaviruses	SI
Crypt Degeneration	
Canine parvovirus	Primarily SI
Feline panleukopenia virus	Primarily SI

*SI = small intestine.

tion or their failure to obtain sufficient colostrum may further predispose these puppies to infection. E. coli is also able to cross the intestinal epithelial barrier until 48 to 72 hours after birth, after which the cells also cease to absorb immunoglobulins. Puppies appear to be completely resistant to intestinal exposure to E. coli at 2 weeks of age.

Group D streptococcal overgrowth, caused by an enterococcal species (Enterococcus [Streptococcus] durans), was found in the small intestine of an 11-day-old pup.[27] The pup was one of three that died in a litter affected with acute diarrhea. Microscopically, bacterial colonization of the enterocytes in the jejunum was diffuse with mild inflammatory changes. A mixed growth of E. coli and Enterococcus (S. durans) 2 was cultured. Although bacterial attachment has been seen in the ileum and colon of healthy pups, it is not usually seen in the upper small intestine. Although enterococci have been shown to produce malabsorption and diarrhea in other animals, their exact role in the diarrhea or death in three puppies was

uncertain. Concurrent infection with another undetected organism may have been possible.

Bacterial overgrowth in the small intestine is a syndrome accompanied by chronic or recurrent diarrhea that has been observed in German shepherds.[28] Affected dogs have generally been between 5 months and 2 years of age. They are usually bright and alert but show variable weight loss, which becomes apparent with time, and consistently have foul smelling, watery feces of weeks' to months' duration. Results of quantitation of bacteria in duodenal secretions from affected animals have revealed increased numbers of E. coli and enterococci, typically normal flora of this site, and proliferation of anaerobes such as clostridia, which are unusual inhabitants.[28]

Although disordered motility and hypochlorhydria are possible causes of bacterial overgrowth, a secretory antibody (IgA) immune deficiency may be present (see Chapter 3).[29] Duodenal bacterial overgrowth also occurs in German shepherd dogs with pancreatic exocrine insufficiency (PEI). Furthermore, similar clinical features of PEI and bacterial overgrowth make these syndromes difficult to differentiate. Anaerobic bacterial overgrowth in the proximal small intestine leads to increased serum folic acid concentrations. Increased serum folate results from increased synthesis of this compound by the large numbers of intestinal bacteria with greater amounts available for absorption. In addition, reduced serum B_{12} in these dogs is thought to be caused by bacterial binding of the vitamin within the intestine, preventing its absorption. Xylose absorption has been variably reduced in affected dogs, presumably as a result of bacterial utilization of xylose in the proximal small bowel, thereby reducing the amount being absorbed. In some cases, abnormal xylose absorption may be corrected by prior administration of antibiotics. Serum trypsin-like immunoreactivity and absorption of bound para-aminobenzoic acid (PABA) have been within reference ranges unless concurrent PEI is present. Minimal histologic abnormalities have been found in affected dogs, and the activities of some brush border intestinal enzymes have been altered depending on whether anaerobic or aerobic bacteria predominate and whether PEI is present.[30–32]

Quantitative examination of duodenal fluid shows bacterial counts greater than

10^5 organisms/ml. Proliferating organisms often consist of normal flora such as *E. coli* and *Enterobacter*, but sometimes unusual species for that location, such as clostridia, predominate.

Response to antimicrobial therapy supports the theory of bacterial overgrowth. For dosages, see Table 9–5. Animals with PEI require enzyme supplementation. Because of the development of overgrowth in some dogs with PEI, antimicrobial therapy may be required in dogs that do not respond to enzyme supplementation alone. In addition, a bland diet, such as cottage cheese or chicken and boiled rice, or specialized diets (I/D, Hills Foods, Topeka, KS) have often been needed during the treatment interval to obtain more consistent responses.

Lymphocytic-plasmacytic enteritis, an inflammatory small bowel condition, characterized by diffuse mucosal infiltration of lymphocytes, plasma cells, eosinophils, and neutrophils has been described in dogs[33,34] and cats.[35,36] The disease may or may not involve the colon. Unlike bacterial overgrowth, no dog breed is predisposed to this syndrome, and affected animals are usually older than 2 years. Similarly, generally older cats are affected. Chronic or intermittent intractable diarrhea is seen in dogs. This may vary in consistency, but gross evidence of hemorrhage is usually lacking. When longstanding and severe, weight loss and hypoproteinemia develop. In contrast, vomiting is the major sign in affected cats; it is often unrelated to eating and may occur in sporadic episodes. Diarrhea is less common and variable and can occur in the small or large bowel or both. Appetite may be reduced, corresponding to the episodic nature of vomiting and diarrhea. Some dogs and cats with significant weight loss have a voracious appetite similar to PEI. Thickening or discomfort may be found on palpation of the intestine. Edema, hyrothorax, or ascites may be found in animals with severe hypoproteinemia. With the exception of hypoalbuminemia, clinical laboratory evaluation for malabsorption or maldigestion is within reference ranges, and contrast radiographic findings are variable. Biopsy by endoscopy or exploratory laparotomy of the large bowel is the only means of definitive diagnosis. Diagnosis and therapy of lymphocytic enteritis are very similar to that for large intestinal syndrome and are covered under Colitis, later. Bacterial overgrowth, especially in long-standing cases, may be a potential cause of both syndromes. Other organisms or food ingredients may be associated with the pathogenesis, since it can be seen with other enteropathies. Since immune-

Table 9–5. Systemic Therapy for Lower Alimentary Infections[a]

DRUG	SPECIES	DOSE[b] (mg/kg)	ROUTE	INTERVAL (hours)	DURATION (days)
Colitis					
Sulfasalazine	D	12.5	PO	6	21–28
	D	10–25	PO	8	21–28
	C	5–10	PO	8	14–21
	C	25	PO	24	14–21
Metronidazole	B	10–20	PO	12	14–21
	B[c]	7.5–10	PO	8	14–21
	B	30	PO	24	14–21
Tylosin	D	10–25	PO	8	14–21
Prednisolone	B	0.5–1.5	PO	12	14–21
Azathioprine	D	2–2.5[d]	PO	24	14–21
	C	0.3	PO	48	14–21
Clidinium and chlordiazepoxide[e]	D	0.1	PO	6–12	prn
Diphenoxylate	D	0.5–1	PO	8–12	prn
Loperamide	D	0.1	PO	6	prn
Bacterial Overgrowth and Lymphoplasmacytic Enteritis					
Oxy(tetracycline)	D	10–20	PO	12	7–28

[a]D = dog, C = cat, B = dog and cat, IV = intravenous, SC = subcutaneous, PO = oral, IL = intralesional, prn = as needed.
[b]Dose per administration at specified interval, expressed as mg/kg unless otherwise stated.
[c]Most cats get one quarter of a 250-mg tablet per day.
[d]Dose also expressed as 40 mg/m², based on body surface area.
[e]Librax, Roche Products Inc, Marrati, PR.

mediated and infectious causes may be involved, both antimicrobial and immunosuppressive therapy have been used. When the diagnosis is uncertain, antimicrobial therapy should be instituted first because of potential complications of immunosuppression of dogs with bacterial overgrowth.

Hemorrhagic gastroenteritis (HGE), a syndrome characterized by the sudden onset of vomiting and production of profuse, mucoid, bloody diarrhea, was primarily described in small house dogs between 2 and 4 years of age.[37] The syndrome is also marked by hematologic findings that include polycythemia, hyperproteinemia, and coagulation test results suggestive of disseminated intravascular coagulation (DIC) and, occasionally, acute oliguric renal failure.

The pathogenesis of the syndrome of acute HGE is unknown, but many clinical and laboratory findings are similar to those produced by experimental administration of endotoxin, irreversible hemorrhagic shock, or DIC in dogs. Whether a cause or an effect, DIC may explain many of the clinical features that have been observed in dogs. Allergic, hereditary, autoimmune, and infectious etiologies for HGE have been proposed. The high prevalence of the syndrome in certain breeds, such as schnauzers and miniature poodles, has been explained by their hereditary predisposition to such causative factors. The influence on microbial flora of the highly digestible meat-protein diets commonly fed to well-cared-for house dogs should be examined. Diagnosis of the syndrome of HGE is based on historic, clinical, and laboratory findings. Treatment is essentially similar to that for endotoxemia (see Chapter 44); however, antimicrobial agents are usually not required.

Diagnosis of Acute Infectious Gastroenteritis

Collection of fecal samples for culture of aerobic bacteria is easier when commercially prepared, sterile, cotton-tipped applicators are used. These are supplied with transport media or enrichment broth in which the swab is placed immediately following specimen collection (see Chapter 42). Care should be taken to clean the anus with 70% alcohol or dilute organic iodine solution before inserting the cotton-tipped applicator. Special cultural methods may be necessary

when organisms such as *Campylobacter* are suspected (see Diagnosis, Chapter 50).

Cytologic examination of fecal mucus or exudates can be an effective way to determine the integrity of the bowel mucosa. Infectious processes that cause damage to mucosal surfaces result in the appearance of large numbers of neutrophils and macrophages in feces. Diarrhea caused by parvoviruses and invasive bacteria can be distinguished by the presence of inflammatory cells.

Like cultures of specimens from the oral cavity, cultures of feces or other intestinal contents yield ambiguous results. Disturbances in the composition of microflora will not be detected unless quantitative cultures are performed. Primary pathogens such as *Salmonella* and *Shigella* require selective media if they are to be isolated. Enterotoxigenic strains of bacteria require specific identification techniques that are not routinely available to most veterinarians. Finding a potentially pathogenic organism is not the same as identifying the cause of diarrhea, because there is a high prevalence of subclinical carriers of *Salmonella*, *Campylobacter*, and other enteropathogenic bacteria in dog and cat populations. Cultures should always be performed when zoonotic exposure to these latter pathogens is suspected.

Therapy for Acute Infectious Gastroenteritis

Antibiotic therapy is indicated only when episodes of diarrhea or vomiting are accompanied by signs of systemic illness, including fever, depression, impending shock, and the presence of leukopenia or leukocytosis with a marked left shift, findings that indicate there has been absorption of microbes or, more likely, their toxins.[38] In some instances, routine use of antimicrobials may be harmful, altering the composition and number of intestinal microorganisms that normally serve to inhibit the growth of pathogenic varieties. The choice of drugs depends on a knowledge of the susceptibilities of both the usual pathogens and the normal intestinal flora. For further information, see the discussion of therapy for intra-abdominal sepsis that appears later in this chapter. See also Appendices 13 and 14 for appropriate choice and dosages of antimicrobial drugs.

Antimotility agents have been routinely used in the treatment of infectious diarrhea. However, slowing intestinal transit may be counterproductive to the defense mechanism of diarrhea, which acts to eliminate harmful microorganisms and their toxins. The use of antimotility drugs has resulted in increased morbidity and persistence of infection in people with bacterial enteritis (see Therapy, Chapter 50).

Fluid therapy is probably one of the most important symptomatic treatments of the diarrheic animal. Fluids should be given IV when severe shock and hypotension, semicoma, or persistent vomiting or ileus accompanies the diarrheal episode. Less affected animals with these complications should receive subcutaneous fluids. The vast majority of animals with acute nonhemorrhagic diarrheas without vomiting can be treated with specific oral fluid preparations. Oral fluid therapy is based upon the observation that glucose is actively absorbed by the normal small bowel and that sodium is carried with it in about an equimolar ratio. Hypertonic oral antidiarrheal fluid replacement solutions can be prepared that contain sodium and glucose in an equimolar ratio, in addition to bicarbonate and potassium in a composition similar to that of the fluid lost in diarrheic stool (Table 9–6). In most situations, amino acids commercially marketed for veterinary use such as glycine have been added to facilitate absorption. Solutions containing glucose or sodium, either alone or in an imbalanced ratio or of lesser concentration, are **not** effective in reversing fluid and electrolyte flux across the intestinal mucosa. Similarly, polyionic, isotonic fluids such as lactated Ringer's solution, Pedialyte (Ross Laboratories, Columbus, OH) and Gatorade (Stokely VanCamp Co., Indianapolis, IN) are useful only for oral fluid maintenance or electrolyte supplementation and do little to reverse ongoing or existing losses. Oral antidiarrheal solutions are only effective when the integrity of the intestinal mucosa is intact. This can easily be assessed in practice by looking for gross and microscopic evidence of blood and leukocytes in stools.

Promoted by the World Health Organization (WHO) for treating human cholera, "WHO juice" can easily be made by veterinarians or their clients (Table 9–7).[38a,e,f] The ingredients can be mixed and stored in a powdered state and reconstituted when necessary. Unused portions can be stored in a refrigerator for several days or weeks. WHO juice is voluntarily accepted by most dogs and some cats, although some animals require gavage by syringe or stomach tube. The volume of WHO juice to be administered depends on the circumstances, but a range of 50 to 100 ml/kg/day is usually given, according to the fluid losses, until the diarrhea stops. Vomiting, which may occur when use of these hypertonic solutions begins, can usually be obviated by giving small amounts more frequently. Although they facilitate fluid absorption, large volumes of hypertonic fluids may cause a transient increase in stool water volume because of residual unabsorbed electrolytes in the feces. Hypertonic oral fluids can also cause serum hyperosmolality and hyperosmolar coma when adequate volumes of water or isotonic fluids are not concurrently provided free choice. Parenteral isotonic fluid therapy may have to be given concurrently with hypertonic fluids in small or young animals.

The use of kaolin and pectin is limited because they are relatively ineffective in absorbing toxins produced by enteropathogenic bacteria. Kaolin is a potent coagulation activator and may be of some benefit in treating diarrhea associated with mucosal disruption and hemorrhage.

Nonsteroidal anti-inflammatory drugs such as aspirin have been shown to be beneficial in the management of infectious diarrhea. Clinical studies in people and experimental studies in dogs and cats have shown that salicylates interfere with the mechanism of enterotoxin-induced intestinal hypersecretion, presumably by blocking production of cyclic AMP. Subsalicylate preparations (Pepto Bismol, Norwich Eaton Pharmaceuticals, Norwich, NY) that are commonly used in the treatment of diarrhea are thought to work in a similar manner.[39] Further studies have shown that bismuth subsalicylate has antibacterial activity owing to binding and killing of exposed pathogenic bacteria.[39a] Administration of these compounds, at a dose of 1 to 7 ml/kg of Pepto Bismol, early in the course of disease may be helpful in treating diarrhea that results from the mechanism of increased secretion.

LARGE INTESTINE

Microflora

The cecum and colon are the richest source of intestinal microflora, and a single

Table 9–6. Chemical Composition of Various Fluids for Infectious Diarrhea[a]

FLUID (Manufacturer)	Na (mEq/L)	K (mEq/L)	Cl⁻ (mEq/L)	HCO₃⁻ (mEq/L)	GLUCOSE (g/L)[b]	AMINO ACIDS[c] (mM/L)	ENERGY (Kcal/L)	OSMOLARITY (mOsm/L)
Body Fluids								
Normal plasma[d]	142	4.5	105	25	1.0	ND	ND	300
Cholera stool[d]	140	13	104	44	ND	ND	ND	ND
Replacement								
WHO juice[d]	90	20	80	30	20	0	80	330
Rehydrate solution (Ross)	75	20	65	30[e]	25	0	90	ND
Pedialyte RS (Ross)	75	20	ND	ND	25	0	ND	285
Gastrolyte Oral (USV)	90	20	80	30[e]	20	0	80	ND
Ion-Aid[f] (Diamond)	89	28	ND	0	24	125	133	480
Entrolyte[f] (Beecham)	80	17	ND	1.6[e]	23	45	95	350
Life-guard[f] (Norden)	118	28	ND	80	30	110	170	490
Electro-PlusA[f] (Pitman-Moore)	100	15	ND	40[e]	11	60	58	350
Maintenance								
Pedialyte (Ross)	45	20	35	30[e]	25	0	90	250
Infalyte (Pennwalt)	50	20	40	30	20	0	64	260
Supplementation								
Gatorade[g] (Stokely VanCamp)	21	3	11	0	20	0	80	330
Apple juice[h]	1.7	26	0	0	ND	0	ND	ND

[a]ND = no data.
[b]Multiply by 5.5 to get mM/L glucose.
[c]Supplied primarily as glycine.
[d]Data from Pierce and Hirschhorn, 1977[38a] and Sack et al, 1970.[38b]
[e]Anion supplied as citrate instead of bicarbonate.
[f]Data from Lewis and Phillips, 1980.[38c]
[g]Stokely VanCamp Co, Indianapolis, IN, personal communication, December 1982.
[h]Data from Dupont and Pickering, 1979.[38d]

gram of feces contains up to 10¹¹ organisms, approximately 100 times the human population of the world. Organisms that inhabit the lower bowel are primarily gram-negative aerobes and spore- and nonspore-forming anaerobes (see Table 9–3). Anaerobic bacteria, which usually compose more than 90% of the colonic microflora, include clostridia, lactobacilli, *Bifidobacterium*, and *Bacteroides*. Aerobic bacteria primarily consist of streptococci and members of the Enterobacteriaceae.

Table 9–7. Composition of WHO Juice

DRY INGREDIENTS[a]	AMOUNT		SUBSTITUTES
	Grams	Teaspoons	
Sodium chloride (table salt)	3.5	0.64	None
Sodium bicarbonate (baking soda)	2.5	0.55	None
Glucose powder (dextrose)	20.0	4.0	Sucrose (table sugar): 40.0 g (8 tsps) or equivalent amount of honey or corn syrup
Potassium chloride	1.5	0.31	Apple juice: 0.47 liter (1 US pint)

Data modified from World Health Organization: *Treatment and Prevention of Dehydration in Diarrheal Diseases*, Geneva, WHO, 1976; Gangarosa EJ: *Postgrad Med* 62:113–117, 1977; and Pierce NF, Hirschhorn N: *WHO Chron* 31:87–93, 1977.[38a]
[a]In 1 liter of water (1.05 U.S. quarts).

Acute Colitis

A number of acute inflammatory diseases of the colon have been described in dogs and cats. Colitis, whether acute or chronic, usually involves the microflora as a secondary phenomenon. As with stomatitis, many cases of acute colitis in dogs and cats can be associated with stressful circumstances or immunosuppressive diseases. Acute colitis has been reported in cats experimentally infected with panleukopenia virus, although the colonic lesions were milder than those in the small intestine.[40] One case of mycotic colitis in a cat was assumed to be a sequela to panleukopenia virus infection.[41] Acute ulcerative colitis of undetermined cause has been recognized in young cats.[42-44]

Chronic Colitis

Chronic colitis is a common syndrome recognized in dogs, characterized by chronic diarrhea with hematochezia and tenesmus, weight loss, occasional vomiting, and abdominal pain. Fever is not a consistent finding. The colitis that occurs in boxers is frequently granulomatous but is thought to be a secondary result of chronic ulceration and a reaction to intestinal microflora. Chronic ulcerative colitis does not appear to be associated with primary bacterial pathogens but probably results from stress, debilitation, or immunosuppression. That the lesions are invaded by intestinal microflora following mucosal disruption may explain the apparent beneficial effect of antibiotics and the occasional deleterious effect of glucocorticoids in treating this disease.

Older cats appear to be affected by a chronic ulcerative colitis similar to that of dogs.[45] Cats infected with FeLV or FIV can develop chronic ulcerative colitis, presumably as an immunosuppressive phenomenon. Lymphocytic-plasmacytic colitis, a chronic inflammatory bowel disease, has been described in cats with chronic large bowel diarrhea[46] and in cats with feline infectious peritonitis.[35, 43, 44]

Acute or chronic colitis should be suspected in any animal presented with large bowel diarrhea. A stained fecal smear and rectal scraping and a parasite examination are helpful in eliminating parasitism, neoplasia, and algal and fungal disorders as causes of the diarrhea and, in many cases, will confirm a diagnosis. A presumptive diagnosis of colitis should be confirmed by proctoscopy and biopsy when possible.

The antibiotics that have been useful in treating canine and feline ulcerative colitis are primarily those that are effective against anaerobic bacteria (see Table 9–5). The lesions usually do not resolve spontaneously. Dietary management is usually attempted first in dogs and cats. Food should be withheld for 24 to 48 hours, and then the animal should be started on a bland diet in multiple small feedings. A nonallergenic diet low in fat, such as boiled rice, meat, and potatoes, is satisfactory.[47] For dogs, prescription diets (I/D or D/D, Hills, Topeka, KS) are indicated. Drugs that have been most effective in dogs and cats include oral salicylazosulfapyridine (sulfasalazine), oral chloramphenicol, and oral metronidazole. After several weeks of therapy, the dosage should be reduced, and in animals requiring long-term therapy, the minimum effective dose should be determined. Cats with lymphocytic-plasmacytic colitis have responded to sulfasalazine with or without concurrent metronidazole and glucocorticoid therapy or to dietary management using lamb and rice, or a prescription diet (c/d DIET, Hills, Topeka, Kansas).[46] Glucocorticoids should be used at anti-inflammatory doses with caution and only if relapses have occurred after clinical improvement has been noted with antimicrobial therapy. When stress is suspected to be a problem, clidinium and chlordiazepoxide or diazepam may be be added to the regimen. Since colonic motility is already depressed in colitis, there is no need for the routine use of anticholinergic or opiate drugs, unless for relief of acute straining. Antispasmodic drugs, such as diphenoxylate or loperamide, must be used with caution in invasive bacterial infections of the bowel.

INTRA-ABDOMINAL INFECTIONS

Etiology and Clinical Findings

Peritonitis and intra-abdominal abscess formation are frequent complications of intestinal perforation caused by postsurgical wound dehiscence of the GI tract, foreign bodies or severe ulcerative enteritis, penetrating abdominal wounds, or rupture of abscesses of intra-abdominal organs.[47a] Animals may become depressed, weak, and hypotensive following GI illness or abdominal wounds. Fever, abdominal distention, and abdominal pain are variable findings.

Diagnosis

Peritonitis should be suspected when a severe, inappropriate left shift in the leukogram is found. Radiography may be misleading in early or localized disease. Confirmation of intra-abdominal sepsis is best achieved through abdominal paracentesis.

Abdominal Paracentesis. The skin of the abdomen is clipped free of hair and prepared as if for surgery from the umbilicus to the inguinal region. An 18-gauge, 1-inch needle fitted to a 20-ml syringe can be used to make the tap. Plastic IV catheters or metal-teat cannulas are less likely to accidentally penetrate intra-abdominal structures and also allow sampling at greater depths. The use of needles or IV catheters is frequently unrewarding owing to occlusion, too small a volume of abdominal fluid being recovered, or localization of the inflammatory process. Multiple collection attempts in each of the four abdominal quadrants are recommended.

Peritoneal lavage should be attempted if no material can be aspirated.[48, 49] Use of peritoneal dialysis catheters or cutting fenestrated openings in flexible teflon vascular catheters facilitates administration and withdrawal of fluid (Fig. 9–7). Lavage is performed by inserting the large catheter through the caudal ventral abdominal wall in the direction of the pelvic canal. A negative aspiration is followed by rapid infusion of isotonic saline through an IV drip set at a volume of 20 ml/kg. After the animal has been gently rotated, the fluid can be removed by placing the still-connected fluid bottle on the floor to allow gravity drainage. A portion of the fluid that runs back into the bottle should be analyzed for protein concentration and examined cytologically, and if an inflammatory exudate is detected, an aliquot should be submitted for culture. The presence of degenerative neutrophils with nucleated cell counts greater than 9000 cells/μl, intracellular bacteria, or organic debris indicates bacterial peritonitis. A portion of the fluid should be kept in a sealed syringe to preserve anaerobes during transport to the laboratory.

Therapy

Antibiotic therapy is important in the management of intra-abdominal infections (Table 9–8).[50] Mixed infections caused by indigenous flora are associated with bowel leakage. Bacteria that enter tissues owing to leakage from the stomach to the level of the mid small intestine are usually gram-positive organisms or anaerobes that are susceptible to penicillin derivatives or chloramphenicol.

Therapy against facultative gram-negative bacteria and anaerobes is essential when leakage occurs from the small intestine, cecum, or colon. Facultative aerobes are important in producing bacteremia and early mortality in intra-abdominal infections, whereas the anaerobes are instrumental in leading to abscess formation. Drugs such as aminoglycosides have been recommended because of their effect against gram-negative bacteria.[51] It has been found in animals with experimentally induced intra-abdominal sepsis that the administration of aminoglycosides alone greatly reduces the mortality associated with gram-negative sepsis, although the prevalence of postoperative adhesions and abscess formation is unaffected. Under similar experimental circumstances, the use of drugs effective against anaerobic bacteria resulted in death from gram-negative septicemia, even though the prevalence of intra-abdominal abscesses was reduced. This finding indicates that antimicrobial drugs or combinations used in treating intra-abdominal sepsis must be effective against both aerobic and anaerobic intestinal flora to decrease both mortality and abscess formation following peritonitis. A summary of antimicrobial drugs and their effects on experimental abdominal sepsis is presented in Table 9–7.

Timing of Antimicrobial Prophylaxis for Surgery

Preoperative and intraoperative administration of cephalosporins or penicillin deriv-

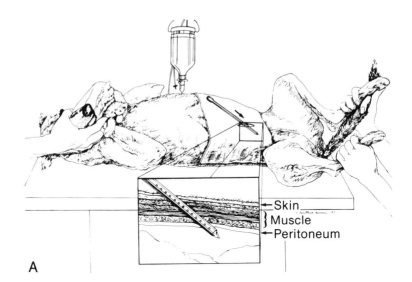

A

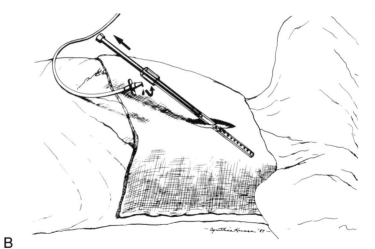

Figure 9–7. A, For peritoneal lavage, the fenestrated catheter with internal metal stylet is thrust through the abdominal wall through a skin incision. B, The stylet is removed and fluids are connected. C, After the prescribed amount of fluid has been infused and the animal has been rotated, the bottle is lowered below the level of the animal to collect large portions of infusate for analysis. Alternatively, for sample collection, a syringe can be attached to the catheter.

B

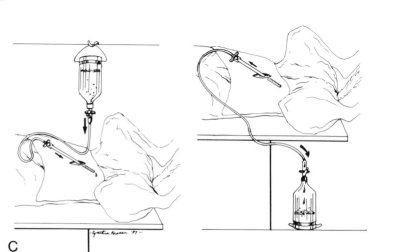

C

Table 9–8. Summary of Antimicrobial Therapy in Experimental Intra-abdominal Sepsis

ANTIMICROBIAL THERAPY	MORTALITY RATE (%)	SURVIVORS WITH ABSCESSES (%)	SURVIVORS WITHOUT ABSCESSES (CURED) (%)
Untreated controls	37	100	0
Gentamicin	4	98	2
Amikacin	7	96	3
Penicillin	13	92	7
Sulfamethoxazole-trimethoprim	0	77	23
Penicillin + amikacin	0	73	27
Chloramphenicol	3	59	40
Cefazolin (L)	7	50	47
Cefamandole (L) + tobramycin	13	38	54
Doxycycline	23	30	54
Clindamycin	42	6	55
Cefamandole (L)	13	35	57
Cephalothin (L)	3	38	60
Erythromycin	27	14	63
Carbenicillin	18	14	70
Cefazolin (H)	0	27	73
Cefamandole (H)	3	24	73
Cephalothin (H)	16	10	76
Metronidazole	10	13	78
Doxycycline + gentamicin	7	14	80
Cefamandole (L) + erythromycin	12	4	85
Rosaramicin + gentamicin	7	7	87
Spectinomycin	2	12	87
Clindamycin + gentamicin	7	5	90
Carbenicillin + gentamicin	3	7	90
Moxalactam (L)	3	7	90
Cefoxitin (L)	0	7	93
Cefotaxime (L)	3	4	93
Spectinomycin + clindamycin	0	4	96
Cefamandole (H) + erythromycin	3	0	97

aL, low-dose regimen; H, high-dose regimen.
(From Bartlett JG: Intra-abdominal abscess. *In* Zak O, Sande MA [eds]: *Experimental Models in Antimicrobial Chemotherapy.* Academic Press, 1986, pp 91–114, with permission.)

atives combined with aminoglycosides has been effective in reducing complications of intestinal leakage and peritoneal contamination in people. Total sterilization of the bowel prior to surgery, however, is impossible in a conventional environment. Bowel sterilization has been achieved only experimentally in dogs that have been kept in a germ-free environment, fed sterilized food, and given combination therapy with large dosages of nonabsorbable antibiotics.[52] Even with these elaborate procedures, decontamination was incomplete, and the microflora was reestablished within 1 week following termination of therapy. Administration of prophylactic antimicrobial therapy for GI surgery should begin 12 to 24 hours prior to the operation and terminate on the day of surgery if the bowel contents are not spilled. One week of therapy is indicated if contamination occurs during the surgical procedure.

Management of Surgical Contamination

Spillage of intestinal contents during experimental surgery in dogs has been best controlled by rinsing the peritoneal cavity with an irrigation solution of neomycin (500 mg), polymyxin (500,000 U), and bacitracin (50,000 U) mixed in 1 liter of saline.[52, 53] Similar broad-spectrum antimicrobial activity can be achieved by rinsing the peritoneal cavity with organic iodine solutions diluted 1:10 to 1:20 with physiologic saline. Intra-abdominal instillation of povidone-iodine solutions can cause peritonitis and hepatotoxicity in dogs.[53a] Dosages of 3.5 ml/kg of a 10% solution caused neutrophilic leukocytosis, increased hepatic enzyme activity, icterus, and death. Lower dosages (2 ml/kg) had less side effects. Although beneficial when used with antimicrobial therapy or drainage, saline alone used to rinse the abdominal cavity has been less successful in preventing infection, despite its diluting effect on the spilled material.

Management of Established Peritonitis

Antimicrobial therapy is essential in animals with acute septic peritonitis. Broadspectrum antimicrobial therapy is less important than lavage in the management of established peritonitis. This procedure involves the placement of intra-abdominal tubes and daily infusion and removal of isotonic saline solutions. Antimicrobial agents can be placed in the infusion fluid and reach higher concentrations than when they are given orally or parenterally. Only small amounts of many systemically administered antibiotics reach the peritoneal cavity, whereas most of the drug introduced into the abdominal cavity enters the systemic circulation.

Open peritoneal drainage has been generally successful for treatment of established generalized peritonitis in dogs and cats.[54] The technique involves exploratory laparotomy, surgically correcting the cause, lavaging the abdominal cavity, and incomplete closure of the ventral midline incision with supportive wraps. Closure of the peritoneal cavity was usually done 3 to 4 days after surgery. Antimicrobial therapy was continued until the time of final closure.

Aminoglycosides, such as gentamicin given IM, and cephalosporins, given orally or IM, result in minimal peritoneal concentrations. Since aminoglycosides are toxic and readily adsorbed by the peritoneal surfaces, they should be added in restricted doses to the peritoneal lavage fluid. When given orally, metronidazole, a relatively effective drug for anaerobic infections, reaches a higher concentration in peritoneal effusions than most other antimicrobial agents.[55]

References

1. Smith JE: The aerobic bacteria of the nose and tonsils of healthy dogs. J Comp Pathol 71:428–433, 1961.
2. Clapper WE, Meade GH: Normal flora of the nose, throat, and lower intestines of dogs. J Bacteriol 85:643–648, 1963.
3. Breenan PC, Simkins RC: Throat flora of a closed colony of beagle dogs. Proc Soc Exp Biol Med 134:566–570, 1970.
4. Sapher DA, Cox GR: Gingival flora of the dog with special reference to bacteria associated with bites. J Clin Microbiol 3:344–349, 1976.
5. Nyby MD, Gregory DA, Kuhn DA, et al: Incidence of Simonsiella in the oral cavity of dogs. J Clin Microbiol 6:87–88, 1977.
5a. Baldrias L, Frost AJ, O'Boyle D: The isolation of Pasteurella-like organisms from the tonsillar regions of dogs and cats. J Small Anim Pract 29:63–68, 1988.
5b. Marretta SM: The common and uncommon clinical presentations and treatment of periodontal disease in the dog and cat. Semin Vet Med Surg 2:230–240, 1987.
5c. Isogai E, Isogai H, Miura H, et al: Oral flora of mongrel and beagle dogs with periodontal disease. Jpn J Vet Sci 51:110–118, 1989.
6. Reed JH: A review of the experimental use of antimicrobial agents in the treatment of periodontitis and gingivitis in the dog. Can Vet J 29:705–708, 1988.
7. Williams RC, Jeffcoat MK, Goldhaber P: Tetracycline treatment of periodontal disease in the beagle dog. J Periodont Res 17:358–365, 1982.
8. Nuki K, Soskolne WA, Raisz LG, et al: Bone resorbing activity of gingiva from beagle dogs following metronidazole and indomethacin therapy. J Periodont Res 16:205–212, 1981.
9. Hamp S, Lindhe J, Loe H: Long-term effect of chlorhexidine on developing gingivitis in the beagle dog. J Periodont Res 8:63–70, 1973.
10. Saxe SR, Greene JC, Bohannan HM, et al: Oral debris, calculus and periodontal disease in the beagle dog. Periodontics 5:217–225, 1967.
11. Black AP, Crichlow AM, Saunders JR: Bacteremia during ultrasonic teeth cleaning and extraction in the dog. J Am Anim Hosp Assoc 16:611–616, 1980.
11a. Russell RG, Slattum MM, Abkowitz J: Filamentous bacteria in oral eosinophilic granuloma of a cat. Vet Pathol 25:249–250, 1988.
11b. Tannock GW, Webster JR, Dobbinson SS: Feline gingivitis. NZ Vet J 36:93–94, 1988.
12. Evermann JF, Bryan GM, McKeirnan AJ: Isolation of a calicivirus from a case of canine glossitis. Canine Pract 8:36–39, 1981.
13. McKeever PJ, Klausner JS: Plant awn, candidal, nocardial and necrotizing ulcerative stomatitis in the dog. J Am Anim Hosp Assoc 22:17–22, 1986.
14. Johnson RP, Povey RC: Effect of diet on oral lesions of feline calicivirus infection. Vet Rec 110:106–107, 1982.
15. Thompson RR, Wilcox GE, Clark WT: Association of calicivirus with chronic gingivitis and pharyngitis in cats. J Small Anim Pract 25:207–210, 1984.
15a. Knowles JO, Gaskell RM, Gaskell CJ, et al: Prevalence of feline calicivirus, feline leukemia virus and antibodies to FIV in cats with chronic stomatitis. Vet Rec 124:336–338, 1989.
16. Johnessee JS, Hurvitz AI: Feline plasma cell gingivitis pharyngitis. J Am Anim Hosp Assoc 19:179–181, 1983.
17. Campbell CB: Comparison of treatments for canine tonsillitis. Canine Pract 10(2):39–43, 1983.
17a. Clapper WE, Meade GH: Normal flora of the nose, throat, and lower intestine of dogs. J Bacteriol 85:643–648, 1963.
17b. Smith HW: Observations on the flora of the alimentary tract of animals and factors affecting its composition. J Pathol Bacteriol 89:95–122, 1965.

17c. Smith HW: The development of the flora of the alimentary tract in young animals. *J Pathol Bacteriol* 90:495–513, 1965.

17d. Strombeck DR: *Small Animal Gastroenterology.* Davis, CA, Stonegate Publishing, 1979.

17e. Hirsch DC: Microflora, mucosa, and immunity. *In* Anderson NV (ed): *Veterinary Gastroenterology.* Philadelphia, Lea & Febiger, 1980, pp 199–219.

18. Warner NS, Van Kruiningen HJ: The incidence of clostridia in the canine stomach and their relationship to acute gastric dilation. *J Am Anim Hosp Assoc* 14:618–623, 1978.

19. Isikawa H, Baba E, Matsumoto H: Studies on bacterial flora of the alimentary tract of dogs. III. Fecal flora in clinical and experimental cases of diarrhea. *Jpn J Vet Sci* 44:343–347, 1982.

20. Henry GA, Long PH, Burns JL, et al: Gastric spirillosis in beagles. *Am J Vet Res* 48:831–836, 1987.

21. Kato E, Kaji Y, Kaneko K: Enterotoxigenic staphylococci of canine origin. *Am J Vet Res* 39:1771–1773, 1978.

22. Wasteson Y, Olsvik O, Skancke E, et al: Heat stable enterotoxin producing *Escherichia coli* strains isolated from dogs. *J Clin Microbiol* 26:2564–2566, 1988.

23. Olson PA, Hedhammer Å, Wasström T: Enterotoxigenic *Escherichia coli* infection in dogs with acute diarrhea. *J Am Vet Med Assoc* 185:982–983, 1984.

23a. Olson PA, Hedhammer Å, Faris K, et al: Enterotoxigenic *Escherichia coli* and *Klebsiella pneumoniae* isolated from dogs with diarrhoea. *Vet Microbiol* 10:577–589, 1985.

24. Pospischill A, Mainol JG, Balger G, et al: Attaching and effacing bacteria in the intestines of calves and cats with diarrhea. *Vet Pathol* 24:320–334, 1987.

25. Fox MW, Haynes E: Neonatal colibacillosis in the dog. *J Small Anim Pract* 7:599–603, 1966.

26. Broes A, Drolet R, Jacques M, et al: Natural infection with an attaching and effacing *Escherichia coli* in a diarrheic puppy. *Can J Vet Res* 52:280–282, 1988.

27. Collins JE, Bergeland ME, Lindeman CJ, et al: Enterococcus (Streptococcus) durans adherence in the small intestine of a diarrheic pup. *Vet Pathol* 25:396–398, 1988.

28. Batt RM, Needham JR, Carter MW: Bacterial overgrowth associated with a naturally occurring enteropathy in the German shepherd dog. *Res Vet Sci* 35:42–46, 1983.

29. Whitbread TJ, Batt RM, Garthwaite G: Relative deficiency of IgA in the German shepherd dog: a breed abnormality. *Res Vet Sci* 37:350–352, 1984.

30. Williams DA, Batt RM, McLean L: Bacterial overgrowth in the duodenum of dogs with exocrine pancreatic insufficiency. *J Am Vet Med Assoc* 191:201–206, 1987.

31. Batt RM, McLean: Comparison of the biochemical changes in the jejunal mucosa of dogs with aerobic and anaerobic overgrowth. *Gastroenterology* 93:986–993, 1987.

32. Batt RM, McLean L, Riley JE: Response of the jejunal mucosa of dogs with aerobic or anaerobic bacterial overgrowth to antibiotic therapy. *Gut* 29:473–482, 1988.

33. Tams TR: Chronic canine lymphocytic plasmacytic enteritis. *Compend Cont Educ Pract Vet* 9:1184–1194, 1987.

34. Rutgers HC, Batt RM, Kelly DF: Lymphocytic plasmacytic enteritis associated with bacterial overgrowth in a dog. *J Am Vet Med Assoc* 192:1739–1742, 1988.

35. Tams TR: Chronic feline inflammatory bowel disorders. Part I. Idiopathic inflammatory bowel disease. *Compend Cont Educ Pract Vet* 8:371–376, 1986.

36. Tams TR: Chronic feline inflammatory bowel disorders. Part II. Feline eosinophilic enteritis and lymphosarcoma. *Compend Cont Educ Pract Vet* 8:464–470, 1986.

37. Burrows CF: Canine hemorrhagic gastroenteritis. *J Am Anim Hosp Assoc* 13:451–458, 1977.

38. Papa M, Halperin Z, Rubinstein E, et al: The effect of ischemia of the dog's colon on transmural migration of bacteria and endotoxin. *J Surg Res* 35:264–269, 1983.

38a. Pierce NF, Hirschhorn N: Oral fluid–a simple weapon against dehydration in diarrhoea: how it works and how to use it. *WHO Chron* 31:87–93, 1977.

38b. Sack RB, Cassells J, Mitra R, et al: The use of oral replacement solutions in the treatment of cholera and other severe diarrheal disorders. *Bull WHO* 43:351–360, 1970.

38c. Lewis LD, Phillips RW: New information on fluid therapy for diarrheic calves. *Norden News* 55(2):4–8, 1980.

38d. Pickering LK: *Infections of the Gastrointestinal Tract.* New York, Plenum Medical, 1979, pp 247–267.

38e. World Health Organization: *Treatment and Prevention of Dehydration in Diarrheal Diseases.* Geneva, WHO, 1976.

38f. Gangarosa EJ: Recent developments in diarrheal diseases. *Postgrad Med* 62:113–117, 1977.

39. Papich MG, Davis CA, Davis LE: Absorption of salicylate from an antidiarrheal preparation in dogs and cats. *J Am Anim Hosp Assoc* 23:221–226, 1987.

39a. Sox TE, Olson CA: Binding and kill of enteropathogenic bacteria by bismuth subsalicylate. Abstr 28th Intersci Conf Antimicrob Agents Chemother, Los Angeles, Am Soc Microbiol, 1988, pp 178.

40. Shindel NM, Van Kruiningen HJ, Scott FW: The colitis of feline panleukopenia. *J Am Anim Hosp Assoc* 14:783–474, 1978.

41. Bolton OR, Brown TT: Mycotic colitis in a cat. *VM SAC* 67:978–981, 1972.

42. Erbeck DH, Hagee JH: A successful course of therapy for necrotic colitis, a newly recognized disease entity of cats. *VM SAC* 69:603–605, 1974.

43. Leib MS, Sponenberg DP, Wilcke JR, et al: Suppurative colitis in a cat. *J Am Vet Med Assoc* 188:739–741, 1986.

44. Van Kruiningen HJV, Ryan MJ, Shindel NM: The classification of feline colitis. *J Comp Pathol* 93:275–294, 1983.

45. Wilkie JSN: Necrotic colitis in two cats–a description of the lesion. *Can Vet J* 23:197–199, 1982.

46. Nelson RW, Dimperio ME, Long GG: Lymphocytic-plasmacytic colitis in a cat. *J Am Vet Med Assoc* 184:1133–1136, 1984.

47. Ridgway MD: Management of chronic colitis in the dog. *J Am Vet Med Assoc* 185:804–806, 1984.

48. Bjorling DE, Crowe DT, Kolata RJ, et al: Penetrating abdominal wounds in dogs and cats. *J Am Anim Hosp Assoc* 18:742–748, 1982.

49. Bjorling DE, Latimer KS, Rawlings CA, et al: Diagnostic peritoneal lavage before and after abdominal surgery in dogs. *Am J Vet Res* 44:816–820, 1983.

50. Bartlett JG: Intra-abdominal abscess. *In* Zak O, Sande MA (eds): *Experimental Models in Antimicrobial Chemotherapy.* New York, Academic Press, 1986, pp 91–114.

51. Ho JL, Barza M: Role of aminoglycoside antibiotics in the treatment of intraabdominal infection. *Antimicrob Agents Chemother* 3:485–491, 1987.

52. Walker RI, MacVittie TJ, Sinha BL, et al: Antibiotic decontamination of the dog and its consequences. *Lab Anim Sci* 28:55–61, 1978.

53. Rakower SR, Keyes J, Miethaner WL: The protective role of intraperitoneal antibiotic irrigation in contaminated penetrating wounds of the cecum. *Surgery* 80:405–410, 1976.

53a. Ndikuwera J, Winstanley EW, Binta-mushi G, et al: Haematology and serum biochemistry in the racing greyhound following intraperitoneal povidone iodine. *Vet Res Comm* 12:77–86, 1988.

54. Greenfield CL, Walshaw R: Open peritoneal drainage for treatment of contaminated peritoneal cavity and septic peritonitis in dogs and cats: 24 cases (1980–1986). *J Am Vet Med Assoc* 191:100–105, 1987.

55. Gerding DN, Kromhout JP, Sullivan JJ, et al: Antibiotic penetrance of ascitic fluid in dogs. *Antimicrob Agents Chemother* 10:850–855, 1976.

10

HEPATOBILIARY INFECTIONS

S. A. Center

NORMAL FLORA

Bacteriologic studies of portal vein blood in the dog have shown that alimentary flora, especially anaerobic organisms, in low quantities commonly circulate to the liver.[1, 2] It is suspected but has not been proved that this is also true for the cat. Liver disorders associated with ischemic tissue injury or impaired hepatic artery perfusion encourage an anaerobic environment conducive to the growth of such bacteria as *Clostridium* or *Bacteroides*. The high probability of anaerobic infection requires special clinical attention in order that specimens be collected and transported using techniques that ensure survival of anaerobic organisms.

The hepatic mononuclear phagocyte system (MPS) is the largest source of fixed macrophages in the body. These cells phagocytize blood-borne microorganisms, particulate matter, and endotoxins. Because of the dual origin of the hepatic blood supply from the portal and systemic circulations, the hepatobiliary system is uniquely susceptible to involvement in systemic infectious disease. Abnormal liver enzyme activity and hepatic dysfunction seem to develop most often in response to the secondary effects of infection rather than to the infectious agent itself. Pyrexia, anoxia, nutritional deficits, toxic by-products from infectious agents, and released inflammatory mediators each may play a role in the development of clinicopathologic abnormalities. Suspicion of primary hepatobiliary disease may cause misdiagnosis when the liver is secondarily involved or is an innocent bystander. On occasion, a self-perpetuating form of chronic, persistent, or active hepatitis may develop as a complication of systemic infection with bacterial or viral agents. Notable examples include chronic active hepatitis in dogs after infection with *Leptospira* or adenovirus (infectious canine hepatitis).[3, 4]

Hepatic Infections

HEPATIC RESPONSE TO SEPSIS AND ENDOTOXEMIA

The hepatic MPS, composed largely of Kupffer cells, provides a major component of the systemic phagocytic clearance capacity. In addition, it serves as an important barrier to the passage of intestinal microorganisms and their toxins into the systemic circulation. Bacteria or their by-products enter the portal circulation in massive quantities when abnormalities such as hemorrhagic shock or bowel ischemia occur.

Between 60% and 90% of bacteria extracted from the circulation are collected by the MPS of the liver or spleen and are either destroyed or eliminated in bile.[5] If hepatobiliary function is compromised, failure to clear these organisms may result in hepatic infection with or without systemic complications.

The response of the liver to systemic sepsis has been studied in dogs experimentally infused with endotoxin or live gram-negative bacteria.[6-8] Acute morphologic changes include dilation and congestion of sinusoids and hepatic veins, necrosis of hepatocytes in central and midzonal areas, fatty vacuolation, an acute diffuse influx of inflammatory cells (neutrophils and monocytes) and microabscess formation. Kupffer cell hyperplasia occasionally develops. With chronicity, canalicular biliary stasis becomes apparent. Hepatocellular dysfunction results in a shift to anaerobic metabolism, impaired hepatic gluconeogenesis, and mobilization of lipids from peripheral stores. Acute increases in the serum concentrations of triglycerides and cholesterol may develop in dogs, as a result of energy dependency on fat metabolism.

Clinical Findings

Hepatomegaly, splenomegaly, fever, and depression are common clinical signs. The hemogram may depict leukopenia, degenerative left shift, and nonregenerative anemia. Hyperglobulinemia, hyperfibrinogenemia, hypoalbuminemia, and hypoglycemia may develop rapidly, as do marked increases in serum ALT (formerly SGPT) and AST (formerly SGOT) activities. In the dog, serum ALP activity increases after several days. Hyperbilirubinemia develops after 36 to 48 hours of septicemia. Jaundice has developed in severe systemic infections and portends a poor prognosis. DIC, acute renal failure, and myocardial dysfunction may also develop as a result of endotoxemia.

Therapy

Treatment consists of the provision of adequate fluid therapy, parenteral antibiotics effective against the causative organism, glucose supplementation, and identification and correction of any underlying disease process (see Endotoxemia, Chapter 44).

PYOGENIC ABSCESS

Bacterial infections of the liver are uncommon as compared with systemic infections and may produce discrete unifocal suppuration and necrosis or multifocal abscesses. Fatal hepatic abscesses may develop as a result of trauma or as an extension of sepsis from adjacent viscera, the peritoneal cavity, hematogenous distribution, or from an as-

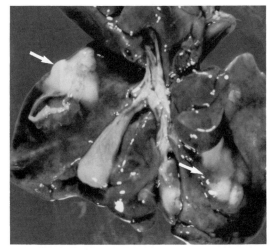

Figure 10–1. Hepatic abscesses (*arrows*) associated with a *Staphylococcus* omphalitis in a neonatal puppy.

cending biliary tract infection. Hepatic abscesses have been reported in neonates with omphalogenic infections,[9] in which the most common isolate has been *Staphylococcus* in dogs and *Streptococcus* in cats (Fig. 10–1, or see Fig. 56–2).

Multifocal microabscess formation has been described in conjunction with a variety of organisms associated with systemic infection, such as *Listeria*, *Salmonella*, *Brucella*, *Escherichia coli*, *Yersinia pseudotuberculosis*, *Bacillus piliformis*, *Actinobacillus lignieresii*, *Actinomyces*, *Nocardia*, and *Pasteurella* (Fig. 10–2).

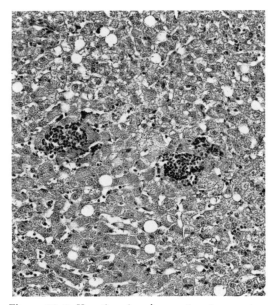

Figure 10–2. Hepatic microabscessation in a mature dog associated with an *Escherichia coli* septicemia.

Clinical Findings

Early diagnosis is difficult due to vague physical abnormalities that may include hepatomegaly, abdominal tenderness, abdominal effusion, fever, and depression. Animals with systemic infections will demonstrate signs attributable to the organ systems involved.

Clinical Laboratory Findings

Clinicopathologic abnormalities may include an inflammatory leukogram with a left shift, marked increases in serum ALT and AST activities, hyperglobulinemia, mild hyperbilirubinemia, hypoglycemia, and detection of a septic abdominal effusion. Abscess formation with gram-negative organisms may produce signs of endotoxemia. Ultrasonographic examination of the liver may detect a fluid-filled parenchymal defect associated with liquefaction necrosis or a hyperechoic lesion associated with caseated material. In some cases, abdominal radio-graphic findings may include an emphysematous nidus associated with a gas-producing organism. Microabscesses are usually not detected by radiography or sonography. Blood or urine culture results may identify the causative organism.

Therapy

Successful treatment of unifocal abscess formation requires early diagnosis, aggressive surgical drainage, and long-term (6- to 8-weeks') administration of an appropriate antibiotic. Broad-spectrum antibiotics should be selected prior to return of culture and susceptibility results. Combination therapy is recommended if cytology or Gram-stained smears display multiple organisms. Body temperature, hemogram, liver enzyme activity, and abdominal ultrasonography may be used to monitor the response to therapy.

Treatment of hepatic microabscess is similar. An underlying immunocompromised condition, such as FeLV or FIV infections or neoplasia, must be investigated with disseminated sepsis.

Biliary Infections

Severe cholestasis is associated with reduced ability to eliminate bacteria in bile, although hepatic uptake of enteric organisms from the portal circulation continues unabated. Cholestasis in itself predisposes the patient to biliary tract infection. Resolution of cholestasis allows mobilization of bacteria from sites of hepatic sequestration and results in the sudden appearance of bacteria in bile. This phenomenon must be considered when surgically treating patients with major bile duct obstruction, as failure to give effective antibiotics during corrective surgery increases the risk of postoperative infection.

FELINE CHOLANGITIS-CHOLANGIOHEPATITIS

The cholangitis-cholangiohepatitis syndrome is one of the most common hepatobiliary disorders diagnosed in cats. Inflammation of intrahepatic bile ducts (cholangitis) frequently is associated with chronic interstitial pancreatitis owing to the anatomic fusion of the common bile and pancreatic ducts of the cat. Infectious agents that are known to cause biliary tree inflammation in cats include trematodes, *Toxoplasma*-like organisms, an organism similar to *Hepatozoon canis*, gram-negative intestinal bacteria, and *Bacillus piliformis* (Fig. 10–3). Although infectious agents may initiate the process, hepatobiliary inflammation may become self-perpetuating owing to activation of immunologic processes. Cholangiohepatitis develops when cholangitis progresses to involve the surrounding hepatic parenchyma. Cholangitis has been separated into two forms for ease of discussion.

Nonsuppurative Cholangitis

Nonsuppurative cholangitis is commonly diagnosed in middle-aged to old cats. It is associated with variable clinical signs, in-

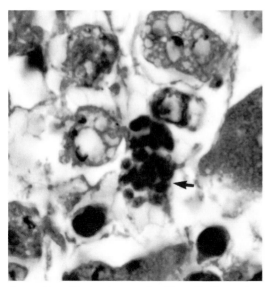

Figure 10–3. Photomicrograph of hepatic tissue demonstrating *Toxoplasma*-like organisms *(arrow)* in a cat with cholangiohepatitis (× 960).

cluding intermittent anorexia, vomiting, diarrhea, depression, fever, weight loss, and with chronicity, jaundice. Many cats remain asymptomatic, and the disorder is diagnosed at necropsy as an incidental observation. **Feline chronic lymphocytic cholangitis** has been described in young longhaired cats.[10, 11] Additional unique clinical signs have included polyphagia, hepatomegaly, peripheral lymphadenopathy, and ascites. This disorder is characterized by bile duct hyperplasia, biliary fibrosis, lymphoid aggregates in the portal triads, and cirrhosis. **Sclerosing cholangitis** is a histologically distinct form characterized by segmental fibrosing inflammatory changes of bile ducts resulting in ductal narrowing and obstruction.[12] Only in rare instances has nonsuppurative cholangitis been proved to be associated with infection.

Suppurative Cholangitis

Suppurative cholangitis has been less commonly diagnosed than has nonsuppurative cholangitis, but it must be distinguished clinically.[13] Affected cats are usually older than 8 years and demonstrate severe clinical illness characterized by jaundice, intermittent GI signs, depression, anorexia, weight loss, and fever. Pathogenic mechanisms involve abnormalities of the biliary system associated with bile stasis, such as choleli-

thiasis, periductal pancreatic and biliary duct fibrosis associated with ascending infection or pancreatitis, trematode infection, or congenital biliary tract malformation. Stasis of bile flow seems to potentiate the development of bacterial infection. Culture of tissue, bile, and choleliths has revealed bacterial infections, especially *E. coli* in some cases. When an organism is isolated by bacterial culture, the question remains whether its presence has caused or is a result of the disorder. The process of biliary infection and cholestasis becomes self-perpetuating. Many affected cats have histories of intermittent vomiting and diarrhea that could be associated with portal bacteremia or reflux of duodenal flora into the bile duct. Once enteric organisms gain access to bile, they may cause the formation of lithocholic acid, a hepatotoxin capable of producing cholestasis and hepatobiliary inflammation.

Suppurative cholangitis is characterized by a neutrophilic infiltration around and within intrahepatic bile ducts, hepatocellular cholestasis, and eventually, periportal fibrosis. It is possible that suppurative cholangitis precedes the development of chronic nonsuppurative cholangitis. If this is true, biliary tract infection may be an early initiating process of the cholangitis syndrome.

Clinical Laboratory Findings

The clinicopathologic features of feline cholangitis are variable. The hemogram may reveal a mild, nonregenerative anemia, a normal leukogram, or a neutrophilic leukocytosis, sometimes accompanied by a left shift. Suppurative cholangitis is more commonly associated with a moderate-to-severe neutrophilic leukocytosis accompanied by a left shift. Increased serum activities of ALT, AST, ALP and γ-glutamyl transferase (GGT) vary, depending on the degree of tissue inflammation and cholestasis. Hyperglobulinemia and mild prerenal azotemia are common. Bilirubinuria in the cat is a sensitive measure of mild hyperbilirubinemia. Obvious hyperbilirubinemia causing jaundice is more consistently present and usually is moderate to severe in cats with suppurative cholangitis. Evaluation of liver function, using serum bile acid quantification, may detect cholestasis before hyperbilirubinemia becomes overt. Bleeding tendencies as a result of impaired vitamin K absorption are only observed when cholangitis is severe and chronic or is accompanied by major bile duct occlusion.

Therapy

See General Treatment Considerations for Hepatobiliary Infections for appropriate surgical and medical support. Suppurative cholangitis should be treated with antibiotics for at least 6 to 8 weeks. Periodic reevaluation (every 2 to 3 weeks) of liver enzyme activity, bilirubin concentration, and hepatic function is advised. The response to treatment is based on improvement in clinical and laboratory abnormalities. Reevaluation of hepatic biopsy is desirable but often cannot be justified when the patient has improved.

Cats with nonsuppurative cholangitis should be treated prophylactically with antibiotics for presumed bacterial infections (Table 10–1). Metronidazole may be useful because of its good hepatobiliary tissue penetration and its effectiveness against anaerobic organisms. If peribiliary fibrosis is observed, cultures are negative, and the cat fails to improve with supportive care and antibiotics, then prednisolone may be indicated (Table 10–1). An initial dose of 1 to 2 mg/kg given orally once a day is recommended. This dose is tapered after the first 1 to 2 weeks if the animal demonstrates improvement. Chronic, continuous, or intermittent anti-inflammatory therapy may be

necessary to control this form of feline cholangitis.

CHOLECYSTITIS

Septic inflammation of the bile ducts and gallbladder occurs in dogs and cats. The pathogenesis of acute cholecystitis is not clearly understood, although a variety of associated etiologic events have been defined. Acute cholecystitis can be experimentally produced by introduction of pepsin, activated proteolytic pancreatic enzymes, neutrophils, or bacteria into the bile duct.[14] Spontaneous reflux of such initiating factors into the bile duct is probably more common in the cat than in the dog. Biliary tract obstruction and septicemia have been implicated as major causes of biliary infection. Cholelithiasis and choledocholithiasis have been associated with septic and nonseptic cholangitis, cholecystitis, and choledochocystitis (duct inflammation) in both dogs and cats. Bile stasis, biliary inflammation, or infection and changes in bile composition are associated with bile stone formation. Insidious duct occlusion by choleliths or slow-growing biliary neoplasia can result in septic inflammation since cholestatic jaundice impairs the biliary elimination of portal vein–derived bacteria.

Clinical Findings

Infection involving the bile ducts and gallbladder is associated with fever, anorexia,

Table 10–1. Commonly Used Drugs for Treatment of Hepatobiliary Infections[a]

DRUG	SPECIES	DOSE[b] (mg/kg)	ROUTE	INTERVAL (hours)	DURATION (weeks)	INDICATIONS
Vitamin K₁	B	5–15 (total)	SC	24	prn	Biliary obstruction, hepatic insufficiency
Metronidazole	B	15[c]	IV, PO	8–12	prn	Anaerobic hepatic or biliary infections, biliary or hepatic inflammation
Gentamicin	B	1–2	IV, SC	8	prn[d]	Gram-negative aerobic hepatobiliary infections
Amp(Amox)icillin	B	11–22	IV, SC, PO	8	prn	Anaerobic hepatobiliary infections
Dehydrocholic acid	D	15–20	PO	8–12	2–4[e]	Hydrocholeresis
	C	10–15	PO	8–12	2–4	

[a]See text for appropriate indications for each drug. B = dog and cat, D = dog, C = cat, PO = oral, SC = subcutaneous, IV = intravenous, prn = as needed.

[b]Dose per administration, given at specified interval, expressed as mg/kg unless otherwise stated.

[c]Dose should be reduced in patients with insufficient hepatic function to avoid neurotoxicity; 7.5 mg/kg given orally two to three times daily has been used with apparent clinical success.

[d]Must monitor for nephrotoxicity.

[e]If use is prolonged, monitor for hepatotoxicity.

vomiting, abdominal tenderness, hepato-megaly, and jaundice. These signs can be persistent, intermittent, or episodic. If complete occlusion of the biliary tract is chronic (>2 weeks), pale acholic feces, absence of urinary urobilinogen, and bleeding tendencies due to vitamin K depletion may also be observed. Six to eight weeks of chronic bile duct occlusion may result in the development of portal hypertension, hepatic fibrosis, and ascites.

Clinical Laboratory Findings

Cholecystitis is frequently associated with clinicopathologic abnormalities typical of major bile duct occlusion. A nonregenerative anemia associated with chronic inflammation may develop. A regenerative anemia may develop in animals that have experienced substantial GI hemorrhage from pyloric or duodenal ulcers. Alimentary ulcerations commonly develop in patients with compromised hepatic function and severe cholestasis due to hypergastrinemia, increased serum bile acid concentrations, and impaired mucosal perfusion and repair. A marked leukocytosis with a regenerative left shift is also common. Serum liver enzyme activities, especially ALP and GGT, are markedly increased (5- to 10-fold reference values). Severe cholestasis is common in animals having cholecystitis, with hyperbilirubinemia reaching as much as 20-fold reference values. Serum concentrations of total cholesterol may be increased 2- to 4-fold reference values. Increased prothrombin time, activated partial thromboplastin time or activated clotting time, may develop owing to vitamin K depletion. Septic bile peritonitis may prevail if the biliary system ruptures. Abdominocentesis yielding yellowish-orange fluid containing bile or bacteria indicates the need for immediate surgical intervention. Abdominal radiography may indicate the presence of abdominal effusion. In exceptional cases, radiodense calcium containing choleliths may be observed (Fig. 10–4). In most instances, choleliths in dogs and cats are radiopaque and cannot be visualized on survey abdominal radiographs.

Ultrasonography can provide important diagnostic information since it can reveal biliary tract thickening or distention and choleliths within the gallbladder. Care must

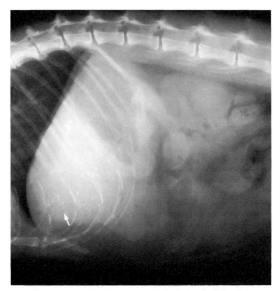

Figure 10–4. Radiodense microcholedocholithiasis (arrow) within the intrahepatic biliary tree in a mature cat that had 2 years previously undergone cholecystotomy for cholelith removal. Chronic cholangitis, biliary infection, and sludged bile were contributing causes of cholelith development.

be taken to avoid confusion of commonly visualized bile sediment within the gallbladder that is due to anorexia with clinically significant cholelithiasis. Ultrasonography can also detect the presence of small quantities of abdominal effusion associated with sepsis or bile peritonitis.

Therapy

Laparotomy is the usual treatment for septic cholecystitis. Follow-up medical management requires the prolonged administration of antibiotics effective against aerobic and anaerobic organisms. E. coli has been a common bacterial isolate from biliary tissue and bile from affected dogs and cats. Chronic cholecystitis has also been associated with Salmonella (dogs) and Pasteurella (cats). Hydrocholeresis may be used in conjunction with fluid therapy and antibiotics to diminish bile stasis. See General Treatment Considerations, later.

EMPHYSEMATOUS CHOLECYSTITIS

Emphysematous cholecystitis is an uncommon medical problem observed in dogs with and without diabetes mellitus.[15, 16] Diagnosis in the cat is rare. The most common precipitating factor is believed to be cystic duct obstruction. Ischemia of the gallbladder wall caused by tense distention allows an anaerobic environment to become established. Gas-producing organisms gaining access to the hepatic circulation or parenchyma can proliferate in the wall of the gallbladder and spread to the pericholangiocystic tissues. Left untreated, the gallbladder may rupture, and the organism may gain access to the abdominal cavity. Pneumoperitoneum associated with septic peritonitis follows (Fig. 10–5).

Clinical Findings

Clinical signs associated with emphysematous cholecystitis include abdominal tenderness, fever, jaundice, anorexia, and vomiting. A neutrophilic leukocytosis, hyperbilirubinemia, increased serum ALP, GGT, ALT, and AST activities and prerenal azotemia are common. When the gallbladder ruptures, the abdomen may become tympanic. Initially, radiographic features of emphysematous cholecystitis consist of gas infiltrates in the gallbladder wall that spread to completely fill the gallbladder lumen and then involve the pericholecystic tissues. A sufficient volume of gas for radiographic detection will accumulate in 24 to 48 hours. The most common bacteria isolated from humans and dogs with emphysematous cholecystitis are clostridia.[16]

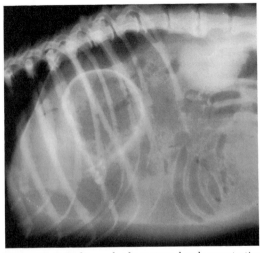

Figure 10–5. Radiograph of a mature dog demonstrating pneumoperitoneum associated with septic bile peritonitis. A clostridial organism was identified on Gram stain and by anaerobic bacterial culture.

Therapy

Management of emphysematous cholecystitis usually includes cholecystectomy combined with the prolonged administration of antibiotics effective against anaerobic organisms, but even then the prognosis is poor (see General Treatment Considerations, later). Only rarely have people and dogs with emphysematous cholecystitis survived without surgical intervention. Medical and surgical treatment for septic peritonitis is usually also indicated.

BILE PERITONITIS

Bile peritonitis is a serious complication of biliary tree infection, inflammation, ischemia, or trauma. The toxicity of bile on tissues and hypovolemic shock associated with pooling of fluid in the peritoneal cavity are responsible for the major clinical signs. Bacterial sepsis is the usual cause of death. Bacterial contamination, usually by anaerobes, of biliary ascites may spontaneously develop.[17, 18] Bile-induced permeability changes in the intestinal wall permit the passage of enteric flora into the peritoneal effusion.

Clinical Findings

Animals with bile peritonitis usually present with histories of anorexia, vomiting, abdominal tenderness and distention, and lethargy. Most patients demonstrate jaundice and fever. Emphysematous peritonitis may develop if gas-producing bacteria contaminate the peritoneal effusion (see Fig. 10–5). Palpation will reveal a tense tympanic abdomen.

Diagnosis

Usual hematologic abnormalities are a neutrophilic leukocytosis with a regenerative left shift, although in some cases a degenerative left shift has been observed. Biochemical abnormalities are characteristic of the underlying disease process. Increased liver enzyme activities and moderate-to-severe hyperbilirubinemia are expected. Hypercholesterolemia may exist if complete bile duct occlusion precedes rupture of the biliary tree. Hypoalbuminemia may develop owing to the loss of protein into the abdominal cavity. Prerenal azotemia is common owing to the hypovolemic shock that frequently accompanies the syndrome. Prolonged hypovolemia may result in renal azotemia.

The primary abnormality observed on abdominal radiography is a diffuse lack of visceral detail owing to the presence of peritoneal fluid. Cholangiography rarely delineates the site of biliary rupture because the competition between bilirubin and iodinated contrast prohibits adequate dye concentration in the biliary tree. Free gas within the peritoneal cavity or migrating within the biliary tree usually indicates anaerobic bacterial infection.

Abdominocentesis reveals a yellowish-orange or greenish-gold fluid. Cytologic examination reveals neutrophils, macrophages, erythrocytes, and bilirubin pigment (Fig. 10–6). The presence of bacteria is easily detected using Wright's Giemsa or new methylene blue stain. Gram staining may be used to aid in the examination of the morphology of the organisms as well as the effusion for the presence of spores. Aerobic and anaerobic cultures should be initiated regardless of whether bacterial organisms are visualized on cytologic examination.

Therapy

Whenever bile peritonitis is suspected, surgical intervention is indicated. See General Treatment Considerations for appropriate surgical and medical support measures.

GENERAL TREATMENT CONSIDERATIONS FOR HEPATOBILIARY INFECTIONS

Supportive Care

Initial management of the animal with hepatobiliary infection involves thorough supportive care, consisting of fluid therapy and provision of a calorically and nutritionally adequate diet. Polyionic isotonic fluids should be given to correct dehydration and contemporary losses and to provide for maintenance needs. If hypoglycemia is detected, isotonic fluids should be supplemented to 2.5% or 5.0% with dextrose. When hepatic insufficiency, ascites, and a tendency for sodium retention are present, a solution of 2.5% dextrose in water should be combined with 50% strength lactated Ringer's or 0.45% sodium chloride. If bile peritonitis exists, especially with concurrent sepsis, aggressive fluid administration at shock volumes (90 ml/kg/hr) may be required prior to general anesthesia and laparotomy.

Anorexia must be corrected by forced alimentation by mouth, nasogastric intubation, pharyngostomy tube, or gastrostomy. Parenteral or enteral alimentation may be required if vomiting becomes a persistent problem. Caloric intake should achieve at least 45 to 55 kcal/kg. The use of benzodiazepines in cats to stimulate the appetite will not ensure adequate caloric intake in most instances. Hepatic insufficiency and hepatoencephalopathy contraindicate the use of these drugs.

Vitamin K_1 should be administered by SC injection in animals with prolonged coagulation times, hemorrhage, or icterus in the event that chronic complete bile duct occlusion exists (Table 10–1). If bleeding tendencies are recognized during surgery, a compatible fresh blood transfusion should be administered.

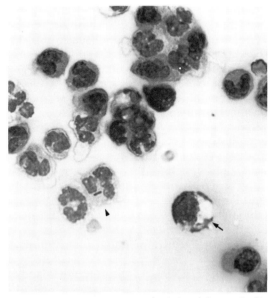

Figure 10–6. Photomicrograph of the abdominal effusion observed in the dog shown in Figure 10–4 with septic bile peritonitis. Neutrophils, macrophages, erythrocytes, intracytoplasmic large gram-positive, rod-form bacteria *(arrowhead)*, and golden bilirubin crystals *(arrow)* characterized the cytologic features (Wright's Giemsa stain; × 680).

Antibiotics

Antibiotics used for hepatobiliary infections should possess the relevant spectrum of activity against organisms commonly cultured from liver tissue and bile. *E. coli*, *Clostridium* spp., *Staphylococcus*, and *Pasteurella* are representative organisms that have been encountered clinically. Culture and susceptibility of the involved organism from liver or biliary tissue remains the best measure for correct antibiotic selection. Aerobic gram-negative organisms commonly associated with hepatobiliary infections are generally most susceptible in vitro, in decreasing order, to kanamycin, gentamicin, chloramphenicol, streptomycin, cephalosporins, tetracyclines, and ampicillin. The drugs most effective against anaerobes are clindamycin, chloramphenicol, and metronidazole. Drugs that achieve good bile concentrations include ampicillin, amoxicillin, metronidazole, tetracycline, and cephalothin. Care should be taken to avoid administration of tetracycline to cats with liver disease since this antibiotic is known to induce hepatic lipidosis in other species. Although good drug penetration into the biliary tract has been recommended, systemic activity of the antibiotic may be more important. It is desirable to have satisfactory tissue antibiotic levels before surgery. Antibiotics administered during complete bile duct occlusion may not attain therapeutic levels in bile owing to the cessation of biliary flow. Therefore, in patients with extrahepatic cholestasis, it is also essential that bile flow be reinstated surgically or by the administration of a hydrocholeretic after bile duct patency has been verified. When bacterial sepsis is suspected, antibiotics should initially be administered IV and should be continued for 4 to 6 weeks.

In the absence of culture and susceptibility results, selected antibiotics should be effective over the expected range of aerobic and anaerobic enteric organisms. Metronidazole is a good first choice antibiotic. Unfortunately, it relies on hepatic biotransformation for elimination and may cause anorexia, vomiting, and serious neurologic signs in patients with insufficient hepatic function. Alternatively, gentamicin can be used as an antiaerobic combined with ampicillin as an antianaerobic antibiotic. Aminoglycosides should not be used until the patient's hydration status and prerenal azo-temia are corrected. Aminoglycoside nephrotoxicity should be monitored by urine sediment examination for granular casts on an alternate day schedule.

Antibiotics that require extensive hepatobiliary activation, biotransformation, or excretion or those that have been associated with adverse effects on the hepatobiliary system are considered poor first-choice selections for patients with compromised hepatic function. These drugs include hetacillin, tetracycline, lincomycin, erythromycin, sulfonamide, trimethoprim-sulfonamide, and chloramphenicol. Furthermore, severe icterus contraindicates the use of antibiotics such as chloramphenicol, erythromycin, doxycycline, rifampin, clindamycin, and nafcillin that are excreted predominantly in the bile.

Surgery

Laparotomy is indicated in most cases of hepatobiliary sepsis. Surgical intervention is imperative if hepatobiliary abscesses, septic peritonitis, bile peritonitis, or major bile duct occlusion are suspected. Hepatic biopsy is the only way to confirm an infectious process localized within the hepatobiliary system and to provide a definitive diagnosis of cholangitis, cholangiohepatitis, cholecystitis, or choledochocystitis.

At surgery, the abdominal viscera should be inspected for a primary disease process. Mesenteric and hepatic lymph nodes should be examined and biopsied if a diagnosis remains uncertain. The liver should be biopsied at one or more sites. Because of hepatic regenerative capacity, entire lobes of liver should be resected if they seem to be involved in an abscess or appear to be necrotic. The biliary tract should be assessed for patency and the bile should be checked for fluidity by gentle compression on the gallbladder and observation of the ease with which bile can be expelled into the duodenum. The gallbladder and major bile ducts should be carefully palpated for choleliths, intraluminal or mural masses, and for sludged bile. If abnormalities are detected, a cholecystotomy should be done, the gallbladder should be biopsied, and any abnormality should be inspected. Choleliths and inspissated bile should be removed. Extrahepatic bile ducts may be surgically flushed with a soft rubber catheter and sterile saline solution to remove choleliths and sludged bile, taking care to avoid peritoneal contamination. Cholecystectomy is advised if the gallbladder wall appears devitalized or has neoplastic involvement.

An alternative route of bile drainage may be indicated in cases of extrahepatic biliary obstruction. If a portion of the common bile duct is damaged, a biliary diversion to the bowel, such as cholecystoduodenostomy or cholecystojejunostomy, may be appropriate. If the cystic duct is damaged, placement of a T-tube or a choledochoenterostomy may be appropriate. Such procedures are often associated with complications of chronic biliary stasis and infection.

Samples of tissue and bile should be cultured anaerobically and aerobically. Bile for culture and cytology should be collected by fine-needle (22-gauge) aspiration into a syringe. The needle should enter the gallbladder at an oblique angle to reduce the chance of bile leakage following collection. If cholecystitis or cholangitis are suspected, biopsy and culture of a portion of the gallbladder wall and liver is frequently more reliable than culture of bile alone. Choleliths should also be submitted for culture.

If peritoneal sepsis is present, the abdominal cavity may generate a fetid foul odor at surgery. Lavage with sterile saline is recommended prior to abdominal closure. The placement of abdominal drains should be considered.

Cytologic smears should be made from each biopsied tissue, lesion, and sample of bile. Bacteria may be more easily visualized on cytologic than on histologic examination. Gram staining will help to identify the organism, thereby assisting in the selection of initial antibacterial therapy. Aerobic and anaerobic bacterial cultures should be requested on representative samples. Strict attention must be paid to the methods of handling and transporting specimens for anaerobic bacterial cultures (see Chapter 42). These should be collected and inserted into an oxygen-depleted transport vial for delivery to the laboratory. If bile is collected into a syringe, the syringe should be capped to preserve the anaerobic environment. Cytology is an important quality control indicator of transport and culture procedures. If organisms are identified on smears made at the time of surgery yet are not grown, transport or culture methods were probably inadequate. If trematode infection is possible, bile and feces should be examined cytologically for trematode eggs. Hepatic tissue should always be submitted for routine histologic evaluation, and the pathologist should be prompted to reexamine tissues for infectious agents.

Hydrocholeresis

After the patency of the biliary tract has been established at surgery, hydrocholeresis can be used to improve the flow of bile in patients having considerable cholestasis, cholelithiasis, or inspissated bile. The resolution of bile stasis seems to assist in the clearance of biliary infection and to prohibit further stone formation. Hydrocholeresis can be accomplished with dehydrocholic acid, a synthetic bile acid that increases the liquid or water component of ductular secretions. Dehydrocholic acid should be used in conjunction with fluid therapy to ensure adequate patient hydration, which will optimize hydrocholeresis in dogs with cholecystitis and cats with cholangitis or cholangiohepatitis (see Table 6–1). Long-term therapy must involve follow-up laboratory testing as dehydrocholic acid can be metabolized to lithocholic acid, a hepatotoxic secondary bile acid. Chronic therapy may be instituted with a reduced dosage on a once-daily schedule when antibiotic therapy has been discontinued.

References

1. Dineen P: The importance of the route of infection in experimental biliary tract obstruction. *Surg Gyn Obstet* 1001–1008, 1978.
2. Cobb LM, McKay KA: A bacteriological study of the liver of the normal dog. *J Comp Pathol* 72:92–96, 1962.
3. Bishop L, Strandberg JD, Adams RJ, et al: Chronic active hepatitis in dogs associated with leptospires. *Am J Vet Res* 40:839–844, 1979.
4. Gocke DJ, Morris TQ, Bradley SE: Chronic hepatitis in the dog. The role of immune factors. *J Am Vet Med Assoc* 156:1700–1705, 1970.
5. Cardoso V, Pimenta A, da Fonseca JC, et al: The effect of cholestasis on hepatic clearance of bacteria. *World J Surg* 6:330–334, 1982.
6. Groves AC, Woolf LI, O'Regan PJ, et al: Impaired gluconeogenesis in dogs with *E. coli* bacteremia. *Surgery* 76:533, 1974.
7. Filkins JP, Cornell RP: Depression of hepatic gluconeogenesis and the hypoglycemia of endotoxic shock. *Am J Physiol* 227:778, 1974.
8. Griffiths J, Groves AC, Leung FY: Hypertriglyceridemia and hypoglycemia in gram-negative sepsis in the dog. *Surg Gynecol Obstet* 136:897, 1973.

9. Hargis AM, Thomassen RW: Hepatic abscesses in beagle puppies. *Lab Anim Sci* 30:689–693, 1980.

10. Prasse KW, Mahaffey EA, DeNovo R, et al: Chronic lymphocytic cholangitis in three cats. *Vet Pathol* 19:99-108, 1982.

11. Lucke VM, Davies JD: Progressive lymphocytic cholangitis in the cat. *J Small Anim Pract* 25:249–260, 1984.

12. Edwards DF, McCracken MJD, Richardson DC: Sclerosing cholangitis in a cat. *J Am Vet Med Assoc* 182:710–712, 1983.

13. Hirsch VM, Doige CE: Suppurative cholangitis in cats. *J Am Vet Med Assoc* 182:1223–1226, 1983.

14. Gonciarz A, Trusz-Gluza M, Kusmierski S, et al: Leukocytic proteases in gallbladder pathology. Experimental acute cholecystitis in dogs. *Digestion* 10:65–72, 1974.

15. Lord PR, Wilkins RJ: Emphysema of the gallbladder in a diabetic dog. *J Am Vet Radiol Soc* 13:49–52, 1972.

16. Burk RL, Johnson GF: Emphysematous cholecystitis in the nondiabetic dog: three case histories. *Vet Radiol* 21:242–245, 1980.

17. Cain JL, Labat JA, Cohn I: Bile peritonitis in germ-free dogs. *Gastroenterology* 53:600–603, 1967.

18. Nora PF, Bransfield JJ, Laufman H: Hyperbaria in experimental bile peritonitis. *Arch Surg* 98:235–238, 1969.

11

GENITOURINARY INFECTIONS

Jeanne A. Barsanti
Cheri A. Johnson

Urogenital bacterial infections are among the most frequently encountered clinical problems in small animal practice. Such infections range in severity from asymptomatic to life threatening.

NORMAL FLORA

The clinical importance of the normal genitourinary microflora is that it must be considered when the results of cultures of clinical specimens such as urine, semen, and vaginal discharges are interpreted. Urine from clinically healthy animals, collected sterilely by cystocentesis, contains no bacteria because the bladder and upper urinary tract do not have resident microflora. However, voided urine usually contains bacteria, occasionally in high numbers, because of preputial, urethral, or vaginal contamination. Catheterized urine samples also may be contaminated by resident urethral and vaginal bacteria, especially in female dogs. Semen samples are also often contaminated by urethral or preputial organisms.

Dog

In clinically healthy male dogs, the usual commensal organisms cultured from the dis-

Table 11–1. Bacteria Isolated from the Distal Urethra of Clinically Healthy Male Dogs

Staphylococcus intermedius	Klebsiella spp.
Staphylococcus epidermidis	Streptococcus canis
Corynebacterium spp.	Streptococcus viridans
Escherichia coli	Mycoplasma spp.
Flavobacterium spp.	Ureaplasma spp.
Haemophilus spp.	

Table 11–2. Bacteria Isolated from the Prepuce of Clinically Healthy Male Dogs[1,2]

Staphylococcus intermedius	Acinetobacter spp.
Staphylococcus epidermidis	Proteus spp.
Corynebacterium spp.	Pasteurella spp.
Escherichia coli	Bacillus spp.
Flavobacterium spp.	Streptomyces spp.
Haemophilus spp.	Streptococcus equisimilis
Klebsiella spp.	Streptococcus canis
Moraxella spp.	Streptococcus viridans
	Mycoplasma spp.
	Ureaplasma spp.

tal urethra and the prepuce are gram-positive bacteria, although gram-negative organisms have been isolated from some dogs (Tables 11–1 and 11–2).[1] Variations in reported organisms isolated are probably due to the method of sampling and the number of dogs examined. Bacteria are not normally found in the proximal urethra and the bladder. Mycoplasmas are common in the distal urethra and the prepuce and have also been isolated from the canine prostate (see Chapter 41).

Table 11–3. Bacteria Isolated from the Vagina of Clinically Healthy Bitches[1,5]

Staphylococcus intermedius	Micrococcus spp.
Staphylococcus epidermidis	Neisseria spp.
Streptococcus viridans	Bacteroides spp.
Streptococcus canis	Bacillus spp.
Streptococcus faecalis	Enterobacter spp.
Streptococcus zooepidemicus	Klebsiella spp.
Escherichia coli	Citrobacter spp.
Pasteurella spp.	Enterococcus spp.
Proteus spp.	Mycoplasma spp.
Haemophilus spp.	Ureaplasma spp.
Acinetobacter spp.	Corynebacterium spp.
Moraxella spp.	Pseudomonas spp.
Flavobacterium spp.	

The normal flora of the vagina of the bitch includes the same types of bacteria (Table 11–3).[1] Mycoplasmas have also been isolated from the vaginas of clinically healthy bitches.[2, 3] Few changes in the microflora occur with stages of the estrous cycle or with neutering.[2, 4, 5] Staphylococci have been isolated more frequently from prepuberal bitches than from postestral bitches.[4] While the same type of organisms are found throughout the vagina, the nearer the site of sampling to the cervix, the fewer vaginal organisms are found.[4] The uterus is normally sterile. Mycoplasmas and ureaplasmas are also normal inhabitants of the canine vagina. There was no difference in the prevalence of *Mycoplasma* between clinically healthy and infertile bitches. The role of *Mycoplasma* or *Ureaplasma* in canine and feline vaginitis is unknown (see Chapter 41).

Cat

The normal flora of the feline urogenital tract has not been extensively studied. Bacterial species isolated from voided or catheterized urine samples from clinical healthy cats that did not have bacteria in bladder urine were, in decreasing order of frequency, *Escherichia coli*, *Staphylococcus* spp., *Streptococcus* spp., *Corynebacterium* spp., *Pasteurella* spp., and *Flavobacterium* spp.[6]

Urinary Tract Infections
Jeanne A. Barsanti

ETIOLOGY

Urinary tract infection (UTI) refers to microbial colonization of the urine or of any urinary tract organ except the distal urethra, which has a normal bacterial flora. Infection of directly adjacent structures such as the prostate gland is included.[7] Infecting organisms are usually bacteria. Infection of the urinary tract may be localized to the kidney (bacterial pyelonephritis) or to the bladder (bacterial cystitis) or prostate (bacterial prostatitis), or it may involve more than one organ. It must be recognized that the entire system is at risk whenever any part is infected. It has been estimated that 14% of all dogs develop a urinary tract infection during their lifetime.[8] Infection rate in 237 dogs submitted for autopsy was 6% in males and 27% in females, most of which were reproductively intact. Infection rates were highest in those less than 2 years of age and in those older than 6 years of age.[9]

Infection of the urinary tract is usually caused by bacterial organisms that are microfloral constituents of the intestinal or lower urogenital tracts. The usual method of infection is by organisms ascending the urethra.[10] Hematogenous spread of infection is less common but is possible, especially in the kidney with its extensive blood supply.[7]

Each infection is usually caused by a single bacterial species, except in complicated infections secondary to severe anatomic or functional abnormalities of the urinary tract. *E. coli* is the most common genitourinary tract pathogen in dogs.[11–14] *Proteus*, *Klebsiella*, *Pseudomonas*, and *Enterobacter* are less frequently found gram-negative genitourinary pathogens. Gram-positive organisms account for approximately 25% of naturally occurring UTI.[12, 14] Infection with staphylococci or *Proteus* is often associated with struvite calculi because of urine alkalinization by the organisms' metabolism of urea. Although mycoplasma have been reported as a cause of UTI, their significance remains obscure since most of the cases reported were complicated by multiple disease processes (see also Chapter 41).[15]

Bacterial UTI is much less common in cats than in dogs. Numerous studies have shown that cats presenting with signs of dysuria or hematuria rarely have bacterial UTI.[16] Bacterial UTI may develop secondary to indwelling urinary catheterization[17] or urinary tract surgery such as perineal urethrostomy.[18] When bacterial infection occurs in cats, the organisms most frequently involved have been *E. coli*, *Pasteurella* spp., *Proteus* spp., staphylococci, and streptococci.[12]

PATHOGENESIS

Development of UTI indicates an alteration in the host and bacterial flora interrelationship.[19,20] In order to accomplish infection, bacteria must colonize the area of the urethral orifice and transport themselves up the urethra, adhering to the uroepithelium. Host antiadherence defense mechanisms include the normal bacterial flora of the vagina, periurethral area, and urethra; Tamm-Horsfall protein; urinary oligosaccharides; urinary immunoglobulins; bladder glycosaminoglycan; rapid epithelial turnover; and mechanical effects of flushing.[20] Bacteria adhere poorly to normal bladder epithelium owing to the presence of a glycosaminoglycan coating.[21, 21a] This coating, which can be replaced within 24 hours if injured, is extremely hydrophilic, so that a layer of water forms at the surface. This aqueous layer provides a barrier between the transitional epithelium and the urine, explaining in part why the bladder epithelium can tolerate constant exposure to a substance as irritating as urine. Infection is likely to occur if this surface coating is damaged as by uroliths, neoplastic transformation, or exposure to irritants such as cyclophosphamide. Women with recurrent UTI have been found to have vaginal epithelium that permits increased bacterial adherence.[22, 23]

Precipitating causes for infection include underlying disease of the urinary system, alterations in host immune competence, and an increase or change in bacterial virulence. An important host factor in resistance to infection is the normal, frequent emptying of the urinary bladder. Any condition that impairs normal micturition or obstructs urine flow will predispose to infection. The high osmolality of normal dog and cat urine is inhibitory to bacterial growth. Urine osmolality values greater than 1200 mOsm (approximately a specific gravity of 1.040) are inhibitory to growth of E. coli.[24] Conditions lowering urine osmolality result in urine that is less resistant to infection. Examples of the importance of host immunocompetence are the high prevalence of urinary tract infections in dogs with Cushing's disease and in those on chronic glucocorticoid therapy.[25]

Infection can also occur in the absence of such host factors. Virulence properties of urinary tract infecting agents, particularly E. coli, may be important since typical urinary tract pathogens constitute only a small percentage of the normal genital and fecal flora. Differences in virulence properties have also been found among strains of E. coli causing pyelonephritis, acute cystitis, or asympto-

matic bacteriuria in people.[26,27] These properties include resistance to the bactericidal properties of serum, ability to produce hemolysin, and ability to attach to urinary tract epithelium.[26, 28] The ability of E. coli to produce hemolysin has been related to UTI in dogs.[29, 30] The presence of P-fimbriae, bacterial adherence structures, on E. coli was only found in one of the reports.[29] E. coli associated with UTI were also found to cluster in certain serotypes, as in people, and to be of probable fecal origin.[30] In direct comparison with human urinary isolates, canine E. coli were more likely than human isolates to produce hemolysins,[31] to be antibiotic-resistant, and to have a higher R-plasmid transmissibility rate.[31] This latter factor may reflect indiscriminate antibiotic use in pet dogs.

One predisposing iatrogenic cause for UTI is catheterization, especially if the catheter is left in place (indwelling).[17] There are a few valid indications for use of an indwelling urinary catheter: following relief of urethral obstruction, when rapid reobstruction would compromise patient survival; in the pre- and postoperative management of lower urinary tract trauma; in animals with neurologic bladder dysfunction; and as a means of monitoring urine output in animals at risk of or suspected of having oliguric renal failure. Unfortunately, placement of such a catheter puts the patient at high risk for UTI. Bacteria can readily ascend either around or through the catheter. Use of closed, sterile systems can prevent bacterial access within the catheter lumen, but no method to date has been effective in preventing bacterial access around the sides of the catheter. Urinary catheterization should be performed intermittently, if possible. Indwelling catheters should be used only when absolutely necessary and for the minimum time period. Consequences of bacteriuria arising from indwelling catheterization include pyelonephritis, bacteremia, prostatitis, and epididymitis (see also Nosocomial Urinary Tract Infections, Chapter 1).

CLINICAL FINDINGS

Asymptomatic Bacteriuria

Urinary tract infections are often asymptomatic. Because of the lack of historic and physical signs, such infections can be difficult to localize. In humans asymptomatic infections are considered relatively benign unless they are caused by underlying urinary tract abnormalities or immunodeficiency states.[32]

The significance of asymptomatic bacteriuria in companion animals is unknown. In one study,[33] six of twelve clinically asymptomatic female dogs with UTI had infection localized to one or both kidneys; however, three dogs had no associated renal inflammation, whereas the others had mild to moderate inflammation. In the other six dogs with asymptomatic infection localized to the bladder, three also had little or no inflammation of the bladder wall. Yet clinical cases with few historic signs may develop severe tissue injury, such as renal or prostatic abscess formation. Duration of asymptomatic infection or other host factors may be important in determining the degree of tissue injury.

Pyelonephritis

In acute bacterial pyelonephritis, dogs may be systemically ill with fever, depression, anorexia, renal pain, and leukocytosis. These signs are inconsistent, however, and in experimentally induced disease, very transient. Chronic pyelonephritis may be associated with no abnormal clinical signs or with polyuria and secondary polydipsia. Polyuria can occur prior to the onset of renal lesions and can resolve with eradication of the infection. Its cause is unknown. With bilateral pyelonephritis, signs of renal failure may eventually occur, especially if infection is associated with other structural abnormalities such as urolithiasis.

Cystitis and Urethritis

The bladder and proximal urethra are so closely associated that inflammation in the bladder usually affects the proximal urethra. Infection of the distal urethra unassociated with infection in the rest of the lower urinary tract is uncommon unless an anatomic abnormality exists in that region.

Urethrocystitis is characterized by dysuria (straining) and pollakiuria (frequent voiding of small amounts of urine). The urine is often cloudy and hemorrhagic and has a foul odor. Gross hematuria at the end of urination

suggests that the blood is from the bladder. Gross hematuria at the beginning of urination or a urethral discharge may be associated with urethral or prostatic disease. In general, prostatic disease is a more common cause of a urethral discharge independent of urination than is urethral disease in dogs. Signs of systemic illness, such as fever and leukocytosis, are not associated with bacterial urethrocystitis. The bladder is often contracted and painful on abdominal palpation, and with chronic infection the wall is thickened.

DIAGNOSIS

Examination of bladder urine is the method by which UTI is confirmed. However, the presence of bacteria in urine collected from the bladder does not localize the infection to the bladder wall. It is incorrect to use the term *cystitis* whenever bacteria are isolated from urine. The bacteria could be originating from the kidney(s) or prostate gland. Diagnostic tests in addition to history and physical examination that are used to localize infection are discussed under Bacterial Pyelonephritis, Bacterial Cystitis, and Prostatitis. At the present time, there is no definitive localizing test that can be used without surgical biopsy. Tests such as antibody coating of bacteria in urine, originally thought to localize infection, have been found unreliable in dogs.[33] The extensiveness of the diagnostic evaluation required on each case varies with severity of illness, duration of signs, and response to initial antimicrobial therapy (Table 11–4).

Urine Collection

Because the distal urethra, vagina, and prepuce have a normal bacterial flora, the method of urine collection is important for accurate assessment of the results of urinalysis and urine culture. Whenever a urine sample is collected, the method of collection should be recorded.

Cystocentesis. Cystocentesis is the preferred method of urine collection for culture, since lower genitourinary tract contamination is avoided. Any bacteria present in such samples can be considered indicative of infection unless inadvertent bowel penetration or

Table 11–4. Guidelines to Management of Urinary Tract Infection in Dogs

CLINICAL CHARACTERISTIC	DIAGNOSIS	THERAPY
Female		
No or few previous episodes; not immunosuppressed; may be asymptomatic	Urinalysis, urine culture	Antimicrobial agent for 10 days (initial choice ampicillin or trimethoprim-sulfonamide)
Rapidly relapsing	Urinalysis, urine culture, radiography (survey, possibly contrast)	Antimicrobial agent for 21–28 days; treatment for underlying disease process if identifiable; prophylactic therapy may need to be considered
Persistent	Urinalysis, urine culture, survey and contrast radiography	Try to identify an effective antimicrobial agent, continue for 6 wks; treatment for underlying disease process if identifiable; if relapses, suppressive therapy may be required
Male		
No or few previous episodes; may be asymptomatic	Urinalysis, urine culture	Antimicrobial agent for 21 days (initial choice, trimethoprim-sulfonamide)
Rapidly relapsing	Urinalysis, urine culture, ejaculate cytology and culture, survey radiography, prostatic ultrasonography	Antimicrobial agent (with prostatic penetrance) for 6 wks, based on culture and susceptibility; treatment for underlying disease process if identifiable
Persistent	Urinalysis, urine culture, ejaculate cytology and culture, survey and contrast radiography, prostatic ultrasonography	Antimicrobial agent—be sure effective by recheck cultures; if effective—continue for 3 mos; if rapidly relapses, consider suppressive therapy; treat underlying disease process if identifiable
Male or Female		
Neurogenic bladder or indwelling urinary catheter	Urinalysis, urine culture	Use only intermittent catheterization in males or closed indwelling catheters in either sex; avoid antimicrobials if possible until normal bladder function returns

skin contamination occurs. Because of the possibility of inadvertent contamination, diagnosis is more certain if urine is cultured quantitatively (with evaluation of the number of organisms found) as well as qualitatively (identification of the infecting species).

Before cystocentesis is performed, a small area of skin around the site of needle insertion should be clipped free of hair and cleansed. The bladder should be palpated and immobilized against the pelvis with one hand. A 21-gauge or smaller needle is inserted into the bladder at an oblique angle, and urine is withdrawn into a syringe. The palpating hand releases pressure on the bladder, negative pressure on the syringe is discontinued, and the needle is withdrawn. Cystocentesis is performed with the animal in the position in which it seems most comfortable (standing, lying down, or suspended by the front or rear limbs) (Figs. 11–1 to 11–4). The only complication noted to date has been leakage when the bladder is distended secondary to inability to voluntarily void urine in cases of urethral obstruction or neurologic detrusor dysfunction. In animals that are unable to urinate, the bladder should be emptied as soon as possible after cystocentesis.

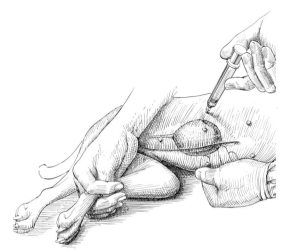

Figure 11–1. Cystocentesis with the dog in lateral recumbency. The thumb of the palpating hand can also be placed along the cranial border of the bladder to push the bladder back toward the pelvis and further immobilize it.

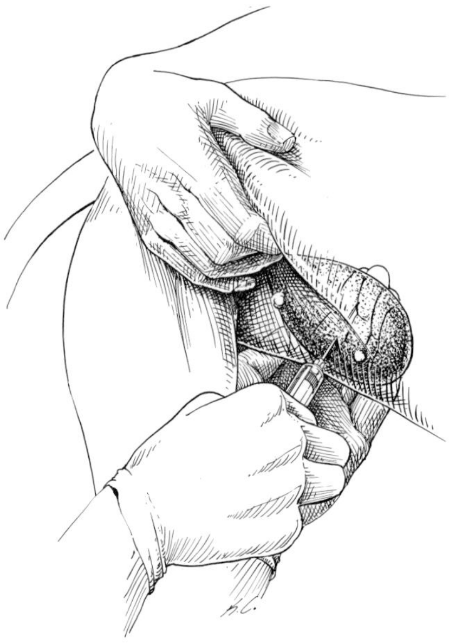

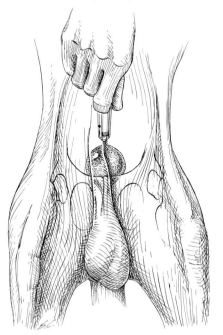

Figure 11–2. Cystocentesis with the dog standing. Again the thumb of the palpating hand can be placed on the cranial border of the bladder to further immobilize it.

Catheterization. If the bladder is not palpable or if blind cystocentesis fails, urine should be collected for culture in male dogs by catheterization. Catheterization techniques should always be performed as asep-

Figure 11–3. Cystocentesis with the dog in dorsal recumbency or suspended by the front limbs. Cystocentesis using the blind technique is demonstrated: the needle is inserted perpendicular to the body wall, 1 to 2 inches cranial to the cranial edge of the pubic bone.

tically and gently as possible. In males the prepuce should be retracted and the penis cleansed and dried. A sterile, disposable catheter should be used. The catheter should be passed using only sterile instruments or gloves. Catheterization done in this way rarely results in introducing bacteria into urine and then only in low ($<10^3$/ml) numbers.[34, 35]

In contrast, catheterization of female dogs, using as aseptic a technique as possible, introduces bacteria approximately 50% of the time and then occasionally with large (10^5/ml) numbers of organisms.[34] Experimentally, introduction of large numbers of bacteria into the bladders of normal female dogs by catheterization does not usually result in persistent UTI unless a complicating factor, such as a bladder foreign body, was present.[35] Because of the difficulty in distinguishing infection from contamination and because of the small risk of inducing UTI, catheterization is not an adequate substitute for cystocentesis in female dogs. Use of diuretics such as furosemide to distend the bladder for cystocentesis is preferable to evaluate UTI, although the effect on specific gravity must be noted.

If an indwelling urinary catheter is placed in a female or male dog, samples may be obtained through this catheter for quantitative culture. Even low numbers of bacteria suggest infection in this situation, since bacterial numbers tend to increase if the catheter is left in place.[17] However, antimicrobials should not be given until the catheter is removed (see Urinary Tract Infection Associated with Catheterization).

In cats, contamination of catheteried samples was with fewer than 10^3 bacteria/ml in both males and females.[6] However, unsedated cats are difficult to catheterize atraumatically. As in female dogs, diuretics may be needed to distend the bladder so that cystocentesis can be accomplished.

Midstream Collection. Midstream collection during voluntary voiding has been found to introduce bacteria with numbers occasionally more than 10^5 bacteria/ml.[34] Because of the chance of significant contamination during voiding, midstream collection should not be utilized to obtain urine for culture from dogs. Because bacterial contamination of urine is expected to occur with midstream collection, ambiguities in interpretation may occur. A certain percentage of animals with

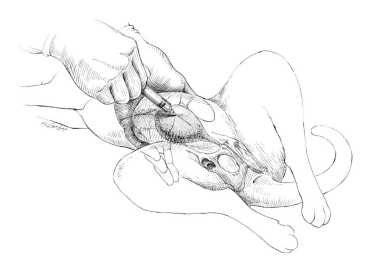

Figure 11–4. Cystocentesis with the cat in dorsal recumbency. The bladder is stabilized by abdominal compression applied cranially as the bladder wall is entered at a 45-degree angle. Physical restraint (not shown) is also necessary.

urine bacterial concentrations of 10^2 to 10^4 probably have UTI.[19]

Midstream-collected urine occasionally must be used for culture in severely dysuric cats. Such cats may not allow the bladder to fill sufficiently for successful cystocentesis, even following administration of diuretics. In these cases, urine should be expressed as cleanly as possible into a sterile container. The urine should be cultured quantitatively. A urinalysis should also be performed so that the sediment findings can be correlated with culture results.

Handling of Urine Samples

Once urine is collected for culture, it must be handled properly to prevent changes in bacterial numbers. Specimens should be refrigerated and cultured within 6 hours.[36] However, tubes with preservatives for urine holding (Becton-Dickenson Co., Cockeysville, MD) have been shown to maintain type and numbers of bacteria in urine for up to 72 hours with refrigeration.[37] Prior to culture, urine should not be incubated, kept at room temperature, or frozen because these practices may induce changes in bacterial numbers.

Although standard quantitative cultures are preferred, when urine is collected by cystocentesis, screening for infection can be performed with dip-strip methods (Microstix, Ames Co., Elkhart, IN), miniature agar plates (Testuria, Ayerst, New York, NY), agar cups (Bacturcult, Wampole, Cranberry, NJ), and dip slides (Uricult, Medical Technology Corp., Hackensack, NJ).[38]

Interpretation of Urinalysis

In order to evaluate a dog or cat for infection by urinalysis, a complete urinalysis, *including sediment examination*, must be performed. Findings on a dipstick that may occur with infection are positive occult blood and protein, but these findings indicate only hemorrhage, which has many potential causes. Infection can also occur without hemorrhage and can be associated with a normal dipstick evaluation. Dipstick leukocyte assays[39] and dipstick assays for bacteria[38] have been found to be inaccurate in companion animals.

Findings on a urine sediment examination that suggest UTI are pyuria, hematuria, and bacteriuria. Of these, the most specific is bacteriuria. Knowing the method of urine collection is essential in accurately interpreting the results. False-positive bacteriuria on cystocentesis can only arise as a consequence of contamination or misinterpretation of brownian movement or amorphous debris. False-negative results are possible since large numbers of organisms, particularly with cocci, must be present in order to be consistently visualized. Correlation of Gram-stained smears of canine urine with culture results was good,[27] whereas that of unstained smears was poor.[34, 40] As a general rule, a urine culture is definitive evidence as to the presence or absence of infection if the sample is correctly handled and transported.

Pyuria is often, but not always, present in association with bacteriuria. Pyuria without bacteriuria indicates inflammation, and a culture of urine is necessary to determine if bacterial or fungal infection is the cause of the inflammation. Bacteria are more difficult to detect than WBC. Infection with minimal tissue invasion may not induce pyuria. Hypercortisolemia inhibits pyuria.[25] In dogs treated with glucocorticoids or with canine Cushing's disease, urine culture is essential to evaluate for infection.

Red blood cells in urine indicate hemorrhage. Hemorrhage may or may not occur with infection, depending on site and severity. Mild, fresh hemorrhage may occur secondary to cystocentesis. Subsequent evaluation of a voided sample is recommended to eliminate this possibility.

Protein can be present in urine as a consequence of hemorrhage or inflammation.

Interpretation of Urine Culture Results

Any bacteria are considered significant in a properly collected cystocentesis sample. Since most UTIs involve a single bacterial species and since numbers of bacteria are usually high, results of multiple types or low (<1000/ml) numbers should be reevaluated. Artifactual contamination of urine with intestinal contents leads to presence of multiple bacterial species. Contamination from the skin or in the laboratory leads to low numbers of organisms.

Dogs. Catheterization can be used as an alternative method to collect urine for culture in male dogs as long as the procedure is atraumatic and aseptic. In most cases in male dogs, more than 10^5 bacteria/ml in a catheterized sample indicates infection. Fewer than 10^3 bacteria/ml usually indicates contamination. Intermediate (10^3 to 10^5/ml) numbers may indicate either contamination or infection. Other case information such as history, physical examination, urinalysis results, and the degree of potential contamination during catheterization can help guide a decision as to whether infection exists when culture results are inconclusive. Catheterization of female dogs to collect urine for culture is not recommended.

In an animal with an indwelling urinary catheter, any number of bacteria collected through the catheter is considered possibly significant, since in both people and animals, small numbers of organisms will in-

crease to large numbers within a few days if the catheter remains in place.[17,41,42]

Midstream or expressed urine samples should not be used for culture in dogs because of the great likelihood of contamination.

Cats. Interpretation of results of cystocentesis is the same as in dogs. In samples of urine obtained by catheterization, bacterial counts greater than 10^3/ml are considered indicative of infection in both male and female cats.[6] In cats with indwelling catheters, any number or type of bacteria may be significant. If midstream samples must be used in a dysuric cat, $>10^5$ bacteria/ml would be suggestive of infection if contamination during collection was minimal. Even counts $>10^5$ bacteria per ml would not confirm infection, since counts this high were found in a small number of urine specimens from cats with negative culture results by cystocentesis.[6] Results of urinalysis should be correlated with culture results in making a final determination as to whether the bacteria cultured are due to infection or contamination.

Bacterial Pyelonephritis

The diagnosis of bacterial pyelonephritis is usually made by finding UTI and localizing the origin of this infection to the kidney by history, physical examination, laboratory tests, excretory urography, pyelocentesis, or renal biopsy.

Clinical Laboratory Findings. A CBC may show a neutrophilic leukocytosis with or without a left shift in acute or severe chronic pyelonephritis, especially with renal abscess formation. As a general rule, an inflammatory leukogram in association with UTI suggests the UTI is of renal or prostatic origin. However, a normal CBC does not eliminate the possibility of pyelonephritis.

Abnormalities in renal function (abnormal creatinine clearance, inadequate urine concentrating ability in spite of demand or azotemia) in association with UTI suggest that the UTI may be of renal origin. However, further tests are indicated, since the abnormality in renal function and the UTI may be unrelated.

On urinalysis, hematuria, pyuria, and bacteriuria are often noted but are not specific for pyelonephritis. Consistently low urine specific gravity readings should increase the suspicion of pyelonephritis. Concentrated urine (>1.035) does not rule out pyelonephritis, because the infection may be unilateral and the degree of concentrating defect depends on how diffusely and severely the renal medulla is affected. The presence of leukocyte or erythrocyte casts with bacteriuria suggests renal infection. The absence of casts, however, does not eliminate the possibility of bacterial pyelonephritis.

Excretory Urography. Within 10 days of inducing experimental pyelonephritis in dogs, decreased opacity of the vascular nephrogram and of diverticula of the renal pelvis, and renal pelvic and ureteral dilation were found.[43] The size of infected kidneys progressively decreased over 8 weeks. In one of two dogs, the collecting system remained dilated. Similar renal changes have been noted in clinical cases in dogs with suspected bacterial pyelonephritis.

Pyelocentesis. Percutaneous nephropyelocentesis allows collection of urine for culture directly from the renal pelvis.[44] The renal pelvis is visualized by means of excretory urography and fluoroscopy and dilated by application of an abdominal compression band. A 20-gauge disposable arterial needle is then directed through the skin of the lateral flank into the dilated renal pelvis. A positive culture result confirms renal pelvic infection.

Renal Biopsy. Culture and histologic examination of tissue samples obtained by renal biopsy can be used to confirm a diagnosis of bacterial pyelonephritis. Tissue culture is important since histologic evidence of inflammation does not necessarily correlate with infection.[33] The keyhole technique of renal biopsy used in dogs and the percutaneous technique used in cats have been well described.[45]

Bacterial Cystitis

The diagnosis of acute bacterial cystitis is usually based on history and clinical signs of dysuria and pollakiuria and on confirming UTI by results of urinalysis and urine culture. A CBC is usually normal with cystitis.

Chronic cystitis is usually confirmed radiographically by finding thickening of the bladder wall on cystography. Radiography is also useful to detect uroliths or other space-occupying masses such as neoplasms, which can be underlying causes of chronic infection. Biopsy of the bladder wall can be performed in difficult cases. Biopsy specimens should be cultured for bacteria as well as processed for histologic evaluation.

THERAPY

Urine Concentration of Antimicrobial Agents

The major difference between therapy for UTIs and for infections in other organ systems is that antimicrobials reach the urine in high concentrations as a result of renal excretion (Table 11–5).[7, 46] Standard Kirby-Bauer disk susceptibility tests for most antimicrobials are based on blood concentrations of drugs (see Chapter 42). Exceptions are nitrofurantoin, sulfonamides, and trimethoprim, with which disks used usually contain urine concentrations.[47] Because most antimicrobial disks contain achievable serum concentrations, routine antimicrobial susceptibility results should be used only as rough guidelines for treatment of UTIs. If the infecting organism is reported to be susceptible to a certain antimicrobial agent, that agent will probably be effective if it is excreted in active form by the kidney and if renal function is normal. However, an antimicrobial to which the organism is reported to be resistant may also give good results in vivo because of significantly higher urine than serum concentrations.

A more accurate method of choosing an effective therapeutic agent for UTIs is to determine the minimum inhibitory concentration (MIC) of antimicrobials for the infective agent (see Chapter 42). The use of manufactured kits is making this determination more feasible for the commercial laboratory. Rather than absolute susceptibility or resistance, the concentration of antimicrobial that will inhibit the growth of the organism is reported. The MIC is then compared with the concentration reached by that antimicrobial in urine. If the mean urine concentration (Table 11–6) exceeds the MIC by at least four times, the antimicrobial agent should be effective.

As a general rule, resolution of UTI is

Table 11–5. A Comparison of Antimicrobial Concentrations in Serum and Urine of Adult Humans with Normal Renal Function[a]

DRUG	DOSE GIVEN ORALLY EVERY 6 HOURS (mg)	AVERAGE SERUM CONCENTRATION (μg/ml)	AVERAGE URINE CONCENTRATION (μg/ml)
Penicillin G	500	1	150
Nitrofurantoin	100	1	100
Oxytetracycline	250	1–2	150
Chloramphenicol	500	3–4	100
Ampicillin	250	1–2	300
Cephalexin	1000	15–25	2000–3000
Streptomycin	500[b]	6–8	400
Gentamicin	0.8[c]	2–3	100

[a]Data compiled from Stamey TA: *Urinary Infections.* Baltimore, Williams & Wilkins, 1980.
[b]Given intramuscularly every 12 hours.
[c]Dosage expressed as mg/kg given intramuscularly every 8 hours.

more directly related to urine than serum concentrations of antimicrobial agents.[48] In renal parenchymal and prostatic infections, special considerations apply to antimicrobial penetration, which is discussed under Bacterial Pyelonephritis and Prostatitis, respectively.

Based on the MIC determinations of antimicrobials for common urinary tract pathogens, some general rules have been formulated (Table 11–7). Penicillin G or ampicillin is usually effective against UTI caused by staphylococci, streptococci, or *Proteus*. Trimethoprim-sulfonamide is often effective against UTIs caused by *E. coli*, and tetracycline is often successful in treating UTIs caused by *Pseudomonas*. *Klebsiella* infec-

tions are the most difficult UTIs for which to predict antibiotic efficacy. Trimethoprim-sulfonamide or cephalosporins are most frequently successful, although cure rates for trimethoprim-sulfonamide have not exceeded 60% for *Klebsiella pneumoniae*.[49a] Highly resistant *E. coli* infections may require amoxicillin-clavulanic acid, enrofloxacin, or drugs only approved for human use such as other quinolones, third generation cephalosporins, or extended spectrum penicillin derivatives.[50–52] One quinolone, pipemidic acid, has been found to be successful in dogs and cats for the treatment of recurrent UTI due to multiresistant strains of *E. coli*.[53]

Although selection of an antimicrobial

Table 11–6. Mean Urine Concentrations of the Antimicrobial Agents Commonly Used in the Management of Canine Urinary Tract Infections[a]

AGENT	DAILY DOSAGE (mg/kg)	FREQUENCY OF ADMINISTRATION	ROUTE[b]	MEAN URINE CONCENTRATION (± 1 SD)
Penicillin G	37,000[c]	t.i.d.	PO	294.9 (± 210.7) U/ml
Penicillin V	26	t.i.d.	PO	148.3 (± 98.5) μg/ml
Ampicillin	26	t.i.d.	PO	309.1 (± 55.1) μg/ml
Hetacillin	26	t.i.d.	PO	300.3 (± 156.1) μg/ml
Amoxicillin	11	t.i.d.	PO	201.5 (± 93.2) μg/ml
Tetracycline	18	t.i.d.	PO	137.9 (± 64.6) μg/ml
Chloramphenicol	33	t.i.d.	PO	123.8 (± 39.7) μg/ml
Sulfisoxazole	22	t.i.d.	PO	1466.3 (± 832.4) μg/ml
Nitrofurantoin	4.4	t.i.d.	PO	100.0 (?) μg/ml
Trimethoprim-sulfonamide	13	b.i.d.	PO	55.0 (± 19.2) μg/ml
Kanamycin	4	b.i.d.	SC	529.6 (± 150.5) μg/ml
Gentamicin	2	t.i.d.	SC	107.4 (± 33.0) μg/ml
Amikacin	5	t.i.d.	SC	342.0 (± 143.0) μg/ml
Tobramycin	1	t.i.d.	SC	66.0 (± 39.0) μg/ml

[a]Values were determined in hydrated dogs with normal renal function. To determine the efficacy of a drug, multiply the MIC of the bacteria isolated from the infection by 4. If the total is less than the mean urine concentration for that drug, the drug has about a 95% efficacy.
[b]PO = orally; SC = subcutaneously.
[c]In U/kg.

(Data supplied courtesy of Dr. Gerald Ling, University of California, Davis, California. Permission to reproduce these data granted by Dr. Ling.)

Table 11–7. Guideline to Antimicrobial Choice in UTI Based on Identification of the Causative Bacteria[a, 8, 49]

MICROBE	ANTIMICROBIALS RECOMMENDED
Staphylococci	Amp(amox)icillin, trimethoprim[b], nitrofurantoin, cephalexin, chloramphenicol, penicillin
Streptococci	Amp(amox)icillin, trimethoprim, penicillin
Escherichia coli	Trimethoprim, nitrofurantoin, cephalexin
Proteus	Amp(amox)icillin, trimethoprim, cephalexin, penicillin
Pseudomonas[c]	Tetracycline, trimethoprim, gentamicin
Klebsiella	Cephalexin, trimethoprim
Enterobacter	Trimethoprim

[a]Highly antibiotic-resistant UTI can be a problem in animals that have received antibiotic therapy. Organisms involved are usually *E. coli, Enterobacter, Klebsiella,* or *Pseudomonas*. Alternative drugs that can be considered in resistant infections are combination drugs with clavulanic acid, norfloxacin, ciprofloxacin, carbenicillin, and third generation cephalosporins.

[b]Trimethoprim as used in this table refers to trimethoprim-sulfonamide combinations.

[c]It is difficult to predict susceptibility of *Pseudomonas*. Although aminoglycosides are usually effective, they are not generally used for UTI because of nephrotoxicity and need for injection. Repeated urine evaluation is essential to determine response to therapy with this organism.

agent by organism identification and susceptibility testing usually correlates with success of therapy in vivo, the correlation is not 100%.[8] Various factors such as location of infection (as noted earlier), renal function, polyuric states, and urine characteristics will influence antimicrobial urine concentrations and response to therapy. The only way to be certain that the chosen drug is effective is to reexamine the urine during and following therapy. Urine should be recultured, or the sediment should be examined cytologically after a few days of therapy. If the antibiotic eliminates bacteria from the urine within a few days, the drug's efficacy against that bacterial species is confirmed. However, a much longer course of therapy is usually necessary to eliminate the organism from infected bladder, renal, or prostatic tissues. Urine should also be examined cytologically or cultured a few days to a week after conclusion of therapy to be sure the infection was eliminated and not merely suppressed.

Asymptomatic Bacteriuria

A diagnostic effort should be made to determine whether an underlying cause of immunosuppression exists, such as glucocorticoid therapy or hyperadrenocorticism. Asymptomatic infections should be treated with at least a 14-day course of an antimicrobial agent based on urine culture results (see Table 11–4). A urine culture should be repeated approximately one week after concluding therapy. If the infection remains, a diagnostic effort should be made to localize the tissue source (kidney, bladder, prostate). Treatment should be reinstituted and urine cultured during therapy. If the chosen drug is effective during therapy, duration of therapy should be extended to at least 6 weeks. Lack of resolution of infection should prompt further diagnostic efforts to determine why the organism persists despite appropriate therapy.

Pyelonephritis

Acute. Urine should be cultured to determine the causative organism. Antibiotic therapy should be started pending the culture result. Trimethoprim-sulfonamide or chloramphenicol is better able to diffuse into the renal interstitium than other drugs and should be considered initially. Norfloxacin also penetrates well into the renal parenchyma,[54] as do the aminoglycosides. Short-term (3 days) use of gentamicin plus ampicillin for several weeks achieved the best results in experimental rats.[55] The nephrotoxic potential of the aminoglycosides must always be considered prior to their use. Gentamicin should be used only if serum creatinine and serum urea nitrogen (BUN) are within reference limits.

If the animal is systemically ill, initial therapy should consist of parenteral antibiotics as well as IV fluid support. Parenteral therapy should be continued until response is indicated by normalization of body temperature and appetite. When the results of urine culture and susceptibility are obtained, antibiotic therapy should be reevaluated. Especially when the organism is reported resistant to the chosen antimicrobial, urine should be rechecked to determine if the drug is efficacious in vivo. If the drug is not efficacious in vivo, therapy should be changed. If the drug is efficacious, therapy should be continued for at least 4 to 6 weeks, with follow-up cultures made during and 1 to 2 weeks after the conclusion of treatment. Urine cultures should be performed monthly for several months to detect recurrence.

Chronic. Chronic pyelonephritis requires therapy for at least 6 weeks. Antibiotic choice should be based on identification of the causative organism. In general, chloramphenicol and trimethoprim have the best renal tissue penetration. Although aminoglycosides also have excellent renal tissue penetration, nephrotoxicity makes them unacceptable choices for long-term therapy. Efficacy of the chosen antimicrobial agent should be checked by urinalysis and urine culture after the first few 2 weeks of therapy. If the urine is not sterile at this point, drug therapy should be reconsidered. If the urine is sterile, the antimicrobial agent should be continued for a total of at least 6 weeks. Urine cultures should be performed 1 to 2 weeks and 1 month after the conclusion of therapy to ensure the infection has been eliminated and not merely suppressed.

If conservative therapy is unsuccessful and if the infection appears to be unilateral (usually determined by contrast radiographic abnormalities), nephrectomy can be considered if the remaining kidney appears to be able to maintain normal renal function. Crude indicators are BUN, creatinine, urine specific gravity, and radiographic appearance. At surgery the kidney that is to remain should be examined and palpated prior to removal of the diseased kidney. Since chronic infection of one kidney can result in infection of the other kidney, nephrectomy should be considered only if the remaining kidney is normal and uninfected. Nephrectomy is indicated if the infected kidney has become an abscessed kidney.

Cystitis

Acute Initial Episode. Acute, uncomplicated bacterial cystitis in female dogs and cats should be treated with a broad-spectrum antimicrobial for approximately 10 days. Although some studies in women have shown success with single, high-dose therapy, studies to date in dogs of both sexes[40, 56] and other studies in women[51, 57] have shown better success with conventional 10-day therapy. Antimicrobial therapy is best chosen on the basis of organism identification

as discussed above. Empirically chosen antimicrobials that are usually effective include amoxicillin, ampicillin, and trimethoprim-sulfonamide. The efficacy of ampicillin and amoxicillin may be less than predicted if the animal has received these drugs within the previous 2 months because of the development of resistance in the intestinal flora, the usual source of infecting organisms. Combining amoxicillin with clavulanic acid (augmentin, clavamox) increases efficacy against *E. coli*, *Klebsiella*, and *Proteus*, but is more expensive.[58] *Enterobacter*- and *Pseudomonas*-UTI are usually resistant to the combination.[51]

Because clinical signs often improve within 48 hours, the client must be instructed to give all medication as directed. Three to 5 days after therapy is concluded, a urine sample should be collected for cytology of sediment with or without culture to ensure that therapy has been effective. Follow-up is important to prevent chronic infections and to prompt an early search for an underlying predisposing cause for treatment failure, such as calculi, pyelonephritis, abnormal bladder or urethral function, renal failure, urinary tract neoplasia, or hyperadrenocorticism. Uncomplicated bacterial cystitis in female dogs and cats should respond rapidly to an appropriate antimicrobial agent. If it does not, further diagnostic tests should be performed.

In intact male dogs, prostatitis often occurs in conjunction with cystitis. Thus, in male dogs treatment should be continued for at least 3 weeks and follow-up evaluations should include evaluation of prostatic fluid as well as urine. Drugs with prostatic penetrance such as trimethoprim or chloramphenicol are preferred (see Prostatitis, Therapy). However, one study indicated no difference in clinical response between ampicillin (little prostatic penetrance) and trimethoprim-sulfonamide (good prostatic penetrance) in UTI in male dogs.[8]

Recurrent Infections. In some dogs, acute cystitis recurs frequently. The causative organism should be determined by urine culture. If the organism has been of the same species with a similar antibiotic susceptibility spectrum, the infection may be relapsing. Without serotyping, it is uncertain whether infection is from a new or different organism. Since serotyping is not clinically available, antibiotic susceptibility is used as a rough guideline as to whether the organism is of the same strain. Recurrence by the same organism should prompt a diagnostic investigation to determine the site of tissue infection that is leading to reinfection of the urine. Possibilities are chronic pyelonephritis, chronic cystitis, and in males, chronic prostatitis. Treatment should be directed toward the underlying condition.

If the organism is different during the episodes of cystitis, reinfection is occurring. This suggests a problem with genitourinary anatomy or function or with other host immune defenses. A careful history should be taken and complete physical examination performed to determine whether micturition and urinary tract anatomy are normal. Consideration should also be given to hyperadrenocorticism or glucocorticoid therapy. Some bitches have recurrent cystitis with no other discernible abnormality.

Each episode of reinfection is treated individually. If infections recur frequently, low-dose, once daily antibiotic therapy can be used for 6 to 12 months as prevention. Infections should be treated until urine is sterile before prophylactic therapy is begun. Drugs usually recommended are trimethoprim-sulfonamide, first generation cephalosporins, or nitrofurantoin at 33% to 50% of the normal daily dose, given one time just prior to a 6- to 12-hour period when urine will be retained in the bladder, such as at night in house dogs.[59] Research is continuing on the use of glycosaminoglycans, substances that coat the uroepithelium of the lower urinary tract to prevent bacterial adherence, as preventative therapy.[60]

Chronic Cystitis. Chronic bacterial cystitis requires protracted treatment. Urine should always be cultured to determine the causative agent, and treatment should be guided by MIC determinations if possible. If not, the Kirby-Bauer susceptibility disk method can be used in conjunction with the general guidelines discussed in Urine Concentration of Antimicrobial Agents. Urine should be recultured or checked with screening tests (e.g., Microstix, Ames Co., Elkhart, IN) approximately 7 days after therapy is begun. If the antimicrobial is potentially effective, the urine should be sterile at this time. If the urine is sterile, that antimicrobial should be continued for 4 to 6 weeks. If it is not sterile, another antimicrobial should be chosen and culturing should be repeated after approxi-

mately 7 days of treatment until an effective agent is found. Urine should be recultured or rechecked by screening tests prior to and 1 to 2 weeks after the conclusion of therapy. It is also recommended that monthly urine cultures be made for several months to determine whether infection has recurred.

Persistent UTIs

Persistent UTIs are those in which either bacteriuria does not resolve while on an appropriately chosen antimicrobial or bacteriuria with the same organism recurs within a short time of discontinuing the antimicrobial agent. Persistent UTIs are also referred to as relapsing or unresolved infections.

In such an infection, an effort should be made to localize the infection and to determine whether any predisposing factors exist. Such factors include disease states such as hypercortisolism or chronic glucocorticoid administration, urolithiasis, chronic bacterial prostatitis, pyelonephritis, residual urine in the bladder after micturition, and an anatomic abnormality such as a persistent urachus. Diagnostic evaluation might include survey and contrast radiography, ultrasonography, examination of prostatic fluid, and tissue biopsy and culture.

Treatment of such infections should be directed toward correcting any underlying factors. Antimicrobial therapy should be based on culture and susceptibility results. Therapy should be continued at least 6 weeks (see Table 11–4). Urine cultures should be evaluated during and 1 and 4 weeks after discontinuing therapy. If antimicrobial therapy eliminates bacteriuria during therapy but bacteriuria recurs with discontinuation of therapy, a longer course of therapy for 4 to 6 months should be considered. When using antimicrobials for this duration of time, consideration must be given to long-term side effects. Prolonged use of drugs with potentially serious side effects, such as chloramphenicol, should be avoided. The risk of keratoconjunctivitis sicca or folate deficiency anemia with long-term use of trimethoprim-sulfonamide should be conveyed to the owner (see Trimethoprim-sulfonamide, Chapter 43).

If antimicrobials fail, use of antiseptics such as methenamine mandelate or methenamine hippurate should be considered, although the efficacy of these products is controversial.[22] Such drugs have the advantages of low toxicity, as long as renal function is normal, and of failing to induce antimicrobial resistance. Relatively high doses may be required since these drugs are most efficacious at a urine pH of 5.5 or less. Acidemia is a potential adverse effect. Whether the efficacy of these drugs is due to methenamine or the acid component is controversial. Methenamine acts by conversion to formaldehyde, which requires incubation in the bladder. Thus, methenamine is ineffective in renal or prostatic infections or in animals with indwelling urinary catheters.

If the infection cannot be eliminated, suppressive therapy can be considered to prevent extension of the infection and to control symptoms. Suppressive therapy consists of administration of a single dose of an antimicrobial per day, preferably at a time when the animal will be confined so that urination is prevented for several hours. An example would be administration of the drug just prior to confining the animal in the house for the night. Preferred drugs for suppressive therapy in people are trimethoprim, nitrofurantoin, cephalexin, cinoxacin, or norfloxacin. Risks include antimicrobial toxicity and induction of bacterial resistance. Supplementation with B vitamins will help prevent folic acid deficiency from long-term use of trimethoprim-sulfonamide (see Chapter 43).

UTI Associated with Catheterization

Systemic treatment of UTIs developing during indwelling urinary catheterization should be delayed until the catheter is removed, unless systemic signs of infection develop. Antibiotics should not be used prophylactically to prevent UTI developing during catheterization. Although use of antibiotics may delay onset of bacteriuria, such use will not prevent infection if the catheter remains in place and will predispose to infection with resistant organisms.[17, 22, 42] Use of antibiotics in this situation leads to emergence of organisms with resistance to multiple antibiotics.

Removal of the catheter as soon as possible is the best preventive measure. Whether any local therapy into the bladder is beneficial during catheterization is controversial. In general, the short contact time plus the necessity of disconnecting the closed catheter system to infuse the antimicrobial substance abrogates any beneficial effect. Any disconnection of closed systems of urinary catheterization can rapidly lead to infection, even if the system is disconnected only for a short time.[61]

When a urinary catheter is removed and the animal is again urinating normally, the urine should be cultured and appropriate antimicrobial therapy should be started if infection is found. Treatment should continue at least 10 days with reculture of urine approximately 1 week after therapy is discontinued.

Catheter-induced infections may involve more than one bacterial species that may have varied antimicrobial susceptibility patterns. In these cases, one species is generally treated first. Urine is reevaluated following treatment, and if infection persists with another species, that infection is treated. Except for trimethoprim-sulfonamide, simultaneous administration of two or more antimicrobial agents is generally avoided in UTI.

Preoperative Prophylaxis

If surgery or genitourinary tract manipulation is to be performed on an animal with a urogenital infection, antibiotics should be administered prior to and during surgery to reduce the possibility of sepsis. If the animal's condition permits, determination of the causative organism and its susceptibility prior to surgery is recommended.

Male Genital Infections   Jeanne A. Barsanti

The most common species of bacteria associated with male genital infection in dogs are the same as those associated with UTI. Anaerobes are occasionally associated with abscess formation. Genital infections in male cats are uncommon, with the exception of those following scrotal injury during fighting.

PROSTATITIS

Etiology and Pathogenesis

In male dogs, the prostate gland is the closest genital organ to the normal flora of the distal urethra. Normally, the prostatic urethra and prostate itself are sterile. Migration of bacteria up the urethra to the prostate is inhibited by nonspecific defense mechanisms such as urine flow during micturition, urethral pressure, characteristics of the urethral mucosa, normal secretion of prostatic fluid, and the antibacterial nature of normal prostatic fluid. The prostate gland can also produce specific IgA as a local response to bacterial infection. The higher prevalence of UTI in castrated male dogs than in intact ones, both receiving glucocorticoids,[25] may be reflective of the importance of prostatic antibacterial factor.

The sequential pathogenesis of prostatic infections is incompletely understood. The close anatomic relationship between the bladder, proximal urethra, and prostate gland is reflected in the high frequency with which all three are simultaneously infected. Prostatic fluid normally refluxes into the bladder, and urine can enter prostatic ducts during micturition. Whether prostatic infection usually precedes or follows or develops simultaneously with bladder infection cannot be answered currently. Any condition that increases bacterial numbers in the prostatic urethra predisposes to infection. Examples include urethral urolithiasis, neoplasia, trauma, or strictures, or lower urinary tract infection. Diseases that interfere with normal prostatic fluid formation and excretion also predispose to infection. Examples are squamous metaplasia of the prostate and cystic hyperplasia.

Clinical Findings

Bacterial prostatitis occurs in sexually mature male dogs. Clinical signs associated with acute bacterial prostatitis include fever, depression, anorexia, urethral discharge, and pain on prostatic palpation. Vomiting is possible owing to an associated localized peritonitis. Less common signs are constipation from avoidance of defecation because of pain and a stiff, stilted rear-limb gait.

Chronic bacterial prostatitis is usually not associated with signs of systemic illness, although a purulent or hemorrhagic urethral discharge may be present. In some dogs, the only indication of chronic bacterial prostatitis is recurrent UTI. However, with prostatic abscess formation, the prostate may become enlarged and asymmetric, causing tenesmus and constipation. Dysuria can occur as a result of interference with normal urethral function. If the abscess is deep within the gland, palpable abnormalities may be absent. Pain on palpation may not be present. Rupture of a prostatic abscess can cause localized or diffuse peritonitis with signs of abdominal pain and vomiting, progressing to endotoxic or septic shock. Icterus due to hepatic compromise may be present (see Clinical Findings, Enterotoxemia, Chapter 44).

Diagnosis

The main diagnostic techniques used to determine whether bacterial prostatitis is present are history and prostatic palpation, CBC, urinalysis and urine culture, semen evaluation, prostatic massage, and prostatic aspiration and biopsy. Associated clinical signs and physical examination findings in conjunction with CBC and urinalysis and urine culture results are often sufficient to establish a tentative diagnosis of acute prostatitis. Further diagnostic tests are necessary in cases of chronic prostatitis to localize the site of infection to the prostate gland since clinical signs are minimal. Prostatic ultrasonography or surgical biopsy is often necessary to determine the possibility of abscess formation.

Clinical Laboratory Findings. An inflammatory leukogram with or without a left shift is often associated with acute bacterial prostatitis and with prostatic abscess formation. The CBC is usually normal in dogs with chronic prostatitis without abscess formation.[62]

Urinalysis and urine culture indicate UTI in most, but not all, cases. Some cases of prostatic infection have normal urine test results.

Semen Evaluation. An ejaculate is valuable in evaluating for chronic prostatic infection because its largest component is prostatic fluid. The prostatic fluid is the last fraction of the ejaculate, following the sperm-rich fraction. In collecting the ejaculate, the dog is allowed to urinate to remove any stagnant urethral contents, then returned to his run or to a quiet environment. Any preputial discharge is removed from the sheath by gentle, minimal cleansing with moistened, sterile gauze sponges. The area is gently dried. The ejaculate is collected using a sterile funnel and tube, a large, sterile plastic syringe case, or a sterile urine cup. If a dog's semen cannot be collected after manual manipulation, he can be teased using a bitch in estrus or an anestrous bitch to whose vulva dog pheromone, p-methyl hydroxybenzoate (Eastman Kodak, Rochester, NY), has been applied. Part of the ejaculate is used for cytologic study and part for quantitative culture. The latter procedure is essential because of the normal flora of the distal urethra.

Both ejaculate cytology and culture results must be considered. Normal dogs occasionally have leukocytes and positive culture results. Bacteria number fewer than 10^5/ml and are usually gram-positive. High numbers ($>10^5$/ml) of gram-negative organisms with large numbers of leukocytes indicate infection. Large numbers of gram-positive organisms with large numbers of leukocytes also indicate infection if preputial contamination did not occur. Lower numbers of gram-negative or gram-positive organisms must be correlated with clinical signs and ejaculate cytologic findings to determine their significance. If results of culture and cytology are questionable, a second sample should be evaluated.

Prostatic Massage. Because of the animal's discomfort, inexperience, or temperament, it is not possible to collect ejaculates from all male dogs. An alternative method for collecting prostatic fluid is prostatic massage. The dog is allowed to empty the bladder by normal voiding. A urinary catheter is then passed to the bladder using aseptic technique. The bladder is flushed several times with sterile saline to ensure that all urine is removed. The last flush of 5 to 10 ml is saved as the premassage sample. The catheter is then retracted distal to the prostate, as determined by rectal palpation, and the prostate is massaged rectally or per abdomen for 1 to 2 minutes. Sterile physiologic saline is injected slowly while the urethral orifice is occluded around the catheter to prevent reflux of the fluid. The catheter is slowly advanced to the bladder with repeated aspiration in the prostatic urethra. The bulk of the fluid will be aspirated from the bladder. Both the premassage and postmassage samples are examined by cytology and quantitative culture. It is most important to compare the postmassage sample with the premassage sample to ensure that any abnormality arose in the prostatic fluid and did not preexist in the bladder or urethra. Prostatic massage in normal dogs yields only a few erythrocytes and transitional epithelial cells.

The disadvantage of collection of prostatic fluid by prostatic massage in cases of infection is that abnormalities in urine will obscure those in prostatic fluid. If UTI is present, an antibiotic (e.g., ampicillin) that enters urine but not prostatic fluid is administered for a few days prior to massage. The prostatic fluid samples then obtained must be cultured immediately so that the antibiotic in the urine does not kill any bacteria in the prostatic fluid.

Radiography. The only radiographic sign of acute prostatitis is an indistinct cranial prostatic border. This is not noted in all cases. A change associated with some cases of chronic prostatitis is prostatic mineralization, but the prostate is often radiographically normal with chronic infection, and prostatic mineralization also occurs with prostatic neoplasia.[63] Infection without abscessation does not cause marked prostatomegaly. With abscess formation, the prostate is usually enlarged and irregular, and the prostatic urethra may be narrowed.[63] Similar changes may also be seen with neoplasia or cystic hyperplasia. The sublumbar lymph nodes may be enlarged.

On retrograde urethrography, greater than normal urethroprostatic reflux may be noted, but this is again not specific for abscess formation, occurring with most other prostatic diseases. However, distortion or destruction of the prostatic urethra strongly suggests neoplasia as opposed to abscess formation.[63]

The principal use of radiography is to localize and characterize the prostate gland when it cannot be thoroughly palpated. Use of distention retrograde urethrocystography may be useful to help differentiate an abscess from a neoplasm. Results of radiography should be correlated with results of prostatic fluid examination, urinalysis, and if possible, ultrasonography, to reach the most likely definitive diagnosis.

Ultrasonography. Acute bacterial prostatitis has not yet been characterized by ultrasonography in dogs. Diffuse, multifocal, or focal hyperechoic prostatic parenchyma has been associated with chronic bacterial prostatitis.[64] This finding is not definitive of infection, since increased echogenicity is also noted with neoplastic prostatic disease. Fluid-filled parenchymal cavities can be identified in dogs with prostatic abscesses, but these cavities cannot be distinguished from noninfected prostatic cysts. Ultrasound is primarily useful in identifying cystic cavities within the prostate gland. Correlation of results of ultrasonography with results of prostatic fluid evaluation is useful in identifying the underlying prostatic disease.

Needle Aspiration or Biopsy. Diagnosis of prostatic disease can also be approached by needle aspiration or biopsy by the perirectal or transabdominal route, depending on the location of the prostate. Needle aspiration is done aseptically using a long (21-gauge, 1½- to 2½-inch) needle with a stylet, such as a spinal needle. In the perirectal approach, the needle is guided by rectal palpation (Figs. 11–5 and 11–6). The procedure can be performed in most dogs with mild tranquilization. Needle aspiration is best avoided in dogs with suspected abscesses, as bacteria may be seeded along the needle track. In general, aspiration is not performed in dogs with fever or leukocytosis or before examining prostatic fluid obtained by ejac-

ulation or massage. In spite of these precautions, abscess formation has been inadvertently diagnosed by aspiration in dogs. The screening procedures did not indicate infection, because the abscessed areas were apparently not communicating with the urethra. After aspiration of occult abscesses, some dogs have developed signs of localized peritonitis that required parenteral antibiotic therapy to resolve. Because of the possibility of an occult abscess, fine-needle aspiration should always be performed prior to a closed-needle biopsy. Cytology should be performed on all aspirates. If pus is aspirated, aerobic and anaerobic bacterial cultures are indicated.

Closed prostatic biopsy can be performed perirectally, transabdominally, or via a caudal abdominal surgical exposure. It requires tranquilization and local anesthesia, and a needle such as the Tru-Cut (Travenol Laboratories, Deerfield, IL) is used. Closed biopsy can be directed by palpation or by ultrasound. The only complication reported from blind prostatic biopsy is mild hematuria, although significant hemorrhage is possible in any blind biopsy procedure. The dog should always be monitored closely for several hours after biopsy. Biopsy samples can be cultured for bacteria as well as examined histologically.

Therapy

Acute Bacterial Prostatitis. In acute bacterial prostatitis, an antibiotic should be administered for 21 to 28 days. The choice of anti-

Figure 11–5. Technique of perirectal aspiration of the prostate gland showing the point of needle insertion. The dog is sedated or anesthetized, placed in lateral recumbency, and the prostate is simultaneously palpated rectally with a gloved finger of the other hand.

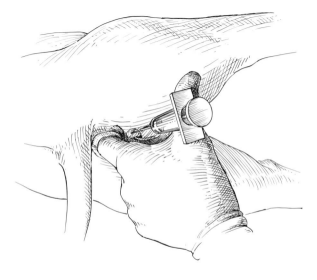

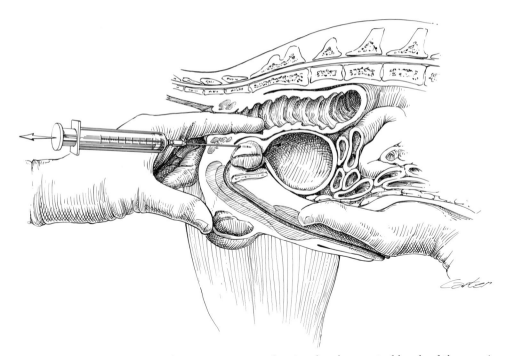

Figure 11–6. Lateral view of the procedure in Figure 11–5 showing the placement of hands of the examiner and assistant to stabilize the prostate gland. The assistant applies caudal and dorsal pressure to the abdomen to force the gland caudally while the index finger of the examiner's hand presses downward.

biotic can be based on urine culture, as the organism in the urine probably originated from the prostate. Since the blood–prostatic fluid barrier is usually damaged in acute inflammation, a wide choice of antibiotics, similar to that for UTI, may be considered for treatment. Supportive therapy should be given as necessary for systemic illness. Because acute infections may become chronic, reexamination should be performed 3 to 4 days after the antibiotic therapy is finished. This examination should include physical examination, urinalysis, urine culture, and prostatic fluid cytology and culture.

Chronic Bacterial Prostatitis. Cases of chronic bacterial prostatitis are very difficult to treat effectively because of a blood–prostatic fluid barrier. This barrier is related to the pH difference between the blood and prostatic interstitium and the prostatic fluid, the characteristics of the prostatic acinar epithelium, and the plasma protein-binding characteristics of antibiotics.

The pH of the blood and the prostatic interstitium is 7.4, whereas the pH of normal and infected prostatic fluid in dogs is less than 7.4.[62] When prostatic fluid is acidic, basic antibiotics (pKA >7) such as erythromycin, oleandomycin, clindamycin, norflox-

acin, and trimethoprim will cross the barrier more readily than other antibiotics (Table 11–8; Fig. 11–7).[65] If infected prostatic fluid is alkaline as in human males, these drugs would be much less effective, and acidic drugs such as carbenicillin and some of the quinolones (amifloxacin) would be more effective.[66] Thus, drug efficacy in people cannot be directly extrapolated to that in dogs.

The distribution of chloramphenicol is not affected by pH because it is un-ionized and lipid soluble. Lipid solubility is also an important factor in determining drug movement across the prostatic epithelium. Drugs with low lipid solubility, such as penicillin, ampicillin, cephalosporins, oxytetracycline, and the aminoglycosides, cannot cross into the prostatic acini. Chloramphenicol, the macrolide antibiotics, trimethoprim, quinolones, and carbenicillin are examples of lipid-soluble drugs that can cross the barrier effectively.

Protein binding in plasma also determines the amount of drug that enters prostatic fluid. The more protein-bound the drug is, the less of it is available to cross the prostatic epithelium. This factor is probably less important than lipid solubility or ionization, as biologic systems rarely reach equilibrium. Examples of drugs with significant protein

Table 11–8. Pharmacologic Characteristics of Certain Antibiotics

ANTIBIOTIC	LIPID SOLUBLE?	ACID OR BASE?	pKA[a]
Erythromycin	Yes	Base	8.8
Oleandomycin	Yes	Base	8.5
Tetracycline	Yes	Amphoteric	3.3, 7.7, 9.7
Kanamycin	No	Base	7.2
Penicillin G	No	Acid	2.7
Ampicillin	No	Acid	2.5
Cephalothin	No	Acid	2.5
Trimethoprim	Yes	Base	7.3
Chloramphenicol	Yes	NA[b]	NA[b]
Clindamycin	Yes	Base	7.6
Lincomycin	Fair	Base	7.6
Sulfisoxazole	Yes	Acid	Low
Sulfamethoxazole	Yes	Acid	Low

[a]pKA = the negative logarithm of the ionization constant (K) of an antibiotic.
[b]Not applicable.

binding are clindamycin and chloramphenicol.

In general, diffusion of tetracyclines into canine prostatic fluid is minimal. Although clinical studies in human males with prostatitis demonstrated efficacy of minocycline and doxycycline, these drugs did not penetrate well into canine prostatic fluid.

Current recommendations for the treatment of chronic bacterial prostatitis are based on whether a gram-positive or gram-negative organism is the infective agent. If the causative organism is gram-positive, erythromycin, clindamycin, oleandomycin, chloramphenicol, or trimethoprim-sulfonamide can be used, depending on the organism's susceptibility. If the causative organism is gram-negative, chloramphenicol or trimethoprim-sulfonamide is best. If a gram-negative organism fails to respond to these drugs, carbenicillin or the quinolones (norfloxacin, enrofloxacin, or ciprofloxacin) should be considered. Determination of the efficacy of quinolones in prostatic infections in dogs requires further study (see Quinolones, Chapter 43). Efficacy in people is considered at least as good as other available agents and perhaps better in relation to *E. coli*.[67] Measurement of prostatic fluid pH may help in choosing a potentially effective drug in difficult cases.

Antibiotic therapy should be continued for at least 6 weeks. If UTI is present, urine should be reevaluated by culture during therapy to be sure the administered drug has eliminated the UTI. Urine and prostatic fluid should be recultured 3 to 4 days and 1 month after discontinuing antibiotics to ensure that the infection has been eliminated, not merely suppressed. If initial therapy fails, a 3-month course of therapy shoud be instituted, bearing in mind potential adverse effects of the drug chosen. For such long-term therapy, trimethoprim, norfloxacin, and carbenicillin are the best current choices. Trimethoprim is the most cost effective. However, trimethoprim-sulfonamide can result in keratoconjunctivitis sicca or mild anemia due to folate deficiency. Folic acid should be supplemented when using trimethoprim-sulfonamide at full dosage for longer than 6 weeks. The prognosis for cure, based on experience in human medicine, is only fair. The long-term cure rate in humans is only about 40% to 60%.[67] If the prostatic infection cannot be eliminated, antibiotics must be used continuously to prevent recurrent UTI (see Therapy of Persistent UTI).

Prostatic Acinus

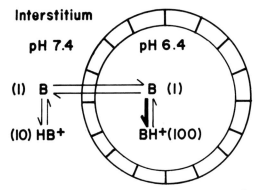

Figure 11–7. The diffusion into the prostate of an antibiotic that is a weak base (ionization constant pKA of 8.4) is shown at equilibrium. At a more acid pH within the prostate, the drug becomes more ionized and hence cannot leave the prostatic fluid. The prostatic fluid:plasma ratio is 101:11. (B = basic drug [pKA > 7]; BH, HB = ionized drug) (From Barsanti JA, Finco DR: *Vet Clin North Am* 9:679–699, 1979.)

Castration is recommended as adjunctive therapy to control infection. Limited studies indicate that castration in dogs is beneficial in resolution of prostatic infection.[68] Use of estrogens as chemical castration is not currently recommended as therapy for prostatitis. The major reason is that estrogens can induce squamous metaplasia and thus predispose to infection.[69] Also, estrogen therapy can be associated with significant bone marrow toxicity.

Prostatic Abscesses. Prostatic abscesses require surgical drainage, needle aspiration, tube or Penrose drains, or marsupialization for definitive therapy. Alternatively, the entire prostate may be removed. Complications are common with all methods, and postoperative survival of at least 1 year was approximately 50% in one survey.[70] Regardless of the surgical therapy elected, the dog should be treated with antibiotics as described previously for chronic prostatitis. IV antimicrobials should be used if the dog is systemically ill and during surgery. Initial antibiotic choice is empiric pending culture results. Final antibiotic choice should be based on culture and susceptibility and the dog's response to empiric therapy. If possible, surgery should be delayed until after culture results are obtained.

If prostatic enlargement has resulted in partial urethral obstruction, bladder and urethral function should be carefully assessed. It is especially important to assess bladder and urethral function prior to prostatectomy, since abnormalities prior to surgery increase the likelihood of postoperative incontinence. Prolonged bladder overdistention can result in bladder atony, leading to overflow incontinence. An indwelling urinary catheter may be necessary to let the detrusor muscle recover. If the bladder has been chronically distended and infected, it may be irreversibly damaged.

Polyuria and polydipsia, similar to that expected with nephrogenic diabetes insipidus, has been noted in a few dogs after surgical treatment for prostatic abscess formation.[70] This resolved within 1 month after surgery. Evidence of hepatopathy also resolved postoperatively.

Castration is recommended along with antibiotic and surgical therapy. Castration without abscess drainage leads to reduction of prostatic tissue but continuation of abscess pocket(s).

If the owners decline surgery, the dog can be managed with long-term suppressive antibiotic therapy after the UTI is controlled with at least 6 weeks of standard, full-dose therapy. The owners must realize that the abscess will persist and will potentially result in life-threatening infection.

EPIDIDYMITIS AND ORCHITIS

Etiology

Although bacterial infection is the most common cause of epididymo-orchitis, up to 20% of human cases have no identifiable causative organism.[71] Similar studies in dogs are lacking. Infection of the epididymis and testicles can occur secondary to UTI in both men and dogs.

Clinical Findings

In dogs, both the testicle and the epididymis are usually involved in inflammatory disease. The infection may be unilateral or bilateral. Clinical signs include pain, heat, and swelling in acute infections. The affected testicle or epididymis is often swollen and is doughy to firm in consistency. The dog will often lick the edematous scrotum. Systemic signs, such as fever, are variable. With chronic infection, fibrosis will produce increased firmness and contracture. Localized areas of abscess formation may feel softer. Bacterial infections of the testicles and epididymides are rare in cats, except secondary to fight wounds.

Diagnosis

Orchitis or epididymitis is usually strongly suspected on the basis of physical examination. Diagnostic tests should include a CBC, urinalysis, urine culture, and testing for canine brucellosis. If the dog will ejaculate, cytologic examination and quantitative culture of semen should be performed. Because of the public health hazard, semen should be evaluated only if *Brucella* test results are negative (see Diagnosis, Chapter 52). With semen, the cytologic finding of bacteria and neutrophils and the culture of more than 10^5 gram-negative organisms/ml suggest infection. Because of the urethral microflora, quantitative cultures are mandatory for rational assessment of results. If semen samples cannot be obtained because of the dog's discomfort and urinalysis and urine culture indicate UTI, treatment can be based on identification and antibiotic susceptibility of the organism isolated from urine. If the urine is not infected, testicle or epididymal aspiration using a 21- to 23-gauge needle and a 12-ml syringe can be performed for cytologic, histologic, and culture studies. Various testicular biopsy techniques can be performed. Ultrasound can be used to differentiate primary inflammatory disease from testicular torsion and traumatic rupture.[70]

Therapy

Bilateral orchidectomy is the treatment of choice for orchitis and epididymitis. If the dog is a valuable sire and the condition is unilateral, the testicle on the affected side should be removed to save the other from thermal degeneration. A bilateral infection has the potential to reduce fertility markedly.

Antibiotics should be given whether or not surgery is performed. Isolation of the causative organism and antimicrobial susceptibility testing should be used to guide therapy. Therapy should be continued at least 2 weeks. While culture results are pending, broad-spectrum antibiotics such as ampicillin, amoxicillin, chloramphenicol, or trimethoprim-sulfonamide should be started. Adjunctive soaks in cool water may help to reduce testicular degeneration from the hyperthermia of inflammation.

BALANOPOSTHITIS

Balanoposthitis is usually caused by bacteria normally present in the prepuce. Herpesvirus infections and blastomycosis also have caused balanoposthitis.

Mild balanoposthitis is extremely common and may be considered normal in male dogs. It is characterized by a purulent exudate within or dripping from the prepuce with variable degrees of inflammation of the preputial mucosa. There are no signs of systemic illness. Dogs usually are nonsymptomatic, but some will lick the prepuce.

There is no specific diagnostic test for balanoposthitis except cytologic examination of preputial exudate. Bacteria and large numbers of degenerate and nondegenerate neutrophils are seen. A culture of pus can be performed, but results may be difficult to interpret because of the abundant normal flora. Culture is not required for successful management of most cases.

Balanoposthitis is not a serious medical problem but may be an annoyance to the owner. Cleansing antiseptic douches or local antibacterials may be of benefit. Neutering affected animals may help reduce the amount of secretion produced.

Female Genital Infections   *Cheri A. Johnson*

VAGINITIS

Etiology

Bacteria, mycoplasmas and ureaplasmas, and viruses have been associated with vaginitis. Vaginitis is much more common in bitches than in queens. So-called "juvenile" or "puppy" vaginitis is not uncommon in otherwise normal, healthy prepubertal bitches and resolves spontaneously with the first estrous cycle in most affected bitches. Bacterial vaginitis in cats is uncommon.

Viral infections of the canine or feline vagina are less commonly a clinical problem than are bacterial infections. Herpesviruses (canine herpesvirus, feline rhinotracheitis virus) cause vesicular lesions and erythema when inoculated intravaginally.[72, 73] Although genital tract infection readily occurs after experimental inoculation, genital herpesvirus infection has been an uncommon clinical entity. Vaginal lymphoid follicular hyperplasia, which could result from any inflammatory process, may be mistaken for vesicle formation. Confirmation of genital herpesvirus infection should include viral isolation and histologic examination of the vesicular lesions (see Diagnosis and Pathologic Findings, Chapter 18).

Clinical Findings

The most common historic and clinical findings associated with vaginitis are licking of the vulva and the presence of a vulvar discharge in an otherwise healthy animal. The discharge may attract male dogs. Signs of systemic illness such as fever, malaise, anorexia, or changes in water consumption are not expected. The perineal hair may be discolored by saliva and the exudate. The animal may appear to be uncomfortable during micturition and during examination of the vulva or vagina. Cystitis may accompany vaginitis, in which case, pollakiuria or discolored urine may also be found.

Diagnosis

The diagnosis of vaginitis is strongly suggested by the historical and physical abnormalities, vaginal cytology, and vaginoscopy. The most important diagnostic considerations are whether the vulvar discharge is truly abnormal and whether an existing inflammatory process is confined to the vagina.

To avoid contamination from skin and the vestibule, samples for bacterial culture from the cranial vagina should be obtained with a guarded swab or through a sterile speculum. The results of vaginal cultures must be interpreted cautiously, because the most common pathogens of the vagina and uterus are E. coli, Streptococcus, and Staphylococcus, which are also commensal organisms. Diseased animals had greater numbers of these bacteria when compared with normal bitches.[1] Bacterial cultures will not confirm the diagnosis of vaginitis, since some bacterial growth is expected. Nevertheless, bacterial culture and susceptibility testing are often performed, because the results will help determine the choice of antibiotics as well as help differentiate persistent from recurrent infections.

Cytologic evidence of inflammation (WBC) with or without sepsis (bacteria) is expected from animals with vaginitis. Vaginal cytology must be interpreted in light of the stage of the estrous cycle. WBC are often very numerous during the first few days of diestrus. This normal phenomenon can be distinguished from inflammation because the number of WBC declines markedly in 24 to 48 hours of diestrus, whereas it persists with vaginitis. A mucoid vulvar discharge is normal during the early postpartum period in the bitch and queen. A hemorrhagic vulvar discharge is normal during proestrus and estrus in the bitch. Cytologic evidence of endometrial cells or uteroverdin indicates uterine involvement.

Vaginoscopy is used to evaluate the source of the discharge and the nature and extent of vaginal lesions and to obtain specimens for biopsy and culture. Sedation or general anesthesia may be necessary to adequately examine animals with severe vaginitis. The vaginal mucosa will be hyperemic. There is likely to be an exudate in the vaginal lumen. The inciting cause of the vaginitis may be identified during vaginoscopy. Vaginal cultures are easily obtained during vaginoscopy. Vaginal biopsies are usually obtained only when discrete, focal lesions are seen.

Abnormalities such as vaginal strictures, vaginal septa, vaginal neoplasia, or clitoral hypertrophy may be predisposing causes of vaginitis. The diagnosis is established by physical, endoscopic, and radiographic examinations. The presence of foreign substances, such as suture material or urine, may cause vaginitis. Urine may accumulate in the vagina because of vaginal, urethral, or ureteral anomalies. The latter are best evaluated by excretory urography.

The prognosis of vaginitis in normal, cycling bitches may vary with the stage of the estrous cycle. If vaginitis is concurrent with pregnancy, the possible teratogenic or abortifacient effects of therapy must be considered. If vaginitis occurs in proestrus or estrus, the possibility of transmission of a potential pathogen to the stud should be considered. The effects of therapy on sperm survival should also be considered. The prognosis for recovery from vaginitis in intact bitches is usually good.

Therapy

Antiseptic douches, instillation of antibiotic suppositories, ointments, or solutions, and systemic antibiotic therapy have been used with apparent success to treat vaginitis.[1] Using solutions that alter pH, such as vinegar (0.25% to 0.50%) or most commercial douches, discourages the overgrowth of vaginal bacteria. The relative efficacy of these treatments has yet to be investigated in small animals. Surgical correction of anatomic abnormalities, surgical excision of vaginal masses, and removal of androgenic stimuli in cases of clitoral hypertrophy will help to eliminate predisposing causes of vaginitis. Treatment of puppy vaginitis is usually conservative. Often perineal hygiene is sufficient to control clinical signs and prevent secondary dermatitis. The prognosis for recovery from juvenile vaginitis is excellent, provided the animal is allowed to experience an estrous cycle. When no inciting cause can be found in neutered bitches, vaginitis may persist despite aggressive medical therapy.

UTERINE INFECTION

Etiology

Metritis and pyometra are two distinctly different clinical bacterial infections of the canine and feline uterus. **Metritis** is an acute ascending bacterial infection of the uterus,[74] usually in a postpartum female. It may follow dystocia, obstetric manipulations, or retention of fetal or placental parts. Rarely, metritis may occur after natural or artificial insemination or abortion. **Pyometra**, on the other hand, is a bacterial infection secondary to hormonally induced uterine pathology.[75] Progesterone causes cystic endometrial hyperplasia and fluid accumulation within endometrial glands and the uterine lumen and decreases myometrial activity. Ascending bacterial infection then occurs. Because progesterone initiates the sequence of events, pyometra occurs during the luteal (diestrus) phase of the cycle or following the administration of progestins. Though bacteria do not initiate pyometra in the bitch, the secondary infection is the cause of most of the morbidity and mortality. Since the vagina is the probable source of uterine bacteria, it is not surprising that *E. coli*, *Streptococcus*, and *Staphylococcus* are the most commonly isolated organisms in both metritis and pyometra.[74–76]

Many organisms cross the canine placenta and infect fetuses but do not infect the uterus per se. They may however be transiently recovered from uterine or vaginal cultures of parturient or periparturient bitches. These organisms include canine herpesvirus, adenovirus, distemper virus, *Brucella canis*, and *Toxoplasma gondii*.[77] Experimental, intrauterine inoculation of *Mycoplasma canis* can cause uterine pathology in bitches,[78] but the role of mycoplasmal infection in spontaneous disease is uncertain (see Chapter 41). In cats, feline leukemia and herpesviruses can be transmitted to the fetuses of viremic queens. Pyometra involving the uterus masculinus of hermaphrodites can occur in dogs and cats.[78a]

Clinical Findings

Most of the clinical signs of pyometra and metritis—lethargy, anorexia, and dehydration—are referable to bacterial infection. Fever is common with metritis but not with pyometra. Septicemia or endotoxemia may develop at any time, in which case, animals may have tachycardia, tachypnea, poor peripheral perfusion, and subnormal body temperature. A purulent, malodorous vulvar discharge is present in metritis because the postpartum cervix is usually "open." The cervix may or may not be open and draining in animals with pyometra. Other findings are uterine enlargement, neglect of neonates, and polydipsia-polyuria.

Diagnosis

The diagnosis of bacterial uterine infection is established by the history, the stage of the estrous cycle, physical examination, and laboratory and radiographic abnormalities.[74, 76] Abnormalities on vaginal cytology include degenerate neutrophils and bacteria. Endometrial cells may also be found.[79] The results of CBC are variable, although a leukocytosis with a left shift is usually present and is most dramatic, with "closed" pyometra. Leukopenia with a degenerative left shift and neutrophil toxicity may be found in animals with septicemia. Anemia, hyperglobulinemia and hyperfibrinogenemia, and azotemia may be detected. Isosthenuria and proteinuria are found in 30% of bitches with pyometra. Isosthenuria is thought to be a result of endotoxin-induced unresponsiveness to antidiuretic hormone and tubular injury. Mild tubulointerstial nephritis is the most consistent pathologic finding.[79a] Impaired tubular concentrating ability contributes to the polyuria, with compensatory polydipsia, often seen in bitches with pyometra. Most affected bitches, with or without azotemia, have reduced glomerular filtration rates that are not correlated with structural alterations in glomeruli.[79a] Glomerular lesions characteristic of immune-complex deposition have been identified in some bitches with pyometra. Concurrent urinary tract infection has been detected in 22% of affected bitches.[79a] CBC, biochemical profile, and urinalysis are essential to detect the metabolic abnormalities associated with septicemia or toxemia and to evaluate renal function. Urine collection should be done carefully because of the risks of perforating the enlarged uterus during cystocentesis and introducing organisms from the reproductive tract into the bladder during catheterization.

The most important diagnostic consideration for pyometra is differentiating it from pregnancy. The vulvar discharge of metritis must be differentiated from the normal postpartum discharge, lochia. Abdominal radiography will confirm the presence of uterine enlargement, but the nature of the uterine contents cannot be determined from radiographs unless calcified fetal structures are present. Ultrasonography is useful in differentiating fetal structures, solid masses, and luminal fluid. Cystic endometrial hyperplasia has also been identified by ultrasonography.[80]

Therapy

Treatment should be prompt and aggressive because rapid deterioration is common in animals with septicemia. Therapy consists of administration of IV fluids, antibiotics, and evacuation of uterine contents. Fluid therapy should be continued throughout surgical or medical management to ensure adequate tissue perfusion. Glucocorticoids may be indicated for animals in septic shock.

Antibiotic therapy is clearly indicated for animals with uterine infection. The antibiotics should be chosen on the basis of culture and susceptibility testing of the uterine exudate. Samples should be obtained directly from the uterine lumen at the time of ovariohysterectomy. If surgery is not performed, culture specimens should be obtained from the cranial vagina as discussed earlier. Pending the return of culture results, an antibiotic effective against E. coli should be administered.

Ovariohysterectomy is the definitive treatment for metritis or pyometra for dogs and cats. However, it may be unacceptable to some owners, even though it is the treatment of choice. Prostaglandin $F_2\alpha$ ($PGF_2\alpha$) has been successfully used in treating pyometra and metritis in the bitch and queen. For medical treatment, naturally occurring $PGF_2\alpha$ (Lutalyse and Prostin, both, Upjohn Co, Kalamazoo, MI) is given at a dose of 0.1 to 0.25 mg/kg SC for 3 to 5 days until the uterus is empty and the vaginal discharge is resolving.[81–83] The need for longer therapy may be associated with a poorer prognosis. Some have recommended repeating the $PGF_2\alpha$ regimen if the vaginal discharge persists after 2 weeks.[83] This could also be associated with a poorer prognosis and should prompt reevaluation of the patient and the choice of antibiotics. The most common side effects of the prostaglandin therapy are restlessness, pacing, hypersalivation, panting, vomiting, abdominal discomfort, tachycardia, and fever.

The beneficial effects of prostaglandins apparently are solely due to evacuation of uterine contents, rather than to changes in the endometrium or ovarian function. Oxytocin may be useful for the treatment of postpartum metritis,[74] but not for pyometra.[75] Hysterotomy with curettage may be considered for animals with metritis, especially if retained fetuses or other debris are known to be present. When diffuse uterine disease exists, as is the case with pyometra, hysterotomy has not been helpful.

Intrauterine infusion of antiseptic or antibiotic solutions is of questionable value. The canine cervix is extremely difficult to cannulate; therefore, most infusions are probably intravaginal rather than intrauterine. Intrauterine infusion of nitrofurazone may actually decrease subsequent fertility in some species.[74] Surgical placement of drains within the uterus and subsequent flushing is usually not successful.[75] If ovariohysterectomy is not performed, antibiotic therapy should continue for 2 to 4 weeks.

The prognosis for recovery from metritis and pyometra is very good when ovariohysterectomy is performed. There is, of course, mortality associated with the diseases as well as with the surgical procedure.[75, 76] The prognosis for recovery from clinical illness is also good for animals treated medically, if the cervix is open. Only 42% of bitches with closed-cervix pyometra were treated successfully with $PGF_2\alpha$.[81]

There are no reports of successful medical

management of closed-cervix pyometra in the queen. Of the bitches and queens successfully treated for pyometra, subsequent conception rates have ranged from 40% to 90%.[81, 82] Recurrence of pyometra can be expected in most bitches after medical treatment. Less is known about subsequent fertility in animals treated medically for metritis, but at least some of them are likely to conceive.[83]

References

1. Barsanti JA: Genitourinary tract infections. *In* Greene CA (ed): *Clinical Microbiology and Infectious Diseases of the Dog and Cat.* Philadelphia, WB Saunders Co, 1984, pp 269–283.
2. Ling GV, Ruby AL: Aerobic bacterial flora of the prepuce, urethra and vagina of normal adult dogs. *Am J Vet Res* 39:695–698, 1978.
3. Doig PA, Ruhnke HL, Bosu WTK: The genital mycoplasma and ureaplasma flora of healthy and diseased dogs. *Can J Comp Med* 45:233–238, 1981.
4. Olson PNS, Mather EC: Canine vaginal and uterine bacterial flora. *J Am Vet Med Assoc* 172:708–711, 1978.
5. Hinman F: Meatal recolonization in bitches. *Trans Am Assoc Genitourin Surg* 68:73–77, 1977.
6. Lees GE, Simpson RB, Green RA: Results of analyses and bacterial cultures of urine specimens obtained from clinically normal cats by three methods. *J Am Vet Med Assoc* 184:449–454, 1984.
7. Kunin CM: Detection, prevention, and management of urinary tract infections. Philadelphia, Lea & Febiger, 1987.
8. Ling GV: Therapeutic strategies involving antimicrobial treatment of the canine urinary tract. *J Am Vet Med Assoc* 185:1162–1164, 1984.
9. Kivisto AK, Vasenius H, Sandholm M: Canine bacteruria. *J Small Anim Pract* 18:707–712, 1977.
10. Sobel JD: Pathogenesis of urinary tract infections. *Infect Dis Clin North Am* 1:751–772, 1987.
11. Hirsh DC: Multiple antimicrobial resistance in *E. coli* isolated from the urine of dogs and cats with cystitis. *J Am Vet Med Assoc* 162:885–887, 1973.
12. Wooley RE, Blue JL: Quantitative and bacteriological studies of urine specimens from canine and feline urinary tract infections. *J Clin Microbiol* 4:326, 1976.
13. Weaver AD, Pillinger R: Lower urinary tract pathogens in the dog and their sensitivity to chemotherapeutic agents. *Vet Rec* 101:77–79, 1977.
14. Ling GV, Biberstein EL, Hirsh DC: Bacterial pathogens associated with urinary tract infections. *Vet Clin North Am* 9:617–630, 1979.
15. Jang SS, Ling GV, Yamamoto R, et al: Mycoplasma as a cause of canine urinary tract infection. *J Am Vet Med Assoc* 185:45–57, 1984.
16. Barsanti JA, Finco DR, Shotts EB, et al: Feline urologic syndromes: further investigation into etiology. *J Am Anim Hosp Assoc* 18:387–390, 1982.
17. Barsanti JA: Urinary tract infections due to indwelling bladder catheters in dogs and cats. *J Am Vet Med Assoc* 187:384–388, 1988.
18. Gregory CR, Vasseur PB: Electromyographic and

19. Stamm WE, Hooten TM, Johnson JR, et al: Urinary tract infections: from pathogenesis to treatment. *J Infect Dis* 159:400–406, 1989.
20. Reid G, Sobel JD: Bacterial adherence in the pathogenesis of urinary tract infection: a review. *Rev Infect Dis* 9:470–487, 1987.
21. Parsons CL: Bladder surface glycosaminoglycan: efficient mechanism of environmental adaptation. *Urology (Suppl)* 27:9–14, 1986.
21a. Parsons CL: Pathogenesis of urinary tract adherence, bladder defense mechanisms. *Urol Clin North Am* 13:563–568, 1986.
22. Nicolle LE, Ronald AR: Recurrent urinary tract infection in adult women: diagnosis and therapy. *Infect Dis Clin North Am* 1:793–806, 1987.
23. Stamey TA: Recurrent urinary tract infection in female patients: an overview of management and treatment. *Rev Infect Dis (Suppl)* 9:S195–S210, 1987.
24. Lees GE, Osborne CA: Antibacterial properties of urine: a comparative review. *J Am Anim Hosp Assoc* 15:125–132, 1979.
25. Ihrke PJ, Norton AL, Ling GV, et al: Urinary tract infection associated with long-term corticosteroid administration. *J Am Vet Med Assoc* 186:43–46, 1985.
26. Eden CS, deMan P: Bacterial virulence in urinary tract infection. *Infect Dis Clin North Am* 1:731–750, 1987.
27. O'Hanley P, Low D, Romero I, et al: Gal-Gal binding and hemolysin phenotypes and genotypes associated with uropathogenic *Escherichia coli.* *N Engl J Med* 313:414–420, 1985.
28. Uehling DT: Future approaches to the management of urinary tract infection. *Urol Clin North Am* 13:749–758, 1986.
29. Westerlund B, Pere A, Korhonen TK, et al: Characterisation of *Escherichia coli* strains associated with canine urinary tract infections. *Res Vet Sci* 42:404–406, 1987.
30. Wilson RA, Keefe TJ, Davis MA, et al: Strains of *Escherichia coli* associated with urogenital disease in dogs and cats. *Am J Vet Res* 49:743–746, 1988.
31. Nolan LK, Wolley RE, Brown J, et al: Comparison of virulence factors and antibiotic resistance profiles of *Escherichia coli* strains from humans and dogs with urinary tract infections. *J Vet Intern Med* 1:152–157, 1987.
32. Boscia JA, Kaye D: Asymptomatic bacteriuria in the elderly. *Infect Dis Clin North Am* 1:893–905, 1987.
33. Ling GV, Cullen JM, Kennedy PC, et al: Relationship of upper and lower urinary tract infection and bacterial invasion of uroepithelium to antibody-coated bacteria test results in female dogs. *Am J Vet Res* 46:499–504, 1985.
34. Comer KM, Ling GV: Results of urinalysis and bacterial culture of canine urine obtained by antepubic cystocentesis, catheterization and the midstream voided methods. *J Am Vet Med Assoc* 179:891–895, 1981.
35. Biertuempfel PH, Ling GV, Ling GA: Urinary tract infection resulting from catheterization in healthy adult dogs. *J Am Vet Med Assoc* 178:989–991, 1981.
36. Padilla J, Osborne CA, Ward GE: Effects of storage time and temperature on quantitative culture of canine urine. *J Am Vet Med Assoc* 178:1077–1081, 1981.

37. Allen TA, Jones RL, Purvance J: Microbiologic evaluation of canine urine: direct microscopic examination and preservation of specimen quality for culture. *J Am Vet Med Assoc* 190:1289–1291, 1987.

38. Klausner JS, Osborne CA, Stevens JB: Clinical evaluation of commercial reagent strips for detection of significant bacteriuria in dogs and cats. *Am J Vet Res* 37:719–722, 1976.

39. Vail DM, Allen TA, Weiser GA: Applicability of leukocyte esterase test strip in detection of canine pyuria. *J Am Vet Med Assoc* 189:1451–1453, 1986.

40. Rogers KS, Lees GE, Simpson RB: Effects of single-dose and three-day trimethoprim-sulfadiazine and amikacin treatment of induced *Escherichia coli* urinary tract infection in dogs. *Am J Vet Res* 49:345–349, 1988.

41. Starck RP, Maki DG: Bacteruria in the catheterized patient. What quantitative level of bacteriuria is relevant? *N Engl J Med* 311:560–564, 1984.

42. Warren JW: Catheter-associated urinary tract infections. *Infect Dis Clin North Am* 1:823–854, 1987.

43. Barber DL, Finco DR: Radiographic findings in induced bacterial pyelonephritis in dogs. *J Am Vet Med Assoc* 175:1183–1190, 1979.

44. Ling GV, Ackerman N, Lowenstine LJ, et al: Percutaneous nephropyelocentesis and nephropyelostomy in the dog: a description of technique. *Am J Vet Res* 40:1605–1612, 1979.

45. Osborne CA, Finco DR, Low DG: Renal failure: diagnosis, treatment, and prognosis. In Ettinger SJ (ed): *Veterinary Internal Medicine*. Philadelphia, WB Saunders Co, 1975, pp 1465–1534.

46. Stamey TA: *Urinary Infections*. Baltimore, Williams & Wilkins, 1980.

47. Antimicrobial susceptibility tests. *Med Lett Drugs Ther* 28:2–4, 1986.

48. Stamey TA, Fair WR, Timothy MM, et al: Serum versus urinary antimicrobial concentration in cure of urinary tract infections. *N Engl J Med* 291:1159–1163, 1974.

49. Rohrich PJ, Ling GV, Ruby AL, et al: In vitro susceptibilities of canine urinary bacteria to selected antimicrobial agents. *J Am Vet Med Assoc* 183:863–867, 1983.

49a. Ling GV, Rohrich PJ, Ruby AL, et al: Canine urinary tract infection: a comparison of in vitro antimicrobial susceptibility test results and response to oral therapy with ampicillin or with trimethoprim-sulfa. *J Am Vet Med Assoc* 185:277–281, 1984.

50. James JR, Stamm WE: Diagnosis and treatment of acute UTI. *Infect Dis Clin North Am* 1:773–791, 1987.

51. Lawrence RM: Current therapy of urinary tract infections and pyelonephritis. *Semin Nephrol* 6:241–249, 1986.

52. Cox CE, Corrado ML: Safety and efficacy of imipenem/cilastatin in treatment of complicated urinary tract infection. *Am J Med* 78:92–94, 1985.

53. van Oosterom RA, Hartman EG: Pipemidic acid, a new treatment for recurrent urinary tract infection in small animals. *Vet Q* 8:2–5, 1986.

54. Lee C, Roanld AR: Norfloxacin: its potential in clinical practice. *Am J Med* 82:27–34, 1987.

55. Bergeron MG, Marois Y: Benefit from high intrarenal levels of gentamicin in the treatment of *E. coli* pyelonephritis. *Kidney Int* 30:481–487, 1986.

56. Turnwald GH, Gossett KA, Cox HU, et al: Comparison of single-dose and conventional trimethoprim-sulfadiazine therapy in experimental *Staphylococcus intermedius* cystitis in the female dog. *Am J Vet Res* 47:2621–2633, 1986.

57. Fihn SD, Johnson C, Roberts PL, et al: Trimethoprim-sulfamethoxazole for acute dysuria in women: a single dose or 10-day course. *Ann Intern Med* 108:350–357, 1988.

58. Senior DF, Gaskin JM, Buergelt CD, et al: Amoxicillin and clavulanic acid combination in the treatment of experimentally induced bacterial cystitis in dogs. *J Am Anim Hosp Assoc* 22:227–233, 1986.

59. Stamey TA: Recurrent urinary tract infections in female patients: an overview of management and treatment. *Rev Infect Dis* 9 (Suppl):S195–S210, 1987.

60. Senior DF: Bacterial urinary tract infections: invasion, host defenses, and new approaches to prevention. *Compend Cont Educ Pract Vet* 7:334–344, 1985.

61. Nickel JC, Grant SK, Costerton JW: Catheter-associated bacteruria: an experimental study. *Urology* 26:369–375, 1985.

62. Barsanti JA, Prasse KW, Crowell WA, et al: Evaluation of various techniques for diagnosis of chronic bacterial prostatitis. *J Am Vet Med Assoc* 183:219–224, 1983.

63. Feeney DA, Johnston GR, Klausner JS, et al: Canine prostatic disease–comparison of radiographic appearance with morphologic and microbiologic findings: 30 cases (1981–1985). *J Am Vet Med Assoc* 190:1018–1026, 1987.

64. Feeney DA, Johnston GR, Klausner JS, et al: Canine prostatic disease–comparison of ultrasonographic appearance with morphologic and microbiologic findings: 30 cases (1981–1985). *J Am Vet Med Assoc* 190:1027–1034, 1987.

65. Barsanti JA, Finco DR: Canine bacterial prostatitis. *Vet Clin North Am* 9:679–699, 1979.

66. Frimodt-Moller PC, Dorflinger T, Madsen PO: Amifloxacin distribution in the dog prostate. *Prostate* 6:163–168, 1985.

67. Weidner W, Schiefer HG, Dalhoff A: Treatment of chronic bacterial prostatitis with ciprofloxacin: results of a one-year follow-up study. *Am J Med* 82:280–283, 1987.

68. Cowan LA, Barsanti JA, Garcia M, et al: Effect of castration on experimentally induced chronic prostatic infection in dogs. *Am J Vet Res*, in press, 1989.

69. Klausner JS: Management of canine bacterial prostatitis. *J Am Vet Med Assoc* 182:292–296, 1983.

70. Hardie EM, Barsanti JA, Rawlings CA: Complications of prostatic surgery. *J Am Anim Hosp Assoc* 20:50–56, 1984.

71. Ireton R: Prostatitis and epididymitis. *Urol Clin North Am* 11:83–94, 1984.

72. Hill H, Mare CJ: Genital disease in dogs caused by herpes virus. *Am J Vet Res* 35:669–672, 1974.

73. Hoover EA, Griesemer RA: Comments: pathogenicity of feline viral rhinotracheitis virus and effect on germ-free cats, growing bone and gravid uterus. *J Am Vet Med Assoc* 158:929–930, 1971.

74. Magne ML: Acute metritis in the bitch. In Morrow DA (ed): *Current Therapy in Theriogenology*, ed 2. Philadelphia, WB Saunders, 1986, p 505.

75. Hardy RM, Osborne CA: Canine pyometra: pathophysiology, diagnosis, and treatment of uterine and extrauterine lesions. *J Am Anim Hosp Assoc* 10:245–268, 1974.

76. Kenney KJ, Matthiesen DT, Brown NO, et al: Pyometra in cats: 183 cases (1979–1984). *J Am Vet Med Assoc* 191:1130–1132, 1987.

77. Krakowka S: Transplacentally acquired microbial and parasitic diseases of dogs. *J Am Vet Med Assoc* 171:750–753, 1977.

78. Doig PA, Ruhnke HL, Bosu WTK: The genital mycoplasma and ureaplasma flora of healthy and diseased dogs. *Can J Comp Med* 45:233–238, 1981.

78a. Schulman J, Levine SH: Pyometra involving uterus masculinus in a cat. *J Am Vet Med Assoc* 194:690–691, 1989.

79. Olson PN, Thrall MA, Wykes PM, et al: Vaginal cytology. Part II. Its use in diagnosing canine reproductive disorders. *Compend Cont Educ Pract Vet* 6:385–390, 1984.

79a. Stone EA, Littman MP, Robertson JL, et al: Renal dysfunction in dogs with pyometra. *J Am Vet Med Assoc* 193:457–464, 1988.

80. Poffenbarger EM, Feeney DA: Use of gray-scale ultrasonography in the diagnosis of reproductive disease in the bitch: 18 cases (1981–1984). *J Am Vet Med Assoc* 189:90–95, 1986.

81. Nelson RW, Feldman EC: Pyometra. *Vet Clin North Am [Small Anim Pract]* 16:561–576, 1986.

82. Meyers-Wallen VN, Goldschmidt MH, Flickinger GL: Prostaglandin $F_2\alpha$ treatment of canine pyometra. *J Am Vet Med Assoc* 181:899–903, 1982.

83. Nelson RW, Feldman FC, Stabenfeldt GH: Treatment of canine pyometra and endometritis with prostaglandin F_{2a}. *J Am Vet Med Assoc* 181:899–903, 1982.

12 BACTERIAL INFECTIONS OF THE CENTRAL NERVOUS SYSTEM

William R. Fenner

ETIOLOGY

In comparison with the frequency of infections in other organ systems, CNS infections are uncommon in animals. The usual causes of CNS infections are viruses, protozoa, rickettsia, and bacteria, in decreasing order of involvement. This low prevalence of CNS infections may result from better protection offered to the CNS by its barriers than from the scarcity of infectious agents that can attack the CNS. Infections are usually caused by a flaw in the normal defense barriers instead of resulting from exposure to some organism with a specific neurotropism.[1]

Of the infectious causes of CNS inflammation, bacteria have the best chance for being eliminated by antimicrobial therapy. This chapter will focus on bacterial infections; other infectious causes of CNS inflammation will be covered in other chapters. Bacteria commonly associated with CNS infections in dogs and cats include *Staphylococcus intermedius*, *S. epidermidis*, *S. albus*, *Pasteurella multocida*, *Actinomyces*, *Nocardia*, and various anaerobes, including *Bacteroides*, *Fusobacterium*, *Peptostreptococcus*, and *Eubacterium*.[2]

Meningitis, an inflammation of the meninges, can be localized or diffuse. Diffuse meningitis is common in dogs and cats. Brain abscesses, which result from a focal accumulation of pus, appear to be associated with contiguous infections, such as progression of otitis interna or, rarely, from hematogenous spread of organisms. Brain abscesses are uncommon in the dog and cat.[3, 4] This may in part be due to the inability

of the nervous system to form scar tissue, which in other tissue, restricts the spread of pyogenic infections. Since epidural abscesses develop outside the parenchyma of the nervous system, true abscess formation can occur. Spinal epidural abscesses are more common than are cranial epidural abscesses because of the greater available space in the spinal canal.

PATHOGENESIS

The location(s) of the infection in the CNS will be determined by the interplay of a number of factors, including the etiologic agent and its route of entry into the nervous system, whether the infection remains focal or becomes generalized after entry, and the character of the immune response of the host and its nervous system to the infection.[5] The most common routes of infection include hematogenous, direct invasion, contiguous or parameningeal spread, and entry along a nerve root (Table 12–1).

There are several limiting barriers to the entry of microorganisms into the CNS. The principal barrier to hematogenous entry is the blood-brain barrier (BBB), which provides an anatomic and physiologic barrier between the systemic circulation and the parenchyma of the CNS. The anatomic BBB is created by the CNS capillaries, which have tight junctions between the endothelial cells, lack fenestrations in the basement membrane, and are enveloped by astroglial foot processes (Fig. 12–1).[5a] Hematogenous infections must penetrate this barrier. In viral infections, this occurs when infected lym-

Table 12–1. Source and Localization of Non-neurotropic Infections of the Central Nervous System

POINT OF ENTRY	USUAL LOCATION OR TYPE OF INFECTION
Paranasal sinuses	Frontal lobes Focal epidural abscess Diffuse epidural empyema
Petrous temporal bone (otitis media)	Temporal lobe Cerebellum Brain stem (cerebellopontine angle)
Cranial nerves	Basilar meninges Most frequently cranial nerves VII and VIII
Spinal cord	Diffuse subarachnoid infection
Hematogenous	Diffuse subarachnoid infection Focal parenchymal abscess or granuloma

phocytes are transported across the BBB. In bacterial infections, successful infection generally requires disruption of the BBB.[5] The physiologic barrier, which becomes important in drug entry into the CNS, is discussed under Therapy, later in this chapter.

Barriers to direct spread of infection into the subarachnoid space include the meninges, spinal column, and skull. Direct invasion by microorganisms usually is preceded by some prior trauma that provides access across these protective membranes. Contiguous (parameningeal) spread is a fairly common cause of bacterial infections of the spinal column, e.g., discospondylitis, but the infections rarely invade the CNS itself. Contiguous infections of the brain, such as migration from an inner ear infection, are also common. In dogs and cats, migration of

bacteria along a nerve appears to be a relatively rare method of entry into the CNS. Organisms that may use this route are *Cryptococcus neoformans* and *Listeria monocytogenes*.

Infectious processes may cause CNS dysfunction by several mechanisms. If the signs are the result of destruction of the parenchyma, the chance for recovery is slight. If the signs are from secondary effects, reversing the cause may allow for restoration of neural health. The same anatomic features that served to protect the CNS from infection may increase the damage once infection is present. The meninges and bony indentations of the skull and spine may trap the infection, promoting local abscess formation, creating a local mass effect. This mass will cause pressure necrosis of adjacent healthy tissue. Once an infection has become established, the loose attachments of the dura to the CNS will facilitate rapid local extension. Since the CNS lacks lymphatics, there is no immediate drainage for removal of by-products of inflammation, which are particularly destructive. Finally, the BBB may limit the ingress of phagocytes, antibodies, and antibiotics, thus delaying attempts to control the infection.

Effects of the organism itself include whether or not it produces toxins or vasculitis or is neurotropic. Toxins may produce more injury to the CNS than the infecting organism itself, resulting in severe injury even in the presence of low grade infections. Vasculitis within the CNS produced by some organisms may result in CNS infarction with peracute onset of additional signs. Certain bacteria, especially gram-negative rods, pro-

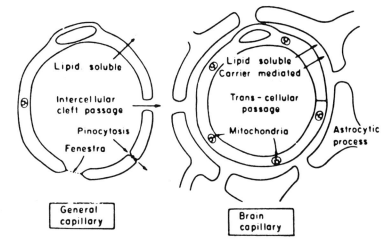

Figure 12–1. Comparison of features of systemic capillaries and the capillary endothelial cells of the brain. (Reproduced from Oldendorf WH: In Bito LZ, Davson H, Fenstermacher JD: Experimental Eye Research. Supplement, Vol 25: The Ocular and Cerebrospinal Fluids. London: Academic Press, 1977, pp 177–190. Reprinted with permission.)

duce more damage to the meninges than gram-positive organisms. Organisms such as *Corynebacterium* spp., *Nocardia*, and *Serratia marcescens* are of low virulence and usually only produce infection in immunocompromised hosts. If the organism is neurotropic, it will cause direct destruction of neural elements. In most cases, bacteria are non-neurotropic and produce secondary neural damage.

Secondary effects are compression of healthy tissue by the accumulation of pyogenic exudates that may produce significant mass lesions. Inflammation results in fibrin deposition, thrombosis of veins, and arteritis, all of which predispose to encephalitis. Degenerating leukocytes release toxins that produce vasospasm, local ischemia, and tissue edema. Brain edema appears to be induced by free unsaturated fatty acids found in membranes of neutrophils. In some cases of encephalitis, there is a significant mass effect, with high risk for brain herniation.[6] The potential for herniation is increased by increases in CSF pressure, which is correlated with the bacterial titers. With meningitis, there is marked resistance to the outflow of CSF through the arachnoid granulations. This resistance is associated with elevations of CSF pressure and may be decreased with the use of glucocorticoids.

During meningitis, the tight junctions of the BBB open. The immunoglobulins that are present in the CSF appear to extravasate across this opening. The majority of the phagocytic cells that are present in inflammations of the CNS originate from the blood. The peak inflammatory response occurs about 72 hours after the infection begins. Local production of antibody in the CSF comes from blood-derived plasma cells that migrate into the CNS. In addition, injury to the BBB will facilitate entry of antibodies into the CSF, as will elevated plasma levels of antibodies.

If an infection does become established in the CNS, isolation of the nervous system from the systemic immune responses by the healed BBB may delay or prevent the control of the infection.

CLINICAL FINDINGS

Systemic Signs

Many patients with CNS infections will have clinical signs of systemic illness in addition to the signs of CNS involvement. Some patients may have concomitant infections of other systems with respective clinical signs. In addition to fever, which may result from the inflammatory process, hyperthermia may be superimposed because of muscle tremors, seizures, or exertional activity. Animals with meningitis may also have signs of ophthalmic inflammation, including retinitis, choroiditis, uveitis, and vasculitis of retinal vessels. There may be abnormalities of heart rate and rhythm, as a result of elevated intracranial pressures or from direct involvement of the brain stem. In advanced disease, with severe brain edema or mass effect, brain herniation with acute respiratory insufficiency may be seen.

CNS Signs

Neurologic signs such as hyperesthesia result from meningeal involvement. Hyperesthesia on muscle palpation or traction on limbs may be seen with radicular irritation. Vomiting, photophobia, nuchal rigidity, and depressed mental status are often associated with meningeal inflammation as well. Neurologic dysfunction varies according to the area(s) of the CNS involved. Forebrain diseases tend to be characterized principally by behavioral or personality changes and seizures. Behavioral changes may include abnormal sleep patterns, changes in eating and voiding habits, and excessive aggression or docility. Other findings with cerebral diseases include normal gait, circling towards the side of the lesion and contralateral menace deficits, partial facial muscle weakness, reduced facial pain sensation, and abnormal postural reactions. Despite the menace and visual deficits, pupillary light reflexes will be normal unless there is secondary compression of the diencephalon or midbrain. Brain stem involvement is manifest by abnormalities in consciousness, head tilt, loss of balance, ataxia, weakness of limbs (abnormal gait), and multiple cranial nerve deficits, especially pathologic nystagmus. Generally, gait dysfunction and ataxia will be profound and involve all limbs. As the disease progresses, the animal becomes stuporous and finally comatose. Brain stem infections have a poor prognosis because of damage to the cardiorespiratory centers. Cerebellar disorders usually are characterized by ataxia, tremor, and nystagmus. Spinal cord inflammation results in ataxia and weakness of limbs. Paraspinal pain is quite common, with meningeal inflammation around the spinal cord, and generally is associated with a "walking-on-eggshells" gait.

In reality, inflammations tend to involve multiple portions of the CNS. Even when the history suggests primarily a focal CNS disease, a careful neurologic examination will reveal involvement of additional portions of the CNS in most patients. Multifocal involvement should make inflammatory disease the most likely consideration.

DIAGNOSIS

Any dog or cat with progressive signs of multifocal CNS dysfunction or meningeal irritation should be suspected of having encephalitis, meningitis, or both. Hematologic or biochemical abnormalities are rare. Generally, the diagnosis of CNS inflammation primarily relies on results of CSF analysis. Serology has primarily been used for nonbacterial infections.

CSF Evaluation

Results of CSF analysis generally are abnormal with bacterial meningitis. Based on the character of the changes in the CSF, the clinician generally can confirm the presence of an inflammatory process, can determine the nature of the inflammation, can often determine a specific etiology for the inflammation, and in some cases, can monitor the effectiveness of therapy.

False-negative results on CSF evaluation occur for several reasons. First, the direction of bulk movement of CSF tends to be from cranial to caudal. For this reason, CSF collected from the cerebellomedullary cistern could be normal in patients with a spinal cord infection. Second, for cells to be shed into CSF, the inflammation must involve the ventricular system or the subarachnoid space. Deeply seated inflammations may result in a disruption of the BBB with protein leakage but no migration of cells into the CSF. Bacterial diseases are more likely to involve the ventricles and subarachnoid regions, so the chance of a missed diagnosis is lessened. With chronic bacterial meningitis, fewer cells and more mononuclear types are found in the CSF. Predominantly

nonsuppurative cytologic findings should not eliminate bacterial infection as a consideration.

Technique. CSF may be collected at the cerebellomedullary cistern or the lumbar space. Comparing collection at both sites, the lumbar space is more difficult to enter, yields smaller volumes, and has a higher rate of blood contamination. Results of analysis of CSF collected at the cerebellomedullary cistern may not always evaluate abnormalities in the lower spinal cord but usually reflect changes in inflammatory conditions. Therefore, the cerebellomedullary cistern is the preferred site of CSF collection.

The equipment needed for both the collection and the analysis includes: a small (20- or 22-) gauge, 1.5- to 2.5-inch spinal needle, a container for the fluid, and if pressure will be measured, a three-way stopcock and manometer. All patients should be anesthetized and intubated during the collection process. The complications of CSF collection include anesthetic accidents, damage to the CNS with the spinal needle, and brain herniation following anesthesia and CSF removal caused by increased intracranial pressure. Any animal that has a deterioration of consciousness prior to CSF collection or papilledema on fundic examination is at increased risk for herniation. If during the CSF collection the pressure appears to be elevated, the collection process should be stopped, and the patient should be allowed to recover. Hyperventilation with O_2 may help decrease the intracranial pressure sufficiently to avoid problems.[7]

For collection from the **cerebellomedullary cistern,** the animal should have the cranial portion of the dorsal neck and back of the skull clipped from between the pinnae caudally to the second or third cervical vertebra. This should be performed prior to anesthesia to shorten the time under anesthesia and help minimize complications. During the anesthesia, hyperventilation will help to minimize increases in CSF pressure. After induction of anesthesia, the animal should be placed in lateral recumbency, and the clipped area should be prepared as for a sterile procedure. The animal's spine should be parallel to the table; if necessary, use padding to straighten the cervical spine. The head should be held at 90 degrees to the long axis of the body (Fig. 12–2).[7a] Overflexion of the neck may obstruct the patient's

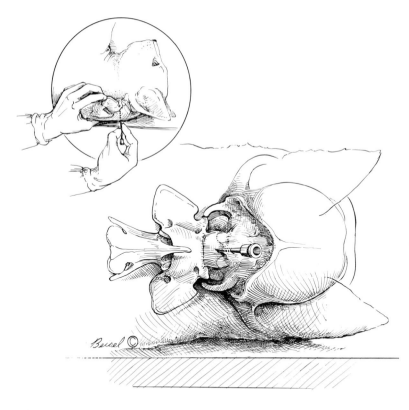

Figure 12–2. One landmark for CSF collection is the intersection of a line drawn transversely between the wings of the atlas on the cranial aspect and a midline drawn through the occipital protuberance. (From Greene CE, Oliver JE: *In*: Ettinger SJ (ed): *Textbook of Internal Medicine: Diseases of the Dog and Cat,* ed 2. WB Saunders Co, 1983, pp 419–460. Reprinted with permission.)

airway as well as occlude the jugular veins. Jugular venous occlusion will artifactually elevate intracranial pressure and increase the potential for brain herniation. The landmarks are the wings of the atlas (C1) and the occipital protuberance. An imaginary T is drawn, using the line between the two wings of the atlas for one bar and the midline of the neck as determined by the occipital protuberance for the other. The point where the two lines cross is the site where the needle is inserted (Fig. 12–2). Prior to advancement of the needle into the CSF space, it is first inserted through the skin that has been pinched up. This will prevent sudden, inadvertent advancement of the needle when the procedure is performed on a tough-skinned animal such as a cat. The bevel of the needle should be facing cranially, toward the occipital protuberance. The needle is then advanced slowly through the muscle layers on a line approximately perpendicular to the long axis of the spine. When the needle advances through the subarachnoid space, there will be a sudden loss of resistance. Rarely, if ever, is muscle twitching noted when the dura is penetrated at this site. As soon as the change in resistance is felt, the stylet is removed to look for CSF. To prevent accidental advancement, the needle should be held with thumb and forefinger each time the stylet is removed. If no CSF appears after a few seconds, the stylet should be replaced and the needle advanced further. If the location feels correct and there is still no CSF flow, the jugular veins should be occluded to increase the flow of CSF. If there is still no flow, there is a possibility that the animal has suffered a brain herniation that is blocking the flow of CSF.

If the needle hits bone, the tip should be moved cranially then caudally a few millimeters. If that does not work, the needle should be removed and the entire collection process started over. The average distance between skin and subarachnoid space will vary with the size of the patient. Distances are 0.5 inch for cats or for dogs <4.5 kg; 0.75 inch for dogs 4.5 to 9.1 kg; 1 inch for dogs 9.1 to 22.7 kg; 1.5 inches for dogs 22.7 to 50.9 kg; and 2 inches for dogs >50.9 kg.[8] When fluid begins to flow, it is best to collect the fluid by allowing it to drip into a container or each drop may be aspirated into a syringe. If the fluid is going to be stored for any length of time, it should be stored in a plastic container to prevent WBC adherence to the glass.

The **lumbar subarachnoid space** is the preferred site to collect CSF in the presence of spinal cord diseases or if it is impossible to collect it from the cerebellomedullary cistern. The collection sites will be the L7 to S1 interspace in the cat and the L6 to L7 interspace in the dog. Prior to anesthesia, the areas on the back between the last rib and the tuber coxae should be clipped for a distance of 2 to 3 inches on each side of the midline. After anesthesia is induced, the animal is placed in lateral recumbency, and the spine is flexed. The forelimbs are drawn back, between the pelvic limbs. The spine should be parallel to the table, using padding if needed to assure a straight line. A 20- or 22-gauge needle is adequate, but for this procedure, it generally should be 2.5 to 3 inches long. The dorsal spinal process of the vertebra should be used for a landmark. The bevel of the needle should be facing cranially, and the needle should be placed just cranial to the dorsal spinous process of the posterior vertebra along a line perpendicular to the long axis of the spine. The needle should be advanced until bony resistance is felt and then moved cranially or caudally a few millimeters to find the interspace. When the needle passes through the interarcuate ligament, there will be a sudden loss of resistance. As the needle penetrates the dura, there usually is a sudden twitching of the pelvic limbs. The stylet of the needle should be removed and observed for CSF to appear. Because the pressures at the lumbar space are often quite low and the needle longer (2.5 inches), the wait is longer than the 4 to 5 seconds needed for the cerebellomedullary collection. If no fluid appears, the stylet should be replaced and the needle advanced until it contacts the bony floor of the spinal canal. The needle should be slightly withdrawn; then, after the stylet is removed, again observe for fluid. Penetration of the spinal cord is not preferred as it may produce cord injury and artifactual hemorrhage in the CSF sample. If pressures are adequate, CSF should be collected by letting it drip into a plastic container. If the pressure is low, the needle is too long, or the gauge of the needle is too small, the flow of fluid will often be insufficient for spontaneous collection. In those cases, a syringe should be used to aspirate the fluid, which will increase the potential for blood contamination. Although CSF pressures can be measured,[9] they are not as helpful as cytologic assessment in the evaluation of CNS infection.

Complications. Blood contamination, the most common problem with accurate CSF evaluation, is generally the result of penetration of meningeal vessels. If the fluid appears bloody at the beginning of the collection process, the stylet should be replaced with the needle left in place. After waiting 30 to 60 seconds, the stylet may be removed with clearing of the fluid. If there are still small traces of blood, the CSF should be collected in at least two portions, with the sample in separate containers. Often, the contamination will diminish during the collection, leaving a second sample that is adequate for interpretation.

The most serious complication of CSF collection is brain herniation. In the face of elevated intracranial pressure, the pressure shift created by the removal of CSF may precipitate a shift in intracranial contents. This sudden movement of intracranial contents (brain herniation) generally results in death of the patient. Brain herniation in dogs and cats has occurred in association with CSF collection or anesthesia.[6] Progressive sensory and motor paralysis, pupillary size, and reflex abnormalities signal brain herniation is occurring.

Analysis. The analysis of the CSF should include a gross visual examination, cytologic analysis, biochemical analysis, and where indicated by cytology, cultural or serologic evaluation. Under most circumstances, fluid from the cerebellomedullary cistern tends to have slightly more cells and lower protein than the fluid from the lumbar space.[10]

Normal CSF should be clear and colorless on gross examination. CSF generally becomes turbid and assumes an offwhite to grayish color from an increase in the number of WBC and protein in the presence of inflammation. If there is evidence of turbidity, it usually indicates an elevation of the cell count above 500/μl. Centrifugation should always be performed before color is evaluated since pink coloration occurs from blood contamination. Persistent pink color after centrifugation indicates free hemoglobin and suggests previous subarachnoid hemorrhage rather than contamination during fluid collection. Fluid that is yellow-orange (xanthochromic) in color generally indicates previous hemorrhage or marked elevations of CSF protein (>100 mg/dl). Xanthochromia may occasionally be seen in some cases of protracted icterus. In some cases, with pigment-producing bacteria such as *Pseudomonas*, the CSF may actually acquire a greenish tint.

The cytologic evaluation should consist of a total cell count on unconcentrated fluid and preparation of a slide from a concentrated fluid sample for evaluation of cell types and differential numbers. The total cell count should be performed as soon as possible, as the cells from CSF begin to undergo degeneration rapidly.[11] After a 2-hour delay, greater than 90% of RBC survive, but fewer than 60% of the WBC survive, greatly altering the interpretation of findings. Refrigeration slows the lysis of WBC, if analysis cannot be done immediately. An aliquot of freshly collected CSF can be mixed with an equal volume of 90% ethanol to help preserve cell morphology for longer periods. For the most accurate interpretation of the differential cell count, some form of cell concentrating technique should be used. In the cytocentrifugation procedure, the CSF is spun at 1500 × g for 10 minutes in a conventional centrifuge[8] or 100 × g for 10 minutes in a cytocentrifuge (Cytospin, Shandon Southern Instruments Inc, Sewickley, PA).[12] Then the supernatant is removed, and the remaining cells are resuspended by adding a drop of normal serum or 20% albumin. This provides better adherence of cells to the slide and also prevents drying artifact in the cells. Staining is generally done with a Wright's or Giemsa stain.

In the sedimentation technique, CSF and normal serum are mixed in equal volumes and put in a cylinder placed on the slide, and time is allowed for the cells to sediment. The liquid is pipetted off, the cylinder is removed, and the slide is stained. In a variation of this technique, filter paper can be used to remove fluid. Sedimentation techniques require larger volumes of the CSF although they preserve the architecture of the cells in the CSF better than the centrifugation methods. For the general practitioner, the sedimentation technique is the easiest and quite reliable.

A third, less commonly used membrane filtration technique allows for good preservation of architecture, but generally uses different stains. The cytologist needs to be experienced in reading membrane filtration cytology for the results to be valid.

Normally, there should be less than 5 WBC/μl in the CSF, regardless of collection site. Typically, with inflammations of the CNS, there is an absolute increase in the concentration of WBC. The type and number of cells present in the CSF will reflect the cause of the meningitis and so will provide etiologic information to the clinician, especially in acute, untreated CNS infections. As the disease becomes more chronic and various therapies are tried, CSF analysis may not reflect the cause as accurately as it did in earlier stages. Because there are some infections that do not cause ventriculitis or meningitis, normal cell counts should not exclude the possibility of an infectious process. In contrast, artifactual increases in cell counts can result with blood contamination. The number of WBC in CSF will increase by approximately 1 WBC/μl and protein by 1 mg/dl for each 500 RBC/μl present.[8, 13] A more accurate correction factor can be determined by taking the patient's own hematologic values. The ratio of the concentration of WBC to RBC in the blood is multiplied by the concentration of RBC in the CSF. The expected WBC from contamination is used to determine the significance of the measured WBC in CSF. The adjusted WBC (observed minus expected) or the ratio of the observed to expected WBC in CSF can be determined. Overall, the ratio of observed to expected count is more accurate than the adjusted method in determining bacterial meningitis. In addition, the observed to expected count is more accurate in determining bacterial meningitis than viral or aseptic meningitis. A ratio of 10 or greater is considered predictive of culture-positive bacterial infections.[13a] Correcting for contamination may allow valid conclusions to be drawn in cases with mild contamination, but marked contamination makes most CSF uninterpretable.

A diagnosis of suppurative meningitis may be made if the number of cells, predominantly neutrophils, in the CSF is increased. Suppurative meningitis is the most common pathologic response to bacterial encephalitis, although it also can be seen with fungal infections; acute, severe viral infections; and idiopathic, glucocorticoid-responsive meningitis or vasculitis of young dogs.[14–16] The number of cells and proportion of neutrophils are generally greater with bacterial disease than with other causes. If phagocytized organisms are noted within neutrophils, a presumptive diagnosis of bacterial encephalitis may be made. Free, nonphagocytized organisms in the CSF may be the result of contamination in the stain used in slide preparation.

A mixed inflammatory process, composed of multiple cell types, including macrophages, lymphocytes, neutrophils, and sometimes plasma cells, generally is the result of a granulomatous inflammation, as occurs with fungal, protozoal, and idiopathic diseases. This cytologic change may also be seen in chronic bacterial infections that are being inadequately treated. Nonsuppurative inflammation is typified by increased numbers of mononuclear cells, especially lymphocytes, in the CSF. It is most characteristic of viral and rickettsial infections but may rarely be seen with bacterial infections.[17]

Because there are normally changes in the cytology of CSF during the progression of any illness, the most reliable diagnostic evaluation would consist of serial CSF collections.[18] The need for anesthesia makes this an unlikely occurrence in the diagnosis of CNS disease of the dog and cat. High initial pretreatment WBC counts have been associated with a favorable prognosis, while continued postreatment pleocytosis carries a poorer prognosis.[19]

If organisms are seen, the cytologic preparation should be Gram stained to aid in further identification. With cytologically evident inflammatory changes, the CSF sample should be inoculated into a culture medium. There is a high prevalence of negative cultures seen even with known bacterial encephalitis. A negative culture may simply be the result of too few organisms in the CSF, improper storage or transport of the sample, improper choice of culture technique, or inadequate nutrients in the culture medium to support growth. There also may be a substance present in CSF that actively inhibits the growth of organisms.[20] Anaerobic cultures should be performed if there is evidence of a mass lesion, since that patient may have a bacterial abscess.[2] Cultures of CSF when there is no evidence of inflammation are probably of little value even if they are positive. The cultured organism is probably a contaminant of the CSF.

Where available, countercurrent immunoelectrophoresis (CIE) may be used to identify the bacteria by detection of bacterial antigens and may also be used to glean prognostic information. Patients with the highest quantity of CSF antigen carry the most guarded prognosis. CIE must be performed prior to therapy, as there appears to be no correlation between antigen quantity and prognosis after drug therapy has been initiated.

CSF is produced both by active transport and by ultrafiltration. As a result, although CSF contains essentially the same constituents as plasma, they are present in differing concentrations. Generally, those levels are lower than the serum levels. Two constituents measured most commonly are protein and glucose. In dogs and cats, protein from a cerebellomedullary cisternal tap is generally less than 25 mg/dl, whereas that from a lumbar puncture may be as high as 45 mg/dl.[10] With all types of inflammation, CSF protein is usually increased. These values are still much lower than the 5 to 8 g/dl of protein seen in plasma. Since storage of CSF does not significantly affect protein content, CSF may be sent to an outside laboratory for protein evaluation.

In encephalitis and meningitis, the CSF protein is generally elevated. This elevation may be the result of increased permeability of the BBB, production of immunoglobulins in the intrathecal space, or a combination of both.[21, 22] Ideally, since many conditions other than inflammations will elevate the CSF protein, quantitative and qualitative analyses using electrophoresis or immunoelectrophoresis are desirable.[23, 24] Unfortunately, routine screening tests used in practice (Pandy and Nonne-Apelt tests) and those used by most commercial laboratories do not allow for quantitation of each constituent of the total CSF protein. If globulins are the primary protein present, an inflammatory disease is likely even if the cytologic examination is inconclusive. A mixed elevation of CSF proteins is less supportive of inflammation as the sole cause of the protein elevation. If the principal protein present is albumin, it is suggestive of a noninflammatory injury to the BBB.[21, 22]

Normal CSF glucose is about 60% to 80% of the serum concentration. In people, the ratio between blood glucose and CSF glucose is routinely lowered in bacterial infections. A similar relationship between bacterial encephalitis and decreased CSF glucose has not been established in dogs and cats. In people, elevated lactic acid dehydrogenase activity in CSF has been used as an indicator of the presence of bacterial infections of the CNS. Although there have been false-negatives, there have been no false-positives, even in the face of blood contamination. Similarly, CSF ferritin concentration has been measured to determine bacterial and fungal meningitis.[25] Whether these procedures will work for evaluation of meningitis in dogs and cats is uncertain.

Other Tests. Detection of the presence of specific antibodies or antigens may be helpful in the diagnosis of viral, fungal, and rickettsial diseases but is less helpful in bacterial encephalitis. In most circumstances, the presence of antibodies is an indication of local immunoglobulin production, which suggests that the organism to which the antibodies are directed is the cause of the encephalitis. Yet, false-positive antibody levels can be caused by leakage of plasma proteins into the CSF as a result of fever or collection. Antibodies may also be the result of previous infections. Increased albumin on CSF electrophoresis would support a false-positive diagnosis, as will measuring simultaneous serum antibody titers. The accuracy of CSF serology can be increased by evaluating paired CSF or corresponding serum titers.

Although measurement of bacterial antigen has been uncertain, cryptococcal antigens can be detected in CSF using the latex agglutination procedure (see Diagnosis, Chapter 67). Viral antigen has been detected in CSF cells using immunofluorescent methods.

Other Diagnostics

Since bacterial infections of the CNS often originate from other sites in the body, a careful examination of the patient for other sites of infection should be undertaken. This should include hemograms, urinalysis, and radiographs of the structures adjacent to the suspected site of CNS infection. The culture of other body fluids in addition to CSF may be helpful in certain systemic bacterial infections. In dogs with discospondylitis, the use of blood and urine cultures has often yielded the causative agent without the need for invasive procedures (see Vertebral Osteomyelitis, Chapter 6).[26]

Electroencephalography (EEG) may be helpful in the recognition of CNS inflammations but not in the diagnosis of a causative agent. Although the EEG is often abnormal in patients with encephalitis and

meningitis, the abnormalities are rarely specific. The use of computerized tomography and magnetic resonance imaging has been of great benefit in the diagnosis of mass effects within the CNS. These two tools appear to be the diagnostic tests of choice in cases of suspected brain abscess; however, they are only available at referral centers.

THERAPY

Treatment of CNS infections involves control of the specific causative agent and provision of supportive care for life-threatening complications such as brain edema. There will be some cases in which presumptive therapy, based on Gram stain or intuition, may be instituted prior to cultures. If the organism can be isolated, subsequent treatment should be based upon the susceptibility results and those agents that penetrate better in the CNS.

Antimicrobial Therapy

The ideal treatment is the single least toxic, most effective, bactericidal drug that achieves therapeutic levels in the CNS in the acute and healing phases of the inflammatory process.[27]

The ability to obtain and maintain therapeutic blood levels is of special consideration in treating CNS diseases because the BBB also limits the entry of therapeutic agents into the CNS. As a result, there are often significant discrepancies between serum and CSF concentrations of drugs. Ideal drugs have low albumin binding, a low degree of ionization at physiologic pH, and high lipid solubility.

Drugs should be chosen that will achieve sufficient concentrations in the CNS to inhibit the infecting microorganism throughout the period of therapy (Table 12–2), because with chronicity the BBB will stabilize and CSF concentrations will drop. Concurrent use of glucocorticoids also will stabilize the BBB, causing a decline in the CSF concentrations of antimicrobials.

Since bacterial encephalitis is occurring in an area of impaired host defenses, a bactericidal drug is preferred for treatment.[5] Previous studies have shown that the CSF of rabbits with pneumococcal meningitis becomes sterile during the first 5 days of treat-

Table 12–2. Antimicrobial Drugs Penetrating Blood-Brain and Blood–Cerebrospinal Fluid Barriers

	GOOD PENETRATION	INTERMEDIATE PENETRATION	POOR PENETRATION
Microbicidal Drugs	Trimethoprim Metronidazole	Penicillin Ampicillin Methicillin Oxacillin Carbenicillin	Cephalosporins Aminoglycosides
Microbiostatic Drugs	Chloramphenicol Sulfonamides	Tetracyclines Flucytosine	Amphotericin B Erythromycin

ment with ampicillin or bactericidal doses of chloramphenicol. When chloramphenicol has been used in bacteriostatic doses, the therapy consistently has failed.[29] Higher antibiotic concentrations may be required in CSF for maximum effect than would be expected from the minimum inhibitory concentration (MIC) determined in vitro. This may be due to lowered pH of CSF in meningitis, which reduces activity of certain antimicrobials. The increased protein levels of the CSF in meningitis may increase the protein binding of drugs such as the cephalosporins, lowering the clinically active free fraction of the drug. Another factor may be the overall slower growth of bacteria in CSF than in broth, where the susceptibility testing was performed.

If possible, a drug that is available in parenteral formulation is recommended because IV therapy for the first few days may allow higher concentrations of the drug to be achieved in the CNS and CSF. The drugs recommended for specific bacterial infections are presented in Table 12–3. The recommended dose and routes of antimicrobials administered for treating CNS infections are listed in Table 12–4. Therapy should initially be started with a drug effective against gram-positive organisms, generally one of the penicillins. After Gram stain or culture results, it may be modified.

The Penicillins. The penicillins reach therapeutic concentrations in CSF in the presence of meningeal inflammation, but penetrate noninflamed meninges poorly. In the absence of meningeal inflammation, the CSF concentrations of penicillin are only 1% to 2% those of serum as contrasted with 10% to 18% in the presence of inflammation.[30, 31] Ampicillin appears slightly different in that there appears to be less need for meningeal inflammation in order to reach high concentrations in CSF.[32]

The high activity of these drugs along with their low toxicity keeps them as the mainstay for the treatment of CNS bacterial infections.[33] Ampicillin and penicillin remain the first choice drugs for treatment of meningitis in dogs and cats.[8, 34, 35] Gram-positive infections such as streptococcal infections are generally treated with penicillin. Anaerobic and gram-negative infections may be treated with other members of the penicillin family (see also Penicillins, Chapter 43).

Vancomycin. This drug is effective against staphylococci and streptococci and is more likely to reach therapeutic CSF concentrations in the presence of meningeal inflammation since it has relatively poor penetration of noninflamed meninges. It is used primarily as an alternative therapy after other drugs have failed.

Chloramphenicol. Chloramphenicol reaches high CSF concentration (45% to 99% of

Table 12–3. Recommended Antimicrobials for Specific Agents or Settings[20, 28]

AGENT	FIRST CHOICES (SECOND CHOICES)
Staphylococcus aureus	Methicillin, nafcillin, ampicillin (vancomycin, trimethoprim-sulfonamide, chloramphenicol)
Streptococcus	Penicillin (erythromycin)
Actinomyces	Ampicillin (minocycline)
Gram-negatives	Cefotaxime, moxalactam, quinolones (gentamicin[a, b])
Pseudomonas aeruginosa	Gentamicin[a] plus carbenicillin or ticarcillin (chloramphenicol, gentamicin,[b] piperacillin, quinolones)
Pasteurella	Ampicillin (trimethoprim)
Brucella	Minocycline (gentamicin[a])
Salmonella	Trimethoprim (chloramphenicol)
Enterococcus	Ampicillin (minocycline)
Bacteroides	Penicillin (carbenicillin)

[a]Parenteral
[b]Intrathecal

Table 12–4. Antimicrobial Drug Dosages for CNS Bacterial and Fungal Infections of Dogs and Cats[a]

DRUG	DOSE[b]	ROUTE	INTERVAL (hours)
Penicillin (aqueous)	$10\text{–}22 \times 10^3$ U/kg	IV	4–6
Ampicillin	5–22	IV	6
Carbenicillin	10–30	IV, IM	4–6
Oxacillin (or cloxacillin)	8.8–20	IV, PO	4–8
Trimethoprim-sulfonamide[c]	15–20	IV, PO	8–12
Gentamicin[c]	2	IV, IM	8
Chloramphenicol	10–15	PO	4–6
Cefalexin	20 (10–30)	PO	8
Cephapirin	20–30	IV, IM	8
Amphotericin B[c]	0.15–0.50	IV	48
Flucytosine	50	PO	8
Rifampin	10–20	PO	8–12
Metronidazole	10–15	PO	8
Cefotaxime	6–40	IM, IV	4–6

[a]See Drug Administration for recommended duration of therapy and precautions. See respective chapters for dosages used in treating viral, protozoal, and some fungal infections.

[b]Expressed as mg/kg unless otherwise stated.

[c]Potential for renal toxicity is greatest in cats and young or dehydrated dogs. Closely monitor renal function, and use lowest dosage under these circumstances.

serum concentrations) regardless of whether or not there is meningeal inflammation.[36] This drug also appears to concentrate in the CNS, reaching levels that exceed those in serum; however, large doses are required for bactericidal effects in the CNS.[27] There is a high relapse rate with this drug, suggesting that it is not bactericidal at dosages used in dogs and cats.[8] This drug is used for treating gram-negative infections but is not the first choice. There appears to be no therapeutic difference between its IV and oral administration.

The Cephalosporins. The earliest generations of cephalosporins did not cross the BBB well, even in the face of inflammation. Some of the third generation cephalosporins, such as moxalactam and cefotaxime, do cross both the normal and inflamed meninges.[37] In addition to these, ceftizoxime, ceftazidime, and ceftriaxone have been shown to be effective in the treament of bacterial meningitis in people. This group of drugs will play an increasing role in the treatment of drug-resistant bacterial meningitis, but the cost for the dosage required may preclude their use in cats and small dogs.

Trimethoprim and Sulfonamides. This drug combination is effective against organisms causing human meningitis, such as pneumococci, meningococci, *Listeria monocytogenes, Haemophilus,* some staphylococci, and many gram-negative organisms. These

drugs penetrate both the normal and inflamed meninges at therapeutic levels. This drug combination has not been widely used for treating CNS infections in veterinary practice, although it probably should be used more regularly.

Metronidazole. Metronidazole has the ability to cross both normal and inflamed meninges in therapeutic concentrations. This drug is primarily indicated for the treatment of anaerobic infections. The drug is bactericidal in concentrations achieved in the CSF.

The Aminoglycosides. Aminoglycosides do not readily cross the normal or inflamed BBB. For the aminoglycosides to be consistently bactericidal in CSF, they must be present in levels that are 10 to 20 times the MIC as determined in vitro. In people, aminoglycosides are effective in neonatal meningitis but not in older human patients; the situation in canine and feline meningitis is uncertain. There are some synergistic combinations of antimicrobials with aminoglycosides for treating bacterial infections (see Table 12–3). The inability of the aminoglycosides to cross the BBB and the diminished effectiveness at low pH may limit the expected synergistic effect of such drug combinations. High CSF concentrations are reported with intrathecal administration of aminoglycosides, but this route is not routinely recommended.

Drug Administration

In treatment of CNS infections, the major variable determining efficacy of an appropriate drug is the peak CSF concentration. If the peak concentration is more than 10 times the minimum bactericidal concentration, a cure will be seen in more than 90% of cases. The frequency of administration is less important than achieving periodic high concentrations of the drug in the CSF. Treatment should be continued for a minimum of 10 to 14 days after the patient becomes asymptomatic. If CSF can be collected before ending therapy, normalization of the glucose and a lowering of both the WBC count and the protein concentration is expected.

Supportive Therapy

Supportive therapy is first directed at treating or preventing brain edema. Initially, fluid restriction is used, unless the patient is hypovolemic or has systemic illness. If the animal is being anesthetized for CSF collection, controlled ventilation may alleviate or prevent brain swelling.[27] If not, then osmotic diuretics such as mannitol (1.25 g/ kg) may be given. The use of other forms of diuretics or the limited use of glucocorticoids may be indicated if the animal's condition worsens. The routine use of glucocorticoids is contraindicated since their use may increase mortality. When used, dexamethasone is more effective in relieving the secondary effects of meningitis than is prednisone.[27] Primarily large breed, young (<2 years old) dogs with suppurative meningitis that do not respond to antimicrobial therapy may be suffering from glucocorticoid-responsive meningitis or vasculitis.[14-16] Only when anti-infective therapy fails should long-term (1 to 2 months or more) therapy with immunosuppressive dosages of prednisolone (2 to 4 mg/kg/day) be instituted.

Hyperthermia from tremors or seizures should be treated with cool water baths, ice packs, or topical application of alcohol. If the patient develops seizures, they should be treated with anticonvulsants. Recumbent animals should be kept on a waterbed, if available. Frequent turning to prevent decubital ulcers and passive pulmonary congestion is essential. If the patient has an altered mental status, the bladder may need to be expressed, and if necessary, suppositories should be used to prevent constipation. Management of systemic infections is covered in Endotoxemia, Chapter 44, and Cardiovascular Infections, Chapter 7.

PROGNOSIS

Prognosis in CNS infections is determined by a number of factors. The most important are the abilities to identify the causative agent and to select an effective antimicrobial that will enter the CNS. The speed with which specific therapy is instituted will play a large role in determining the prognosis. Regardless of etiology, many of the inflammatory diseases of the CNS are expensive to treat, and relapses may occur when treatment is discontinued. Even in those cases where the infection is successfully treated, the potential for residual neurologic deficits may be discouraging to the client.

References

1. Johnson RT: *Viral Infections of the Nervous System.* New York, Raven Press, 1982.
2. Dow SW, LeCouteur RA, Henik RA, et al: Central nervous system infection associated with anaerobic bacteria in two dogs and two cats. *J Vet Intern Med* 2:171–176, 1988.
3. Meric JM: Canine meningitis: a changing emphasis. *J Vet Intern Med* 2:26–35, 1988.
4. Bruyette DS, Tomlinson JL: Canine cerebral abscess: a case report and discussion. *Vet Med/Small Anim Clin* 78:1706–1711, 1983.
5. Tauber MG, Brooks-Fourneier RA, Sande MA: Experimental models of CNS infections. Contributions to concepts of disease and treatment. *Neurol Clin* 4:249–264, 1986.
5a. Fishman RA: *Cerebrospinal Fluid in Diseases of the Nervous System.* Philadelphia, WB Saunders Co, 1980, p 44.
6. Kornegay JN, Oliver JE, Gorgacz EJ: Clinicopathologic feature of brain herniation in animals. *J Am Vet Med Assoc* 182:1111–1116, 1983.
7. Shores A: Neuroanesthesia: a review of the effects of anesthetic agents on cerebral blood flow and intracranial pressure in the dog. *Vet Surg* 14:257–263, 1985.
7a. Greene CE, Oliver JE: Neurologic examination. In Ettinger SJ (ed): *Textbook of Veterinary Internal Medicine: Diseases of the Dog and Cat,* ed 2. Philadelphia, WB Saunders Co, 1983, pp 419–460.
8. Greene CE: Infections of the central nervous system. In Greene CE (ed): *Clinical Microbiology and Infectious Diseases of the Dog and Cat.* Philadelphia, WB Saunders Co, 1984, pp 284–300.
9. Simpson ST, Reed RB: Manometric values for normal cerebrospinal fluid pressure in dogs. *J Am Anim Hosp Assoc* 23:629–632, 1987
10. Bailey CS, Higgins RJ: Comparison of total white

blood cell count and total protein content of lumbar and cisternal cerebrospinal fluid of healthy dogs. *Am J Vet Res* 46:1162–1165, 1985.

11. Chow G, Schmidley JW: Lysis of erythrocytes and leukocytes in traumatic lumbar punctures. *Arch Neurol* 41:1084–1085, 1984.

12. Cristopher MM, Perman V, Hardy RM: Reassessment of cytologic values in canine cerebrospinal fluid by use of cytocentrifugation. *J Am Vet Med Assoc* 192:1726–1729, 1988.

13. Shores A, Coleman ES: Cerebrospinal fluid collection and analysis: indications and techniques. *Texas Vet Med J* 48:27–30, 1986.

13a. Mayefski JH, Roghmann KJ: Determination of leukocytosis in traumatic spinal tap specimens. *Am J Med* 82:1175–1181, 1987.

14. Russo EA, Lees GE, Hall CL: Corticosteroid-responsive aseptic suppurative meningitis in three dogs. *Southwest Vet* 35:197–201, 1983.

15. Meric SM, Perman V, Hardy RM: Corticosteroid-responsive meningitis in ten dogs. *J Am Anim Hosp Assoc* 21:677–684, 1985.

16. Meric SM: Canine meningitis: a changing emphasis. *J Vet Intern Med* 2:26–35, 1988.

17. Powers WJ: Cerebrospinal fluid lymphocytosis in acute bacterial meningitis. *Am J Med* 79:216–220, 1985.

18. Feigin RD, Shackelford PG: Value of repeat lumbar puncture in the differential diagnosis of meningitis. *N Engl J Med* 289:571–574, 1973.

19. Giampaolo C, Scheld M, Boyd J, et al: Leukocyte and bacterial interrelationships in experimental meningitis. *Ann Neurol* 9:328–333, 1981.

20. Agbayani MM, Braun J, Chang CT, et al: Effect of CSF on bacterial growth. *Arch Neurol* 38:43–45, 1981.

21. Bichsel P, Vandevelde M, Vandevelde E, et al: Immunoelectrophoretic determination of albumin and IgG in serum and cerebrospinal fluid in dogs with neurologic disease. *Res Vet Sci* 1:101–107, 1984.

22. Sorjonen DC: Total protein, albumin quota, and electrophoretic patterns in cerebrospinal fluid of dogs with central nervous system disorders. *Am J Vet Res* 48:301–305, 1987.

23. Krakowka S, Fenner W, Miele JA: Quantitative determination of serum origin cerebrospinal fluid protein in the dog. *Am J Vet Res* 42:1975–1977, 1981.

24. Sorjonen DC, Warren JW, Schultz RD: Quantitative and qualitative determination of albumin, IgG, IgM and IgA in normal cerebrospinal fluid of dogs. *J Am Anim Hosp Assoc* 17:833–839, 1981.

25. Campbell DR, Skikne BS, Cook JD: Cerebrospinal fluid ferritin levels in screening for meningism. *Arch Neurol* 43:1257–1260, 1986.

26. Kornegay JN, Barber DL: Diskospondylitis in dogs. *J Am Vet Med Assoc* 177:337–341, 1980.

27. Overturf GD: Pyogenic bacterial infections of the CNS. *Neurol Clin* 4:69–90, 1986.

28. Greenlee JE: Bacterial meningitis. *In* Johnson RT (ed): *Current Therapy in Neurologic Disease.* Philadelphia, WB Saunders Co, 1985, pp 123–128.

29. Scheld WM, Sande MA: Bactericidal versus bacteriostatic therapy of experimental pneumococcal meningitis in rabbits. *J Clin Invest* 71:411–419, 1983.

30. Ruedy J: The concentration of penicillins in the cerebrospinal fluid and brain in rabbits with experimental meningitis. *Can J Physiol Pharmacol* 43:763–772, 1965.

31. Hieber JP, Nelson JD: A pharmacologic evaluation of penicillin in children with purulent meningitis. *N Engl J Med* 297:410–413, 1977.

32. Kaplan JM, McCracken GH Jr, Horton LJ, et al: Pharmacologic studies in neonates given large doses of ampicillin. *J Pediatr* 84:571–577, 1974.

33. Whitby M, Finch R: Bacterial meningitis. Rational selection and use of antibacterial drugs. *Drugs* 31:266–278, 1986.

34. Greene CE: Meningitis. *In* Kirk RW (ed): *Current Veterinary Therapy VIII.* Philadelphia, WB Saunders Co, 1983, pp 735–738.

35. Kornegay JN, Lorenz MD, Zenoble RD: Bacterial meningoencephalitis in two dogs. *J Am Vet Med Assoc* 177:1334–1336, 1978.

36. Friedman CA, Lovejoy FC, Smith AL: Chloramphenicol disposition in infants and children. *J Pediatr* 95:1071–1077, 1979.

37. Bell WE: Treatment of bacterial infections of the nervous system. *Ann Neurol* 9:313–327, 1981.

13 OCULAR INFECTIONS
Charles L. Martin

LOCAL BACTERIAL INFECTIONS

Normal Flora

Despite the fact that all dogs have indigenous conjunctival bacteria in their conjunctival cul-de-sac, positive isolation rates between 46% and 91% of clinically healthy dogs have been reported (Table 13–1). Variables in the type of isolate and the frequency may be due to geography, culturing technique, breed, and season.

In contrast to the dog, the cat has relatively lower isolation rates of cultivable bacteria from its conjunctival flora.[4] In one study, cultures revealed bacteria or *Mycoplasma* from 34% of the conjunctival samples and from 25% of the samples from the lid margins (Table 13–2).

Ocular Surface Infections

Most surface bacterial infections are not strictly primary; other debilitating conditions often potentiate the pathogenicity of organisms that are indigenous to the ocular surface. Correction of underlying factors such as eyelid conformation, reduced tear secretions, UV radiation, ocular irritation, or trauma is important because sterilization of the ocular surface with antibiotics generally is incomplete and relapses may occur. To become established, corneal infections usually require a break in the epithelial surface. Local niduses of infection, such as in the lacrimal sac and meibomian glands or adjacent structures to the eye (ears, lip folds), should be sought and corrected to overcome persistent or recurring infection.

Bacterial conjunctivitis and, to a lesser extent, keratitis are common syndromes in the dog, and the isolated agents are usually similar to the indigenous flora. Isolates in decreasing order of prevalence have included coagulase-positive *Staphylococcus aureus (intermedius)*, α- or β-hemolytic streptococci, *S. epidermidis*, and *Escherichia coli* or *Proteus mirabilis*.[6, 6a] Bacterial keratitis or conjunctivitis should be considered in any animal with a strong leukotactic response. This is recognized as a dense creamy-white infiltrate at a nidus or around the periphery of an ulcer. Bacteria, such as *Pseudomonas aeruginosa*, that have proteolytic enzymes typically produce rapidly progressive corneal ulcers.

The decision to perform bacterial cultures from the ocular surface should be made **before** topical anesthetics are applied to the eye, as they have bactericidal properties. The use of a moist or calcium alginate swab improves the recovery rate.[2, 3] The swab is rolled over the involved ocular surface, taking care to avoid the eyelashes and eyelids.

Table 13–1. Frequency of Isolation of Bacteria from the Conjunctival Sacs of Clinically Normal Dogs[1–3]

ORGANISM	ISOLATION (%)
Staphylococcus (total)	57–70
Coagulase-positive	24–45
Coagulase-negative	46–55
Streptococcus (total)	6–43
Nonhemolytic	12–51
α-Hemolytic	4–34
β-Hemolytic	2–7
Corynebacterium (total)	30–75
Undifferentiated	11
C. pseudodiphtheriticum	9
C. xerosis	13
Neisseria (total)	26
Undifferentiated	4
N. catarrhalis	9
N. pharyngitidis	4
N. sicca	3
N. caviae	3
N. lactamicus	3
N. flavescens	3
Pseudomonas	14
Moraxella	7
Bacillus	6–18

Since the volume of material collected is usually small and subject to drying, swabs should be inoculated quickly onto appropriate media or placed in transport media.

Cytologic examination of conjunctival and corneal scrapings is an important diagnostic aid, particularly in cats with infectious conjunctivitis.[7] A topical anesthetic is applied, and the appropriate surface is scraped with a small flat spatula (Fig. 13–1). Excessive ocular discharges should be removed prior to scraping. Only a small amount of material is collected, and it is tapped directly onto the slides and air dried. Multiple slides should be prepared, as some slides may not have adequate numbers of cells. The slides are stained with a modified Giemsa method for cytologic evaluation and a Gram stain to evaluate the presence of bacteria. An alternate technique is to roll a cotton-tipped applicator over the appropriate surface and then roll it onto a slide. Suitable preparations can be made with this method, but fewer cells are usually obtained.

Intraocular Infections

Intraocular bacterial infections may be exogenous or endogenous in origin. Endogenous infections are discussed further under Systemic Ocular Infections. The source of an exogenous infection from a penetrating ocular injury may be obvious from the history and appearance of the eye or occult, such as a self-sealing cat claw injury through the conjunctiva and sclera. Exogenously induced infections are usually unilateral, whereas endogenous infections are often bilateral.

All recent perforating ocular injuries should be considered septic and treated intensively with bactericidal broad-spectrum antibiotics until susceptibility data is obtained. A surprising number of perforating missiles (BBs, pellets) and cat claw injuries do not result in infection, but since the consequence of ocular infection is so devastating, it is preferable to err by overtreating.

Most active intraocular inflammations associated with perforating injuries should have centesis performed. Anterior chamber centesis for cultures and cytology is safe, easy, and may yield specific information to guide future therapy. Aqueous centesis is not as reliable as vitreous centesis in demonstrating bacterial growth in endophthalmitis; consequently, negative culture results from an aqueous sample are not definitive evidence of sterile inflammation.[8] Sepsis is indicated on oculocentesis by finding degenerate neutrophils and bacteria. Nondegenerate neutrophils may indicate a sterile purulent inflammation such as phacoanaphylaxis (lens-induced inflammation) caused by an ocular injury.

Aqueous Centesis. This procedure is performed under heavy sedation or general anesthesia. A 25- to 27-gauge needle on a tuberculin syringe is used with the "seal" broken so movement of the plunger does not require a jerky effort. The site of centesis is usually in the dorsal or lateral limbus because it is the most accessible. A pair of forceps applied to the conjunctiva close to the limbus will fixate the globe and apply counterpressure to the pushing force of the needle. The needle enters the cornea just rostral to the limbus and parallel to the plane of the iris, the operator being careful to avoid the iris, lens, and corneal endothelium (Fig. 13–2). The diseased cornea may make the procedure more hazardous because the needle point is obscured, and the increased

Table 13–2. Bacterial Isolates from 120 Normal Cats[5]

LOCATION	ORGANISM	PERCENTAGE
Conjunctivae	Staphylococcus albus	16.3
	S. aureus	10.4
	Mycoplasma	5.0
	Bacillus spp.	2.9
	α-Hemolytic Streptococcus	2.5
	Corynebacterium	1.3
Lids	S. albus	13.8
	S. aureus	8.8
	α-Hemolytic Streptococcus	1.7
	Bacillus spp.	1.7
	Escherichia coli	0.4

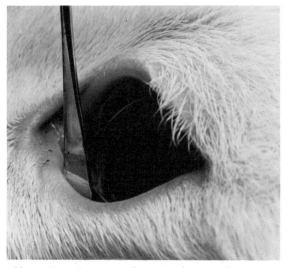

Figure 13–1. Conjunctival scraping being performed on a cat under topical anesthesia with a Kimura spatula.

corneal thickness results in a longer, beveled tract before the needle enters the anterior chamber. The volume that can be removed without excessively collapsing the anterior chamber in the dog is about 0.3 ml and in the cat about 0.5 ml. A culture swab is saturated with a portion of the aspirated aqueous, and the remaining aliquot is prepared for cytology by centrifugation or passed through a fine filter (Millipore Co, Bedford, MA). An antibiotic is frequently injected after aspiration of the aqueous.

Vitreous Centesis. Centesis of the vitreous cavity has more potential complications than aqueous centesis and is usually re-

served for eyes that have lost considerable visual function. Vitreous hemorrhage and retinal hole formation are the two most common complications. A 25-gauge needle with a 3 ml syringe for added suction is utilized. The site of entry is 6 mm caudal to the limbus in the dorsal-lateral quadrant. Forceps are used to apply counterpressure, and the needle point is aimed for the center of the globe (Fig. 13–3). The needle should be short (0.5 inch) so that it is not inadvertently passed completely across the vitreous to tear the opposite retina. If fluid cannot be obtained, minor positioning changes of the needle point are attempted and, if unsuccessful, the procedure is repeated with a 22-gauge needle. The syringe is removed while the needle is kept in place and the aspirated fluid is placed on a culture swab, and the remainder is concentrated by centrifugation for cytology. A bactericidal antibiotic is injected at the appropriate dose if a bacterial endophthalmitis is suspected.

Therapy

The therapeutic routes available for treating ocular infections are topical, subconjunctival, intraocular, retrobulbar, and systemic. The route(s) selected will depend on the location, severity of the infection, and the drug being utilized.

The eye has three rather formidable barriers to drug penetration: the intact cornea

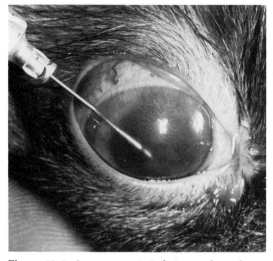

Figure 13–2. Aqueous centesis being performed on a cat with feline leukemia–associated anterior uveitis.

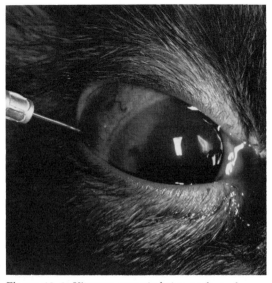

Figure 13–3. Vitreous centesis being performed on a cat. The needle enters 6 mm posterior to the limbus.

for topical penetration and the blood-aqueous and blood-retinal barriers for systemic drug penetration. In general, drugs with a differential solubility in water and lipids and of small molecular size are better able to penetrate these barriers. Inflammation or ulceration will negate these barriers to a variable degree and allow better penetration. Table 13–3 summarizes the ability of a variety of antibacterials to penetrate into the normal eye.[9] The vitreous is a large rather inert structure; this results in low drug levels by any route of drug administration except direct intravitreal injection, in which the vitreous acts as a depot for the relatively slow release of the drug.

Topical Administration. Depending on the drug and whether the cornea is intact, topical therapy may provide adequate drug levels only on the surface or as deep as the iris and ciliary body. Other variables influencing drug concentrations via topical administration are the frequency of application and drug contact time. In general, ointments have a longer contact time than solutions, but some drugs (dexamethasone) bind to the ointments, resulting in decreased drug availability.

When drops are used, about 20 μl of a preparation is adequate. Multiple or rapidly repeated instillations of the same or different preparations simply increase the rate of loss via the nasolacrimal duct or mutually dilute each preparation, thereby reducing the availability of each drug.

Treatment of routine surface infections of the conjunctiva or prophylactic antibacterial therapy of corneal ulcers should utilize topical broad-spectrum antibiotics, such as neomycin-polymyxin-bacitracin, that are not used systemically. This rationale is based on minimizing bacterial resistance to antibiotics that are beneficial in systemic therapy and avoiding sensitization of a patient by topical usage of an antibiotic that might have potential in systemic therapy. In practice, routine bacterial conjunctivitis is not initially cultured owing to the cost and the ambiguous results.

Subconjunctival Administration. Subconjunctival administration is used primarily for anterior segment disease and can achieve therapeutic intraocular levels of water-soluble antibiotics that normally do not penetrate into the eye. The major limitations of subconjunctival injections are drug irritation and ocular manipulation. The means by which a subconjunctivally injected drug reaches the interior of the eye are controversial, but both direct diffusion through the sclera, which has no epithelial barrier, and vascular uptake and leakage through the needle hole with topical absorption have been demonstrated. Except for long-acting drugs, most others must be readministered at 12- to 24-hour intervals to maintain therapeutic levels. Whereas significant posterior segment levels of drugs can be achieved when injecting near the equator of the globe,

Table 13–3. Intraocular Penetration of Antibacterial Agents in the Noninflamed Eye[a]

AGENT	PENETRATION BY ROUTE		
	Systemic	Topical	Subconjunctival
Penicillin	Poor	Poor	Good
Ampicillin	Poor	Poor	Good
Methicillin	Good (with multiple doses)	—	Good
Erythromycin	Poor	Good	Good
Cephalosporins	Poor	Poor	Good
Colistin	Poor	Poor	Good
Gentamicin	Poor	Poor	Good
Tobramycin	Poor	—	Good
Lincomycin	Good	—	—
Neomycin	—	Poor	—
Chloramphenicol	Poor to fair	Good (ointment)	Good
Tetracycline	Poor	Good (ointment)	—
Bacitracin	—	Poor	Poor
Polymyxin B	—	Poor	Poor
Trimethoprim-sulfadiazine	Good	—	—
Sulfonamides (in general)	Good	Good	Good

(Data abstracted from Havener W: *Ocular Pharmacology*, ed 3. CV Mosby Co, 1974.)

[a]Most of the data are derived from the rabbit, and significant species variations in penetration have been demonstrated.

the subconjunctival route is not adequate for bacterial infections of the vitreous or optic nerve. Table 13–4 gives the subconjunctival dosages for various antibiotics.

Intraocular Administration. Intracameral or intraocular injection of antibiotics is a heroic and extremely effective means of achieving high levels of antibiotics. To preserve vision, the decision to utilize the intracameral route must be made early to avoid rapidly devastating inflammation to delicate intraocular structures. As cultures and susceptibility are not initially available, a broad-spectrum bactericidal antibiotic is usually administered. The intraocular injection in itself has an inherent risk; but in addition, the drug concentration is critical owing to toxicity to the retina, lens, and corneal endothelium. Historically, gentamicin (350 to 500 μg), cephaloridine (250 μg), and cephalothin (2 mg), either alone or in combination, have been the drugs recommended for intraocular administration.[11] Intravitreal injection of cephalothin and gentamicin produce therapeutic levels for 32 and 96 hours, respectively. However, the combination of gentamicin and cephalosporins in the vitreous may be of questionable value, as aminoglycosides are inactivated when incubated in vitro with β-lactam antibiotics. With the emergence of gentamicin-resistant organisms, use of other aminoglycosides has been advocated. Amikacin is inactivated by β-lactam antibiotics

to a lesser degree than gentamicin and tobramycin. The retinal toxicity of aminoglycosides in decreasing order is gentamicin, netilmicin, tobramycin, amikacin, and kanamycin. The relative lack of resistant organisms combined with decreased toxicity has resulted in amikacin (400 μg) being advocated over gentamicin for intraocular injection;[12, 13] however, amikacin has a 20% to 50% higher incidence of falsely resistant organisms than gentamicin and tobramycin when tested by the Kirby-Bauer disks.[12, 13]

Systemic and topical antibiotics are often used concurrently with intraocularly administered antibiotics, although it is doubtful that they add to the therapeutic effectiveness. Intraocular injections of dexamethasone in conjunction with antibiotics have been recommended to minimize the inflammation and ocular tissue disruption,[11] although this practice is controversial.

Adjunctive Therapy. In addition to specific antimicrobial therapy, standard nursing care involves cleansing of the ocular surface and lids with warm, moist swabs or by hot packing, if lid and orbital swelling is evident, to remove accumulated discharges. Antiprostaglandin preparations such as flunixin, phenylbutazone, or aspirin provide analgesia and lessen the inflammatory reaction. Topical atropine minimizes ocular pain due to ciliary muscle spasm and pupillary adhesions and is usually standard therapy with intraocular inflammation.

Table 13–4. Concentrations and Dosages of Locally Used Ocular Antibacterial Agents[a]

	TOPICAL	SUBCONJUNCTIVAL	INTRAVITREAL
Ampicillin	. . . . .	50–250 mg	500 ug
Bacitracin	10,000 units/ml	10,000 units	. . . . .
Carbenicillin	4 mg/ml	100 mg	250 ug–2 mg
Cefazolin	50 mg/ml	100 mg	2.25 mg
Cephalothin	50 mg/ml	50–100 mg	. . . . .
Chloramphenicol	5 mg/ml	1–2 mg	2 mg
Clindamycin	. . . . .	15–40 mg	1 mg
Colistin	5–10 mg/ml	15–37.5 mg	. . . . .
Erythromycin	50 mg/ml	100 mg	500 ug
Gentamicin	8–15 mg/ml	10–20 mg	100–400 ug
Lincomycin	. . . . .	150 mg	1.5 mg
Methicillin	. . . . .	20–100 mg	2 mg
Neomycin	5–8 mg/ml	250–500 mg	. . . . .
Penicillin G	100,000 units/ml	0.5–1 million units	. . . . .
Polymyxin B	16,250 units/ml	10 mg	. . . . .
Streptomycin	. . . . .	50–100 mg	. . . . .
Sulfacetamide	100–300 mg/ml	. . . . .	. . . . .
Tobramycin	3 mg/ml	. . . . .	0.2–0.4 mg
Vancomycin	50 mg/ml	25 mg	1 mg

[a]Adapted from Copyright © *Physician's Desk Reference for Ophthalmology* 1989 Edition. Published by Medical Economics Co, Inc, Oradell, NJ 07649. With permission.
For dosage recommendations for systemic administration, see Appendix 14.

SYSTEMIC INFECTIONS

In addition to local ocular infections, the eye frequently is affected by systemic infectious agents. It is not unusual for the presenting complaint to be an ocular lesion, whereas systemic manifestations remain occult. It is important to recognize the systemic involvement to give an accurate prognosis and adequate therapy. Conversely, ocular lesions may provide rapid diagnostic clues in an animal with an undiagnosed systemic infection. Table 13–5 summarizes the involvement of infectious agents with the eye and adnexa.

Canine Distemper

Catarrhal signs of distemper are usually associated with a bilateral conjunctivitis that progresses from serous to mucopurulent in nature. The palpebral conjunctiva is primarily involved, and lacrimal adenitis or dehydration may result in a marked reduction in tear production (sicca), which in turn results in more profound signs of blepharospasm and corneal ulceration. Sicca usually resolves if the animal recovers from systemic infection. Occasionally, conjunctival or lacrimal involvement occurs with such mild systemic signs that distemper is not suspected.

Distemper often produces a multifocal, nongranulomatous chorioretinitis that does not usually cause blindness. The incidence of chorioretinitis is unknown but probably varies, as do the neurologic signs, with strain of virus and immunocompetency of the host. Occasionally, chorioretinitis is diffuse and blinding and may mimic the genetic syndrome of progressive retinal atrophy. Acute focal lesions in the tapetum have hazy or ill-defined borders with mild to moderate disruption of the mosaic texture and color changes. Acute lesions in the nontapetum have hazy borders and are white in color (Fig. 13–4).[14] Chorioretinal scars due to distemper have sharply demarcated borders, are hyperreflective in the tapetum and depigmented in the nontapetum (Fig. 13–5). Histologically, retinal changes are characterized by degeneration of the retina with perivascular cuffing in some instances. Lesions may be focal or diffuse degeneration of ganglion cells, proliferation of retinal pigment epithelium, atrophy of photoreceptors, disorganization of retinal layers, focal gliosis, and distemper inclusion bodies in glial cells.

The most dramatic clinical ocular problem associated with distemper is optic neuritis.[15] This syndrome is characterized by an acute onset of bilateral blindness and mydriasis. If inflammation extends rostrally to the optic papilla, ophthalmoscopic signs of peripapillary hemorrhages and edema, retinal vascular congestion and elevation of the papilla are observed.[15] If the neuritis remains retrobulbar, the diagnosis is made by exclusion, i.e., blind eyes with dilated pupils and normal retinal function as tested by electroretinography. The optic neuritis syndrome may be isolated, prodromal, or concurrent to other neurologic distemper signs. Distemper-associated blindness also may occur with inflammation of the occipital cortex or optic radiations, but pupillary reflexes are usually normal under such circumstances.

Ocular signs are suggestive but not definitive for distemper. Acute lesions of chorioretinitis usually correlate well with concurrent systemic disease, but chorioretinal *scars* do not. Finding distemper inclusions (Fig. 13–6) or positive immunofluorescence on conjunctival scraping may be of diagnostic help early in the course of systemic disease (5 to 21 days postinoculation), but a negative finding is inconclusive. Distemper should be considered in any acute optic neuropathy or acute onset of keratoconjunctivitis sicca.

Since no specific antiviral therapy is available, treatment is mainly symptomatic. Acute optic neuritis syndromes are treated with systemic anti-inflammatory dosages of glucocorticoids if other distemper signs are absent (see also Chapter 16).

Infectious Canine Hepatitis

Canine adenovirus-1 (CAV-1) has been estimated to produce ocular lesions in approximately 20% of dogs recovering from natural infections, whereas a 0.4% or less prevalence has been noted in CAV-1–vaccinated dogs. The lesion, considered to be an immune-complex Arthus reaction, occurs 10 to 21 days after vaccination and requires about an equal time to resolve. The condition is bilateral in 12% to 28% of the cases. The Afghan hound has been reported to have an increased prevalence,[16] and other sight hounds and the Siberian husky may share a simi-

Table 13–5. Possible Ocular Tissue Involvement with Systemic Infectious Diseases

INFECTIOUS AGENT	CONJUNC-TIVA[a]	LACRIMAL SYSTEM[b]	CORNEA[c]	ANTERIOR CHAMBER[d]	ANTERIOR UVEA[e]	LENS[f]	VITRE-OUS[g]	RETINA/CHOROID[h]	OPTIC NERVE[i]
Viruses									
Canine distemper virus	C	M	—	—	—	—	—	M	N
Infectious canine hepatitis virus	—	—	I, E	G	U	—	—	—	—
Canine herpesvirus (neonate)	—	—	K	—	U	C	—	C, R	N
(adult)	C, S	—	—	—	U (rare)	—	—	—	N (rare)
Feline herpesvirus	C, S	E	U, N, S	—	—	—	—	—	—
Feline panleukopenia virus	—	—	—	—	—	—	—	D, A	H
Feline leukemia virus	—	—	I	T, G, H, F	U, P	C	—	I, H, V, X	—
Feline infectious peritonitis virus	—	—	—	G, F	U	C	—	X, C	N
Rabies virus	E	—	—	—	A	—	—	C	—
Rickettsiae									
Chlamydia psittaci	C	—	—	—	—	—	—	—	—
Ehrlichia canis	H	—	—	H	U	—	B	E, P, X	—
Rickettsia rickettsii	C, H	—	I	—	U	—	—	H, L	—
Haemobartonella felis & H. canis	—	—	—	—	—	—	—	P, H	—
Bacteria									
Leptospira	C, H, I	—	I	—	U	C	H	—	—
Brucella canis	—	—	—	—	U	—	—	C	—
Clostridium tetani	E	—	I	—	—	—	—	C, X	—
Mycobacterium bovis	—	—	I	S	U	—	—	C, X	—
Bacterial septicemia	—	—	—	S	U	C	H	C, H	—
Systemic Fungi	—	—	—	S	U	C	H	C, X	N
Algae (*Prototheca*)	—	—	—	—	—	—	—	C, X	N
Protozoa									
Toxoplasma gondii	—	—	—	—	U	—	H	C	N
Leishmania donavani	C	—	K	S	S	—	H	—	—

aC = conjunctivitis, S = symblepharon, E = prolapsed third eyelid, H = hemorrhage, I = icterus.
bM = mucopurulent secretions, E = epiphora.
cI = interstitial keratitis, E = edema, K = keratitis, U = ulcerative keratitis, N = nonulcerative keratitis, S = symblepharon.
dG = glaucoma, T = tumor mass, H = hyphema, F = fibrin, S = secondary glaucoma.
eU = uveitis, P = paradoxical pupil size, A = anisocoria.
fC = cataract.
gB = hemorrhage, H = hyalitis.
hM = multifocal chorioretinitis, C = chorioretinitis, R = retinal dysplasia, D = dysplasia, A = atrophy, I = multifocal infiltrates, H = hemorrhages, V = pale vessels, X = detachment, E = vascular engorgement, P = perivascular infiltrates, L = vasculitis.
iN = neuritis, H = hypoplasia.

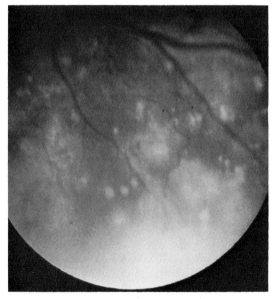

Figure 13–4. Multifocal acute distemper lesions in the nontapetum. Note the hazy, ill-defined borders and lack of retinal vessel deviation over the lesions.

lar high frequency of ocular reactions to CAV-1.

The most visible ocular lesion is stromal corneal edema resulting from inflammatory cell damage to the corneal endothelium (Fig. 13–7). Occasionally, a dog will have blepharospasm, miosis, hypotony, and anterior chamber flare 1 to 2 days before the corneal edema is manifest. Corneal edema may be focal or generalized and is usually transient. In some instances, the edema is permanent, or it may require several months to clear. A

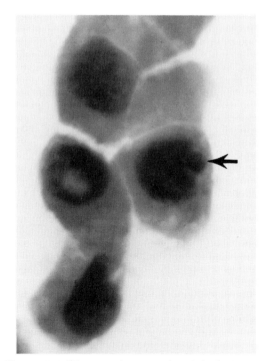

Figure 13–6. Distemper intracytoplasmic inclusion (*arrow*) in conjunctival epithelium. Scraping was taken from a febrile dog with conjunctivitis that developed a neurologic syndrome 2 weeks later.

marked hypotony combined with altered corneal rigidity may result in a keratoconus. Glaucoma, the most significant sequela, usually results in blindness, as it is masked in the early stages by the preexisting corneal edema and conjunctival hyperemia. The syndrome is usually diagnosed by the typical ocular lesions combined with the history

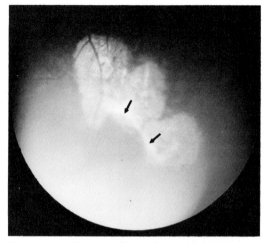

Figure 13–5. Three confluent chorioretinal scars compatible with a diagnosis of prior distemper exposure. Note the sharply demarcated borders of the lesion. Arrows indicate perivascular sheathing of a retinal vessel.

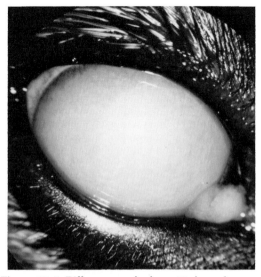

Figure 13–7. Diffuse corneal edema 10 days after vaccination with a modified live hepatitis virus vaccine.

of recent vaccination or illness in a puppy or young (<2 years of age) dog. Other causes of corneal edema, such as a congenital pupillary membrane syndrome, glaucoma, or corneal ulceration, should be ruled out.

There are no data to indicate whether routine uveitis therapy (glucocorticoids and mydriatics) is either beneficial or harmful. Based on the proposed pathogenesis of ocular damage, glucocorticoids theoretically should be beneficial early in the course of the disease to suppress the inflammatory reaction; however, they may retard endothelial healing and interfere in the recovery phase. Mydriatic therapy for uveitis is based on relieving pain from ciliary spasms and minimizing synechia and pupil occlusion. As the uveitis is characterized by minimal adhesions and variable pain, the use of atropine depends on the individual signs. The inflammatory reaction routinely is limited to the anterior uvea; consequently, topical therapy can achieve therapeutic tissue levels without the risk of using systemic glucocorticoids. The eyes should be monitored for secondary glaucoma and should be treated with systemic carbonic anhydrase–inhibiting diuretics if it develops (see also Chapter 17).

Herpesvirus Infections

Canine herpesvirus infection in the adult has produced only a transient conjunctivitis and vaginitis of 4 to 5 days' duration. The suspicions that herpesvirus produces a follicular conjunctivitis and vaginitis syndrome of an apparent contagious nature and that it can cause a keratopathy have been discounted. Occasional dendritic ulceration patterns, typical of herpesvirus infection, are seen in the dog, but their etiology has not been determined. Neonatal herpesvirus infection produces a bilateral panuveitis with keratitis, synechiae, cataracts, retinal necrosis and disorganization, retinal atrophy and dysplasia, and optic neuritis and atrophy.[17]

Feline herpesvirus-1 (rhinotracheitis virus) is responsible for a variety of ocular lesions that often are without overt respiratory signs. A bilateral, serous to mucopurulent conjunctivitis is typically associated with the upper respiratory signs. Neonatal cats may have severe systemic and ocular syndromes resulting in corneal perforations and loss of all visual function (Fig. 13–8).

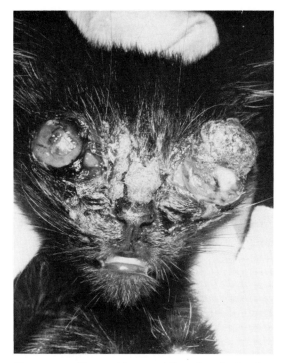

Figure 13–8. Kitten with severe bilateral ocular involvement associated with herpesvirus infection. The left cornea has perforated with a resultant anterior staphyloma, or fibrinous mass, layered over the prolapsed iris.

In young kittens, severe conjunctivitis and concurrent corneal ulceration may lead to symblepharon with conjunctival adhesions to the cornea, obliteration of the lacrimal lake and puncta, and permanent prolapse of the membrana nictitans. In young adults, conjunctivitis with minimal respiratory signs may be produced and must be differentiated from other causes of feline conjunctivitis. In the young adult cat, feline herpesvirus-1 produces a variety of corneal lesions, the most specific being a group of punctate coalescing epithelial erosions that produce linear branching (dendritic) epithelial ulcers (Fig. 13–9). Although the dendritic ulcer is more characteristic of herpesvirus, larger irregular (geographic) epithelial ulcers may also develop and progress into the stroma. Stromal inflammation concurrent with epithelial erosions may occur, but ulcerations may not be present in this stage. Stromal involvement is manifest as vascularization, white infiltrates, and edema. Corneal involvement may be unilateral or bilateral and often is found in otherwise normal cats without a history of respiratory disease or a known febrile episode. Blindness may rarely occur following respiratory disease and is typically sudden, complete, and associated

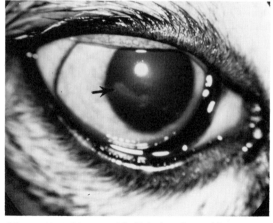

Figure 13–9. Linear epithelial ulcer (arrow) in a young adult cat without obvious respiratory disease. Note the chemosis from the dorsal conjunctiva.

with dilated unresponsive pupils. The retina is normal on ophthalmoscopic and electrophysiologic examination. This syndrome is thought to be a herpesvirus-induced optic neuritis (see also Chapter 27).

The cause of conjunctivitis or dendritic corneal ulceration with upper respiratory signs in cats may be confirmed by viral cultures of the pharynx or conjunctiva or by fluorescent antibody testing for antigen in cytologic smears from mucous membranes. Conjunctival cytology rarely demonstrates inclusion bodies with routine cytologic techniques; however, large bizarre epithelial cells may be observed.[18] Stromal keratitis usually is assumed to be caused by herpesvirus when other etiologies, such as mechanical irritation or injuries, are eliminated.

Specific topical antiviral therapy is available for herpesvirus infections. Herpesvirus conjunctivitis and ulcerative keratitis appear to respond to antiviral therapy, but relapses may occur because no drug to date has eliminated the carrier state. Three drugs are currently available for treating ocular herpesvirus infection: idoxuridine, adenine arabinoside, and trifluthymidine. Therapy is given at least 4 to 6 times daily (see Antiviral Chemotherapy, Chapter 15). In vitro testing of feline herpesvirus susceptibility to antiviral drugs indicated a relative potency in decreasing order of trifluridine, idoxuridine, vidarabine, bromovinyldeoxyuride, and acyclovir. Given the cost and efficacy difference between these commercial preparations, idoxuridine is used initially, and if the herpesvirus infection persists for more than 1

week thereafter, the medication is switched to trifluridine (see Trifluridine, Chapter 15).

Feline Panleukopenia

Feline panleukopenia virus only causes ocular involvement in animals that are less than 3 months of age. The virus has an affinity for rapidly dividing cells and affects the prenatal eye and CNS while they are undergoing differentiation. In utero or early neonatal infection may result in focal retinal necrosis and dysplasia.[19] During an opthalmoscopic examination, these asymptomatic and inactive lesions are visualized as sharply demarcated hyperreflective lesions of the tapetum or as depigmented areas of the nontapetum. Optic nerve hypoplasia and perhaps aplasia may be associated with these early infections and may result in decreased vision. Lesions in older cats are usually incidental. When associated with cerebellar signs, a presumptive diagnosis of panleukopenia can be made. No therapy for the ocular lesions is indicated.

Feline Leukemia Virus Infection

Feline leukemia virus (FeLV) has been associated with a number of ocular syndromes that are often prodromal to systemic signs by weeks to months. Anterior uveitis, the most common FeLV ocular syndrome, is usually bilateral although often is quite asymmetrical in severity. The uveitis is manifest by posterior synechiae, which create irregular fixed pupils, hypotony, fibrin in the anterior chamber that may be blood-tinged, large and small keratic precipitates, prominent conjunctival vessels, and often secondary glaucoma with iris bombé.[20] Cataracts usually develop secondarily, but the posterior ocular segment is usually normal. Large keratic precipitates are produced by aggregations of macrophages and plasma cells and signify a clinical diagnosis of granulomatous anterior uveitis (Fig. 13–10). Experimentally, subcutaneous injection of FeLV and feline sarcoma virus produced anterior uveitis similar to the clinical syndrome.[21]

Isolated lymphoma formation from the iris may occur, creating a mass that invades the anterior chamber. Nodule formation may occur during the course of uveitis or may be

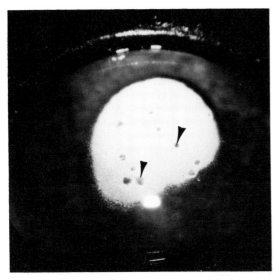

Figure 13–10. Large keratic precipitates (KPs) (mutton fat KPs indicated by *arrows*) and small KPs visualized against the tapetal reflex in a cat with feline leukemia virus–associated anterior uveitis. Note the irregular pupil from posterior synechia.

independent of it. Experimentally, intracamerally inoculated feline sarcoma virus has induced anterior uveal melanomas; however, the clinical significance of this is unknown.[22]

Paradoxical pupil movements in healthy cats with otherwise normal eyes are a unique observation. The syndrome is manifest by irregular periods (hours or days) of anisocoria, bilateral mydriasis, or miosis, without evidence of intraocular inflammation. In the subsequent months, most animals develop systemic signs of FeLV. Unexplained urinary incontinence may accompany the anisocoria.[23] Persistent pupillary dilation and progressive autonomic dysfunction in cats are more characteristic of progressive autonomic ganglioneuropathy (Key-Gaskell syndrome), which is not related to FeLV or other known infectious causes.[24]

Involvement of the posterior ocular segment with FeLV occurs as a result of blood dyscrasias, such as anemia, thrombocytopenia, pancytopenia, or leukemic infiltrates, that are produced. The most common lesions with anemia are hemorrhages of variable size and number and are consistent with hematocrits of 5% to 7% despite adequate platelet numbers. However, the presence of thrombocytopenia with anemia produces the most dramatic hemorrhages (Fig. 13–11). Pale retinal vessels with a dull mottled tapetum are also present. Leukemic infiltrates may manifest as multifocal gray opacities. Exudative retinal detachments occasionally may occur. Rarely, orbital infiltration will occur with exophthalmos and prolapsed membrana nictitans.

The diagnosis of ocular signs related to FeLV is made by determining the presence of viremia or the eventual development of systemic manifestations. Aqueous centesis in uveitis syndromes is usually nonspecific.

Anterior uveitis may respond dramatically to topically or subconjunctivally administered glucocorticoid therapy if systemic signs are absent or there is no objection to maintaining a viremic cat. Glaucoma, which may develop as the inflammation is controlled, is treated with carbonic anhydrase–inhibiting diuretics.

Feline Infectious Peritonitis

The most common ocular syndrome with feline infectious peritonitis (FIP) is bilateral granulomatous anterior uveitis, which is similar to that attributed to FeLV. Since up to 50% of FIP-infected cats are also FeLV-positive, there is often difficulty in determining which is the cause of the uveitis. Anterior uveitis is more common with the

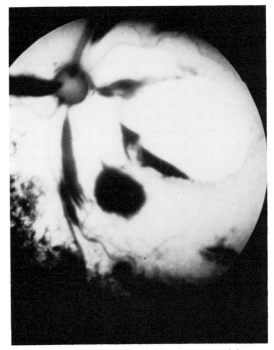

Figure 13–11. Multiple retinal and preretinal hemorrhages in a cat with feline leukemia virus–associated pancytopenia.

noneffusive form of FIP and may be prodromal to obvious systemic signs. Anterior segment pathology may occur without observable posterior segment changes, or may obscure posterior changes. Posterior segment changes vary from complete or focal exudative retinal detachments, diffuse or focal choroiditis, hemorrhages, vasculitis, and optic neuritis (Fig. 13–12). Severe forms are essentially an overwhelming panophthalmitis, and secondary glaucoma is common.[25] Associated systemic manifestations and results of thoracic or abdominocentesis may be diagnostic of effusive FIP. Elevated serum globulin concentration and FIP titers are less definitive tests (see Diagnosis, Chapter 24).

Ocular therapy usually is not attempted when systemic signs are present, but topical, subconjunctival, or systemic glucocorticoid therapy may produce significant improvement in the ocular inflammatory lesions (see also Chapter 24).

Feline Chlamydial Infection

Chlamydia psittaci infection in cats produces a contagious conjunctivitis with minimal respiratory signs. Initially, ocular involvement is often unilateral but progresses to bilateral involvement in about 1 week. Blepharospasm, increased lacrimation, chemosis, and hyperemia of the conjunctiva are

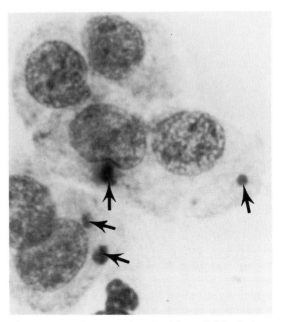

Figure 13–13. Intracytoplasmic chlamydial inclusions *(arrows)* in conjunctival epithelial cells of a cat with conjunctivitis.

early signs, and the animal may be febrile (39.4° to 40.5°C [102.9° to 104.9°F]). The discharge progresses from serous to mucopurulent after 3 to 5 days, with an increased chemosis and hyperemia and hyperplasia of the lymphoid tissue of the membrana nictitans. With chronicity, the discharge diminishes and the chemosis is decreased, and infections of several months' duration and relapses are common.[26] No corneal lesions are produced unless the blepharospasm induces a spastic entropion with mechanical irritation to the cornea. *Chlamydia* may produce conjunctivitis neonatorum in a kitten during the period of physiologic ankyloblepharon. *Chlamydia* may become enzootic in a cattery or similar setting owing to chronic infections and the existence of a carrier state. *Chlamydia* should be considered a zoonosis, and personal hygiene should be observed when examining infected cats.

The presence of chlamydial inclusions on conjunctival cytology is the most rapid diagnostic test (Fig. 13–13), but the frequency of observing inclusions decreases with chronicity. Culturing techniques utilizing embryonated eggs or tissue cultures are often not readily available for diagnosis.

Topical tetracycline is the therapy of choice. Treatment should be continued for a week after a clinical cure to minimize

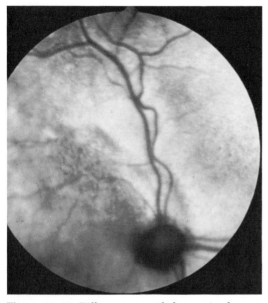

Figure 13–12. Diffuse gray-mottled areas in the tapetum, representing choroidal infiltrates in a cat with feline infectious peritonitis.

relapses. Rapid improvement will be noted in acute cases, but chronic cases will respond gradually and require 2 to 3 weeks of therapy. Response to topical tetracycline therapy is often used to differentiate the clinical syndrome from herpesvirus infection. In multiple-cat households or catteries, a vaccination program should be instituted (see Prevention, Chapter 27, and Vaccination Recommendations for Feline Respiratory Disease, Chapter 2).

Canine Ehrlichiosis and Rocky Mountain Spotted Fever

Ocular findings in canine ehrlichiosis may result from thrombocytopenia-induced hemorrhages or by an inflammatory reaction. Hemorrhages vary from petechiae to massive orbital or ocular hemorrhage with ehrlichiosis. Experimentally, large perivascular retinal infiltrates have been observed during the first 2 months of infection, but these resolved, leaving a hyperreflective tapetal reflex.[27] Additional ocular signs are bilateral anterior uveitis, secondary glaucoma, rhegmatogenous and exudative retinal detachments, chorioretinitis, and papilledema.[28]

Rickettsia rickettsii has produced ocular lesions that are similar to, albeit milder than, *Ehrlichia canis*. Initial signs of conjunctivitis, chemosis, and petechiae of the conjunctiva and retina may be followed in 14 to 28 days by an anterior uveitis.[29]

Diagnosis and antimicrobial therapy of these diseases are discussed in Chapters 37 and 38. The inflammatory lesion of the anterior ocular segment should be treated with topical or subconjunctival glucocorticoids in addition to systemic antibiotics.

Systemic Bacterial Infections

Septicemias caused by a variety of bacteria may localize in the eyes. Examples are embolization from local infections such as bacterial endocarditis and oral or dental infections. Contagious bacterial infections such as canine brucellosis, leptospirosis, tuberculosis, and salmonellosis may also manifest with ocular lesions. The ocular lesions may remain occult if embolization to the posterior segment occurs. In some instances, blindness from an overwhelming endophthalmitis may be the presenting sign.

Brucella canis has been a documented cause of unilateral or bilateral anterior uveitis and endophthalmitis (see also Chapter 52).[30] Although tuberculosis is rare today, anterior and posterior uveitis, retinal detachment, keratitis, and blepharitis have been observed in the cat. *Mycobacterium bovis* has been the most common species involved with ocular disease (see also Chapter 51). In the Pacific Northwest, an acid-fast organism has occasionally been associated with a proliferative keratitis[31] and may be an atypical *Mycobacterium* similar to those associated with feline leprosy. This organism seems to be confined to that coastal region. Salmonella may localize intraocularly in septicemic stages and has produced a conjunctivitis in asymptomatic cats that were fecal shedders.[32]

The diagnosis of intraocular bacterial infections is usually based on cultures of centesis samples from the eye in association with systemic signs and serology. Therapy consists of systemic and often intraocular antibiotics as the inflammatory reaction is rapidly devastating to ocular morphology. Refer to respective chapters to determine the proper drugs.

Systemic Fungal Infections

The systemic mycoses in North America are frequently associated with a granulomatous anterior and posterior uveitis or endophthalmitis in the dog and to a lesser extent in the cat. Ocular syndromes are a part of systemic infections, which may otherwise be inapparent. The ocular syndromes associated with the different organisms are clinically similar. Systemic mycoses are important rule-outs if bilateral uveitis-endophthalmitis and systemic signs are seen simultaneously. With the exception of cryptococcosis, these diseases have been more commonly seen in dogs than cats.

In indigenous regions of the Mississippi and Ohio Rivers and the central Atlantic states, *Blastomyces dermatitidis*–induced ocular infections are common. Ocular involvement may vary from a relatively occult focal granulomatous chorioretinitis to a panophthalmitis syndrome (Fig. 13–14).[33] Secondary glaucoma is a frequent complication (see also Chapter 65).

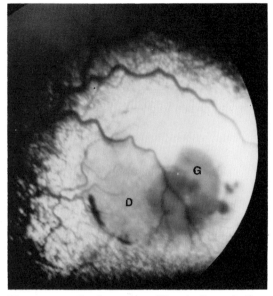

Figure 13–14. Focal granuloma (G) and adjacent bullous detachment (D) in a dog with blastomycosis.

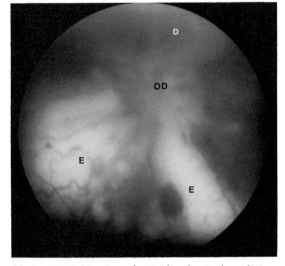

Figure 13–15. Massive subretinal and retinal exudation (E) in a dog with protothecosis. Exudative retinal detachment (D) has occurred, and the optic disc (OD) is obscured by the inflammatory haze. The opposite eye had multiple small granulomas but was functional.

Judging from a published report, ocular involvement with histoplasmosis is relatively rare in dogs.[34] In the cat, the ocular syndrome of histoplasmosis occurs in association with a systemic wasting or neurologic disease and will mimic the more common syndromes of FIP and FeLV infection. In the cat, the predominant lesion is a granulomatous choroiditis with minimal anterior segment inflammation (see also Chapter 66).[35]

Coccidioides immitis is endemic in the southwestern United States. It produces a characteristic granulomatous posterior uveitis that frequently extends to the anterior segment. Organisms are found predominantly in the retina and choroid. The lesions are usually unilateral, and ocular signs may be present without systemic signs (see also Chapter 67).[36]

Ocular infection with *Cryptococcus neoformans* has occurred in the dog and cat via direct extension from nasal or CNS involvement. However, hematogenous spread appears to be the most important route. Posterior uveitis is the predominant lesion, and the organisms are readily demonstrable. Anterior uveal inflammation is less frequent, and when present, the organisms may not be demonstrable at this site, resulting in speculation that the lesion may be a sterile immune-mediated inflammation.[37] Orbital and optic nerve granulomatous inflammation may also occur (see also Chapter 67).

Bilateral granulomatous chorioretinitis or endophthalmitis should suggest the possibility of systemic mycoses. Associated systemic signs of fever and respiratory, skeletal, dermatologic, or CNS involvement are usually present. The specific diagnosis is often made by finding the organism in tissue aspirates. With most of the systemic mycoses, ocular involvement is often confirmed by

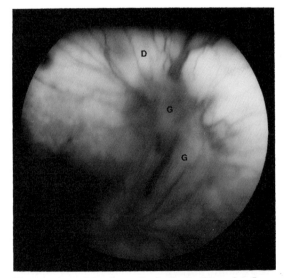

Figure 13–16. Massive retinal gliosis (G) and inflammation in a dog with neurologic disease and subsequently diagnosed on postmortem as toxoplasmosis. Retinal detachment (D) has occurred in the upper half of the tapetum.

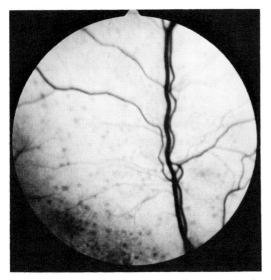

Figure 13–17. Multifocal acute toxoplasmic retinochoroidal lesions. (Courtesy of Dr. S. Vainisi, Oneida, WI.)

vitreal centesis, which may be the method of making the systemic diagnosis.

The main therapy for ocular involvement with the systemic mycoses is either systemic amphotericin B or ketoconazole as discussed in Chapter 63. Subconjunctival injections of 125 μg or intraocular injection of 1 to 5 μg of amphotericin B may augment systemic therapy but are of questionable value. Most ocular conditions that are considered desperate enough for local ocular therapy have such severe structural alterations that blindness results no matter how intensively they are treated. In some instances, the ocular inflammatory reaction continues to worsen despite systemic therapy, and intraocular injection of amphotericin B has arrested the progressive worsening although the end result was still blindness. Enucleation may be required to ensure effective elimination of infection where the eye has become severely damaged.

Protothecosis

Prototheca are ubiquitous algae in soil and water that are occasionally pathogenic to animals (see Chapter 75). More than 50% of affected animals may have ocular involvement.[38] Most ocular syndromes are associated with systemic signs, but in some instances, the systemic signs are occult. Lesions include a granulomatous posterior uveitis (Fig. 13–15) or panuveitis that is usually bilateral and blinding. Lesions may

be dramatic but will have to be differentiated from more common causes of granulomatous uveitis. Definitive diagnosis is usually made by finding the organism on aspirates, exudates, excretions, or biopsy. No efficacious therapy has been reported.

Toxoplasmosis

The most common ocular lesion is a multifocal posterior retinochoroiditis that may result in retinal detachment (Figs. 13–16 and 13–17).[39] Ocular disease, more commonly seen in cats than in dogs, may be the only overt manifestation of the disease. The lesions may be granulomatous or nongranulomatous. Anterior uveitis may be seen as well with mononuclear cell infiltration.[40] The possibility of a sterile immune-mediated inflammation exists.[39] The extraocular muscles may also be involved with a more generalized *Toxoplasma*-induced myositis.

Because of the ubiquitous presence of *T. gondii*, it should be considered in the differential diagnosis of endogenous anterior uveitis and chorioretinitis whether or not systemic signs are present. A diagnosis of toxoplasmosis is usually based on serologic testing (see Chapter 86).

Toxoplasmosis may be a self-limiting disease that does not require therapy, but if systemic signs or active intraocular inflammation are present, systemic therapy is usually advised. Traditional therapy consists of systemic sulfonamides and pyrimethamine with folinic acid supplementation. Clindamycin may be more effective. In experimental infections in rabbits, minocycline has been successful in ameliorating the clinical disease and sterilizing the ocular tissues.[41]

References

1. Bistner SI, Roberts SR, Anderson RP: Conjunctival bacteria: clinical appearances can be deceiving. *Mod Vet Pract* 50:45–47, 1969.
2. Hacker DV, Jensen HE, Selby LA: A comparison of conjunctival culture techniques in the dog. *J Am Anim Hosp Assoc* 15:223–225, 1979.
3. Urban M, Wyman M, Rheins M, et al: Conjunctival flora of clinically normal dogs. *J Am Vet Med Assoc* 161:201–206, 1972.
4. Shewen PE, Povey RC, Wilson MR: A survey of the conjunctival flora of clinically normal cats and cats with conjunctivitis. *Can Vet J* 21:231–233, 1980.
5. Campbell LH, Fox JG, Snyder SB: Ocular bacteria and mycoplasma of the clinically normal cat. *Feline Pract* 3:10–12, 1973.

6. Murphy JM, Lavach JD, Severin GA: Survey of conjunctival flora in dogs with clinical signs of external eye disease. *J Am Vet Med Assoc* 172:66–68, 1978.

6a. Gerding PA, McLaughlin SA, Troop MW: Pathogenic bacteria and fungi associated with external ocular disease in dogs: 151 cases (1981–1986). *J Am Vet Med Assoc* 193:242–244, 1988.

7. Lavach JD, Thrall MA, Benjamin MM, et al: Cytology of normal and inflamed conjunctivas in dogs and cats. *J Am Vet Med Assoc* 170:722–727, 1977.

8. Forster RK, Abbott RL, Gelender H: Management of infectious endophthalmitis. *Ophthalmology* 87:313–319, 1980.

9. Havener WH: *Ocular Pharmacology*, ed 3. St Louis, CV Mosby Co, 1974.

10. *Physician's Desk Reference for Ophthalmology*. Oradell, NJ, Medical Economics Co, 1989.

11. Peyman GA, Carroll CP, Raichand M: Prevention and management of traumatic endophthalmitis. *Ophthalmology* 87:320–324, 1980.

12. D'Amico D, Caspers-Velu L, Libert J, et al: Comparative toxicity of intravitreal aminoglycoside antibiotics. *Am J Ophthalmol* 100:264–275, 1985.

13. Talamo J, D'Amico D, Kenyon K: Intravitreal amikacin in the treatment of bacterial endophthalmitis. *Arch Ophthalmol* 104:1483–1485, 1986.

14. Fischer CA: Retinal and retinochoroidal lesions in early neuropathic canine distemper. *J Am Vet Med Assoc* 158:740–752, 1971.

15. Fischer C, Jones G: Optic neuritis in dogs. *J Am Vet Med Assoc* 160:68–79, 1972.

16. Curtis R, Barnett K: The ocular lesions of infectious canine hepatitis. II. Field incidence. *J Small Anim Pract* 14:737–745, 1973b.

17. Albert DM, Lahav M, Carmichael L, et al: Canine herpes-induced retinal dysplasia and associated ocular anomalies. *Invest Ophthalmol* 15:267–278, 1976.

18. Cello RM: Clues to differential diagnosis of feline respiratory infections. *J Am Vet Med Assoc* 158:968–973, 1971.

19. Percy D, Scott F, Albert D: Retinal dysplasia due to feline panleukopenia virus infection. *J Am Vet Med Assoc* 167:935–937, 1975.

20. Williams LW, Gelatt KN, Gwin RM: Ophthalmic neoplasms in the cat. *J Am Anim Hosp Assoc* 17:999–1008, 1981.

21. Lubin JR, Albert DM, Essex M, et al: Experimental anterior uveitis after subcutaneous injection of feline sarcoma virus. *Invest Ophthalmol Vis Sci* 24:1055–1062, 1983.

22. Albert DM, Shadduck SJ, Craft JL, et al: Feline uveal melanoma model induced with feline sarcoma virus. *Invest Ophthalmol* 20:606–624, 1981.

23. Barsanti JA, Downey R: Urinary incontinence in cats. *J Am Anim Hosp Assoc* 20:979–982, 1984.

24. Rochlitz I: Feline dysautonomia (the Key-Gaskellor dilated pupil syndrome): a preliminary review. *J Small Anim Pract* 25:587–598, 1984.

25. Doherty M: Ocular manifestations of feline infectious peritonitis. *J Am Vet Med Assoc* 159:417–424, 1971.

26. Shewen PE, Povey RC, Wilson MR: Feline chlamydial infection. *Can Vet J* 19:289–292, 1978.

27. Ellett E, Playter R, Pierce K: Retinal lesions associated with induced canine ehrlichiosis: a preliminary report. *J Am Anim Hosp Assoc* 9:214–218, 1973.

28. Swanson JF: Uveitis associated with *Ehrlichia canis* infection. *Proc Am Coll Vet Ophthalmol* 13:102–115, 1982.

29. Davidson MG, Breitschwerdt EB, Walker DH, et al: Experimental *Rickettsia rickettsii* vasculitis in the canine eye. *In* Proceedings. Int Congr Rickettsiologists. Palermo, Italy, 1987, p 137.

30. Gwin RM, Kolwalski JJ, Wyman M, et al: Ocular lesions associated with *Brucella canis* infection in a dog. *J Am Anim Hosp Assoc* 16:607–610, 1980.

31. Dice P: Intracorneal acid-fast granuloma resembling feline leprosy. *Proc Am Coll Vet Ophthalmol* 8:91–92, 1977.

32. Fox J, Galus C: Salmonella associated conjunctivitis in a cat. *J Am Vet Med Assoc* 171:845–847, 1977.

33. Buyukmihci N: Ocular lesions of blastomycosis in the dog. *J Am Vet Med Assoc* 180:426–431, 1982.

34. Gwin RM, Makley TA, Wyman M, et al: Multifocal ocular histoplasmosis in a dog and cat. *J Am Vet Med Assoc* 176:638–642, 1980.

35. Quinn AJ: Granulomatous chorioretinitis of disseminated histoplasmosis in cats. *Proc Am Soc Vet Ophthalmol*, Las Vegas, NV, April 25–28, 1982, pp 159–163.

36. Angell JA, Merideth RE, Shively JN, et al: Ocular lesions associated with coccidioidomycosis in dogs: 35 cases (1980–1985). *J Am Vet Med Assoc* 190:1319–1322, 1987.

37. Blouin P, Cello R: Experimental ocular cryptococcosis—preliminary studies in cats and mice. *Invest Ophthalmol* 19:21–30, 1980.

38. Migaki G, Font RL, Sauer RM, et al: Canine protothecosis: review of the literature and report of an additional case. *J Am Vet Med Assoc* 181:794–797, 1982.

39. Vainisi SJ, Campbell LH: Ocular toxoplasmosis in cats. *J Am Vet Med Assoc* 154:141–152, 1969.

40. Piper RC, Cole CR, Shadduck JA: Natural and experimental ocular toxoplasmosis in animals. *Am J Ophthalmol* 69:662–668, 1970.

41. Rollins DF, Tabbara KF, Ghosheh R, et al: Minocycline in experimental ocular toxoplasmosis in the rabbit. *Am J Ophthalmol* 93:361–365, 1982.

VIRAL, RICKETTSIAL, AND MYCOPLASMAL INFECTIONS

SECTION II

14 LABORATORY DIAGNOSIS OF VIRAL AND RICKETTSIAL INFECTIONS

James F. Evermann

INTRODUCTION AND JUSTIFICATION

The diagnosis of viral and rickettsial diseases historically has relied upon a combination of clinical criteria, including recognition of symptoms and laboratory analysis of antemortem or postmortem specimens (Fig. 14–1).[1–3] Over the past decade, this pattern of clinical observation and laboratory analysis has been redefined. The needs of the veterinarian have expanded to include the use of a laboratory diagnosis for confirmation of the clinical diagnosis and assistance in making a differential diagnosis. In addition, clients require up-to-date information on how to manage infectious diseases in a single-pet household or a multiple-animal facility and how to monitor animals for zoonotic infections.[3, 4]

Pursuing a laboratory diagnosis to confirm a clinical diagnosis is essential in cases when an animal has clinical symptoms that may be caused by any one of a number of infectious agents, such as those causing feline upper respiratory diseases or canine enteric infections. A laboratory diagnosis can aid in conveying to the client the impact the infection is having on the affected animal and others with which it has contact.[5] This is especially true of diseases for which it is difficult to vaccinate, such as feline infectious peritonitis and canine herpesvirus infection.

Laboratory diagnosis of zoonotic infections is essential for patient management and client well being. Rabies and the tick-borne rickettsial infections are examples of well-recognized zoonotics. Of increasing

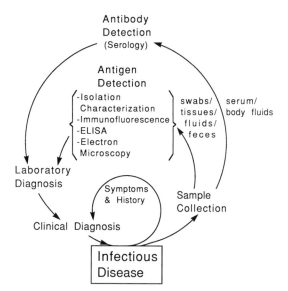

Figure 14–1. Scheme depicting the relationship between a laboratory diagnosis and a clinical diagnosis. The ultimate objective is for the laboratory diagnosis to confirm the clinical diagnosis on the basis of either antigen/antibody detection or both.

concern to physicians and veterinarians is the potential role of zoonoses of pet animals maintained at convalescent centers and facilities for immunocompromised people. Screening pets for zoonotic infections prior to placement into high-risk areas for human infection demands the highest priority by veterinarians and public health officials.[4–6]

LABORATORY ANALYSES AND INTERPRETATION OF RESULTS

Sample Collection

Laboratory diagnosis of viral and rickettsial infections requires proper sample selec-

Table 14–1. Samples to Collect for Laboratory Diagnosis of Viral and Rickettsial Diseases

SITE(S) OF CLINICAL SIGNS	ANTEMORTEM[a]	POSTMORTEM[b]
Respiratory and ocular tissues	Nasal swabs, conjunctival scraping, serum, whole blood[c]	Selected tissues[d] and bronchiolar lymph nodes
Gastrointestinal tract	Feces, vomitus, serum, whole blood	Selected sections of small intestine, intestinal contents, mesenteric lymph nodes
Skin and mucous membranes	Swabs, scrapings of lesions, serum, whole blood	Selected tissues[d] and regional lymph nodes
Central nervous system[e]	CSF, serum, whole blood, feces	Selected sections from brain
Genitourinary tract	Urogenital swabs, vaginal mucus, urine, serum, whole blood	Selected sections from placenta, fetal lung, liver, kidney, and spleen

Modified from Fenner F, et al: *In* Fenner F, Bachmann PA, Gibbs EPJ, et al (eds): *Veterinary Virology.* Academic Press, 1987, pp 237–264, with permission.

[a]Samples to be kept moist and chilled.

[b]Fresh samples to be collected for viral or rickettsial analysis, and fixed samples (10% buffered formalin) for histologic analysis.

[c]Whole blood collected in EDTA.

[d]Selected tissues include the hematogenous organs: lung, liver, kidney, and spleen.

[e]Neurologic suspects should be handled with extreme caution and cleared for rabies virus through the Public Health Laboratory prior to further diagnostic pursuit.

Table 14–2. Specimen Collection, Processing, and Shipment

PROCEDURE (SPECIMEN)	COLLECTION AND PROCESSING	SHIPMENT
Organism isolation (tissue, secretions)	Collect aseptically to prevent bacterial contamination, and store at ≤10° C to prevent inactivation; do not freeze or fix	Use swabs,[a] commercial transport media, or sterile Hanks's balanced salt solution with 10% bovine albumin or 0.5% lactalbumin hydrolysate; add penicillin (100 U/ml) and streptomycin (2 µg/ml) to inhibit bacterial growth; pack on wet ice to last 48–72 hrs
Serology (serum)	Collect aseptically to prevent contamination and handle gently to prevent hemolysis; remove needle from syringe before dispensing; allow to clot at room temperature; rim clot and centrifuge at 650 × G for 20 min; although paired samples (10–14 days apart) are preferred, single samples may be diagnostic, e.g., canine distemper virus IgM	Refrigerate until shipping
Histology (tissue)	Collect aseptically to prevent contamination, 5 mm thick; fix in 10% buffered formalin (10 × volume); make tissue impression prior to fixation	Ship in leakproof container with adequate fixative
Direct immunofluorescent testing (tissue, tissue impression)	As for isolation; make impression on clean dry microscope slide, air dry; fix with alcohol for cytology or with acetone for immunofluorescence[b]	Pack on wet ice and ship as for isolation; smears can be shipped unrefrigerated
Electron microscopy (tissue)	Collect aseptically, 1 × 2 mm thick; fix in 2%–4% glutaraldehyde (10 × volume) for 24 hrs at 20° C	Ship in leakproof container with adequate fixative
(Feces or body fluids)	Collect fresh, do not freeze or fix	Refrigerate until shipping; pack on wet ice to last 48–72 hrs

[a]Culturettes, Marion Scientific, Kansas City, MO.

[b]Michel's fixative (see Appendix 12) is used to preserve tissue specimens for antibody testing by IFA. For antigen detection, other fixatives may be used.

Table 14–3. *Techniques for Detection and Identification of Viruses at Various Taxonomic Levels*

TAXONOMIC LEVEL	TECHNIQUES OF CHOICE
Family (group)	Cytopathology in cell culture, electron microscopy, hemagglutination, complement fixation, agar gel precipitation, immunofluorescence, ELISA
Species type and/ or subtype	Virus neutralization, monoclonal antibody serology
Variants (genomic)	Restriction endonuclease patterns, oligonucleotide fingerprints, nucleic acid hybridization
Mutants	Nucleic acid sequencing, monoclonal antibody serology

Modified from Fenner F, et al. *In* Fenner F, Bachmann PA, Gibbs EJ, et al (eds): *Veterinary Virology.* Academic Press, 1987, pp 237–264, with permission.

tion, collection, and submission.[1, 2, 7–9] Samples should be obtained whenever an animal has clinical signs. Although postmortem samples may be of value, the degree of diagnostic precision is reduced owing to degradation of the antigens or antibodies in the samples. Samples to collect to determine the cause of an infectious disease are listed in Table 14–1 and are presented according to the site(s) of clinical signs. Table 14–2 presents information about collection, processing, and shipping of specimens to the diagnostic laboratory.

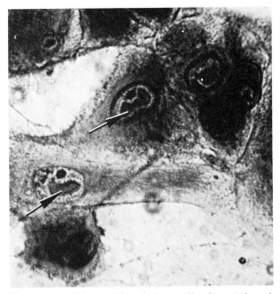

Figure 14–2. Primary feline kidney cell culture infected with feline herpesvirus showing intranuclear inclusions *(arrows)* 48 hours postinoculation. (Courtesy of Dr. P. D. Lukert, University of Georgia, Athens, GA.)

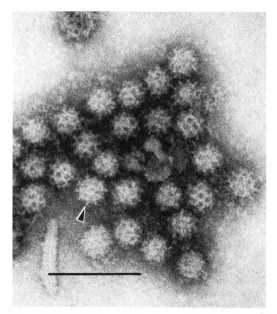

Figure 14–3. Electron photomicrograph of canine calicivirus. Note characteristic spikes on virus *(arrow).* Bar represents 100 nm. (From Crandell R: *Arch Virol* 98:67, 1988. Reprinted with permission.)

Surveillance Programs

When the laboratory is being used to monitor clinically normal animals for infections such as feline leukemia virus (FeLV) or canine coronavirus, the laboratory should be consulted prior to sample collection and submission (see Appendix 8). In some cases, the laboratory may offer a panel of tests that can be run on a single sample of whole blood, serum, or feces.

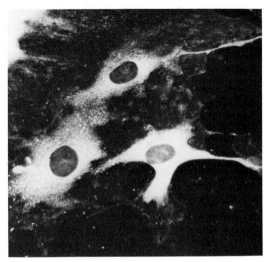

Figure 14–4. Cheetah kidney cells infected with feline infectious peritonitis virus showing cytoplasmic fluorescence (20 hours postinoculation).

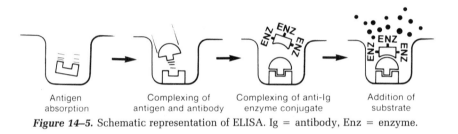

| Antigen
absorption | Complexing of
antigen and antibody | Complexing of anti-Ig
enzyme conjugate | Addition of
substrate |

Figure 14–5. Schematic representation of ELISA. Ig = antibody, Enz = enzyme.

Laboratory Analyses

Table 14–3 presents various techniques that may be used in the detection and identification of the major viruses affecting cats and dogs.[8] Most laboratories have the capacity to determine what family group of viruses or rickettsia is causing the infection. However, specialized laboratories may be required for more specific analysis if a case warrants (i.e., if there are unusual clinical signs or suspected new variants of preexisting viruses, such as canine parvovirus).[7, 10] The detection of viruses and rickettsia may generally be classified as either antigen or antibody detection. Both may be employed to determine the cause of infection.

The major methods of antigen detection currently used in veterinary medicine can be further divided into (1) conventional viral or rickettsial isolation in cell cultures or embryonating eggs (Fig. 14–2); (2) viral detection by electron microscopy (Fig. 14–3);[11] (3) antigen detection in tissue sections and cell culture by immunodiagnostic tests (immunofluorescence and immunoperoxidase)(Fig. 14–4); and (4) antigen detection in body secretions, excretions, blood, or serum by ELISA (Fig. 14–5).

Advances being made in diagnostic techniques will increase the specificity and sensitivity of currently available antigen-detection tests such as the FeLV-ELISA, which incorporates monoclonal antibodies for increased specificity and shorter test time. The use of complementary DNA (C-DNA) probes for the detection of more fastidious viruses such as canine distemper virus and feline infectious peritonitis virus will enable clinicians to make rapid in-clinic diagnostic assessments of their patients.[12–15]

The second approach of diagnosis involves the testing of serum or body fluids for the presence of specific antibody. These serologic techniques are able to provide definitive proof of a rise or fall in antibody levels coincident with the clinical episode. In more recent years, serology has been used extensively to determine the **prevalence** of one point-in-time assessment of an infection in a population of animals irrespective of disease.[16] In contrast, when serum samples are collected and tested from the same group of animals over a period of time, the **incidence** of infection in a population of animals can be determined. Seroepidemiology (spread and occurrence of an infection in a population) of viral and rickettsial infections has proved useful in defining populations of animals at risk of infection or as potential threats to susceptible animals.[16–18] Seroepidemiology has been of particular value in monitoring natural sentinel populations for zoonotic infections such as *Rickettsia rickettsii* and for tracing the divergence of canine parvovirus in domestic and wild Canidae.[16, 17, 19]

Table 14–4. Interpretation of Laboratory Analysis in a Case in Which Canine Parvovirus Enteritis Was Suspected on the Basis of Clinical Signs and History[a]

CLINICAL INQUIRY	TEST(S)	LEVEL OF INTERPRETATION
1. Is dog infected with parvovirus?	ELISA	Yes/no
2. When was dog exposed?	Serology (IFA for IgM) EM/virus isolation	7–10 days Rotaviruses, coronaviruses, and caliciviruses
3. Are other infectious agents present?	ELISA Bacteriology Parasitology	Rotavirus *Salmonella* sp., *Campylobacter* sp. *Giardia* sp.

[a]Interpretation is dependent upon the level of clinical inquiry and the types of laboratory tests used.

Interpretation of Laboratory Results

Interpretation of results presents the greatest interface between the clinician and diagnostician. The interpretation of a laboratory test has at least two levels of significance: (1) the type of test that is conducted and the recognition of the limitations of the test and (2) how the interpretation of the test results influences patient management and client information. An example of how the levels of interpretation are influenced by the level of the questions asked and laboratory tests run is presented in Table 14–4.

The limitations of interpreting results from certain laboratory tests should be recognized by both the diagnostician and the clinician. The value of certain tests may be that they are additive in terms of an overall laboratory analysis rather than providing a definitive one-test type diagnosis. Examples of vague tests are serum IgG antibody tests for feline infectious peritonitis virus and canine distemper virus. In the case of feline infectious peritonitis, serum titers are useful for determining prior exposure to the feline coronavirus group but should not be used as the sole criteria for making a clinical diagnosis. This is in contrast to other tests for canine distemper, in which a positive immunofluorescence for viral antigen on conjunctival scrapings or a positive canine distemper virus antibody titer from the CSF is considered definitive of canine distemper virus infection.

APPLICATIONS OF MOLECULAR BIOLOGY AND BIOTECHNOLOGY TO IMPROVE VETERINARY DIAGNOSTICS

One of the benefits of molecular biology and biotechnology has been the increased emphasis on improvement of diagnostic assays and on making these assays directly available to the clinician.[12, 13, 20] Since there are examples of diagnostic tests that lack specificity (the ability to distinguish closely related strains) or sensitivity (the ability to detect low levels of antigen or antibody), it now appears that with the techniques currently available, many of the problems that are encountered will be solved by the use of highly specific monoclonal antibodies that recognize individual epitopes and by tests that utilize C-DNA probes for the more fastidious viruses such as canine distemper virus, canine herpesvirus, and feline immunodeficiency virus.[14, 17, 21–23]

The accessibility of viral diagnostic test kits for the small animal clinician in practice has been somewhat restricted in the past, and these kits have included ELISA tests for feline leukemia virus, canine parvovirus, and feline immunodeficiency virus infections (see Appendix 8). It is anticipated that the new generation of diagnostic tests will not only be more specific and more sensitive but will also be more available to the clinician as in-office kits. This will provide the clinician with more information with which to make decisions regarding patient management and client information.[24–26]

References

1. Guy JS: Diagnosis of canine viral infections. *Vet Clin North Am* 16:1145–1156, 1986.
2. Ott RL: Diagnosis of feline viral infections. *Vet Clin North Am* 16:1157–1170, 1986.
3. Marchette N: The distribution and relationships of rickettsiae. In Marchette NJ (ed): *Ecological Relationships and Evolution of the Rickettsiae*, vol 1. Boca Raton, FL, CRC Press, 1982, pp 11–28.
4. Elliot DL, Tolle SW, Goldberg L, et al: Pet-associated illness. *N Engl J Med* 313:985–995, 1985.
5. Reif JS: The epidemiology of viral infections in dogs and cats. *Vet Clin North Am* 16:1029–1040, 1986.
6. Ristic M: Pertinent characteristics of leukocytic rickettsiae of humans and animals. In Leive L (ed): *Microbiology 1986*. Washington, DC, Am Soc Microbiol, 1986, pp 182–187.
7. England JJ: Nature and classification of viruses affecting small animals. *Vet Clin North Am* 16:1015–1028, 1986.
8. Fenner F, Bachmann PA, Gibbs EPJ, et al: Laboratory diagnosis of viral diseases. In Fenner F, Bachmann PA, Gibbs EPJ, et al (eds): *Veterinary Virology*. New York, Academic Press, 1987, pp 237–264.
9. Wooley RE: Laboratory diagnosis of viral and rickettsial diseases. In Greene CE (ed): *Clinical Microbiology and Infectious Diseases of the Dog and Cat*. Philadelphia, WB Saunders, 1984, pp 113–120.
10. Parrish CR, O'Connell PH, Evermann JF, et al: Natural variation of canine parvovirus. *Science* 230:1046–1048, 1985.
11. Crandell RA: Isolation and characterization of caliciviruses from dogs with vesicular genital disease. *Arch Virol* 98:65–71, 1988.
12. Haase AT: In situ hybridization and covert virus infections. In Notkins AL, Oldstone MBA (eds): *Concepts in Viral Pathogenesis II*. New York, Springer-Verlag, 1986, pp 310–316.
13. Richman DD, Wahl GM. Nucleic acid probes to detect viral diseases. In Notkins AL, Oldstone MBA (eds): *Concepts in Viral Pathogenesis II*. New York, Springer-Verlag, 1986, pp 301–309.

14. Oglesbee M, Jackwood D, Perrine K, et al: In vitro detection of canine distemper virus nucleic acid with a virus-specific C-DNA probe by dot-blot and in situ hybridization. *J Virol Meth* 14:195–211, 1986.

15. DeGroot, FJ, Maduro J, Lenstra JA, et al: C-DNA cloning and sequence analysis of the gene encoding the peplomer protein of feline infectious peritonitis virus. *J Gen Virol* 68:2639–2646, 1987.

16. Breitschwerdt EB, Moncol DJ, Corbett WT, et al: Antibodies to spotted fever–group rickettsiae in dogs in North Carolina. *Am J Vet Res* 48:1436–1440, 1987.

17. Parrish CR, Have P, Foreyt WJ, et al: The global spread and replacement of canine parvovirus strains. *J Gen Virol* 69:1111–1116, 1988.

18. O'Brien SJ, Roelke ME, Marker L, et al: Genetic basis for species vulnerability in the cheetah. *Science* 227:1428–1434, 1985.

19. Thomas NJ, Foreyt WJ, Evermann JF, et al: Seroprevalence of canine parvovirus in wild coyotes from Texas, Utah and Idaho (1972–1983). *J Am Vet Med Assoc* 185:1283–1287, 1984.

20. Kurstak E, Tijssen P, Kurstak C, et al: Enzyme immunoassays and related procedures in diagnostic medical virology. *Bull WHO* 64:465–479, 1986.

21. Evermann JF: Diagnosis of canine herpetic infections. *In* Kirk RW (ed): *Current Veterinary Therapy X.* Philadelphia, WB Saunders, 1989, pp 1313–1316.

22. Pedersen NC, Ho EN, Brown ML, et al: Isolation of a T-lymphotropic virus from domestic cats with an immunodeficiency-like syndrome. *Science* 235:790–793, 1987.

23. Harbour DA, Williams PD, Gruffydd-Jones TJ, et al: Isolation of a T-lymphotropic lentivirus from a persistently leucopenic domestic cat. *Vet Rec* 122:84–86, 1988.

24. Eisenstein BI, Engleberg NC: Applied molecular genetics: new tools for microbiologists and clinicians. *J Infect Dis* 153:416–430, 1986.

25. Caskey CT: Disease diagnosis by recombinant DNA methods. *Science* 236:1223–1229, 1987.

26. Tenover FC: Impact of DNA probes on clinical microbiology. *In* Tenover FC (ed): *DNA Probes for Infectious Diseases.* Boca Raton, FL, CRC Press, 1989, pp 32–41.

15

ANTIVIRAL CHEMOTHERAPY

Craig E. Greene

The development and clinical use of antiviral drugs have been much slower than those of antibiotics. It is difficult to achieve selective interference with antiviral chemotherapy because viral replication is more dependent on and related to host cell metabolism than is bacterial replication. Unlike antibacterial therapy, antiviral chemotherapy usually involves prophylactic drug administration. Viruses, usually inhibited only during their replicative cycle, may be resistant to therapy during a latent or nonreplicative phase of infection. Acute viral infections are difficult to treat because diagnosis cannot be made before the course of infection is terminated. Antiviral agents are more effective in treating chronic viral infections and in preventing reactivation of latent infections.

Few antiviral drugs are licensed for use at present because most have proved to be too toxic during preliminary screening. The properties of clinically useful antiviral compounds are summarized in Table 15–1 and below.

IDOXURIDINE

Idoxuridine is a synthetic nucleoside containing deoxyribose, the natural sugar that closely resembles thymidine. As a thymidine analog, it is incorporated into DNA structure and inhibits enzymes used in DNA synthesis. As with most clinically used antiviral drugs, it does not affect latent virus infections. It is active against herpesviruses, having been used topically to treat keratitis and dermatitis (see Herpesvirus Infections, Chapter 13). Because of toxicity, it is rarely used systemically for herpesvirus encephalitis. Prolonged topical use may cause irritation or nonhealing corneal ulcers; hepatotoxicity is common with systemic administration. Some strains of herpesvirus are resistant to this drug.

VIDARABINE

Vidarabine, a purine nucleoside, also inhibits DNA synthesis by being incorporated into the nucleic acid and by inhibiting DNA-synthetic enzymes. It is effective in vitro against herpesviruses, poxviruses, and oncoviruses, but its clinical use in humans has been restricted to the treatment of smallpox and herpesviral keratitis and encephalitis. Vidarabine must be administered IV because of its low solubility, and it must be given in relatively large volumes of fluid over extended periods during the day. Toxic effects include local irritation at the site of infusion, nausea, vomiting, and diarrhea. The drug also causes depression of the bone marrow, resulting in anemia, leukopenia, and thrombocytopenia. Vidarabine monophosphate, a new form, can be given IM without the need for large fluid volumes.

AMANTADINE

Amantadine is a highly stable cyclic amine with a narrow spectrum that primarily inhibits penetration and uncoating of RNA viruses. It is rapidly and completely absorbed following oral administration and is widely distributed throughout the body. About 90% is excreted unchanged in the urine. It has been used only in the prophylaxis of human influenza and is most efficacious when administered early in the course of infection. Commonly encountered side

221

Table 15–1. Dosages of More Commonly Used Antiviral Drugs[a]

DRUG	CLINICALLY AVAILABLE PREPARATION	BRAND (MANUFACTURER)	ROUTE	DOSE[b] (mg/kg)	INTERVAL (hours)	DURATION (days)
Idoxuridine	0.1% ophthalmic solution	Dendrid (Alcon)	Ocular, topical	Solution	5–6	3–5
	0.5% cutaneous ointment	Herplex (Allergan) Stoxil (SKF)		Ointment	1–2	3–5
Vidarabine	3% ophthalmic ointment	Vira-A (Parke-Davis)	Ocular, topical IV	1 cm ointment	5–6	prn
	Injection 200 mg/ ml suspension			10–30	24[c]	5–10
Amantadine	Capsules (100, 500 mg)	Symmetrel (Endo) (Dupont)	PO	100 mg (total)[d]	12–24 (adult)	5–7
	Syrup (50 mg/5 ml)				24 (juvenile)	
Rimantadine	NA	NA	PO	100–200 mg total[d]	24 (juvenile)	5–7
				200–300 mg total[d]	24 (adult)	5–7
Acyclovir	5% cutaneous ointment	Zovirax (Burroughs Welcome)	Topical	1 cm/25 cm² area	8–12	prn
	200 mg capsules, 500 mg/vial		PO	50–100 mg (total)[d]	5–6	7
	powder for IV injection		IV IV	80 mg/m² 5–12.5[d]	8 8	7 10–14
Ganciclovir	NA	NA	IV	2–5[d]	8	14–30
Ribavirin	6 g/100 ml vial powder	Virazole (ICN Pharmaceuticals)	PO, IV[e]	330–500 mg total[d]	8	10
Trifluridine	1% ophthalmic solution	Viroptic (Burroughs Welcome)	Topical, IV	1.5 (2.9 mg/kg)[d]	4–8 (4)	prn
IFN-α2b	3 × 10⁶ IU/vial[f]	Intron A (Schering)	SC, IM	3 × 10⁶ IU (total)[d, g]	24	112–168
IFN-α2a	3 × 10⁶ IU/vial	Roferon-A (Roche)	SC, IM	3 × 10⁶ IU (total)[d, g]	24	112–168
Zidovudine[h]	100 mg capsules	Retrovir (Burroughs Welcome)	PO	10–20	12–24	42
Suramin	1 g vial powder	Centers for Disease Control, Atlanta, GA	IV	1 g (total)[d]	Once weekly	prn

[a]IU = international units, NA = not available, SC = subcutaneous, IM = intramuscular, IV = intravenous, PO = oral, IFN = interferon.
[b]Dose per administration at specified interval, expressed as mg/kg unless otherwise stated.
[c]Given as continuous drip for 12–24 hours.
[d]Human doses.
[e]Over 8–18 hour period daily.
[f]Stronger strengths also available.
[g]Diluted in sterile albumin preparations, IFN-α has been given orally to feline leukemia virus–infected cats at a dose of 1 U/animal/day (see also text).
[h]Azidothymidine.

effects include CNS toxicity, nausea, and vomiting in people, although dogs have been given high daily doses for over 2 years without ill effects. Rimantadine, a closely related analog of amantadine, has equal or greater efficacy with reduced CNS side effects but more GI irritation. However, it is not currently licensed for use in the United States.

ACYCLOVIR

This acyclic purine nucleoside is more potent in vitro against certain herpesviruses than idoxuridine and vidarabine and is becoming the agent of choice for treating herpesvirus infections.[1] In its unique antiviral mechanism, it is metabolized by viral-directed enzymes of infected cells to an intermediate that inhibits viral DNA polymerase. Because it interferes only with actively replicating virus, it does not cure latent viral infections. It is not metabolized by uninfected cells and is not toxic to cellular DNA. It has been used parenterally, orally, and topically in people for the treatment of genital and mucocutaneous herpesviral infections and parenterally in people and experimental animals for the treatment of herpesviral encephalitis.[2] It has also been given to cats.[2a] Systemic chemotherapy in people is most effective for genital infections. CSF concentrations are approximately 50% of plasma values. It is incompletely absorbed when administered orally, and more than 45% of the dose appears in the urine unmetabolized. Excretion of the drug is delayed in renal failure.

Acyclovir has a relatively low toxicity because it selectively interferes with viral DNA synthesis. However, when given parenterally or orally, it may precipitate in the renal tubules, causing obstructive nephropathy if diuresis is inadequate. This renal failure is reversible with adequate rehydration. IV administration may produce phlebitis and local irritation. It has potential benefits for treatment of herpesviral infections in domesticated animals. A number of derivatives have been synthesized that have potent antiviral activity.[1] One, 6-deoxyacyclovir, is well absorbed orally and is converted to acyclovir in the body. The main advantage of its use is the high dosage levels achieved with oral dosing. Ganciclovir, another structural analog, has activity against all the herpesviruses. Its effect, again, is highly specific for viral-infected cells. It is an investigational drug that has been given only IV. Resistance of human herpesviruses to acyclovir and ganciclovir has been reported.[2b, 2c]

Bromovinyl deoxyuridine is a halogenated thymidine analog with a similar mechanism of action as acyclovir. It has relatively low toxicity and increased antiviral activity as compared with acyclovir.

RIBAVIRIN

Ribavirin is a broad-spectrum triazole nucleoside that has marked in vitro antiviral activity against a variety of DNA and RNA viruses. It primarily interferes with protein synthesis, and in animal studies, its strongest antiviral activity is against RNA respiratory viruses and herpesviruses. Ribavirin has been effective in treating people with Lassa fever, an arenavirus infection,[3] and people with human immunodeficiency virus (HIV) infection.[4] It is marketed and has been used for aerosol therapy of people with respiratory syncytial viral infection.[5] By the aerosol route, only low concentration appears in the systemic circulation, whereas concentration in the respiratory secretions can be much higher when it is given orally. Although not currently marketed for oral use in humans, it has been given orally to cats experimentally infected with calicivirus.[6] Treated cats have had increased severity of clinical illness, depressed bone marrow, weight loss, increased hepatic enzymes, and icterus. None of these abnormalities were found in beagle dogs given 60 mg/kg of ribavirin for 2 weeks,[6a] although nonregenerative anemia develops in people and other animals given similar dosages. Side effects may limit the systemic use of ribavirin in veterinary practice.

TRIFLURIDINE

Trifluridine (trifluorothymidine), a synthetic nucleoside, blocks DNA synthesis through inhibiting enzyme production by becoming incorporated in the structural framework of the viral nucleic acid. When given systemically, it causes many toxic side effects, including leukopenia and GI signs. It has been used most often as a topical agent to treat ocular herpesviral infections.

INTERFERONS

Interferons are polypeptide molecules produced by vertebrate cells in response to viral infections or certain inert substances, such as double-stranded RNA, and other microbial agents. There are at least three types of interferon: α-interferon (IFN-α), formerly leukocyte interferon; β-interferon (IFN-β), formerly fibroblast interferon; and γ-interferon (IFN-γ). IFN-α and IFN-β are structurally similar and are produced in response to viral infections or polyribonucleotide administration. IFN-γ is structurally distinct, being produced by T lymphocytes in response to specific antigenic stimulus. Human IFN-α has been manufactured by recombinant DNA technology and is commercially available for clinical use (Table 15–1). Interferons have been marketed for treatment of hairy cell leukemia. IFN-γ has been cloned, which will allow large scale production in the future.

Interferons bind to specific cell receptors that activate enzymes that in turn inhibit synthesis, assembly, and release of virus.

They are not virucidal but merely inhibit viral nucleic acid and protein synthesis. Interferons are not species-specific in their effects, although their biologic activity is greater in cells of genetically related species. They are active against many DNA and RNA viruses, although the in vitro sensitivities vary. Myxoviruses are susceptible, whereas adenoviruses are not. Interferons have been shown to inhibit oncogenic transformation induced by retroviruses.

Interferons are usually given IM and IV, whereas intranasal and oral administration of these drugs is not widely accepted. Approximately 80% is absorbed after IM injection. They are not absorbed topically and are inactivated when administered in body fluids. Interferon is usually administered parenterally. Clearance from the circulation is rapid, occurring within 4 hours, and penetration into CSF, brain, and eye is poor.[7] Although interferons are cleared rapidly, their antiviral activity persists. Given intracisternally, their activity lasts for up to 24 hours.

Human IFN-α has been given orally in low doses (0.5 or 5 U/day) and has been beneficial in ameliorating the clinical course of feline leukemia virus–positive cats when given simultaneously with experimental inoculation of virus (see Table 15–1).[8] Treated cats had improved survival rates, less weight loss, and increased appetite compared with untreated cats, although there was no effect on the viremia.

In people, interferons given parenterally at high dosages have shown some efficacy against infections such as influenza, rhinoviruses, herpesviruses, and papilloma viruses. Interferons have been given topically, intranasally, and ocularly to control rhinovirus respiratory and papilloma virus infections.

Side effects of IFN-α, which occur within 2 to 4 hours after parenteral administration, include fever, nausea, vomiting, and myalgia. Hematologic alterations include leukopenia, thrombocytopenia, and reticulocytopenia with high dosages and relatively impure preparations.

REVERSE TRANSCRIPTASE INHIBITORS

In an attempt to control the retroviruses affecting people and animals, a number of compounds that interfere with RNA-dependent polymerase (reverse transcriptase) have been evaluated. Distamycin A and netropsin bind to single-stranded viral DNA. Rifamycins, streptovaricin, and alkaloids bind to the viral enzyme. Oligothymidylate derivatives, vinyl analogs and Poly C are template-primer analogs.

Zidovudine (azidothymidine, AZT), an inhibitor of reverse transcriptase, shows the most promise in treatment of retroviral (AIDS) infection in people. It is 100 times more active against HIV-transcriptase than mammalian cell DNA-polymerases. It has activity against other mammalian retroviruses in addition to HIV. AZT has been shown to be somewhat effective in treating cats experimentally infected with feline leukemia virus when treatment is initiated before 3 weeks after infection.[9, 10] When treated before 1 week after challenge, cats are protected from bone marrow infection and persistent viremia. If the infection is already established, there may be some reduction in the amount of antigen in the blood with therapy, although viremia persists. The probability of infection is reduced when treatment is initiated soon after infection and when higher doses of zidovudine are used.

AZT can be given orally or IV. Following oral administration, it is rapidly absorbed from the GI tract. It has a short serum half-life and is rapidly metabolized by the liver and excreted by the kidney. It has wide tissue distribution, including the CNS. Bone marrow suppression is the major side effect. Other adverse effects include fever, malaise, GI signs, myalgia, and rash.

SURAMIN

This derivative of naphthalene trisulfonic acid is an antiparasitic agent used to treat African trypanosomiasis. In addition, it inhibits viral reverse transcriptase. It is not absorbed orally, but because it is too painful when given IM, it must be given IV. It is highly protein bound and has a prolonged serum half-life. It does not enter the CNS or CSF and is primarily renally excreted. Its use has been associated with a high degree of side effects such as fever, proteinuria, azotemia, myelosuppression, and hepatotoxicity. Although it has been shown to inhibit feline leukemia virus in tissue culture, it has not been effective in treating infected cats. It suppresses HIV viremia but has no effect on reversing immunologic deficits.

PHOSPHONOFORMIC ACID

This pyrophosphate analog (foscarnet) has a wide spectrum of effect against DNA and RNA viruses. It is administered IV and continuously because of its short half-life. Most of the drug is eliminated from tissues and excreted in urine. It accumulates in bone matrix, but penetration of the blood-brain barrier is controversial. It has been used in treating HIV infection, but significant nephrotoxicity has limited its use. Certain herpesvirus infections in people, resistant to acyclovir, have been treated successfully with foscarnet.[11]

References

1. Laskin OL: Acyclovir, pharmacology and clinical experience. Arch Intern Med 144:1241–1246, 1984.
2. Whitley RJ, Alford CA, Hirsch MS: Vidarabine versus acyclovir therapy in herpes simplex encephalitis. N Engl J Med 314:144–149, 1986.
2a. Hirschberger J: Administration of acyclovir to cats. Tierarztl Prax 16:427–430, 1988.
2b. Erlich KS, Mills J, Chatis P, et al: Acyclovir-resistant herpes simplex virus infections in patients with acquired immunodeficiency syndrome. N Engl J Med 320:293–296, 1989.
2c. Erice A, Chou S, Biron KK, et al: Progressive disease due to ganciclovir-resistant cytomegalovirus in immunocompromised patients. N Engl J Med 320:289–293, 1989.
3. McCormick JB, King IJ, Webb PA, et al: Lassa fever, effective therapy with ribavirin. N Engl J Med 314:20–26, 1986.
4. Reines ED, Gross PA: Antiviral agents. Med Clin North Am 72:691–715, 1988.
5. Hall CB, Walsh EE, Hruska JF, et al: Ribavirin treatment of experimental respiratory syncytial viral infection. JAMA 249:2666–2670, 1983.
6. Povey RC: Effect of orally administered ribavirin on experimental feline calicivirus infection in cats. Am J Vet Res 39:1337–1341, 1978.
6a. Canonico PG: Efficacy, toxicity and clinical application of ribavirin against virulent RNA viral infections. Antiviral Res (Suppl)1:75–81, 1985.
7. Cantell K, Pyhala L: Pharmacokinetics of human leukocyte interferon. J Infect Dis 133(Suppl):A6–A12, 1976.
8. Cummins J, Tomplins M, Olsen R, et al: The oral use of human interferons in cats. J Biol Response Mod 7:513–523, 1988.
8a. Turner RB, Durcan FJ, Albrecht JK, et al: Safety and tolerance of ocular administration of recombinant alpha interferon. Antimicrob Agents Chemother 33:396–397, 1989.
9. Macy DW: Management of the FeLV-positive patient. In Kirk RW (ed): Current Veterinary Therapy X. Philadelphia, WB Saunders Co, 1989, pp 1069–1076.
10. Tavares L, Roneker C, Johnston K, et al: 3'azido-3-deoxythymidine in feline leukemia virus–infected cats: a model for therapy and prophylaxis of AIDS. Cancer Res 47:3190–3194, 1987.
11. Chatis PA, Miller CH, Schrager LE, et al: Successful treatment with foscarnet of an acyclovir-resistant mucocutaneous infection with herpes simplex virus in a patient with acquired immunodeficiency syndrome. N Engl J Med 320:297–300, 1989.

16

CANINE DISTEMPER

Craig E. Greene
Max J. Appel

ETIOLOGY

Canine distemper virus (CDV) is a member of the genus *Moribillivirus* of the Paramyxoviridae and is closely related to measles and rinderpest viruses. CDV is relatively large (150 to 250 nm) with single-stranded RNA wound in helical symmetry. It is surrounded by a lipoprotein envelope derived from viral glycoproteins incorporated into the cell membrane. Viruses such as CDV that code for proteins capable of integrating in the cell membrane make infected cells susceptible to damage by immune-mediated cytolysis. CDV also may induce cellular fusion as a means of direct intercellular spread.

CDV is susceptible to UV light, although protein or antioxidants help to protect it from inactivation. Extremely susceptible to heat and drying, CDV is destroyed by temperatures greater than 50° to 60°C for 30 minutes. However, it survives for at least an hour at 37°C and is viable at room temperature (20°C) in tissue suspensions for 3 hours and in exudates for at least 20 minutes.[1] In warm climates, CDV does not persist in kennels after infected dogs have been removed. Storage and survival times of CDV are longer at colder temperatures. At near-freezing temperatures (0° to 4°C), it survives in the environment for weeks. Below freezing the virus is stable, surviving at −65°C for at least 7 years. Lyophilization reduces the lability of the virus and is an excellent means of preserving it for commercial vaccines and laboratory use.

CDV remains viable between pH of 4.5 and 9.0. As an enveloped virus it is susceptible to ether and chloroform, dilute (<0.5%) formalin solutions, phenol (0.75%), and quaternary ammonium disinfectants (0.3%). Use of routine disinfection procedures is usually effective in destroying CDV in a kennel or hospital.

The disease and natural host ranges of CDV include certain species of terrestrial carnivores (see Table 2–9), and various other species can be infected experimentally. A virus indistinguishable from CDV has caused severe morbidity in seals and porpoises and may have spread to them from dogs or other susceptible carnivores.[2, 3, 3a] CNS signs have been produced in mice and hamsters by intracerebral inoculation. Rabbits and rats are resistant to parenteral inoculation. Inapparent, self-limiting infections, produced in cats, nonhuman primates, and humans by parenteral inoculation of virulent CDV, resemble those in dogs that have been given modified live virus (MLV) vaccines. Pigs infected with the virus develop bronchopneumonia.[4] Recently, CNS infections in exotic Felidae have been attributed to infection with CDV (see Feline Paramyxovirus Encephalomyelitis, Chapter 29). Similarly, a naturally infected nonhuman primate was reported to have developed encephalitis.[4a]

EPIDEMIOLOGY

CDV, most abundant in respiratory exudates, is commonly spread by aerosol exposure; however, it can be isolated from other body tissues and secretions, including urine. Virus can be excreted up to 60 to 90 days following infection, although shorter periods of shedding are more typical. Contact between recently infected (subclinical or diseased) animals maintains the virus in a population, and a constant supply of puppies helps to provide a susceptible population for infection. Although immunity to canine distemper is prolonged, it is not necessarily solid or lifelong. Dogs that do not receive periodic immunization may lose their protection and become infected following stress, immunosuppression, or contact with diseased individuals. The infection rate is higher than the disease rate, which reflects a certain degree of natural and vaccine-induced immunity in the general dog population. Estimates are that between 25% and 75% of susceptible dogs become subclinically infected but clear the virus from the body without showing signs of illness.

The prevalence rate of spontaneous distemper in cosmopolitan dogs is greatest between 3 to 6 months of age, correlating with the loss of maternal antibodies in puppies following weaning. In contrast, in susceptible, isolated populations of dogs, the disease is severe and widespread, affecting all ages. Increased susceptibility among breeds has been suspected but not proved. Brachiocephalic dogs have been reported to have a lower incidence of disease, mortality, and sequelae compared with dolichocephalic breeds. Breeds most commonly and severely affected include greyhounds, Siberian huskies, Weimaraners, Samoyeds, and Alaskan malamutes.

Viral virulence is another parameter that may affect the severity and extent or type of clinical disease. Certain isolates, such as Snyder Hill or R252 strain, are highly virulent and neurotropic. Others vary in ability to cause CNS lesions.

PATHOGENESIS

Systemic Infection

During natural exposure, CDV spreads by aerosol droplets and contacts epithelium of the upper respiratory tract (Fig. 16–1). Within 24 hours, it multiplies in tissue macrophages and spreads in these cells via local lymphatics to tonsils and bronchial lymph nodes.[5] By 2 to 4 days postinoculation (PI), virus numbers increase in tonsils and retropharyngeal and bronchial lymph nodes, but low numbers of CDV-infected mononuclear cells are found in other lymphoid organs. By days 4 to 6 PI, virus multiplication occurs within lymphoid follicles in the spleen; in the lamina propria of the stomach and small

intestines; in the mesenteric lymph nodes; and in Kuppfer's cells in the liver. Widespread virus proliferation in lymphoid organs corresponds to an initial rise in body temperature and leukopenia. The leukopenia is primarily a lymphopenia caused by viral damage to lymphoid cells, affecting both T and B cells.[6]

Further spread of CDV to epithelial and CNS tissues on days 8 to 9 PI probably occurs hematogenously, as a cell-associated and plasma-phase viremia, and depends on the dog's humoral and cell-mediated immune status. By day 14 PI, animals with adequate CDV antibody titers and cell-mediated cytotoxicity clear the virus from most tissues and show no clinical signs of illness.[7] Specific IgG-CDV antibody has been shown to be effective in neutralizing extracellular CDV as well as in inhibiting its intercellular spread.[8]

Dogs with intermediate levels of cell-mediated immunoresponsiveness with delayed antibody titers by days 9 to 14 PI have virus spread to their epithelial tissues. Clinical signs that develop may eventually resolve as antibody titer increases. Virus is cleared from most body tissues as antibody titers increase but may persist for extended periods as complete virus in uveal tissues, neurons, and integument such as foot pads. Spread and persistence of virus in these tissues may be responsible for delayed CNS signs and digital hyperkeratosis (hard pads) that occur in some dogs.

Dogs with poor immune status by days 9 to 14 PI undergo virus spread to many tissues, including skin, exocrine and endocrine glands, and epithelium of the GI, respiratory, and genitourinary tracts. Clinical signs of disease in these dogs are usually dramatic and severe, and virus usually persists in their tissues until death. The sequence of pathogenetic events depends on the virus strain and may be delayed by 1 to 2 weeks.

Studies on serologic response to CDV in gnotobiotic dogs confirm that serum antibody titers vary inversely with the severity of the disease. Antibody response in dogs has been separated into envelope and core determinants of the virus. Only dogs producing anti-envelope antibodies appear to be able to ward off persistent infection of the CNS with CDV. To be predictive of recovery, tests for virus neutralizing antibody must be done for IgG rather than IgM and must be done in other than dog lung

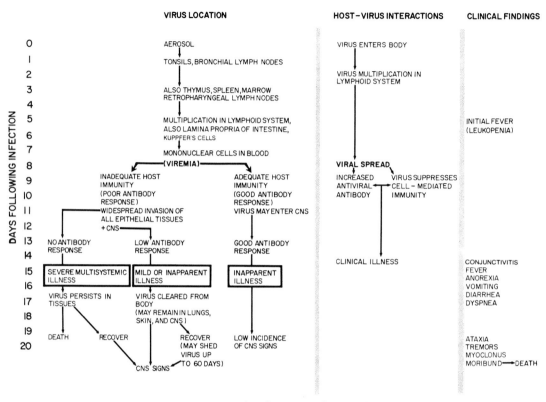

Figure 16–1. Sequential pathogenesis of canine distemper.

macrophages.[8, 9] Mortality in gnotobiotic dogs approaches that of naturally infected animals, de-emphasizing the role of secondary bacterial infection in influencing the severity of CNS disease; however, bacteria are probably important in complicating the signs of disease in the respiratory and GI tracts.

CNS Infection

As previously discussed, the spread of virus to the CNS depends upon the degree of systemic immune responses mounted by the host. Virus probably enters the nervous system of many viremic CDV-infected dogs whether or not neurologic signs are observed. Antiviral antibody and resultant immune-complex deposition may facilitate the spread of virus to vascular endothelium in the CNS.[9a] Virus, either free or platelet- and leukocyte-associated, may enter vascular endothelial cells in the meninges, choroid plexus epithelial cells of the fourth ventricle, and ependymal cells lining the ventricular

system.[9b] Viral antigen is first detected in CNS capillary and venular endothelium and perivascular astrocytic foot processes.[9c] The infection of choroid plexus epithelium has been shown to be productive throughout the course of infection, in that virus is continually being produced.[10] From these sites, free or lymphocyte-associated virus may enter the CSF, where it spreads to periventricular and subpial structures. Spread of virus through CSF pathways probably explains the frequent distribution of lesions in subependymal areas such as the cerebral cortex (primarily archicortex and paleocortex), optic tracts and nerves, rostral medullary velum, cerebral peduncles, and spinal cord.

The type of lesion produced and the course of infection within the CNS depend upon a number of factors, including the age and immunocompetence of the host at the time of exposure and the neurotropic and immunosuppressive properties of the virus. Different viral strains have been shown to produce variable severity and location of lesions within the CNS.[11] Either acute or chronic encephalitis can occur independently, or acute-phase lesions may progress to those of the chronic form in animals that survive.

Acute encephalitis, which occurs early in the course of infection in young or immunosuppressed animals, is characterized by direct neuronal infection and necrosis. White matter lesions, characterized by myelin damage, are secondary to neuronoaxonal degeneration rather than to primary demyelination. Inflammatory changes are minimal, presumably because of immunodeficiency resulting from the physiologic immaturity of the immune system and viral-induced immunosuppression or because of the early phase of illness being studied.

In contrast, infections in slightly older or immunocompetent puppies or in later phases of disease are characterized by nonsuppurative encephalomyelitis with segmental internodal primary demyelination.[12] Noninflammatory demyelination in early lesions appears to be associated with viral infection of astroglial rather than oligodendroglial cells, with secondary edema and myelin degeneration.[13, 13a, 13b]

Chronic distemper encephalitis is probably a progression of the acute lesion that develops in immunocompetent hosts that survive initial infection. Immunologic recovery in infected dogs usually corresponds to the development of chronic encephalitis and is characterized by more severe and nonselective demyelination and perivascular mononuclear cell infiltration. Research has clarified the pathogenesis of demyelination in this chronic inflammatory phase of encephalomyelitis. Increased concentration of antimyelin antibodies, which have been found in dogs with chronic encephalomyelitis, is more likely a secondary reaction to the inflammatory process.[14] Intrathecal administration of antimyelin antibodies to dogs in the absence of CDV infection can produce demyelination and subsequent perivascular inflammation. However, the lesions of allergic encephalomyelitis in dogs sensitized to myelin have been shown to be substantially different from distemper.[15] Myelin damage and corresponding inflammatory cell infiltration in chronic distemper encephalitis appear to correlate with increased intrathecal virus-neutralizing antibodies and the immunopathologic response by the body to the virus.[16, 17] If viral spread through the CNS has been extensive by the time the host responds to the virus, then widespread damage occurs. Still, certain areas of virally infected brain tissue are spared the inflammatory process, presumably because of noncytolytic infections or reduced expression of CDV proteins on the surface of inflammatory cells, both of which have been identified in cell culture.[18, 19] Viral antigen is no longer detected in the CNS of dogs that recover or have static neurologic deficits, but it persists in those suffering from chronic progressive encephalitis.[18, 20]

Bilaterally symmetric ischemic necrosis of the pyriform cortex, hippocampus, and deep temporal lobe structures has been characterized as a specific form of distemper encephalitis.[21] Selective polioencephalomalacia involving these particular CNS structures can be explained by the relatively high blood flow with hematogenous entry of virus, susceptibility to hypoxia caused by seizures, or the mode of spread of virus into the CNS along CSF pathways. Vascular lesions produced from the inflammatory process also may be involved.

CLINICAL FINDINGS

Systemic Signs

Clinical signs of canine distemper vary, depending on virulence of the virus strain, environmental conditions, and host age and immune status. More than 50% to 70% of CDV infections are probably subclinical. Mild forms of clinical illness are also common, with signs including listlessness, decreased appetite, fever, and upper respiratory tract infections. Bilateral serous oculonasal discharge can become mucopurulent with coughing and dyspnea. Many mildly infected dogs develop clinical signs that are indistinguishable from those due to other causes of "kennel cough" (see Chapter 19). Keratoconjunctivitis sicca may develop following systemic or subclinical infections in dogs. Persistent anosmia was reported as a sequela in dogs that had recovered from canine distemper.[21a]

Severe generalized distemper is the commonly recognized form of the disease. It can occur in dogs of any age with poor immune status but most commonly affects unvaccinated, exposed puppies 12 to 16 weeks of age that have lost their maternal immunity or younger puppies that received inadequate concentrations of maternal antibody. The initial febrile response in natural infections is probably unnoticed. The first sign of infection is a mild, serous-to-mucopurulent conjunctivitis (Fig. 16–2), which is followed within a few days by a dry cough that rapidly becomes moist and productive. Increased lower respiratory sounds from the thorax can be heard upon auscultation. Depression and anorexia are followed by vomiting that is commonly unrelated to eating. Diarrhea subsequently develops, varying in consistency from fluid to frank blood and mucus. Tenesmus can be present and intussusceptions may occur. Severe dehydration and emaciation can result from adipsia and fluid loss. Animals can die suddenly from systemic illness, but adequate therapy in many cases can reduce the mortality rate.

Neurologic Signs

These manifestations usually begin 1 to 3 weeks after recovery from systemic illness; however, there is no way to predict which dog will develop neurologic disorders. On an empirical basis, certain features of the systemic disease can be predictive of the incidence of neurologic sequelae. Impetiginous dermatitis in puppies is rarely associated with CNS disease, while dogs developing nasal and digital hyperkeratosis usually have various neurologic complications (Figs. 16–3 and 16–4). Mature or immune dogs can develop neurologic signs without prior history of systemic disease.

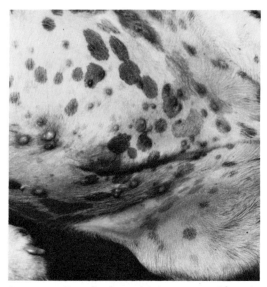

Figure 16–3. Pustular dermatitis in a puppy with canine distemper. Rarely associated with neurologic complications, this is usually a favorable prognostic sign.

Neurologic signs, whether acute or chronic, are typically progressive. Chronic relapsing neurologic deterioration with intermittent recovery and a later superimposed acute episode of neurologic dysfunction was reported in a dog.[21b]

Neurologic complications of canine distemper are the most significant factors concerning prognosis and recovery from infection. Neurologic signs vary according to the area of the CNS involved. Hyperesthesia and cervical rigidity can be found as a result of meningeal inflammation. Seizures, cerebellar and vestibular signs, paraparesis or tetra-

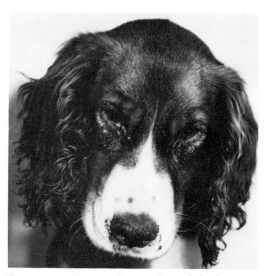

Figure 16–2. Mucopurulent oculonasal discharge in a dog with systemic distemper.

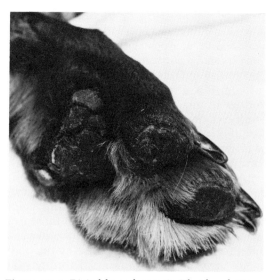

Figure 16–4. Digital hyperkeratosis ("hard pads") in a dog dying of distemper encephalomyelitis.

paresis with sensory ataxia, and myoclonus are common. Seizures can be of any type, depending upon the region of the forebrain that is damaged by the virus. The "chewing gum" type of seizures, classically described for CDV infection, often occurs in dogs developing polioencephalomalacia of the temporal lobes. However, lesions from other causes in the same region can produce similar seizures.

Myoclonus, the involuntary twitching of muscles in a forceful simultaneous contraction, can be present in the absence of other neurologic signs. It reflects irritation of the particular lower motor neuron segment involved. With more extensive spinal cord damage, there may be upper motor neuron paresis of the affected limb associated with myoclonus. The rhythmic contractions can be present while the dog is awake or, commonly, while it is sleeping. The neural mechanisms for myoclonus originate with local irritation of the lower motor neurons of the spinal cord or cranial nerve nuclei. Although considered specific for CDV infection, myoclonus can also be seen in other paramyxovirus infections of the dog and cat (see Chapter 29).

Transplacental Infection

Young puppies infected transplacentally may develop neurologic signs during the first 4 to 6 weeks of life.[22] Mild or inapparent infections are seen in the bitch. Depending on the stage of gestation at which infection occurred, abortions, stillbirths, or the birth of weak puppies may be noted. Puppies that survive such infections may suffer from permanent immunodeficiencies.[23]

Neonatal Infections

Young puppies infected with CDV prior to the eruption of permanent dentition may have severe damage to the enamel of their teeth. An irregular appearance may be noted (Fig. 16–5). Enamel hypoplasia may be present as an incidental finding in an older dog, with or without neurologic signs and is relatively pathognomonic for prior infection with CDV.

Neonatal (<7 days old) gnotobiotic puppies have developed viral-induced cardiomyopathy following experimental infection

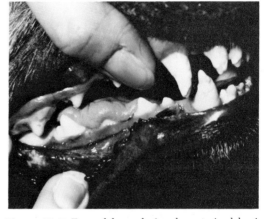

Figure 16–5. Enamel hypoplasia, characterized by irregularities in the dental surface, in an older dog that survived neonatal distemper.

with CDV.[24] Clinical signs, including dyspnea, depression, anorexia, collapse, and prostration, developed between days 14 to 18 PI. Lesions were characterized by multifocal myocardial degeneration, necrosis, and mineralization, with minimal inflammatory cell infiltration. The clinical significance of this process following natural infection is uncertain at the present time. Whether there is a relationship to onset of adult cardiomyopathy in dogs remains to be determined.

Ocular Signs

Dogs with CDV encephalomyelitis often have a mild anterior uveitis that is clinically asymptomatic.[25] More obvious ophthalmologic lesions in canine distemper have been attributed to an effect of the virus on the optic nerve and the retina (see also Canine Distemper, Chapter 13). Optic neuritis can be characterized by a sudden onset of blindness, with dilated, unresponsive pupils. Degeneration and necrosis of the retina produce gray-to-pink irregular densities on the tapetal or nontapetal fundus or both. Bullous or complete retinal detachment can occur where exudates dissect between the retina and choroid. Chronic inactive fundic lesions are associated with retinal atrophy and scarring. These are circumscribed, hyperreflective areas termed gold medallion lesions, which are considered characteristic of previous canine distemper infection.

DIAGNOSIS

Clinical diagnosis of canine distemper is primarily based on clinical suspicion. A characteristic history of a 3- to 6-month-old, unvaccinated puppy is supportive. Dogs with severe disease in most cases have clinical signs distinctive enough to make the diagnosis. Missed are the large number of upper respiratory infections in older dogs that are labeled infectious tracheobronchitis. Specific laboratory tests are not always available to confirm the suspicion of CDV infection, and the practicing veterinarian must instead rely on nonspecific findings of routine laboratory procedures.

Clinical Laboratory Findings

Abnormal hematologic findings include an absolute lymphopenia caused by lymphoid depletion that is viral-strain dependent. This frequently persists in very young dogs with rapidly progressive systemic or neurologic signs. Thrombocytopenia (as low as 30,000 cells/μl) and a regenerative anemia have been found in experimentally infected neonates (<3 weeks) but have not been consistently recognized in older or spontaneously infected dogs. Distemper inclusions can be detected on examination of stained peripheral blood films, in low numbers in circulating lymphocytes, and with even less frequency in monocytes, neutrophils, and erythrocytes. Inclusions in lymphocytes stained with Wright-Leishman stain are large

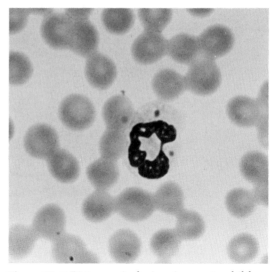

Figure 16–7. Distemper inclusions in a neutrophil from a peripheral blood film (Wright's stain; × 1000). (Courtesy of Dr. Ken Latimer, University of Georgia, Athens, GA.)

(up to 3 μm), singular, oval, gray structures, whereas erythrocytic inclusions, most numerous in polychromatophilic cells, are round and eccentrically placed and appear light blue (Figs. 16–6 and 16–7).[26] Erythrocytic inclusions are intermediate in size between metarubricyte nuclei and Howell-Jolly bodies. Buffy coat and bone marrow examination and use of phloxinophilic stains can improve the chances of detecting inclusions. Electron microscopy has confirmed that these inclusions consist of paramyxovirus-like nucleocapsids.

The magnitude and type of serum biochemistry changes in acute systemic infection are nonspecific. Total protein analysis includes decreased albumin and increased α- and γ-globulin concentration in non-neonates. Marked hypoglobulinemia has been found in puppies infected prenatally or neonatally with CDV from persistent immunosuppression caused by the virus.[23]

Radiology

Thoracic radiography demonstrates an interstitial lung pattern in early cases of distemper. An alveolar pattern is seen with secondary bacterial infection and more severe bronchopneumonia (Figs. 16–8).

CSF

Abnormalities are detectable in dogs with neurologic signs of distemper; however,

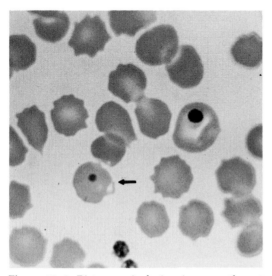

Figure 16–6. Distemper inclusion in an erythrocyte from a peripheral blood film *(arrow)*. Compare its appearance with that of a Howell-Jolly body (Wright's stain; × 1000). (Courtesy of Dr. O. W. Schalm, deceased, formerly of University of California, Davis, Davis, CA.)

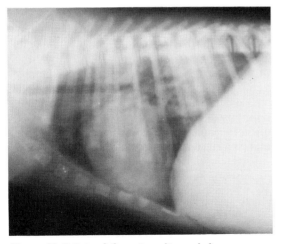

Figure 16–8. Lateral thoracic radiograph from a puppy with canine distemper bronchopneumonia.

false-negative results can be anticipated. The CSF may flow more rapidly than normal during collection because of increased intracranial pressure caused by inflammation. Increases in protein (>25 mg/dl) and cell count (>10 cells/μl with a predominance of lymphocytes) have been characteristic. Increased protein in CSF has been identified primarily as IgG with specific anti-CDV activity.[27, 28] Differences in the humoral immune response in CSF and sera to the H and F envelope proteins have been noted between some dogs with chronic progressive encephalitis, as compared with other forms of distemper encephalitis.[29] Increased anti-CDV antibody in CSF offers definitive evidence for distemper encephalitis because antibody is locally produced, and these increases have not been present in vaccinated dogs or those with systemic distemper without CNS disease.[29a, 29b] CSF antibody may be artifactually increased owing to traumatic collection procedure causing contamination by whole blood. Although the test for CSF antibodies is sensitive and specific for canine distemper, it can be performed only by properly equipped diagnostic or research laboratories (see Appendix 8).

Immunocytology

Immunofluorescent techniques have added a new dimension to the specific diagnosis of canine distemper; however, these tests also require special equipment and are usually run by regional diagnostic laboratories. In clinically affected dogs, immunofluores-cence is usually performed on cytologic smears prepared from conjunctival, tonsillar, and respiratory epithelium. Smears should be made on precleaned slides, air-dried thoroughly, and preferably fixed in acetone for 5 minutes prior to transport to the laboratory. At the laboratory, they are stained directly or indirectly with fluorescein-conjugated CDV antibody and examined by fluorescent microscopy.

Antigen, first detected in buffy coat smears from 2 to 5 days PI, decreases as antibody titer increases by 8 to 9 days PI. Since clinical signs are becoming apparent shortly after this time (day 14), positive results would not be recognized except in dogs that do not mount a sufficient immune response and succumb to infection. Positive fluorescence in conjunctival and genital epithelium is usually detected only within the first 3 weeks PI, at a time when systemic illness is apparent. Virus also disappears in these tissues after the first 1 to 2 weeks of clinical illness (21 to 28 days PI) as antibody titers rise in association with clinical recovery. Beginning with the recovery stage, antibody may bind and mask antigen in infected cells. Consequently false-negative results will be obtained. Virus can sometimes be detected for longer periods of time in epithelial cells and macrophages from the lower respiratory tract and transtracheal washings can be obtained for diagnosis. Virus also persists for periods of at least 60 days in the skin, uveal tissues, foot pad, and CNS. Direct fluorescent antibody examination of cells in CSF or blood films is helpful in acute phases of illness but in chronic cases is usually unrewarding because antibody coating of viral antigen interferes with diagnostic immunofluorescence. Foot pad biopsy has been recommended as a premortem diagnostic technique.

Fluorescent antibody techniques can also be performed on frozen sections of biopsy or necropsy specimens. Tissues collected from dogs that died from distemper should include spleen, tonsils, lymph nodes, stomach, lung, duodenum, bladder, and brain. Animals dying of generalized infection frequently have abundant quantities of virus in these tissues. Fluorescent antibody techniques can also be adapted to paraffin-embedded sections if special cold (4°C) ethanol (95%) fixation is used.[30]

An immunoperoxidase technique, developed for histologic detection of distemper antigen in formalin-fixed and paraffin-embedded tissues,[31] has also been applied to ultrastructural localization of CDV antigens within cells.[32] Similarly, nucleic acid hybridization studies, using single-stranded RNA probes, have been used to detect virus in tissue sections.[32a]

Immunologic Testing

A microneutralization method has further simplified the use of neutralizing antibody testing in diagnostic laboratories. The more sensitive ELISA has been used to detect serum IgG and IgM antibodies to CDV.[33, 34] Increased titers of serum IgM neutralizing antibody can be measured in dogs that survive the acute phase of infection. Although detection of IgM is specific for recent infection with CDV, this test is cumbersome and must be performed by specialized laboratories. Increased serum IgG titers are ambiguous and can indicate either recent, past, or present infection with or vaccination for distemper virus. Analysis of CSF-specific IgG is more reliable in detecting chronic progressive CDV infections of the nervous system (see CSF).

Cell-mediated immunosuppression has been documented following CDV infection. Lymphocyte transformation testing of experimentally infected neonates has shown profound depression of lymphocyte response to phytomitogens at a time corresponding to acute viremia and lymphopenia.[6] This depressed response persisted for more than 10 weeks in convalescing puppies and never returned to baseline values in those that died acutely. Prenatal and neonatal distemper infections are causes of immunodeficiency in surviving puppies. Immunosuppression caused by CDV may make concurrent infections by other viruses such as parvovirus more virulent.

Viral Isolation

Isolation of virulent CDV has been difficult in routine cell cultures. The most successful viral replication occurs during direct cultivation of target tissues of lymphocytes and macrophages from the infected host. Alveolar macrophage cultures detect the virus in 24 to 48 hours. Giant cell (syncytia) formation is a characteristic cytopathic effect of CDV in many tissue cultures. Giant cell formation is detected within 2 to 5 days, at which time the virus can be isolated by overlays made on other cells. Growth in pulmonary macrophages was once considered an essential feature of virulent CDV isolates; however, virulent CDV was isolated in bovine kidney cell and primary bladder epithelial cell cultures without the need for adaptation or loss of virulence of the virus.[35] Cultures can be examined for virus with fluorescent antibody when cytopathic effects are not observed within 48 to 72 hours PI.

PATHOLOGIC FINDINGS

Young dogs prenatally or neonatally infected with CDV usually have thymic atrophy. Pneumonia and catarrhal enteritis are present in older puppies with systemic disease (Fig. 16–9). Upper respiratory tract lesions include conjunctivitis, rhinitis, and inflammation of the tracheobronchial tree. Hyperkeratosis of the nose and foot pads is common in dogs suffering from neurologic disease. Gross lesions in the CNS are minimal except for occasional meningeal congestion, ventricular dilation, and increased CSF pressure due to brain edema.

A typical histologic finding in dogs with systemic illness is lymphoid depletion. Diffuse interstitial pneumonia is characterized by thickened alveolar septa and proliferation of alveolar epithelium. Alveoli contain desquamated epithelial cells and macrophages; transitional epithelium of the urinary system

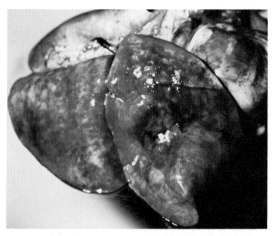

Figure 16–9. Gross appearance of lungs from a puppy with canine distemper bronchopneumonia. An antero-ventral distribution of lesions is more characteristic than the diffuse pattern observed here.

is swollen. Puppies developing distemper may have defects in enamel of the teeth, and necrosis and cystic degeneration of ameloblastic epithelium are usually present. Ophthalmic lesions are described in Chapter 13.

In acute fatal encephalitis of neonates, neuronal and myelin degeneration or primary demyelination can occur without significant perivascular inflammation. In surviving animals, patchy areas of necrosis are replaced by hypertrophic astrocytes that form a network for macrophages ingesting myelin. The most severe white matter changes in the CNS can be found in the lateral cerebellar peduncles, the dorsolateral medulla adjacent to the fourth ventricle, and the deep cerebellar white matter. Lesions are also present in the midbrain, basal ganglia, and temporal lobes of the cerebral cortex. Superficial areas such as the optic tracts, crus cerebri, cranial nerve pathways, and infundibulum also can be affected.

Lesions in older dogs or in those surviving to develop chronic ("old dog") encephalitis are characterized by widespread perivascular lymphoplasmacytic infiltration in areas of demyelination and neuronal degeneration. In more chronic cases, the lesion may progress to sclerosing panencephalitis characterized by infiltration and replacement of nervous tissue by a dense astrocytic network.

On histologic examination, CDV inclusions are most commonly cytoplasmic and acidophilic staining. They are 1 to 5 μm in diameter and can be found in epithelial cells of mucous membranes, reticulum cells, leukocytes, glia, and neurons. Inclusions can be found up to 5 to 6 weeks PI in the lymphoid system and urinary tract. Intranuclear inclusions are most common in lining or glandular epithelium and ganglion cells.

The morphologic significance of distemper inclusions is not completely understood. Histochemically, they are composed of aggregates of viral nucleocapsids and cellular debris as a result of viral infection. Caution must be used when absolutely confirming a diagnosis of canine distemper based on the presence of inclusions alone. Cytoplasmic inclusions typical for CDV infection have been identified in the urinary bladder of normal dogs. Unfortunately, inclusion bodies not only are nonspecific but may appear too late in the disease to be routinely useful. On the other hand, use of inclusion bodies alone to detect CDV infection can lead to a false-negative diagnosis in dogs as compared with more sensitive immunocytochemical methods for CDV detection in tissues that have been developed.[31, 36]

Formation of giant cells primarily in CNS white matter, anterior uvea of the eye, and secondarily in lymph nodes, lung and leptomeninges is peculiar to paramyxoviruses such as CDV and can be used to substantiate CDV infection.[37]

THERAPY

Despite vast advances in research on canine distemper, only minor changes have been made in therapeutic recommendations. Aims in treatment, while supportive and nonspecific, are frequently beneficial in that mortality is reduced. The only reason for refusing to initiate treatment at an owner's insistence is the presence of neurologic signs that are incompatible with life. Even in the absence of neurologic signs, owners should always be warned that neurologic sequelae may develop at a later time. The spontaneous improvement seen in many dogs with symptomatic management of non-neurologic systemic distemper has fostered inappropriate credits to the success of certain treatment regimens. However, unlike the systemic signs, neurologic signs in themselves are not usually reversible and frequently are progressive.

Dogs with upper respiratory infections should be kept clean, warm, and free of drafts. Oculonasal discharges should be cleaned from the face. Pneumonia is frequently complicated by secondary bacterial infection, usually with *Bordetella bronchiseptica*, which requires the use of broad-spectrum antibiotic therapy. Good initial antibiotic choices for bronchopneumonia include ampicillin, tetracycline, and chloramphenicol (Table 16–1). However, because of dental staining, tetracycline must be avoided in puppies. Parenteral therapy is essential when gastrointestinal signs are present. Antimicrobial therapy should be altered when dictated by susceptibility testing based on transtracheal washing or when there is a lack of response to the initial antibiotics used.

Food and water should be discontinued if vomiting and diarrhea are present. Supplementation with polyionic isotonic fluids such as lactated Ringer's solution should be

Table 16–1. Drug Therapy for Canine Distemper[a]

DRUG	DOSE[b] (mg/kg)	ROUTE	INTERVAL (hours)	DURATION (days)
Antimicrobial				
Amp(amox)icillin	20	PO, IV, SC	8	7
Tetracycline[c]	22	PO, IV	8	7
Chloramphenicol	15–25	PO, SC	8	7
Cephapirin	10–30	IM, IV, SC	6–8	3–5
Anticonvulsive				
Phenobarbital	1–2	PO, IV, IM	12	prn
Anti-inflammatory				
Dexamethasone				
CNS edema	1–2	IV	24	1
Optic neuritis[d]	0.1–0.2	PO	24	3–5

[a]PO = oral, IV = intravenous, SC = subcutaneous, IM = intramuscular, prn = as needed.
[b]Dose per administration at specified interval, expressed as mg/kg unless otherwise stated.
[c]Avoid in dogs less than 6 months of age because of dental staining.
[d]Equivalent glucocorticoid dosage of prednisolone in mg/kg is five times this dose.

given IV or SC, depending on the hydration status of the patient. B vitamins should be administered to replace those lost from anorexia and diuresis and to stimulate the appetite nonspecifically. Historically, benefits have been described with administration of IV ascorbic acid; however, its use is controversial and without proven efficacy.

Therapy for neurologic disturbances in canine distemper is less rewarding. Progressive multifocal encephalitis usually leads to tetraplegia, semicoma, and incapacitation so great that euthanasia should be recommended. Despite ineffective therapy, dogs should not be euthanatized unless the neurologic disturbances are progressive or incompatible with life. There may be variable or temporary success in halting neurologic signs in some dogs with single anti–CNS edema doses of dexamethasone.

Seizures, myoclonus, or optic neuritis are three neurologic manifestations in dogs that can be tolerated by many owners. Myoclonus is untreatable and irreversible; many forms of therapy have been attempted without success. Recommendations have been made to administer anticonvulsants after the onset of systemic disease but prior to the development of seizures. No evidence shows that anticonvulsants prevent entry of the virus into the CNS; however, they may suppress irritable foci from causing seizures, which, in turn, may prevent seizure circuits from becoming established. Glucocorticoid therapy at anti-inflammatory dosages may have variable success in controlling the blindness and pupillary dilation caused by optic neuritis.

PREVENTION

Chapter 2 and Appendices 1 and 3 should be consulted for overall recommendations on vaccination for canine distemper. The following discussion describes features that are unique to protection against this disease. Immunity to CDV infection is considered long-term, and lasting immunity and immunologic homogeneity of the virus have made disease prevention possible through vaccination. Maternal antibodies, received both in utero and in colostrum from the dam, block adequate immunization in puppies for a period of time after birth and weaning, respectively. Maternal antibody to CDV decreases with a half-life of 8.4 days. Three percent of antibody transfer for CDV occurs in utero and 97% in the colostrum, resulting in an initial titer in nursing newborn puppies that is usually equal to 77% of that in the bitch (see Tables 2–2, 2–3, and 2–4). In the absence of ingestion of colostrum, the puppy is probably protected for at least 1 to 4 weeks.[1, 38] In nursing puppies, nomograms based on the bitch's titer can be used to determine when immunization should be done, although this is not routinely practical. Vaccines for CDV are given every 3 to 4 weeks between 6 to 16 weeks of age in puppies that have received colostrum.

Following a single distemper vaccination, naive puppies do not generally develop immunity that lasts at least 1 year. For this reason, despite the lack of maternal antibody interference, at least two distemper vaccines should be given at 2- to 4-week intervals in first presentation of colostrum-deprived neonates or in dogs older than 16 weeks of age. Similarly, and because older vaccinated dogs can still develop distemper, periodic boosters are recommended for this disease, despite the relatively long-lived immunity afforded by vaccination.

Humoral immune mechanisms do not totally explain resistance to canine distemper. IV vaccination with attenuated virus appears to protect dogs when it is given prior to or within 4 days of exposure to virulent distemper virus.[39] Because of allergic reactions that may develop, use of canine adenovirus-1 and leptospiral antigens should be avoided with IV vaccination. This rapid protection against distemper may relate to immune interference, interferon, or cell-mediated immune mechanisms. Despite a decrease in antibody titer, immunity to distemper following booster or anamnestic vaccination is known to last as long as 7 years, as demonstrated in isolated challenged dogs.[1] The duration of protection is much greater than that predicted from antibody titer alone and also demonstrates that challenge with virulent organisms is more meaningful than neutralizing antibody titer for predicting the duration of immunity.

Inactivated canine distemper vaccines do not produce sufficient immunity to prevent illness following challenge exposure, but vaccinates show an anamnestic immunity response and less severe disease as compared with unvaccinated controls.[40] Although inactivated whole-virus vaccines have been unsuccessful, purified fusion (F) antigen, a surface glycoprotein of CDV, has been used to protect dogs against subsequent experimental challenge with virulent virus.[41] Similarly, an inactivated subunit vaccine containing membrane F antigen and a hemagglutinating glycoprotein (H) modified into immune stimulating complexes (ISCOMs) has been effective in protecting dogs from challenge by virulent virus.[42] Similar inactivated vaccines have been used to protect seals against infection with phocine distemper virus.[41a]

Despite the success with subunit vaccine, MLV vaccines are presently used to protect dogs against CDV; however, vaccine-induced immunity is never as long-lasting as the immune response that occurs following natural or experimental infection with virulent virus. Required use of MLV vaccines for distemper has led to questions concerning both vaccine stability and safety.

Vaccine Stability

Viability of canine distemper vaccines is an important consideration with respect to vaccination failures. Lyophilized tissue-culture vaccines are stable for 16 months under refrigeration (0° to 4°C), 7 weeks at 20°C and 7 days when exposed to sunlight at 47°C. When reconstituted, tissue culture virus remains stable for 3 days at 4°C and 24 hours at 20°C. Therefore, vaccine should be used immediately once it is reconstituted for injection or refrigerated if the delay until usage will be longer than an hour.

Postvaccinal Complications

Efficacy and safety of MLV-distemper vaccination in dogs with compromised immune systems are important considerations. Dogs on folic acid deficient diets and methotrexate therapy had no response to MLV distemper vaccine. Although the vaccine virus could be isolated from the lymphoid system, no postvaccinal signs or epithelial tissue infection was detected.[1] In contrast, dogs receiving one dose of antithymocyte serum in conjunction with methotrexate for 5 days developed systemic and neurologic signs of vaccine-induced distemper.[43]

Unlike virulent virus, MLV does not appear to suppress cell-mediated immunity. Modified live vaccine viruses have not reverted to virulence under natural conditions and do not spread to other dogs. However, reversion to virulence has been experimentally demonstrated in attenuated vaccine virus passed serially in dogs and ferrets or in pulmonary macrophages in tissue culture. Vaccine-induced distemper infections have been reported in numerous exotic carnivores, including the lesser panda, black-footed ferrets, and gray foxes. Postvaccinal distemper can be prevented in ferrets by using chick embryo rather than canine cell–propagated vaccines.[44, 44a, 44b]

Encephalitis has been reported in dogs following vaccination with MLV distemper vaccines (see Postvaccinal Encephalomyelitis, Chapter 2). CDV vaccine–induced encephalomyelitis has been documented in 3-week-old puppies simultaneously infected with virulent canine parvovirus;[45] however, similar findings could not be reported in 11- to 15-week-old puppies.[46]

Vaccine Interference

Adverse environmental influences can affect the response to distemper vaccination in dogs. High humidity (85% to 90%) and high temperature that caused dogs to have rectal temperatures averaging 39.8°C (103.6°F) reduced the immune response following distemper vaccination.[47]

Dogs subjected to anesthesia (barbiturate induction with halothane maintenance) followed by surgery were studied for their response to distemper vaccination.[48] There was no demonstrable impairment in the humoral antibody response to vaccination, although challenge studies were not performed. There was some depression of the peripheral blood lymphocyte response to phytohemagglutinin.

Glucocorticoid therapy, given at immunosuppressive dosages for 3 weeks, did not suppress the normal humoral response to distemper vaccine, although treated dogs developed depressed responses to phytohemagglutinin stimulation of lymphocytes.[49] These dogs also survived subsequent challenge with virulent CDV.

Concurrent parvoviral infection has been suspected in reducing the antibody response of dogs vaccinated against canine distemper.[50] Simultaneous vaccination against parvoviral infection was suspected of inhibiting the response of dogs to vaccination against CDV infection, although adequate control data were lacking[51] and this has not been substantiated in older dogs.[46] For a further discussion of canine parvovirus–induced immunologic interference with CDV vaccination, the reader should consult Chapters 2 and 21.

Measles Vaccination

Canine distemper and human measles viruses are antigenically related, and experimental infection of dogs with measles virus protected dogs from subsequent infection with CDV. Distemper virus antibody titers are minimally elevated following measles vaccination despite adequate protection. Cell-mediated immunity and other factors are thought to be the primary factor involved in the protective response. Measles vaccine virus produces a self-limiting, noncontagious infection in the lymphoid system of dogs similar to that of MLV-CDV vaccines.

There is probably little danger of reversion to virulence and probably no danger to humans when proper vaccination procedures are followed. Only measles vaccines licensed for use in dogs (not human products) should be used by veterinarians. Higher antigen mass in canine products is required owing to the heterologous nature of this product.

Measles vaccination offers the theoretic advantage of protection in young puppies with high concentrations of maternal antibodies to distemper.[52] It should only be used as a replacement for the first vaccination in 6- to 12-week old puppies. Dogs younger than 6 weeks of age with very high maternal antibody concentrations do not respond well to either distemper or measles vaccination. If female puppies are vaccinated with measles vaccine after 12 weeks of age, passive transfer of measles antibody will occur to their offspring, especially if they are bred on the first heat cycle.

Immunity to distemper acquired from measles vaccination is not only transient but weaker than that derived from a successful vaccination with MLV distemper vaccine.[9] SC inoculation of measles vaccine is not as effective as the initially recommended IM route. However, puppies over 6 weeks of age immunized with measles virus vaccine are protected within 72 hours from challenge with CDV. During an initial vaccination series, measles vaccination alone or in combination with distemper vaccination should be followed by at least two distemper vaccinations to produce adequate long-term immunity of at least 12 months' duration.[52]

Environmental Control

CDV is extremely susceptible to commonly used disinfectants. Infected animals are the primary source of the virus, and they should be segregated from other healthy dogs. Dogs usually shed the virus in secretions for 1 to 2 weeks following the acute systemic illness. Those recovering from systemic illness or with later developing neurologic signs (without systemic disease) may still be shedding some virus.

PUBLIC HEALTH CONSIDERATIONS

Multiple sclerosis (MS) is a neurologic affliction of humans that resembles both subacute sclerosing panencephalitis (SSPE, an encephalitis of humans thought to be caused by a chronic infection with defective or latent measles virus) and chronic progressive distemper encephalitis in dogs. Both of the latter diseases are pathologically similar, with demyelination, glial proliferation, and other findings characteristic of a chronic persistent nonsuppurative encephalitis. The cause of MS is still uncertain, but evidence has focused on an association with human measles virus. This speculation is based on elevated serum and CSF antibody titers to measles virus in MS patients. It is proposed that a persistent or latent measles infection might result in this disease. Attention has been directed at the possibility that canine distemper virus might cause MS. An excellent review of the literature on this subject has been provided.[53] Several reports have made an epidemiologic association between MS patients and previous dog ownership or contact and the incidence of canine distemper in local dogs. Cross-reactivity between antibody to canine distemper and measles viruses makes cautious interpretation of immunologic studies necessary. Based on current evidence, there is no proof that canine distemper is associated with MS.[54, 55] A better case can be made for the relationship between measles virus and MS patients. A positive association has been found between MS in people having measles at a later than usual age.[56]

Chronic distemper encephalitis of dogs appears to be analogous to SSPE in humans. Studies have shown that an incompletely replicating measles virus or a measles-like paramyxovirus can be isolated from affected SSPE patients,[57] and that this agent can produce similar neurologic signs following intracerebral inoculation in dogs.[58] However, the exact relationship of this agent to measles and canine distemper viruses is presently being determined. Although the measles-like virus isolated from humans with SSPE is defective and requires co-cultivation techniques for its isolation, the CDV in dogs with chronic progressive encephalomyelitis can be more readily detected in and isolated from brain tissue because of its complete replication during chronic CNS infection.[59]

A suggestion has been made that Paget's disease, an inflammatory bone disorder in people, might be related to CDV acquired from exposure to dogs.[60] Evidence has accumulated that the disease may be caused by chronic paramyxovirus infection of osteoclasts. Ownership of dogs was found to have a high correlation with Paget's disease patients, although the indirect relationship between these factors should not be overstated.[61]

References

1. Appel M, Gillespie JH: Canine distemper virus. *In* Gard S, Hallauer C, Meyer KF (eds): *Virology Monographs, II.* New York, Springer-Verlag, 1972, pp 1–96.
2. Distemper found in Soviet seals in April. *New Scientist* 119:29, 1988.
3. Osterhaus AD, Vedder EJ: Identification of virus causing recent seal deaths. *Nature* 335:20, 1988.
3a. Kennedy S, Smyth JA, Cush PF, et al: Viral distemper now found in porpoises. *Nature* 336:21, 1988.
4. Appel M, Sheffy BE, Percy DH, et al: Canine distemper virus in domesticated cats and pigs. *Am J Vet Res* 35:803–806, 1974.
4b. Yoshikawa Y, Ochikubo F, Matsubara Y, et al: Natural infection with canine distemper virus in a Japanese monkey *(Macaca fuscata). Vet Microbiol* 20:193–205, 1989.
5. Appel M: Pathogenesis of canine distemper. *Am J Vet Res* 30:1167–1182, 1969.
6. Krakowka S, Higgins RJ, Koestner A: Canine distemper virus: review of structural and functional modulations in lymphoid tissues. *Am J Vet Res* 41:284–292, 1980.
7. Appel MJG, Shek WR, Summers BA: Lymphocyte-mediated immune cytotoxicity in dogs infected with virulent canine distemper virus. *Infect Immun* 37:592–600, 1982.
8. Winters KA, Mathes LE, Krakowka S, et al: Immunoglobulin class response to canine distemper virus in gnotobiotic dogs. *Vet Immunol Immunopathol* 5:209–215, 1984.
9. Appel MJG, Mendelson SG, Hall WM: Macrophage Fc receptors control infectivity and neutralization of canine distemper virus–antibody complexes. *J Virol* 51:643–649, 1984.
9a. Krakowka S, Cork LC, Winkelstein JA, et al: Establishment of central nervous system infection by canine distemper virus: breach of the blood-brain barrier and facilitation by antiviral antibody. *Vet Immunol Immunopathol* 17:471–482, 1987.
9b. Krakowka S: Canine distemper virus infectivity of various blood fractions for central nervous system vasculature. *J Neuroimmunol* 21:75–80, 1989.
9c. Axthelm M, Krakowka S: Canine distemper virus: the early blood-brain barrier lesion. *Acta Neuropathol (Berl)* 75:27–33, 1987.
10. Higgins RJ, Krakowka SG, Metzler AE, et al: Experimental canine distemper encephalomyelitis in neonatal gnotobiotic dogs. A sequential ultrastructural study. *Acta Neuropathol (Berl)* 57:287–295, 1982.
11. Summers BA, Greisen HA, Appel MJG: Canine distemper encephalomyelitis: variation with virus strain. *J Comp Pathol* 94:65–75, 1984.
12. Higgins RJ, Krakowka SG, Metzler AE, et al: Primary demyelination in experimental canine distemper virus induced encephalomyelitis in gnotobiotic

dogs. Sequential immunologic and morphologic findings. *Acta Neuropathol (Berl)* 58:1–8, 1982.

13. Vandevelde M, Zurbriggen A, Dumas M, et al: Canine distemper virus does not infect oligodendrocytes in vitro. *J Neurol Sci* 69:133–137, 1985.

13a. Summers BA, Appel MJ: Demyelination in canine distemper encephalomyelitis: an ultrastructural study. *J Neurocytol* 16:871–881, 1987.

13b. Mutinelli F, Vandevelde M, Groit C, et al: Astrocytic infection in canine distemper virus–induced demyelination. *Acta Neuropathol (Berl)* 77:333–335, 1988.

14. Vandevelde M, Higgins RJ, Kristensen B, et al: Demyelination in experimental canine distemper virus infection: immunological, pathological, and immunohistological studies. *Acta Neuropathol (Berl)* 56:285–293, 1982.

15. Summers BA, Greisen HA, Appel MJG: Canine distemper and experimental allergic encephalomyelitis in the dog: comparative patterns of demyelination. *J Comp Pathol* 94:575–589, 1984.

16. Bollo E, Zurbriggen A, Vandevelde M, et al: Canine distemper virus clearance in chronic inflammatory demyelination. *Acta Neuropathol (Berl)* 72:69–73, 1986.

17. Vandevelde M, Zurbriggen A, Steck A, et al: Studies on the intrathecal humoral immune response in canine distemper encephalitis. *J Neuroimmunol* 11:41–51, 1986.

18. Kimoto T: In vitro and in vivo properties of the virus causing natural canine distemper encephalitis. *J Gen Virol* 67:487–503, 1986.

19. Zurbriggen A, Vandevelde M, Dumas M: Secondary degeneration of oligodentrocytes in canine distemper virus infection in vitro. *Lab Invest* 54:424–431, 1986.

20. Vandevelde M, Zurbriggen A, Higgins RJ, et al: Spread and distribution of viral antigen in nervous canine distemper. *Acta Neuropathol (Berl)* 67:211–218, 1985.

21. Finnie JW, Hooper PT: Polioencephalomalacia in dogs with distemper encephalitis. *Aust Vet J* 61:407–408, 1984.

21a. Myers LT, Hanrahan LA, Swango LJ, et al: Anosmia associated with canine distemper. *Am J Vet Res* 49:1295–1297, 1988.

21b. Higgins RJ, Child G, Vandevelde M: Chronic relapsing demyelinating encephalomyelitis associated with persistent spontaneous canine distemper virus infection. *Acta Neuropathol (Berl)* 77:441–444, 1988.

22. Krakowka S, Hoover EA, Koestner A, et al: Experimental and naturally occurring transplacental transmission of canine distemper virus. *Am J Vet Res* 38:919–922, 1977.

23. Stevens DR, Osburn BI: Immune deficiency in a dog with distemper. *J Am Vet Med Assoc* 168:493–498, 1976.

24. Higgins RJ, Krakowka S, Metzler AE, et al: Canine distemper virus–associated cardiac necrosis in the dog. *Vet Pathol* 18:472–486, 1981.

25. Summers BA, Greisen HA, Appel MJG: Does virus persist in the uvea in multiple sclerosis, as in canine distemper encephalomyelitis? *Lancet* 2:372–375, 1983.

26. McLaughlin BG, Adams PS, Cornell WD, et al: Canine distemper viral inclusions in blood cells of four vaccinated dogs. *Can Vet J* 26:368–372, 1985.

27. Cutler RWP, Averill DR: Cerebrospinal fluid gamma globulins in canine distemper encephalitis. *Neurology* 19:1111–1114, 1969.

28. Imagawa DT, Howard EB, Van Pelt LF, et al: Isolation of canine distemper virus from dogs with chronic neurological diseases. *Proc Soc Exp Biol Med* 164:355–362, 1980.

29. Rima BK, Baczko K, Imagawa DT, et al: Humoral immune response in dogs with old dog encephalitis and chronic distemper meningoencephalitis. *J Gen Virol* 68:1723–1735, 1987.

29a. Johnson GC, Fenner WR, Krakowka S: Production of immunoglobulin G and increased antiviral antibody in cerebrospinal fluid of dogs with delayed-onset canine distemper viral encephalitis. *J Neuroimmunol* 17:237–251, 1988.

29b. Potgieter LND, Ajidagba PA: Quantitation of canine distemper virus and antibodies by enzyme-linked immunosorbent assays using protein A and monoclonal antibody capture. *J Vet Diagn Invest* 1:110–115, 1989.

30. Kristensen B, Vandevelde M: Immunofluorescence studies of canine distemper encephalitis on paraffin-embedded tissue. *Am J Vet Res* 39:1017–1021, 1978.

31. Miry C, Ducatelle R, Thoonen H, et al: Immunoperoxidase study of canine distemper virus pneumonia. *Res Vet Sci* 34:145–148, 1983.

32. Higgins RJ, Krakowka S, Metzler AE, et al: Immunoperoxidase labeling of canine distemper virus replication cycle in Vero cells. *Am J Vet Res* 43:1820–1824, 1982.

32a. Mitchell NJ, Russell SE, Clark DK, et al: Identification of negative strand and positive strand RNA of canine distemper virus in animal tissues using single stranded RNA probes. *J Virol Methods* 18:121–131, 1987.

33. Noon KF, Rogul M, Binn LN, et al: Enzyme-linked immunosorbent assay for evaluation of antibody to canine distemper virus. *Am J Vet Res* 41:605–609, 1980.

34. Bernard SL, Shen DT, Gorham JR: Antigen requirements and specificity of enzyme-linked immunosorbent assay for detection of canine IgG against canine distemper viral antigens. *Am J Vet Res* 43:2266–2269, 1982.

35. Bui HD, Tobler LH, Van Pelt LF, et al: Canine bladder epithelial cells in culture: susceptibility to canine distemper and measles viruses. *Am J Vet Res* 43:1268–1270, 1982.

36. Axthelm MK, Krakowka S: Immunocytochemical methods for demonstrating canine distemper virus antigen in aldehyde-fixed paraffin-embedded tissue. *J Virol Methods* 13:215–229, 1986.

37. Summers BA, Appel MJG: Syncytia formation: an aid in the diagnosis of canine distemper encephalomyelitis. *J Comp Pathol* 95:425–435, 1985.

38. Krakowka S, Long D, Koestner A: Influence of transplacentally acquired antibody on neonatal susceptibility to canine distemper virus in gnotobiotic dogs. *J Infect Dis* 137:605–608, 1978.

39. Appel M: Canine distemper. *In* Kirk RW (ed): *Current Veterinary Therapy VI*. Philadelphia, WB Saunders, 1977, pp 1308–1313.

40. Appel MJG, Shek WR, Shesberadaran H, et al: Measles virus and inactivated canine distemper virus induce incomplete immunity to canine distemper. *Arch Virol* 82:73–82, 1984.

41. Norrby E, Utter G, Orvell C, et al: Protection against canine distemper virus in dogs after immunization with isolated fusion protein. *J Virol* 58:536–541, 1986.

41a. Osterhaus AD, Uytdehaag FG, Visser IK, et al: Seal vaccination success. *Nature* 337:21, 1989.

42. De Vries P, Uytdehaag FGC, Osterhaus ADME: Canine distemper virus (CDV) immune-stimulating complexes (iscoms), but not measles virus iscoms, protect dogs against CDV infection. *J Gen Virol* 69:2071–2083, 1988.

43. Slater EA: The response to measles and distemper virus in immuno-suppressed and normal dogs. *J Am Vet Med Assoc* 156:1762–1766, 1970.

44. Davidson M: Canine distemper virus infection in the domestic ferret. *Compend Cont Educ Pract Vet* 8:448–453, 1986.

44a. Appel MJG, Harris WV: Antibody titers in domestic ferret jills and their kits to canine distemper virus vaccines. *J Am Vet Med Assoc* 193:332–333, 1988.

44b. Gill JM, Hartley WJ, Hodgkinson NL: An outbreak of post-vaccinal suspected distemper-like encephalitis in farmed ferrets (*Mustela putorius furo*). *NZ Vet J* 36:173–176, 1988.

45. Krakowka S, Olsen RG, Axthelm M, et al: Canine parvoviruses potentiate canine distemper encephalitis attributable to modified live-virus vaccine. *J Am Vet Med Assoc* 180:137–139, 1982.

46. Swango LJ: Frequently asked questions about CPV disease. *Norden News* 58:4–10, 1983.

47. Webster AC: The adverse effect of environment on the response to distemper vaccination. *Aust Vet J* 51:488–490, 1975.

48. Kelly GE, Webster AC: The effect of surgery in dogs on the response to concomitant distemper vaccination. *Aust Vet J* 56:556–557, 1980.

49. Nara PL, Krakowka S, Powers TE: Effects of prednisolone on the development of immune responses to canine distemper virus in beagle pups. *Am J Vet Res* 40:1742–1747, 1979.

50. Glickman LT, Appel MJ: Parvovirus infection and distemper vaccination. *J Am Vet Med Assoc* 178:1029–1031, 1981.

51. Kesel ML, Neil SH: Combined MLV canine parvovirus vaccine: immunosuppression with infective shedding. *VM SAC* 78:687–691, 1983.

52. Wilson JHG, Pereboom WJ, Leemans-Dessy S: Combined distemper-measles vaccine. *Vet Rec* 98:32–33, 1976.

53. Burridge MJ: Multiple sclerosis, house pets and canine distemper: critical review of recent reports. *J Am Vet Med Assoc* 173:1439–1444, 1978.

54. Parton D, Murray TJ, Love J: No increase in multiple sclerosis among veterinarians. *N Engl J Med* 305:894, 1981.

55. Anderson LJ, Kibler RF, Kaslow RA, et al: Multiple sclerosis unrelated to dog exposure. *Neurology* 34:1149–1154, 1984.

56. Sullivan CB, Visscher BR, Detels R: Multiple sclerosis and age at exposure to childhood diseases and animals: cases and their friends. *Neurology* 34:1144–1148, 1984.

57. Koestner A: Subacute sclerosing panencephalitis, multiple sclerosis animal model: distemper-associated demyelinating encephalomyelitis. *Am J Pathol* 78:361–364, 1975.

58. Notermans SLH, Tijl WFJ, Willems FTC, et al: Experimentally induced subacute sclerosing panencephalitis in young dogs. *Neurology* 23:543–553, 1973.

59. Hall WW, Imagawa DT, Choppin PW: Immunological evidence for the synthesis of all canine distemper virus polypeptides in chronic neurological diseases in dogs. Chronic distemper and old dog encephalitis differ from SSPE in man. *Virology* 98:283–287, 1979.

60. O'Driscoll JB, Anderson DC: Past pets and Paget's disease. *Lancet* 2:919–921, 1985.

61. Barker DJP, Detheridge FM: Dogs and Paget's disease. *Lancet* 2:1245, 1985.

17 INFECTIOUS CANINE HEPATITIS AND CANINE ACIDOPHIL CELL HEPATITIS

Craig E. Greene

Infectious Canine Hepatitis

ETIOLOGY

Infectious canine hepatitis (ICH), caused by canine adenovirus 1 (CAV-1), has worldwide serologic homogenicity, as well as immunologic similarities to human adenoviruses. It is antigenically and genetically distinct from canine adenovirus 2 (CAV-2), which produces respiratory disease in the dog (see Etiology and Pathogenesis, Chapter 19).[1] Genetic variants of CAV-2 have been isolated from the intestine of a puppy with hemorrhagic diarrhea[2] and from kenneled dogs with diarrhea.[2a]

As with other adenoviruses, CAV-1 is resistant to environmental inactivation, surviving disinfection with various chemicals such as chloroform, ether, acids, and formalin, and is also stable when exposed to certain frequencies of UV radiation. CAV-1 survives for days at room temperature on soiled fomites and remains viable for months at temperatures below 4°C. CAV-1 is inactivated after 5 minutes at 50° to 60°C, which makes steam cleaning a plausible means of disinfection. Chemical disinfection has also been successful when iodine, phenol, and sodium hydroxide are used.

CAV-1 causes clinical disease in dogs, foxes, and other Canidae and in Ursidae.[2b] The high prevalence of naturally occurring neutralizing antibodies in the unvaccinated dog population suggests that subclinical infection is widespread. CAV-1 has been isolated from all body tissues and secretions of dogs during the acute stages of the disease. By 10 to 14 days postinoculation (PI), it can be found only in the kidneys and is excreted in the urine for at least 6 to 9 months. Aerosol transmission of the virus via the urine is unlikely insofar as susceptible dogs housed 6 inches apart from virus shedders do not become infected. Viral spread can occur by contact with fomites, including feeding utensils and hands. Ectoparasites can harbor CAV-1 and may also be involved in natural transmission of the disease.

PATHOGENESIS

Following natural oronasal exposure, the virus initially localizes in the tonsils (Fig. 17–1), where it spreads to regional lymph nodes and lymphatics before reaching the blood through the thoracic duct. Viremia, which lasts 4 to 8 days PI, results in rapid dissemination of the virus to other tissues and body secretions including saliva, urine, and feces. Hepatic parenchymal cells and vascular endothelial cells of many tissues are prime targets of viral localization and injury.

Initial cellular injury of the liver, kidney, and eye is associated with cytotoxic effects of virus. A sufficient antibody response by

242

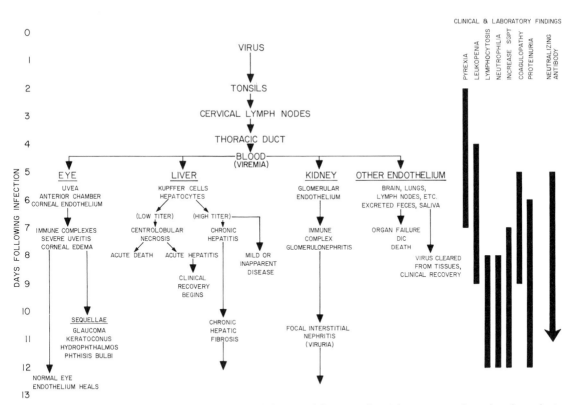

Figure 17–1. Sequential pathogenesis of ICH. Solid vertical bars on the right correspond to the chronologic occurrence of and the duration of the respective clinical or laboratory findings associated with ICH.

day 7 PI clears the virus from the blood and liver and restricts the extent of hepatic damage. Widespread centrolobular to panlobular hepatic necrosis is often fatal in experimentally infected dogs with a persistently low (<1:4) antibody titer.[3] Acute hepatic necrosis can be self-limiting and restricted centrolobularly, so that hepatic regeneration occurs in dogs that survive this phase of the disease. Dogs demonstrating a partial neutralizing antibody titer (>1:16, <1:500) by day 4 or 5 PI develop chronic active hepatitis and hepatic fibrosis. Persistent hepatic inflammation continues, probably as a result of chronic latent hepatic infection with virus.[4] Dogs with sufficient antibody titers (≥1:500) on the day of infection usually show little clinical evidence of disease. Dogs immune to parenteral challenge with CAV-1 are still susceptible to respiratory disease via aerosolized viral particles.

Both virulent and modified live strains of CAV-1 produce renal lesions.[5] Virus detected by positive immunofluorescence and ultrastructural evaluation initially localizes in the glomerular endothelium in the vi-

remic phase of disease and produces initial glomerular injury. An increase in neutralizing antibody at approximately 7 days PI is associated with the glomerular deposition of circulating immune complexes (CIC) and transient proteinuria. CAV-1 is not detected in the glomerulus after 14 days PI; however, it persists in renal tubular epithelium. Tubular localization of the virus is primarily associated with viruria, and only a transient proteinuria is noted. A mild focal interstitial nephritis is found in recovered dogs; however, unlike the liver disease, there is no evidence to suggest that chronic progressive renal disease results from ICH infection.[5]

Clinical complications of ocular localization of virulent CAV-1 occur in approximately 20% of naturally infected dogs and less than 1% of dogs following SC-MLV CAV-1 vaccination. The development of ocular lesions begins during viremia, which develops 4 to 6 days PI; the virus enters the aqueous humor from the blood and replicates in corneal endothelial cells.

Severe anterior uveitis and corneal edema develop 7 days PI, a period corresponding to an increase in neutralizing antibody titer. CIC deposition with complement fixation results in chemotaxis of inflammatory cells into the anterior chamber and extensive corneal endothelial damage. Disruption of the intact corneal endothelium causes accumulation of edematous fluid within the corneal stroma.

Uveitis and edema are usually self-limiting unless additional complications or massive endothelial destruction occur. Clearing of corneal edema coincides with endothelial regeneration and restoration of the hydrostatic gradient between the corneal stroma and aqueous humor. Normal recovery of the eye is usually apparent by 21 days PI. If the inflammatory changes are severe enough to block the filtration angle, increased intraocular pressure may result in glaucoma and hydrophthalmos.

Complications are often associated with the pathogenesis of ICH. Dogs are more prone to develop pyelonephritis due to renal damage following ICH infection. Disseminated intravascular coagulation (DIC), a frequent complication of ICH, begins in the early viremic phase of the disease and may be triggered by endothelial cell damage with widespread activation of the clotting mechanism or by the inability of the diseased liver to remove activated clotting factors. Decreased hepatic synthesis of clotting factors in the face of excessive consumption compounds the bleeding defect.

Although the cause of death in ICH is uncertain, the liver is a primary site of viral injury. Hepatic insufficiency and hepatoencephalopathy may result in a semicomatose state and death. Some dogs die so suddenly that liver damage with resulting hepatic failure does not have time to occur. Death in these dogs may result from damage to the brain, lungs, and other vital parenchymal organs or from the development of DIC.

CLINICAL FINDINGS

ICH is most frequently seen in dogs less than 1 year of age, although unvaccinated dogs of all ages can be affected. Peracutely affected dogs become moribund and die within a few hours after the onset of clinical signs. Owners frequently believe that their dog was poisoned. Clinical signs in dogs that survive the acute viremic period include vomiting, abdominal pain, and diarrhea with or without evidence of hemorrhage.

Abnormal physical findings in the early phase of infection include increased rectal temperature (39.4° to 41.1°C [103° to 106°F]) and accelerated pulse and respiratory rates. Fever may be transient or biphasic early in the course of the disease. Tonsillar enlargement, usually associated with pharyngitis and laryngitis, is common. Coughing and ausculted harsh lower respiratory sounds are manifestations of pneumonia. Cervical lymphadenopathy is frequently found with subcutaneous edema of the head, neck, and dependent portions of the trunk. Abdominal tenderness and hepatomegaly are usually apparent in the acutely ill dog. A hemorrhagic diathesis that is manifested by widespread petechial and ecchymotic hemorrhages, epistaxis, and bleeding from venipuncture sites may occur. Icterus is uncommon in acute ICH, but it is found in some dogs that survive the acute fulminant phase of the disease. Abdominal distention is caused by accumulation of serosanguine fluid or hemorrhage. CNS signs, including depression, disorientation, seizures, or terminal coma, may develop at any time following infection.

Clinical signs of uncomplicated ICH frequently last 5 to 7 days prior to improvement. Persistent signs may be found in dogs with a concurrent viral infection such as canine distemper or in those dogs that develop chronic active hepatitis.

Corneal edema and anterior uveitis usually occur when clinical recovery begins and may be the only clinical abnormalities seen in dogs with inapparent infection (also see Infectious Canine Hepatitis, Chapter 13). Dogs with corneal edema show blepharospasm, photophobia, and serous ocular discharge. Clouding of the cornea usually begins at the limbus and spreads centrally (Fig. 17–2). Ocular pain, present during the early stages of infection, usually subsides when the cornea becomes completely clouded. However, pain may return with the development of glaucoma or corneal ulceration and perforation. In uncomplicated cases, clearing of the cornea begins at the limbus and spreads centrally.

DIAGNOSIS

Early hematologic findings in ICH include leukopenia with lymphopenia and neutro-

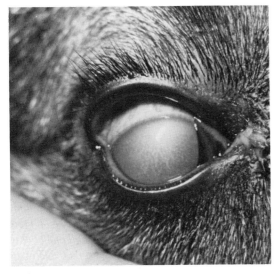

Figure 17–2. Complete clouding of the cornea ("blue eye") in a dog with ICH.

penia. Neutrophilia and lymphocytosis occur later in dogs with uncomplicated clinical recovery. Increased numbers of dark staining (activated) lymphocytes and nucleated erythrocytes may be found. Serum protein alterations, detectable only on serum electrophoresis, are a transient increase in α_2-globulin by 7 days PI and by a delayed increase in γ-globulin which peaks 21 days PI.[6]

The degree of increased activities of ALT (formerly SGPT), AST (formerly SGOT), and serum ALP depends on the time of sampling and the magnitude of hepatic necrosis. These enzyme increases gradually increase until day 14 PI, after which they decline, although persistent or recurrent elevations may be found in dogs that develop chronic active hepatitis. Moderate to marked bilirubinuria is frequently found owing to the low renal threshold for conjugated bilirubin in the dog; hyperbilirubinemia is uncommon. Sulfobromophthalein retention at 30 minutes may be increased during the acute course of ICH or later in dogs that develop chronic hepatic fibrosis. Hypoglycemia may be found in dogs in the terminal phases of the disease.

Coagulation abnormalities characteristic of DIC are most pronounced during the viremic stages of the disease. Thrombocytopenia with or without altered platelet function is usually apparent. One-stage prothrombin time (PT), activated partial thromboplastin time (APTT), and thrombin time (TT) are variably prolonged. Early prolongation of the APTT probably results from Factor VIII consump-

tion. Factor VIII activity is decreased, and fibrinogen degradation products (FDPs) are increased. Platelet dysfunction and later prolongation of the APTT probably result from increased FDPs. Prolongation of the PT is usually less noticeable.

Proteinuria (primarily albuminuria) is a reflection of the renal damage caused by the virus and can usually be detected on random urinalysis because the concentration is greater than 50 mg/dl. The increase in glomerular permeability can result from localization of the virus in initial stages of infection, or as the disease progresses, glomeruli become damaged by CICs or as an effect of DIC. Abdominal paracentesis yields a fluid that varies in color from clear yellow to bright red, depending on the amount of blood present. It is usually an exudate with a protein content ranging from 5.29 to 9.3 g/dl (specific gravity from 1.020 to 1.030).

Bone marrow cytology reflects the dramatic change in leukocytes in the peripheral circulation. Megakaryocytes are absent or decreased during the viremic stage of the disease, and those that are present may have altered morphology.

CSF is normal in dogs with neurologic signs caused by hepatoencephalopathy; it is usually abnormal in dogs that develop a nonsuppurative encephalitis from localization of the virus within the brain. There is an increase in protein concentration (>30 mg/dl) with mononuclear pleocytosis (>10 cells/mm^3). The aqueous humor also has increased concentrations of protein and cells associated with anterior uveitis.

Results of laboratory procedures previously discussed are all suggestive of ICH and are the primary means of making a diagnosis in clinical practice. Antemortem confirmation, although not essential for appropriate therapy, can be obtained by serologic testing, virus isolation, and immunofluorescent evaluation. Serologic tests include indirect hemagglutination, complement fixation, immunodiffusion, and ELISA.[7] ELISA tests usually show higher IgG titers following infection with virulent virus in contrast with MLV vaccines.

CAV-1 can be easily isolated because it readily replicates in cell cultures of several species, including dogs. Typical adenovirus-induced cytopathology includes clustering of host cells and detachment from the monolayers with the formation of intranuclear inclusions. When viremia begins, on day 5

PI, CAV-1 can be cultured from any body tissue or secretion. The virus is isolated in the anterior chamber during the mild phase of uveitis prior to antibody infiltration and immune-complex formation. It is often difficult to culture virus from the liver of dogs because hepatic arginase inhibits viral nucleic acid replication.[8] The virus has not been isolated from the liver later than 10 days PI, even in dogs with chronic active hepatitis, perhaps because viral latency develops. The kidney is the most persistent site of virus localization, and CAV-1 can be isolated from the urine for at least 6 to 9 months after the initial infection.

Immunofluorescent techniques are used experimentally to confirm the presence of virus within various tissues. This method has helped to locate the sites of viral replication, the spread of the virus within the cells, and the presence of viral antigen in inclusion bodies. Immunoperoxidase procedures, used on formalin-fixed, paraffin-embedded tissues, have detected virus in liver tissues stored for up to 6 years.[4] See Appendix 8 for a listing of available tests and the laboratories that perform them.

PATHOLOGIC FINDINGS

Findings on necropsy or biopsy examination of tissues from dogs can usually confirm a diagnosis of ICH. Dogs that die during the acute phase of the disease are often in good flesh, with edema and hemorrhage of superficial lymph nodes and cervical subcutaneous tissue. Icterus is not usually apparent. The abdominal cavity may contain fluid that varies in color from clear to bright red. Petechial and ecchymotic hemorrhages are present on all serosal surfaces. The liver is enlarged, dark, and mottled in appearance, and a prominent fibrinous exudate is usually present on the liver surface and in the interlobar fissures (Fig. 17–3). The gallbladder is thickened and edematous and has a bluish-white opaque appearance. Fibrin may be deposited on other abdominal serosal surfaces, giving them a ground glass appearance. Intraluminal GI hemorrhage is a frequent finding. The spleen is enlarged and bulges on the cut surface.

Variable gross lesions in other organs include multifocal hemorrhagic renal cortical infarcts. The lungs have multiple, patchy, gray-to-red areas of consolidation. Hemor-

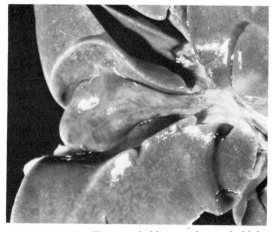

Figure 17–3. Swollen, mottled liver with rounded lobar edges and gallbladder edema characteristic of ICH.

rhagic and edematous bronchial lymph nodes are found. Scattered hemorrhagic areas, present on coronal section of the brain, are primarily located in the midbrain and caudal brain stem. Ocular lesions, when present, are characterized by corneal opacification and clouding of the aqueous humor.

Dogs surviving the acute phase of the disease may have lesions that can be found on subsequent necropsy examination. The liver of those with chronic hepatic fibrosis may be small, firm, and nodular. The kidneys of many dogs that recover are studded with multiple white foci (0.5 cm diameter), extending from the renal pelvis to the outer cortex. Ocular sequelae from the acute disease can include either glaucoma or phthisis bulbi.

Histologic changes in the liver of dogs that die of acute hepatitis include widespread centrolobular to panlobular necrosis. With mild hepatocellular necrosis, the margin between necrotic and viable hepatocytes is sharply defined within the liver lobule (Fig. 17–4). The preservation of the underlying support stroma allows for eventual hepatic regeneration. Only in severe cases does coagulation necrosis of entire hepatic lobules prevent regeneration of the liver. Neutrophilic and mononuclear cell infiltrates are associated with the removal of underlying necrotic tissue. Bile pigment rarely accumulates in most cases because of the transient nature of hepatocellular necrosis and the frequent lack of peripherolobular involvement of portal radicles. Intranuclear inclusions are initially found in Kupffer's cells and later in viable hepatic parenchymal cells.

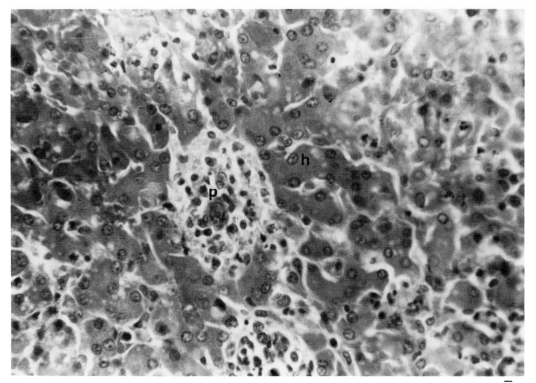

Figure 17–4. Histologic appearance of massive centrolobular necrosis in a fatal case of ICH, showing a few remaining viable hepatocytes (h) around a portal vein (p) in the peripheral lobular area (H and E; × 250).

Subacute to chronic hepatic disease is marked by sporadic foci of necrosis with neutrophilic, mononuclear, and plasma cell infiltration and is found in dogs with partial immunity that survive initial stages of infection.

Widespread histologic alterations occur in other organs as a result of endothelial injury caused by the virus. The gallbladder has marked subserosal edema, but the epithelium remains intact. Viral inclusions are first detected in the renal glomeruli but later are found in renal tubular vascular endothelium. Focal interstitial accumulations of neutrophils and mononuclear cells are found in the renal cortex and medulla. These mild changes often progress to focal interstitial fibrosis. Lymphoid organs, including the lymph nodes, tonsils, and spleen, are congested with neutrophilic and mononuclear cell infiltrates. Lymphoid follicles are dispersed with central areas of necrotic foci. Intranuclear inclusions are present in vascular endothelial cells and histiocytes. The lungs have thickened alveoli with septal cell and peribronchial lymphoid accumulations. Alveoli in consolidated areas are filled with an exudate consisting of erythrocytes, fibrin,

and fluid. Mucosal and submucosal edema with focal subserosal hemorrhage are found in the intestinal tract. Widespread vascular degeneration and tissue hemorrhage and necrosis is associated with the presence of intravascular fibrin thrombi.

Swollen, desquamated endothelial cells in meningeal vessels contain intranuclear inclusions. Mononuclear cuffing is present around small vessels throughout the parenchyma of the CNS. Mild endothelial proliferation and mononuclear perivascular infiltration persist for at least 3 weeks following clinical recovery.

Ocular changes are characterized by granulomatous iridocyclitis with corneal endothelial disruption and corneal edema. Iridial and ciliary vessels are congested with inflammatory cells that are also present in the iris and filtration angle.

The inclusion bodies seen in ICH have been classified as Cowdry type A and are present in both ectodermal and mesodermal tissues. That they are abundant in the liver makes this the most logical tissue for impression smears obtained by biopsy or at necropsy. Initial hypertrophy of the cell nucleus is followed by peripheral margination of the chromatin network and nucleolus, which forms a central, dark-staining nuclear remnant surrounded by a halo of chromatin (Fig. 17–5). The initial inclusions are acidophilic but become basophilic as the chromatin marginates. Care must be taken to distinguish inclusions from faintly staining hepatocyte nucleoli.

THERAPY

Clinical management of dogs developing ICH is primarily symptomatic and supportive. Fulminant hepatic failure from hepatocellular necrosis is a common cause of death in dogs that do not survive the acute stages of the disease. In the absence of complicating factors, clinical recovery and hepatocellular regeneration can occur with centrolobular necrosis. Therapy is supportive until there is adequate time for hepatocellular repair. Since the dogs are frequently semicomatose, it is impossible to predict whether the neurologic signs relate to hepatoencephalopathy or viral encephalitis. However, this can partially be resolved by

evaluating blood glucose or ammonia concentrations at the time therapy is instituted.

Immediate placement of an indwelling IV catheter is a necessity in severely affected dogs, but because of incoagulability, care must be taken to avoid excessive hemorrhage. Fluid therapy with a polyionic isotonic fluid such as Ringer's solution is used to correct losses from vomiting and diarrhea and to assist in lowering the body temperature. Animals that are too depressed to drink or that continue to vomit must be given daily maintenance fluid requirements (45 ml/kg) by parenteral route.

Treatment of DIC depends on the stage of the clotting deficit. Removal of the inciting stimulus is the initial aim of therapy, but this is not possible in viral diseases. Owing to insufficient hepatic synthesis, replacement of clotting factors and platelets by fresh plasma or whole blood may be necessary in conjunction with anticoagulant therapy when marked incoagulability is present.

Since the possibility exists that hypoglycemia is responsible for the comatose state, an IV bolus of 50% glucose (0.5 ml/kg) should be given over a 5-minute period.

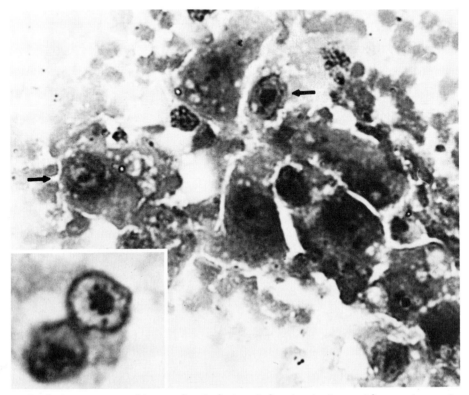

Figure 17–5. Cytologic appearance of intranuclear inclusions in hepatocytes (arrows) from an impression smear of liver tissue at necropsy (Wright's stain; × 400). Inset shows histologic appearance of inclusions (H and E; × 400). Samples were taken from the liver of a puppy that died of ICH.

Hypoglycemia is likely to recur if continuous infusion of hypertonic glucose is not maintained. Hypertonic glucose infusion should be continued at a rate not greater than 0.5 to 0.9 gm/kg/hour for efficient utilization. Therapy to decrease the blood ammonia concentration is directed at reducing protein catabolism by colonic bacteria and ammonia resorption in the renal tubules. Ammonia production from protein degradation in the bowel can be reduced by decreasing the quantity of protein intake and by stopping GI hemorrhage. The colon can be evacuated by cleansing and acidifying enemas that relieve bowel stasis and retard ammonia absorption. The use of nonabsorbable oral antibiotics such as neomycin has been advocated to reduce ammonia-producing bacteria in the intestine, but their effectiveness is questionable. Acidification of the colonic contents can also be achieved by feeding oral lactulose in nonvomiting animals. Renal reabsorption of ammonia can be reduced by administration of parenteral or oral potassium and correction of the metabolic alkalosis. Urinary acidification with a nontoxic acidifier such as ascorbic acid may greatly reduce ammonia reabsorption by the kidney.

Polyinosinic-polycytidylic acid, an interferon inducer, has been experimentally used to reduce the mortality of dogs experimentally infected with ICH virus, but its clinical use is impractical (see Interferon, Chapter 2).

PREVENTION

Maternal Immunity

The duration of passively acquired immunity in the pup is dependent on the antibody concentration of the bitch. The half-life of ICH antibodies is 8.6 days compared with 8.4 days for antibodies to distemper virus, and these values correlate well with the half-life for canine globulin (see Maternal Immunity, Chapter 2 and Tables 2–2, 2–3, and 2–4). Immunization for ICH is usually successful when maternal antibody titers decrease below 1:100, which may occur beginning at 5 to 7 weeks of age. The level of ICH maternal antibodies in the newborn pup declines to negligible concentrations by 14 to 16 weeks.

Vaccinations

Inactivated CAV-1 vaccines do not produce any lesions in vaccinated dogs, but they must be given frequently to equal the protection afforded by MLV vaccines. Adjuvants must be added to inactivated products, making them potentially more allergenic than MLV vaccines. Annual revaccination against ICH with an inactivated CAV-1 vaccine provides continuous protection against infection.[9] These products are not available in the United States.

An inactivated CAV-2 vaccine was tested for use in dogs against challenge infection with CAV-2 infection.[10] Dogs received two doses of vaccine at a 14-day interval and were challenged 14 days following the second dosage. All dogs became seropositive following vaccination but had mild clinical signs of infection compared with challenged unvaccinated dogs. The clinical usefulness of this vaccine remains to be determined, and long-term protection studies are needed.

In contrast to inactivated vaccines, modified live CAV-1 vaccines can produce lifelong immunity with a single dose. A potential disadvantage with the use of MLV vaccines, however, has been that vaccine virus localizes in the kidney and causes mild subclinical interstitial nephritis and persistent shedding of vaccine virus. Increased passage of the virus in cell culture can reduce the incidence of urinary shedding. Ocular localization with associated anterior uveitis occurs in approximately 0.4% of dogs following IV and SC injection. IV CAV-1 vaccination produces a transient systemic illness characterized by pyrexia, tonsillar enlargement, and a 20% incidence of anterior uveitis. A summary of the pathogenicity of modified live CAV-1 vaccine and a comparison with that for CAV-2 vaccine are listed in Table 17–1.

Some CAV-1 and CAV-2 strains are known to be oncogenic in hamsters, but those used in commercial vaccines do not appear to produce this side effect. Oncogenic reactions in dogs have not been reported in more than 20 years of field use of these products.

CAV-2 vaccines have been developed as an alternative in the prevention of ICH. Modified live CAV-2 vaccine rarely, if ever, produces ocular or renal disease when given IM or SC, although the vaccine virus may localize in and be shed from the upper respiratory tract. It produces ocular lesions only when

Table 17–1. Comparison of Pathogenicity of Modified Live Canine Adenovirus Vaccines

ROUTE ADMINISTERED	CLINICAL SIGNS OBSERVED	
	CAV-1[a]	CAV-2[b]
Intravenous	Fever Uveitis (20%) Urinary shedding	Fever Mild respiratory disease Tonsillitis
Intranasal	None	Mild respiratory disease
Intraocular (anterior chamber)	Uveitis (100%)	Uveitis (100%)
Intramuscular or subcutaneous	Uveitis rare (0.4%), urinary shedding (some strains)	None

[a]Canine adenovirus 1.
[b]Canine adenovirus 2.

experimentally injected into the anterior chamber. Given IV and intranasally, modified live CAV-2 vaccine may produce a mild respiratory disease with associated coughing and tonsillar enlargement, although such infections have been shown to be subclinical and self-limiting. More severe respiratory signs might develop with CAV-2 vaccine with secondary bacterial infections. Care should be taken to avoid aerosolizing vaccine when it is given by the IM or SC routes. Dogs are adequately protected by the heterotypic antibody titer against CAV-1 infection if CAV-2 vaccine is used; however, the homotypic antibody response is usually greater. CAV-2 vaccine was experimentally given to 3- to 4-week old pups in an attempt to break through the heterotypic maternal antibodies to ICH virus.[11] Although parenteral vaccination at this age was ineffective, intranasal vaccination produced a delayed antibody response to CAV-2 and a weak response to CAV-1 4 to 8 weeks later. Modified live CAV-2 probably localized in the respiratory tract until maternal antibody declined and then spread systemically stimulating an immune response.

The recommended schedule with any vaccine for ICH involves the use of at least two vaccinations, 3 to 4 weeks apart at 8 to 10 and 12 to 14 weeks of age. This is most commonly accomplished through the combination of this antigen with the canine distemper vaccination protocol (see Vaccination Recommendations, Chapter 2, and Appendix 1). Earlier and more frequent vaccination may be advised in areas of high prevalence. Sporadic ICH infection will be noted in puppies when their vaccinations are delayed. Annual vaccination is often recommended but is probably not essential because of the long-standing immunity produced by MLV vaccines.

Canine Acidophil Cell Hepatitis

A hepatitis distinct from ICH and characterized by acute, persistent, or chronic forms was described in Great Britain.[12] Evidence implying this syndrome has an infectious nature came from the high prevalence of hepatocellular carcinoma in dogs. The agent, suspected to be a virus, has not been identified, although the disease can be reproduced by inoculating bacteriologically sterile liver homogenates not containing CAV-1 or CAV-2 from spontaneously affected animals into experimental dogs.

Presumably, acute infections with this agent lead to acute to chronic hepatitis, cirrhosis with multilobular hyperplasia, and in some cases, hepatocellular carcinoma.[13]

Clinical findings in the early phase of the illness can be vague and include variable fever, inappetence, vomiting, and abdominal pain, but fever is usually lacking. Terminal clinical signs include abdominal distention with ascites, episodes of seizures, mental status abnormalities, and semicoma.

The only consistent laboratory abnormalities include episodic increased ALT and ALP activities. Diagnosis involves gross and microscopic examination of liver tissue. Gross biopsy or necropsy findings include hepatomegaly with rounded lobe edges and enlarged tonsils, regional lymph nodes, and Peyer's patches. Chronically affected dogs may have reduced hepatic size with exaggerated delineation of the portal radicles or nodular proliferation. Increased fibrous tissue is apparent histologically, both centrally and peripherally. Acidophil cells are scattered throughout hepatic lesions and are characterized by angular cytoplasm with acidophil cytoplasm and a hyperchromatic nucleus.

Therapy for this condition is uncertain, and it appears to progress with time. Prevention would not seem plausible until the nature of the suspected infectious agent is determined. Although reported only in Great Britain, the disease may be more widespread and should be suspected when a high frequency of chronic active hepatitis or hepatic fibrous or hepatocellular carcinoma is reported.

References

1. Assaf R, Marsolais G, Yelle J, et al: Unambiguous typing of canine adenovirus isolates by deoxyribonucleic acid restriction–endonuclease analysis. Can J Comp Med 47:460–463, 1983.
2. Hamelin C, Jouvenne P, Assaf R: Genotypic characterization of type-2 variants of canine adenovirus. Am J Vet Res 47:625–630, 1986.
2a. McCartney L, Cavanaugh HM, Spibey N: Isolation of canine adenovirus-2 from the faeces of dogs with enteric disease and its unambiguous typing by restriction endonuclease mapping. Res Vet Sci 44:9–14, 1988.
2b. Whetstone CA, Draayer H, Collins JE: Characterization of canine adenovirus type 1 from American black bears. Am J Vet Res 49:778–780, 1988.
3. Gocke, DJ, Morris TQ, Bradley SE: Chronic hepatitis in the dog: the role of immune factors. J Am Vet Med Assoc 156:1700–1705, 1970.
4. Rakich PM, Prasse KW, Lukert PD, et al: Immunohistochemical detection of canine adenovirus in paraffin sections of liver. Vet Pathol 23:478–484, 1986.
5. Wright NG: Canine adenovirus: its role in renal and ocular disease; a review. J Small Anim Pract 17:25–33, 1976.
6. Beckett SD, Burns MJ, Clark CH: A study of the blood glucose, serum transaminase, and electrophoretic patterns of dogs with infectious canine hepatitis. Am J Vet Res 25:1186–1190, 1964.
7. Noon KF, Rogul M, Binn LN, et al: An enzyme-linked immunosorbent assay for the detection of canine antibodies to canine adenoviruses. Lab Anim Sci 29:603–609, 1979.
8. Carmichael LE: Identification of a canine adenovirus (infectious canine hepatitis virus) inhibitor in dog liver extracts as arginase. Infect Immun 6:348–354, 1972.
9. Miller ASH, Curtis R, Furminger IGS: Persistence of immunity to infectious canine hepatitis using a killed vaccine. Vet Rec 106:343–344, 1980.
10. Curran JM, Cunningham CK: Efficacy of an inactivated canine adenovirus-type 2 vaccine. VM SAC 78:51–59, 1983.
11. Appel M, Carmichael LE, Robson DS: Canine adenovirus type 2–induced immunity to two canine adenoviruses in pups with maternal antibody. Am J Vet Res 36:1199–1202, 1975.
12. Jarrett WFH, O'Neil BW: A new transmissible agent causing acute hepatitis, chronic hepatitis and cirrhosis in dogs. Vet Rec 116:629–635, 1985.
13. Jarrett WFH, O'Neil BW, Lindholm I: Persistent hepatitis and chronic fibrosis induced by canine acidophil cell hepatitis virus. Vet Rec 120:234–235, 1987.

18 CANINE HERPESVIRUS INFECTION

Leland E. Carmichael
Craig E. Greene

ETIOLOGY

Canine herpesvirus (CHV) has biologic and pathogenetic properties similar to herpesviruses affecting other species. An antigenic relationship to human herpes simplex virus has not been confirmed. CHV is inactivated by exposure to most disinfectants and to lipid solvents (e.g., ether, chloroform) and by heat (56°C for 5 to 10 minutes, 37°C for 22 hours). Like other herpesviruses, CHV is readily inactivated at 20°C but is stable at −70°C. It is stable at pH between 6.5 and 7.6 but is rapidly destroyed below pH 5.0.

CHV has a restricted host range and appears to infect only domestic and wild Canidae or canine cell cultures. The virus causes a rapidly spreading, highly destructive cytopathic effect in cell cultures with formation of intranuclear inclusions.

The replication of CHV is similar to that of other herpesviruses. Synthesis of viral DNA and nucleocapsids occurs within the host cell nucleus, with the viral envelope being acquired at the nuclear membrane. Virus is transported through the endoplasmic reticulum and Golgi apparatus to the cell surface, where it is released, but most virus remains intracellular.

PATHOGENESIS

Newborn puppies can acquire CHV infection in utero, or from passage through the birth canal, or from contact with infected littermates, oronasal secretions of the dam, or fomites. Neonatal puppies experimentally infected when they are less than 1 week of age are particularly susceptible to fatal gen-

eralized infections; dogs older than 2 weeks are relatively resistant and generally develop mild or inapparent clinical illness. Virus growth in older dogs is usually restricted to the nasopharynx, genital tract, tonsils, retropharyngeal lymph nodes, bronchial lymph nodes, and lungs.

In Utero Infection

Although neonatal infection usually is acquired at or soon after birth, the possibility of transplacental transmission in late gestation should not be overlooked. The effects of transplacental infection with CHV depend upon the stage of gestation in which infection occurs. Infertility and abortion of stillborn or weak pups with no clinical signs in the dam have been reported.[1, 2] Although some puppies can survive such in utero infections and appear normal on caesarean section, some harbor the virus inapparently in their tissues. Others, however, develop systemic herpesvirus infection within 9 days of birth.[2]

Systemic Neonatal Infection

Following oronasal exposure, CHV is first detected in the nasal epithelium and pharyngeal tonsils (Fig. 18–1). Primary replication occurs in epithelial cells and mucosa within 24 hours postinoculation (PI). Then the virus enters the blood stream by way of macrophages. Intracellular viremia results in viral spread throughout the body within 3 to 4 days PI. Localization in the mononuclear phagocytic cells of the lymph nodes

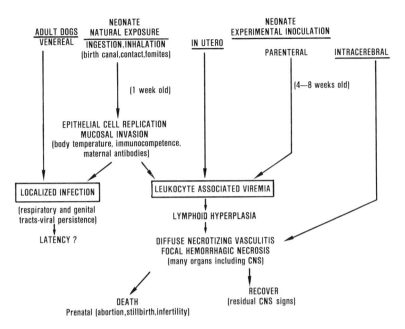

Figure 18–1. Pathogenesis of CHV infection.

and spleen results in cell-to-cell spread and lymphoid hyperplasia and necrosis. Progressive multifocal necrosis occurs in several parenchymal organs, with highest concentrations of virus being found in the adrenals, kidneys, lungs, spleen, and liver.

Multifocal hemorrhage associated with the necrosis may relate to the marked thrombocytopenia that occurs during infection.[3] Thrombocytopenia may result from DIC associated with widespread vascular endothelial damage and tissue necrosis.

Meningoencephalitis occurs in oronasally infected neonatal puppies, but CNS signs are not always apparent. Intracerebral inoculation, however, produces acute fatal meningoencephalitis.[4] Under normal circumstances, puppies generally die from systemic illness before neurologic signs are manifest. Ganglioneuritis of the trigeminal nerve is a frequent lesion in puppies infected by oronasal exposure.[5] CHV may travel up the nerve axons to the CNS as occurs with human herpes simplex virus.

Several factors, including temperature regulation and immune status, are involved in the abrupt development of resistance to infection that develops between 1 and 2 weeks of age. Optimal growth of CHV in cell cultures has been shown to occur between 35° and 36°C. The normal rectal temperature of adult dogs, 38.4° to 39.5°C (101° to 103°F), is above the range. Temperature regulation

of the newborn pup is not developed until 2 to 3 weeks of age, and rectal temperature is usually 1° to 1.5°C (2° to 3°F) lower than that of adult dogs. Besides having a reduced capacity for temperature regulation, neonatal pups are incapable of adequate fever production. Cell-mediated immune functions are also suppressed at temperatures lower than 39°C, rendering hypothermic pups more susceptible not only to CHV but also to vaccinal distemper and canine adenoviruses.[6] Puppies of 4 to 8 weeks of age are normally clinically asymptomatic following challenge but will develop systemic CHV infection if their body temperatures are artificially reduced.[7] Conversely, elevation of the environmental temperature and, subsequently, of the rectal temperature of CHV-infected puppies less than 1 week of age reduces the severity of infection but does not eliminate it.[7, 8]

The amount of immunity acquired from the dam also appears to be important in the survival of infected puppies. Pups nursing seronegative bitches develop a fatal multisystemic illness when they are infected with CHV. On the other hand, puppies suckling seropositive bitches become infected but remain nonsymptomatic, and the virus is recovered primarily from their oropharyngeal region.[9] Maternal antibody or immune lymphocytes acquired through the milk may explain why naturally infected bitches having diseased puppies, with rare exceptions, subsequently give birth to normal litters. Serum antibody titers in previously infected pregnant bitches may also suppress viremia and spread of infection to the fetus.

Adult Genital Infection

Herpesviruses have been isolated occasionally from papulovesicular lesions of the canine genital tract, and such lesions have been described as possible recurrent episodes in previously infected bitches.[2] With CHV, localized genital or respiratory infections, restricted intracellular infections, and viral shedding can occur in the presence of circulating antibody titers. Infection of the genital tract generally appears to be asymptomatic or limited to vaginal hyperemia with hyperplastic lymphoid follicles. Genital localization of the virus in adult dogs may be an important means of venereal transmission of the virus, as well as a source of infection for pups at birth.

Adult Respiratory Infection

Field evidence suggests that CHV might be a cause of respiratory disease, but studies have failed to incriminate CHV as a primary cause of respiratory illness.[10] Of uncertain significance, CHV was recovered from the lungs of dogs with distemper and from dogs with acute conjunctivitis.[11] Neonates that recover from CHV infections or older dogs that have subclinical infections have periodic episodes of viral recrudescence in their oronasal secretions. Viral latency has been demonstrated in intranasally infected dogs for as long as 6 months PI, with recrudescence occurring within 1 week following treatment with glucocorticoids or antilymphocyte serum.[12] Recrudescence of latent virus has also been demonstrated in seropositive adults after their exposure to seronegative juveniles, suggesting a stress mechanism for transmission of CHV in a manner similar to that occurring with feline herpesvirus infection.

CLINICAL FINDINGS

No premonitory sign of illness or prior history of neonatal mortality is seen in bitches that lose litters of puppies to CHV. This can occur at any stage of gestation and can result in abortion of mummified or dead fetuses, premature or stillborn pups, or weak or runted newborn puppies. Some pups within the same litter may not be affected, and gestational age of illness may vary within a litter. Death of neonatal puppies less than 1 week of age appears to be less common and probably indicates in utero infection of virus.[2]

CHV infection in postnatally infected puppies is associated with an acutely fatal illness primarily occurring between 1 to 3 weeks of age. If affected when older than 3 weeks of age, pups had disseminated herpesvirus infection that was thought to be exacerbated by concurrent infections or immunosuppression.[13, 14] Infected puppies appear dull and depressed, lose interest in nursing, and pass soft, yellow-green feces. They cry persistently and show discomfort during abdominal palpation. Despite the continued muscular activity associated with crying, restlessness, and shivering, there is no elevation in body temperature. A rhinitis is frequently manifest by serous to mucopurulent or hemorrhagic nasal discharges. Petechial hemorrhages are widespread on the mucous membranes. An erythematous rash consisting of papules or vesicles and subcutaneous edema of the ventral abdominal and inguinal region are occasionally noted. Vesicles are sometimes present in the vulva and vagina of female puppies, prepuce of the males, and buccal cavity. Puppies lose consciousness and show opisthotonus and seizures just before death. Rectal temperatures become subnormal prior to death, which usually occurs within 24 to 48 hours after the onset of clinical illness.

Some puppies develop mild clinical disease with subsequent recovery. Animals that survive the systemic infection are likely to develop persistent neurologic signs. Ataxia, blindness, and cerebellar vestibular deficits are most commonly seen.

Dogs older than 3 to 5 weeks of age develop a mild or inapparent upper respiratory infection due to CHV. Signs of systemic infection are rare; however, vomiting, anorexia, depression, serous ocular discharge, hepatomegaly, and sudden death have been reported in naturally infected 8- to 10-week-old coyote pups.[15] For a discussion of ocular lesions see Chapter 13.

Primary genital infections in older female

dogs are characterized by lymphofollicular lesions on the vaginal mucosa.[2] No discomfort or vaginal discharge is noted in affected pregnant dogs, even those who had abortions or stillbirths. Vesicular lesions have been noted during the onset of proestrus and regress during anestrus. Male dogs, with similar lesions over the base of the penis and preputial reflection, may have a preputial discharge.

DIAGNOSIS

Clinical Laboratory Findings

The determination of CHV infection in neonatal pups usually depends upon information obtained from the clinical history, physical examination, and pathologic changes seen in affected puppies. Hematologic and biochemical abnormalities are nonspecific, but marked thrombocytopenia may be observed. A marked increase in the ALT (formerly SGPT) activity can be found in infected neonates.

Viral Isolation

CHV can be isolated from several parenchymal organs of puppies dying of acute systemic infection but most likely from the adrenals, kidneys, lungs, spleen, and liver. In recovered or older animals, growth of CHV is usually restricted to the oral mucosa, upper respiratory tract, and external genitalia. Viral isolation has not been demonstrated longer than 2 to 3 weeks PI, following primary infection. However, viral recrudescence may be provoked by stress.

CHV grows only in cells of canine origin, primarily in dog kidney cells at an optimal temperature range of 35° to 37°C. Infected cells become rounded and detach from the glass surfaces, leaving clear plaques surrounded by necrotic cells. Plaque formation is best observed when monolayers are overlaid with semisolid media such as agar or methylcellulose. Plaque morphology has been used as a marker for virus pathogenicity.[16] CHV produces Cowdry type A intranuclear inclusions, which can be difficult to demonstrate but are best revealed in tissues that have been fixed in Bouin's solution before staining (see Appendix 12). Multinucleation of infected cells is unusual with

CHV but has been observed with an isolate from the canine genital tract.[17]

Serologic Testing

Serologic testing for CHV antibodies is based upon viral neutralization tests which rely on reduction in cytopathogenicity or plaque formation. Test procedures and their limitations have been described.[12, 18] Neutralizing antibodies increase following infection, and low (1:2 to 1:8) titers can be detected for at least 2 years. Fluorescent antibody techniques and electron microscopy can be used to detect CHV in tissues and cell cultures (Fig. 18–2).[19] See Appendix 8 for a listing of commercial laboratories that perform these tests.

PATHOLOGIC FINDINGS

Gross lesions of fatal CHV infection in neonates include diffuse multifocal hemorrhage and gray discoloration in a variety of parenchymal organs, especially the kidney (Fig. 18–3), liver, and lungs. Serous to hemorrhagic fluid is usually present in the pleural and peritoneal cavities. The lungs are usually firm and edematous with marked enlargement of the bronchial lymph nodes. Splenomegaly and generalized lymphade-

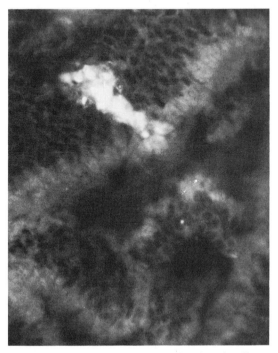

Figure 18–2. Focus of herpesviral infected cells in spleen of a neonatal puppy. (FA method; × 125.) (From Appel MJG et al: *Am J Vet Res* 30:2067–2073, 1969. Reprinted with permission.)

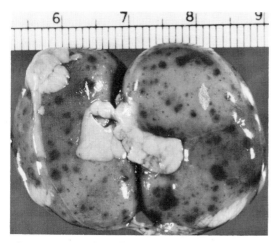

Figure 18–3. Kidney from a puppy inoculated with CHV. Hemorrhagic areas consist of necrotic foci packed with erythrocytes. (From Kakuk TJ, Conner GH: *Lab Anim Care* 20:69–79, 1970. Reprinted with permission.)

nopathy are consistent findings. Petechial hemorrhages are usually numerous throughout the serosal surfaces of the intestinal tract. Icterus has been only rarely reported.[20]

Histologic findings in disseminated infections of neonates are characterized by foci of perivascular necrosis with mild cellular infiltration in the lung, liver, kidney, spleen, small intestine, and brain. Less severe lesions occur in the stomach, pancreas, adrenals, omentum, retina, and myocardium. The lymph nodes and spleen show reactive hyperplasia of mononuclear phagocyte elements. Multifocal necrotizing lesions were also described in the placenta from pregnant bitches and in the pups that acquired infection in utero.[1] The characteristic histologic cutaneous or mucosal lesion, which is the primary lesion in older infected animals, consists of various-sized vesicles produced by profound degeneration of the epithelial cells resulting in marked acantholysis. Basophilic or acidophilic inclusions, depending on the stage of the cellular infection and method of fixation, may be seen but are less common than in other herpesvirus infections. They are more readily seen in the nasal epithelium or kidney than in areas of widespread necrosis such as occur in the lungs or liver.

Histologic lesions in the CNS of recovered puppies are characterized by a nonsuppurative ganglioneuritis and meningoencephalitis. A multifocal granulomatous encephalitis characterized by increased pericapillary cellular proliferation occurs primarily in the brain stem and cerebellum. Cerebellar and retinal dysplasia are frequent histologic findings.

THERAPY

Once a diagnosis has been made, treatment of puppies suffering CHV infection is unrewarding because of the rapidly fatal progression of the disease. However, mortality may be reduced during an epizootic and also in some pups in infected litters treated at a time prior to appearance of generalized signs by injecting them intraperitoneally with 1 to 2 ml of hyperimmune sera.[13] Only one injection is required because of the short susceptibility period. Once systemic infection has occurred, antiserum is ineffective. This prophylactic treatment seems to be beneficial in reducing losses within an exposed litter. Immune sera can be obtained by pooling sera from bitches that have recently lost litters to CHV infection.

Elevating the environmental temperature and subsequently the rectal temperature of already affected puppies is ineffective. Newborn puppies kept at 36.6° to 37.7°C (98° to 100°F) and 45% to 55% humidity have been able to maintain their rectal temperatures at 38.4° to 39.5°C (101° to 103°F). Under such experimental conditions, puppies have reduced mortality, severity of clinical signs, pathologic changes, and viral growth in tissues as compared with puppies having naturally subnormal rectal temperatures. However, body temperatures were elevated prior to exposure to the virus, which is not possible in naturally infected cases.

Treatment of systemic CHV infection with antiviral drugs such as 5-iodo-2-deoxyuridine has been reported to be unsuccessful.[21] Newer antiviral agents such as vidarabine (adenine arabinoside) and acyclovir (acycloguanosine) have been found to be effective in treating localized and CNS infections of herpes simplex virus in people and in laboratory animals by topical and systemic administration, but similar trials have not been reported for CHV infection (see Chapter 15). In one instance, two 15-day-old pups died of confirmed CHV; five littermates, given a course of vidarabine as soon as the deaths were noted, survived and had high (>1:64) neutralizing antibody titers 2 months later, indicating that they had been infected.[22] Antiviral treatment may spare life, but residual damage to the CNS and myocardium may occur, and this possibility must be discussed with owners before undertaking antiviral treatment of an infected litter.

PREVENTION

The low frequency of clinical outbreaks and poor immunogenicity of CHV reduces the incentive to produce a commercial vaccine for this disease. Reports from Europe and the United States have demonstrated a prevalence of anti-CHV antibodies in 6% of the random dog population, whereas it may be as high as 100% in kennels with a high prevalence of infection.[23, 24]

Immunization with a commercially inactivated vaccine in Europe has been shown to increase neutralizing titers fourfold in most dogs[24] but does not appear to provide long-term protection. Live virus vaccines would probably be required for serviceable immunity in puppies, but such vaccines have the potential disadvantage of establishing latent infections. There is no current vaccine that can be claimed to be truly effective.

If a problem exists in a kennel, prophylactic protection for puppies may be achieved with the administration of hyperimmune globulin during the first few days of life. Other methods have been of little value, although administration of an interferon inducer (avian poxvirus) to bitches prior to breeding and whelping and to newborn puppies in problem kennels was claimed to induce nonspecific protection against fatal CHV infection.[18] On a practical basis, eradication of CHV from a kennel is not possible at the present time. Screening for infected animals is impractical (see Diagnosis), and owners should be advised that subsequent litters from an affected bitch have much less risk of developing any complications. Accordingly, use of caesarean delivery or artificial insemination (AI) are not justified to reduce further spread of infection. AI might be used when a known or suspected infected male is bred to a primiparous bitch, but the benefit of such a practice has not been studied.

Care should be taken to ensure that the environmental temperature of newborn puppies is kept warm. This can be achieved with heated whelping boxes, heat lamps, or other warming devices that do not cause excessive dehydration.

Inapparent infections are common in recovered CHV-infected dogs with occasional mild rhinitis, vaginitis, or balanoposthitis as the only clinical signs. Such dogs may act as reservoirs of infection for neonates and should be separated from new litters. Clinically affected puppies shed large quantities of virus in their secretions for 2 to 3 weeks following recovery.[13] Virus persists for only short periods of time in respiratory or vaginal secretions, so that spread is most common by way of immediate direct contact with infected animals or through fomites.

References

1. Hashimoto A, Hirai K, Yamaguchi T, et al: Experimental transplacental infection of pregnant dogs with canine herpesvirus. Am J Vet Res 43:844–850, 1982.
2. Hashimoto A, Hirai K, Suzuki Y, et al: Experimental transplacental transmission of canine herpesvirus in pregnant bitches during the second trimester of gestation. Am J Vet Res 44:610–614, 1983.
3. Kakuk TJ, Conner GH: Experimental canine herpesvirus in the gnotobiotic dog. Lab Anim Care 20:69–79, 1970.
4. Huxsoll DL, Hemelt IE: Clinical observations of canine herpesvirus. J Am Vet Med Assoc 156:1706–1713, 1970.
5. Percy DH, Munnel JF, Olander HJ, et al: Pathogenesis of canine herpesvirus encephalitis. Am J Vet Res 31:145–156, 1970.
6. Schultz RD: Ambient temperature affects canine immune response. Norden News Winter/Spring:36, 1984.
7. Carmichael LE, Barnes FD, Percy DH: Temperature as a factor in resistance of young puppies to canine herpesvirus. J Infect Dis 120:669–678, 1969.
8. Percy DH, Carmichael LE, Albert DM, et al: Lesions in puppies surviving infection with canine herpesvirus. Vet Pathol 8:37–53, 1971.
9. Carmichael LE: Herpesvirus canis: aspects of pathogenesis and immune response. J Am Vet Med Assoc 156:1714–1725, 1970.
10. Carmichael LE: Unpublished data. Cornell University, Ithaca, NY, 1974.
11. Appel MJG: Unpublished data. Cornell University, Ithaca, NY, 1980.
12. Carmichael LE: Canine herpesvirus infection in puppies. In Kirk RW (ed): Current Veterinary Therapy VI. Philadelphia, WB Saunders Co, 1977, pp 1296–1297.
13. Carmichael LE: Herpesvirus canis: aspects of pathogenesis and immune response. J Am Vet Med Assoc 156:1714–1725, 1970.
14. Kraft S, Evermann JF, McKiernan AJ, et al: The role of neonatal canine herpesvirus infection in mixed infections in older dogs. Compend Cont Educ Pract Vet 8:688–697, 1986.
15. Evermann JF, Leamaster BR, McElwain TF, et al: Natural infection of captive coyote pups with a herpesvirus antigenically related to canine herpesvirus. J Am Vet Med Assoc 185:1288–1289, 1984.
16. Carmichael LE, Medic BLS: Small-plaque variant

of canine herpesvirus with reduced pathogenicity for newborn pups. *Infect Immun* 20:108–114, 1978.

17. Poste G: Characterization of a new canine herpes virus. *Arch Gesamte Virusforsch* 36:147–157, 1972.

18. Bibrack B, Schaudinn W: Investigation into the occurrence of canine herpes in West Germany with the help of a quick neutralization test. *Zentralbl Veterinarmed* [B] 23:384–390, 1976.

19. Appel MJG, Menegus M, Parsonson et al: Pathogenesis of canine herpesvirus in specific-pathogen–free dogs: 5- to 12-week-old pups. *Am J Vet Res* 30:2067–2073, 1969.

20. Durham PJK, Poole WSH: Experimental canine her-

pesvirus infection in newborn puppies, using a New Zealand isolate. *N Z Vet J* 27:14–16, 1979.

21. Wright NG, Cornwell HJC: Further studies on experimental canine herpesvirus infection in young puppies. *Res Vet Sci* 11:221–226, 1970.

22. Carmichael LE: Unpublished observations. Cornell University, Ithaca, NY, 1988.

23. Fulton RW, Ott RL, Duenwald JC, et al: Serum antibodies against canine respiratory viruses: prevalence among dogs of eastern Washington. *J Am Vet Med Assoc* 35:853–855, 1974.

24. Engels M, Mayr-Bebrack B, Ruckstuhl B, et al: Seroepizootiology of canine herpes in Switzerland and preliminary trials of a vaccine. *Zentralbl Veterinarmed* [B] 27:257–267, 1980.

19 CANINE INFECTIOUS TRACHEOBRONCHITIS

Richard B. Ford
Shelly L. Vaden

Infectious tracheobronchitis (ITB) is the term used by veterinarians to describe an acute, highly contagious respiratory disorder in dogs affecting the larynx, trachea, bronchi, and occasionally the nasal mucosa, lower airways, and pulmonary interstitium. "Kennel cough" is the layperson's designation for this disease. Mild to severe episodes of cough and respiratory distress are characteristic clinical features recognized in affected dogs. Most infections are self-limiting. ITB has worldwide distribution and is recognized as one of the most prevalent infectious diseases of dogs.

ETIOLOGY AND PATHOGENESIS

Multiple agents, bacterial as well as viral, are implicated in the etiopathogenesis; in nature it is likely that infection by two or more organisms is commonplace. Although many agents have been incriminated, canine parainfluenza virus, *Bordetella bronchiseptica*, and mycoplasmas are the agents most frequently associated with ITB.

Parainfluenza virus is the most common viral isolate from dogs with upper respiratory disease. Following aerosol exposure, the virus replicates in the epithelial cells of the nasal mucosa, trachea, bronchi, bronchioli, and peribronchial lymph nodes. Clinical signs develop 9 days postinoculation (PI). The clinical signs of a pure parainfluenza infection are mild and of short duration (<6 days). Histologic examination of tissue from experimentally infected dogs reveals lymphocytic, plasmacytic, neutrophilic, and histiocytic infiltrates of the larynx and large bronchi. Squamous metaplasia and denuda-

tion of cilia may also be evident in the larger airways. Cellular infiltrates are present in up to 57% of the nonrespiratory bronchioles and in 25% of the alveoli.

B. bronchiseptica is the most common bacteria isolated from canine respiratory disease. Initial damage of the tracheobronchial mucosa by viral agents may facilitate the colonization of this organism in the respiratory tract. In certain cases, *Bordetella* is thought to be of primary pathogenic significance. The bacterium forms fibrillar attachments to the respiratory cilia, overcoming the primary local defense mechanism of the respiratory tract and allowing colonization of the bacteria. In vitro, complete ciliostasis of respiratory epithelium is evident within 3 hours of contact with metabolically active *B. bronchiseptica*. The bacterium also secretes an extracellular adenylate cyclase that may decrease the killing capacity of the alveolar macrophages, overcoming the local immune response of lower airways. Histologic findings in experimentally infected dogs reveal neutrophilic exudate in the epithelium and connective tissue of the respiratory tract, with few animals demonstrating lesions in the lower airways.[1]

Clinical signs of *B. bronchiseptica* infection develop 3 to 4 days PI and last approximately 10 days. Recovery corresponds to the appearance of secretory IgA (sIgA) in the respiratory secretions and reduction of bacterial counts. The clearance of *B. bronchiseptica* from the lower respiratory tract takes an average of 6 to 14 weeks (compared to 3 to 4 days for other bacteria) resulting in the formation of nonsymptomatic carriers.[1]

Bacterial-viral synergism is seen when combined *B. bronchiseptica* and parainfluenza infections occur. The clinical signs are more severe and of longer duration (average, 18.6 days). Acute bronchopneumonia may occur in combined infections with bacteria evident in the lower airways.[2, 2a]

Mycoplasma spp. have been isolated from dogs with clinical signs of ITB. The role of mycoplasmas as primary pathogens is uncertain (see Chapter 41). However, it is known that *Mycoplasma cynos* can be a primary pathogen of the respiratory tract. Like *Bordetella* sp., this agent is capable of attaching to the respiratory cilia, thereby escaping the mucociliary clearance apparatus, and colonizes the upper respiratory tract.[3] Concurrent viral infections may allow for more severe clinical signs of infection by permitting colonization of the organism in the lower airways. Once *M. cynos* colonizes the airways, it may persist and become resident.

Infection with either **canine adenovirus-1** (CAV-1) and **canine adenovirus-2** (CAV-2) causes clinical signs of ITB.[3a] Vaccination does not prevent infection by these organisms but may reduce the severity of clinical signs. **Canine herpesvirus** and **reovirus-1, -2,** and **-3** have rarely been reported as isolates from dogs with kennel cough but are not thought to play a major role in the disease complex.[4] **Canine distemper virus**, which produces respiratory signs that can be confused with ITB as well as systemic infection, is discussed in Chapter 16.

CLINICAL FINDINGS

Two forms of ITB have been described. The uncomplicated form, perhaps most common, is characterized as a dry, hacking cough followed by retching. Affected dogs usually have a history of current vaccination against canine distemper and infectious canine hepatitis. They are affected by a self-limiting, primarily viral, infection of the trachea and bronchi. A complicated form of ITB is described in puppies or immunocompromised dogs with an uncertain vaccination history. Secondary bacterial infections and involvement of pulmonary tissue complicate the viral process in a majority of cases. The cough is associated with a mucoid discharge with or without nasal or ocular discharges. The condition may progress to bronchopneumonia and, in the most severe instances, death.

Uncomplicated ITB

The clinical signs in dogs associated with ITB vary, depending on the type of agent(s) involved, the patient's environment, overall physical condition, and age. Cough of sudden onset, which is frequently paroxysmal, is the hallmark clinical sign recognized in the majority of infected dogs. The high-pitched cough, frequently described as "honking," is attributed to laryngitis and vocal fold swelling (Fig. 19–1). Tracheobronchial inflammation provides the principal stimulus for cough. Rhinitis, with associated serous to mucopurulent nasal discharge, and conjunctivitis may also be apparent. In most cases, affected dogs continue to eat well and remain alert and active throughout the course of infection. Clinical signs in uncomplicated cases usually resolve spontaneously within 2 weeks or less.

Production of excessive, viscous respiratory secretions is common. Dogs with ITB may attempt to expel secretions from the trachea following a coughing episode. Outwardly, the dog will arch its back, open its mouth, retch, and discharge a white, often foamy, mucoid discharge. Owners may misinterpret such behavior and, in fact, may present a dog with ITB for the primary complaint of vomiting or choking. There appears to be little clinical value in defining the cough associated with ITB as productive or nonproductive. The production of excessive respiratory secretions is a variable finding in dogs with ITB, because they frequently swal-

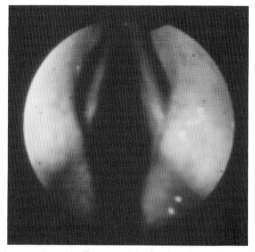

Figure 19–1. Swollen vocal folds in a dog with acute infectious tracheobronchitis; increased airway resistance generates a high-pitched "honk" during coughing episodes.

low tracheal secretions following expectoration. Furthermore, when visualized endoscopically, the amount of secretions varies in each case.

Complicated ITB

Although ITB is generally self-limiting, significant life-threatening complications can be expected in neonates or dogs with underlying airway or immunosuppressive disorders. Miniature and toy breeds with congenital tracheobronchial collapse, dogs with chronic bronchitis, and dogs with primary ciliary dyskinesia (immotile cilia syndrome) are at greatest potential risk of complications induced by ITB. Chronic bacterial bronchopneumonia, manifested by dyspnea, weight loss, fever, lethargy, and decreased appetite, is characteristic of complicated ITB. Radiographic features of pneumonia in addition to leukocytosis support the diagnosis of bacterial lung disease (also see Chapter 8).

DIAGNOSIS

The diagnosis of canine ITB is primarily based on clinical signs and a history of recent exposure to other dogs. Results of laboratory analyses are often within reference limits. If abnormalities are present, they may be nonspecific. A stress leukogram with mature neutrophilia, lymphopenia, and eosinopenia may be evident. Less frequently, an inflammatory leukogram with marked leukocytosis or left shift is present owing to lower airway disease or lobar pneumonia. Radiographic abnormalities associated with uncomplicated parainfluenza infection include pulmonary hyperinflation and segmental atelectasis. Dogs with combined *B. bronchiseptica* and parainfluenza infections may have lobar consolidation evident on thoracic radiographs.[2] A neutrophilic exudate will often be evident on cytologic analysis of transtracheal wash fluid obtained from dogs with either form of ITB.

It is rarely necessary to pursue the diagnosis of ITB with more specific tests. Bacterial culture and susceptibility testing in animals with prolonged infections may allow for confirmation of *B. bronchiseptica* infections and selection of appropriate antibiotic therapy. *B. bronchiseptica* usually can be isolated from nasal swabs whenever tracheal exudates also contain organisms.[5] Viral isolation can be performed on nasopharyngeal or laryngeal swabs and, less preferably, transtracheal wash fluid when attempting to determine the cause of the outbreak. Serum may be submitted to screen animals for the presence of antibodies (IgG) to *B. bronchiseptica* and parainfluenza virus. However, serotesting may yield erroneous results because sIgA is the major antibody elicited during infection. A negative result of a serum IgG titer does not rule out infection, and many dogs will have positive serum titer results caused by vaccination. Results of paired serum samples revealing a rising IgG titer are necessary to confirm concurrent infection with either organism.

THERAPY

Antimicrobials

In uncomplicated cases of ITB, the value of antimicrobial therapy appears limited. Antibiotics have not been shown to reach significant levels in tracheobronchial secretions, nor do they shorten the clinical course of the infection. Although there is no evidence that antimicrobials prevent development of systemic signs, prophylactic antibiotic therapy has been recommended.[3] Indications for treatment of ITB are listed in Table 19–1.

Antimicrobial therapy is indicated if deeper respiratory or systemic bacterial infection develops, particularly bacterial bronchopneumonia or interstitial pneumonia.[3] The drug used should be selected on the basis of bacterial culture and susceptibility testing of blood or intratracheal exudates and should be administered for 10 to 14 days. Since the prevalence of *B. bronchiseptica* infection is high in complicated ITB, it may be necessary to initiate therapy without culture results; tetracycline is the preferred antimicrobial for the treatment of bordetellosis. Dosages for antimicrobials having potential for controlling ITB complicated by bacterial pneumonia are outlined in Table 19–2. Antimicrobials have been administered by local (transtracheal) and aerosol routes but with variable success in managing ITB.[1]

Table 19–1. Treatment Recommendations for Infectious Tracheobronchitis

	UNCOMPLICATED	COMPLICATED[a]
Antimicrobials	Optional	Tetracycline or trimethoprim-sulfonamide or cephalexin or ampicillin and gentamicin
Glucocorticoids	Prednisolone	No
Antitussives	Hydrocodone or butorphanol	No
Bronchodilators	Aminophylline or theophylline elixir	Aminophylline or theophylline elixir
Aerosol therapy	No	Gentamicin

[a]Implies pulmonary involvement or secondary bacterial infections.

Antivirals

Although the availability and potential for clinical application of antiviral compounds in veterinary medicine has increased in the past 3 years, specific antiviral drugs for agents causing canine ITB are not available at this writing.[6] New compounds are currently being investigated for possible use in animals, but their role in treating viral respiratory disease appears limited.

Glucocorticoids

Anti-inflammatory doses of glucocorticoids are highly effective in ameliorating the cough associated with uncomplicated ITB; glucocorticoids may also reduce the volume of respiratory secretions produced during active infection. Glucocorticoids do not appear to shorten the clinical course of ITB. Orally administered prednisolone can be used as needed to suppress coughing. Although long-term glucocorticoid therapy should be avoided, there are no data to support concerns over their short-term use.[7] They may worsen the illness in immunosuppressed animals with complicated ITB.

In addition to anecdotal, unpublished reports on the efficacy of intratracheal administration of methylprednisolone, at least one article supported the use of intratracheal dexamethasone in the management of ITB in dogs.[8] However, there are no published studies supporting the use of intratracheal over orally administered glucocorticoids.

Antitussives

Antitussives, alone and in combination with bronchodilators, have been recom-

Table 19–2. Drug Dosages for Treating Canine Infectious Tracheobronchitis[a]

DRUG	DOSE[b] (mg/kg)	ROUTE	INTERVAL (HOURS)	DURATION (DAYS)
Antimicrobials				
Tetracycline	20	PO	8	7
Trimethoprim-sulfonamide	15	PO, SC	12	7
Cephalexin	30	PO	12	7
Glucocorticoids				
Prednisolone	0.25–0.5	PO	12	5–7
Antitussives				
Hydrocodone bitartrate	0.22	PO	6–24	prn
Butorphanol tartrate	0.05–0.1	SC	6–24	prn
Bronchodilators				
Aminophylline dihydrate	11	PO, IV	6–12	5–10
Theophylline elixir	5–10	PO	6–12	5–10
Aerosol therapy				
Gentamicin	200 mg total[c]	nebulized	6–24	5

[a]PO = oral, SC = subcutaneous, prn = as needed, IV = intravenous.
[b]Dose per administration at specified interval, expressed as mg/kg unless otherwise stated.
[c]Diluted in a total volume of 4 to 6 ml of isotonic saline.

mended as the principal therapy in the management of ITB. Objectively, these drugs are intended to interrupt the cough cycle; however, certain limitations to antitussive therapy should be noted. Over-the-counter cough suppressant drugs appear to offer little or no relief from the cough associated with ITB. Narcotic cough suppressants such as hydrocodone are generally effective in attenuating or eliminating cough. However, excessive use of these products may not only suppress cough but may compromise ventilation, thereby predisposing the patient to retention of respiratory secretions and diminished clearance of bacteria. In ITB complicated by bacterial pneumonia, suppression of cough with narcotic antitussives is not recommended.

Bronchodilators

The methylxanthine bronchodilators theophylline and aminophylline (theophylline ethylenediamine) prevent bronchospasm and therefore may be effective cough suppressants. However, it should be noted that bronchospastic disease such as occurs with human asthma has not been reported in dogs. Therefore, ITB patients can be expected to derive little benefit from bronchodilator therapy alone.

Aerosol Therapy

In contrast to humidification therapy, aerosol therapy, or nebulization, refers to the production of a liquid particulate suspension within a carrier gas. Patients with ITB that derive the most benefit from aerosol therapy are those with excessive accumulations of bronchial and tracheal secretions and those with secondary bronchial infections, particularly B. bronchiseptica. Small, disposable, hand-held jet nebulizers are inexpensive and are commercially available (Fig. 19–2). Patients must be treated in the hospital. Four to 6 ml of sterile saline solution is nebulized over 15 to 20 minutes from one to four times daily. Oxygen is delivered at flow rates of 3 to 5 L/minute to nebulize the saline solution. Most patients tolerate aerosol therapy well and generally do not require physical restraint.

Currently, most authors agree there is no value in nebulizing mucolytic agents. These

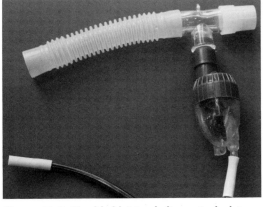

Figure 19–2. Hand-held jet nebulizer attached to an oronasal cone can be used to administer aerosol therapy to dogs with infectious tracheobronchitis.

compounds can be irritating and may induce bronchospasm. Furthermore, liquefying tenacious respiratory secretions may not be an effective means of facilitating clearance of mucus from the lower airways. Nebulization of glucocorticoid solutions has not been examined in veterinary medicine. However, in acute paroxysms of cough leading to respiratory distress, such therapy has interesting potential. Dogs that are unresponsive to oral or parenteral administration of antibiotics may respond to nebulized antibiotics. Aerosolized kanamycin, gentamicin, or polymyxin B have been shown to be effective at reducing the population of B. bronchiseptica in the trachea and bronchi of infected dogs for up to 3 days following discontinuation of drug.[9] Although clinical signs are not eliminated, the severity of signs may be reduced.

Expectorants

Saline expectorants, guaifenesin, and volatile oils that are inhaled as a vapor are intended to stimulate the secretion of less viscous bronchial mucus, thereby enhancing clearance of viscous respiratory secretions from the trachea and bronchi. However, the value of expectorant therapy in dogs with ITB has not been established, nor is it recommended.

Supportive Care

Treatment of canine ITB in the individual animal is directed at maintaining adequate caloric and fluid intake during the acute infection, preventing systemic (secondary) bacterial infection, and suppressing the cough. However, successful management of ITB outbreaks in kennels necessitates additional considerations.

PREVENTION

Following natural exposure to infectious agents via the respiratory tract, sIgA constitutes the primary immune response in both the upper and lower airways. The sIgA response is of shorter duration than that of the systemic IgG response. Serum neutralizing antibodies (IgG) are protective against systemic disease but not in infections localized to the upper respiratory tract.[10] In kennels, ITB often develops in dogs shortly after weaning suggesting that maternal immunity is short lived.

A comprehensive vaccination program against the agents known to cause ITB is the single most important factor in reducing the prevalence and severity of infectious respiratory disease in a kennel environment. The choice of vaccines and vaccination schedules should be flexible enough to meet the need of the individual animals at risk within a given population. Also see Chapter 2 and Appendix 1 for a summary of combined vaccination protocols.

Maternal antibody will effectively interfere with parenteral vaccination against B. bronchiseptica. Intranasal vaccine stimulates the production of both sIgA and IgG, is not affected by maternal antibody, and is associated with less viral shedding after virulent virus challenge than in dogs given parenteral vaccines.

Following experimental inoculation with B. bronchiseptica, dogs are protected against rechallenge for up to 16 weeks.[1] Extracted antigen and whole-cell B. bronchiseptica parenteral bacterins are available that are less toxic than earlier vaccines, produce high serum agglutinating titers, and protect against the development of severe bronchopneumonia. However, they do not significantly alter the course of the disease following challenge and are susceptible to neutralization by maternal antibody. Live avirulent intranasal vaccine administration is associated with production of sIgA within 4 days and significantly reduces clinical

signs and bacterial counts by 95% of those in controls.[10] Serum titers are detectable for 10 to 12 months following vaccination, but twice yearly vaccination is probably needed to induce adequate local immunity.

Active immunization (by vaccination) against ITB is directed against B. bronchiseptica and parainfluenza virus. Parenteral and intranasal attenuated canine parainfluenza virus vaccines are available. Two initial doses of canine parainfluenza virus parenteral vaccine with annual revaccination are necessary to provide adequate systemic immunity.

Combined canine parainfluenza virus and B. bronchiseptica intranasal vaccines are available and are associated with significantly higher titers than those following immunization with monovalent vaccines. There is also a further reduction in clinical signs evident following postvaccinal challenge suggesting a bacterial-viral vaccinal synergism.[11]

Infection with CAV-1 and CAV-2 is prevented by use of a parenteral MLV–CAV-2 vaccine. Adequate immunity is obtained after one dose, and annual revaccination is necessary. CAV-2 antigen is often combined with canine distemper vaccine.

As an adjunct to a vaccination program, endemic respiratory disease can be reduced by minimizing population density and maximizing ventilation to more than 12 air changes/hour. In addition to direct contact, aerosol transmission via infectious microdroplets can be a highly effective means of exposing susceptible dogs; therefore, segregation of dogs suspected of or known to have ITB is essential. Use of disposable dishware is recommended in kennels that cannot reliably wash and disinfect metal utensils. In confined outbreaks within kennels, personnel handling coughing dogs should wear clean, disposable gloves. Infected dogs should be isolated from other animals to avoid spread of the disease.

The best virucide for routine disinfection of premises is household bleach (5.6% sodium hypochlorite) diluted with water by adding 1 part bleach to 32 parts water to create a 0.175% sodium hypochlorite solution. This solution can be combined with a quaternary ammonium compound (A-33 Dry, Ecolab Inc, St. Paul, MN) for cleansing without loss of virucidal activity.

Public Health Considerations

Despite the multiple agents known to be associated with ITB in dogs, none of these organisms are regarded as pathogenic for people. Canine ITB is not a zoonotic disease.

References

1. Bemis DA, Greisen HA, Appel MJG: Pathogenesis of canine bordetellosis. *J Infect Dis* 135:753–762, 1977.
2. Wagener JS, Sobonya R, Minnich L, et al: Role of canine parainfluenza virus and *Bordetella bronchiseptica* in kennel cough. *Am J Vet Res* 45:1862–1866, 1984.
2a. Wagener JS, Minnich L, Sobonya R, et al: Parainfluenza type II infection in dogs. *Am Rev Resp Dis* 127:771–775, 1983.
3. Bemis DA: Current strategies for the control of canine infectious tracheobronchitis. *Proceedings.* 5th Annu East States Vet Conf, Orlando, FL, January:22–35, 1988.
3a. Azetaka M, Konishi S: Kennel cough complex: confirmation and analysis of outbreaks in Japan. *Jpn J Vet Sci* 50:851–858, 1988.
4. Appel MJG: Canine infectious tracheobronchitis (kennel cough): a status report. *Compend Cont Educ Pract Vet* 3:70–81, 1981.
5. Bemis DA, Carmichael LE, Appel MJG: Naturally occurring respiratory disease in a kennel caused by *Bordetella bronchiseptica*. *Cornell Vet* 67:282–293, 1977.
6. Gustafson DP: Antiviral therapy. *Vet Clin North Am Small Anim Pract* 16:1181–1189, 1986.
7. Ford RB: Concurrent use of corticosteroids and antimicrobial drugs in the treatment of infectious diseases in small animals. *J Am Vet Med Assoc* 185:1142–1144, 1984.
8. Hutchison RV: Intratracheal gentamicin and dexamethasone for treatment of canine infectious tracheobronchitis in the dog. *VM/SAC* 70:843–945, 1975.
9. Bemis DA, Appel MJG: Aerosol, parenteral and oral antibiotic treatment of *Bordetella bronchiseptica* infections in dogs. *J Am Vet Med Assoc* 170:1082–1086, 1977.
10. Bey RF, Shade FJ, Goodnow RA, et al: Intranasal vaccination of dogs with live avirulent *Bordetella bronchiseptica*: correlation of serum agglutination titer and the formation of secretory IgA with protection against experimentally induced infectious tracheobronchitis. *Am J Vet Res* 42:1130–1132, 1981.
11. Konter EJ, Wegrzyn RJ, Goodnow RA: Canine infectious tracheobronchitis: effects on an intranasal live canine parainfluenza-*Bordetella bronchiseptica* vaccine on viral shedding and clinical tracheobronchitis (kennel cough). *Am J Vet Res* 42:1694–1698, 1981.

20 NONRESPIRATORY PARAINFLUENZA VIRUS INFECTIONS OF DOGS

Craig E. Greene

ETIOLOGY

Canine parainfluenza virus (CPiV) is a member of the family Paramyxoviridae, which contains canine distemper virus, simian virus-5 (SV-5), and human measles and mumps viruses. Human, simian, and canine type 2 parainfluenza viruses have all been termed SV-5 viruses in the past because of their close antigenic relationship. Monoclonal antibody studies have shown minor antigenic differences between SV-5 isolates.[1] Whether different SV-5 isolates are transmitted between people, nonhuman primates, and dogs remains to be established. The virus associated with respiratory disease in dogs has been designated CPiV.[2] It causes acute, self-limiting cough in the syndrome of infectious tracheobronchitis (see Chapter 19) and is now recognized worldwide as an important cause of respiratory disease in dogs.[3,4] Serologic studies indicate that the overall prevalence of CPiV in the canine population is high but variable. There is evidence that related but distinct paramyxoviruses may cause systemic or nonrespiratory infections in dogs.[5]

CLINICAL FINDINGS

A parainfluenza virus variant was isolated from the CSF of a 7-month-old dog with ataxia and paraparesis of 3 to 4 days' duration.[6] The dog had been vaccinated against canine distemper at 7.5 weeks of age. Gnotobiotic puppies inoculated intracerebrally with this virus isolate developed two forms

of clinical illness.[7,8] Some developed acute encephalitis characterized by seizures, myoclonus (involuntary rhythmic muscle contractions), and progressive neurologic signs within a few days postinoculation. Five of six inoculated dogs observed for 6 months postinoculation developed internal hydrocephalus, although clinical signs were not noted at this time. The hydrocephalus was thought to result from ependymitis with decreased absorption of CSF with or without aqueductal obstruction. Seven-week-old seronegative ferrets intracerebrally inoculated have also been found to develop a self-limiting nonsuppurative ependymitis and choroiditis.[8a]

A 6-week-old puppy was found in extremis as a result of acute hemorrhagic enteritis.[9] Although a paramyxovirus variant was isolated, it is too early to say it was responsible for the clinical illness.

At present it is uncertain whether the CNS or GI forms of disease caused by paramyxoviral variants occur with any frequency under natural circumstances. Neurologic illness has been more commonly recognized as a complication of other paramyxovirus infections, such as with canine distemper in dogs (Chapter 16) and in people with measles and mumps viruses (Chapter 34). In laboratory rodents, other paramyxoviruses have been shown to produce encephalitis and hydrocephalus that are very similar to those that result when the paramyxoviral-variant was injected into dogs. Naturally occurring encephalitis, periventriculitis, and hydrocephalus of a suspected bacterial origin have been discribed in young dogs (see Periventricular Encephalitis, Chapter 90).

266

DIAGNOSIS

Paramyxoviral-induced encephalitis or hydrocephalus may be confirmed serologically by the hemagglutination-inhibition assay; however, owing to the high prevalence of antibody in canine populations and the routine use of a vaccine for CPiV, confirmation requires demonstration of a rising serum antibody titer. CSF antibody titer to this variant virus was shown to remain persistently high in dogs following experimental infection.[6] Viral isolation can be performed on CSF or brain tissue of infected dogs. In addition, immunofluorescence can be used to detect viruses in nervous tissue. For cases of enteritis, virus isolation and electron microscopy of feces would be most valuable. Serologic techniques such as virus neutralization or hemagglutination inhibition must be used to distinguish these variant paramyxoviral strains from CPiV.

PATHOLOGIC FINDINGS

Gross pathologic findings have been identified only in experimentally infected dogs that became hydrocephalic. Moderately enlarged lateral and third ventricles are present. Microscopically, acute meningoencephalitis was characterized by multifocal neuronal necrosis, lymphoplasmacytic cellular infiltrates, and reactive gliosis. Focal ependymitis was also apparent. Flattening and discontinuities of the ependymal cells lining the ventricles were seen in dogs developing hydrocephalus. Ultrastructurally, the virus could not be found in the brains of dogs developing hydrocephalus and encephalitis that were examined 1 to 6 months after experimental infection.

In the puppy with enteritis, the intestinal and gastric contents were blood tinged. Atrophy of small intestinal villi, mucosal congestion, and lymphoid necrosis were noted.

THERAPY AND PREVENTION

The prevalence of paramyxoviral variant diseases is unknown at present. There is no known treatment. It is possible that the CPiV vaccine, developed for tracheobronchitis, may help to prevent these other paramyxoviral diseases.

References

1. Randall RE, Young DF, Goswami KK, et al: Isolation and characterization of monoclonal antibodies to simian virus 5 and their use in revealing antigenic differences between human, canine and simian isolates. J Gen Virol 68:2769–2780, 1987.
2. Binn LN, Eddy GA, Lazar EC, et al: Viruses recovered from laboratory dogs with respiratory disease. Proc Soc Exp Biol Med 126: 140–145, 1967.
3. Moloney MB, Pye D, Smith HV, et al: Isolation of parainfluenza virus from dogs. Aust Vet J 62:285–286, 1985.
4. Ajiki M, Takamura K, Hiramatsu K, et al: Isolation and characterization of parainfluenza 5 virus from a dog. Jpn J Vet Sci 44:607–618, 1982.
5. Evermann J: Paramyxovirus infections of dogs. Vet Rec 117:450–451,1985.
6. Evermann JF, Lincoln JD, McKiernan AJ: Isolation of a paramyxovirus from the cerebrospinal fluid of a dog with posterior paresis. J Am Vet Med Assoc 177: 1132-1134, 1980.
7. Baumgärtner WK, Krakowka S, Koestner A, et al: Acute encephalitis and hydrocephalus in dogs caused by canine parainfluenza virus. Vet Pathol 19: 79–92, 1982.
8. Baumgärtner WK, Krakowka S, Koestner A, et al: Ultrastructural evaluation of acute encephalitis and hydrocephalus in dogs caused by canine parainfluenza virus. Vet Pathol 19:305–314, 1982.
8a. Baumgärtner W, Krakowka S, Gorham JR: Canine parainfluenza virus–induced encephalitis in ferrets. J Comp Pathol 100:67–76, 1989.
9. Macartney L, Cornwell HJ, McCandlish IA, et al: Isolation of a novel paramyxovirus from a dog with enteric disease. Vet Rec 117:205–207, 1985.

21

CANINE VIRAL ENTERITIS

Roy V.H. Pollock
Leland E. Carmichael

Since the appearance of canine parvoviruses in the late 1970s, viral enteritis has become recognized as one of the most common causes of vomiting and diarrhea in dogs, especially in those less than 1 year of age. Canine parvoviruses (CPV) 1 and 2, coronaviruses, and rotaviruses have been incriminated as primary pathogens. Astrovirus, herpesvirus, enteroviruses, calicivirus, and parainfluenza viruses have been isolated from dogs with diarrhea, but their pathogenicity is uncertain.

Canine Parvoviral Enteritis

ETIOLOGY

The parvoviruses are small, nonenveloped, single-stranded DNA viruses (Fig. 21–1). The adeno-associated parvoviruses replicate only in cells simultaneously infected by an adenovirus. The nondefective parvoviruses, which include the closely related feline panleukopenia virus (FPV), mink enteritis virus (MEV), and CPV type 2 (CPV-2), replicate only in dividing cells such as those of the intestine, lymphoid system, bone marrow, and fetal tissues. Their effects in these tissues are especially severe. Although CPV-2 is commonly referred to as simply canine parvovirus, this term is imprecise because there are two other known canine parvoviruses, canine adeno-associated virus, which is apparently non-pathogenic, and CPV-1, the minute virus of canines (MVC), of uncertain pathogenicity.

There is ample evidence that CPV-2 is truly a new canine pathogen. Retrospective serologic studies worldwide have failed to detect specific antibodies in serum samples collected prior to 1976.[1] Presently, high seroprevalence exists in privately owned, stray dogs and wild Canidae.[2]

It is likely that CPV-2 has mutated from FPV or a closely related parvovirus of wildlife.[3,4] All CPV-2 isolates collected before 1980 have been of a single antigenic type. A second antigenic type arose about 1980 and has largely supplanted the original type strain, perhaps because it replicates more efficiently in dogs.[5] The differences between the two strains are small, however, and they fully cross-immunize.[6]

Parvoviruses are resistant to inactivation. Virus can remain infectious in ground contaminated with fecal material for 5 months or more if conditions are favorable.[7] Most common detergents and disinfectants fail to inactivate parvoviruses, although chlorine bleach and Quatricide PV (Pharmical Research Laboratories, Naugatuck, CT) have been shown to be effective and inexpensive disinfectants.

Under proper conditions of pH and tem-

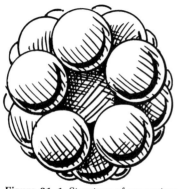

Figure 21–1. Structure of parvovirus.

perature, CPV hemagglutinates RBCs from a number of species; hemagglutinating activity may be lost during prolonged passage in tissue culture. However, hemagglutination tests can be performed directly on fecal specimens to indicate the presence of CPV-2.

EPIDEMIOLOGY

Host Range

CPV-2 infections have been reported in the domestic dog, bush dogs, coyotes, crab-eating foxes, maned wolves, and raccoon dogs.[8] Serologic evidence of infection has been detected in blue foxes and gray wolves. It is probable that most, if not all, Canidae are susceptible.

Limited infections can be produced in domestic cats by parenteral inoculation.[3,9,9a] Viral replication occurs in lymphoid organs, and infected cats develop high levels of serum antibody. However, cats are not believed to play an important role in the epidemiology of CPV-2.

Despite an early report, raccoons do not appear to be susceptible to CPV-2. Rather, there is a distinct raccoon parvovirus that shares antigenic cross-reactivity with both CPV-2 and FPV. In addition, Mustelidae do not appear to be susceptible to CPV-2, although results are inconclusive.

Serologic evidence of infection must be interpreted with caution because standard serologic tests do not clearly distinguish antibody to CPV-2 from that to FPV, MEV, or raccoon parvovirus. Thus, serosurveys of wild species without confirmatory viral isolation or experimental infection studies could produce a misleading picture of the host range.

Transmission

CPV-2 is transmitted principally by the fecal-oral route. Viral organisms in excess of 10^9 median tissue culture dose $(TCID_{50})/g$ of feces are shed during the period of acute illness, and susceptible dogs are readily infected by oral inoculation with infected feces or tissue culture fluids.

Experimental infection can be produced by a number of routes, including oral, nasal, or oronasal exposure, and by IM, IV, or SC inoculation. The minimum infectious dose is believed to be very small; IM inoculation of as few as 16 $TCID_{50}$ of an attenuated stain has been sufficient to initiate infection.[10] Whether there are other natural routes of transmission is unresolved. It has been postulated that insects or rodents could carry the virus from one location to another,[11] but studies to substantiate this speculation have not been done.

The persistence of virus in the environment is believed to be more important than chronic carriers in perpetuating the disease. In most instances, active shedding of virus in feces is confined to the first 2 weeks postinoculation (PI). Once shed, however, CPV-2 remains infectious for days to months.[7] There is evidence that some dogs may shed virus periodically, perhaps for as long as 1 year, but this does not appear to be common. In general, recovered dogs fail to transmit disease to susceptible kennel mates even when they have been housed together for several months.

Subclinically infected animals probably play a significant role in the epidemiologic chain. Serologic evidence has suggested that the majority of infections are mild or subclinical. In several kennels, virtually universal seroconversion has been documented during periods in which the number of clinical cases of enteritis was relatively small.[12] Since even subclinically affected dogs shed substantial quantities of virus, these inapparent infections are important sources of contagion for dogs in kennels, shows, humane shelters, and veterinary hospitals.

Subclinical infection is also prevalent in stray dogs and wild Canidae.[1,2] Feral dogs, coyotes, and other canines are important reservoirs of infection. Eradication would be impossible. The occurrence of outbreaks of CPV-2 enteritis in several closed dog colonies suggests that transport by people or fomites contributes to the spread of infection.[13]

Natural History

Because CPV-2 was a previously unknown pathogen when it emerged in the late 1970s, all dogs were susceptible. Early outbreaks were characterized by high morbidity and mortality. There was an inverse relationship between age and case fatality. Outbreaks occurred throughout the year, although they were more frequent in the spring and summer months. Seasonal variations in the birth rate of dogs probably contributed to the observed seasonality.

The majority of adult dogs are now immune by virtue of immunization or prior infection, and large outbreaks of disease are rare. Parvoviral enteritis has become almost exclusively a disease of puppies between weaning and about 6 months of age. Unless adequately immunized, most pups become infected soon after their maternally derived antibody drops below protective levels, usually between 6 and 18 weeks of age.[12] Those that survive the infection are thereafter immune, probably for life.

In contrast to the continued episodes of parvoviral enteritis, acute parvoviral myocarditis is now extremely rare.[14] Apparently, myocarditis develops only if pups are infected in utero or within a few days of birth.[15,16] Since nearly all dams are now immune, perinatal infection of pups is prevented, and the myocardial form of the disease has virtually disappeared.

Predisposing Factors

One of the impediments to early research on CPV enteritis was the difficulty of reproducing the typical clinical syndrome by experimental infection. Various hypotheses have been advanced to explain the difference between laboratory and natural infections as well as the wide range of outcomes observed under field conditions. The key determinants may be the rates of lymphoid and intestinal epithelial cell turnover. Since parvoviruses depend on cell division for their own replication, it follows that higher rates of cell turnover would favor more extensive viral replication and cytolysis. This explanation might account for the increased pathogenicity of CPV-2 seen with concurrent intestinal parasitism or viral infections[17] (see also Prevention, Canine Coronaviral Infection). In addition, recent isolates appear to be more virulent, causing an often fatal hemorrhagic enteritis in exposed pups.[18]

A second, but not necessarily exclusive, hypothesis is that the duration and magnitude of viremia may be key predictors of the severity of clinical illness.[19] Dogs that have mounted a more rapid immune response may have been able to limit the extent of the viremic period and have less severe clinical disease.

Whatever the reason, clinical experience strongly suggests that crowding, stress, concurrent disease, or general ill-health favors the development of clinical disease.[17] Certain breeds, especially the Rottweiler and Doberman pinscher, also are at higher risk of severe illness.[20] The reasons for this predisposition are not known.

PATHOGENESIS

Although CPV-2 infection is seen most often as clinical enteritis, the disease is systemic.[21,22] Hence, generalized infection[23] and vasculitis[24] should be considered part of the normal spectrum of disease, rather than as distinct syndromes. The myocardial form is a special case because of its dramatic presentation and very restricted target population.

Myocardial Disease

Age appears to determine whether CPV-2 infection results in myocarditis or enteritis. Cardiac myocyte replication is sufficiently rapid to support parvoviral replication only until approximately 2 weeks of age. Older dogs develop enteritis but not myocarditis. Although CPV-2–induced myocarditis most often appears clinically as acute heart failure in 6- to 8-week-old pups, it is the end result of infection begun several weeks earlier.[15,16] Myocardial fiber loss and scarring can lead to chronic heart failure weeks to months later in pups that survive the acute infection.

The age-related shift in the clinical manifestation of infection from myocarditis to enteritis is believed to reflect the decreasing rate of myocardial cell proliferation and increasing rate of intestinal epithelial turnover that occur in the first few weeks after birth.

Intestinal Form

Following ingestion, primary replication occurs in the lymphoid tissues of the oropharynx, mesenteric lymph nodes, and thymus (Fig. 21–2). Virus apparently generalizes from its initial sites of replication by way of the blood stream. A primary plasmaphase viremia of low magnitude has been detected on the first or second day PI.[19,20] Replication in secondarily infected sites

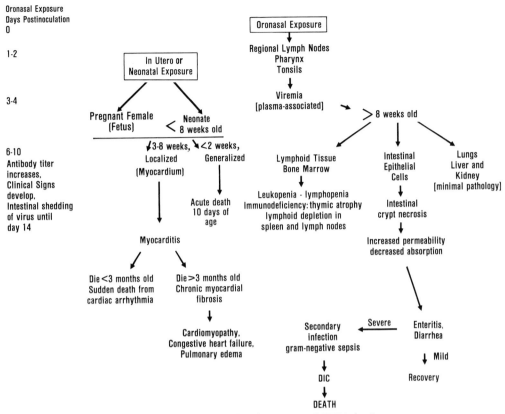

Figure 21–2. Sequential pathogenesis of CPV infection.

leads to marked (up to 10^6 $TCID_{50}$/ml) mostly plasma-phase viremia on the third and fourth day PI.[25] Immunoperoxidase and immunofluorescent studies demonstrate widespread viral replication in lymphoid organs at this time.

The development of histologic lesions parallels the replication of virus.[22,25,26] On the second day PI, there is histologic evidence of necrosis within the germinal centers of the tonsil and the retropharyngeal and mesenteric lymph nodes. On the third day, lymphoid necrosis is more widespread, and cell loss is evident in the thymus of young dogs. A few infected cells can be detected in the lymphoid follicles of the intestinal tract, but infection of the intestinal epithelium is not observed until the fourth day PI.[25] Even then, infected epitheliocytes are usually restricted to areas adjacent to infected lymphoid tissue, suggesting that infection spreads to the epithelium from infected lymphocytes rather than directly from the GI lumen. Later, areas of the mucosa are involved that are not associated with lymphoid aggregations, suggesting that spread

through the epithelium with or without hematogenous infection also occurs.

Active excretion of CPV-2 in the feces usually begins on the third day after oronasal exposure, often before overt clinical signs commence. The amount of infectious virus in the feces increases rapidly until the fifth or sixth day PI, at which time there may be more than 10^9 $TCID_{50}$/g of stool.[10,21] During this period, which usually corresponds to the period of illness in clinically affected dogs, virus is detected readily in the stool by several methods (see Diagnosis). The amount of virus that can be recovered from stool specimens is sharply lower the seventh or eighth day, and only rarely can virus be demonstrated in the feces of dogs more than 12 days PI.[27] Local intestinal antibody may be important in the termination of virus excretion in the feces.

Necrosis of the germinal epithelium of the intestinal glands results in the inability to replace the normal turnover of intestinal epithelium. Intestinal villi become blunted, fused, and covered by immature, cuboidal epithelium. Diarrhea results from loss of absorptive and digestive capabilities; inflammation may contribute a secretory component to the diarrhea as well. In severe cases, there is complete denuding of the lamina propria with hemorrhage into the intestine. Rapid regeneration of the intestinal epithelium occurs in animals that survive the acute infection. Even in fatal cases, there are areas of germinal epithelial hyperplasia and regeneration. When dogs recover from the intestinal form, they do so completely; no long-term effects have been documented.

Reproductive Performance

Whether CPV-2 affects reproductive performance is still a matter of debate. The conception rate among bitches, the number of stillborn pups, the average litter size, and the average number of pups weaned per litter were not significantly different after CPV-2 became established in one kennel.[28] However, other investigators have claimed a decrease in reproductive efficiency coincident with the introduction of CPV-2.[29] Despite the conflicting evidence, CPV-2 does not appear to be an important or frequent cause of reproductive failure, in contrast to the effects of porcine parvovirus in pigs. However, CPV-1 may be a cause of abortion and birth defects in dogs (see CPV-1 Infection).

Effect on Bone Marrow

CPV-2 also infects the bone marrow, resulting in necrolysis of both myeloid and erythroid stem cells. The endotoxemia and septicemia that accompany severe enteric lesions may be partially responsible for the marrow changes. Because of the long half-life of RBCs, changes in the peripheral blood red cell indices have seldom been observed clinically.

The peripheral blood leukocyte count, however, reflects both peripheral consumption and myeloid destruction. In severe cases, there is progressive reduction in the number of circulating leukocytes, beginning on days 3 to 5 PI. The earliest change, relative lymphopenia, probably is the direct result of lymphocytolysis[25] that may progress to an absolute lymphopenia. In severe cases, neutropenia, accompanied by a degenerative left shift and toxic neutrophils, appears concurrent with the onset of intestinal damage approximately 6 days PI.[25] Leukocytosis and marrow hyperplasia are common during recovery.

Effect on Immune System

There has been great speculation about the effects of CPV-2 infection on the immune system, but limited data. During acute infection, there is widespread destruction of lymphocytes in the GI-associated lymphoid tissues, lymph nodes, and thymus. It is tempting, although erroneous, to take this as prima facie evidence of immunosuppression. Severely affected dogs do appear to be at increased risk of opportunistic infections, such as bacterial septicemia, intestinal candidiasis, and haemobartonellosis.[30] Direct evidence of reduced lymphocyte blastogenesis has been reported in naturally infected dogs,[31] although this finding may be nonspecific. Another study concluded that CPV-2 does not cause immunosuppression.[32]

Distemper-induced encephalitis in 3-week-old pups challenged with CPV-2 3 days following distemper vaccination was attributed to viral "immunosuppression."[33] Although immunosuppression caused by the CPV-2 infection might have occurred, alternate explanations are possible, such as disruption of blood-brain barrier, which is normally impermeable to vaccinal distemper virus. Subsequent investigators have been unable to reproduce distemper vaccine–induced encephalitis in older (11- to 15-week-old) dogs infected with CPV-2,[17] and direct investigation of the effects of CPV-2 on the immune system revealed no evidence of immune suppression.[32]

CLINICAL FINDINGS

Intestinal Form

The signs of CPV-2 enteritis are extremely variable, even within a single litter. The classic presentation is a 6- to 20-week-old puppy with an acute onset of fever, vomiting, and diarrhea (Fig. 21–3). Fever may exceed 41°C (106°F) in young dogs. Depression, anorexia, and lethargy are common prodromal signs. The character of the vomitus and diarrhea are variable and do not distinguish CPV-2 infection from other en-

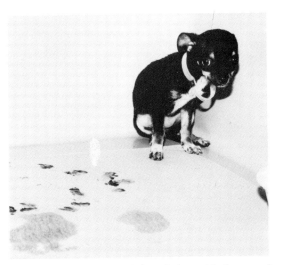

Figure 21–3. Parvovirus-infected dog with fever and depression. Watery vomitus and blood-streaked diarrhea are visible on the cage paper. This dog was from a herd of Chihuahuas that developed an epizootic infection in 1978; 19 dogs died.

teritides. Hematochezia is present in up to 50% of cases.

Animals that survive the first 3 to 4 days of intestinal disease usually make a rapid recovery, generally within 1 week in uncomplicated cases. Severely ill pups that develop secondary septicemia or other complications may require prolonged hospitalization.

Myocardial Form

Puppies with parvoviral myocarditis are often found dead, or they succumb after a very short episode of dyspnea, crying, and retching. Mortality commonly exceeds 50% in an affected litter. Surviving puppies may appear clinically normal but have EKG changes and histologic lesions indicative of myocarditis. Such pups may develop signs of congestive heart failure (exercise intolerance, coughing, dyspnea) months or even years later, apparently as a result of secondary myocardial fibrosis.

DIAGNOSIS

The clinical diagnosis of CPV-2 enteritis is confounded by its unpredictable clinical presentation. The classical signs of CPV-2 enteritis may be mistaken for salmonellosis or the enteric form of distemper. Leukopenia is a distinguishing, although variable, find-ing. A single WBC count performed soon after the onset of diarrhea will detect leukopenia in about one third of CPV-2–infected dogs. If serial leukograms are performed during the clinical course of the disease, leukopenia may be detected in 85% of field cases. Severe leukopenia usually corresponds to severe clinical signs and a poor prognosis. In less severe cases, or when the WBC count is normal or marginal, CPV-2 enteritis is indistinguishable from a large number of other acute enteritides. Neither the biochemical nor the radiographic findings of acute CPV-2 enteritis are unique. Definitive diagnosis depends on the demonstration of virus or viral antigen with or without specific antibody responses.

Virus Detection

Evidence of active viral shedding or the demonstration of viral antigen in tissue samples is unequivocal evidence of current infection. Methods available for detecting CPV-2 in feces or intestinal contents include electron microscopy, fecal hemagglutination, viral isolation, latex agglutination, and ELISA tests.[34,35] All appear adequate for diagnosis of acute cases since the amount of virus present in the stool is great. Until recently, these tests have been available only at commercial diagnostic laboratories. The advent of a solid-phase ELISA test for parvovirus (CITE Test, IDDEX, Inc, Portland, ME) has made in-office testing practical. The in-office test requires a small stool sample or rectal swab and takes approximately 10 minutes to complete. Both sensitivity and specificity appear to be high.

Samples submitted to diagnostic laboratories should be taken during the acute phase of infection and submitted cold but not frozen, since freezing may preclude electron microscopic examination for other agents (e.g., coronavirus). Immunofluorescent antibody, immunoperoxidase, or radioimmunoassay methods can be used to positively identify virus in tissue samples.

Serologic Testing

Various serologic techniques have been developed to test for antibody to CPV-2. These include hemagglutination inhibition (HI), radial hemolysis, virus neutralization (VN), IFA, and radioimmune assay (RIA) techniques. There is no standard method, and variations of all of the above techniques are in use by different laboratories. When different methods have been compared, they have generally yielded parallel results, although some techniques are more sensitive than others.[36] In the absence of standardization, comparison of antibody titers between studies or laboratories is potentially misleading. The titer of a single sample can vary from 20 to 1,000 depending on the specific test, antigen, and technique used.[37] Thus, titers from different laboratories cannot be used to compare vaccine-induced responses.

Because antibodies to CPV-2 are prevalent, serologic diagnosis of active infection requires evidence of seroconversion or IgM-class antibody. The latter method is more practical, since it can be accomplished on a single serum sample, either by pretreatment with 2-mercaptoethanol or by the use of IFA with specific anti-IgG and anti-IgM conjugates. Failure to observe seroconversion cannot be used to rule out infection; many dogs have already produced substantial quantities of IgG by the time they are presented for veterinary care. See Appendix 8 for listings of available diagnostic tests and the laboratories that perform them and for commercially available test kits.

PATHOLOGIC FINDINGS

In fatal cases, the histologic lesions are distinct and diagnostic. Fresh samples of jejunum, mesenteric lymph nodes, and thymus are most important in cases of enteritis; sections of myocardium are essential in suspected CPV-2 myocarditis.

Intestinal Form

The gross lesions of CPV-2 enteritis are variable and nonspecific. Early lesions are most pronounced in the distal duodenum; later, the jejunum is the most severely affected. Lesions, if present, are frequently segmental and consist of discoloration and subserosal hemorrhage and congestion (Fig. 21-4). Mesenteric lymph nodes are often enlarged and edematous with multifocal petechial hemorrhages in the cortex. Thymic cortical necrosis and a small thymus are

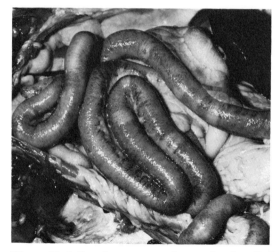

Figure 21–4. Bowel at necropsy from a dog that died suddenly of parvoviral enteritis. Note the discoloration of the bowel wall and fibrin on the serosal surface.

found in young dogs. In the severe cases, only a thin, lacy remnant of the thymus may remain.

The microscopic lesions of CPV-2 infection are most prominent in areas of proliferating cell populations and resemble severe radiation damage. The early lesions consist of necrosis of the intestinal gland (crypt) epithelium. The crypts may be dilated and filled with necrotic debris (Fig. 21–5). Amphophilic intranuclear inclusion bodies are occasionally present in intact epithelial cells, but surprisingly few inflammatory changes are associated with these early lesions.

By damaging the gland epithelium, CPV-2 destroys the source of epithelial cells. Hence, as the disease progresses, the villi become blunted and covered by thin immature epithelial cells. Adjacent villi may fuse. The loss of crypt epithelium is not permanent, and evidence of intestinal epithelial regeneration is often present, even in fatal cases. Remaining intestinal crypts become elongated and lined by hyperplastic epithelium with a high mitotic index. Lesions occasionally are present in the large bowel, but they are usually mild, consisting mainly of an increase of dark amphophilic cells in the proliferative areas of the intestinal glands.

There is widespread necrosis and depletion of lymphocytes in the GI-associated lymphoid tissue, the germinal centers of mesenteric lymph nodes, and the splenic nodules. Diffuse cortical necrosis of the thymus occurs in young dogs.

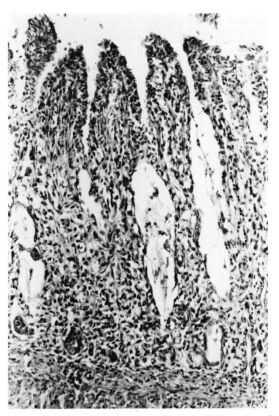

Figure 21–5. Photomicrograph of the small intestine of a dog that died of parvoviral enteritis. Villi are collapsed, and crypt lumina are dilated and filled with necrotic debris (H and E; × 100). (Courtesy of Dr. Ed Mahaffey, University of Georgia, Athens, GA.)

Myocardial Form

The gross lesions of CPV-2 myocarditis are those of heart failure. The cardiac chambers are dilated and flaccid, and there is pulmonary edema and passive congestion of the liver. Ascites, hydrothorax, and hydropericardium may be present. Pale white streaks associated with myocardial necrosis and cellular infiltrates are often grossly visible in the ventricular myocardium (Fig. 21–6). The left ventricle is usually more severely affected.

Microscopically, a nonsuppurative myocarditis is observed. Edema and myofiber loss are present, together with a locally extensive lymphocytic infiltrate. A small number of intranuclear inclusion bodies are present, which stain intensely with anti-CPV-2 or anti-FPV fluorescein-antibody conjugate. Healing occurs by interstitial fibrosis and scarring; extensive areas of fibrosis develop in chronic cases.

Cerebellar hypoplasia occurs with parvo-

viral infection in kittens or hamsters but has not been reported in association with CPV-2 infection in the dog.

THERAPY

Treatment of CPV-2 enteritis is nonspecific and supportive.[38] The general guidelines for treatment of acute nonspecific gastroenteritis should be followed. The principal objectives are to rest the GI tract, to restore and maintain fluid and electrolyte balance, and to minimize continuing fluid losses. In general, pups with enteritis can be treated as outpatients unless they have clinical findings that suggest a life-threatening condition, such as severe dehydration or blood loss, seizures, high fever, or marked depression. These pups and others that have failed to respond to conservative treatment should be hospitalized and an intensive therapeutic and diagnostic program should be instituted. Young puppies dehydrate rapidly and are more likely to require hospitalization and close monitoring than adults.

Fluids

Fluid therapy is probably the single most important aspect of clinical management of CPV-2 infection. It should be initiated promptly and continued for as long as the vomiting or diarrhea persist. Oral electrolyte solutions are the simplest form of therapy, provided that they can be tolerated. Com-

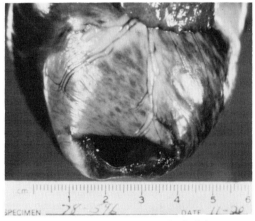

Figure 21–6. Heart from a dog that died of the myocardial form of CPV infection. Pale streaking of the myocardium is apparent. (Courtesy of Norden Laboratories, Lincoln, NE.)

mercial preparations, such as those for calves (for example, Resorb, Beecham Laboratories, Bristol, TN) or people (Gatorade, Stokely VanKamp Co, Indianapolis, IN), are excellent, but a homemade formula of 3.5 g NaCl (table salt), 3.5 g $NaHCO_3^-$, 1.5 g KCl, and 20 g glucose dissolved in 1 liter of water can also be used (see also Chapter 9, Table 9–7).[38] Maintenance requirements are about 70 ml/kg/day, but more will be necessary if the patient continues to have diarrhea or to vomit.

SC fluid administration is appropriate in mildly to moderately dehydrated animals that cannot tolerate oral electrolyte solutions. Care should be exercised in the SC administration of fluids, however, as cellulitis and even necrosis of the skin can occur if this route is overused or if an excessive amount is instilled in a single site. Dogs with CPV-2 enteritis seem especially prone to complications following SC fluid administration.

IV fluid therapy should be initiated promptly for severely ill or dehydrated patients. Ideally, acid-base and electrolyte imbalances should be monitored and corrected, but even if this is not possible, simple volume expansion with a balanced electrolyte solution is often life-saving. Alkalinization with $NaHCO_3^-$ has been recommended, based on assumed losses due to diarrhea. More recent studies, however, suggest that dogs with CPV-2 enteritis are only rarely acidotic.[39] In the absence of acid-base data, bicarbonate supplementation is probably not warranted.

Although only a relatively small proportion of dogs with CPV-2 enteritis are hypokalemic, potassium supplementation is advised whenever glucose-containing solutions are administered parenterally, because they cause an intracellular shift of the electrolyte. Anorexia and food restriction can lead to potassium depletion, which further exacerbates intestinal ileus. IV potassium supplementation should be given at a maximum of 40 mEq/L in isotonic fluids whenever serum potassium drops below 3.5 mEq/L. SC potassium supplementation is much safer and easier; it can be given more rapidly at higher concentrations with less danger of causing cardiac arrhythmias.

Fluids containing 2.5% to 5% dextrose may be valuable in counteracting the endotoxic shock and hypoglycemia observed in some cases (see also Chapter 44). In a con-

trolled study, the administration of antiendotoxin hyperimmune plasma was shown to decrease both mortality and the length of hospitalization in dogs with CPV-2 enteritis.[40]

Symptomatic Therapy

Withholding food for 12 to 24 hours is a simple but important part of symptomatic therapy. Water should also be withheld if vomiting is severe; otherwise, animals may initiate a vicious cycle of drinking and vomiting that only exacerbates the problem. SC or IV fluids should be used to prevent dehydration.

Food, in the form of a warm bland gruel, should be gradually reintroduced after enteric signs have subsided. Commercially available bland diets (for example, Prescription Diet i/d, Hills Co, Topeka, KS) are convenient, but cottage cheese and boiled rice are a satisfactory homemade substitute. If feeding causes a recurrence of vomiting or diarrhea, the fast should be continued for an additional 12 to 24 hours. After food can be tolerated, frequent meals of the bland diet, given in small amounts, should be continued for 2 to 3 days, with gradual reintroduction of the regular diet.

Antibiotics

Routine use of antibiotics for simple enteritis is poor practice. Oral antibiotics may alter the intestinal flora in favor of enteric pathogens. They may also prolong shedding of enteropathogens like *Salmonella* and favor the development of resistant strains. Parenteral antibiotics, on the other hand, probably have a place in the management of severe CPV-2 enteritis because affected animals are at risk of secondary pneumonia and generalized bacterial infection.[38] A combination of ampicillin and gentamicin has been recommended because it provides a broad spectrum of activity against both aerobes and anaerobes (Table 21–1). Care must be taken to ensure adequate hydration if any of the aminoglycosides are used, because they can cause fatal nephrotoxicity, especially in dehydrated or very young patients. Urine sediment should be monitored frequently to detect tubular casts that herald the onset of tubular nephrosis.

Motility Modifiers and Intestinal Protectants

The value of many traditional medicaments for vomiting and diarrhea has been questioned. In controlled trials in people, kaolin-pectin preparations, for example, have failed to reduce either the duration or severity of diarrhea.[41] Likewise, the routine use of motility modifiers, such as anticholinergics and opiate agonists is discouraged. Anticholinergics, in particular, can be detrimental because they decrease segmental contractions to a greater extent than propulsive movements and can therefore actually reduce resistance to the flow of ingesta. Opiate agonists increase segmentation and slow the passage of ingesta but in so doing, may lead to a fatally increased absorption of endotoxin.

Antiemetic drugs are indicated when vomiting is severe and persistent, although their efficacy is limited in cases of CPV-2 enteritis. Metoclopramide has proven useful in otherwise intractable cases (Table 21–1). SC dosing can be given every 8 hours, or in very severe cases, the drug can be given as a continuous IV drip. Phenothiazines such as thiethylperazine or trimethobenzamide, which do not produce CNS depression, may be helpful to control persistent vomiting.

PREVENTION

Immunity After Infection

Recovery from CPV-2 infection confers long-lived immunity. Dogs challenged orally with CPV-2 up to 20 months after recovery have been completely immune to reinfection,[42] and it is probable that this immunity is life-long. The mechanisms by which immunity is achieved and maintained remain to be elucidated. In general, there is a direct correlation between serum antibody titer and resistance to infection. Antibody titers remain very high for prolonged periods after infection, even in the absence of reexposure.[42] In the presence of low levels of humoral antibody, localized infection can still occur, but viremia and generalized illness do not. The role of intestinal IgA is uncertain. Secretory antibody may have a role in elimination of the virus from the host but probably is not vital to long-lived immunity, since coproantibody titers reportedly declined to undetectable levels within 15 days PI.

Immunization

A number of effective vaccines are available for parvoviral prophylaxis, but there is no agreement about the optimal immunization strategy. The disagreement arises from inadequate or biased experimental designs, different doses and routes of administration, differences in serologic methodology, differing definitions of immunity, and variable risk of exposure. Results of field trials are particularly difficult to interpret because clinical disease is infrequent in older animals. Nevertheless, most commercially available vaccines seem to perform satisfactorily in routine practice. For additional information besides that provided below, see Canine Vaccination Recommendations, Ca-

Table 21–1. Drug Dosages for Treating Canine Viral Enteritis[a]

DRUG	DOSE[b] (mg/kg)	ROUTE	INTERVAL (hours)	DURATION (days)
Antibiotics				
Amp(amox)icillin	10–20	IV, SC	6–8	3–5
Gentamicin[c]	2	IV, IM, SC	8	3–5
Antiemetics				
Metoclopramide[d]	0.2–0.4	PO, SC	6–8	prn
	1–2	IV	24	prn
Thiethylperazine[e]	0.05–0.5	IM, SC	8	prn
Trimethobenzamide	3	IM	8	prn

[a]IV = intravenous, SC = subcutaneous, IM = intramuscular, PO = oral, prn = as needed.
[b]Dose per administration at specified interval, expressed as mg/kg unless otherwise stated.
[c]Renal function (BUN, urine casts) should be closely evaluated and the drug not used for longer than 7–10 days.
[d]Total dose IV not to exceed 1–2 mg/kg/day, given as bolus infusions throughout the day.
[e]Should not be given with other motility modifiers.

nine Parvoviral Enteritis, Chapter 2, and Appendices 1 and 3.

Inactivated Vaccines. Inactivated FPV, MEV, and CPV vaccines of sufficient antigenic mass immunize dogs against challenge with CPV-2.[43,44] Certain adjuvants may enhance the immune response.

If immunity is defined as absolute resistance to infection, then that produced by most inactivated vaccines is short-lived; subclinical infection has been shown to occur as little as 2 weeks after vaccination. However, prior sensitization with inactivated vaccines allows dogs to mount a rapid secondary response, thereby suppressing generalized viremia, which appears to be a critical determinant of clinical disease.[19] Thus, if immunity is taken to mean resistance to clinical disease, then some inactivated vaccines appear capable of providing protection for as long as 15 months.[43] Most studies, however, including those required for licensure, have been of short duration, with challenge only 2 to 4 weeks after vaccination. No adequately controlled field trials of vaccine efficacy have been reported.

Up to 60% of pups successfully vaccinated with inactivated vaccines had serologic evidence of subclinical CPV-2 infection during the following year.[14] The high frequency of subclinical infection following killed vaccine administration probably contributes significantly to their apparent effectiveness in the field. However, since subclinically infected dogs excrete large amounts of virus, they serve as an important source of infection for other dogs.

MLV-FPV Vaccines. Attenuated FPV also has been used to immunize dogs against CPV-2 challenge, but the principal disadvantage of live FPV vaccines is that the response varies markedly.[45] Some animals demonstrate the high and persistent antibody titers typically induced by a live vaccine, whereas others show immune reactions more typical of those to inactivated or nonreplicating agents. Since attenuated CPV-2 vaccines produce more uniform results, they have largely replaced live FPV in commercial vaccines.

MLV-CPV-2 Vaccines. Attenuated CPV-2 vaccines appear to provide the most protection against infection.[10,42,45–47] Several strains of virus have been developed for use in commercial vaccines, but detailed studies have been published on only a few; differences may exist with respect to degree of attenuation.

The events following inoculation of attenuated virus parallel those that result from wild-type viral infection. There is a viremia and systemic distribution of the attenuated strain on the second day after parenteral inoculation. Viral shedding from the intestinal tract occurs on days 3 to 7 postinoculation, but in amounts 10^2 to 10^4 times lower than that observed in wild-type viral infections.[10] Susceptible contacts are immunized by the virus shed by vaccinates. The attenuated strains appear genetically stable, and vaccinal virus has remained nonpathogenic through up to six sequential back-passages in dogs.[46,47]

Humoral immune responses to the attenuated CPV-2 strains studied have been similar to those observed with wild-type virus infection.[43,46,47] Antibody is usually detectable on day 3 after inoculation, rising rapidly to levels comparable to those observed after natural infection. High titers persist in the absence of reexposure for at least 2 years, and dogs challenged 24 months after vaccination could not be infected.[10]

There is no persuasive evidence that significant immunosuppression or other illness is caused by vaccinal CPV.[17] Studies that have hypothesized immunosuppression by vaccinal CPV-2 were based on indirect evidence or faulty experimental design. Well-controlled studies[48] failed to reveal immunosuppression by vaccinal CPV-2. However, there was significant suppression with polyvalent vaccines that contained canine distemper virus combined with canine adenovirus-1 or -2. Although a slight reduction in the number of circulating lymphocytes often occurs on days 3 to 5 after CPV-2 vaccination, this cannot be assumed to indicate immunosuppression without further evidence.[17] Preliminary studies have failed to detect changes in lymphocyte responsiveness in the 2 weeks following vaccination.[17,49] Antibody titers to other viral agents administered simultaneously with attenuated CPV-2 have generally been similar to those obtained to the agents alone.[45,46] In one study, decreased lymphocyte blastogenesis followed revaccination of some previously immune dogs.[50] Since CPV-2 does not replicate in immune dogs, it is probable that the observed immunosuppression had other causes.

Effect of Maternally Derived Antibody. The most important cause of vaccination "failure" in puppies appears to be suppression of an active immune response by maternally derived antibodies.[49] The age at which pups will respond to vaccination depends upon the antibody titer of the dam. After ingestion of colostrum, titers in pups are usually equal to that of the bitch. Thereafter, maternal antibody is lost, with a half-life of approximately 9 days (see Tables 2–2, 2–3, and 2–4). In litters born to bitches with high titers, pups may not respond to commercial vaccines until as late as 18 weeks of age.[42] Exposure to virulent parvovirus such as in endemically contaminated premises may accelerate the decline in maternal antibody titer in pups.[49a]

Inactivated vaccines appear to be particularly susceptible to maternal antibody interference, although adjuvant may partially offset this tendency by increasing the persistence of antigen. Attenuated CPV-2 vaccines appear to be less susceptible to interference by maternal antibody than inactivated virus or attenuated FPV vaccines.[46,49] Highly attenuated CPV-2 strains are more liable to maternal antibody suppression than less highly attenuated strains, but no vaccine consistently immunizes pups in the face of high levels of maternal antibody. In several kennels, attenuated CPV-2 vaccines have been substantially more effective than attenuated FPV or unadjuvanted inactivated vaccines in reducing puppy mortality.[46,51]

The principal problem in the prevention of CPV-2 enteritis is that levels of maternal antibody that are too low to provide resistance to infection can suppress response to vaccination. Thus, as their maternal antibody titers decline, all pups born to immune bitches experience a period during which they are susceptible to infection but refractory to immunization. Most CPV-2 infections now occur during this critical period, despite otherwise effective vaccines and rigorous immunization schedules.

Immunization success rates are inversely correlated with the amount of maternal antibody at the time of vaccination. In one study, fewer than 40% of dogs with reciprocal HI titers of 20 responded to vaccination, and fewer than 60% of dogs with titers of 10 responded. A successful immunization rate of 90% has been observed only in pups that were seronegative by the HI test.[42,49]

PUBLIC HEALTH CONSIDERATIONS

Studies have failed to find any evidence of human infection by CPV-2, even among kennel workers in heavily contaminated premises,[12,52] although people apparently can act as a passive transport vehicle for virus. It has been suggested, however, that CPV-2 enteritis may increase the likelihood of kennel workers being exposed to *Campylobacter* or *Salmonella* in the feces of infected dogs. This may account for the increased incidence of human diarrhea reported during some canine outbreaks. Thus, although CPV-2 is not itself a human pathogen, extra care should be practiced in handling fecal materials from diarrheic animals.

Canine Parvovirus-1 Infection

ETIOLOGY

CPV-1, originally isolated from fecal specimens of healthy dogs, was named the minute virus of canines (MVC). It appears to be widespread in the dog population but is not presently considered an important cause of clinical disease.

Physical and chemical properties of the MVC are typical of parvoviruses. The virus has been propagated successfully in only one cell line, the Walter Reed canine (WRC) cell line, and this has impeded research. In addition, MVC has been shown to replicate in primary canine fetal lung cell cultures.[53]

By HI tests, the MVC is serologically distinct from parvoviruses of a number of other species. Recent data indicate that the MVC and CPV-2 are different viruses; no homology in DNA restriction sites between the 2 viruses has been demonstrated using several restriction enzymes.[54]

EPIDEMIOLOGY

The dog is the only known host; it is likely but not proved that other Canidae are susceptible. Specific HI antibody has been found in sera of up to 85% of dogs tested and in commercial canine globulin preparations. Information concerning other aspects of the epidemiology of CPV-1 is lacking. It seems reasonable to assume that spread is similar to that of CPV-2.

PATHOGENESIS

The pathogenicity of CPV-1 for dogs is unclear at present. The virus has been identified by immunoelectron microscopy in the feces of normal pups and in dogs with mild diarrhea. Four to 6 days following oral exposure, virus can be recovered from the small intestine, spleen, mesenteric lymph nodes, and thymus. Histologic changes in lymphatic tissues are similar to those observed in pups infected with CPV-2 but are much less severe.[54] In addition, there is preliminary experimental evidence that CPV-1 is capable of crossing the placenta and producing early fetal deaths and birth defects.[53] Whether this is common with natural infections is uncertain. Characterization of the true pathogenic potential of the virus awaits further study.

CLINICAL FINDINGS

CPV-1 has been observed occasionally in field dogs with mild diarrhea as well as in the feces of clinically healthy animals. Experimental infections have been subclinical, although there is clear evidence of viral replication and tissue destruction in the intestine and lymphoid tissues.[54] The potential exists for CPV-1 to exacerbate concurrent infections.

PATHOLOGIC FINDINGS

Principal macroscopic changes in pups euthanatized at 4 to 6 days PI have included thymic edema and atrophy and enlarged lymph nodes.[54] Microscopic changes were most prominent in the thymus and lymph nodes and consist of cortical thymic lymphocytolysis. Occasional thymocytes had amphophilic intranuclear inclusion bodies typical of parvoviruses that stained positively with fluorescein-labeled anti–CPV-1 antiserum. There has been extensive interlobular and interstitial thymic edema. Moderate depletion of the germinal centers of the lymph nodes has been evident, and the histiocytic reticulum cell framework has been prominent. Small pyknotic, amphophilic cells have also been present in the splenic white pulp.

Necrosis of individual crypt cells and a few darkly staining amphophilic cells occurred in the duodenum. Villi were normal, although prominent intranuclear inclusions were observed in some enterocytes. Inclusions have been prominent in the lymphocytes of the GI-associated lymphoid tissue, but there has been little change in the mucosal surface. Changes were absent in other areas of the small intestine in the pups studied.

DIAGNOSIS

CPV-1 infection should be considered in young dogs with mild diarrhea that are CPV-2–negative or in unexplained fetal abnormalities or abortions.

CPV-1 has been observed in fecal and rectal swab samples from field dogs by electron microscopy. Immunoelectron microscopy is necessary to distinguish CPV-1 from CPV-2. Inhibition of hemagglutinating activity in stool suspensions by specific antiserum also is diagnostic for CPV-1.

Sera can be tested for specific antibody by use of VN or HI tests. Since only a few cell lines support growth of CPV-1, the availability of virus isolation and serum VN tests is limited.

IMMUNITY

Little is known about the immune responses to CPV-1. Dogs have developed substantial HI antibody titers ($> 1:640$) within 3 weeks of infection; VN antibody titers have been two- to fourfold higher.[53] Dogs with HI antibody titers $\geq 1:1280$ failed to shed virus in their feces or to develop increased HI titers following challenge with CPV-1.

It should be possible to develop effective vaccines, but the present understanding of the disease suggests that vaccination is unwarranted.

PUBLIC HEALTH CONSIDERATIONS

There is no known public health concern, although the question has not been adequately investigated.

Canine Coronaviral Enteritis

ETIOLOGY

Canine coronavirus (CCV) belongs to a group of closely related single-stranded RNA viruses that include transmissible gastroenteritis virus of swine and the feline enteric coronaviruses (see Chapter 24). Coronaviridae are pleomorphic, enveloped viruses, 60 to 180 nm in diameter, named for the corona of leaf-shaped peplomers that project from the viral envelope (Fig. 21–7). The envelope is derived from the lipid membrane of the endoplasmic reticulum and hence is readily disrupted by most detergents and lipid solvents. An intact viral envelope is necessary for infectivity, so that Coronaviridae are more readily inactivated than parvoviruses.

EPIDEMIOLOGY

The true importance of CCV as a cause of enteritis in dogs is not known. Serologic studies suggest that most adult dogs, especially those in group housing, have been exposed to the virus and have recovered from infection.[12] Few studies have attempted to document the incidence of CCV among cases of acute enteritis. Available data suggest that CCV has been present indefinitely in the dog population and is a less frequent cause of enteritis than is generally supposed.[55,55a]

Detailed studies of the transmission of infection are lacking, although the spread is almost certainly fecal-oral. In contrast to CPV infection, chronic carriers probably play an important role in the perpetuation of the disease. Infected dogs have been shown to shed the virus intermittently for months following clinical recovery. Within a kennel, CCV infection spreads rapidly, and high seroprevalence rates are common among dogs housed in groups.[12] Immunity to coronaviruses appears short-lived in most species, and repeated infections by the same or related strains also may help propagate the disease.

PATHOGENESIS

Following oral ingestion, CCV invades the mature epitheliocytes on the luminal aspect of the villi in the small intestine. The infection spreads distally over the next 24 to 48 hours until the entire small intestine is involved. In contrast to CPV-2 enteritis, infection of the intestinal epithelium is limited to the mature epitheliocytes of the intestinal villi. Viremia and systemic spread are not prominent aspects of CCV enteritis.

Viral replication causes death and desquamation of mature epithelial cells, resulting in villous blunting. The loss of absorptive and digestive capacity leads to diarrhea. Since the germinal epithelium of the intestinal glands is spared, healing is relatively rapid and is usually complete within 1 week.

CLINICAL FINDINGS

As with CPV-2 enteritis, the signs of CCV infection are variable and nonspecific. Although much has been written about the clinical presentation, there is no pattern of clinical features that reliably distinguishes it from other causes of acute enteritis in dogs. Leukopenia is not a feature of CCV enteritis.

DIAGNOSIS

Definitive diagnosis depends on serologic tests or the demonstration of virus or viral antigens in the intestine or feces. There are no discriminating clinical pathologic or radiographic findings.

Virus can be detected in feces or intestinal contents by electron microscopy or viral isolation. The principal identifying feature of CCV in electron micrographs is their characteristic fringe. False-positive electron microscopic findings commonly occur because there are many artifactually fringed particles in fecal specimens that may be difficult to differentiate from true coronaviruses.[55] Conversely, false-negative results occur because the fringe on true virions deteriorates rapidly as the sample ages. Virus can also be destroyed by freezing-thawing. Thus, electron microscopic findings for coronavirus must be interpreted with caution. Positive results are meaningful only when large numbers of well-preserved virions are observed. In one study of more than 1000 fecal samples submitted for electron microscopic examination, 50% were positive for parvoviruses; approximately 1% had particles with CCV morphology.[56] Negative findings are of little value except when obtained after thorough examination of fresh specimens. Immunoelectron microscopy increases the specificity and sensitivity of the test.

CCV can be isolated relatively easily in feline cell culture. Identification of virus in feces confirms the presence of infection but not necessarily that CCV is responsible for the clinical illness. Coronaviruses, rotaviruses, and parvoviruses have been found in fecal specimens from healthy dogs from many parts of the world.[57]

Several commercial laboratories offer serologic tests for CCV (see Appendix 8). Diagnosis must depend upon demonstrating seroconversion, since the seroprevalence of CCV antibody may be as high as 80% in some populations.[12] Titers increase more slowly with CCV enteritis than in CPV-2 infection; hence, seroconversion is easier to detect. Seroconversion, generally considered ≥ fourfold increase in titer, can be demonstrated between acute samples collected at the time of illness and convalescent samples collected 2 to 6 weeks later.[12]

As with all canine viral enteritides, laboratory confirmation of CCV enteritis is undertaken principally for academic or epidemiologic reasons in a disease outbreak, since treatment is supportive only and since test results are not generally available until after the diagnostic work-up and treatment have been completed.

PATHOLOGIC FINDINGS

Gross necropsy findings on cases of CCV enteritis are nonspecific. There may be dilated loops of bowel filled with gas and watery ingesta. The intestinal mucosa may be congested or hemorrhagic and the mesenteric lymph nodes enlarged and edematous.

Microscopic lesions of CCV enteritis are less pronounced and specific than those of CPV-2 infection. Because they are rapidly obscured by postmortem autolysis, it is difficult to obtain histologic confirmation of CCV enteritis in field cases. In fresh specimens, shortening and fusion of the intestinal villi are seen, together with deepening of the crypts, increased goblet cells, and increased cellularity of the lamina propria.

THERAPY AND PREVENTION

Treatment is supportive only and should follow the general guidelines given for CPV-2 enteritis. Antibiotics are not indicated unless there is independent evidence of sepsis.

The basis and duration of immunity to CCV are not known. Because it is a surface infection, secretory antibody (IgA) is probably more important than circulating antibody. Dogs that have recovered from CCV are immune to reinfection for at least 1 month, but the nature and duration of this immunity have not been established.

Two inactivated vaccines against CCV are commercially available (see Coronaviral Infection, Chapter 2). An attenuated vaccine was marketed briefly but was withdrawn because of a substantial number of fatal adverse effects.[58] (See also Postvaccinal Complications, Chapter 2.)

Dogs challenged 2 weeks after vaccination have shown a marked reduction in the amount of viral replication in the intestinal

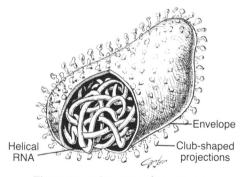

Figure 21–7. Structure of coronavirus.

Helical RNA

Envelope

Club-shaped projections

tract, although they are not completely re-fractory to infection.[59] Protection from clini-cal disease has been more difficult to assess, because most experimental CCV infections are subclinical. Appropriately controlled field trials have not been reported. Combined CCV/CPV-2 infections have been shown to be much more severe than either virus alone,[60] and it may be that even partial protection against CCV is of value in reducing the severity of mixed infections. Valid studies of the cost-benefit ratio for CCV vaccination remain to be done.

PUBLIC HEALTH CONSIDERATIONS

The public health aspects of CCV have not been thoroughly investigated. Coronaviruses are not strictly host-specific, so the possibility of human infection cannot be entirely ruled out. A study of over 1000 veterinary students, however, failed to detect serologic evidence of infection. Thus, CCV is not believed to pose an important threat to human health.

Canine Rotaviral Infection

ETIOLOGY

The rotaviruses belong to the family Reoviridae (Fig. 21–8).[61] A remarkable feature of the viruses of this family is that the genome is divided among 10 or 11 separate pieces of double-stranded RNA, hence resortment can occur if a cell is simultaneously infected by two different viruses. The virions are also distinguished by their unique double capsid. The viruses are unenveloped, and resistant to acid and lipid solvents. The double-capsid appears to be an adaptation to protect the virus from inactivation in the upper GI tract. Indeed, in vitro culture attempts were unsuccessful until it was discovered that proteolytic enzyme digestion of the outer capsid is a prerequisite for infectivity of most strains.[61]

In the past decade, rotaviruses have been recognized as important causes of neonatal diarrhea in many domestic species and in people. In people, they are the leading causes of sporadic acute enteritis in infants and young children. A canine rotavirus has been isolated,[62,63] but evidence to date suggests that it is rarely a cause of illness in dogs.

Rotaviruses from a wide range of species share a common group antigen that is a component of the inner capsid. Originally, all pathogenic rotaviruses were believed to share this antigen, but a group of antigenically distinct rotaviruses has been recognized.[64]

EPIDEMIOLOGY

Rotaviruses are transmitted by fecal-oral contamination. The viruses are well adapted for survival outside the host and for passage through the upper GI tract.

Serologic surveys reveal that the majority of adult dogs have been infected by canine rotavirus.[65] Since serologic surveys are, in essence, measures of survivorship, the disease appears to have a low case fatality. It is probable that canine rotavirus occurs throughout the world.

PATHOGENESIS

Rotaviruses infect the most mature epithelial cells on the luminal tips of the intestinal villi.[62,66,67] Infected cells swell, degenerate, and desquamate into the bowel lumen, where they release large numbers of virions that become sources of infection for lower

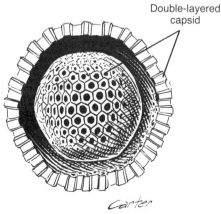

Double-layered capsid

Carter

Figure 21–8. Structure of reovirus.

bowel segments and for other animals. The denuded villi contract, resulting in villous atrophy. Necrosis of rotavirus-infected cells is most pronounced 18 to 48 hours after oral infection.[67] Necrotic cells are rapidly replaced by immature crypt epithelium. Clinical signs result principally from the loss of disaccharidases and other brush border enzymes, leading to an osmotic diarrhea.

CLINICAL FINDINGS

Rotaviral diarrhea has been reported exclusively in pups less than 12 weeks old and most often in pups less than 2 weeks of age. Experimentally, it has not been possible to reproduce the disease in animals more than 6 months old. Oral inoculation of 2-day-old, gnotobiotic puppies has resulted in severe diarrhea and dehydration, but hematologic changes have not been detected.[62] Most natural infections appear to be subclinical or to be limited to relatively mild, nonspecific diarrhea, anorexia, and lethargy.

DIAGNOSIS

Most pathogenic rotaviruses share a common group antigen that can be detected by a number of methods,[64] including a commercial ELISA test (Rotazyme, Abbott Laboratories, North Chicago, IL). Rotaviruses can also be identified in fecal specimens by electron microscopy, although care must be taken to differentiate rotaviruses from the apparently nonpathogenic reoviruses occasionally present in dog feces. Immunoelectron microscopy improves specificity of the test. Testing for evidence of seroconversion is possible[65] but not widely available. See Appendix 8 for a listing of commercially available test kits and laboratories that assist in the diagnosis of rotaviral infections.

PATHOLOGIC FINDINGS

Pathologic changes are limited to the small bowel, consisting of mild to moderate villous blunting.[67] In natural cases, these changes are usually obscured by autolysis, so that the diagnosis can seldom be confirmed by histology. Virus can be detected in frozen sections by fluorescent antibody techniques.

THERAPY AND PREVENTION

Treatment consists solely of symptomatic therapy as described for CPV-2 enteritis.

The duration and nature of immunity to canine rotavirus have not been adequately investigated. The principal source of protection for neonatal puppies is probably antibodies present in the milk of immune bitches. Given that the infection is confined to the surface epithelium of the digestive tract, it is probable that secretory antibody is more important in protection than humoral immunity. No vaccine is available, and current estimates of the frequency and severity of disease do not appear to justify vaccine development.

PUBLIC HEALTH CONSIDERATIONS

Rotaviruses do not appear to be host-specific. For example, human rotavirus can be serially propagated in dogs. Thus, puppies with rotaviral enteritis may pose a potential human health hazard, particularly for infants. Care should be exercised when handling fecal material from diarrheic dogs in general, although the risk of contracting campylobacteriosis is probably a more significant reason for caution than the danger of rotaviral enteritis.

Other Viral Enteritides

A number of other viruses have been observed in the feces of dogs both with and without diarrhea. For the most part, their pathogenicity and importance as causes of clinical disease remain unknown. Based on work in other species, some (e.g., astrovirus) may be true enteric pathogens, while others (e.g., reovirus) are most likely incidental findings.

Astrovirus-like particles have been reported in the stools of clinically healthy and diarrheic dogs.[55,68] Astroviruses are known to cause enteritis in other species, such as swine, but whether this is either true or common in the dog is not known.

A herpesvirus antigenically related to feline rhinotracheitis virus has been isolated from a dog with diarrhea,[69] but Koch's postulates have not been fulfilled. Likewise, the importance of serologic reactivity of some dogs to human echoviruses and coxsackieviruses is unclear (see Chapter 33).

An apparently specific canine calicivirus has been isolated on several occasions from the feces of dogs with enteritis, sometimes alone and sometimes in conjunction with other known enteric pathogens.[70,71] Likewise, an antigenically distinct parainfluenza virus, isolated from a dog with bloody diarrhea, was believed to be causal (see Chapter 20).

The study of viral enteritis in dogs is in its infancy; there are undoubtedly other viruses that affect the canine GI tract, but they remain to be discovered and characterized.

References

1. Schwers A, Pastoret P-P, Bortonboy G, et al: Frequence en Belgique de l'infection a Parvovirus chez le chien, avant et aprés l'observation des premiers cas cliniques. Ann Med Vet 123:561–566, 1979.
2. Thomas NJ, Foreyt WJ, Evermann JF, et al: Seroprevalence of canine parvovirus in wild coyotes from Texas, Utah and Idaho (1972 to 1983). J Am Vet Med Assoc 185:1283–1287, 1984.
3. Parrish CR: Canine Parvovirus and Feline Panleukopenia Virus: Structure and Function. Ph.D. dissertation, Cornell University, Ithaca, NY, 1984.
4. Parrish CR, Carmichael LE: Antigenic structure and variation of canine parvovirus type-2, feline panleukopenia virus, and mink eneteritis virus. Virology 129:401–414, 1983.
4a. Reed AP, Jones EV, Miller TJ: Nucleotide sequence and genome organization of canine parvovirus. J Virol 62:266–276, 1988.
5. Parrish CR, O'Connell PH, Evermann JF, et al: Natural variation of canine parvovirus. Science 230:1046–1048, 1985.
6. Appel MJG, Carmichael LE: Can a commercial vaccine protect pups against a recent field isolate of parvovirus? Vet Med 82:1091–1093, 1987.
7. Gordon JC, Angrick EJ: Canine parvovirus: environmental effects on infectivity. Am J Vet Res 47:1464–1467, 1986.
8. Pollock RVH, Parrish CR: Canine parvovirus. In Olsen RG, Krakowka S, Blakeslee JR (eds): Comparative Pathobiology of Viral Diseases, Vol 1. Boca Raton, FL, CRC Press, 1985, 145–177.
9. Goto H, Uchida E, Ichijo S, et al: Experimental infection of canine parvovirus in specific pathogen-free cats. Jpn J Vet Sci 46: 729–731, 1984.
9a. Uchida E, Ichijo S, Goto H, et al: Clinical hema-

10. Carmichael LE, Joubert JC, Pollock RVH: A modified live canine parvovirus strain with novel plaque characteristics. I. Viral attenuation and dog response. Cornell Vet 71: 408–427, 1981.
11. Studdert MJ, Oda C, Riegl CA, et al: Aspects of the diagnosis, pathogenesis and epidemiology of canine parvovirus. Aust Vet J 60:197–200, 1983.
12. Binn LN, Marchwicki RH, Eckermann EH, et al: Viral antibody studies of laboratory dogs with diarrheal disease. Am J Vet Res 42:1665–1667, 1981.
13. Mason MJ, Gillett NA, Muggenburg BA: Clinical, pathological and epidemiological aspects of canine parvoviral enteritis in an unvaccinated closed beagle colony: 1978–1985. J Am Anim Hosp Assoc 23:183–192, 1987.
14. Sabine M, Feilen C, Herbert L, et al: Canine parvovirus—five years later. Aust Vet Practit 14:24–27, 1984.
15. Meunier PC, Cooper BJ, Appel MJG, et al: Experimental viral myocarditis: parvoviral infection of neonatal pups. Vet Pathol 21:509–515, 1984.
16. Lenghaus C, Studdert MJ: Acute and chronic viral myocarditis. Am J Pathol 115:316–319, 1984.
17. Brunner CJ, Swango LJ: Canine parvovirus infection: effects on the immune system and factors that predispose to severe disease. Compend Cont Educ Pract Vet 7:979–989, 1985.
18. Parrish CR, Have P, Foreyt WJ, et al: The global spread and replacement of canine parvovirus strains. J Gen Virol 69:1111–1116, 1988.
19. Meunier PC, Cooper BJ, Appel MJG, et al: Pathogenesis of canine parvovirus enteritis: the importance of viremia. Vet Pathol 22:60–71, 1985.
20. Glickman LT, Domanski LM, Patronek GJ, et al: Breed-related risk factors for canine parvovirus enteritis. J Am Vet Med Assoc 187:589–594, 1985.
21. Meunier PC, Cooper BJ, Appel MJG, et al: Pathogenesis of canine parvovirus enteritis: sequential virus distribution and passive immunization studies. Vet Pathol 22:617–624, 1985.
22. Macartney L, McCandlish IAP, Thompson H, et al: Canine parvovirus enteritis 2: pathogenesis. Vet Rec 115:453–460, 1984.
23. Lenghaus C, Studdert MJ: Generalized parvovirus disease in neonatal pups. J Am Vet Med Assoc 181:41–45, 1982.
24. Johnson BJ, Castro AE: Isolation of canine parvovirus from a dog brain with severe necrotizing vasculitis and encephalomalacia. J Am Vet Med Assoc 184:1398–1399, 1984.
25. Macartney L, McCandlish IAP, Thompson H, et al: Canine parvovirus enteritis 1: clinical, haematological and pathological features of experimental infection. Vet Rec 115:201–210, 1984.
26. Macartney L, McCandlish IAP, Thompson H, et al: Canine parvovirus enteritis 3: scanning electron microscopical findings of experimental infection. Vet Rec 115:533–537, 1984.
27. Mochizuki M, Hida S, Hsuan SW, et al: Fecal examination for diagnosis of canine parvovirus infection. Jpn J Vet Sci 46:587–591, 1984.
28. Meunier PC, Glickman LT, Appel MJG, et al: Canine parvovirus in a commercial kennel: epidemiologic and pathologic findings. Cornell Vet 71:96–110, 1981.
29. Gooding GE, Robinson WF: Maternal antibody, vac-

cination and reproductive failure in dogs with parvovirus infection. *Aust Vet J* 59:170–174, 1982.

30. Anderson PG, Pidgeon G: Candidiasis in a dog with parvoviral enteritis. *J Am Anim Hosp Assoc* 23:27–30, 1987.

31. Olsen CG, Stiff MI, Olsen RG: Comparison of the blastogenic response of peripheral blood lymphocytes from canine parovirus-positive and -negative outbred dogs. *Vet Immunol Immunopathol* 6:285–290, 1984.

32. Phillips TR, Schultz RD: Failure of vaccine or virulent strains of canine parvovirus to induce immunosuppressive effects on the immune system of the dog. *Viral Immunol* 1:135–144, 1987.

33. Krakowka S, Olsen RG, Axthelm MK, et al: Canine parvovirus infection potentiates canine distemper encephalitis attributable to modified live-virus vaccine. *J Am Vet Med Assoc* 180:137–139, 1982.

34. Veijalainen PML, Neuvonen E, Niskanen A, et al: Latex agglutination test for detecting feline panleukopenia virus, canine parvovirus, and parvoviruses of fur animals. *J Clin Microbiol* 23:556–559, 1986.

35. Mathys A, Mueller R, Pedersen NC, et al: Comparison of hemagglutination and competitive enzyme-linked immunosorbent assay procedures for detecting canine parvovirus in feces. *Am J Vet Res* 44:152–154, 1983.

36. Luff PR, Wood GW, Hebert CN, et al: Canine parvovirus serology: a collaborative assay. *Vet Rec* 120:270–273, 1987.

37. Pollock RVH: Canine parvovirus: host response and immunoprophylaxis. Ph.D. dissertation, Cornell University, Ithaca, NY, 1981.

38. Pollock RVH, Zimmer JF: Canine enteric infections. In Scott F (ed): *Contemporary Issues in Small Animal Practice 3: Infectious Diseases.* New York, Churchill Livingstone, 1986, pp 55–80.

39. Heald RD, Jones BD, Schmidt DA: Blood gas and electrolyte concentrations in canine parvoviral enteritis. *J Am Anim Hosp Assoc* 22:745–748, 1986.

40. Wessels BC, Gaffin SL: Anti-endotoxin immunotherapy for canine parvovirus endotoxaemia. *J Small Anim Pract* 27:609–615, 1986.

41. Watkinson M: A lack of therapeutic response to kaolin in acute childhood diarrhoea treated with glucose electrolyte solution. *J Trop Pediatr* 28:306–310, 1982.

42. Carmichael LE, Joubert JC, Pollock RVH: A modified live canine parvovirus vaccine II. Immune response. *Cornell Vet* 73:13–29, 1983.

43. Povey RC, Carman PS, Ewert E: The duration of immunity to an inactivated adjuvanted canine parvovirus vaccine. A 52- and 64-week postvaccination challenge study. *Can Vet J* 24:245–248, 1983.

44. Wallace BL, Salsbury DL, McMillen JK: An inactivated canine parvovirus vaccine: protection against virulent challenge. *Vet Med* 80:41–48, 1985.

45. Murray RW: A comparative study of the effectiveness of four "combined" vaccines for dogs. *Aust Vet Practit* 15:151–155, 1985.

45a. Thompson H, McCandlish AP, Cornwell HJC, et al: Studies of parvovirus vaccination in the dog: the performance of live attenuated feline parvovirus vaccine. *Vet Rec* 122:378–385, 1988.

46. Churchill AE: Preliminary development of a live attenuated canine parvovirus vaccine from an isolate of British origin. *Vet Rec* 120:334–339, 1987.

47. Carmichael LE, Pollock RVH, Joubert JC: Response of puppies to canine-origin parvovirus vaccines. *Mod Vet Pract* 65:99–102, 1984.

48. Phillips TR, Jensen JL, Rubino MJ, et al: Effects of vaccines on the canine immune system. *Can J Vet Res* 53:154–160, 1989.

49. Carmichael LE: Immunization strategies in puppies—why failures? *Compend Cont Educ Vet Pract* 5:1043–1052, 1983.

49a. Macartney L, Thompson H, McCandlish IAP, et al: Canine parvovirus, interaction between passive immunity and virulent challenge. *Vet Rec* 122:573–576, 1988.

50. Mastro JM, Axthelm M, Mathes LE, et al: Repeated suppression of lymphocyte blastogenesis following vaccinations of CPV-immune dogs with modified-live CPV vaccines. *Vet Microbiol* 12:201–211, 1986.

51. Glickman LT, Appel MJG: A controlled field trial of an attenuated canine origin parvovirus vaccine. *Compend Cont Educ Vet Pract* 4:888–894, 1982.

52. Toma B, Chappuis G, Eloit M: Recherche des anticorps du parvovirus et du coronavirus canins chez l'homme. *Rec Med Vet* 158:607–610, 1982.

53. Carmichael LE, Parrish CR: Unpublished results, Cornell University, Ithaca, NY, 1987.

54. Macartney L, Parrish CR, Binn LN, et al: Characterization of minute virus of canines (MVC) and its pathogenicity for pups. *Cornell Vet* 78:131–145, 1988.

55. Hammond MM, Timoney PJ: An electron microscopic study of viruses associated with canine gastroenteritis. *Cornell Vet* 73:82–97, 1983.

55a. Evermann JF, McKeirnan AJ, Eugster AK, et al: Update on canine coronavirus infections and interactions with other enteric pathogens of the dog. *Companion Anim Pract* 19(2):6–12, 1989.

56. Styer E: Unpublished observations. University of Georgia Diagnostic Lab, Tifton, GA, 1988.

57. Roseto A. Lema F, Cavalieri F, et al: Electron microscopy and characterization of viral particles in dog stools. *Arch Virol* 66:89–93, 1980.

58. Martin ML: Canine coronavirus enteritis and a recent outbreak following modified live virus vaccination. *Compend Cont Educ Pract Vet* 7:1012–1017, 1985.

59. Edwards BG, Fulker RH, Acree WM, et al: Evaluating a canine coronavirus vaccine through antigen extinction and challenge studies. *Vet Med* 80:28–33, 1985.

60. Appel MJG: Does canine coronavirus augment the effects of subsequent parvovirus infection? *Vet Med* 83:360–366, 1988.

61. Tzipori S: The relative importance of enteric pathogens affecting neonates of domestic animals. *Adv Vet Sci Comp Med* 29:103–206, 1985.

62. England JJ, Poston RP: Electron microscopic identification and subsequent isolation of a rotavirus from a dog with fatal neonatal diarrhea. *Am J Vet Res* 41:782–783, 1980.

63. Fulton RW, Johnson CA, Pearson NJ, et al: Isolation of a rotavirus from a newborn dog with diarrhea. *Am J Vet Res* 42:841–843, 1981.

64. Eiden J, Vonderfecht S, Theil K, et al: Genetic and antigenic relatedness of human and animal strains of antigenically distinct rotaviruses. *J Infect Dis* 154:972–982, 1986.

65. Mochizuki M, Minami K, Sakamoto H: Seroepizootiologic studies on rotavirus infections of dogs and cats. *Jpn J Vet Sci* 48:957–964, 1986.

66. Johnson CA, Fulton RW, Henk WG: Inoculation of neonatal gnotobiotic dogs with a canine rotavirus. *Am J Vet Res* 44:1682–1686, 1983.

67. Johnson CA, Snider TG, Fulton RW, et al: Gross

and light microscopic lesions in neonatal gnotobiotic dogs inoculated with a canine rotavirus. *Am J Vet Res* 44:1687–1693, 1983.

68. Marshall JA, Healey DS, Studdert MJ, et al: Viruses and virus-like particles in the faeces of dogs with and without diarrhoea. *Aust Vet J* 61:33–38, 1984.

69. Evermann JF, McKeirman AJ, Ott RL, et al: Diarrheal condition in dogs associated with viruses antigenically related to feline herpesvirus. *Cornell Vet* 72:285–291, 1982.

70. Evermann JF, McKeirnan AJ, Smith AW, et al: Isolation and identification of caliciviruses from dogs with enteric infections. *Am J Vet Res* 46:218–220, 1985.

71. Schaffer FL, Soergel ME, Black JW, et al: Characterization of a new calicivirus isolated from feces of a dog. *Arch Virol* 84:181–195, 1985.

22

CANINE VIRAL PAPILLOMATOSIS

Clay A. Calvert

ETIOLOGY

Multiple canine papillomas are benign mucocutaneous tumors caused by infectious papillomavirus of the Papovaviridae family.[1] Members of this family are small, ether-resistant, double-stranded, DNA-containing viruses that are similar in structure to, but larger than, parvoviruses (see Fig. 21–1). Papillomaviruses are naturally oncogenic but are usually species specific. Serologic cross-reactivity has not been detected among papillomaviruses of different species. Papillomaviruses of humans, cattle, and dogs, although antigenically distinct, share at least one group-specific determinant. Inoculation of canine oral papillomavirus (COPV) into kittens, mice, rats, guinea pigs, rabbits, and nonhuman primates has failed to produce papillomas.

EPIDEMIOLOGY

Papillomas may be either naturally occurring, noninfectious, solitary tumors or transmissible, viral-induced, multiple tumors. Although solitary nonviral papillomas do occur in older dogs, infectious papillomas are usually multiple and occur in young dogs in oral, ocular, and cutaneous forms. Oral papillomas occur on the oral, labial, and pharyngeal mucosae, as well as the tongue and rarely in the esophagus (Fig. 22–1). Ocular papillomas occur on the conjunctivae, cornea, and eyelid margins (Fig. 22–2). Ocular papillomas are less common than oral papillomas. Viral particles identical to COPV that have been taken from ocular papillomas can produce oral papillomas in dogs.[2,3]

Cutaneous papillomas, presumably of viral origin, are uncommon, with variable site distribution. COPV inoculated into the skin of the face may produce papilloma, but attempts to produce a tumor by inoculating the skin of the abdomen or back with COPV have usually failed. Papillomas have been produced following local inoculation of COPV into brain, bladder, stomach, and rectal tissues.[2]

Dogs older than 2 years seldom develop oral papillomas, and older dogs are resistant to COPV infection. Ocular papillomas occur most often in dogs 6 months to 4 years of age but have been reported in dogs as old as 9 years.[4] The age range of dogs with cutaneous papillomas of presumed viral etiology is unclear but apparently is broader.[2] In Australia, cutaneous papillomas of the distal limbs in racing greyhounds occur in dogs 12 to 18 months of age.[5]

Papovavirus has been observed in cutaneous papillomas, and viral inclusions have been seen in the superficial layers of the epithelium.[5,6] A spectrum of proliferative cutaneous lesions occurred in dogs inoculated with COPV. Group-specific papillomavirus antigen was detected in some of the lesions.[7]

Most infectious papillomas undergo spontaneous regression. Malignant transformation to squamous cell carcinoma has been reported in some species.[8] However, progression to carcinoma has been reported only in a dog with oral papillomas and a dog with a corneal papilloma.[9, 10]

PATHOGENESIS

COPV infects the basal cells of the stratum germinativum. The first tissue response to COPV infection is an increase in mitotic

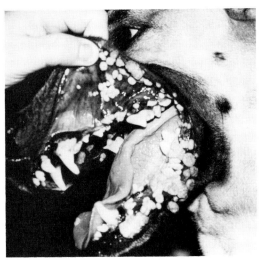

Figure 22–1. Typical canine oral papillomatosis.

activity resulting in acanthosis and hyperkeratosis.[8] As the disease progresses, some infected cells are diverted to a role of virus production. These cells develop inclusion material but do not undergo cytoplasmic differentiation. Cytoplasmic degeneration and cell death ensue with viral persistence in strands of keratin. The majority of basal layer cells, however, differentiate into keratogenic normal cells.[8]

The incubation period of COPV is usually 4 to 8 weeks postinoculation. Tumor growth usually lasts 1 to 5 months before spontaneous regression begins and subsequent immunity develops. When COPV was inoculated into the eyelid, only 50% of dogs

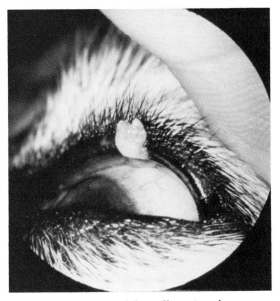

Figure 22–2. Eyelid papilloma in a dog.

developed papillomas, the incubation period was longer, and tumors persisted longer than in the oral cavity.

The mechanism resulting in spontaneous regression of papillomas is unknown. Virus-neutralizing antibody inactivates COPV in sensitized animals but does not inhibit established virus or papillomas.

Serum from dogs whose papillomas have undergone spontaneous regression not only fails to produce tumor regression but enhances tumor growth. This effect may be the result of the induction of blocking antigen-antibody factors that impeded cytotoxic lymphocyte action on target cells. Cellular immune mechanisms may be more important in inhibiting the development of early papillomas in dogs.

Concentration of COPV in the inoculum may variably influence subsequent tumor growth and regression. Dogs given small dosages of virus develop more papillomas, and regression is delayed relative to dogs given larger dosages of virus.

When inoculated into puppies, COPV has produced hyperplastic and neoplastic lesions at the sites other than the oropharyngeal mucosa.[7] Lesions have included epidermal hyperplasia, epidermal cysts, squamous papilloma, basal cell epitheloma, and squamous cell carcinoma. However, only a very small number of inoculations were associated with these extraoral lesions.

CLINICAL FINDINGS

The oral mucosa, labial margins, tongue, palate, pharynx, and epiglottis are most often affected by COPV. Oral papillomas initially are pale, smooth, elevated lesions but soon become cauliflower-like with fine, white, stringy projections. Early tumors appear to "seed" the rest of the susceptible oral tissues.

Recognition of the lesions usually occurs while the numbers of tumors are still increasing. Halitosis, ptyalism, hemorrhage, and host discomfort are variably observed by the owners of affected dogs. As many as 50 to 100 tumors are often present at the time of diagnosis. Regression usually begins after 4 to 8 weeks of tumor growth. Occasionally, incomplete regression occurs, and a few papillomas persist indefinitely. Oral papillomatosis may occasionally persist for 6 to 24 months or longer. Dogs affected by persistent papillomas often have many large tumors and may become malnourished. Secondary bacterial infection of some lesions may result in a purulent discharge.

Ocular papillomas tend to persist longer than oral papillomas. There has been no clinical association of ocular papillomas with oral or cutaneous papillomas under natural conditions.

DIAGNOSIS

The diagnosis of papillomatosis is based on the epidemiology and gross appearance of the tumors. Ocular papillomas are usually examined histologically because they are not as morphologically distinct as oral papillomas. Cutaneous papillomas, usually morphologically distinct, are often excised for aesthetic reasons and examined microscopically. Cutaneous papillomas have been found on the lower extremities, often in the interdigital areas, foot pads, and occasionally, subungually.

THERAPY

Treatment is often not recommended if only a few papillomas are present. However, the patient should be re-examined in order to determine if tumor numbers are increasing. In such cases, clients often opt for treatment.

Therapy is usually unnecessary because of spontaneous regression but may be indicated if tumors persist, when large, multiple tumors produce pharyngeal obstruction, and for esthetic reasons when clients are particularly concerned.

Surgical excision, cryosurgery, and electrosurgery are acceptable modes of treatment of oral tumors. Surgical removal, freezing, or simply crushing 5 to 15 of the tumors may induce spontaneous regression, presumably resulting from antigenic stimulation.

Surgical excision or cryosurgery is effective for papillomas of the conjunctiva or eyelid. Cryosurgery is not recommended for corneal papillomas. Care should be taken to prevent spread of the virus to adjacent ocular tissues, and cryosurgery has an advantage in this regard.[11]

The prevalence of spontaneous regression of oral papillomatosis makes the interpretation of treatment difficult. Although commonly recommended, the efficacy of autogenous wart vaccines in dogs is questionable. Vaccines are usually not effective against persistent papillomatosis.

The author has observed that systemic chemotherapy utilizing single-agent vincristine, cyclophosphamide, doxorubicin, or bleomycin in persistent oral papillomatosis has produced variable results. Chemotherapy may be reserved for tumors that have persisted for longer than 2 months, especially those remaining for 5 months or longer. Interferon has been given IM to humans at a dose of 1×10^6 units daily until a response causing regression of persistent viral papillomas is noted.[12] See Interferons, Chapters 2 and 15, for additional information on administration and precautions.

References

1. Pfister H: Biology and biochemistry of papillomaviruses. Rev Physiol Biochem Pharmacol 99:111–181, 1984.
2. Tokita H, Konishi S: Studies on canine oral papillomatosis. II. Oncogenicity of canine oral papilloma virus to various tissues of dog with special reference to eye tumor. Jpn J Vet Sci 37:109–120, 1975.
3. Hare CL, Howard EB: Canine conjunctiva-corneal papillomatosis. J Am Anim Hosp Assoc 13:688–690, 1977.
4. Bonney CH, Koch SA, Conter AW, et al: Case report: a conjunctivocorneal papilloma with evidence of a viral etiology. J Small Anim Pract 21:183–188, 1980.
5. Davis PE, Huxtable CRR, Sabcine M: Dermal papillomas in the racing greyhound. Aust J Dermatol 17:13–16, 1976.
6. Allison AC: Viruses inducing skin tumors in animals. In Rook AJ, Walton CS (eds): Comparative Physiology and Pathology of the Skin. Philadelphia, FA Davis, 1965, pp 615–636.
7. Bregman CL, Hirth RS, Sundberg JP, et al: Cutaneous neoplasms in dogs asociated with canine oral papillomavirus. Vet Pathol 24:477–487, 1987.
8. Theilen GH, Madewell BR: Papillomatosis and fibromatosis. In Theilen GH, Madewell BR (eds): Veterinary Cancer Medicine. Philadelphia, Lea and Febiger, 1987, pp 267–281.
9. Watrach AM, Small E, Case MT: Canine papilloma: progression of oral papilloma to carcinoma. J Natl Cancer Inst 45:915–920, 1970.
10. Belkin PV: Ocular lesions in canine oral papillomatosis. Vet Med Small Anim Clin 74:1520–1524, 1979.
11. Bonney CH, Koch SA, Dice PF, et al: Papillomatosis of conjunctiva and adnexa in dogs. J Am Vet Med Assoc 176:48–52, 1980.
12. Bomholt A: Interferon therapy for laryngeal papillomatosis in adults. Arch Otolaryngol 109:550–552, 1983.

23 FELINE PANLEUKOPENIA

Craig E. Greene
Fredric W. Scott

ETIOLOGY

Feline panleukopenia is caused by a small, serologically homogeneous parvovirus with single-stranded DNA (see Fig. 21–1). Feline panleukopenia virus (FPV) is extremely stable; it is able to survive for 1 year at room temperature in organic material on solid fomites. It resists heating to 56°C for 30 minutes and remains viable for longer periods at lower temperatures. The virus survives disinfection with 70% alcohol, various dilutions of organic iodines, phenolics, and quaternary ammonium compounds. It is inactivated by bleach (6% sodium hypochlorite), 4% formaldehyde, and 1% glutaraldehyde in 10 minutes at room temperature.[1]

EPIDEMIOLOGY

FPV can cause disease in all members of the family Felidae. Some Viverridae, Procyonidae, and Mustelidae, including the binturong, raccoon, coatimundi, ringtail cat, and mink, are also susceptible (see Table 2–8). The virus is ubiquitous because of its contagious nature and capacity for persistence in the environment, and virtually all susceptible cats are exposed and infected within the first year of life. Unvaccinated kittens that acquire maternal immunity through colostrum are usually protected for up to 3 months of age. Most infections are subclinical, inasmuch as 75% of unvaccinated, clinically healthy cats have demonstrable antibody titers by 1 year of age. Seasonal variations in the incidence of panleukopenia and disease outbreaks presumably parallel increases in the numbers of susceptible newborn kittens.

FPV is most commonly transmitted by direct contact of susceptible animals with infected cats or their secretions. It is shed from all body secretions during active stages of disease but is most consistently recovered from the intestine and feces. Cats shed virus in their urine and feces for a maximum of 6 weeks after recovery. FPV is maintained in the population by its environmental persistence rather than by the prolonged carrier state. Virus has been isolated for a maximum of 1 year from the lungs and kidneys of neonatally infected kittens, but shedding does not occur. Owners who lose a kitten to feline panleukopenia should *not* introduce a new kitten into the household without having it vaccinated before bringing it on the premises.

Fomites play a relatively important role in disease transmission because of prolonged survival of the virus on contaminated surfaces. Vehicles for exposure include contaminated clothing, hands, food dishes, bedding, and infected cages. Transmission also probably occurs via flies and other insect vectors during warm periods.

PATHOGENESIS

FPV, as a parvovirus, requires rapidly multiplying cells for successful infection, and the distribution of lesions within a prospective feline host occurs in tissues with the greatest rate of mitotic activity (Fig. 23–1). Lymphoid tissue, bone marrow, and intestinal mucosal crypts (intestinal glands) are most commonly invaded in adult animals. Late prenatal and early neonatal infections in cats result in some lymphoid and bone marrow lesions, but the CNS, including the cerebrum and cerebellum and the retina and optic nerves, can be affected.

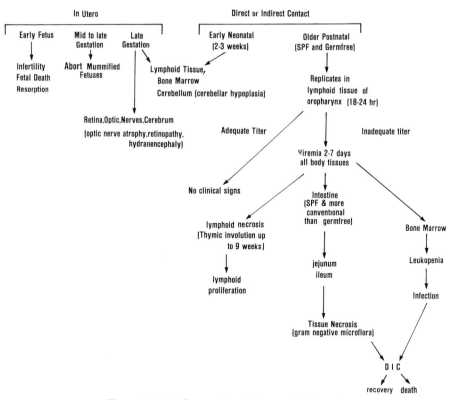

Figure 23–1. Pathogenesis of feline panleukopenia.

In Utero Infection

Early in utero infection can produce a spectrum of reproductive disorders in the pregnant queen, including early fetal death and resorption with infertility, abortions, or the birth of mummified fetuses. In utero inoculation of FPV produces variable effects on animals from the same litter. Some kittens are apparently unaffected, owing to either innate resistance or the acquisition of maternal antibody, but may harbor virus subclinically for up to 8 or 9 weeks in some cases.[2]

Systemic Infections

Experimental infections have been produced in specific pathogen–free (SPF) and germ-free kittens.[3] Clinical severity of infection is milder in these animals as compared with that in field cases and in experimentally infected conventional cats, suggesting that copathogenic factors may play a role in the natural disease. The virus undergoes replication in lymphoid tissues of the oro-

pharynx 18 to 24 hours following intranasal or oral infection. A plasma-phase viremia, occurring between 2 and 7 days, disseminates the virus to all body tissues, although pathologic lesions primarily occur in tissues with the highest mitotic activity. Lymphoid tissue undergoes initial necrosis, followed by lymphoid proliferation. Thymic involution and degeneration are found in germ-free and SPF cats infected up to 9 weeks of age. Decreased T cell responsiveness has been reported in FPV-infected cats,[4] but there is no interference in humoral immune responses.[5] Cats surviving infection have a decrease in viremia corresponding to a rapidly rising viral neutralizing serum antibody titer by 7 days postinoculation.[6]

SPF cats have more severe intestinal lesions, compared with germ-free kittens. The proliferation rate of crypt epithelium is faster in SPF kittens as a result of indigenous microflora or their metabolic by-products, which stimulate the turnover rate of intestinal epithelial cells. The extent of damage throughout the intestinal tract parallels the presence of the virus, and lesions are milder in the colon, where epithelial mitotic rates are slower than in the small intestine. The jejunum and ileum are more affected than is the duodenal segment, which may reflect lower numbers of indigenous microorganisms in the proximal small bowel.

During intestinal infection, the virus selectively damages replicating cells deep in the crypts of the intestinal mucosa. Differentiated absorptive cells on the surface of the villi are nondividing and are not affected. Shortening of the intestinal villi results from damage to the crypt cells, which normally migrate up the villi, replacing absorptive cells. Damage to the intestinal villi results in diarrhea caused by malabsorption and increased permeability (see Fig. 9–8C).

SPF and conventional cats with panleukopenia are also susceptible to secondary bacterial infections with enteric microflora. Gram-negative endotoxemia, with or without bacteremia, is a common complication of systemic FPV infection. DIC, a frequent complication of endotoxemia, can also develop with feline panleukopenia.

CNS Infection

The CNS, optic nerve, and retina are only susceptible to injury by FPV during prenatal or early neonatal development, and of CNS lesions, cerebellar damage has been most commonly reported. This predilection for cerebellar disease may be explained by the fact that the cerebellum develops during late gestation and early neonatal periods of cats. FPV interferes with cerebellar cortical development, resulting in reduced and distorted cell layers. It can be affected from infections occurring as late as 9 days of age. Other CNS lesions can be produced by earlier prenatal infections. Lesions of the spinal cord and cerebrum, including hydrocephalus and hydranencephaly and retinal abnormalities can occur (see Clinical Findings).

CLINICAL FINDINGS

The frequency with which cats show evidence of clinical disease with FPV is much less than the number of cats infected with the virus. This fact is supported by the high prevalence of FPV antibodies in the cat population. Subclinical cases, more common in older susceptible cats, go unrecognized. Severe clinical illness is the rule in young unvaccinated kittens, with the highest morbidity and mortality occurring between 3 and 5 months.

Fever (40° to 41.6°C [104° to 107°F]), depression, and anorexia are the most common findings and usually occur 3 to 4 days prior to presentation. Vomiting, which develops during the illness in most cats, is frequently bile-tinged and occurs unrelated to eating. Extreme dehydration, sometimes manifest by the cat crouching with its head over the water dish, may occur as a nonspecific feature of this disease. Diarrhea is seen with less frequency, and when it is present, it usually occurs somewhat later in the course of illness.

On abdominal palpation, the intestinal loops have a thickened, "rope-like" consistency, and discomfort is commonly noted. Mesenteric lymphadenomegaly is usually present, whereas peripheral lymph nodes are not enlarged. Oral ulceration, bloody diarrhea, or icterus may be noted in complicated infections. Petechial and ecchymotic hemorrhages may be found in cats with complicating DIC, although cats do not frequently show overt signs of hemorrhage, even with marked thrombocytopenia.

Severe dehydration associated with anorexia, vomiting, and diarrhea can lead to progressive weakness, depression, and semicoma, and cats become hypothermic during the terminal stages of the illness. They can die suddenly from complications associated with secondary bacterial infection, dehydration, and DIC. Animals that survive infection for longer than 5 days without developing fatal complications usually recover, although frequently it takes several weeks.

Queens infected during pregnancy may show infertility or abortion of dead or mummified fetuses, but there are never any clinical signs in the aborting female. Some kittens in a litter may be born with ataxia, incoordination, tremors, and normal mental status typical of cerebellar disease (Fig. 23–2). They walk with a broad-based stance with hypermetric movements, and they frequently fall to either side and show intention tremors of the head. Tremors and incoordination are absent when kittens are at rest. Not all kittens in a litter are affected or have the same degree of neurologic deficits.

Retinal lesions may be visible on fundic examination of kittens affected with neurologic signs or as an incidental finding in clinically normal cats. These areas of retinal

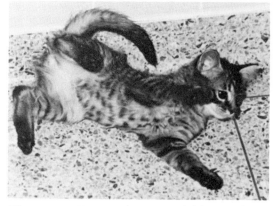

Figure 23–2. Kitten with congenital feline panleuko-penia and cerebellar hypoplasia showing marked ataxia.

degeneration appear as discrete, gray foci with darkened margins, and retinal folding or streaking may be seen (Fig. 23–3).

DIAGNOSIS

Clinical Laboratory Findings

A presumptive diagnosis of feline panleu-kopenia is usually made on the basis of clinical signs and the presence of leuko-penia. Leukocyte counts during the height of infection (day 4 to 6 of infection) are usually between 50 and 3000 cells/μl.[7] Leu-kopenia, from which the disease gets its name, is not pathognomonic for FPV infec-tion alone and may not occur in all cases of FPV. The degree of leukopenia usually par-allels that of clinical illness, and leukopenia

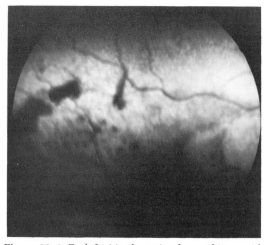

Figure 23–3. Dark foci in the retina from a kitten with hydranencephaly and optic nerve hypoplasia as a result of in utero FPV infection.

also develops in infected germ-free and SPF cats. Subsequent examination of the leuko-cyte count in 24 to 48 hours in recovering FPV-infected cats will show a rebound in leukocyte numbers. Repeated examinations should be made since diseases such as feline leukemia cause a more protracted illness and persistent leukopenia. Lymphopenia is less common with FPV infection than is neutro-penia, and concurrent lymphopenia and neutropenia are more suggestive of feline leukemia virus infection. Feline salmonel-losis with overwhelming septicemia may mimic feline panleukopenia with the pres-ence of leukopenia and acute GI illness. Fecal culture may be helpful under these circumstances.

A transient decrease in absolute reticulo-cyte count and mild (5% to 10%) decrease in hematocrit have been found during the viremic period in experimentally infected kittens.[8] Because of the sudden onset of the disease and relatively long life span of eryth-rocytes, marked anemia is also less common in panleukopenia unless intestinal blood loss is severe. A persistent, nonregenerative anemia and leukopenia are more suggestive of feline leukemia infection (see Diagnosis, Chapter 26).

Thrombocytopenia is a variable feature of feline panleukopenia and may be found with other coagulation abnormalities in cats that develop DIC. Thrombocytopenia, resulting from direct bone marrow injury, can also occur in association with leukopenia early in the course of infection.[8]

Biochemical findings in FPV infections are usually nonspecific. Increases in ALT (for-merly SGPT) and AST (formerly SGOT) ac-tivities or bilirubin can reflect hepatic in-volvement, but elevations are mild to moderate and icterus is rare. Azotemia is frequently present from prerenal or nonrenal causes such as dehydration, although the virus can produce minimal renal pathology.

Serologic Testing

These procedures are available for the properly equipped diagnostic and research laboratories, although they are rarely indi-cated for clinical practice. Serum neutrali-zation is the most commonly used method. Twofold serial dilutions of antisera are per-formed against precalculated amounts of FPV. Virus and sera are incubated prior to inoculation of the cell culture. Cultures can be examined for specific cytopathic changes and inclusion bodies produced by the virus. Complement fixation titers also can be performed. Hemagglutination-inhibition and hemagglutination tests can be used for some strains of FPV. FPV, like canine parvovirus, will variably agglutinate porcine erythrocytes at 0°C. The variation usually relates to individual variation among pig erythrocytes used in the test.[9] Direct fluorescent antibody testing can be used to detect virus in cell cultures and from tissues of infected cats within 2 days after infection.

Viral Isolation

Feline cells are required to support viral replication in cell cultures, and frequent mitosis is needed to ensure a continuing infection, although FPV has been shown to replicate in cells in which DNA synthesis has been blocked.[10] Cytopathic effects, required to substantiate the presence of the virus, are more easily demonstrated in young, rapidly multiplying cells. Plaque detection methods are possible when certain cell types and cell synchronization are used.[11] Virus can be isolated from the urine and feces of kittens surviving experimental in utero inoculation at 3 and 6 weeks after birth, respectively. Direct culture from trypsinized lung and kidney tissues allows improved isolation of virus for up to 70 days. Virus has been isolated by direct culture for up to 1 year from the lungs and kidneys of prenatally infected kittens, despite a high level of circulating antibody. Virus can be found in the CNS for at least 22 days following neonatal infection and thereafter persists in Purkinje's cells.

PATHOLOGIC FINDINGS

Gross pathologic changes in naturally infected cats are usually minimal. The intestinal tract is obviously dilated; the bowel loops are firm and may be hyperemic with petechial and ecchymotic hemorrhages on the serosal surfaces. The feces frequently have a fetid odor when blood is present. Prenatally infected cats may have a small cerebellum, hydrocephalus, or hydranencephaly (Fig. 23–4). Thymic atrophy, pres-

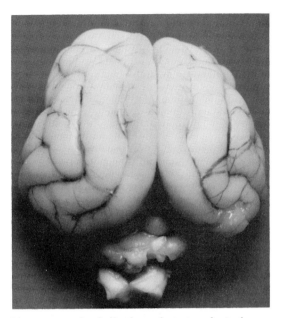

Figure 23–4. Cerebellar hypoplasia in a brain from a cat with in utero FPV infection.

ent in all neonates, is the only gross finding in germfree kittens.

Histologic abnormalities in the intestine include dilated crypts (intestinal glands), with sloughing of epithelial cells and necrotic debris into the lumen (Fig. 23–5). Crypt-lining cells may slough completely in some cases so that only the basement membrane remains. Shortening of villi occurs secondary to the necrosis of crypt cells. The most severe histologic lesions are found in the jejunum and ileum; the duodenum and colon are less severely affected. Focal damage is most prominent around lymphoid follicles in the submucosa of the small intestine. Lymphocytic infiltrations are conspicuously absent from all tissues, and lymphocyte depletion is present in the follicles of lymph nodes, Peyer's patches, and spleen. Lymphoid atrophy is present, with concomitant mononuclear phagocyte hyperplasia.

Histologic abnormalities in the cerebrum of prenatally or neonatally infected kittens can include dilation of the ventricles and disruption of ependymal cells with malacia of subcortical white matter. Cerebellar degeneration is marked by disorientation and reduced population of the granular and Purkinje's cell layers. Myelin degeneration can be found predominantly in the lateral funiculi of the spinal cord.

Eosinophilic intranuclear inclusions can be found in FPV infection, although they are

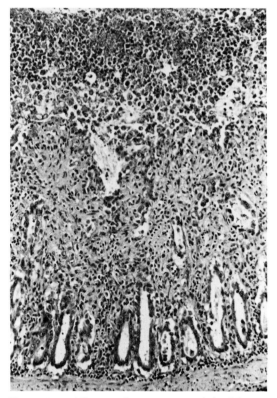

Figure 23–5. Microscopic appearance of the jejunum from a cat with FPV infection. Dilated crypt lumina and collapsed villi are visible in the lower part of the figure; there is sloughing of epithelial cells. Necrotic debris and overlying inflammatory exudate are present in the intestinal lumen in the upper part of the figure (H and E; × 100).

transient and are frequently absent with routine formalin fixation. Bouin's or Zenker's fixatives must be used. Electron microscopic findings indicate that the inclusions correspond with sites of viral replication.

THERAPY

Mortality caused by FPV infection can be avoided with appropriate symptomatic therapy and nursing care. Cats that can be kept alive for several days by using supportive measures usually develop adequate immune defense mechanisms to overcome the infection. Parenteral fluid therapy is used to replace lost electrolytes, counteract dehydration, and replace daily maintenance needs. Oral intake of food and water should be withheld during this time to lessen vomiting and because reducing oral intake slows the bowel mitotic activity necessary for viral replication. Fluid volumes that must be re-

placed as a result of vomiting and diarrhea can be calculated by evaluating the cat's state of hydration. Additional maintenance needs from insensible losses are administered at a rate of 44 ml/kg/day. Balanced isotonic fluid replacement with lactated Ringer's solution is desirable. Fluids can be administered SC unless there is severe dehydration associated with reduced peripheral vascular circulation for which IV therapy is required.

Antiemetics (Table 23–1) may be required to control persistent vomiting. The use of anticholinergic medications is controversial and is contraindicated because they produce sustained ileus of the bowel. GI protectants such as kaopectate or bismuth subsalicylate have been recommended to coat the bowel but cannot be used in vomiting animals. Bismuth compounds have the added theoretic advantage of reducing increased intestinal secretion and resulting diarrhea. Glucocorticoid therapy should not be used routinely at anti-inflammatory or higher dosages because of its immunosuppressive effects.

Plasma or blood transfusion therapy may be required in cats that develop severe anemia, hypotension, or hypoproteinemia (plasma protein < 5.0 g/dl). A platelet count and activated coagulation time should be evaluated prior to administration of blood products in cases of ongoing DIC. Low-dose SC heparin therapy (50 to 100 U/kg, given every 8 hours) can be used simultaneously with transfusion if thrombocytopenia and severe incoagulability are present.

Broad-spectrum antibiotics, such as ampicillin or chloramphenicol, are used to control secondary bacterial infection resulting from virus injury to the intestinal mucosa (Table 23–1). However, the latter drug may suppress the bone marrow regenerative response. Parenteral therapy is preferred because of continued vomiting. A combination of a penicillin or cephalosporin derivative with parenteral aminoglycosides may be required for cats that are septic or moribund. One rationale for antibiotic therapy in this disease is to reduce the mitotic activity of the bowel epithelium by decreasing intestinal microflora, since germ-free animals have been shown to have a mild form of disease.

Combination B vitamin therapy should be given parenterally to all cats with feline panleukopenia because of decreased food intake from anorexia, high requirements for

Table 23–1. Drug Dosages for Treating Feline Panleukopenia[a]

DRUG	DOSE[b] (mg/kg)	ROUTE	INTERVAL (hours)	DURATION (days)
Antiemetics				
Metoclopramide	0.2–0.4[c]	PO, SC	6–8	prn
	1–2	IV	24[d]	prn
Thiethylperazine	0.5–5	IM, SC	8	prn
Trimethobenzamide	3	IM, SC	8	prn
Antimicrobials				
Amp(amox)icillin	15–20	IV, SC	6–8	prn
Cephapirin	10–30	IV, SC, IM	6–8	prn
Gentamicin	2	IV, SC, IM	8	prn[e]

[a]PO = oral, SC = subcutaneous, IV = intravenous, prn = as needed.
[b]Dose per administration at specified interval, expressed as mg/kg unless otherwise stated.
[c]Should not be given in conjunction with other motility modifiers.
[d]Total dose IV not to exceed 1 to 2 mg/kg/day; this dose may be divided as multiple bolus infusions throughout the day.
[e]Renal function (BUN, urine casts) should be closely evaluated, and the drug should not be continued for longer than 7 to 10 days at this dosage.

B vitamins, and loss in diuresis, to prevent development of thiamine deficiency. Low-dose oral or parenteral diazepam (2.5 mg total) can be used intermittently, a few minutes prior to feeding, to stimulate the appetite of anorectic cats that are not vomiting.

Response to therapy can be followed by monitoring the total and differential leukocyte count since there is a resurgence of leukopoiesis within 24 to 48 hours. Bizarre forms of leukocytes can be detected in the blood and bone marrow.

Following the nursing period, the cat can be started on oral alimentation by frequent feedings of small quantities of bland baby food, broth, or blended foods. Eventually, the cat may be fed larger quantities of solid foods. Semimoist foods have lower residue and help to firm the feces of cats with persistent diarrhea. Rarely, cats that refuse to eat after several days should be force fed by mouth or by pharyngostomy or gastrostomy tube or given diazepam.

PREVENTION

Colostral antibodies to feline panleukopenia have a half-life of 9.5 days (see Tables 2–2, 2–3, and 2–4). Both MLV and inactivated tissue culture-origin vaccines are ineffective when maternal-derived antibody virus neutralization titers as measured by some laboratories are greater than 1:10. Successful vaccination without maternal antibody interference can be achieved by 12 weeks of age in most cases (range, 6.8 to 18.8 weeks), depending on the antibody titer in the queen.[12] Kittens with virus neutralization titers from 1:10 to 1:30 cannot be successfully vaccinated but are susceptible to infection with FPV.[12] Therefore, as with canine parvovirus, kittens can still be infected with FPV prior to the time they are immunized, although this problem has not been as widely recognized. Recovery from natural infection with virulent virus probably results in lifelong immunity.[13]

Therapeutic passive immunity has been used to prevent panleukopenia. Homologous antisera from cats with a high titer to infection will provide immunity according to the titer of the product and the amount administered. The recommended dosage is 2 ml/kitten, given SC or intraperitoneally. Since administered immunoglobulins persist for up to 2 to 4 weeks, the neonatal vaccination series must be delayed. Passive administration of antisera is recommended for use *only in exposed susceptible* (unvaccinated) cats that require immediate protection or in colostrum-deprived kittens, with subsequent vaccinations at 2 to 3 or 4 to 5 weeks of age with inactivated or MLV vaccines, respectively. Newborn kittens are immunologically competent to FPV and can respond with neutralizing antibodies at 7 to 12 days of age.

Active immunization against FPV has been the most important factor in reducing the incidence of the disease. Both inactivated and MLV products have been effective in preventing this disease. Tissue culture–origin inactivated products can break through maternal immunity as early as MLV vaccines. Unlike MLV products, they have the advantage of being safe to use in pregnant queens and in kittens less than 4 weeks of age. Inactivated vaccines may be given to febrile kittens when an effective immune response is doubtful. There is no danger of postvaccinal virus spread or clinical illness as a result of reversion to virulence, although there has been suspicion that inactivated products can contain live virus.[14-16] The major disadvantage of these products is that in the absence of maternal antibody, two injections are required to achieve a titer that can be obtained from one injection of MLV product. Antibody titers to inactivated vaccine have been adequate for protection by 2 weeks following the first vaccination but have been greatly boosted by the second injection.[17] Protection with inactivated vaccines does not consistently occur until 3 to 7 days following the second vaccination. Cell-mediated immune responses to FPV were stimulated as early as 3 days following the second of two doses of adjuvanated inactivated FPV vaccine.[17] The inactivating agents used in some of these vaccines are also irritating to cats. With cloning of FPV into bacterial plasmids,[18] it may be possible to develop a more purified subunit vaccine against this infection.

MLV vaccines produce more rapid and effective immunity than do inactivated virus vaccines. In the absence of maternal antibodies, one injection of any of the currently available MLV products for panleukopenia will produce a protective titer greater than 1:8 to 1:10 in a previously unvaccinated cat; however, a second vaccination is recommended. Oral vaccination with MLV vaccine is ineffective, whereas intranasal or aerosol exposure to vaccine produces an active immune response.[19, 20]

Colostrum-deprived kittens can be vaccinated regardless of age, but MLV products should be avoided in kittens less than 4 weeks of age because of the danger of producing cerebellar degeneration. Colostrum-deprived kittens less than 4 weeks old at first presentation should receive at least 2 inactivated FPV vaccines 2 to 3 weeks apart. If 4 weeks or older they can receive one MLV-FPV vaccine with an optional one given 2 to 3 weeks later.

Initial vaccinations for nursing kittens are generally begun at 8 to 9 weeks of age and are followed by at least one more MLV product or 2 more inactivated vaccines, depending on which type of antigen is used. Subsequent vaccines should be given 2 to 4 weeks thereafter, with the last vaccine being given at 12 to 14 weeks of age. Panleukopenia vaccines are usually given SC. Combined vaccines that contain FPV and rabies or feline respiratory viruses have been marketed.

Annual vaccination against panleukopenia is recommended and performed by most veterinarians, although it is probably not essential. Actually, one MLV product or two inactivated vaccines may produce lifelong immunity. It is probable that revaccination produces an anamnestic response and presumably is not harmful.

References

1. Scott FW: Virucidal disinfectants and feline viruses. Am J Vet Res 41:410–414, 1980.
2. Csiza CK, Scott FW, deLahunta A, et al: Feline viruses. XIV. Transplacental infections in spontaneous panleukopenia of cats. Cornell Vet 61:423–439, 1971.
3. Hosokawa S, Ichijo S, Goto H: Clinical hematological and pathological findings in specific pathogen–free cats experimentally infected with feline panleukopenia virus. Jpn J Vet Sci 49:43–50, 1987.
4. Schultz RD, Mendel H, Scott FW: Effect of feline panleukopenia virus infection on development of humoral and cellular immunity. Cornell Vet 66:324–332, 1976.
5. Carlson JH, Scott FW, Duncan JR: Feline panleukopenia. III. Development of lesions in the lymphoid tissues. Vet Pathol 15:383–392, 1978.
6. Goto H, Hosokawa S, Ichijo S, et al: Experimental infection of feline panleukopenia virus in specific pathogen–free cats. Jpn J Vet Sci 45:109–112, 1983.
7. Wosu LO: Feline panleukopenia—in vivo infectivity studies. Vet Microbiol 16:137–143, 1988.
8. Prasse KW: Personal communication. University of Georgia, Athens, GA, 1983.
9. Wosu LO: In vitro studies on feline panleucopaenia virus. Standardisation of haemagglutination-inhibition test for feline panleucopaenia virus antibody. Comp Immun Microbiol Infect Dis 7:201–206, 1984.
10. Lenghaus C, Mun TK, Studdert MJ: Feline panleukopenia virus replicates in cells in which cellular DNA synthesis is blocked. J Virol 53:345–349, 1985.
11. Tham KM, Studdert MJ: Parvovirus (feline panleukopenia virus) plaque formation. Arch Virol 84:261–268, 1985.
12. Scott FW, Csiza CK, Gillespie JH: Maternally derived immunity to feline panleukopenia. J Am Vet Med Assoc 156:439–453, 1970.
13. Gaskell RM: The natural history of the major feline viral diseases. J Small Anim Pract 25:159–172, 1984.

14. Pollock RVH: The parvoviruses. Part I. Feline panleukopenia and mink enteritis virus. *Compend Cont
Educ Pract Vet* 6:227–241, 1984.

15. Milwright RDP: Enteritis in kittens associated
with feline panleukopenia virus. *Vet Rec* 114:51,
1984.

16. Rivera E, Karlsson KA, Bergman R: The propagation
of feline panleukopenia virus in microcarrier cell
culture and use of the inactivated virus in the
protection of mink against viral enteritis. *Vet Microbiol* 13:371–381, 1987.

17. Tham KM, Stoddart MJ: Antibody- and cell-mediated immune responses to an inactivated feline

panleukopenia virus vaccine. *Zentralbl Veterinarmed [B]* 34:701–712, 1987.

18. Carlson JH, Rushlow K, Maxwell I, et al: Cloning
and sequence of DNA encoding structural proteins
of the autonomous parvovirus feline panleukopenia
virus. *J Virol* 55:574–582, 1985.

19. Schultz RD, Scott FW: Absence of an immune
response after oral administration of attenuated
feline panleukopenia virus. *Infect Immun* 7:547–
549, 1973.

20. Scott FW, Glauberg AF: Aerosol vaccination against
feline panleukopenia. *J Am Vet Med Assoc* 166:
147–149, 1975.

24 FELINE CORONAVIRAL INFECTIONS

Jeffrey E. Barlough
Cheryl A. Stoddart

ETIOLOGY AND PATHOGENESIS

The coronaviruses are a large and diverse family of enveloped, single-stranded RNA viruses that cause disease in a number of avian and mammalian species. Cats are susceptible to infection with several closely related viruses in this family, including porcine transmissible gastroenteritis virus (TGEV), canine coronavirus (CCV), and the feline coronaviruses. These viruses may be closely related and may have evolved from common stock. Both TGEV and CCV produce asymptomatic infections in cats under experimental conditions; the prevalence of natural infection with these agents is unknown. The feline coronaviruses, however, display a broad spectrum of virulence, thereby producing disease in cats that varies in severity from asymptomatic infection with only seroconversion to a lethal, disseminated pyogranulomatous vasculitis known as feline infectious peritonitis (FIP).[1-5]

Feline coronavirus strains that can cause FIP in cats have been termed FIP virus (FIPV) (Fig. 24–1).[6] Those strains that are capable of inducing enteritis have been designated feline enteric coronavirus (FECV).[7] A number of experimental and clinical observations, however, blur the distinction between FIPV and FECV strains. First, although originally obtained from cats with FIP, FIPV strains vary dramatically in their ability to cause disease. Thus, some FIPV strains are avirulent (strain UCD2, for example) or of low virulence (UCD3, UCD4), whereas others (UCD1, 79-1146, Nor15) consistently produce FIP. The FECV strains typically are of low virulence and produce enteritis in only a minority of infected cats,

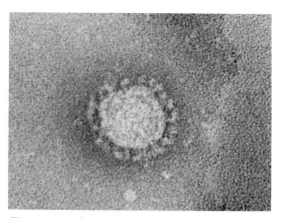

Figure 24–1. Electron photomicrograph of FIPV, illustrating the thick peplomer fringe or "corona" characteristic of the Coronaviridae (× 261,000). (From Stoddart et al: *Arch Virol* 79:85–94, 1984. Reprinted with permission.)

especially very young kittens. Second, intestinal lesions have been demonstrated in some cats with FIP, and at least one FIPV strain (Yayoi) is capable of producing both FIP and enteritis.[8,9] Third, virulent FIPV strains can convert to less virulent or avirulent strains during passage in cell culture.[10] In light of these and other newer data, it may be more useful to consider all strains under the general category of feline coronaviruses, that is, divergent strains of virus that are closely related but that vary in their pathogenicity for cats.

Among cats, coronavirus infections appear to be limited to domestic breeds and to certain exotic species, including the cheetah, cougar, bobcat, sand cat, caracal, serval, lynx, jaguar, leopard, and lion. The devastation wrought by introduction of FIPV into a captive population of the genetically depauperate cheetah species has been the subject of much research interest.[11,12]

The routes by which feline coronaviruses are spread from cat to cat have not been identified with certainty, but it is most likely that initial infection results from ingestion or inhalation of virus, and in all probability is dependent on the tissue tropism of the infecting strain. Strains producing enteritis are spread primarily by the fecal-oral route,[7-10] but FIP-producing strains may be excreted in other ways because they produce systemic infections. Close contact with infected cats or their excreta is usually required for effective virus transmission, although the possibility of spread by fomites (on clothing, bedding, feeding bowls, litter pans, etc.) also exists. Transmission of virus by hematophagous arthropods is unproven and probably unlikely. In utero transmission is suggested by observations of FIP in stillborn kittens, but the frequency of this type of transmission is not known.[13] In common with many other enveloped viruses, feline coronaviruses are relatively unstable outside the host, especially when subjected to drying, and are rapidly inactivated by detergents and disinfecting agents such as bleach.

Experimental studies performed over the past several years have succeeded in identifying some of the major host-virus interactions of FIPV in the domestic cat.[14,15] Following infection of large mononuclear cells in regional lymphoreticular tissue at or near the site of initial virus penetration, a primary viremia involving virus and virus-infected cells occurs within one week of exposure. In this way, virus is transported throughout the body, particularly to the liver, spleen, and lymph nodes. These organs contain sizable populations of macrophages, which are the primary target cells for virulent FIPV infection. This is in contrast to the situation for FECVs, which appear to infect primarily enterocytes in the intestines. Hematogenous dissemination of FIPV also results in infection of circulating mononuclear cells (monocytes) and, importantly, in localization of virus and virus-infected cells within the walls of small blood vessels, particularly venules and small veins. A secondary cell-associated viremia may occur after initial infection of target tissues and results in further systemic spread of the virus. Deposition of virus-infected mononuclear cells and virus-antibody immune complexes within blood vessel walls produces an intense vas-culitis, with complement-dependent damage of vessels and subsequent escape of fibrin-rich serum components into the intercellular space. This exudate accumulates as characteristic "FIP fluid" within body cavities, resulting in effusive, or "wet," FIP. Leukotriene B_4, prostaglandin E_2, and interleukin 1 appear to be involved in mediating this inflammatory response.[16,17] DIC may result from widespread vascular damage and activation of terminal complement components by virus-antibody immune complexes. Development of the rarer noneffusive or, "dry," form of FIP is believed to involve a number of similar mechanisms, although the accumulation of fluid does not occur.[18]

Studies have revealed that some cats with preexisting coronavirus antibody, when experimentally infected with FIPV, experience a more rapid and fulminating onset of disease ("accelerated" FIP) than do seronegative cats similarly infected.[10,14,15,19,20] Accelerated FIP can be induced in seronegative cats by passive transfer of hyperimmune serum, suggesting an antibody-mediated enhancement or hypersensitivity phenomenon. Feline coronavirus strains appear to predominate as sensitizing coronaviruses; neither TGEV, CCV, nor human coronavirus 229E (a related human pathogen) has produced significant sensitization in experiments reported thus far.[21-23, 23a] Sensitization appears to be dependent on the identity of both the sensitizing and the challenge coronavirus. The genesis of this sensitization phenomenon and its restriction to certain coronavirus strains appear to be linked to an unknown factor at the molecular level that makes feline coronavirus strains virulent.

A correlation has been shown to exist between virulence and the ability of a coronavirus strain to infect feline macrophages in vitro.[24] Moreover, infection of macrophages is enhanced if coronavirus antibody is added to the culture system, a possible in vitro analog to the in vivo sensitization phenomenon.[25] Macrophages may be more susceptible to infection with virus by uptake of virus-antibody immune complexes via their cell receptors for the Fc portion of IgG. Avirulent strains do not appear to show this enhancement and infect macrophages only poorly.

Sensitivity to the action of proteolytic enzymes and pH fluctuations in the bowel may be other correlates of virulence. Virulent feline coronavirus strains appear to be more resistant to trypsin degradation and higher pH in vitro than less virulent strains.[26,27]

There is also some evidence that underlying immune defects in the host, either intrinsic or acquired, may contribute to the development of FIP. First, reduced T lymphocyte function appears to enhance uptake of FIPV into macrophages and results in more severe disease, particularly if coronavirus antibody is provided by passive serotherapy.[28,29] Second, cheetahs appear to be highly susceptible to FIPV infection and disease, possibly owing to the loss of relevant resistance factors such as major histocompatibility loci from their restricted gene pool.[12] Third, experimental infection of healthy FIPV-exposed, seropositive cats with feline leukemia virus (FeLV), can result in reactivation of a latent FIPV infection with development of fulminant FIP.[10] This latter phenomenon may also occur with some frequency in nature; approximately 20% of cats with spontaneous FIP are also infected with FeLV.[30]

It has been proposed that cell-mediated immune functions may be of greater importance in protecting cats against FIP than humoral antibody and that this protection may be maintained by a persistent coronavirus infection (premunition).[3,10,31,31a] However, considerable protection of 4 or 5 months' duration is also transferred by some seropositive queens to their kittens.[10,31] The exact nature of this protection has not been elucidated.

There are several possible explanations for the widespread exposure of cats to coronaviruses in the absence of widespread disease outbreaks. First, healthy seropositive cats may have been exposed to feline coronavirus strains but have developed resistance that is perhaps mediated by premunition immunity. Second, most healthy seropositive cats may have been exposed only to avirulent or less virulent feline coronavirus or to other coronavirus strains, some of which are more prevalent than virulent strains in the cat population. Third, infection with avirulent or less virulent feline coronavirus strains may induce only minimal cross-protection against other, more virulent strains. A fourth explanation may be that although many cats are exposed to a virulent strain, only those with an underlying immune defect may develop disease. Last, perhaps only those cats exposed to FIPV by an aberrant route or to massive doses of the agent, develop clinical illness.

There is no recognized environmental reservoir for feline coronaviruses, and no other natural host animals are known other than Felidae; thus the natural reservoir is assumed to be infected cats. Cats infected with less virulent coronavirus strains (FECV) have been shown to shed virus in feces for at least 2 to 3 weeks, whereas cats infected with FIPV can harbor the virus without showing clinical signs for at least 4 to 5 months.[7,10,19,31] Healthy seropositive cats or cats in the incubatory stages of the disease are a likely source of virus, because cats with FIP are usually short-lived, and many cases of the disease occur in animals with no known history of exposure to a cat with FIP.[10,31] It has been suggested that a persistent coronavirus infection may be responsible for maintaining protective immune responses, and that when this infection is lost, immunity wanes.[31]

Several important epidemiologic questions remain. How long are "immune carrier" cats infectious? What is the most important route by which they excrete virus? Is excretion continuous or intermittent? Is FIP possibly stress-related? In nature, what is the extent of the role of triggering cofactors such as FeLV or the feline immunodeficiency virus (FIV)? What percentage of cats infected with feline coronaviruses actually become carriers? To what extent is a seropositive cat with an unknown history a potential disease threat to other cats with which it may come into contact, and how might those that shed virulent virus be detected?

CLINICAL SIGNS

Most cases of FIP are seen in young (3 to 4 years of age) adult cats. No statistically significant sex or breed predisposition has been established. Cases of the disease occur sporadically; "outbreaks" involving large numbers of cats housed jointly are uncommon. The onset of clinical signs may be sudden, especially in kittens, or it may be slow and insidious, with the severity of signs increasing gradually over a period of weeks. The earliest signs are usually nonspecific. Anorexia is variable; some affected cats continue to eat and remain alert and responsive for a considerable period of time. Weight loss, lethargy, depression, and dehydration also may be seen. Antibiotic-unresponsive fever (39.5° to 40.6°C [103.1 to 105.1°F]), however, is a more consistent finding and usually persists until the last few hours of life. The temperature will often wax and wane during the daytime, steadily rising overall as evening approaches, and then falling during the night.

Three forms of FIP are recognized, of which effusive (wet) FIP and noneffusive or parenchymatous (dry) FIP are more common. The third form of FIP, which occasionally is seen, represents a combination of the other two forms and usually involves only small quantities of effusion fluid. There is some experimental evidence that in a small percentage of cats, a mild, localized upper respiratory disease, characterized by conjunctivitis and rhinitis, may precede development of FIP. It has been further proposed that many cats experience this localized upper respiratory infection (primary FIP) without developing the lethal, disseminated disease.[3]

Effusive FIP

Accumulation of fibrin-rich fluid within the peritoneal cavity, with progressive, usually painless, enlargement of the abdomen, is probably the most common clinical manifestation of effusive FIP (Fig. 24–2).[32] Effusive FIP is the more fulminant form of the disease, with a more rapid onset and shorter clinical course than the noneffusive form. Many affected cats, especially those among the shorthair breeds, will be presented relatively early in the course of the disease because swelling of the abdomen and weight loss have become readily apparent to the owner. Other animals, especially longhair cats in whom abdominal distension and weight loss may be more difficult for an owner to discern, will be presented later and in a correspondingly more deteriorated condition.

Respiratory difficulty may be seen if abdominal fluid accumulation becomes excessive or, more commonly, when serositis involves the pleura and accumulation of fluid occurs within the thorax. Many cats will develop both thoracic and abdominal effusion; in most of these, one or the other site of involvement will predominate clinically. In general, 40% to 50% of cases show some evidence of pleural involvement at necropsy, whether or not clinical signs of res-

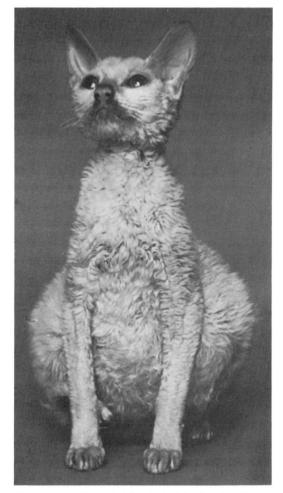

Figure 24–2. Marked abdominal distention in a Rex cat with effusive FIP. (Courtesy of Feline Advisory Bureau, England.)

piratory disease were manifest. Dyspnea usually results from compression of the lungs, but exudation of fluid into the airways may occur as a result of vasculitis. Respiratory signs of effusive FIP include dyspnea (especially upon handling), tachypnea, muffled heart sounds, extreme reluctance to move, and mucous membrane pallor. In addition, pericardial effusion with corresponding clinical signs may be present.

Other, less consistent signs of effusive FIP include icterus (especially in the later stages of the disease, secondary to hepatic involvement), vomiting, fluctuating bouts of diarrhea and constipation, bleeding gums, and ventral edema. Affected lymph nodes and kidneys may feel enlarged and irregular when palpated, suggesting a diagnosis of lymphosarcoma rather than FIP. Rarely, the inflammatory process in the abdomen damages the pancreas, so that clinical pancreatitis, pancreatic exocrine deficiency, or even diabetes mellitus develops. Intact male cats with peritoneal involvement may have scrotal enlargement, resulting from direct extension of fibrinous serositis from the peritoneal cavity. Clinical involvement of other organs such as the eyes or CNS is apparent in only a small percentage of cats with effusive disease.

The clinical course of effusive FIP can be quite variable, but the usual survival time after onset of signs is about 5 to 7 weeks. Some young kittens may survive for no longer than a few days, while some adults may live for 6 to 8 months with smoldering clinical disease.

Noneffusive FIP

The onset of noneffusive FIP is often insidious, with clinical signs reflective of involvement of specific organ systems in the disease process. Weight loss, depression, anemia, and fever are almost always seen, but fluid accumulation is usually minimal. These nonspecific signs may be present for several weeks prior to manifestation of organ-specific localizing signs. In other cases, localizing signs may be apparent from the onset. Abdominal palpation may reveal mesenteric lymphadenopathy or nodular irregularities of the viscera, both suggestive of lymphosarcoma. Involvement of the lungs may be manifest as a pyogranulomatous pneumonia, producing a persistent cough without noticeable signs of dyspnea. Clinical signs of renal or hepatic insufficiency, pancreatic disease, or ocular and nervous system disease may be observed in cats with severe organ impairment. Neurologic and ocular abnormalities are more common in this form of the disease.

The most frequent neurologic signs are posterior paresis and ataxia progressing to tetraparesis. Other possible signs include paraspinal or generalized hyperesthesia, tremors, increased muscle rigidity, head-tilt, circling, nystagmus, anisocoria, behavioral changes, cranial nerve deficits, paralysis, and seizures. The neuroanatomic distribution of lesions will govern the clinical manifestation of the disease process. Lesions in the nervous system, as in other areas of the body, are surface-oriented and associated with blood vessels, affecting most frequently the meninges of the brain and spinal cord, the choroid plexus, and the subependymal region. With chronicity, deeper parenchymal lesions will cause progressive sensorimotor dysfunction. Hydrocephalus can develop secondary to ependymal involvement, with inflammatory exudate obstructing the normal flow of CSF.[32a]

Ocular signs in FIP usually are bilateral and commonly manifest as an anterior uveitis (iridocyclitis with a miotic pupil, aqueous flare, hypopyon, keratic precipitates, hyphema, corneal edema, and synechiae). The iris may be edematous and misshapen and may show a loss of striations, and a mild conjunctivitis may accompany corneal edema. If clouding of the anterior chamber is incomplete, other abnormalities may be visualized in the posterior portion of the globe: pyogranulomatous chorioretinitis with perivascular exudates such as characteristic sheathing of retinal vessels with exudate, flame-shaped retinal hemorrhages, and retinal detachments (see Fig. 13–12). The sheathing of retinal vessels is a characteristic sign of FIP. Ocular disease can occur in conjunction with CNS disease or peritoneal involvement or may appear alone as the sole sign of FIP. The uveal lesions are vascular in orientation and are characterized primarily by necrotizing pyogranulomatous inflammation of the vessels of the iris and ciliary body.

The clinical course of noneffusive FIP is generally more protracted than that of the effusive form. A few cats, especially those with primary ocular involvement and little systemic involvement, may survive for as long as a year or more, with or without glucocorticoid therapy.

Reproductive Disorders

"Kitten mortality complex" (KMC) is a general term that has been used to describe a specific cluster of disease conditions in catteries and breeding colonies with which FIPV was once thought to be etiologically associated. The complex has been divided into two major disease problems: (1) reproductive failure in queens such as repeat breeding, fetal resorption, abortion, stillbirths, and congenital birth defects and (2) neonatal mortality variously attributed to acute congestive cardiomyopathy, FIP, or nonspecific illness ("fading kitten" syndrome). In addition to these, respiratory disease, recurrent fever spikes, endometritis, and cardiovascular disease have been reported in some adult cats within affected catteries. The cause of KMC has not been determined. A single FIPV isolation was reported from a neonate born to a queen experiencing reproductive problems; however, subsequent inoculation experiments with this isolate failed to reproduce any component of KMC except FIP itself.[19]

Feline Coronaviral Enteritis

FECV strains can produce an enteritis that clinicopathologically resembles those produced by TGEV in pigs and by CCV in dogs.[3,7] The severity of the infection is age-related, being greater in young kittens; most infected adults remain essentially asymptomatic. Signs in kittens include a low-grade fever and a mild to moderately severe diarrhea lasting from 2 to 5 days. Concurrent with the onset of diarrhea, there may be a transient depression in leukocyte numbers primarily owing to a decrease in neutrophils. The most severe lesions are produced in the mature columnar epithelium of the ileum and jejunum. The mortality rate is negligible; virtually all affected kittens recover.

DIAGNOSIS

FIP

The diagnosis of FIP is made by evaluation of the history, presenting signs, and results of appropriate laboratory tests. Clinicopathologic and serologic procedures useful in diagnosis include analysis of thoracic or abdominal fluid, hemogram, serum protein electrophoresis, clinical biochemistry profiles, serum coronavirus antibody titers, and histology.

Effusive Fluid. Evaluation of effusive fluid remains one of the most useful diagnostic aids for differentiating the effusive form of FIP from other disease conditions; it is of obviously lesser significance in the diagnosis of noneffusive FIP. The volume of fluid present is variable and generally is a reflection of disease chronicity. In most cases, between 15 to 1000 ml will be found; in chronic cases, more than a liter may accumulate.

Typically, this fluid is clear or slightly clouded and straw-colored to bright yellow or amber in appearance; occasionally, it may have a greenish or reddish tinge. It is thick and viscous, serum-like in consistency, rich in fibrin, and may clot upon exposure to air. It is odorless and occasionally contains a small amount of flocculent material, consisting of fibrin strands and flakes, which may be visible on a stained smear. The fluid is a modified transudate or exudate of high specific gravity (1.017 to 1.047, median 1.032), high protein content (5 to 12 g/dl or more), and usually low leukocyte cellularity (in contrast to the high numbers found in septic peritonitis or pyothorax). In acute cases, the differential leukocyte count consists primarily of neutrophils, with smaller numbers of mononuclear cells. In chronic cases, mononuclear and mesothelial cells predominate. In contrast to the degenerate and toxic neutrophils seen in cases of septic disease, the majority of leukocytes in FIP effusive fluid are relatively normal in appearance. The protein electrophoretic pattern of the fluid roughly parallels that of the serum in affected animals, being enriched in globulins (γ in particular). A γ-globulin content $\geq 32\%$ is highly predictive for a diagnosis of FIP, whereas an albumin content $> 48\%$ or an albumin:globulin (A:G) ratio > 0.81 are highly predictive for ruling out FIP.[33]

Hematologic Findings. Alterations in the hemogram tend to be similar in both the effusive and noneffusive forms but are variable and nonspecific for FIP. Commonly observed changes include leukocytosis caused by an absolute neutrophilia, with or without a modest left shift to bands, eosinopenia, and lymphopenia. Some circulating neutrophils may contain intracytoplasmic inclusion bodies, which probably represent phagocytosed virus-antibody immune complexes rather than replicating virus. Occasionally, a leukopenia will be seen, particularly in cats with more fulminating effusive FIP or in those in the final stages of the disease. About 40% of cats with FIP also develop a mild to moderate normocytic, normochromic anemia that tends to be progressive, becoming more severe toward termination of the illness. The anemia may be exacerbated by concurrent infection with *Haemobartonella felis* or FeLV.

DIC has been observed in cats with experimentally induced FIP[20] and in some spontaneous cases. Clotting abnormalities, including prolonged prothrombin and partial thromboplastin times; depression of coagulation factors VII, VIII, IX, XI, and XII activities; elevation of fibrin-fibrinogen degradation products; and thrombocytopenia have been documented in these cases.

Serum Protein Analysis. Hyperproteinemia (range usually 7.8 to 12.0 g/dl or more) is seen in about 50% of cats with effusive FIP and about 70% of cats with noneffusive FIP. This usually is the result of a polyclonal (very rarely monoclonal) hypergammaglobulinemia with accompanying elevations of α_2 (fibrinogen, haptoglobin) and β globulins. Frequently, there is a reversal of the A:G ratio. Fibrinogen concentrations are elevated above 400 mg/dl in about 45% to 60% of FIP cases. Although these changes are suggestive of FIP, they are not diagnostic but rather are a reflection of chronic inflammation and antibody production and thus may also be seen in other inflammatory disease processes associated with persistent antigenic stimulation.

Clinical Biochemistry. In general, abnormalities in clinical chemistry profiles reflect the extent of involvement of different organ systems. Hyperbilirubinemia may be seen in about 40% of cases and is a reflection of multifocal hepatic necrosis. Despite the presence of hepatic necrosis, serum ALP and ALT (SGPT) activities are often not elevated as they are with cholangiohepatitis or hepatic lipidosis. A proteinuria with or without increased BUN and serum creatinine and electrolyte disturbances may be seen in cases with renal impairment. Analysis of CSF from cats with severe meningeal lesions may reveal elevated protein (90 to 2000 mg/dl or more) and leukocytes (90 to 9250 cells/μl), the latter predominantly neutrophils. Similar changes may be seen in aqueous humor from cats with extensive involvement of the uveal tract.[3]

Serologic Tests and FIP

Most cats with FIP have moderate to high titers of coronavirus antibody. A number of laboratory test procedures have been developed to detect this antibody, the most popular being indirect fluorescent antibody (IFA) and ELISA. Either FIPV itself or one of the other closely related, cross-reacting coronaviruses such as TGEV or CCV can be

used as the target antigen in these assays. Coronaviruses other than FIPV were used extensively in the past because of longstanding difficulties in propagating FIPV in vitro. Because these procedures have not been standardized and because some laboratories modify the tests they use, results on a given serum sample often differ from one laboratory to another. For this reason, testing laboratories should provide their clients with information on the clinical significance of the titers they report. Similar considerations apply to the manufacturers of test kits. See Appendix 8 for a listing of diagnostic tests and laboratories that perform them, as well as commercially available test kits.

Nonspecificity of Tests. The ability of several different cross-reacting coronaviruses to detect FIPV antibodies in cat serum highlights one of the great problems of the current serologic test methodology, namely, its nonspecificity. Studies using monoclonal antibodies have pinpointed antigenic differences among certain feline coronavirus isolates;[34,35] however, there is as yet no serologic test available that can make strategic use of these observed differences to distinguish cats with FIP or cats subclinically infected with FIPV from cats infected with less virulent feline coronavirus strains. Interpretation of coronavirus antibody titers often is not clear-cut.[36,36a]

Seropositive Cats. Excluding cats in catteries and multiple-cat households, approximately 10% to 40% of cats tested in the general population will be seropositive. A special situation is encountered when cats are clustered in catteries, in which case most cats are either seronegative, indicating no coronavirus exposure, or are seropositive, suggesting efficient spread of the virus among animals. The presence of seropositive cats in a cattery does not necessarily correlate with its FIP history; e.g., antibody may be found in healthy cats in catteries that have experienced losses to FIP as well as in catteries that have never seen the disease.

The occurrence of serum coronavirus antibody in any cat, whether healthy or diseased, is indicative of only one thing: exposure to a coronavirus in the FIPV antigenic cluster. It does not provide information on the nature of the infection, i.e., whether the cat is actively diseased, a healthy carrier, or simply has been exposed at some time in the past. The percentage of exposed cats that become carriers is unknown. Neither, however, does a positive titer indicate that a cat is protected from developing FIP, because most cats with FIP are antibody-positive.

Seronegative Cats with FIP. A small minority of cats with FIP that do not have detectable serum coronavirus antibody at the time of testing can be found. Detectable antibody can sometimes disappear from the circulation during the terminal stages of disease. This phenomenon has been seen repeatedly in experimentally induced cases of FIP and is undoubtedly responsible for a percentage of the seronegative FIP cats seen in the field. It is probably related to formation of immune complexes with an apparent disappearance of antibody from the circulation. Repeated draining of effusions may accelerate this phenomenon.

Peracute disease, as can be seen in some young seronegative kittens, may limit the amount of time available for the development of antibody responses and hence the capability of a serologic test to detect them. This problem may be compounded by use of a coronavirus other than FIPV by the testing laboratory, since these heterotypic viruses are not as sensitive at detecting lower levels of FIPV antibody.

False-Positive Reactions. Antibody against bovine serum components occasionally found in cat serum reacts with similar components present in cell cultures used to propagate target viruses for coronavirus antibody tests.[37,38] One possible explanation for this antibovine reactivity is parenteral vaccination. Viral vaccines frequently contain extraneous cell culture material that is probably the source of much of this noncoronavirus reactivity. Supportive studies have shown further that this nonspecific reactivity dissipates with time. The probability of encountering this false-positive result can be minimized if serum samples for elective testing are obtained no sooner than 3 to 4 months following the most recent parenteral vaccination.

When to Test. Despite the difficulties with current feline coronavirus antibody testing methods, there remain certain select situations in which the test can be of assistance.

First, the major use of antibody titers is for screening purposes, to detect the presence of seropositive cats in a previously untested household and to detect possible virus carriers when introducing new cats into an antibody-negative household. Only about 10% to 20% (or minimum of three cats) in a previously untested household need to be evaluated, because antibody will either be totally absent or present in a majority of the resident cats. While the identification of seropositive cats in such households will not diagnose the problem, knowledge that coronavirus antibody is absent will be helpful in ruling out an FIPV-group coronavirus as the culprit. Unfortunately, available coronavirus antibody tests have absolutely *no predictive value*, i.e., a positive test in no way indicates that a cat is doomed to develop FIP at some time in the future.

Determination of serum coronaviral antibody titers should only be used as an aid in diagnosis and should be given no more weight than any of the other clinical laboratory procedures. Fluid cytology and analysis will often be most consistent when effusion is present, even in cats where the serum antibody titer is low. If a conflict occurs between clinical or laboratory findings and the coronaviral antibody titer, the diagnosis should be based on the other relevant data, regardless of the titer value. In cats with prolonged illness suggestive of FIP, a fourfold or greater increase in titer over a period of 4 to 6 weeks is highly suspicious for active FIP. Elevated titers in some cats may vary about a certain fixed level for months to years or may show a progressive decline. Perhaps those that maintain high titers represent the elusive immune carriers, whereas those whose titers eventually disappear are cats that have cleared the infection.

Feline Coronaviral Enteritis

A definitive diagnosis of coronaviral enteritis in kittens is difficult when using currently available methods, and the clinical resemblance to other enteritides may confound the diagnosis. Electron microscopy of stool specimens to search for coronavirus particles is an expensive and time-consuming procedure fraught with false-negative and false-positive results; furthermore, true-positive results can only provide presumptive evidence of the cause of diarrhea. There is a widely accepted misconception that coronavirus antibody titers can be used to discriminate between FIP and infection with coronavirus strains of lesser virulence. In reality, currently available coronavirus antibody tests are unable to provide a definitive diagnosis of feline coronaviral enteritis. Similarly, histologic lesions seen in affected kittens are not specific enough for diagnosis. Viral isolation is currently impractical for use on a routine basis.

PATHOLOGIC FINDINGS

At necropsy, the serosal surfaces of the abdomen or thorax or both are covered by a diffuse or multifocal, necrotic fibrinous exudate that frequently is most apparent on the spleen and liver (Fig. 24–3). The omentum, mesentery and mesenteric lymph nodes, liver, spleen, kidneys, and pancreas are most often involved. Pyogranulomatous lesions appear as multifocal, white to gray, plaque-like nodules that are 1 to 10 mm in diameter and have a noticeable surface orientation. Often, the mesentery is thickened and has a watery or gelatinous consistency. The omentum may appear as a contracted mass of fibrinous adhesions in the ventral abdomen. In long-standing cases, these adhesions may be extensive and involve more of the abdominal viscera. Corresponding thoracic lesions can involve the pleura, lungs, pericardium, epicardium, myocardium, or thymus.

Granulomatous or pyogranulomatous lesions in the abdominal and thoracic viscera of cats with noneffusive FIP appear grossly as raised, white foci, 1 to 20 mm in diameter. They tend to be subcapsular and surface oriented but may extend deeper into the parenchyma and are usually distributed along the meandering course of the smaller blood vessels. The dissemination of these lesions may be quite widespread throughout the body, both at the macroscopic and microscopic levels.

Histologic examination of tissues taken from biopsy or necropsy specimens remains the only accepted test procedure available that can provide a *definitive* diagnosis of FIP.[39] There are many "FIP look-alike" diseases producing similar clinical signs or grossly visible lesions that affect cats, including lymphoma and other neoplasms (especially those involving the liver, biliary tract, kidneys, lungs, brain), cardiomyopathy, nephrotic syndrome, liver disease (including cholangitis and cholangiohepatitis), septic peritonitis, diaphragmatic hernia, pyothorax, chylothorax, internal abscesses, pansteatitis, toxoplasmosis, cryptococcosis, and tuberculosis.

Although simpler, percutaneous needle biopsy is not always recommended for obtaining tissue specimens in cats with FIP owing to the friability of affected viscera and the potential for serious hemorrhage, especially in cases with clotting abnormalities. However, postoperative fluid leakage from an incision site is avoided with this method. If percutaneous biopsy is performed, the

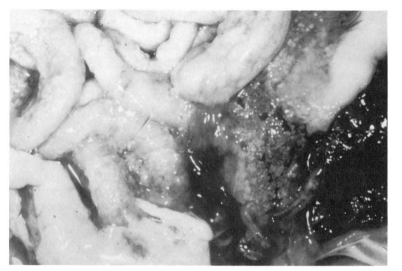

Figure 24–3. Abdominal viscera in a case of effusive FIP. Note the characteristic fibrinous coating on the surfaces of the viscera and the presence of effusion fluid. (Courtesy of Dr. James L. Carpenter, Angell Memorial Animal Hospital, Boston, MA.)

kidney is usually selected because of its common involvement. Exploratory laparotomy with organ biopsy is the preferred method for obtaining FIP tissue specimens.[39] Light general anesthesia with an inhalant such as halothane is preferred over barbiturates or ketamine in patients with compromised hepatic and renal function. Collected tissues may be fixed in 10% buffered neutral formalin and should include samples of omentum, liver, spleen, mesenteric lymph node, and kidney. Typical histologic lesions of FIP include a disseminated pyogranulomatous and fibrinonecrotic reaction oriented around small veins, necrotizing phlebitis and thrombosis, and lymphoreticular and mesothelial cell hyperplasia.

THERAPY

FIP

No curative therapy for FIP currently exists, and the disease is virtually always fatal once clinical signs of effusion or severe organ involvement have appeared. Although there is some evidence that cats with mild FIP occasionally experience spontaneous remission,[3] this does not seem to be a widespread phenomenon. On the basis of serologic data, it appears that cats are frequently exposed to coronavirus strains of the FIPV-antigenic group. Many of these cats that are diagnosed on the basis of seropositivity as suffering from FIP but later improve may actually be suffering from another disease that resolves spontaneously.

Current therapy for cats with FIP remains an exercise in palliation. There are no effective antiviral compounds and no methods for eliminating the virus from affected animals. However, some treatment regimens may induce temporary, short-term remissions of weeks to months in a small percentage of carefully chosen patients. The best candidates for palliative therapy are cats that are still in good physical condition, are still eating, are not showing severe anemia, neurologic signs, or other significant organ dysfunction, and are not also infected with FeLV. The FeLV and FIV status of all FIPV-infected cats should be determined prior to treatment because the prognosis for cats with concurrent infections is exceedingly grave.

The basic aim of palliative therapy in FIP is to ameliorate the disseminated, self-destructive inflammatory reactions that represent the immune system's unsuccessful efforts at eliminating the virus from the cat's body. The most effective treatment protocols combine high levels of glucocorticoids, cytotoxic drugs, and broad-spectrum antibiotics with maintenance of nutrient intake and fluid and electrolyte balance (Table 24–1). Drainage of significant quantities of peritoneal exudate, followed by instillation of isotonic fluids twice daily may be of benefit in some cases of effusive FIP. Cats receiving cytotoxic drugs need to be routinely monitored for evidence of bone marrow suppression and kidney dysfunction. If the cat shows a positive response to therapy over the first few weeks, treatment should be continued for at least 3 months. Rarely, if a cat appears to be in complete remission, glucocorticoids and cytotoxic drugs may be slowly withdrawn. Treatment should be reinstated, however, if signs of FIP reappear. Progressive physical deterioration in the face of treatment is a poor prognostic indicator.

A possible exception to this gloomy overall picture of FIP therapy is the cat with primary ocular involvement. Cases of FIP in which the disease process is restricted to the eyes may respond to topical therapy with ophthalmic glucocorticoid preparations, perhaps supplemented with periodic retrobulbar injections or systemic medication. Some of these cats will present with extraordinarily elevated coronavirus antibody titers, which may gradually decline as treatment progresses. Often the disease can be kept under control for many months to a year or more; however, a percentage of these long-term remissions do eventually collapse, with either spread of virus to the brain and manifestations of neurologic disease or the development of classic effusive or noneffusive FIP.

It has been suggested that the use of certain immunomodulatory compounds affecting primarily T cell and macrophage activities may have some beneficial effect early in the course of FIP. Some of these compounds include thioproline, isoprinosine, thymosin, and interferon. To date, however, controlled studies have not been published. Likewise, there is no documented scientific evidence that supplemental multivitamin therapy is of any benefit in treating FIP.

Table 24–1. Drug Therapy for FIP[a]

DRUG	DOSE[b] (mg/kg)	ROUTE	INTERVAL (hours)	DURATION (weeks)
Prednisolone	4	PO	24	3–9[c]
Cyclophosphamide (Cytoxan)	2	PO	24	3–9[c,d]
OR				
Melphalan (Alkeran)	1 (Total)	PO	72	3–9[c]
Ampicillin	20	PO	8	3–6[c]
Stanozolol (Winstrol-V)	1 (Total)	PO	12	prn

[a]PO = oral, prn = as needed.
[b]Dose per administration, expressed as mg/kg unless otherwise stated.
[c]Duration of therapy is empirical and is based on the ill cat's needs and clinical response.
[d]Treatment given on 4 consecutive days each week.

Feline Coronaviral Enteritis

Treatment of feline coronaviral enteritis is purely supportive, but most kittens will recover with or without treatment. Fluid and electrolyte balance need to be maintained to correct dehydration in severely affected kittens. Antibiotic therapy is usually not required.

PREVENTION

A safe and effective feline coronavirus vaccine is still unavailable.[40,41] Studies in this area have been under way for several years, but because of the antibody-dependent sensitization phenomenon, the inconsistent protection delivered by homotypic feline coronavirus strains, and the lack of cross-protection afforded by heterotypic coronaviruses, attempts to produce a uniformly safe and effective broad-spectrum vaccine have proven unsuccessful. The ideal FIP vaccine would contain an FIPV strain capable of inducing cell-mediated immunity without producing FIP, even following stress or infection by immunosuppressive agents such as FeLV or FIV. Such a strain of virus may be difficult to find, and even if identified, its use in a vaccination program might provide little added benefit to immunity derived from natural exposure. Recently an MLV vaccine employing an attenuated strain of FIPV has been described.[41] Although the data are still preliminary, most cats vaccinated intranasally with this experimental vaccine have thus far resisted challenge with virulent virus. Additional studies exploring the safety and efficacy of this new vaccine are currently in progress (see also Vaccination for FIP, Chapter 2).

Until a vaccine is available, control of coronavirus infections must be based on accurate identification and isolation of diseased animals and on maintenance of coronavirus antibody–negative catteries and households when possible. Veterinarians should advise breeders to eliminate FeLV antigen-positive and FIV antibody-positive cats, reduce cattery crowding, avoid inbreeding, and stop breeding particular pairs of cats that tend to produce kittens with FIP, or eliminate problem breeding stock from the cattery altogether. However, a test-and-removal program for coronavirus antibody–positive cats similar to that utilized for control of FeLV infection cannot be recommended on the basis of current knowledge. Because there is no available diagnostic test that can specifically identify the seropositive immune carriers, there is no medical reason for destroying healthy seropositive cats. Euthanasia of such cats to achieve antibody-negative status in a cattery thus cannot be justified; instead, control must be exerted at the level of admission. *All* cats ideally should test negative both before and after a 4- to 6-week quarantine period before entry into an antibody-negative population of cats. In addition, routine testing at periodic 3- or 6-month intervals should be performed in negative households that send cats to show or stud. Feline coronaviruses do not appear to represent a health hazard for human beings.

References

1. Barlough JE, Stoddart CA: Feline infectious peritonitis. In Scott FW (ed): *Contemporary Issues in Small Animal Practice 3: Infectious Diseases.* New York, Churchill Livingstone, 1986, pp 93–108.
2. Lutz H, Hauser B, Horzinek MC: Feline infectious

peritonitis (FIP)—the present state of knowledge. *J Small Anim Pract* 27:108–116, 1986.

3. Pedersen NC: Coronavirus diseases (coronavirus enteritis, feline infectious peritonitis). *In* Holzworth J (ed): *Diseases of the Cat*, vol 1. Philadelphia, WB Saunders Co, 1987, pp 193–214.

4. Scott FW: Feline infectious peritonitis and other feline coronaviruses. *In* Kirk RW (ed): *Current Veterinary Therapy IX*. Philadelphia, WB Saunders Co, 1986, pp 1059–1062.

5. Stoddart ME, Gaskell CJ: Feline coronavirus infection. *In* Chandler EA, Hilbery ADR, Gaskell CJ (eds): *Feline Medicine and Therapeutics*. Oxford, Blackwell Scientific Publications, 1985, pp 284–289.

6. Stoddart CA, Barlough JE, Scott FW: Experimental studies of a coronavirus and coronavirus-like agent in a barrier-maintained feline breeding colony. *Arch Virol* 79:85–94, 1984.

7. Pedersen NC, Boyle JF, Floyd K, et al: An enteric coronavirus infection of cats and its relationship to feline infectious peritonitis. *Am J Vet Res* 42:368-377, 1981.

8. Hayashi T, Watabe Y, Nakayama H, et al: Enteritis due to feline infectious peritonitis virus. *Jpn J Vet Sci* 44:97–106, 1982.

9. Hayashi T, Watabe Y, Takenouchi T, et al: Role of circulating antibodies in feline infectious peritonitis after oral infection. *Jpn J Vet Sci* 45:487–494, 1983.

10. Pedersen NC, Floyd K: Experimental studies with three new strains of feline infectious peritonitis virus: FIPV-UCD2, FIPV-UCD3, and FIPV-UCD4. *Compend Cont Educ Pract Vet* 7:1001–1011, 1985.

11. Evermann JF, Roelke ME, Briggs MB: Feline coronavirus infections of cheetahs. *Feline Pract* 16(3):21–30, 1986.

12. O'Brien SJ, Roelke ME, Marker L, et al: Genetic basis for species vulnerability in the cheetah. *Science* 227:1428–1434, 1985.

13. Pedersen NC: Feline infectious peritonitis and feline enteric coronavirus infections. Part 2. Feline infectious peritonitis. *Feline Pract* 13(5):5–20, 1983.

14. Pedersen NC, Boyle JF: Immunologic phenomena in the effusive form of feline infectious peritonitis. *Am J Vet Res* 41:868–876, 1980.

15. Weiss RC, Scott FW: Pathogenesis of feline infectious peritonitis: pathologic changes and immunofluorescence. *Am J Vet Res* 42:2036–2048, 1981.

16. Goitsuka R, Hirota Y, Hasegawa A, et al: Release of interleukin 1 from peritoneal exudate cells of cats with feline infectious peritonitis. *Jpn J Vet Sci* 49:811–818, 1987.

17. Weiss RC, Vaughn DM, Cox NR: Increased plasma levels of leukotriene B$_4$ and prostaglandin E$_2$ in cats experimentally inoculated with feline infectious peritonitis virus. *Vet Res Commun* 12:313–323, 1988.

18. Hayashi T, Utsumi F, Takahashi R, et al: Pathology of non-effusive type feline infectious peritonitis and experimental transmission. *Jpn J Vet Sci* 42:197–210, 1980.

19. Pedersen NC, Evermann JF, McKeirnan AJ, et al: Pathogenicity studies of feline coronavirus isolates 79-1146 and 79-1683. *Am J Vet Res* 45:2580–2585, 1984.

20. Weiss RC, Dodds WJ, Scott FW: Disseminated intravascular coagulation in experimentally induced feline infectious peritonitis. *Am J Vet Res* 41:663-671, 1980.

21. Barlough JE, Johnson-Lussenburg CM, Stoddart CA, et al: Experimental inoculation of cats with human coronavirus 229E and subsequent challenge with feline infectious peritonitis virus. *Can J Comp Med* 49:303-307, 1985.

22. Barlough JE, Stoddart CA, Sorresso GP, et al: Experimental inoculation of cats with canine coronavirus and subsequent challenge with feline infectious peritonitis virus. *Lab Anim Sci* 34:592-597, 1984.

23. Stoddart CA, Barlough JE, Baldwin CA, et al: Attempted immunisation of cats against feline infectious peritonitis using canine coronavirus. *Res Vet Sci* 45:383–388, 1988.

23a. Toma B, Duret C, Chappuis G, et al: Échec de l'immunisation contre la péritonite infectieuse féline par injection de virus de la gastro-entérite transmissible du porc. *Recl Méd Vét* 155:799–803, 1979.

24. Stoddart CA, Scott FW: Intrinsic resistance of feline peritoneal macrophages to coronavirus infection correlates with in vivo virulence. *J Virol* 63:436-440, 1988.

25. Stoddart CA, Scott FW: Antibody-mediated enhancement of in vitro infection of feline peritoneal macrophages with feline infectious peritonitis virus. *J Virol.* In press, 1989.

26. McKeirnan AJ, Evermann JF, Davis EV, et al: Comparative properties of feline coronaviruses *in vitro*. *Can J Vet Res* 51:212–216, 1987.

27. Fiscus SA, Teramoto YA: Functional differences in the peplomer glycoproteins of feline coronavirus isolates. *J Virol* 61:2655–2657, 1987.

28. Hayashi T, Sasaki N, Ami Y, et al: Role of thymus-dependent lymphocytes and antibodies in feline infectious peritonitis after oral infection. *Jpn J Vet Sci* 45:759–766, 1983.

29. Takenouchi T, Ami Y, Hayashi T, et al: Role of T cells in feline infectious peritonitis virus infection of suckling mice. *Jpn J Vet Sci* 47:465–468, 1985.

30. Reinacher M: Infections with feline leukaemia virus detected upon post-mortem examination. *J Small Anim Pract* 28:640–646, 1987.

31. Pedersen NC: Virologic and immunologic aspects of feline infectious peritonitis virus infection. *Adv Exp Med Biol* 218:529–550, 1987.

31a. Weiss RC, Cox NR: Delayed-type hypersensitivity skin responses associated with feline infectious peritonitis in two cats. *Res Vet Sci* 44:396–398, 1988.

32. Horzinek MC, Osterhaus ADME: The virology and pathogenesis of feline infectious peritonitis. *Arch Virol* 59:1–15, 1979.

32a. Tamke PG, Petersen MG, Dietze AE, et al: Acquired hydrocephalus and hydromyelia in a cat with feline infectious peritonitis: a case report and brief review. *Can Vet J* 29:997–1000, 1988.

33. Shelly SM, Scarlett-Kranz J, Blue JT: Protein electrophoresis on effusions from cats as a diagnostic test for feline infectious peritonitis. *J Am Anim Hosp Assoc* 24:495–500, 1988.

34. Baines JD: Molecular analyses of feline coronaviruses. PhD dissertation. Cornell University, Ithaca, NY, 1988.

35. Fiscus SA, Teramoto YA: Antigenic comparison of feline coronavirus isolates: evidence for markedly different peplomer glycoproteins. *J Virol* 61:2607–2613, 1987.

36. Barlough JE: Cats, coronaviruses and coronavirus antibody tests. *J Small Anim Pract* 26:353–362, 1985.

36a. Ingersoll JD, Wylie DE: Comparison of serologic assays for measurement of antibody response to coronavirus in cats. *Am J Vet Res* 49:1472–1479, 1988.

37. Barlough JE, Jacobson RH, Pepper CE, et al: Role of recent vaccination in production of false-positive coronavirus antibody titers in cats. *J Clin Microbiol* 19:442–445, 1984.

38. Barlough JE, Jacobson RH, Scott FW, et al: Effect of recent vaccination on feline coronavirus antibody test results. *Feline Pract* 15(5):17–26, 1985.

39. Weiss RC, Scott FW: Laboratory diagnosis of feline infectious peritonitis. *Feline Pract* 10(2):16–22, 1980.

40. Scott FW: Immunization against feline coronaviruses. *Adv Exp Med Biol* 218:569–576, 1987.

41. Scott FW: Immunization of cats against feline infectious peritonitis. *Proc 4th Annu Kal Kan Infect Dis Seminar*, Eastern States Vet Conf, Orlando, FL, 1988, pp 3–8.

25 FELINE ASTROVIRAL AND ROTAVIRAL INFECTIONS

Feline Astroviral Infections David A. Harbour

ETIOLOGY

Astroviruses were first described in feces from cases of human infantile gastroenteritis.[1] They have since been identified in the feces in several other species, including dogs (see Other Viral Enteritides; Chapter 21)[2,3] and cats.[4–7] When negatively stained and examined by transmission electron microscopy, astroviruses appear as unenveloped, spherical particles approximately 28 to 30 nm in diameter, with a characteristic 5- or 6-pointed star-shaped surface pattern, depending on the orientation (Fig. 25–1).

CLINICAL FINDINGS

Only two cases of a natural astrovirus infection in cats have been reported in de-

tail.[4,6] In both cases the illness was characterized by persistent green, watery diarrhea, dehydration, and anorexia. No hematologic abnormalities were noted, and the only biochemical abnormalities were mild acidosis and hypokalemia in one of the cats. Other variable signs were gas-distended loops of the small intestine, pyrexia, depression, poor body condition, and vomiting. Vomiting and diarrhea have been reported in another infected cat, although no further clinical details were given.[7]

In a recent outbreak of diarrhea in a breeding colony, astrovirus was seen by electron microscopy in the feces of 25% of affected kittens.[8] Initial signs in these kittens were inappetence, depression, and prolapse of the third eyelid. Other litters in the colony previously had developed a similar syndrome,

Figure 25–1. Negatively stained astrovirus particles. Arrows indicate particles with 5- and 6-pointed star-shaped surface patterns. (Courtesy of Charles Ashley, Bristol Public Health Laboratory, Bristol, U.K.)

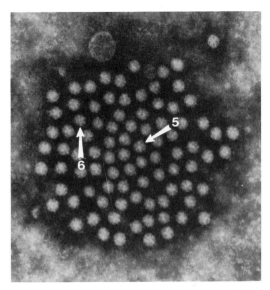

with diarrhea that persisted 4 to 14 days. A number of adults were also affected. Sera from several of these animals had antibody to astrovirus.

Experimental oral administration of an astroviral isolate to specific pathogen–free kittens resulted in mild diarrhea 11 to 12 days later.[6] This coincided with a period of pyrexia and virus shedding with subsequent seroconversion. The kittens remained otherwise well.

in cell culture, although no cytopathic effect is produced and virus-infected cells must be located by specific immunofluorescence. It is not known whether all isolates are cultivable.

A limited serologic and virologic survey of United Kingdom cats with diarrhea suggests that the infection is not very common, less than 10% of animals tested having antibody to the Bristol isolate.[9] However, more than one serotype may exist, as in people.

DIAGNOSIS

Astrovirus infection is most conveniently diagnosed by electron microscopy of negatively stained preparations of diarrheic stools. It may be possible to isolate the virus

THERAPY

Treatment of affected animals probably is not necessary, other than to replace lost fluids and electrolytes if the diarrhea is severe or prolonged.

Feline Rotaviral Infections   Craig E. Greene

Rotaviruses are included in the family Reoviridae. They have been implicated as the cause of diarrhea in neonates of many mammalian species. Serologic studies indicate that exposure to the animal population is widespread. Canine rotaviral infection is discussed under that heading in Chapter 21. Although rotaviruses of different hosts can infect other species, these infections are self-limiting. Rotaviral infections, as with the astroviral infections, are restricted to the GI mucosa. The spread of infection is by fecal-to-oral means. As unenveloped viruses, they are relatively resistant to environmental destruction.

Rotaviral infections in cats are primarily subclinical. There is a high prevalence of seropositivity without clinical illness. Diarrhea was found in a 6-week-old orphaned kitten[10] and an 8-month-old cat[11] that were excreting rotavirus in their feces. The diarrhea lasted less than 1 week and was of liquid to semiformed consistency. A 3-day-old, colostrum-deprived cat was inoculated with the isolated virus, and it developed anorexia and diarrhea.[10]

Electron microscopy can be used to detect the virus in the feces. ELISA tests developed for identifying rotaviral antigen in the feces of other hosts could be used in testing cat feces. Histologic findings include swollen intestinal villi with mild infiltration by macrophages and neutrophils. Viral antigen can be detected by FA or electron microscopy in epithelial cells. See Appendix 8 for listing of commercial laboratories and diagnostic tests that assist in the diagnosis of rotaviral infections.

Treatment is symptomatic for diarrhea. Signs are mild and transient and there is not impairment of mucosal integrity. Fluids can be given IV or SC, depending on the severity of dehydration. There is presently no vaccine available.

References

1. Madeley CR, Cosgrove BP: 28nm particles in faeces in infantile gastroenteritis. Lancet ii:451–452, 1975.
2. Williams FP: Astrovirus-like, coronavirus-like and parvovirus-like particles detected in the diarrhoea stools of beagle pups. Arch Virol 66:215–226, 1980.
3. Hammond MM, Timoney PJ: An electron microscopic study of viruses associated with canine gastroenteritis. Cornell Vet 73:82–97, 1983.
4. Hoshino Y, Zimmer JF, Moise NS, et al: Detection of astroviruses in feces of a cat with diarrhea. Arch Virol 70:373–376, 1981.
5. Marshall JA, Kennett ML, Rodger SM, et al: Virus and virus-like particles in the faeces of cats with and without diarrhoea. Aust Vet J 64:100–105, 1987.
6. Harbour DA, Ashley CR, Williams PD, et al: Natural and experimental astrovirus infection of cats. Vet Rec 120:555–557, 1987.
7. Herbst W, Krauss H: Electron microscopy in the

diagnosis of enteritis in cats. *J Small Animal Pract* 29:5–11, 1988.

8. Harbour DA, Baxter CP: Unpublished observation, University of Bristol, U.K., 1987.

9. Harbour DA: Unpublished observation, University of Bristol, U.K., 1988.

10. Snodgrass DR, August KW, Gray EW: A rotavirus from kittens. *Vet Rec* 104:222–223, 1979.

11. Chrystie IL, Goldwater PN, Banatvala JE: Rotavirus infection in a domestic cat. *Vet Rec* 105:404–405, 1979.

26 FELINE VIRAL NEOPLASIA

Feline Leukemia Virus Infection
Susan M. Cotter

ETIOLOGY

Feline leukemia virus (FeLV) is an exogenous retrovirus (previously oncornavirus), 115 nm in diameter, containing a protein core with single-stranded RNA protected by a lipoprotein envelope. Based on similarities in nucleotide sequences, it has been determined that the evolutionary source of the virus was from an ancestor of the rat. Unlike endogenous retroviruses, FeLV is a horizontally transmitted agent and is not transferred by germ cells. The virus replicates within many tissues, including bone marrow, salivary glands, and respiratory epithelium. The virus is noncytopathic and escapes from the cell by budding from the cell membrane (Figs. 26–1 and 26–2). As is characteristic of C-type viruses, nucleocapsid cores are only visible as the virus forms at the cell surface.

Genetic Map and Viral Subgroups

The genetic map of FeLV, similar to that of the murine leukemia viruses, is summarized in Table 26–1. Three virus subgroups have been identified on the basis of interference testing, virus neutralization, and ability to replicate in nonfeline tissues (Table 26–2).[1] All viremic cats carry subgroup A virus, either alone or in combination with subgroup B or C or both. Although subgroup A may cause malignancy by itself, combination with subgroup B may have a synergistic effect on oncogenicity. Group B viruses may have arisen by recombination between FeLV-A and endogenous proviral elements contained in normal cat DNA.[2]

Viral Proteins

Feline viral core proteins are immunogenic, and many infected cats produce antibodies to them; however, these antibodies are not effective in virus neutralization. They share group-specific antigens with other related retroviruses. Core protein is not regularly expressed in the intact virion because it is masked by the presence of the envelope. However, viremic cats rarely have high circulating levels of anti-p27 antibody. Core proteins, especially p27, may be produced in excess within the cell and may be detected by indirect fluorescent antibody (IFA) testing. They may also circulate free in the plasma or be excreted in tears or saliva where they can be detected by ELISA technique.

The major envelope glycoprotein (gp70) varies with the subgroup (A, B, or C) and thus is type-specific rather than group-specific. Antibody to gp70 is also type-specific and results in neutralization of and immunity to reinfection by the specific subgroup of FeLV. Thus, gp70 is important in natural resistance and as a target for vaccine production.

Reverse transcriptase (RT; RNA-dependent DNA polymerase) is an enzyme characteristic of the retrovirus that allows the virus to enter a cell and make a DNA copy, referred to as provirus, which integrates in a stable fashion into the host cell genome (Fig. 26–3).

An antigen designated feline oncornavirus cell membrane antigen (FOCMA) is present on the membrane of malignant cells but absent on all other cells of the body, even those infected with FeLV. Cats with high antibody titers to FOCMA are resistant to

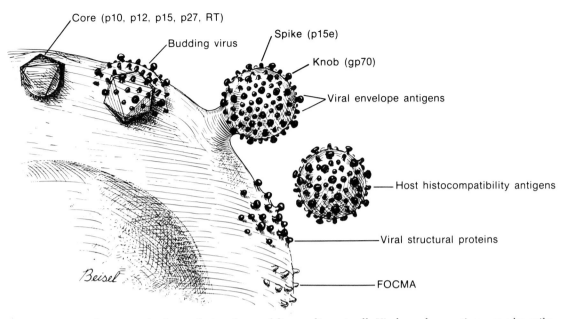

Core (p10, p12, p15, p27, RT)

Budding virus

Spike (p15e)

Knob (gp70)

Viral envelope antigens

Host histocompatibility antigens

Viral structural proteins

FOCMA

Beisel

Figure 26–1. Production and release of virus from a feline malignant cell. Viral envelope antigens can be spike-shaped or knob-shaped. Host histocompatibility antigens may appear on the virus; viral structural proteins may appear on the host cell. Virus replication can also occur in nonmalignant cells, but feline oncornavirus cell membrane antigen (FOCMA) is not on the surface of those cells.

the development of leukemia and lymphoma, regardless of whether they test positive or negative for FeLV. In the presence of complement, FOCMA antibody lyses tumor cells and plays a role in immune surveillance against tumor development. Cats with increased FOCMA antibody titers may be viremic, since FOCMA antibody does not neutralize virus. FOCMA titers may change with time, and immunity may decline in the absence of continued immune stimulation.

FOCMA is apparently a virally coded portion of endogenous FeLV-C gp70, expressed when FeLV integrates in some fashion to activate the latent endogenous sequence.[3]

EPIDEMIOLOGY

FeLV is now considered to be the most prevalent cause of severe illness and death in domestic cats. The virus, which spreads

Figure 26–2. Ultrastructural view of FeLV budding from cell surface *(arrow)*. (Courtesy of Norden Laboratories, Lincoln, NE.)

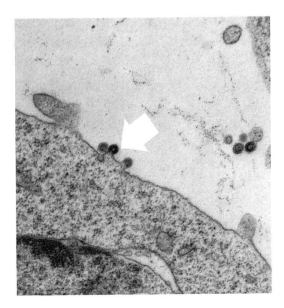

Table 26–1. Summary of Genetic Map and Function of Feline Leukemia Virus Proteins[a]

| GENE | VIRAL PROTEINS | | |
	Location	Type	Function
gag	Core	p15 p12 p27 p10	Basis for IFA and ELISA tests, immune complex disease, and cytotoxic effects
pol	Core	RT	Copies viral protein into complementary DNA strand
env	Envelope	gp70	Type-specific antigens, A,B,C; responsible for neutralizing or protective antibody against viral infection
		p15e	Viral immunosuppression

[a]As listed in chart, genes are located from 5' to 3' end with long terminal repeat sequences at each end. RT = reverse transcriptase.

in a contagious manner among cats, has no sex or breed predisposition. Approximately 33% of all cancer deaths in cats are caused by FeLV. The incidence of feline leukemia and lymphoma has been estimated at 200 cases/100,000 population/year. An even greater number of FeLV-infected cats die of anemia and infectious diseases caused by suppressive effects of the virus on bone marrow and the immune system.

Transmission of FeLV from one cat to another occurs primarily via the saliva, and the concentration of virus in salivary secretions is higher than that in plasma. Large amounts of virus are also present in respiratory secretions. Viremic cats shed virus constantly; the levels of virus in the saliva and blood of healthy viremic cats are just as high as those in viremic cats with leukemia or lymphoma. Urine, feces, and fleas are less likely routes of spread. The virus is maintained in nature because viremic cats may live for several years and because shedding of virus appears to be constant. Close, prolonged, direct contact is required for spread of virus between cats because the virus is unable to survive in the environment for any

extended period. If virus is kept moist and at room temperature, it may survive for as long as 24 to 48 hours.[4] Thus a prolonged waiting period is not needed before introducing a new cat in a household after removal of a viremic one. The viral envelope is lipid-soluble and susceptible to disinfectants, soaps, heating, and drying. It is not a hazard in a veterinary hospital or boarding kennel as long as infected cats and their secretions are not in direct contact with uninfected cats and routine equipment disinfection and hand washing are performed.

PATHOGENESIS

Sequential pathogenesis of FeLV infection has been determined by experimental studies and is summarized in Figure 26–4. The initial infection may be characterized by malaise and lymphadenopathy from lymphocytic hyperplasia. If the immune response does not intervene within several weeks, the virus then spreads to the bone marrow to infect hematopoietic precursor

Table 26–2. Subgroups of Feline Leukemia Virus (FeLV)

VIRUS SUBGROUPS	FREQUENCY OF ISOLATION IN FeLV-POSITIVE CATS	ASSOCIATED DISEASE	COMPARISON BY SPECIES OF IN VITRO REPLICATION
A	100% viremic cats	Hematopoietic neoplasia, experimentally may cause hemolysis	Cat
B	Occurs with subgroup A in approximately 50% of cats with neoplastic disease	Not pathogenic alone, finding with A may indicate chronic viremia	Cat, dog, cow, human
C	Rarely isolated; possibly replication-defective	Nonregenerative anemia	Cat, dog, guinea pig, cow, human

(Data from Jarrett O: Feline leukemia virus subgroups. *In* Hardy WD et al: *Feline Leukemia Virus.* Elsevier, 1980, pp 473–479.)

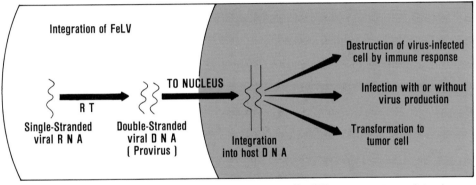

Figure 26–3. Formation of FeLV and integration into cells. (RT = reverse transcriptase).

cells. Most cats probably acquire the virus as kittens, perhaps from the queen since middle-aged viremic cats are sometimes found that have lived indoors in isolation for their entire lives. Even though kittens are most susceptible to infection, adults may become viremic after long-term exposure to FeLV-positive cats, representing either a recent infection or stress-induced reactivation of a previous infection.

Viral Persistence

Cats that are transiently viremic with FeLV may actually develop persistent infec-

tion of the bone marrow while neutralizing antibody prevents viral expression. Virus has been isolated from the marrow of 30% to 60% of a group of experimentally infected cats from 1 to 90 days after recovery from viremia.[5] Whether or not this latent infection develops depends upon whether the viremia was terminated before hematopoietic precursor cells were infected. Once the marrow has been infected, virus could remain integrated in a small number of cells for a long time. Latent infection can be present even though the blood and marrow are negative for virus by IFA, ELISA, or viral infectious assay (Table 26–3). The presence of latent virus can be demonstrated by in vitro culti-

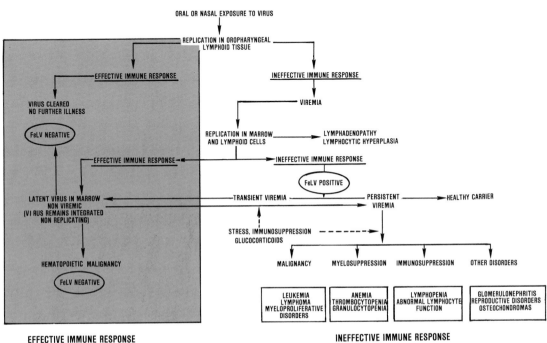

Figure 26–4. Pathogenesis of FeLV infection.

Table 26–3. Classification of FeLV Infection Based upon Viral and Immune Testing[a]

FeLV STATUS	FeLV ANTIGEN TEST RESULTS[b]			VIRUS-POSITIVE BONE MARROW CULTIVATION	ELEVATED SERUM NEUTRALIZING ANTIBODY	ELEVATED SERUM FOCMA ANTIBODY
	Blood ELISA	IFA	Marrow IFA			
Never exposed	−	−	−	−	−	−
Recovered	−	−	−	−	±	±
Latent	−	−	−	+	+	±
Immune carrier	+	−	−	+	+	+
Persistently viremic	+	+	+	+	+	+

[a] + = results positive, − = results negative, ± = results variable.
[b] ELISA = enzyme-linked immunosorbent assay, IFA = immunofluorescent antibody assay.

vation of marrow cells, eliminating the effects of the immune system and allowing virus to grow. These findings help explain relapsing viremias, protracted incubation periods, persistent high titers of antiviral and anti-FOCMA antibodies, and some discrepancies between ELISA and IFA tests. Latent infections may also explain how my-, elodysplasia or hematopoietic malignancy could be FeLV-related in FeLV-negative cats. Latently infected queens have been shown to transmit FeLV to their kittens in the milk[6] and rarely to their kittens in utero. The latent virus was probably activated to produce a transient viremia by the stress of pregnancy.

A small number of virus-producing myeloid and lymphoid cells in the marrow are probably kept in check by the immune response. As the antibody concentration increases, virus production decreases. When the number of virus-producing cells is small, antibody production decreases, permitting proliferation of virus-infected cells. This fluctuation continues, and the cat remains healthy unless the immune response fails to keep up with virus production or until a transformed clone of cells causes a virus-negative tumor. A focal infection of the marrow also may result in viremia if the immune system is suppressed by glucocorticoids or stress (Fig. 26–4). It is not known whether glucocorticoids increase the risk of infection or malignancy in viremic cats, but one might speculate that further immunosuppression of these cats could be detrimental.

Latent infection with FeLV is usually not of clinical significance since the virus is not reactivated in most circumstances. The prevalence of latent infections in transiently viremic cats becomes lower as the time interval since the termination of their viremia becomes longer. Viral latency is probably a

stage in the elimination process of the virus from its feline host. Only 0.05% of experimentally transiently infected cats had long-term detectable latent infections.[5] So long as the infection remains latent, these cats are not contagious.

Cats that mount a partial immune response may suppress FeLV before marrow infection becomes established. These cats are known as immune carriers and have a positive or weakly positive ELISA result and a negative IFA test result (Table 26–3). They are more likely to eliminate the infection than persistently infected cats that test positive for both IFA and ELISA. Immune carrier cats may shed virus in their secretions as a source of infection for other cats.

Environmental Factors

Studies of households with many infected cats have provided information on the immune response of cats to FeLV exposure. The prevalence of leukemia, lymphoma, anemia, FeLV infection, as well as other infectious disease is higher in cats from these households than in the general population. Prospective studies have shown that viremic cats develop FeLV-related disorders much more frequently than do FeLV-negative cats in the same household. Healthy unexposed kittens placed in multicat ("cluster") households become either infected or immune within 5 months of entry. Removal of viremic cats from these households has been effective in preventing further seroconversion. Prospective studies of viremic cats in several households have shown that the death rate of healthy, persistently FeLV-positive cats is approximately 50% in 2 years and 80% in 3 to 5 years, with most of the deaths caused by non-neoplastic disorders.[7] A majority of nonviremic cats in similar circumstances remain alive during the same interval.

Many cats in cluster households have antibody titers to FOCMA, indicating recent exposure to FeLV. Cats with the highest titers against FOCMA are the ones most likely to remain healthy over long periods of time. Correlation between FOCMA antibody and virus-neutralizing antibody titer is not absolute; however, many cats rejecting FeLV have high FOCMA antibody titers as well. Neither FOCMA nor virus-neutralizing antibodies remain protective indefinitely, so these tests have minimal long-term prognostic significance (Table 26–4). In cluster households, some cats that were initially viremic with a high FOCMA antibody titer have been observed to develop leukemia or lymphoma months to years later, after the titer declined.

When virus buds from the cell membrane, some host histocompatibility antigens become incorporated into the viral envelope. These antigens appear to play some role in the natural immune response when this virus enters a new host. These cellular antigens may serve as targets for antibody neutralization of FeLV. Immune-complex inflammatory disorders have been described in viremic cats (e.g., glomerulonephritis, polyarthritis). These are more likely related to antibodies to viral proteins than to histocompatibility antibodies.

Prevalence of Viremia

Approximately 1% to 2% of normal cats are positive for FeLV, but this percentage is higher in crowded catteries or cluster households where infected cats are allowed to roam free. The prevalence of viremic cats in multicat households may be over 50%, particularly if kittens are born or added to the group periodically. Kittens less than 4 months of age are highly susceptible to natural and experimental infection with FeLV.

Approximately 70% of all cats with leukemia or lymphoma are viremic with FeLV. There are several reasons for the absence of viremia in some cases. First, the major difference between viremic and nonviremic cats with leukemia and lymphoma is that cats with FeLV-negative disease are older than the FeLV-positive cats. Most persistently viremic cats have become infected at a young age, remain viremic, and die of hematopoietic malignancy within 3 years, so that few of the persistently viremic cats survive to develop malignancy later. In older cats, FeLV could cause virus-negative tumors by previous infection and transformation of cells with subsequent virus elimination or by sequestration of the virus as in latent infections. Therefore, the great majority of cats that live to develop leukemia or lymphoma over 8 years of age would not be viremic. Second, tumors involving the stomach or intestinal tract are less likely to be associated with replicating virus. Over 90% of feline leukemias and lymphomas are of T cell origin. Most alimentary lymphomas are of B cell origin and are unassociated with virus. Last, certain types of FeLV may be capable of producing cell transformation but are defective and unable to replicate without helper virus, as occurs with feline sarcoma virus (FeSV).

In conclusion, most FeLV-negative malignancy is probably caused by FeLV, even though virus is not detectable. Epidemiologic studies have shown that cats from

Table 26–4. Comparison of Diagnostic Tests Related to Feline Leukemia Virus (FeLV)

TEST	SUBSTANCE DETECTED	SIGNIFICANCE	PROGNOSTIC VALUE OF TEST
FeLV test (IFA, ELISA)	Antigen p30	Detects viremia	Valuable: positive test indicates increased risk of leukemia, lymphoma, marrow suppression, anemia, immunosuppression
FOCMA antibody test	Antibody against malignant cell	Protects against leukemia/lymphoma	Poor: titer can change with time. FeLV-positive cats with positive titers can die of nonmalignant disease
Neutralizing antibody test	Antibody against virus envelope	Protects against viremia	Poor: titer can change with time

IFA = immunofluorescent antibody assay; ELISA = enzyme-linked immunosorbent assay; FOCMA = feline oncornavirus cell membrane antigen.

FeLV-cluster households had a 40-fold higher rate of development of FeLV-negative malignancy than did cats from the general population.[8] Lymphomas have also been FeLV-negative in laboratory cats known to have been infected previously with virus. When FeLV-negative malignant cells are tested for FOCMA, they are uniformly positive, which indicates specific involvement of FeLV or FeSV.

Newer techniques may be needed to demonstrate the existence of hidden retroviruses. Cats with FeLV-negative lymphomas or leukemias have been shown not to be FeLV-infected by standard research methods such as viral isolation from blood, electron microscopy, IFA, and radioimmunoassay. Nucleic acid hybridization, probably the most sensitive means to determine the presence of latent virus, has been done with equivocal results. Some investigators report no evidence of viral nucleic acid sequences, whereas others have found evidence of short sequences in common with part of an FeSV genome. Occasionally, FeLV-negative cats with lymphoma have been found to have latent infections when their marrow was cultured.

Cell Transformation

The mechanism by which FeLV causes malignancy is under study. It may be that when FeLV randomly inserts into the genome of the cat, it sometimes inserts near a cellular oncogene, which is then activated. In some lymphomas, FeLV has incorporated the cellular oncogene c-myc into the virus, resulting in a recombinant virus containing oncogene sequences that are then rearranged and activated.[9]

CLINICAL FINDINGS

Neoplastic Diseases

Any cell of the myeloid, erythroid, lymphoid, or platelet series can be affected in viral-induced transformation with resultant clinical illness depending on the involved cell type.

Lymphoma. Lymphoma is a malignant tumor composed of abnormal lymphocytes at various stages of maturity (Fig. 26–5). Feline

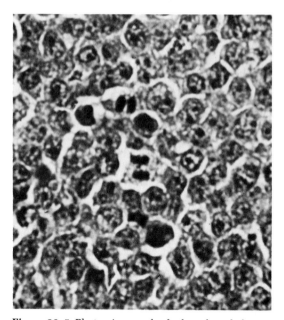

Figure 26–5. Photomicrograph of a lymph node biopsy specimen from a cat with lymphoblastic lymphoma. The architecture of the node has been replaced by a diffuse population of large lymphocytes, many of which contain nucleoli (H and E, × 400).

lymphomas are most commonly lymphoblastic, but they may be mixed lymphoblastic and lymphocytic or histiocytic. No definitive clinical differences between these forms are noted except that lymphocytic lymphoma may occur more frequently in older cats and may progress more slowly. Histiocytic lymphoma, usually a rapidly progressive disease, can arise in extralymphatic sites such as skin and is less likely to involve blood or marrow than is the lymphoblastic form.

Feline lymphoma has been classified by the primary site of involvement.[10] The most frequent form has been mediastinal lymphoma, which arises in the area of the thymus, grows rapidly, and eventually causes a malignant pleural effusion (Fig. 26–6). Cytologic evaluation of this fluid is usually sufficient to confirm the diagnosis (Fig. 26–7). The fluid nucleated cell count is usually over $8000/\mu l$, with the majority of the cells being abnormal lymphocytes. The most frequent presenting sign is dyspnea, but sometimes dysphagia from pressure on the esophagus or Horner's syndrome from pressure on sympathetic nerves is present.

Alimentary lymphoma has been commonly reported in older cats in Europe, but it is less common in the United States. Clinical signs of alimentary lymphoma include

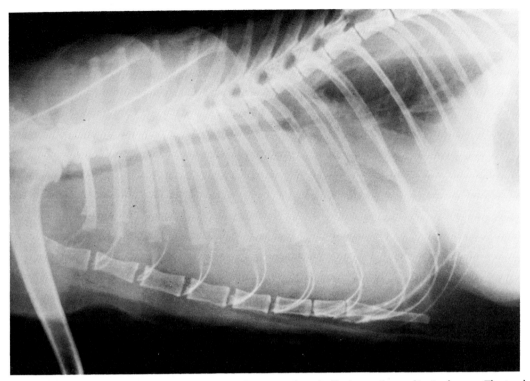

Figure 26–6. Lateral thoracic radiograph of a cat with severe pleural effusion and a mediastinal mass. The trachea is displaced dorsally, and the cardiac shadow is not visualized.

vomiting or diarrhea with weight loss. In cases of mesenteric lymph node involvement, the tumor may grow quite large without signs of illness except for lethargy and weight loss.

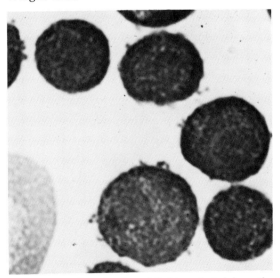

Figure 26–7. Examination of fluid aspirated from the cat in Figure 26–6 showed > 15,000/μl immature lymphocytes. The majority of the cells were lymphoblasts, confirming the diagnosis of lymphoma (Wright's stain, × 1000).

Lymphoma is classified as multicentric if there is major involvement of several sites, such as mediastinal mass and leukemia. Lymphoma can involve any organ such as retrobulbar area, nasal cavity, gingiva, skin, liver, urinary bladder, brain, and lungs. Clinical signs reflect the organ of involvement when the neoplasms become large enough to alter organ function. Renal lymphoma is usually bilateral and does not cause signs of illness until the kidneys are heavily infiltrated and renal failure occurs. Kidneys are enlarged and usually irregular but may be smooth. Epidural lymphoma may cause sudden or gradual onset of posterior paralysis (Fig. 26–8). The bone marrow is involved in about 50% of these cats even though a CBC may be normal. If the marrow is normal, the diagnosis may be confirmed only by myelography and laminectomy.

Although attempts are made to classify leukemias and myeloproliferative disorders, the predominant cell type may be difficult to identify even with cytochemical stains and may vary within a given cat over a period of time. This is more likely to occur among the nonlymphocytic myeloproliferative disorders. This tendency to change or

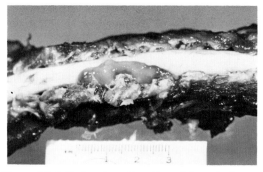

Figure 26–8. Postmortem dissection of the spinal canal reveals a cream-colored gelatinous mass in the epidural space. Histologic findings were diagnostic of lymphoma.

overlap probably indicates that transformation occurs at or very close to the stem cell level, so that several cell lines may be affected.

Leukemias and Myeloproliferative Diseases. All hematopoietic cell lines are susceptible to transformation by FeLV; thus, lymphocytic, myelogenous, erythroid, and megakaryocytic malignancies have all been reported. Clinical signs with acute leukemia of any cell line are related to anemia, sepsis (granulocytopenia), or bleeding (thrombocytopenia).

Lymphoblastic Leukemia. Acute lymphoblastic leukemia is one of the most prevalent forms of lymphoid malignancy. Most cats with leukemia have primary involvement of the bone marrow, usually with some circulating lymphoblasts, although the total lymphocyte count is usually normal or low. Severe lymphocytosis with large numbers of blast cells is seen occasionally. Anemia is generally severe at the time of diagnosis. Infections are common at presentation because of granulocytopenia and immunosuppression associated directly with FeLV or secondary to leukemic invasion of the marrow. Thrombocytopenia is present in some leukemic cats but is less common than in human leukemia. Some have gross lesions of lymphoma in other organs, but most have only microscopic infiltration. Splenomegaly occurs frequently in leukemic cats.

Diagnosis of lymphoblastic leukemia, as with myeloproliferative syndromes, is made by blood count and bone marrow aspiration. In cats with large numbers of circulating lymphoblasts (>50,000 cells/μl), the blood count may in itself be diagnostic. Transient abnormalities in peripheral blood lymphocyte numbers or maturation occur in some cats, especially viremic cats. A diagnosis of leukemia should not be made on the basis of these abnormalities alone, because they may result from antigenic stimulation or from other infections or they may be preleukemic. The diagnosis should be made only when there is marrow infiltration by these cells.

Erythroleukemia. Peripheral blood smears from cats with erythroleukemia often contain large numbers of nucleated erythrocytes of varying degrees of maturity (Fig. 26–9). Evidence of regeneration (reticulocytosis, polychromasia) is absent in spite of the presence of anemia and nucleated erythrocytes. The marrow is infiltrated by erythroid precursors of varying degrees of maturity. Megaloblastic changes in erythrocytes, asynchrony of nuclear and cytoplasmic maturation, and large cells are often seen in blood or marrow of cats with erythroleukemia. The term erythremic myelosis is sometimes used to describe malignancy limited to erythroid cells. Erythroleukemia refers to abnormalities both of erythroid and myeloid cells. Reticuloendotheliosis, an undifferentiated leukemia, may also be of red cell origin. These disorders are probably variations of

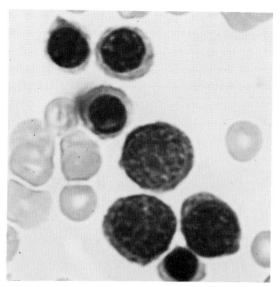

Figure 26–9. Peripheral blood film of a cat with erythroleukemia. At presentation, the cat had severe anemia without reticulocytosis. More than 95% of the circulating nucleated cells were erythroid precursors of varying degrees of maturity. Severe granulocytopenia was noted (Wright's stain, × 1000).

the same condition, and differentiating them has no practical clinical significance.

Myelogenous Leukemia. Acute myelogenous (granulocytic) leukemia is characterized by a proliferation of myeloblasts or promyelocytes or by occasional myelocytes in the marrow and blood. Monocytic or myelomonocytic leukemia occurs in cats and appears morphologically similar to myelogenous leukemia, except that the monocyte nucleus may be characteristically folded or indented.

Eosinophilic leukemia probably exists in cats, but the differentiation between hypereosinophilic syndromes and malignancy is unclear. Some reported cases of eosinophilic leukemia may represent an eosinophilic response to some unrecognized stimulus. Both disorders have been associated with large numbers of morphologically normal eosinophils in the marrow, peripheral blood, and other organs, such as intestine and liver. Neither syndrome responds well to glucocorticoids, as might be expected with an eosinophilia from allergic or parasitic stimuli. Although most cats with eosinophilic leukemia are FeLV-negative, a virally associated case was described in a cat that had been inoculated with FeLV.[11]

Other Myeloproliferative Diseases. Myelofibrosis, classified as a myeloproliferative disease, has been described in viremic cats. This has occurred most frequently in chronically anemic cats and is usually associated with severe extramedullary hematopoiesis (myeloid metaplasia) of the liver and spleen to the point of destroying the normal structure of these organs. Rarely, malignancy of megakaryocytes has been reported in cats with very high blood platelet counts.

Myelodysplasia (dysmyelopoiesis) is a term used to describe a form of marrow failure sometimes seen in viremic cats.[12] These cats have nonregenerative anemia, sometimes with granulocytopenia or thrombocytopenia. Examination of the marrow reveals abnormalities of maturation of one or more cell lines. There may be nuclear or cytoplasmic atypia or asynchronous maturation of the nucleus and cytoplasm with megaloblastosis of erythroid precursors. Abnormal megakaryocytes are sometimes seen. A few cats may have a disproportionate number of lymphoblasts but too few to make a diagnosis of leukemia. This syndrome is

preleukemic in some cats that eventually develop some form of leukemia. Others eventually die of persistent anemia or infection without developing overt malignancy. A few will improve with supportive care.

Two other malignancies that may occur in the marrow or blood of cats but have not been associated with FeLV are mastocytoma and plasma cell myeloma.

Bone Marrow Suppression Syndromes

Anemia secondary to non-neoplastic bone marrow suppression is one of the most frequent disorders caused by FeLV. The reason for the anemia is not well understood, but the virus may affect erythroid precursors at or just beyond the stem cell level. Evidence for stem cell involvement is that leukopenia, thrombocytopenia, or both may accompany the anemia in some viremic cats. In some cats, cyclic hematopoiesis, manifest by periodic fluctuation in reticulocytes, leukocytes, and platelets, may be noted.[13] The pathogenesis could be a block in differentiation of erythroid precursors or an inhibition of the normal effect of helper T cells on erythroid differentiation. Anemic cats infected with FeLV have increased levels of serum erythropoietin but decreased erythropoiesis on ferrokinetic studies and bone marrow culture.[14] In vitro exposure of normal feline marrow to some strains of FeLV caused suppression of erythrogenesis.[15, 16] Just as FeLV is thought to be the cause of 30% of virus-negative leukemias and lymphoma, approximately 30% of cats with nonregenerative anemia are FeLV-negative without another evident cause. FeLV subgroup C has been found in some cats with FeLV-negative anemias (see Table 26–2).[17]

Anemia. Determining the cause of anemia in cats is a common and perplexing problem. When a viremic anemic cat is seen, a reticulocyte count will categorize regenerative and nonregenerative anemias. Either category may have circulating nucleated erythrocytes so that these are not an accurate indication of regenerative anemia. If the anemia is nonregenerative, a bone marrow aspirate will help to rule out leukemia and to determine whether erythroid precursors are present in adequate numbers and whether the maturation of these cells is normal.

Viremic cats usually have nonregenerative anemia; this is called pure red cell aplasia if the leukocyte and platelet counts are normal. The typical hemogram for FeLV-induced red cell aplasia consists of a normochromic normocytic or macrocytic anemia without evidence of reticulocyte response. Whenever macrocytic anemia (MCV > 60) occurs in the cat in the absence of reticulocytosis, FeLV infection should be suspected. These cats are not folate- or B_{12}-depleted, and the macrocytosis may represent skipped mitoses during erythropoiesis.[18] The bone marrow is usually normocellular but may be hypocellular. The myeloid-to-erythroid (M:E) ratio is increased. Occasionally, invasion of the marrow by leukemic cells is found in the presence of a normal peripheral leukocyte count; however, abnormal cells are usually present in the blood if leukemia is present. Anemia in the viremic cat appears to be a distinct syndrome and not a preleukemic manifestation in most cases.

Occasionally, regenerative anemia may occur in FeLV infection, and prognosis for the latter is usually better than for nonregenerative anemia. The primary cause of regenerative anemia in some cats may be related to haemobartonellosis or autoimmune hemolytic anemia (AIHA). The relationship among FeLV, *Haemobartonella felis*, and AIHA may be confusing, and test results may change during the course of the anemia. Haemobartonellosis most frequently occurs secondary to FeLV-induced anemia (also see Chapter 39). There is no evidence for an immune-mediated cause in most FeLV-induced anemias since Coombs' test results are usually negative. Some viremic cats develop anemia following infection or stress. Therefore, these factors should be identified, if possible, since elimination of stress or symptomatic treatment of infection may allow for recovery from the anemia.

Platelet Abnormalities. Thrombocytopenia may occur in viremic cats secondary to decreased platelet production from marrow suppression or leukemic infiltration. The life span of platelets is shortened in some viremic cats.[19] Although the platelet count is low, the mean platelet volume is increased. Some platelets may approach the size of red cells, falsely raising the red cell count as reported by automated cell counters. In some cats, platelet counts may be increased rather than decreased.

Leukocyte Abnormalities. Viremic cats may have reductions in granulocyte or lymphocyte counts. Cats that have recently become infected with FeLV often have lower lymphocyte counts than those that have been chronically viremic. This may correlate with a higher rate of illness in recently infected cats than in chronically infected ones. Cats with granulocytopenia are usually seen because of recurrent or persistent bacterial infections, such as necrotic gingivitis. The usual signs of inflammation such as hyperemia and purulent exudate may not be evident in oral ulcers, since granulocytes are necessary for the inflammatory response.

A condition known as "panleukopenia-like" syndrome consists of leukopenia with hemorrhagic enteritis. However, anemia and thrombocytopenia are often present, in contrast to typical cases of panleukopenia in which acute transient leukopenia is usually the only hematologic abnormality. Although the FeLV-marrow suppressive disorders may be reversible, cats with granulocytopenia, thrombocytopenia, or pancytopenia often die of uncontrolled infection or primarily of GI hemorrhage. A bone marrow aspirate should be examined to rule out aplastic anemia secondary to malignant cells in marrow. An antibody test for feline immunodeficiency virus (FIV, formerly FTLV) infection should be performed on FeLV-negative cats that have these persistent leukopenic syndromes (see FIV Infection, this Chapter).

Immunosuppression

In addition to anemia, the major cause of death in FeLV-positive cats is infection. These cats are predisposed to infection primarily because of virus-induced immunosuppression, which has been associated with the envelope protein p15. Viremic cats with immunosuppressive syndromes have been found to have a high concentration of unintegrated viral DNA in bone marrow cells, presumably from replication-defective viral variants.[19a] This is in contrast to most viremic cats that have a more typical pattern of integration.[20] This situation is similar to that seen in human AIDS patients infected with the human immunodeficiency virus (HIV).

It appears that T cell function is most disrupted by the presence of FeLV. Decreased rejection of skin grafts, reduced lymphocyte transformation response, and increased suppressor cell activity have been observed in viremic cats. Interleukin-2 suppression has also been found.[20a] Humoral antibody response, both primary and secondary, to specific antigens is delayed and reduced in viremic cats.[21] At the same time, more nonspecific increases of IgG and IgM have been noted in viremic cats than in controls. It is possible that the impaired humoral antibody response was caused by decreased helper T cell function.

In addition to immunosuppression, granulocytopenia is frequently present, increasing the risk of bacterial infections. Granulocytes of viremic cats also have decreased chemotactic and phagocytic function when compared with normal cats.[22, 23] Cats that are transiently viremic continue to have depressed neutrophil function for an unknown period of time after cessation of viremia.

Infections in viremic cats include those that are bacterial (stomatitis, abscesses, pyothorax), rickettsial (haemobartonellosis), viral (feline infectious peritonitis, upper respiratory infection), protozoal (toxoplasmosis), and fungal (aspergillosis and cryptococcosis). Some infections in viremic cats can be treated successfully with aggressive specific and supportive care.

Other Syndromes Associated with FeLV

Cats infected with FeLV develop other disorders in addition to malignancy, myelosuppression, and immunosuppression.

Immune-Complex Diseases. Viremic cats have increased circulating immune complexes. These have been observed after experimental treatment of persistent viremia with monoclonal antibodies to gp70, and in studies of inoculation of complement-depleting factors.[24, 25] Immune complexes predispose to such diseases as glomerulonephritis and polyarthritis. Immune-complex glomerulonephritis may cause clinical or subclinical renal disease. Measurement of FeLV antigens has shown that cats with glomerulonephritis have more circulating viral proteins that do other viremic cats. Some cats with glomerulonephritis have circulating antibody to FeLV but are not viremic. The immune complexes may have

developed during previous viremia or latent infection.

Reproductive Disorders. Reproductive disorders associated with FeLV are infertility in female cats, resorption or abortion of fetuses, and endometritis. The apparent infertility might actually be early absorption of fetuses. Abortions usually occur late in gestation, with expulsion of normal-appearing fetuses. Bacterial endometritis has sometimes accompanied these abortions, particularly in cats with leukopenia. Kittens born to an infected queen may become exposed to virus transplacentally, but heavy exposure also occurs at birth and throughout the nursing period. Some kittens become immune and are uninfected, but most become viremic and die at an early age of "fading kitten syndrome." This poorly defined syndrome consists of failure to nurse, dehydration, hypothermia, and death within the first 2 weeks of life. In addition, young viremic kittens develop thymic atrophy, which is associated with reduced T cell function.

Lymphadenopathy. Some FeLV-positive cats, especially younger cats, have peripheral lymphadenopathy, usually most severe in submandibular nodes. This syndrome may be asymptomatic or associated with fever and anorexia. In a few cats, a biopsy is diagnostic of lymphoma, but the majority are classified as lymphocytic hyperplasia. Cultures of hyperplastic nodes are negative for bacteria. Whether this lesion is a response to FeLV or to some as yet undetermined antigenic stimulus is unknown. Kittens experimentally infected with FeLV have been reported to develop transient lymphadenopathy. A few naturally infected cats with FeLV-associated lymph node hyperplasia subsequently developed lymphoma, but in most the nodes stay the same or decrease in size. In some young cats, a distinctive form of lymphadenopathy occurs with severe hyperplasia of lymphocytes, plasma cells, and immunoblasts to the point of destroying the architecture of the node.[26] This form may be confused with lymphoma cytologically or histologically. Therapy for lymphocytic hyperplasia is not indicated unless the nodes are so large that they interfere with swallowing. In this situation, anti-inflammatory dosages of glucocorticoids might be helpful in reducing the size of the nodes. With minimal clinical signs, glucocorticoids should not be used as they may interfere with an ongoing immune response.

Enteritis. A form of enteritis with intestinal lesions histologically identical to those seen in panleukopenia has been described in cats infected with FeLV but not with feline panleukopenia virus (FPV).[27] The disease is distinguished by the absence of lesions in lymph nodes or marrow as seen in FPV infection. The FeLV-induced enteritis is separate from the previously described panleukopenia-like syndrome of FeLV, which is characterized primarily by pancytopenia with secondary diarrhea. In the FeLV enteritis syndrome, vomiting and diarrhea have been the most frequent clinical signs.

Other Syndromes. Other syndromes associated with FeLV infection include osteochondromas and osteopetrosis,[28] and ocular lesions (see Chapter 13). Polyarthritis has developed in FeLV-positive cats that were also infected with feline syncytium-forming virus (see Chapter 28).

DIAGNOSIS OF FeLV INFECTION

Principles of performing and understanding IFA and ELISA techniques are discussed in Chapter 14. These tests, used clinically to detect FeLV infection, measure the presence of viral antigen. A positive blood test result for FeLV is not diagnostic of leukemia, lymphoma, or any other disease. It merely means that the cat is viremic, not that the virus is necessarily responsible for the illness. Some non-neoplastic disorders such as anemias result directly from suppression of the marrow, but the immunosuppressive nature of the virus also predisposes cats to many other infectious diseases. Thus, the test for FeLV is a presumptive immune function test, and a positive finding carries adverse prognostic significance in cats with secondary infections.

Both IFA and ELISA techniques measure the presence of viral core antigen and are specific for circulating FeLV (see Table 26-3). The ELISA test is somewhat more sensitive than the IFA test, but some false-positive ELISA results have occurred from technical errors. If both are performed properly, there is a good correlation between the two tests.[29] In experimental FeLV infection, cats become positive by ELISA before they are positive by IFA. Cats with transient infections become negative by IFA before they are negative by ELISA. Either test is useful clinically, but cats that have a positive result only on ELISA (immune carriers) have a greater chance of converting to a negative result than those cats with positive results on both tests. The small number of cats with test results that are persistently ELISA-positive and IFA-negative may have focal infections that are kept localized by the immune system (see Immune Carrier, Table 26-3).

Tests are also available to evaluate tears and saliva for FeLV.[30] These are subject to more technical errors or false-negative results in approximately 30% of viremic cats and must be used cautiously. Appendix 8 lists laboratories that perform FeLV tests as well as commercially available test kits.

THERAPY

Principles of management of specific FeLV-related immunosuppressive disorders have been discussed elsewhere in this text. Only treatment of myelosuppressive and neoplastic diseases is briefly covered here.

Lymphoma

Untreated feline lymphoproliferative malignancy is usually fatal within 1 to 2 months. Many cats can be helped transiently with chemotherapy, and a few will have remissions that may last several years. Assuming the cat is not severely debilitated and has a normal bone marrow, the prognosis for complete remission of lymphoma is approximately 75%, with a median duration of remission of 5 months and a 20% chance of still being in remission after 1 year.

Before treatment is considered, the diagnosis of lymphoma must be confirmed. A positive result on a blood test for FeLV alone does not constitute a positive diagnosis. Confirmation is made by identifying neoplastic cells, using histologic or cytologic methods.

Once the diagnosis is confirmed, the condition of the cat must be evaluated to determine whether there is a reasonable chance for sustained remission (Table 26-5). Options for treatment include glucocorticoids or combination chemotherapy. The best

Table 26–5. Prognostic Indicators in Feline Lymphoma

GOOD PROGNOSTIC INDICATORS
Small tumor burden
Peripheral lymph nodes as primary site
Lack of involvement of major organs
Normal or near-normal complete blood count,
    urinalysis, and blood chemistry profile

ADVERSE PROGNOSTIC INDICATORS
Anemia, granulocytopenia, or thrombocytopenia
Leukemic infiltration of the marrow
Major organ involvement with dysfunction (e.g.,
    renal lymphoma with azotemia)
Spinal lymphoma with complete paralysis of more
    than 24 hours' duration
Fever, sepsis, or focal infection (e.g., stomatitis or
    chronic respiratory infection)
Large tumor burden
Skin involvement
Severe debility or emaciation

FACTORS THAT DO NOT APPEAR TO AFFECT PROGNOSIS
FeLV status
Age
Form of lymphoma (i.e., lymphoblastic vs.
    histiocytic); histiocytic lymphoma has been a
    more aggressive human disease but data in dogs
    and cats are lacking

ties, and excretion of these drugs in cats are available.[31, 32]

All these drugs are immunosuppressive, so the owner must be instructed to watch for signs of illness and take the animal's temperature if such signs occur, because fever may be the only sign of an infection that may be otherwise difficult to localize. Infections must be treated quickly and aggressively, especially if they occur at the time of the granulocyte nadir.

In the absence of complications, dosages of drugs must not be decreased nor intervals between treatments lengthened since either would increase the risk of relapse. The rate of relapse becomes less after 1 year of complete remission so therapy may be stopped at that time. Some cats can be expected to relapse after stopping therapy, so owner awareness and periodic checkups are important.

Lymphoblastic Leukemia

Cats with lymphoblastic leukemia are difficult to treat because the bone marrow becomes filled with neoplastic cells. Leukemic cats are usually anemic, granulocytopenic, and sometimes thrombocytopenic. They may also be septic from FeLV-associated immunosuppression and granulocytopenia. The bone marrow first must be cleared of lymphoblasts if remission is to be attained with chemotherapy, and then the normal myeloid and erythroid precursors must regenerate. This may take 3 to 4 weeks, so granulocytopenia and anemia may not be immediately reversible. Prophylactic antibiotics are not used routinely in the treatment of feline leukemia or lymphoma. Bactericidal antibiotics should be given if fever or other signs of infection occur, especially at the time of the nadir of the leukocyte count.

Myeloproliferative Diseases

Nonlymphocytic leukemia, which appears to be a stem cell disorder, is even more

prognosis is with a combination of drugs—each effective by itself—without overlapping toxicities. Single-agent glucocorticoids are minimally effective and should be considered as palliative therapy only after clients have been informed about combination chemotherapy and have rejected this option.

Drugs most frequently utilized in combination include cyclophosphamide (Cytoxan, CTX, Bristol-Myers, Syracuse, NY), vincristine (Oncovin, Eli Lilly, Indianapolis, IN), and prednisone (the combination is abbreviated as COP) (Table 26–6). These drugs have sometimes been combined with cytosine arabinoside (Cytosar, Upjohn, Kalamazoo, MI) and less commonly with doxorubicin hydrochloride (Adriamycin, Adria Laboratories, Dublin, OH), L-asparaginase (Elspar, Merck, Sharp & Dohme, Rahway, NJ), or methotrexate (Methotrexate, Lederle, Wayne, NJ). Detailed descriptions of dosages, efficacy, mechanism of action, toxici-

Table 26–6. Therapy Protocol for Feline Lymphoma

DRUG	WEEK OF THERAPY															
	1	2	3	4	5	6	7	8	9	10	11	12	13	14	15	16
Cyclophosphamide	x			x			x			x			x			x[a]
Vincristine	x	x	x	x			x			x			x			x[a]
Prednisone	Give daily for 1 year or until relapse															

[a]Continue every 3 weeks for 1 year or until relapse.

refractory to treatment than is lymphoblastic leukemia. Included in the nonlymphocytic class are erythroleukemia and myelogenous or myelomonocytic leukemia, all of which respond poorly or not at all to COP therapy.

Treatment of Myelosuppressive Disease

Blood transfusion is the most important part of treatment of nonregenerative anemia. Most cats that respond will do so after the first transfusion. If the packed cell volume (PCV) decreases again, further transfusions are unlikely to be of more than palliative benefit. Of 29 FeLV-positive cats with PCVs less than 20% that were followed for more than 2 weeks, eight cats showed a return to a normal PCV. One cat converted to FeLV-negative test status.[33]

Use of oxymetholone or other testosterone derivatives has been advocated, but objective data are not available to show their efficacy (Table 26–7). Glucocorticoids such as prednisone may increase the life span of erythrocytes and may increase erythrocyte production, especially if any component of FeLV-related anemia is immune mediated. Coombs' positive hemolytic anemia, reported in some viremic cats, may be related to anti-FeLV antibodies on erythrocytes. Any immune-mediated hemolysis related to FeLV is a minor component of FeLV anemia, so glucocorticoids are only occasionally effective clinically.[34] Before glucocorticoid therapy is considered, underlying infection must be ruled out. Anemic cats with treatable infections have the best prognosis because any infection or chronic disease may inhibit hematopoiesis and shorten red cell life span. Since deficiencies of iron, folate, or vitamin B_{12} are rare, replacement therapy is not likely to be helpful. A blood transfusion supplies at least 0.5 mg of iron per ml of blood, so that iron overload and hemosiderosis may occur in a cat that has received multiple transfusions.

Management of the Healthy FeLV-Positive Cat

Most cats persistently infected with FeLV acquired the infection as kittens, although cats exposed as adults may also become infected. Studies in cluster households have shown that neither virus-neutralizing nor FOCMA antibody titers are lifelong, so that a previously immune cat may become viremic or develop malignancy if immunity declines. The viremic cat may remain healthy, but it is highly susceptible to malignancy, anemia, leukopenia, or infections. When a viremic cat is identified, the owner must be informed of the potential danger to other cats in the house. These healthy viremic cats carry and shed just as much virus as do cats with malignancies. A healthy viremic cat should not be removed from the household for the protection of the other cats unless all are tested to be sure that additional carriers are not present. Virus-negative, latently infected cats with leukemia or lymphoma are of no danger to other cats. Because it is almost impossible to separate positive from negative cats within a household, the owner should consider maintaining the status quo or eliminating all viremic cats. In the case of catteries, carriers

Table 26–7. Drug Therapy for Feline Leukemia Virus Infection[a]

DRUG	DOSE[b] (mg/kg)	ROUTE	INTERVAL (hr)	DURATION
Lymphoma				
Cyclophosphamide	300 mg/m²	PO	c	c
Vincristine	0.75 mg/m²	IV	c	c
Prednisolone	2.2	PO	c	c
Diazepam	0.2	IV	d	d
Myelosuppressive Disease				
Prednisolone	2	PO	24	prn
Interferon	0.5–1 U total	PO	24	prn[e]

[a]PO = orally, IV = intravenously, prn = as needed, U = units.
[b]Dose per administration at specified interval, expressed as mg/kg unless otherwise stated.
[c]See also Table 26–6.
[d]Use as needed for appetite stimulation just prior to feeding.
[e]See also Table 15–1.

should be eliminated, since the virus will spread to new cats or kittens. A test-and-removal program is effective in eliminating FeLV from a cattery or household. The testing is repeated in 3 months and any newly infected cats removed. This is continued until all cats test negative.

In a household with a few pet cats, an owner may elect to keep all the cats. The risk of infection in adult FeLV-negative cats is approximately 10% to 15% if they have lived with a viremic cat for more than several months. In this situation, the viremic cats must be kept indoors, not only to protect other cats but also to protect the vulnerable viremic cats from respiratory infections, bite wounds, or other dangers of the outside world. If the household is closed to new animals and viremic cats are kept indoors, the infection will eventually subside, although several years may be required. Viremic cats tend to die before uninfected cats, so that eventually the owner is left with immune, uninfected cats. This may be a reasonable alternative to euthanasia for viremic cats, since some can live a normal life span in a protected environment.

The status of healthy viremic cats should be monitored periodically. A repeat test for FeLV can be done yearly at the time of vaccination. MLV vaccines against panleukopenia and feline upper respiratory viruses can be safely used in viremic cats. MLV rabies vaccines should be avoided because of increased risk of vaccine-induced disease in these immunosuppressed cats.[35] There is no benefit to vaccinating viremic cats against leukemia.

Any illness that develops must be diagnosed and treated as would the same infection in a FeLV-negative cat. Elective surgery such as neutering has occasionally preceded episodes of illness; however, the risk-to-benefit ratio must be considered, and most viremic healthy cats can be neutered without complication. If hospitalization is necessary, the viremic cat should be isolated if possible, primarily for its own protection. Under no circumstances should it be placed in a "contagious ward" with cats suffering from infections such as viral respiratory disease. These cats can be hospitalized in well-marked cages that are not adjacent to other cats. Care should be taken to avoid spread of infection from cats with proper hygienic measures (see Chapter 1).

FeLV by itself does not cause fever, so a search for a concurrent infection must be made in febrile cats. Bacterial infections, such as bite wounds or stomatitis, should be treated aggressively with bactericidal antibiotics. Fevers of unknown origin that are unresponsive to antibiotics may have a viral, protozoal, or fungal origin (see Chapter 4). A work-up for occult infection should include a CBC, thoracic radiography, total serum protein determination, serum chemistry profile, and urinalysis. If a cause is still not evident, blood cultures and serologic testing for FIV, feline infectious peritonitis virus, and *Toxoplasma* may be indicated. Neutropenia secondary to FeLV suppression of the marrow may be the reason for difficulties in eliminating bacterial infections.

Glucocorticoids should be avoided if possible in viremic cats. Although indicated in therapy of lymphoproliferative malignancy, some anemias, and some allergic disorders, glucocorticoids increase the degree of immunosuppression. However, glucocorticoids have been shown to increase neutrophil counts in some cats with FeLV-induced neutropenia.[36] Glucocorticoids also interfere with granulocyte chemotaxis, phagocytosis, and the killing of bacteria, thus compounding the risk of infection. In addition, glucocorticoids may be dangerous in healthy FeLV-negative cats in contact with viremic cats because of the increased risk of infection with FeLV.

PREVENTION

Most cats naturally exposed to FeLV produce antibodies to the major envelope protein gp70 as well as to FOCMA. For the purpose of vaccine production, the emphasis has been to produce immunity against the virus since viremic cats with FOCMA antibody titers shed infectious virus and are still susceptible to non-neoplastic FeLV disorders. Early inactivated pure virus vaccines have not proved effective because of an immunosuppressive protein (p15e) of FeLV. Live virus vaccine is capable of producing better immunity but is not practical. Vaccine virus integrates into the genome and may later cause FeLV-negative lymphomas. The virus could possibly revert to a virulent form, particularly in kittens that may develop clinical disease from "attenuated" FeLV.

A vaccine, Leukocell (Norden Laboratories, Lincoln, NE), produced from a cell line derived from a virus-producing feline lymphoma, has been commercially available since 1985. Three vaccines in a series have been recommended. This vaccine contains both viral and cellular antigens treated to assure that no live virus is present and an adjuvant has been added.[37] A modified vaccine, Leukocell 2, has replaced Leukocell, and two vaccines are recommended in a series. Another vaccine, Covenant (Diamond Scientific, Des Moines, IA) was licensed in 1988. It is a whole-virion vaccine prepared by propagation of FeLV in a nontransformed, chronically infected feline cell line. Despite the fact that the vaccine contains intact p15e, it does not appear to be immunosuppressive.[38] It is similarly inactivated, and an adjuvant has been added.[38] Two vaccines have been recommended in a series. FeLV vaccines show some efficacy in preventing FeLV infection, although challenge studies have been difficult without concurrent immunosuppression because of the natural resistance of cats to experimental infection. Challenge studies for both vaccines are available for only 2 weeks following completion of the vaccination series.

Leukocell has appeared to be less effective and to cause more adverse reactions than other presently available vaccines against feline diseases such as panleukopenia or rabies. It has been reported that 64% of previously unexposed cats developed antibodies after completing the recommended series of vaccinations.[39] Recently a controlled study showed no benefit of two vaccinations for kittens introduced into a colony containing infected cats.[40] Adverse reactions consisting primarily of local pain and fever are relatively common, but anaphylactic deaths have occurred.[41] The prevalence of these reactions has decreased with SC administration.[41a] Testing is recommended before vaccination so that only negative cats are vaccinated. Vaccine should be used for cats likely to be exposed to FeLV.

The manufacturer of Covenant claims that 100% of vaccinated cats in some of their efficacy studies remained protected, whereas persistent viremia and death occurred in 85% of some unvaccinated control cats. Anaphylaxis has been known to occur with this vaccine. Further evaluation of the product will be needed before recommendations can be made (see Feline Leukemia Virus Infection, Efficacy of Vaccines, Chapter 2).

Effective retroviral vaccines are especially difficult to produce. Experimental work continues to find a highly effective and safe vaccine. Recombinant DNA techniques are being tried to produce an envelope (gp70) protein vaccine that will protect against the spectrum of strains of virus and will be immunogenic. One such vaccine is commercially licensed in Europe (Laboratoires Virbac, Nice, France). For a further discussion of FeLV vaccination, see Feline Vaccination Recommendations, Feline Leukemia Virus Infection, Chapter 2.

ANTIVIRAL TREATMENT

Presently, there is no effective antiretroviral treatment. Because the virus integrates into the genome, it is not easily eliminated from the body. Because of similarities of FeLV infection in the cat to HIV infection in people, there has been a major emphasis on research in this area.

Antibody therapy has been used in an attempt to rid viremic cats of virus. Antibodies were derived from immune cats or were developed as murine monoclonal antibodies to epitopes of the gp70 molecule.[24, 42–45] Antibodies have been successful only in experimentally infected cats and only when given within 3 weeks of the time of infection. Naturally infected cats showed no response even though the monoclonal antibodies persisted longer in viremic cats than in normal controls. Viremic cats also developed residual circulating immune complexes that could cause adverse reactions.[24]

Attempts to stimulate the immune response against the virus have been made with interferon, indomethacin, diethylcarbamazine, levamisole, *Corynebacterium parvum* (*Propionibacterium acnes*). No significant clinical benefit has been shown. Some transient responses to extracorporeal staphylococcal protein A therapy have been seen.[46, 47] Interferon therapy (human interferon alpha; see Interferons, Chapter 15) has proved beneficial in preventing disease development when given prophylactically to experimentally infected FeLV-positive cats.[48]

RT inhibitors such as Suramin (available from The Centers for Disease Control, Atlanta, GA) and AZT (Retrovir, Burroughs Wellcome, Research Triangle Park, NC) will transiently decrease viral replication but not eliminate the virus (see Table 15–1 for dosages).[49] For an agent to be effective in treatment of a retroviral infection it must inhibit viral replication and allow for recovery of the immune system. Lifelong treatment may be required, and thus the agent should be effective when given orally and should be relatively nontoxic and inexpensive. So far, no such agent has been found.

PUBLIC HEALTH CONSIDERATIONS

Because FeLV is known to be spread in a contagious manner, concern arose about the possible danger of FeLV to people. A number of facts would tend to suggest that human infection might occur. The virus will grow in human cells in culture.[50] Lymphoma has been experimentally induced by injection of large doses of virus into neonatal pups and marmosets.[51] One epidemiologic study linked prior contact with sick cats to subsequent development of childhood leukemia.[52] Cell-bound antibody believed to be directed towards FeLV-RT has been found on malignant cells of people with chronic myelogenous leukemia in blast crisis.[53] Veterinarians were shown to have a higher death rate from leukemia than a control population of physicians and dentists.[54]

However, serologic studies looking for FeLV or antibody to any of its components in people have been confusing and inconclusive. Some investigators have found antibodies to FeLV in human leukemia patients and owners of FeLV-positive cats, while others using more sensitive radioimmunoassays have obtained negative results. No person has ever been found to be viremic with FeLV. One explanation for the discrepancy between culture of the virus in human cells and the absence of proof of human infection may relate to the lytic action of human complement on the virus. Complement is not active in tissue culture; thus the virus only grows in human cells in vitro. The fact remains that no case of human leukemia has ever been traced to FeLV.

Leukemia viruses have been described in birds, rodents, cattle, primates, and man. Each virus is distinct and does not cross species lines except for evolutionary similarities. Although it is impossible to prove a negative hypothesis, it appears that FeLV is not a human health hazard.

Feline Sarcoma Virus Infection

Susan M. Cotter

ETIOLOGY

Feline sarcoma virus (FeSV) is the cause of multicentric fibrosarcoma in young cats. Several strains of FeSV have been identified from naturally occurring tumors, and all are defective; that is, they are unable to replicate without the presence of FeLV as a helper virus. The helper virus supplies proteins (as those coded by the *env* gene) to FeSV through a process of genetic recombination. The sarcoma viruses contain a cellular gene not present in FeLV, which is referred to as the feline endogenous sequences (*fes*) in Snyder-Theilen and Gardner-Arnstein (GA) strains of virus and feline McDonough sequences (*fms*) in the McDonough virus.[55] These cat cellular oncogene sequences are distinct from the genome of any endogenous viruses. The acute transforming viruses such as FeSV may have evolved from recombination between FeLV and cellular oncogenes, which then allows transformation to occur. The host range for FeSV is dependent upon the helper FeLV. By manipulation of the helper virus in the laboratory, FeSV can enter cells not naturally infected. Experimental inoculation of FeSV has produced tumors in cats, rabbits, dogs, sheep, rats, and nonhuman primates.[56] Many of these tumors regressed spontaneously, even after reaching a large size.

PATHOGENESIS

Fibrosarcoma cells express FOCMA just as lymphoma cells do. Experimental infection with FeSV causes progressive tumors in some cats and none or regressing ones in others. The latter group produces high FOCMA antibody titers. In addition to fibrosarcomas, FeSV (GA) has been experimentally incriminated as a cause of melanomas, showing that FeSV can transform cells of ectodermal as well as of mesodermal origin.[57] Intradermal or intraocular inoculation of the virus into kittens produces melanomas in the skin or anterior chamber of the eye. Similar tumors were produced subcutaneously by local injection of the same strain of virus. So far FeSV has not been associated with naturally occurring melanomas of cats.

CLINICAL FINDINGS

Fibrosarcomas caused by various strains of FeSV tend to be rapidly growing, often with multiple cutaneous or subcutaneous nodules that are locally invasive and metastasize to the lung and other sites. A different syndrome has been observed in old cats with solitary fibrosarcomas apparently not caused by or associated with FeSV or FeLV. These tumors are often slower growing, locally invasive, slow to metastasize, and sometimes curable by excision. In both forms, the skin is usually attached to the mass, and sometimes ulceration occurs.

THERAPY

Treatment of fibrosarcoma is surgical removal if the tumor has not grown too large. Neither chemotherapy nor immunotherapy has proved successful to date, but some responses have occurred with irradiation, sometimes combined with local hyperthermia. Experimentally induced fibrosarcomas in kittens sometimes regress after treatment with anti-FOCMA serum. However, this has not proved true in limited numbers of cats with naturally occurring tumors.

RD114 Infection
Susan M. Cotter

RD114 is an endogenous xenotropic retrovirus, that is present but not replicating in every feline cell. Although there is no evidence of pathogenicity or of any immune response to the virus in cats, the virus may play some role in normal fetal differentiation. The RD114 virus is most closely related to an endogenous baboon retrovirus and only distantly related to FeLV.[58]

Feline Immunodeficiency Virus Infection
E. Elizabeth Sparger

ETIOLOGY

A novel feline retrovirus, isolated in 1986 from ill domestic cats housed within a northern California cattery[59] was initially called the feline T lymphotropic virus (FTLV) because of its isolation from peripheral blood lymphocytes (PBL) from infected cats and its apparent tropism for feline T lymphocytes in vitro. FTLV has since been renamed feline immunodeficiency virus (FIV) because of clinical studies that confirmed the association of FIV infection with acquired immune deficiency states in domestic cats.[60]

Ultrastructural morphology of FIV viral particles, biochemical characteristics of its reverse transcriptase, and nucleotide sequence of its RNA genome support the classification of FIV as a member of the lentivirus subfamily of retroviruses (Fig. 26–10).[59, 61] These same criteria clearly distinguish FIV from FeLV, a member of the oncornavirus subfamily of retroviruses and the feline syncytium-forming virus (FeSFV), a member of the spumavirus subfamily of retroviruses.[62] Other members of the lentivirus subfamily include the ovine lentivirus, Maedi visna virus; caprine arthritis encephalitis virus; equine infectious anemia virus; bovine immunodeficiency-like virus; simian

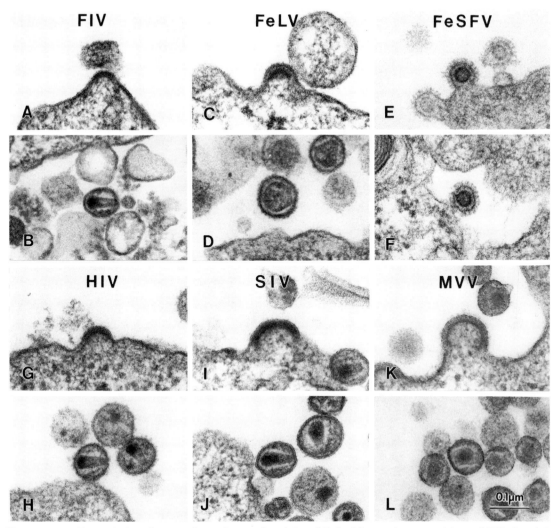

FIV

FeLV

FeSFV

HIV

SIV

MVV

Figure 26–10. Transmission electron photomicrographs of *A* and *B*, budding and mature virions of FIV; *C* and *D*, FeLV; *E* and *F*, FeSFV; *G* and *H*, HIV-1; *I* and *J*, SIV (simian immunodeficiency virus); and *L* and *K*, MVV (Maedi visna virus). (Uranyl acetate and lead citrate stain) (Yamamoto JK et al: *Am J Vet Res* 49:1246–1262, 1988, Reprinted with permission.)

immunodeficiency virus; and the human immune deficiency virus (HIV), the causative agent of AIDS in people.

Lentivirus infections in general have a prolonged nonsymptomatic period of latent infection followed by a period of clinical disease. Clinical disorders commonly associated with lentivirus infections include encephalopathies, pneumonitis, rheumatoid-like arthritis, lymphoproliferative disorders, immune-complex disease with anemia, chronic wasting diseases, and immunodeficiency states.[63] Although cross reactivity between FIV proteins and equine infectious anemia virus proteins has been observed, the clinical disease associated with FIV in-

fection most closely resembles that reported in HIV-infected people suffering AIDS.[64]

FIV has a genome 9.5 of Kd with a gag-pol-env structure as in other retroviruses.[61] The nucleotide sequence of the FIV genome is currently being characterized for additional viral genes that have been identified in other lentiviruses. The sizes of FIV proteins are very similar to the sizes of HIV and other lentiviruses (Table 26–8).

Antigenic variation of the envelope protein among various virus isolates has been well documented for HIV and for other lentiviruses.[63] In fact, antigenic variation exists in isolates from the same host. Preliminary evidence suggests this same phenomenon

Table 26–8. Sizes and Structural Proteins of Human Immunodeficiency Virus (HIV-1) and Feline Immunodeficiency Virus (FIV)[60, 64]

PROTEIN DESIGNATION	SIZE OF PROTEIN (KILODALTONS)	
	HIV-1	FIV
Major envelope	160/120	130/110
Gag precursor	55	47–52
Reverse transcriptase	51/66	54/62?
Transmembrane	41	40–44
Endonuclease	31	32?
Major gag	24	26–28
Small gag	17	15–17
Small gag	10	10

occurs with FIV isolates from different infected cats but has not been evaluated with isolates from the same cat.[65, 66]

EPIDEMIOLOGY

Current knowlege of the epidemiology of FIV infection is based on one study involving over 2765 cats in the United States and Canada[67] and another involving 3323 cats in Japan.[68] Additional reports from the United States,[68a, 68b] the United Kingdom,[68c] and the Netherlands and the Federal Republic of Germany[68d] have corroborated the findings of these two studies. The findings from each study were in general somewhat similar, although neither involved randomly selected cats, and the bias for selection differed in each. Approximately 50% of the Japanese cats evaluated were clinically ill, whereas the remaining cats were healthy. The overall prevalence of infection (seropositivity) rate of Japanese cats including ill and healthy cats was 28.9%, with a prevalence in ill cats of 43.9% and in healthy cats of 12.4%. Approximately 89% of the cats in the United States study were either ill or in a high-risk group for infection, whereas 11% were healthy and were considered in a low-risk group; 14% of the ill, or high-risk, and 1.2% of the healthy, or low-risk, group cats were seropositive. The greater density of free-roaming unneutered cats in Japan may at least partially account for the differing prevalence of infection in the two studies.

Both studies confirmed that the outdoor free-roaming male cats were at greatest risk for FIV infection; the infection rate was two to three times higher in males versus females; and the average age of a FIV-positive cat was 5 to 6 years. Domestic cats versus purebred cats had the highest prevalence of infection. The prevalence of infection in catteries is unknown.

Based on experimental inoculation studies, a major mode of transmission of natural FIV infection appears to be inoculation by bite wound. Healthy cats housed continuously for up to 2 years with experimentally specific pathogen–free (SPF) cats and bred with infected cats have remained seronegative for FIV and virus negative. These cats have remained in a pathogen-free environment and have experienced little or no fighting among themselves. These findings suggest that neither close physical contact nor sexual contact alone are effective modes of transmission. FIV infection was successfully transmitted to healthy cats from naturally infected cats via experimentally induced bite wounds.[69] On the other hand, in the index cattery over a period of a year, two cats seroconverted within a pen housing both seropositive and seronegative cats.[59] Fighting among the cats within this pen may have occurred, since some cats were originally stray and feral cats; however, close contact plus other unidentified factors, such as stage of infection, presence of secondary infectious agents, environmental and genetic factors, and trauma, may also have resulted in transmission of infection.

Three experimentally infected queens have given birth to virus-negative kittens that remained virus-negative despite nursing the infected queens.[60] Virus recovery from infected queens so far has been unsuccessful. The findings from a naturally infected queen were the same. Although preliminary, these findings suggest that in utero and nursing are not effective modes of transmission. Long-term studies of multiple cat households will be necessary to fully understand transmission of FIV infection.

FIV and FeLV infections were not directly associated, since the prevalence (12% to 16%) of FeLV infection in FIV-infected (seropositive) cats was similar to that in FIV-seronegative cats. Those cats infected with both FeLV and FIV were slightly younger and had a shorter life span than cats infected with either virus. The prevalence of FeSFV infection correlated with that of FIV infection. FIV infection was found in 74% of FeSFV-infected cats, whereas only 37% of FeSFV-noninfected cats were FIV-positive. This association of FIV and FeSFV infections in cats may be due to transmission by bite wound. This coinfection of FeSFV in FIV-positive cats significantly complicates FIV isolation, since both viruses latently infect T cells in the host.

Like most lentiviruses, FIV is primarily cell associated, although virus has been isolated from serum, plasma, saliva, and CSF. The ease of recovery from cells and body fluids tends to correlate with the stage of infection.[65] FIV is difficult to isolate from nonsymptomatic cats latently infected with FIV, whereas virus recovery is considerably easier from ill cats in the terminal stages of infection. When there is inflammation of the oral cavity in a FIV-infected cat, there appears to be an increase in virus levels in the saliva, although this correlation has not been exhaustively evaluated.

PATHOGENESIS

Much of what is known of the pathogenesis of clinical disease associated with FIV infection has been gained from studies of the index cattery and from experimental inoculation of SPF cats.[59, 60] Most kittens inoculated by either the intraperitoneal or IV route will seroconvert within 2 to 4 weeks postinoculation (PI). Within this same time period, virus can be cultivated from PBL from inoculated kittens. Serum antibodies to the major gag and transmembrane proteins appear within this same time, and shortly thereafter antibodies to the smaller gag proteins and polymerase appear. Antibodies to the envelope protein also appear early in infection and remain in high concentrations throughout the course of disease. All inoculated cats have remained virus-positive and seropositive during these ongoing studies, several of which are now of 2 years' duration.

Peripheral generalized lymphadenomegaly has been observed 3 to 7 weeks PI in all cats, and during this same period, approximately 72% of the kittens developed fever lasting from 2 to 17 days. The generalized lymphadenomegaly characterized as an exuberant follicular hyperplasia, usually resolved by 7 months PI. Within 6 to 10 weeks PI, approximately 77% of the kittens suffered an absolute neutropenia persisting from 4 to 9 weeks (see Clinical Laboratory Findings). Three inoculated kittens have maintained an unresolved neutropenia up

to 1 year PI that waxes and wanes, and these cats are currently neutropenic.

Less than 50% of the SPF kittens have developed focal facial pyodermas and bacterial cellulitis associated with ear tags. These superficial skin infections resolved with antibiotic therapy, and in most cases, all other clinical signs resolved within 7 months PI and the cats returned to a nonsymptomatic state. This nonsymptomatic period experienced by most of the experimentally inoculated kittens has extended for up to 18 months post acute infection despite the fact that virus can be isolated from their PBL. This nonsymptomatic latent stage of infection has also been observed in a small proportion of the FIV-infected cats in the index cattery; however, the duration of this latent stage has not been well characterized within this setting. The presence of a prolonged disease-free latent stage of infection is a common characteristic of lentivirus infections in general, including HIV infection, in which HIV seropositive people may remain clinically healthy for an average of 5 years before the onset of AIDS or the AIDS-related complex (ARC).[63]

Neutralizing antibodies and cellular immunity to FIV have not been evaluated in infected cats. In lentivirus infections in other species, the presence of cellular immunity and significant neutralizing antibody titers have been observed in the host in the face of latent infection.[63] The onset of AIDS has also been associated with a loss of neutralizing antibody and cellular immunity in HIV-infected people.[70, 71] The average extent of the nonsymptomatic latent stage of FIV infection in field cats has yet to be determined and may be dependent upon environmental, nutritional, immunologic, and genetic factors.

Although most inoculated cats have recovered from the clinical abnormalities of the acute stage of infection and have remained nonsymptomatic, a small proportion have not recovered. Of two inoculated kittens that died within 2 years of inoculation,[60, 72] one developed a myeloproliferative disorder, and the second succumbed to myocardial, brain, and kidney lesions indicative of primary lentivirus infection. Since these cats were maintained in a pathogen-free environment and were not exposed to other cats, the absence of complicating infections would be expected. The presence of clinical disease in FIV infection without the presence of other infectious agents suggests that FIV can act as a primary pathogen. On the other hand, this lack of exposure to secondary pathogens may at least partially account for the prolonged nonsymptomatic state experienced by most experimentally inoculated cats. A pathogen-free environment rarely exists in natural circumstances except for the solitary indoor house cat and certainly is not the environment experienced in the index cattery, where chronic symptomatic stages of FIV infection were well evaluated.

Studies of FIV infection in the index cattery at different time points allowed for evaluation of the chronic and terminal stages of infection.[59, 60] Less than 10% of the infected cats in the cattery were nonsymptomatic, whereas the remaining cats suffered various clinical manifestations typical of an immunodeficient state. This chronic stage of infection, which includes chronic infections, diarrhea, and wasting may persist from 6 months to 3 years, during which time clinical disease waxes and wanes and responds to symptomatic therapy. Eventually, the clinical disease becomes unresponsive to any symptomatic therapy, and the cat frequently succumbs to a nonregenerative anemia.

Secondary pathogens, including various herpesvirus infections such as cytomegalovirus and Epstein-Barr virus infections, have been considered significant cofactors for induction of AIDS or ARC in HIV-infected people.[73] In fact, any infectious agent that activates the T cell arm of the immune system is thought to play a role in activating a latent HIV infection into development of clinical disease.[74] The significance and role of cofactors in the induction of chronic stages of disease in FIV infection must be determined for a better understanding of the pathogenesis of disease in FIV infection.

CLINICAL FINDINGS

Three stages of FIV infection are thought to exist, including the initial acute stage of infection, a nonsymptomatic latent period, and a chronic terminal stage with clinical disease consistent with an immunodeficient state.[60, 67, 68] Since FIV infection is a recently recognized phenomenon, knowledge of the clinical picture of the different stages of FIV infection is incomplete.

Acute Stage

Peripheral generalized lymphadenomegaly is the most consistent clinical feature of acute FIV infection experienced by experimentally inoculated kittens (Table 26–9);[60] fever and malaise are also frequently observed. Bacterial infections of the skin or intestinal tract and bacteremias have been observed in a smaller proportion of these cats. These bacterial infections may be secondary to the absolute neutropenia frequently observed in the acute stage of infection. These same clinical abnormalities are also consistent with acute FeLV infection, generalized lymphosarcoma, systemic lupus erythematosus, primary systemic viral or bacterial infections, or non-neoplastic lymphoproliferative disorders.[72, 75] In most cases, the clinical features of acute FIV infection are of a transient nature; fever resolves within 2 weeks PI, lymphadenomegaly within 6 months PI, and complicating bacterial infections with antibiotic therapy.

Latent Stage

Once the clinical signs of acute infection have resolved, the cat may enter a latent, nonsymptomatic stage of infection. The average duration of this latent stage in naturally or experimentally infected cats has yet to be determined but may range from months to years before the onset of the AIDS phase of infection.

Chronic Stage

The terminal stage of infection may be marked by a variety of clinical signs, alone or in combination (Table 26–10), that usually result from secondary infections from commensal microflora. The most frequently observed clinical findings are severe stomatitis and gingivitis, chronic upper respiratory

Table 26–9. Clinical Abnormalities Associated with Acute FIV Infection

Peripheral generalized lymphadenomegaly
Neutropenia
Fever
Bacterial infections of the skin
Diarrhea
Anemia
Myeloproliferative disease

Table 26–10. Clinical Abnormalities Associated with Chronic FIV Infection

Stomatitis and gingivitis
Diarrhea
Persistent upper respiratory infections
Chronic skin infections
Wasting
Fever of unknown origin
Purulent otitis externa
Lymphadenomegaly
Recurrent bacterial urinary tract infections
Anemia
Neurologic dysfunctions
Lymphosarcoma
Opportunistic infections

disease, chronic diarrhea and wasting, chronic conjunctivitis, and chronic skin infections. Gingivitis and stomatitis are of a purulent necrotizing nature but may also resemble a plasmacytic stomatitis. The chronic upper respiratory disease may be manifest as purulent cyclic conjunctivitis and rhinitis that may or may not be associated with a stomatitis and may partially resolve with antibiotic therapy. Chronic enteritis is often marked by emaciation and may be associated with other clinical signs. Chronic skin infections are frequently bacterial in nature, and purulent necrotizing otitis externa secondary to *Otodectes cyanotis* infection has also been observed. Cats suffering generalized demodecosis often are FIV-positive.[69]

Vague clinical signs observed in a proportion of FIV-positive cats include recurrent fevers of unknown origin, lymphadenomegaly, anemia, recurrent bacterial urinary tract infections, weight loss, and anorexia. Neurologic signs, including behavioral changes or psychotic behavior, dementia, facial twitching movements, and seizures that were reported in FIV-positive cats, mimic the neurologic syndromes observed in human AIDS patients.[76] These clinical abnormalities are probably a direct effect of FIV involvement of the brain. Neurologic disease may also result from secondary infectious agents such as *Toxoplasma* and *Cryptococcus neoformans*.[67, 68, 77] Studies revealed a significant correlation between clinical disease with toxoplasmosis infection and an FIV-seropositive state (see Chapter 86).[77, 77a]

Other opportunistic infections associated with FIV infection include demodectic and notoedric mange, candidiasis, *Pseudomonas* infections, fatal poxvirus infections, atypical mycobacterial infections, and haemobarto-

nellosis.[67, 68, 77b, 77c] The chronic upper respiratory infections observed in FIV-positive cats suggest that feline herpesvirus and calicivirus and perhaps *Chlamydia* may produce opportunistic infections with FIV infection as with other forms of immunosuppression (see also Necrotozing Ulcerative Gingivostomatitis, Chapter 9).[77d] Feline infectious peritonitis, often associated with FeLV infection, has not been observed with any greater frequency in FIV-infected cats.[67, 68] Neoplastic disorders associated with FIV infection include FeLV-negative and FeLV-positive lymphosarcomas, myeloproliferative disorders, fibrosarcomas, and mammary

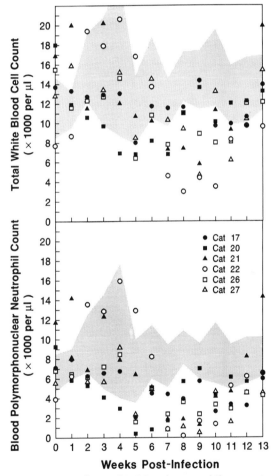

Figure 26–11. The total WBC and neutrophil counts in six cats with experimentally induced FIV infection and in six noninfected contact-control cats. The shaded areas represent the mean and 1 SD of the values obtained from the noninfected contact-control cats. Neutropenia, often associated with some degree of leukopenia, appeared from 4 to 5 weeks after inoculation. The WBC and neutrophil counts for the group were approaching reference ranges at the end of the 13-week observation period. (Yamamoto et al: *Am J Vet Res* 49:1246–1262, 1988. Reprinted with permission.)

gland and squamous cell carcinomas. Lymphosarcomas have almost been exclusively solitary and of the B cell type. Whether these neoplastic disorders are directly related to FIV infection has yet to be proven or even evaluated.

DIAGNOSIS

Clinical Laboratory Findings

Hematologic abnormalities have been observed in cats experimentally and naturally infected with FIV.[60, 67, 68, 77e] More than 75% of the experimentally infected cats have had an absolute neutropenia often asssociated with a leukopenia (Fig. 26–11). The neutropenia has developed during the acute stage of infection—approximately 6 to 9 weeks PI—has persisted from 2 to 8 weeks, and has eventually resolved in most cases when cats entered the nonsymptomatic latent stage of infection. Three of 24 inoculated cats experienced a recurrent neutropenia that persisted during an otherwise nonsymptomatic latent stage of infection.[78] Studies involving bone marrow aspirates from these neutropenic cats, although incomplete, did not reveal evidence of bone marrow suppression.[79] The lack of bone marrow suppression has suggested peripheral consumption or sequestration of mature neutrophils as underlying mechanisms of the neutropenia.

In naturally infected cats, leukopenia associated with both lymphopenia and neutropenia frequently was observed.[69, 67, 68] Depression type, hypoplastic type, and regenerative type anemias were also found. Haemobartonellosis is probably an infrequent cause of anemia in infected cats, since the prevalence of haemobartonellosis in one study was 1.4%, whereas that of anemia was 18%.[68] Thrombocytopenia, frequently observed in FeLV-positive cats and in human AIDS patients, has not been a frequent finding in FIV-positive cats. Myeloproliferative disorders have been rare, with only three cases reported in naturally infected cats and one in an experimentally inoculated cat.

Serologic Testing

In general, diagnosis of lentivirus infections in all species has involved detection of antibody.[63] Because of the permanency of infection once it is established, the presence of antibody to a lentivirus signifies infection. An IFA test utilizes FIV-infected PBL or Crandell feline kidney cells (CRFK), a feline fibroblast cell line, for the detection of FIV antibody.[59, 60, 69] An ELISA method (CITE, IDDEX Corp., Portland, ME) is commercially available.[79a] Western blot is another assay that allows detection of antibodies to specific viral proteins and has been used to confirm results obtained by IFA and ELISA. See Appendix 8 for a list of laboratories that perform these tests and for information on commercially available test kits.

Because the level of viral expression is usually depressed within the host until terminal stages, antigen detection assays have not been useful for routine diagnosis of lentivirus infections.[63] There have only been two instances when antigen can be found in the blood with extremely low or nondetectable levels of antibody.[69] First, in natural infection the average length of time between infection and antibody detection is not known but may be delayed from weeks to months. During this early stage of infection, antigen may be detectable, whereas antibody is not. The second instance occurs in the later stages of infection when a cat is suffering terminal disease. At this time, antibody levels may decrease below the sensitivity of detection methods, whereas viral antigen expression increases. Similarly, in people infected with HIV, viral antigen concentration in blood is inversely proportional to antibody concentration.[80]

Viral Isolation

The most direct approach to diagnosis of FIV infection involves isolating PBLs from a suspect cat and cocultivating them in cell culture with those from a healthy cat. Because of the cost and time involved with this assay, it is only used in the research setting.

Cytopathic effects (CPE) observed in FIV-infected PBL cultures includes cell death, multinucleated giant cells, and balloon formation, also consistent with CPE reported in HIV-infected human PBLs. Electron microscopy, IFA, or ELISA methodology may be used to identify virus in cell culture.

Initial studies suggested that FIV only proliferated in primary feline T cells and feline lymphoid cell lines, just as initial studies with HIV suggested that HIV proliferated only in primary human T cells and T cell lines of the T helper subset. However, additional studies reported a broader tropism for both HIV and FIV. FIV was found to be capable of infecting primary feline macrophages and, after adaptation to cell culture, CRFK.[60, 72] The pathogenicity of virus grown in such nonlymphoid cell lines may be decreased over isolates propagated in lymphoid cells.[69] FIV has not been found to infect primary human, mouse, or dog T cells or T cell lines and, therefore, appears to be species-specific.[60]

PATHOLOGIC FINDINGS

In general, the pathologic abnormalities observed in FIV-positive cats are dependent on the stage of infection. Lesions most frequently involve the oral cavity, respiratory and intestinal tracts, skin, and lymphoid tissues; however, significant variability of lesions within the same tissues from different cats has been observed.[81, 81a] Histologic lesions of the oral cavity may include mucosal ulcerations and erosions, with extensive submucosal plasmacytic infiltrates or nodules and licheniform elevations composed of mucosal plasmacytic infiltrates. The plasmacytic accumulations may extend along vessels to involve underlying muscle, salivary glands, and draining lymph nodes. FIV is thus involved in the syndrome of plasmacytic stomatitis in cats (see Necrotizing Ulcerative Gingivostomatitis, Chapter 9). Infiltrations with neutrophils, lymphoid cells, and mast cells without this intense plasmacytic infiltration have also been observed.

The most frequent lesions in the bowel include small intestinal villous blunting, loss of villi, and crypt dilation, which are changes reported in feline parvovirus-like enteritis and enteritis associated with FeLV infection.[82] Other frequently observed lesions include ulceration or necrotizing pyogranulomatous inflammation of the large intestinal tract with submucosal infiltration of neutrophils, macrophages, and in some cases, histiocytes (Fig. 26–12). FIV-infected cats that experience an acute and fulminating diarrhea often with a fatal outcome, usually have necrotizing typhlitis and colitis. Although infection with commensal microflora is the presumed cause of these in-

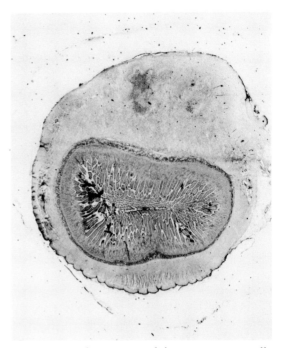

Figure 26–12. Photomicrograph from an experimentally infected kitten suffering severe transmural typhlocolitis 5.5 weeks after inoculation. This focus of mural enteritis was found (at necropsy 3 weeks later) 15 cm craniad to the site of intestinal resection performed previously. (H and E, × 8) (Yamamoto et al: Am J Vet Res 49:1246–1262, 1988. Reprinted with permission.)

testinal lesions, attempts to identify other known pathogens have been unsuccessful.

Abnormalities of the lower respiratory tract have included lymphoplasmacytic cuffing of small bronchioles, diffuse nonsuppurative interstitial pneumonia, and pulmonary abscesses. Lesions from an FIV-infected kitten that developed feline herpesvirus-1 infection, a usual upper respiratory syndrome, had fulminating infection that included hyperplastic and necrotic bronchiolar epithelium, herpesviral inclusions in bronchiolar epithelium, and the presence of syncytia with homogeneous nuclei in the bronchiolar lumina, along with neutrophils and bacteria. Pathologic findings in the upper respiratory tract and skin have been nonspecific and usually reflect chronic or subacute inflammation. Skin lesions have been characterized as folliculitis, ulceration, and multifocal acanthosis.

The most common pathologic finding of lymphoid tissues has been exuberant follicular hyperplasia with the presence of secondary follicles and massive plasmacytic infiltration of the cords and paracortex (Fig. 26–13). Follicular hyperplasia has been a

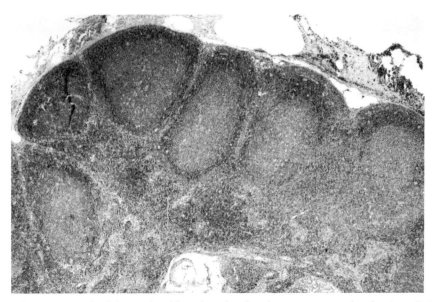

Figure 26–13. Photomicrograph of the popliteal lymph node taken from a cat 16 weeks after inoculation with FIV. There is exuberant follicular hyperplasia with follicular dysplasia. (H and E, × 10) (Yamamoto et al: *Am J Vet Res* 49:1246–1262, 1988. Reprinted with permission.)

consistent finding of the acute and terminal stages of FIV infection and is similar to histologic changes in human AIDS-related complex patients.[83] Another frequent finding has been plasmacytic infiltration of lymph nodes draining the oral cavity of FIV-infected cats with plasmacytic stomatitis (also see Lymphocytic Plasmacytic Stomatitis, Chapter 9). Plasmacytic infiltration and follicular hyperplasia, observed in spleens of infected cats, suggest altered regulation of B cell responses as documented in human AIDS patients.[84] Less frequently, lymphoid depletion has been observed in the terminal stages of FIV infection.

Pathologic changes in the CNS, commonly observed in FIV infection, have not always been associated with clinical neurologic disease. Choroid plexus fibrosis, amphophilic hyaline bodies in the cortex, white matter vacuolation, and perivascular cuffing by macrophages and lymphocytes have been most commonly found. Lesions have primarily involved the cerebral cortex and have produced signs of forebrain dysfunction such as dementia, behavioral changes, or seizures.

THERAPY AND PREVENTION

There is no known therapy to eliminate retroviral infections. However, with the rec-ognition of HIV as the cause of human AIDS, antiviral drug research has become very active. The most effective antiviral drug for this disease, azidothymidine (zivouvidine, AZT) a reverse transcriptase inhibitor (see Therapy, Chapter 23), is of limited value when considering efficacy and toxic side effects.[85] Lymphokines such as interferons and interleukins, also considered antiviral drugs, have not been efficacious when used individually and are plagued with undesirable side effects. Lymphokine combinations may prove more effective and are being evaluated. Until effective drugs are found, symptomatic therapy with antibiotics, fluid therapy, and transfusions, is all that may be offered for the clinically affected cat. Many cats will initially respond to appropriate symptomatic therapy and may survive months longer with good nursing care. Eventually, clinical illness will become refractory to any therapy and the cat will succumb. The long-term (>2 years) prognosis for FIV infection, especially once clinical disease develops, is very poor.

Since transmission of FIV infection is not thoroughly understood, isolation of FIV-infected cats from uninfected cats is recommended. Isolation may be especially important in environments with a high density of cats, where physical interaction is possible and where other cofactors, such as stress of overcrowding or presence of other infectious agents, may predispose to infection and clinical illness. There is no vaccine currently available for FIV, and the development of an effective vaccine may be in the distant future. Vaccine development for other lentivirus infections including HIV in people, Maedi visna virus in sheep, and caprine arthritis encephalitis virus in goats, has been slow and frustrating and major breakthroughs are eagerly awaited.

PUBLIC HEALTH CONSIDERATIONS

There is no current evidence that FIV will infect people or any other nonfeline species. FIV will not infect human primary lymphocytes or human lymphocyte cell lines. In an evaluation of 18 people exposed to infection via either bite wounds from infected cats or virus-infected tissue culture supernatants, all were found seronegative for FIV.[67] Lentiviruses appear to be species-specific.

References

1. Jarrett O: Feline leukemia virus. In Hardy WD, Essex M, McClelland AJ (eds): Feline Leukemia Virus. New York, Elsevier, 1980, pp 473–479.
2. Stewart MA, Warnock M, Wheeler A, et al: Nucleotide sequences of a feline leukemia virus subgroup A envelope gene and long terminal repeat and evidence for the recombinational origin of subgroup B viruses. J Virol 58:825–834, 1986.
3. Ved Brat SS, Rasheed S, Lutz H, et al: Feline oncornavirus-associated cell membrane antigen: a viral and not a cellularly coded transformation-specific antigen of cat lymphomas. Virology 124:445–461, 1983.
4. Francis DP, Essex M, Gayzagian D: Feline leukemia virus: survival under home and laboratory conditions. J Clin Microbiol 9:154–156, 1979.
5. Pedersen NC, Meric SM, Johnson L, et al: The clinical significance of latent feline leukemia virus infection in cats. Feline Pract 14:32–48, 1984.
6. Pacitti AM, Jarrett O, Hay D: Transmission of feline leukemia virus in the milk of a non-viremic cat. Vet Rec 118:381–384, 1986.
7. McClelland AJ, Hardy WD, Zuckerman EE: Prognosis of healthy feline leukemia virus-infected cats. In Hardy WD, Essex M, McClelland AJ (eds): Feline Leukemia Virus. New York, Elsevier, 1980, pp 121–216.
8. Francis DP, Essex M, Cotter SM, et al: Epidemiologic association between virus-negative feline leukemia and the horizontally transmitted feline leukemia virus. Cancer Lett 12:37–42, 1981.
9. Mullins JI, Brody DS, Binari RC Jr, et al: Viral transduction of c-myc gene in naturally occurring feline leukaemia. Nature 308:856–858, 1984.
10. Cotter SM, Holzworth J: Disorders of the hemato-

poietic system. In Holzworth J (ed): Diseases of the Cat. Philadelphia, WB Saunders Co, 1986, pp 755–807.
11. Lewis MG, Kociba GJ, Rojko JL, et al: Retroviral-associated eosinophilic leukemia in the cat. Am J Vet Res 46:1066–1070, 1985.
12. Baker RJ, Valli VE: Dysmyelopoiesis in the cat: a hematological disorder resembling refractory anemia with excess blasts in man. Can J Vet Res 50:3–6, 1986.
13. Swenson CL, Kociba GJ, O'Keefe DA, et al: Cyclic hematopoiesis associated with feline leukemia virus infection in two cats. J Am Vet Med Assoc 191:93–96, 1987.
14. Wardrop KJ, Kramer JW, Abkowitz JL, et al: Quantitative studies of erythropoiesis in the clinically normal, phlebotomized, and feline leukemia virus–infected cats. Am J Vet Res 47:2274–2277, 1986.
15. Rojko JL, Cheney CM, Gasper PW, et al: Infectious feline leukemia virus is erythrosuppressive in vitro. Leuk Res 10:1193–1199, 1986.
16. Abkowitz JL, Holly RD, Grant CK: Retrovirus-induced feline pure red cell aplasia. J Clin Invest 80:1056–1063, 1987.
17. Jarrett O, Golder MC, Toth S, et al: Interaction between feline leukemia virus subgroups in the pathogenesis of erythroid hypoplasia. Int J Cancer 34:283–288, 1984.
18. Weiser MG, Kociba GJ: Erythrocyte macrocytosis in feline leukemia virus–associated anemia. Vet Pathol 20:687–697, 1983.
19. Boyce JT, Kociba GJ, Jacobs RM, et al: Feline leukemia virus-induced thrombocytopenia and macrothrombocytosis in cats. Vet Pathol 23:16–20, 1986.
19a. Poss ML, Mullins JI, Hoover EA: Posttranslational modifications distinguish the envelope glycoproteins of the immunodeficiency disease–inducing feline leukemia virus retrovirus. J Virol 63:189–195, 1989.
20. Mullins JI, Chen CS, Hoover EA: Disease-specific and tissue-specific production of unintegrated feline leukemia virus variant DNA in feline AIDS. Nature 319:333–336, 1986.
20a. Tompkins MB, Ogilvie GK, Gast AM, et al: Interleukin-2 in cats naturally infected with feline leukemia virus. J Biol Response Mod 8:86–96, 1989.
21. Wernicke D, Trainin Z, Ungar-Waron H, et al: Humoral immune response of asymptomatic cats naturally infected with feline leukemia virus. J Virol 60:669–673, 1986.
22. Lafrado LJ, Olsen RG: Demonstration of depressed polymorphonuclear leukocyte function in nonviremic FeLV-infected cats. Cancer Invest 4:297–300, 1986.
23. Kiehl Ar, Fettman MJ, Quackenbush SL, et al: Effects of feline leukemia virus infection on neutrophil chemotaxis in vitro. Am J Vet Res 48:76–80, 1987.
24. Cotter SM, Grant CK, Goldstein MA: Treatment of persistent naturally occurring feline leukemia virus infections with monoclonal antibodies. In Proceedings. Am Coll Vet Intern Med, section 13:3–6, 1986.
25. Tuomari DL, Olsen RG, Kraut EH: Immune complex studies during the preneoplastic stages of feline leukemia virus infection. Proc Am Assoc Cancer Res 25:243, 1984.
26. Moore FJ, Emerson WE, Cotter SM, et al: Distinctive peripheral lymph node hyperplasia of young cats. Vet Pathol 23:386–391, 1986.

27. Reinacher M: Feline leukemia virus-associated enteritis—a condition with features of feline panleukopenia. Vet Pathol 24:1–4, 1987.

28. Cotter SM: Feline viral neoplasia. In Greene CE (ed): Clinical Microbiology and Infectious Diseases of the Dog and Cat. Philadelphia, WB Saunders Co, 1984, pp 490–513.

29. Lutz H, Pedersen NC, Theilen GH: Course of feline leukemia virus infection and its detection by enzyme-linked immunosorbent assay and monoclonal antibodies. Am J Vet Res 44:2054–2059, 1983.

30. Hawkins EC, Johnson L, Pedersen NC, et al: Use of tears for diagnosis of feline leukemia virus infection. J Am Vet Med Assoc 188:1031–1034, 1986.

31. Cotter SM: Treatment of feline lymphoma with cyclophosphamide, vincristine and prednisone. J Am Anim Hosp Assoc 19:166–172, 1983.

32. Theilen GH, Madewell BR: Veterinary Cancer Medicine. Philadelphia, Lea & Febiger, 1987.

33. Cotter SM: Anemia associated with feline leukemia virus infection. J Am Vet Med Assoc 175:1191–1194, 1979.

34. Gasper PW: Studies of feline leukemia virus-induced aplastic anemia. Dissertation Abstr Intern 46:83–84, 1985.

35. Bellinger DA, Chang J, Bunn TD, et al: Rabies induced in a cat by high egg passage Flury strain vaccine. J Am Vet Med Assoc 183:997–998, 1983.

36. Willard MD: Corticosteroid-responsive leukopenia and neutropenia associated with FeLV infection in two cats. Mod Vet Pract 66:729–722, 1985.

37. Sharpee RL, Beckenhaver WH, Baumgartener LE, et al: Feline leukemia vaccine; evaluation of safety and efficacy against persistent viremia and tumor development. Compend Cont Educ Pract Vet 8:267–277, 1986.

38. Covenant, Feline Leukemia Vaccine, Product Information, Diamond Scientific, Des Moines, IA, 1988.

39. Stallman CG, Legendre AM: Field trials of Leukocell™, a commercial subunit feline leukemia vaccine. In Proceedings. Eastern States Veterinary Conference, 1986, pp 20–29.

40. Legendre AM: FeLV vaccinations. In Proceedings. Am Coll Vet Intern Med, 1–2, 1988.

41. Rosenthal RC, Dworkis AS: Adverse reactions to Leukocell^R. J Am Anim Hosp Assoc 23:515–518, 1987.

41a. Lewis MG, Lafrado LJ, Haffer K, et al: Feline leukemia virus vaccine: new developments. Vet Microbiol 17:297–308, 1988.

42. Grant CK, Ernisse BJ, Jarrett O, et al: Feline leukemia virus envelope gp70 of subgroups B and C defined by monoclonal antibodies with cytotoxic and neutralizing functions. J Immunol 131:3042–3048, 1983.

43. Youngren SD, Vukasin AP, de Noronha F: Characterization of monolonal antibodies directed against the envelope proteins of feline leukemia virus. Cancer Res 44:3512–3517, 1984.

44. Haley PJ, Hoover EA, Quackenbush SL, et al: Influence of antibody infusion on pathogenesis of experimental feline leukemia virus infection. J Natl Cancer Inst 74:821–827, 1985.

45. Weijer K, UytdeHaag FG, Jarrett O, et al: Postexposure treatment with monoclonal antibodies in a retrovirus system: failure to protect cats against feline leukemia virus infection with virus neutralizing monoclonal antibodies. Int J Cancer 38:81–87, 1986.

46. Jones FR, Yoshida LH, Ladiges WC, et al: Treatment of feline lymphosarcoma by extracorporeal immunosorption. In Hardy WD, Essex M, McClelland, AJ (eds): Feline Leukemia Virus. New York, Elsevier, 1980, pp 235–243.

47. Engelman RW: Clearance of feline leukemia virus from persistently infected cats during treatment with staphylococcal protein A. Proc Soc Exp Biol Med 181:186, 1986.

48. Cummins J, Tomplins M, Olsen R, et al: The oral use of human interferon-α in cats. J Biol Response Mod 7:513-523, 1988.

49. Cogan DC, Cotter SM, Kitchen LW: Effect of suramin on serum viral replication in feline leukemia virus-infected pet cats. Am J Vet Res 47:2230–2232, 1986.

50. Jarrett O, Laird HM, Hay D: Growth of feline leukemia virus in human cells. Nature 224:1208–1209, 1969.

51. Rickard CG, Post JE, de Noronha F, et al: Interspecies infection by feline leukemia virus: serial cell-free transmission in dogs of malignant lymphoma-induced feline leukemia virus. In Dutcher RM, Chieco-Bianchi L (eds): Unifying Concepts of Leukemia. Basel, Karger, 1972, pp 102–112.

52. Bross IDJ, Gibson R: Cats and childhood leukemia. J Med 1:180–187, 1970.

53. Jaquemin PC, Saxinger SP, Gallo RC, et al: Antibody response in cats to feline leukemia virus under natural conditions of exposure to virus. Virology 91:472–476, 1978.

54. Gutensohn N, Francis DP, Hardy WD, et al: Risk to humans from exposure to feline leukemia virus: epidemiological considerations. In Essex M, Todaro G, Zur Hausen H (eds): Viruses in Naturally Occurring Cancer, vol 7. New York, Cold Spring Harbor Laboratory, 1983, pp 699–706.

55. Coffin JM, Varmus HE, Michael J, et al: Proposal for naming host cell-derived insert in retrovirus genomes. J Virol 40:952–957, 1981.

56. Theilen GH, Snyder SN, Wolfe LG, et al: Biological studies with viral-induced fibrosarcoma in cats, dogs, rabbits and non-human primates. In Comparative Leukemia Research, 1969. Proceedings, 4th International Symposium on Comparative Leukemia Research. Basel, Karger, 1970.

57. McCullough B, Schaller J, Shadduck JA, et al: Induction of malignant melanomas associated with fibrosarcoma in gnotobiotic cats inoculated with Gardner-Arnstein feline fibrosarcoma virus. J Natl Cancer Inst 48:1893–1896, 1972.

58. Todaro GJ, Tevethia S, Meinick J: Isolation of an RD 114-related Type C virus from feline sarcoma virus transformed baboon cells. Intervirology 1:399–404, 1974.

59. Pedersen NC, Ho EW, Brown ML, Yamamoto JK: Isolation of a T-lymphotrophic virus from domestic cats with an immunodeficiency-like syndrome. Science 235: 790–793, 1986.

60. Yamamoto JK, Sparger EE, Ho EW, Anderson PR, et al: Pathogenesis of experimentally induced feline immunodeficiency virus infection in cats. Am J Vet Res 49:1246–1262, 1988.

61. Elder JH: Unpublished results, Scripps Institute, San Diego, CA, 1988.

62. Teich N: Taxonomy of Retroviruses. In Weiss R, Teisch N, Varmus H, Coffin J (eds): RNA Tumor Viruses. Cold Spring Harbor Laboratory, 1982, pp 25–208.

63. Haase AT: Pathogenesis of lentivirus infections. Nature 322:130–136, 1986.

64. O'Connor T, Steinman R, Tonelli Q, et al: Biochemical and immunological characterization of the major structural proteins of feline T-lymphotropic lentivirus. Submitted for publication, 1989.

65. Yamamoto, JK: Personal communication, University of California, Davis, CA, 1988.

66. Elder, JH: Personal communication, Scripps Institute, San Diego, CA, 1988.

67. Yamamoto JK, Hansen H, Ho, EW et al: Epidemiologic and clinical aspects of feline immunodeficiency virus (FIV) infection in cats from the continental United States and Canada and possible mode of transmission. J Am Vet Med Assoc 194:213–220, 1989.

68. Ishida T, Washizu T, Toriyabe K, et al: Feline immunodeficiency virus (FIV) infection in Japan. J Am Vet Med Assoc 194:221–225, 1989.

68a. Shelton GH, Waltier RM, Connor SC, et al: Prevalence of feline immunodeficiency virus and feline leukemia virus in pet cats. J Am Anim Hosp Assoc25:7–12, 1989.

68b. Grinden CB, Corbett WT, Ammerman BG, et al: Seroepidemiologic survey of feline immunodeficiency virus infections in cats of Wade County, North Carolina. J Am Vet Med Assoc 194:226–228, 1989.

68c. Gruffydd-Jones TJ, Hopper CD, Harbour DA, et al; Serologic evidence of feline immunodeficiency virus infection in UK cats from 1975–1976. Vet Rec 123:569-570, 1988.

68d. Weijer K, vanHerwijnen R, Siebelink K, et al: Prevalence of FTLV infections among cats in the Netherlands and West Germany. Tijdschr Diergeneeskd 113:1063–1064, 1988.

69. Pedersen NC: Personal communication, University of California, Davis, CA, 1988.

70. Ranki A, Weiss SH, Sirkka-Liisa V, et al: Neutralizing antibodies in HIV(HTLV-III) infection: correlation with clinical outcome and antibody response against different viral proteins. Clin Exp Immunol 69:321-329,1987.

71. Walker BD, Sekhar C, Moss B, et al: HIV-specific cytotoxic T lymphocytes in seropositive individuals. Nature 328:345–348,1987.

72. Pedersen NC, Yamamoto JK, Ishida T, et al: Feline immunodeficiency virus infection. Vet Immunol Immunopathol. In press, 1988.

73. Gendelman HE, Phelps W, Feigenbaum L, et al: Transactivation of the human immunodeficiency virus long terminal repeat sequence by DNA viruses. Proc Nat Acad Sci USA 83:9759–9763, 1986.

74. Tong-Starksen SE, Luciw PA, Peterlin BM: Human immunodeficiency virus long terminal repeat responds to T-cell activation signals. Proc Nat Acad Sci USA 84: 6845–6849, 1987.

75. Lutz H, Pedersen NC, Theilen GH: Course of feline leukemia virus infection and its detection by enzyme-linked immunosorbent assay and monoclonal antibodies. Am J Vet Res 44:2045–2059, 1983.

76. Snider WD, Simpson DM, Nielson S, et al: Neurological complications of acquired immune deficiency syndrome: analysis of 50 patients. Ann Neurol 14:403–418, 1983.

77. Lappin M, Greene CE, Winston S, et al: Clinical feline toxoplasmosis. Serologic diagnosis and therapeutic management of 15 cases. J Vet Intern Med. In press.

77a. Witt CJ, Moench TR, Gittelsohn CJ, et al: Epidemiologic observations on feline immunodeficiency virus and Toxoplasma gondii coinfection in cats in Baltimore, Md. J Am Vet Med Assoc 194:229–238, 1989.

77b. Chalmers S, Schick RD, Jeffers J: Demodecosis in two cats seropositive for feline immunodeficiency virus. J Am Vet Med Assoc 194:256–257, 1989.

77c. Brown A, Bennett M, Gaskell CJ, et al: Fatal poxvirus infection in association with FIV infection. Vet Rec 124:19–20, 1989.

77d. Knowles JO, Gaskell RM, Gaskell CJ, et al: Prevalence of feline calicivirus, feline leukaemia virus and antibodies to FIV in cats with chronic stomatitis. Vet Rec 124L336–338, 1989.

78. Sparger EE: Personal communication, University of California, Davis, CA, 1988.

79. Mandell CP. Personal communication, University of California, Davis, CA, 1988.

79a. O'Connor TP, Tangvay S, Steinman R, et al: Development and evaluation of an immunoassay for detection of antibodies to feline T-lymphotropic lentivirus (feline immunodeficiency virus). J Clin Microbiol 27:474–479, 1989.

80. Allain JP, Laurian Y, Paul DA, Verroust F, et al: Long-term evaluation of HIV antigen and antibodies to p24 and gp 41 in patients with hemophilia. N Engl J Med 317:1114–1121, 1987.

81. Lowenstine LJ, Pedersen NC, Yamamoto JK, et al: Clinical and pathologic findings in cats naturally infected with feline immunodeficiency virus (FIV). In preparation, 1989.

81a. Dieth V, Lutz H, Hauser B, et al: Pathological findings in lentivirus infected cats. Schweiz Arch Tierheilkd 131:19–25, 1989.

82. Reinacher M: Feline leukemia virus-associated enteritis—a condition with features of feline panleucopenia. Vet Pathol 24:1–4, 1987.

83. Meyer PR, Yanagihara ET, Parker JW, et al: A distinctive follicular hyperplasia in the acquired immune deficiency syndrome (AIDS) and AIDS-related complex. Hematol Oncol 2:319–347, 1984.

84. Lane HC, Masur H, Edgar LC, et al: Abnormalities of B-cell activation and immunoregulation in patients with the acquired immune deficiency syndrome. N Engl J Med 309:453–458, 1983.

85. Yarchoan R, Broder S: Development of antiretroviral therapy for the acquired immune deficiency syndrome and related disorders. N Engl J Med 316:557–564, 1987.

27

FELINE RESPIRATORY DISEASES

R. Charles Povey

ETIOLOGY AND PATHOGENESIS

Respiratory infections in cats have frequently been less severe since the introduction and widespread use of vaccines. Infections in kittenhood still present a major problem for the clinician. Infections are also still common where cats are congregated in breeding or boarding catteries and veterinary hospitals. The epidemiology of the various etiologic agents must be understood before instituting infection management strategies.

The main organisms in order of clinical importance are feline rhinotracheitis virus (FRV = feline herpesvirus-1) and feline calicivirus (FCV), which account for about 80% of the disease problems, and *Chlamydia psittaci* and *Mycoplasma* spp. Although influenza and parainfluenza viruses can infect cats experimentally, they are not naturally important. Reoviruses or reo-like viruses are occasionally isolated from cats, usually from the intestine. Following oral or IV inoculation, one such isolate produced mild conjunctivitis, which spread to other kittens.[1]

Feline Rhinotracheitis Virus

A typical γ-herpesvirus, FRV is also designated feline herpesvirus-1 (FHV-1) (Fig. 27–1). Unlike many other herpesviruses, the DNA genomes of FRV isolates from different countries show considerable homogeneity.[2] Only one serotype is recognized worldwide, although variation in strain virulence does occur. Virus replicates readily in feline cell cultures, causing cytopathic effects of cell swelling, rounding, increased refractility, polykaryocyte formation, and degeneration. Fixed, stained cultures reveal intranuclear

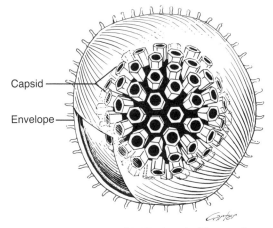

Figure 27–1. Structure of FRV. A typical herpesvirus.

inclusion bodies (see Fig. 14–2). The virus hemagglutinates feline erythrocytes.

FRV is naturally temperature restricted ($\leq 37°C$) in its replication, thereby limiting viremia at normal adult body temperature. Although generalized infection can occur in hypothermic neonatal kittens, FRV has been associated with pancreatitis and viral pneumonia in two older kittens.[3] Most effects of FRV are at the relatively cool mucosal epithelial surfaces such as conjunctiva, turbinates, nasopharynx and, experimentally, vulvovaginal mucosa. Multifocal epithelial cell necrosis occurs at these sites within 24 to 48 hours of droplet or aerosol exposure. Secondary bacterial invasion intensifies the inflammatory response. Extension of viral inflammation to the lower respiratory tract and lungs is unusual; however, secondary bacterial pneumonia is possible. As part of the upper respiratory infection, FRV produces osteolytic effects on turbinate bones.

Intranasal (IN) infection of pregnant cats is followed by abortion, but FRV is not recoverable from the aborted material. IV virus inoculation results in pathologic changes and intranuclear inclusions in uterus, placenta and aborted fetus. Intravaginal instillation of FRV can cause vaginitis resulting in congenitally infected kittens.

Feline Calicivirus

Caliciviruses are small RNA viruses with a characteristic morphology of surface cup-like depressions (calyx = cup) (Fig. 27–2, see also Fig. 14–3). They replicate rapidly in feline cell cultures. Swelling and increased refractility of cells without inclusions are followed by contraction and cell detachment. Caliciviruses do not cause hemagglutination.

FCV shows antigenic and pathogenic strain variation. There is sufficient antigenic cross-reactivity between isolates that only one serotype is recognized. However, antiserum produced against any single FCV isolate will not cross-neutralize all other FCV strains. Sequential inoculation of cats with two or more selected strains can produce broadly cross-neutralizing antisera.[4]

The route of inoculation of FCV has an influence on the pathogenesis of the disease. Direct IN instillation results mainly in upper respiratory and buccal cavity vesiculo-erosive lesions. Viral pneumonia may develop. Aerosol exposure with virulent strains produces acute exudative viral alveolitis with or without buccal and upper respiratory lesions. Viremia is uncommon with most FCV infections, but some strains can cause a "limping syndrome" of uncertain pathogenesis (see Clinical Findings).

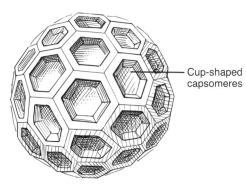

Figure 27–2. Structure of FCV.

Other Organisms

C. psittaci infection primarily produces a catarrhal conjunctivitis and mild rhinitis.[5] The conjunctivitis has a tendency to become chronic or recurrent. The historical name of feline pneumonitis for this infection is a misnomer because there is seldom lower respiratory tract involvement (see Chapter 40).

Mycoplasma spp. are frequently isolated from mucosal surfaces of cats (see Chapter 41). In a survey, 93% of throat swabs of clinically healthy cats yielded one or more *Mycoplasma* spp.[6] *M. felis*, besides being frequently isolated from healthy cats, has been associated with conjunctivitis. Conjunctivitis was reproduced in kittens by ocular instillation of concentrated cultures of *M. felis*, and 2 kittens developed interstitial pneumonia.[7]

Bacteria such as *Bordetella bronchiseptica*, *Pasteurella multocida*, and *Escherichia coli* are often isolated from the upper and lower respiratory tracts of sick cats, but they are found in the upper tracts of healthy cats. They are thought to play only a secondary role in respiratory disease.

EPIDEMIOLOGY

Sources of Infection

FRV is shed in ocular, nasal, and pharyngeal secretions from 1 to 3 weeks during clinical infection. Subclinical infections, reinfections, or re-excretion of virus from carriers result in shorter (1- to 10-day) periods of shedding.[8] Viremia is unusual; however, FRV can occasionally be detected in feces.

FCV is also shed in ocular, nasal, and pharyngeal secretions from several days to several weeks. Some cats remain persistent shedders (carriers) for many months or even years.[9] Subclinical reinfections with reduced duration of viral shedding are common. There is regular fecal shedding, but it is transient. Occasionally, FCV is detected in urine.

Chlamydia is predominantly shed in ocular discharges. Chronic shedding and reinfections are common in endemically infected colonies. Favored sites for harboring *Mycoplasma* spp. are the throat and, to a lesser extent, nose and conjunctiva. Some urogenital and rectal shedding also occurs.

Mode of Transmission

Cats do not produce effective aerosols because of their small tidal volume. Therefore, sneezed macrodroplets containing viruses or organisms are infective, but only over relatively short distances of approximately 4 feet.[10] Direct, close contact is the major mode of transmission for all respiratory pathogens.

The salty moisture film on the hands favors survival of microorganisms. This is an important fomite for indirect transmission from cat to cat by the handler. Clothing, feed bowls, and contaminated surfaces are potential, but less important, means of transmission. The transmission cycles for FRV and FCV are shown in Figure 27-3.

The Carrier State

Persistently infected carriers play a vital role in continually maintaining feline respiratory infections in congregations of cats. The natural history of the carrier state is quite different for FRV and FCV infections.

The FRV-carrier cat is, for the most part, latently infected and only occasionally allows productive viral replication and shedding. This occurs following some natural or simulated stress. Thus, relatively low total daily doses of dexamethasone (0.75 mg) or prednisolone (2.25 mg) given IM in three doses 2 days apart stimulate virus shedding in 80% of FRV-recovered cats between 4 and 18 days later.[11] Natural stresses, boarding in a cattery, or going to a cat show result in shedding after a similar lag period in 50% of cats. Late lactation (4 to 5 weeks postpartum) is another stressful time likely to lead to FRV shedding from carrier queens. Conveniently for the virus, the cycle of infection can be perpetuated, since this coincides with the time kittens are losing maternal antibodies. Following a period of shedding, there is a refractory phase that can last some months. After this the carrier will again shed under stress.

Nerve ganglia such as the trigeminal and those of the ethmoturbinate region may harbor FRV,[12] but in many known carriers, the location of latent virus has not been found.[13]

The FCV-carrier is a persistent shedder.[14]

Quantities of virus shed in nasal and oropharyngeal secretions vary from time to time. The tonsils and lymphoepithelial tissues of the nasooropharynx are the major sites of persistence. Local antibodies appear to be non-neutralizing. Slight antigenic drift is detected in the carrier virus. Termination of the FCV-carrier state usually occurs suddenly from several months to several years after infection. The immunologic basis for this termination is not known.

C. psittaci can be isolated from the conjunctivae of some recovered cats for 2 months after infection. *Mycoplasma* spp. can be isolated from nose, throat, and conjunctiva of some cats over long periods of time.

Environmental Survival

FRV is a typical, fragile herpesvirus. Relative humidity of more than 30% increases lability. FRV is inactivated within 18 hours at 15°C (59°F) in a humid environment. Mycoplasmas and *Chlamydia* are similarly fragile. FCV is the most stable, being viable for several days at room temperatures.

Outcome of Infection

Individual variation between cats in their apparent susceptibility to and severity of respiratory infections is influenced by several factors. For all known pathogens, strain virulence and total exposure dose are important in determining clinical disease and its severity. Young kittens are most often affected with severe clinical signs, and mortality is much higher than in adults. Concurrent infections with potential pathogenic bacteria such as *P. multocida* or immunosuppressive viruses such as feline leukemia or panleukopenia can also influence outcome.

FRV often causes a more severe clinical disease than the other respiratory infections. Mortality rates in young kittens or neonates can reach 70%. Surviving kittens are prone to chronic upper respiratory infection manifested as persistent or recurrent nasal discharge. Even so, many FRV infections, particularly in adults, are mild and transient or subclinical.

FCV causes typically less severe illness than FRV; a high proportion of strains are of

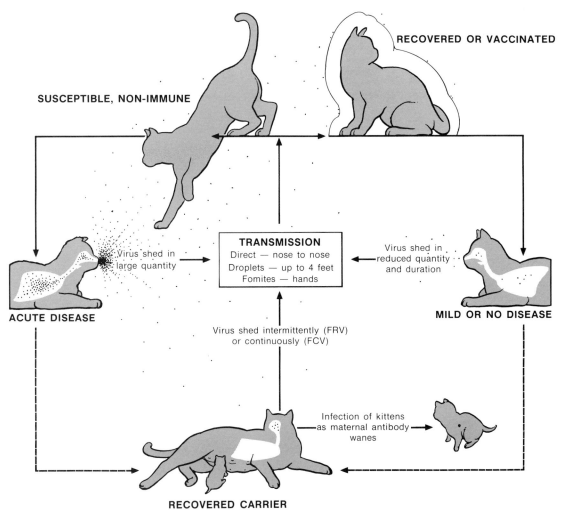

SUSCEPTIBLE, NON-IMMUNE

RECOVERED OR VACCINATED

TRANSMISSION
Direct — nose to nose
Droplets — up to 4 feet
Fomites — hands

Virus shed in
large quantity

Virus shed in
reduced quantity
and duration

ACUTE DISEASE

MILD OR NO DISEASE

Virus shed intermittently (FRV)
or continuously (FCV)

Infection of kittens
as maternal antibody
wanes

RECOVERED CARRIER

Figure 27–3. Cycles of transmission of FRV and FCV.

low virulence and produce asymptomatic infections. However, in some cattery outbreaks, mortality rates in kittens of 30% have been recorded. Acute deaths may occur within 24 to 48 hours.[15]

Chlamydiosis is not usually a fatal disease, although generalized infection may kill young kittens. Many infections are mild and go unnoticed. *Mycoplasma* seldom cause serious clinical infections. Lung involvement in kittens makes prognosis more guarded than in adults.

Immunity

Maternally-derived, primarily colostral antibodies are effective at protecting kittens during the first weeks of life. Serum antibody levels in kittens nursing immune queens rise rapidly in the first 72 hours of birth. During this time, intestinal absorption of immunoglobulin is rapidly curtailed. Exponential decay of this passive antibody occurs, with a half life of FRV antibody of 18.5 days, and antibody is gone by 2 to 10 weeks postpartum.[10] The protective activity of maternally derived immunity cannot be correlated with serum antibody levels. Kittens with antibody titers $> 1:4$ may become infected subclinically and can become latent carriers. Kittens with no detectable antibody can be protected.

Maternal antibody half-life for FCV is 15 days.[16] Most kittens have lost antibody between 10 and 14 weeks. As with FRV, kittens with maternal antibody may still become infected. Kittens born to FCV-carrier queens are often subclinically infected as early as 4 to 8 weeks of age.[17] There is no information

Table 27–1. Clinical Differentiation of Infectious Respiratory Diseases of Cats[a]

	RHINOTRACHEITIS	CALICIVIRUS	CHLAMYDIA	MYCOPLASMA
Incubation (days)	2–6	2–4	5–7	1–10
Severity	Often severe	Often subclinical, can be severe	Mild to moderate	Subclinical or mild
Ocular Signs	Bilateral conjunctivitis, chemosis; keratitis possible, discharge + + +	Mild conjunctivitis; discharge +	Unilateral conjunctivitis becomes bilateral; chemosis, no keratitis; discharge + +	Mild to moderate conjunctivitis; no keratitis; discharge + +
Nasal Signs	Paroxysmal sneezing; discharge + + +	Occasional sneezing; discharge +; ulceration of nasal philtrum	Sneezing; discharge ±	Occasional sneezing; discharge ±
Oral Cavity	Hypersalivation (viscous); occasional small ulcers on tongue, vesicles and ulcers in oropharynx	Lingual vesicles and ulcers, particularly anterior dorsum, also on hard palate	Nil	Nil
Lower Respiratory	Retching cough; dyspnea; pneumonia possible	No cough; pneumonia; with more virulent strains, mouth breathing	Rare pneumonia	Rare secondary pneumonia
Other Signs	Abortion; dehydration; weight loss	Diarrhea & vomiting; "limping syndrome"; interdigital ulceration on paws	Transient fever; anorexia	None
Chronic Signs	Persisting or recurrent keratitis; increased oculonasal discharge	Gingivitis; proliferative oropharyngeal lesions	Recurrent conjunctivitis	Low-grade persistent conjunctivitis; Rhinitis

[a]± = variable, mild; + = often mild; + + = usual, marked; + + + = usual, severe.

on maternally derived immunity to *Chlamydia* or *Mycoplasma*.

The active immune response to FRV involves both systemic and local humoral and cell-mediated factors. FRV-infected cells are lysed by antibody-complement lysis, antibody-dependent cell-mediated cytotoxicity, and direct cell-mediated cytotoxicity. Serum virus-neutralizing and glycoprotein antibodies increase during the course of recovery from infection.[17a] FRV-recovered cats are immune to reinfection for only a few weeks. Within as little as 3 months, reinfection can occur. Such reinfections are mild, or subclinical, with a reduced period of virus shedding. Initial virus-neutralizing antibody titers are low (1:2 to 1:16). Repeated exposure or resheding by carriers boosts titers. Cats with persistently high titers (≥1:256) should be suspected of being carriers. Cats without detectable virus-neutralizing titers may still resist challenge.

Virus-neutralizing antibody to FCV is detectable within 5 days of infection. Maximum (≤1:5000) titers are reached after 5 weeks. Antibody to heterotypic FCV strains is slower to develop and may not be detectable following primary infection. A second infection, particularly with another strain, boosts the heterotypic antibody as well as the antibody to the original infecting strain. A neutralizing titer of 1:16 or greater generally correlates with clinical protection against homologous and many heterologous strains, whereas titers of less than 1:7 are not protective against heterologous strains of FCV. As with FRV, protection is often incomplete. Some virus replication and shedding can still occur upon exposure of the cat. Limited studies on local, nasal antibody to FCV show an IgG rather than IgA component which is neutralizing.[18]

Immunity to *C. psittaci* is incomplete in recovered cats, and infections recur. The presence and level of serum antibody is poorly correlated with resistance. It is likely that cell-mediated and local (mucosal) immunity are more important.

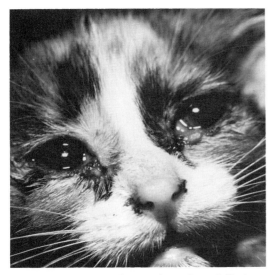

Figure 27–4. Mucopurulent ocular and nasal discharge in a kitten with upper respiratory disease.

Cats infected with M. *felis* develop high (1:10,000) serum titers of hemagglutination-inhibiting antibody or complement fixation (CF) antibody (1:320).[7] The protective significance of this is unknown.

CLINICAL FINDINGS

Clinical features of the various respiratory infections are summarized in Table 27–1.

Feline Rhinotracheitis

The typical case begins with intermittent sneezing that becomes paroxysmal. Fever exceeds 40°C (104°F), the cat is moderately depressed, and appetite is decreased or absent. There is bilateral conjunctival hyperemia and edema and protrusion of the nictitating membrane. Copious, initially serous discharges from eyes and nose become mucopurulent (Fig. 27–4). Crusting of these discharges can seal the eyelids shut and plug the external nares. Hypersalivation and oral ulceration may be present. Recovery begins by the fifth to seventh day and is generally rapid. Prognosis is guarded in cats remaining severely affected for more than 1 week.

Abortion or fetal resorption is expected in pregnant cats. This may be during the acute stage, or delayed by 1 or 2 weeks. In neonatal kittens, the infection can generalize, causing peracute death.

In young kittens, damage to upper respi-

ratory epithelium and osteolysis of nasal turbinates results in persistent or recurrent attacks of rhinitis with or without sinusitis. These kittens have recurrent bouts of sneezing and mucopurulent nasal discharge that are temporarily responsive to antibiotics. Short-nosed breeds have a more severe problem. Nasal deformities may be seen in kittens that develop atrophic rhinitis.

A rare manifestation of FRV is ulcerative dermatitis following ovariohysterectomy.[19, 20] Skin shaved in preparation for surgery was the site affected.[19]

Calicivirus

There is more clinical variation than with FRV. The typical case is less severe. Early signs are lethargy, a hunched appearance, dull and erect haircoat, and anorexia. Fever of up to 41.5°C (106.7°F) may fluctuate or be transient. Exaggerated respiration and open-mouthed breathing are frequent in young kittens.

Oral lesions are usual and begin as small vesicles, particularly on the anterior and lateral margins of the dorsum of the tongue. Rapid rupture leaves red circular erosions or ulcers; some of these coalesce to form large ulcerated areas (Fig. 27–5). These are

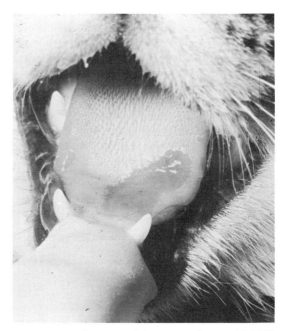

Figure 27–5. Ulceration of the tongue of a cat with FCV infection.

more marked in cats receiving a dry cat food.[21]

A "limping" syndrome characterized by stiffness, hyperesthesia, mild joint pain, and muscle soreness has been observed in naturally and experimentally infected kittens and older cats.[22] Affected cats lose their righting reflexes during the height of their fever. Full recovery occurs within a few days. Occasionally, generalized FCV infections can result in convulsions.[15] FCV antigen deposition has been detected in the joints of cats inoculated with virulent or vaccine virus.[22a] Virus could not be isolated from the synovial membranes, but immunoglobulins and complement deposition was found, suggesting an immune-complex pathogenesis.

The most frequent lesion in the carrier state is a persisting line of gingival reddening at the alveolar margin of the teeth that occurs in the absence of dental plaque accumulation or obvious periodontal disease. In other carriers, focal lymphoproliferative lesions occur on the gums or at the fauces of the throat (see also Necrotizing Ulcerative Gingivostomatitis, Chapter 9). A causal relationship between FCV and these apparently immune-related lesions has been suggested.[23, 23a]

Chlamydia

Conjunctivitis is the main feature of feline chlamydiosis (Fig. 27–6). Initially unilateral, the infection affects the other eye within a few days. The conjunctiva is edematous and chemotic. Close examination of the shining membrane may reveal small vesicles. There is excess lacrimation, and the discharge rapidly becomes purulent. At this time, the conjunctiva is hyperemic. Over several days, the amount of discharge decreases. Relapse is common in the absence of treatment. Chronic mucosal hyperplasia and prominent lymphoid follicle formation is seen. There is no corneal involvement. In neonatal kittens, a more generalized infection with signs of pneumonia is possible.[24]

Mycoplasma

Most often, mycoplasmas play a secondary role in feline respiratory disease. Conjunctivitis, which may persist over several

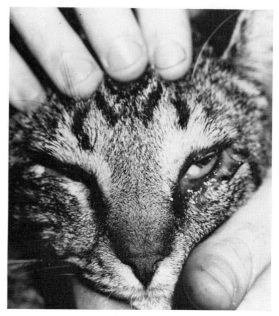

Figure 27–6. Chlamydial conjunctivitis.

weeks, is the most frequent clinical form of feline mycoplasmosis. The conjunctiva may be pale, normal, or hyperemic in appearance. In severe cases, there is papillary hypertrophy of the mucosa with edema and blepharospasm. A pseudodiphtheritic membrane may form. Sneezing and nasal discharge are mainly due to excess ocular discharge draining through the nasolacrimal duct.

DIAGNOSIS

More precise diagnosis usually is not attempted, but it is of relevance to be able to differentiate between the viral infections that are usually vaccinated against—*Chlamydia*, which may be vaccinated against and which requires specific treatment—and other bacterial infections.

There are no specific hematologic abnormalities. A neutrophilic leukocytosis with mild left shift is the most common finding.

Conjunctival smears are taken, under local anesthesia, by vigorous scraping from the inner surface of the nictitating membrane. They can be fixed with a cytologic fixative and stained with Giemsa to demonstrate chlamydial cytoplasmic inclusions as either amorphous or finely particulate initial bodies (3 to 5 μm diam.) or clumps of smaller elementary particles (0.5 to 1 μm) (Fig. 27–7). These may be small in number and require a careful search. Mycoplasmas appear as clusters of coccoid to coccobacillary organisms on or near the surface of epithelial cells. For FRV and FCV, fluorescent antibody techniques can be used. Intranuclear inclusions of FRV are transient and difficult to detect without special fixative (e.g., Bouin's) and hematoxylin and eosin (H and E) staining. For information on staining and fixatives used in the cytodiagnosis of feline respiratory diseases, see Appendix 12.

Laboratory Culture

For FRV and FCV, oropharyngeal swabs should be collected with vigorous rubbing of the tonsillar area. FRV may be found more consistently on nasal swabs.[25] Samples should be collected during the first week of illness. Frozen swabs are submitted in a viral transport media containing antibiotics to prevent bacterial overgrowth. Culture results may be obtained in 1 to 3 days after the inoculation of cell cultures.

Special transport media (e.g., balanced salt solution with 30 μM/ml dextrose, 100 μg/ml streptomycin, 100 μg/ml vancomycin, 10 μg/ml gentamicin, and 10% fetal calf serum) is

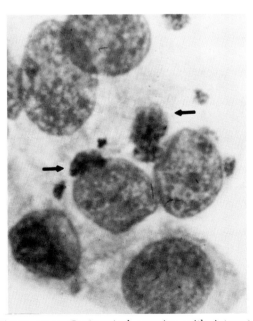

Figure 27–7. Conjunctival scraping with intracytoplasmic inclusions *(arrows)* typical of *Chlamydia* (Giemsa stain; × 1000).

used for *Chlamydia*. Egg or mouse inoculation is performed, and up to 1 week is required for results to be obtained. A genus-specific ELISA has been used to detect chlamydial infections in cats.[26]

Swabs for *Mycoplasma* isolation should be submitted in a bacteriologic transport medium such as Stuart's (Difco, Detroit, MI). Following initial isolation attempts on solid agar and on agar-broth combination, subculture is made to solid agar. Up to 3 weeks is required for results to be obtained.

Serologic Testing

Samples for serologic diagnosis should be collected as early as possible during the acute illness and again 1 to 2 weeks later from the convalescent cat. Microplate techniques have reduced the volume of serum needed to 1 to 1.5 ml. For FRV and FCV, a virus neutralization test in microtitration plates is used. Postinfection antibody titers with FRV are often low (1:8 to 1:64). For FCV, titers are variable (1:8 to 1:8000), depending on the degree of homology between the infecting virus and the virus challenge used in the neutralization test. As with all paired samples, a fourfold or greater rise in antibody between the acute and convalescent sample is diagnostic of active infection. The complement fixation test is used for *Chlamydia*. There is a common complement fixation (CF) antigen amongst all *Chlamydia* species. For *Mycoplasma*, metabolic inhibition, CF, or hemagglutination-inhibition (for *M. felis*) tests can be performed.

PATHOLOGIC FINDINGS

In fatal cases, secondary bacterial complications are likely to be present. Lung consolidation may be extensive in FRV or FCV. FRV produces more severe mucosal damage than FCV, with congestion and exudation that may extend the length of the trachea.

With FCV, apart from oral ulceration, gross upper respiratory tract pathology is minimal. The lungs are diffusely mottled dark red with congestion and edema. Later, foci of firm gray consolidation occur. There are unlikely to be gross pathologic changes with *Chlamydia* or *Mycoplasma*, apart from conjunctivitis.

With experience, microscopic cytologic changes with FRV are characteristic. However, unequivocal intranuclear inclusions are found only early in the infection, predominantly in mucosal epithelial cells of conjunctival, nasal or oropharyngeal mucosa. FCV does not cause inclusions, but the pneumonic lesions it produces are characteristic. There is an early exudative phase with multifocal infiltration of leukocytes between and within alveoli. There is some extravasation of fibrin and proteinaceous fluid. Large macrophages with foamy cytoplasm crowd alveoli. The second phase of FCV pneumonia is proliferative and interstitial. There is hypertrophy of type II alveolar pneumocytes. Alveolar spaces are lined with these polyhedral cells, which are two or more layers thick. During the resolution phase, lymphocytes and plasma cells accumulate adjacent to bronchioles.

Chlamydial conjunctivitis is dominated initially by neutrophilic infiltration and later by mononuclear cell response.[5] There is lymphoid follicular and epithelial hyperplasia. Chlamydial initial or elementary body inclusions are found in epithelial and mononuclear cells.

Mycoplasmal conjunctivitis is characterized by edema and mixed cell infiltrate of polymorphs, lymphocytes, and macrophages. Papillary hyperplasia of the epithelium occurs.

THERAPY

Drug dosages used in the management of feline respiratory diseases are listed in Table 27–2. The acute FVR case, or the severely FCV-affected cat, should be initially assessed for cyanosis and dehydration. Oxygen administration by face mask gives prompt alleviation of cyanosis. Obstructive dyspnea due to blocking of the upper or lower respiratory tract with secretions and exudates may be relieved by phenylephrine hydrochloride (NeoSynephrine, Winthrop, New York, NY) or oxymetazoline hydrochloride (Alfrin, Schering, Kenilworth, NJ) administered by drops or nebulizer (e.g., de Vilbiss hand-held or ultrasonic model) into a closed cage. Mucolytic drugs such as acetylcysteine (Mucomyst, Mead Johnson Laboratories, Evansville, IN) may be helpful in older cats with protracted illness and thick exudates. In most cases, however, conservative aerosol therapy using a vaporizer or nebulizing

0.45% or 0.9% saline solution gives sufficient relief.

Dehydration should be counteracted with lactated Ringer's solution. In severe cases, fluid is given IV, otherwise SC or IP. In mild cases, oral therapy with a glucose-electrolyte formulation is sufficient. ·Benzodiazepines such as diazepam may be used as an appetite stimulant in cats that refuse to eat.

Antibiotics are specifically indicated in treatment of known or suspected chlamydiosis or mycoplasmal infections. Chlamydiae are susceptible to tetracyclines or tylosin. Chlortetracycline or oxytetracycline ophthalmic ointments should be applied for 10 days beyond the remission of clinical signs to prevent recurrence. The use of soluble tetracycline powders in the food at 50 mg/day for 1 month may help to prevent recurrent infection. Mycoplasmas are also susceptible to tetracyclines, as well as to tylosin, chloramphenicol, gentamicin, and spiramycin.

For secondary bacterial complications in FRV or FCV infections, antibiotic therapy should be based on identity and susceptibility of the organisms. Tetracylines and chloramphenicol are useful broad-spectrum antibiotics in mature cats with respiratory disease but should be avoided in kittens. Chloramphenicol should not be given for more than 7 days. Tetracyclines may cause fever, anorexia, and vomiting at higher dosages in cats. Ampicillin is a useful first choice in kittens.

Supportive nursing care is vital in hastening recovery. After acute phase illness, recovery occurs best at home. Inappetence may be overcome by feeding strong-smelling foods and hand-feeding, but stomach-tubing may be necessary. Diazepam or oxazepam, used just prior to feeding, can overcome anorexia. Vitamin B may help stimulate the appetite, and Vitamins A and C may aid in mucosal repair.

Special therapy may be necessary for ocular complications (see Chapter 13). FRV-keratitis responds to local administration of the idoxuridine-containing antiviral drugs, but repeated use is sometimes irritating (see Chapter 15, Idoxuridine and Table 15–1). In cases in which there is descemetocele, symblepharon, ankyloblepharon, or pseudopterygium, surgical measures may be necessary.[27] Although clinically available (see Interferons, Chapter 15), human α-interferon has presently been shown to be effective

Table 27–2. Therapy of Feline Upper Respiratory Syndrome[a]

TOPICAL DRUG[b]	CONCENTRATION	METHOD	AMOUNT	INTERVAL (hours)
Phenylephrine	0.25–0.5%	IN drops, nebulizer	2 drops	8–24
Oxymetazoline	0.25%	IN drops	1 drop	24
Acetylcysteine	10%	Nebulizer for 30 min	20–50 ml/hr	12
Tetracycline	0.5%	Ophthalmic ointment	Small amount OU	8
Idoxuridine	0.1% solution 0.5% ointment	Ocular drops/ Ointment	1–2 drops OU	4–8

SYSTEMIC DRUG	DOSE[c] (mg/kg)	ROUTE	INTERVAL (hours)	DURATION (days)
Tetracycline	20	PO	8	7–10
Chloramphenicol	15	PO	8	7
Amp(amox)icillin	10	PO	8	7
Tylosin	10	PO	8	5
Gentamicin[d]	2	IM	8	5
Diazepam	2.5	PO, IV, IM	24	prn
Vitamin A	5000 U	PO	24	5–10
Vitamin B complex	1–2 ml	IM, IV	72	prn
Vitamin C	250 mg (total)	PO	6–12	5–10
Diazepam	2–5 (total)	IV(PO)	24	prn

[a]IN = intranasal, OU = each eye, PO = oral, IM = intramuscular, IV = intravenous, prn = as needed.
[b]Duration of treatment as needed.
[c]Dose per administration at specified interval, expressed as mg/kg unless otherwise stated.
[d]Avoid in neonates; make sure animal is adequately rehydrated and not azotemic prior to use.

only in reducing the severity of clinical signs in FVR-infected cats when given parenterally, early or prior to infection, and in high (10^8 U/kg) dosages.[28]

PREVENTION

Vaccination

At one time, vaccination against respiratory viruses of cats was regarded as impossible because of the short-term solid immunity following natural infections, particularly with FRV, and the perception of multiple serotypes of FCV. Later, it was recognized that FRV vaccine–induced immunity, although not complete, was effective at controlling reinfections and that FCV isolates shared sufficient antigens to provide a reasonable degree of cross-protection. FRV and FCV antigens are now routine components, along with feline panleukopenia, in feline vaccines. Some combinations also include rabies and chlamydial antigens. A combination with feline leukemia antigen might be anticipated. For information on vaccination additional to that given below, see Feline Respiratory Disease, Chapter 2 and Appendices 2 and 4.

Both MLV and inactivated-virus vaccines have been marketed. MLV vaccines contain FRV strains that grow very poorly at body temperature. Live FRV vaccines inoculated SC or IM replicate very little, and the immune response on respiratory epithelium is not strong. Local, IN administration results in strong and rapid (48 to 96 hours) but short-lived local immunity.[25] Postvaccinal sneezing and ocular discharge often occur with IN vaccine. However, live vaccine, intended for IM or SC use, can initiate upper respiratory infection when inadvertently aerosolized or spilled onto the hair coat during vaccination. Furthermore, spread of MLV-FCV vaccine virus to the oropharyngeal tissues following parenteral inoculation has been demonstrated.[22a] This may occur in cats with pre-existing antibody titers to the virus.

Inactivated-virus respiratory vaccines can be ineffective if not carefully prepared. They must be rich in viral antigen and adjuvanted. Effective inactivated vaccines with these attributes, including a vaccine with two complementary FCV strains, are also available.[14, 28a]

Chlamydial vaccines have been improved, with cell culture vaccine replacing the earlier yolk sac–propagated type. Although reasonably effective, protection is not complete. Vaccines give significant reduction in severity and duration of clinical signs in challenged cats for up to 1 year.[29, 30] Although it is being marketed in combined products, vaccination for *Chlamydia* is only necessary in catteries where the problem has been confirmed.

Most breeding queens have antibodies to FRV and FCV by virtue of vaccination and natural exposure. Therefore, maternally derived antibody will block successful vaccination until the antibody titer has fallen to a low level. Variation in antibody levels between and within litters and in FCV strains make it desirable to boost maternal immunity by prepartum vaccination between 1 to 4 weeks before queening. An inactivated vaccine is preferred for safety. An ideal kitten vaccination program begins at 6 weeks of age with repeat vaccinations at 9 and 12 weeks of age. If only two vaccinations are practical, the 9- and 12-week regime will give the best all-round results (see also Feline Respiratory Disease, Chapter 2, and Appendix 2). Programs can be varied depending on local experience. For best protection, a booster vaccination is given 6 months after the first course, and then at yearly intervals. If the vaccine used contains only a single FCV strain, broader FCV protection may be conferred by switching to a vaccine of a different manufacturer for booster vaccinations. There is no evidence to suggest that parenteral or intranasal vaccination in the presence of infection will reduce acute clinical illness or eliminate a pre-existing chronic carrier state.

Husbandry

Endemic respiratory disease is a frequent problem in any situation where large numbers of cats are housed together. This is a direct consequence of the ease and frequency with which carrier states can establish in cats following FRV and FCV infections.

Control of disease in a closed cat colony is based on preventing its introduction or on containing transmission. Under ideal circumstances, the cat colony that is free of FRV and FCV should be protected by physical barriers such as a clothes-changing room, disinfectant foot bath, use of gloves and mask, and positive–air pressure ventilation. Introduction of new cats should be minimized, and they should be quarantined for 2 weeks, during which time they should be cultured for FCV and FRV following a

course of glucocorticoid therapy (see The Carrier State).

For already infected colonies, the transmission cycle can be interrupted by separating kittens from their possible carrier mothers and other adult cats. Kittens should be weaned at 5 weeks, while they still likely have maternal antibody, and moved to a separate room. They should be vaccinated, beginning at 6 weeks of age. One IN-MLV and two parenteral inactivated vaccines can provide protection in young kittens (<9 weeks of age) that will have maternally derived antibody.[31] At 12 weeks of age, kittens can be moved to new homes or back into the colony.

In hospitals or boarding catteries, transmission is inhibited by preventing direct cat-to-cat contact and importantly, by washing hands, which are preferably gloved, between handling cats. These measures are more helpful than high ventilation rates (>20 air changes/hour) or UV lights.

PUBLIC HEALTH CONSIDERATIONS

Neither FCV nor FRV infects people, although antigenically related calicivirus[32] and herpesvirus[33] infections have been detected in dogs. *C. psittaci* of feline origin can cause conjunctivitis in people that can be chronic and must be treated (see also Public Health Considerations, Chapter 40). No cross-infection occurs between feline and human strains of *Mycoplasma*.

References

1. Scott FW, Kahn DE, Gillespie JH: Feline viruses: isolation, characterization and pathogenicity of a feline reovirus. *Am J Vet Res* 31:11–20, 1970.
2. Herrmann SC, Gaskell RM, Ehlers B, et al: Characterization of feline herpesvirus genome and molecular epidemiology of isolates from natural outbreaks and latent infections. *Curr Top Vet Med Anim Sci* 27:321–336, 1984.
3. Van Pelt CS, Crandell RA: Pancreatitis associated with a feline herpesvirus infection. *Companion Anim Pract* 1:7–10, 1987.
4. Povey RC: The preparation of a polyvalent feline calicivirus antiserum. *Can J Comp Med* 43:187–193, 1979.
5. Hoover EA, Kahn DE, Langlois JM: Experimentally induced feline chlamydial infection (feline pneumonitis). *Am J Vet Res* 39:541–547, 1978.
6. Tan RJS, Lim EW, Ishak B: Ecology of mycoplasmas

in clinically healthy cats. *Aust Vet J* 53:515–518, 1977.

7. Tan RJS: Susceptibility of kittens to *Mycoplasma felis* infection. *Jpn J Exp Med* 44:235–240, 1974.

8. Walton TE, Gillespie JH: Feline viruses VI. Survey of the incidence of feline pathogenic agents in normal and clinically-ill cats. *Cornell Vet* 60:215–232, 1970.

9. Wardley RC: Feline calicivirus carrier state. A study of the host/virus relationship. *Arch Virol* 52:243–249, 1976.

10. Gaskell RM, Povey RC: Transmission of feline viral rhinotracheitis. *Vet Rec* 111:359–362, 1982.

11. Gaskell RM, Povey RC: Experimental induction of feline viral rhinotracheitis virus re-excretion in FVR-recovered cats. *Vet Rec* 100:128–133, 1977.

12. Gaskell RM, Povey RC: Sites of feline viral rhinotracheitis replication and persistence in acutely and persistently infected cats. *Res Vet Sci* 27:167–174, 1979.

13. Ellis TM: Feline viral rhinotracheitis virus: explant and cocultivation studies on tissues collected from persistently infected cats. *Res Vet Sci* 33:270–274, 1982.

14. Povey RC, Wardley RC, Jessen H: Feline picornavirus infection. The in vivo carrier state. *Vet Rec* 92:224–229, 1973.

15. Love DN, Baker KD: Sudden death in kittens associated with feline picornavirus. *Aust Vet J* 48:643, 1972.

16. Johnson RP, Povey RC: Transfer and decline of maternal antibody to feline calicivirus. *Can Vet J* 24:6–9, 1983.

17. Johnson RP, Povey RC: Feline calicivirus infection in kittens borne by cats persistently infected with the virus. *Res Vet Sci* 37:114–119, 1984.

17a. Burgener DC, Maes RK: Glycoprotein-specific immune responses in cats after exposure to feline herpesvirus-1. *Am J Vet Res* 49:1673–1676, 1988.

18. Johnson RP: Immunity to feline calicivirus in kittens. PhD Diss, University of Guelph, Ontario, Canada, 1980.

19. Johnson RP, Sabine M: The isolation of herpesviruses from skin ulcers in domestic cats. *Vet Rec* 89:360–363, 1971.

20. Flecknell PA, Orr CM, Wright AI, et al: Skin ulceration associated with herpesvirus infection in cats. *Vet Rec* 104:313–315, 1979.

21. Johnson RP, Povey RC: Effect of diet on oral lesions of feline calicivirus infection. *Vet Rec* 110:106, 1982.

22. Pedersen NC, Laliberte L, Ekman S: A transient febrile "limping" syndrome of kittens caused by two different strains of feline calicivirus. *Feline Pract* 13(1):26–35, 1983.

22a. Bennett D, Gaskell RM, Mills A, et al: Detection of feline calicivirus antigens in the joints of infected cats. *Vet Rec* 124:329–332, 1989.

23. Thompson RR, Wilcox GE, Clark WT, et al: Association of caliciviruses with chronic gingivitis and pharyngitis in cats. *J Small Anim Pract* 25:207–210, 1984.

23a. Knowles JO, Gaskell RM, Gaskell CJ, et al: Prevalence of feline calicivirus, feline leukaemia virus and antibodies to FIV in cats with chronic stomatitis. *Vet Rec* 124:336–338, 1989.

24. Shewen PE, Povey RC, Wilson MR: Feline chlamydial infection: case report. *Can Vet J* 19:289–292, 1978.

25. Cocker FM, Gaskell RM, Newby TJ, et al: Efficacy of early (48- and 96-hour) protection against feline viral rhinotracheitis following intranasal vaccination with a live temperature sensitive mutant. *Vet Rec* 114:353–354, 1984.

26. Wills JM, Willard WG, Howard PE: Evaluation of a monoclonal antibody based ELISA for detection of feline *Chlamydia psittaci*. *Vet Rec* 119:418–420, 1986.

27. Spiess B: Symblepharon, Pseudopterygium und partielles Ankyloblepharon als Folgen feliner Herpes-Keratokonjunktivitis. *Kleintierpraxis* 30:149–152, 1985.

28. Cocker FM, Howard PE, Harbour DA: Effect of human alpha-hybrid interferon on the course of feline viral rhinotracheitis. *Vet Rec* 120:391–393, 1987.

28a. Tham KM, Studdert MJ: Antibody and cell-mediated immune responses to feline herpesvirus-1 following inactivated vaccine and challenge. *Zentralbl Veterinarmed* 34:585–597, 1987.

29. Shewen PE, Povey RC, Wilson MR: A comparison of the efficacy of a live and four inactivated vaccine preparations for the protection of cats against experimental challenge with *Chlamydia psittaci*. *Can J Comp Med* 44:244–251, 1980.

30. Kolar JR, Rude TA: Duration of immunity in cats inoculated with a commercial feline pneumonitis vaccine. *VM/SAC* 76:1171–1173, 1981.

31. Johnson RP, Povey RC: Vaccination against feline viral rhinotracheitis in kittens with maternally derived feline viral rhinotracheitis antibodies. *J Am Vet Med Assoc* 186:149–152, 1985.

32. Evermann JF, Bryan GM, McKeirnan AJ: Isolation of a calicivirus from a case of canine glossitis. *Canine Pract* 8(2):36–39, 1981.

33. Evermann JF, McKiernan AJ, Ott RL, et al: Diarrheal condition in dogs associated with viruses antigenically related to feline herpesviruses. *Cornell Vet* 72:285–291, 1982.

28 SYNCYTIUM-FORMING VIRUS INFECTION

Craig E. Greene

ETIOLOGY

Feline syncytium-forming virus (FeSFV) has been classified in the Retroviridae family, subfamily Spumavirinae. The prevalence of FeSFV infection is high in both normal and diseased cats; virus has been isolated from primary cultures of tissue and body secretions in up to 90% of a population.[1] More typically, the prevalence of infection in a cat population varies between 4% to 50%, depending on the age, geographic location, and local environment of cats.[2] Fifty percent or more of kittens born to FeSFV-infected queens are infected at birth;[2] and 15% of cultures in fetal cats are positive for the virus, suggesting that it can be transmitted vertically.[3] In utero infection probably occurs by the transfer of infected maternal leukocytes across the placenta but not through milk in lactating animals.[2]

In contrast to most feline infectious diseases, the infection rate in cat colonies is actually lower than that in the random cat population. Roaming or outdoor cats have the highest prevalence, suggesting contact through bite wounds.

FeSFV is a nuisance to virologists and manufacturers of feline vaccines because it is found in many tissues and cell cultures from normal cats that have been subjected to multiple passages. It is not usually present in primary cell cultures.[3a] FeSFV is difficult to distinguish from feline leukemia virus, which is visualized only as it buds from the cell. FeSFV forms a recognizable nucleocapsid within the cytoplasm prior to budding (see Fig. 26–10).

FeSFV derives its name from the fact that it produces multinucleated syncytia within 1 to 2 weeks of growth in certain rapidly multiplying tissue cultures. Cell lysis is rarely if ever noted, and intranuclear inclusions are never seen. Malignant transformation has been noted in tissue culture only in some instances.

PATHOGENESIS

Until very recently, FeSFV was not associated with any disease; many cats were infected both naturally and experimentally without clinical illness. The presence of the virus in 100% of cats affected with chronic progressive polyarthritis has been reported.[4] Concurrent feline leukemia virus infection was found in 70% of these cats. The prevalence of infection with both viruses was 2 to 10 times greater than that in age-matched cats not having chronic progressive polyarthritis. By altering the host immune system, feline leukemia virus may potentiate the ability of FeSFV to produce disease. Other factors must be involved as well since the disease cannot be induced by inoculation of FeSFV alone. Combined infections with FeSFV and feline immunodeficiency virus are also frequently found (see Chapter 26).

Arthritis, thought to result from chronic antigenic stimulation and immune-complex deposition, is characterized histologically by lymphoplasmocytic infiltrates and is temporarily responsive to immunosuppressive therapy. An inherent genetic tendency may explain why certain male cats are more prone to develop disease despite the high prevalence of these viral infections in the general population.

CLINICAL FINDINGS

Most infected cats are nonsymptomatic. Chronic progressive polyarthritis of cats affects males between 1.5 and 5 years of age.[4–7] Two forms of the disease have been described: one with osteoporosis and periarticular periosteal proliferation, the other with periarticular erosions, collapse of the joint space, and joint deformities. Lymphadenopathy, swollen joints, and stiff gait are seen in both types.

DIAGNOSIS

Joint fluid abnormalities consist of increased numbers of neutrophils and large mononuclear cells. That FeSFV stimulates antibody production in infected hosts has been used as the basis for immunodiffusion and IFA testing for antibody.[4, 8] Serology can be used in addition to blood cultures to screen cats for infection. Infected kittens can be detected at birth by culturing buffy coat cells from their peripheral blood. Animals are infected for life and develop persistent, nonprotective antibody titers to the virus. For this reason, cats showing a serologic response to the virus are presumed to be infected. Several strains may exist, and the actual prevalence of infection may be higher than indicated by seropositivity. Neonatal kittens born to infected queens loose their maternal antibody by 6 to 8 weeks of age, if they are not infected. Serum antibody titers will increase after this time if they become infected.[3]

Virus can be isolated from most tissues but requires one to four passages in vitro. FeSFV actually is only detected in vivo in cells and secretions of the oropharynx. Despite genetic material being supplied by the host, viral replication is suppressed. Latency can be expressed by cocultivating buffy coat WBC with fetal cat cells or by exposing cells to oropharyngeal secretions.

THERAPY AND PREVENTION

There is no known cure for chronic progressive polyarthritis, and the clinical and pathologic changes it causes usually are temporarily responsive for weeks to months to immunosuppressive therapy such as prednisolone (10 to 15 mg/day) and cytoxan (7.5 mg/day for 4 days each week). Cats identified as having polyarthritis should be eliminated from research projects and should be removed from vaccine production and specific pathogen-free colonies.

References

1. Hackett AJ, Pfiester A, Arnstein P: Biological properties of a syncytia-forming agent isolated from domestic cats (feline syncytia-forming virus). *Proc Soc Exp Biol Med* 135:899–904, 1970.
2. Pedersen NC: Feline syncytium-forming virus. In Appel MJ (ed): *Virus Infections of Carnivores.* New York, Elsevier, 1987, pp 329–335.
3. Hackett AJ, Manning JS: Comments on feline syncytia-forming virus. *J Am Vet Med Assoc* 158:948–954, 1971.
3a. Kukedi A, Bartha A, Nagy B: Latent infection with feline syncytial virus of cell cultures prepared from the kidneys of newborn kittens. *Vet Microbiol* 16:9–14, 1988.
4. Pedersen NC, Pool RR, O'Brien T: Feline chronic progressive polyarthritis. *Am J Vet Res* 41:522–535, 1980.
5. Pedersen NC, Pool R, O'Brien T, et al: Chronic progressive polyarthritis of the cat. *Feline Pract* 5:42–51, 1975.
6. Wilkinson GT, Robins GM: Polyarthritis in a young cat. *J Small Anim Pract* 20:293–297, 1979.
7. Moise NS, Crissman JW: Chronic progressive polyarthritis in a cat. *J Am Anim Hosp Assoc* 18:965–969, 1982.
8. Gaskin JM, Gillespie JH: Detection of feline syncytia-forming virus carrier state with a microimmunodiffusion test. *Am J Vet Res* 34:245–247, 1973.

29 FELINE PARAMYXOVIRUS ENCEPHALOMYELITIS

Craig E. Greene

Viruses of the family Paramyxoviridae (genera *Paramyxovirus* and *Morbillivirus*) have been shown to cause infections in the CNS of domestic and large exotic Felidae, although none of the viruses in this group are known to be primarily feline viruses. These infections differ from commonly known or suspected viral CNS infections of cats, such as feline panleukopenia (see Chapter 23), feline infectious peritonitis (see Chapter 24), or feline polioencephalomyelitis (see Chapter 90).

Avian Newcastle disease virus (a *Paramyxovirus*) has been experimentally inoculated into the CNS of domestic adult cats and kittens, producing disseminated encephalomyelitis.[1] Neonatal kittens could also be infected by intraocular or intranasal exposure to large quantities of virus. The incubation period of oculonasally administered virus was relatively long (11 to 17 days) compared with that following direct CNS inoculation (3 to 4 days). Clinical signs of encephalomyelitis were seizures, head tilt, and myoclonus. Progressive lower motor neuron paralysis developed in limbs and cranial nerve musculature, and in some affected animals, behavioral alterations were present. A disseminated nonsuppurative meningoencephalitis was found histologically; virus appeared to spread throughout the nervous system along descending and ascending neuronal pathways.

A paramyxovirus-like agent has also been isolated from the CNS of naturally infected cats that had focal demyelinating encephalitis and inclusion body formation.[2] The virus was isolated from affected cats by cocultivating CNS tissue with fetal feline kidney cell lines. The isolated virus, serologically unrelated to known paramyxoviruses, was inoculated into the CNS of neonatal mice that developed a similar encephalitis 5 months later.

Paramyxovirus-like nucleocapsids have also been observed by electron microscopy in explant cultures of CNS tissue from clinically healthy cats or those with demyelinating optic nerve lesions that were cocultured with feline kidney or Vero cell lines.[3] The significance of these ultrastructural findings is uncertain.

Nonsuppurative encephalitis has been reported in an adult Siberian tiger (*Panthera tigris*), in which intranuclear inclusion bodies detected on light microscopy and nucleocapsid material detected on electron microscopy were found to be similar to those of viruses of the family Paramyxoviridae.[4]

Canine distemper virus (a *Morbillivirus*) has been shown to infect a wide variety of terrestrial carnivores.[5] Domestic cats were experimentally inoculated, but clinical signs were absent (see Epidemiology, Chapter 16).[6] A chronic, progressive, nonsuppurative meningoencephalitis, clinically and pathologically similar to that caused by canine distemper virus in dogs, has been described in a Bengal tiger (*P. tigris*).[7] Marked increases in serum and CSF antibodies against canine distemper virus were found. Myoclonus was similar to that seen in other paramyxovirus-type infections in dogs and cats. Use of inactivated distemper virus vaccine has been recommended to protect large exotic Felidae against infection with this virus.[7] However, the efficacy of inactivated vaccines in dogs and other exotic carnivores, not to mention cats, has not been documented.[8]

References

1. Luttrell CN, Bang FB: Newcastle disease encephalomyelitis in cats. I. Clinical and pathological fea-

tures. *AMA Arch Neurol Psychiatr* 79:647–657, 1958.

2. Cook RD, Wilcox GE: A paramyxovirus-like agent associated with demyelinating lesions in the CNS of cats. *J Neuropathol Exp Neurol* 40:328, 1981.

3. Wilcox GE, Flower RLP, Cook RD: Recovery of viral agents from the central nervous system of cats. *Vet Microbiol* 9:355–366, 1984.

4. Gould DH, Fenner WR: Paramyxovirus-like nucleo-capsids associated with encephalitis in a captive Siberian tiger. *J Am Vet Med Assoc* 183: 1319–1322, 1983.

5. Appel MJ: Canine distemper virus. *In* Appel MJ (ed):

Virus Infections of Carnivores. New York, Elsevier, 1987, pp 133–159.

6. Appel M, Sheffy BE, Percy DH, et al: Canine distemper virus in domesticated cats and pigs. *Am J Vet Res* 35:803–806, 1974.

7. Blythe LL, Schmitz JA, Roelke M, et al: Chronic encephalomyelitis caused by canine distemper virus in a Bengal tiger. *J Am Vet Med Assoc* 183: 1159–1162, 1983.

8. Montali RJ, Bartz CR, Teare JA, et al: Clinical trials with canine distemper vaccines in exotic carnivores. *J Am Vet Med Assoc* 183: 1163–1167, 1983.

30 FELINE COWPOX VIRUS INFECTION

Malcolm Bennett
Rosalind M. Gaskell
Derrick Baxby

ETIOLOGY AND EPIDEMIOLOGY

Cowpox virus and the closely related cowpox-like viruses are members of the genus *Orthopoxvirus*, which includes smallpox virus (now eradicated), vaccinia virus (smallpox vaccine), and ectromelia virus (mousepox virus).[1,2] Cowpox virus is relatively resistant and can remain infective in dry conditions for several years. However, it is readily inactivated by most disinfectants, especially hypochlorites.

Cowpox and the cowpox-like viruses appear to be geographically limited to Europe,[1,2] where cowpox virus infection has been described sporadically in domestic cats,[3–6] cheetahs,[7] cattle, and people.[8,9] Cowpox-like viruses have been isolated from zoo-kept cats, wild rodents, and exotic herbivores.[2] The natural reservoir hosts in Western Europe are not known, but the epidemiologic evidence strongly indicates small wild mammals.[2,3,9,10] In Eastern Europe, a cowpox-like virus has been isolated from wild rodents.[2] Cats probably become infected while hunting, and most affected cats come from rural areas. However, occasional instances of cat-to-cat transmission may also occur.[3] There appears to be no sex or age predisposition to infection in cats.[3]

PATHOGENESIS

The most frequent route of infection in domestic cats is probably skin inoculation, possibly through a bite wound,[3] although experimental oronasal inoculation may also lead to clinical disease.[11] Following viral entry, local viral replication results in development of a primary skin lesion. Viral spread to the draining lymph nodes gives rise to a leukocyte-associated viremia and the subsequent development of widespread secondary skin lesions.[11]

During the viremic period, large amounts of virus also can be isolated from the respiratory tract. Mild upper respiratory disease is observed in approximately 20% of infected domestic cats,[3] and fatal pneumonia frequently develops in cheetahs.[7]

CLINICAL FINDINGS

Cowpox virus infection in cats typically causes widespread skin lesions, but most cats have a history of a single primary skin lesion, usually situated on the head, neck, or a forelimb. Since primary lesions often are complicated by concurrent bacterial infection and may vary from a small superficial scabbed-over wound to a large abscess or cellulitis of an entire limb, cowpox is rarely suspected at this stage of the disease.

The characteristic secondary skin lesions generally develop 1 to 3 weeks after appearance of the primary lesion. First apparent as small epidermal nodules randomly distributed over the body, the secondary lesions increase in size over 3 to 5 days to form well-circumscribed ulcers (1 cm diameter), which soon become scabbed (Fig. 30–1). The scabs gradually dry and after 3 to 4 weeks, begin to exfoliate to reveal small areas of healing epithelium beneath.[3,4] New hair growth soon occurs, although some lesions

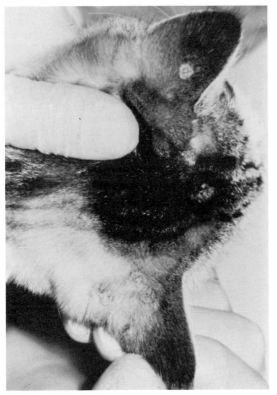

Figure 30–1. Scabbed secondary cowpox lesions on the head of a cat.

may result in small, permanently bald patches.

Many cats show no clinical signs other than skin lesions. When signs of systemic illness occur, they are usually mild and are first observed during the viremic period just prior to development of secondary skin lesions. Cats may be pyrexic, inappetent, or depressed; a few may have coryza or transient diarrhea. More severe disease, including clinical pulmonary disease, is rare and is often associated with either severe bacterial infection or immune dysfunction resulting from some preexisting debilitating disease, such as feline leukemia virus, feline immunodeficiency virus (FIV; feline T lymphotropic virus, FTLV) infection, or glucocorticoid treatment.[3,12] Severely ill cats have a poor prognosis, and euthanasia may be advised.

DIAGNOSIS

A laboratory diagnosis can be reached by viral isolation, serologic methods, or histologic examination. Dried scab material can safely be sent to the laboratory by mail without any need for transport medium. Cowpox virus can be readily isolated in a variety of cell cultures. Viral isolation is the most sensitive means of establishing a diagnosis. In at least 70% of cases, a presumptive diagnosis can be made by examining scab homogenates with an electron microscope.[12] Serum antibodies can be detected by hemagglutination inhibition (HI), virus neutralization (VN), complement fixation, and ELISA. HI antibody is detectable earlier in infection than VN and is also more indicative of recent infection. See Appendix 8 for a listing of diagnostic tests and the laboratories that perform them.

The histologic appearance of feline cowpox virus infection is quite characteristic.[4,11] Epithelial hyperplasia and hypertrophy is seen at the lesion periphery, with multilocular vesicle formation and ulceration toward the center. Many infected cells contain intracytoplasmic, eosinophilic inclusion bodies. Typical histologic changes may be difficult to see following extensive bacterial infection or in healing lesions, but immunostaining techniques can often make diagnosis possible in these cases.[4,11,13]

TREATMENT AND PREVENTION

There is no specific treatment for feline cowpox virus infection. Broad-spectrum antibiotics are recommended to control secondary bacterial infection, and general supportive therapy, including fluids, may sometimes be necessary. Glucocorticoids are contraindicated, as they have been associated with exacerbation of the condition.[3]

No vaccine is currently available, but the use of vaccinia virus may be considered for valuable zoo collections. Vaccinia virus has been used to vaccinate elephants in zoos, and appears to be of low pathogenicity in cats,[11] but its effects in other feline species have not been investigated.

PUBLIC HEALTH CONSIDERATIONS

Cowpox virus is infectious to people and in addition to a painful skin lesion, may cause severe systemic illness requiring hospitalization.[9] The very young, the elderly, and those with a preexisting skin condition or immune deficiency seem particularly at risk. In several recent human outbreaks, cats have been implicated as the source of infection.[8,14,15] Smallpox vaccination may not provide protection against formation of the primary lesion of cowpox virus infection, although it might help prevent more severe disease. However, if basic hygienic precautions are taken, the risk of cat-to-human transmission is small and, with a few exceptional cases, does not warrant euthanasia of the infected cat.

References

1. Baxby D: Poxviruses. In Brown F, Wilson GT (ed): *Topley and Wilson's Principles of Bacteriology, Virology, and Immunology*, vol 4, ed 7. Baltimore, Williams & Wilkins, 1984, pp 163–182.
2. Marennikova SS, Shelukhina EM, Efremova EV: New outlook on the biology of cowpox virus. *Acta Virol (Praha)* 28:437–444, 1984.
3. Bennett M, Gaskell CJ, Gaskell RM, et al: Poxvirus infection in the domestic cat: some clinical and epidemiological observations. *Vet Rec* 118:387–390, 1986.
4. Gaskell RM, Gaskell CJ, Evans RJ, et al: Natural and experimental poxvirus infection in the domestic cat. *Vet Rec* 112:164–170, 1983.
5. Schonbauer M, Schonbauer-Langle A, Kobl S: Pockeninfektion bei einer Hauskatze. *Zentralb Veterinarmed B* 29:434–440, 1982.
6. Thomsett LRM, Baxby D, Denham EMH: Cowpox in the domestic cat. *Vet Rec* 103:567, 1978.
7. Baxby D, Ashton DG, Jones DM, et al: An outbreak of cowpox in captive cheetahs: virological and epidemiological studies. *J Hyg (Camb)* 89:365–372, 1982.
8. Anonymous. What's new pussycat? Cowpox. *Lancet* 2:668, 1986.
9. Baxby D: Is cowpox misnamed? A review of 10 human cases. *Br Med J* 1:1379–1381, 1977.
10. Baxby D, Gaskell RM, Gaskell CJ, et al: The ecology of orthopoxviruses and use of recombinant vaccinia vaccines. *Lancet* 2:850–851, 1986.
11. Bennett M, Gaskell CJ, Gaskell RM, et al: Studies on poxvirus infection in cats. *Arch Virol* 104:19–33, 1989.
12. Brown A, Bennett M, Gaskell CJ: Fatal poxvirus infection associated with FIV infection. *Vet Rec* 124:19–20, 1989.
13. Bennett M, Baxby D, Gaskell RM, et al: The laboratory diagnosis of *Orthopoxvirus* infection in the domestic cat. *J Small Anim Pract* 26:653–661, 1985.
14. Willemse A, Egberink HF: Transmission of cowpox virus infection from domestic cat to man. *Lancet* 1:1515, 1985.
15. Casemore DP, Emslie ES, Whyler DK, et al: Cowpox in a child acquired from a cat. *Clin Exp Dermatol* 12:286-287, 1987.

31 RABIES

Craig E. Greene
David W. Dreesen

ETIOLOGY

The virus of rabies is a member of the genus *Lyssavirus* in the family Rhabdoviridae. They are enveloped, bullet-shaped RNA viruses that usually measure 75 × 180 nm (Fig. 31–1). Rabies viruses that have been isolated worldwide were originally considered to belong to one common antigenic type. However, techniques using monoclonal antibodies produced against nucleocap-

sid or glycoprotein moieties have provided evidence for antigenic differences among various isolates among major wildlife hosts within a given geographic region.[1] Glycoprotein G, a surface antigen that elicits the production of serum-neutralizing antibody, which affords protection against the disease, is measured by virus neutralization testing and is contained in subunit vaccines. Slight changes in amino acid substitution in the glycoprotein cause the virulent virus to be-

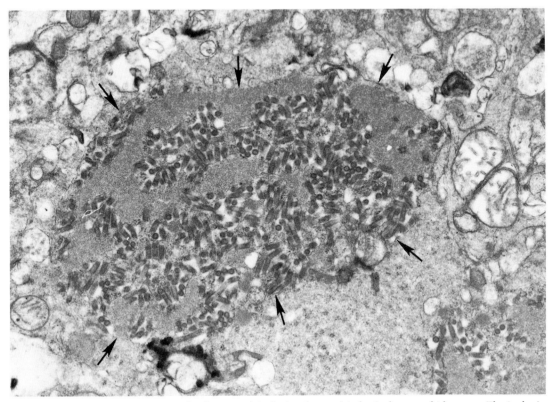

Figure 31–1. Electron photomicrograph of neuronal inclusion (*arrows*) in brain from a rabid mouse. The inclusion contains numerous bullet-shaped rhabdovirus particles (uranyl acetate and lead citrate, × 30,480). (Courtesy of Carey Callaway, Centers for Disease Control, Atlanta, GA.)

come nonpathogenic and to produce milder CNS lesions because of loss of neutralizing activity by antibody to this protein.[2, 3]

Rabies virus replicates by budding from the host cell membranes, and viral nucleocapsid develops in the cytoplasm. Complete viral particles may be formed at the cell surface, but more commonly, they bud from intracytoplasmic membranes. Free virus particles infect new or adjacent cells by fusing their envelopes with the host cell membrane, which allows direct entry of viral genetic material.

As an enveloped virus, rabies is destroyed by various concentrations of formalin, phenol, halogens, mercurials, mineral acids, and other disinfectants. It is extremely labile when exposed to UV light and heat.

Rabies virus remains viable in a carcass for less than 24 hours at 20°C, although it survives much longer (days) when the body of the victim is refrigerated. Immunofluorescent testing, commonly used for rabies diagnosis, does not depend on the presence of viable viral particles; thus, viral antigen may be detected for periods beyond the presence of viable virus. Virus survival can be greatly increased in unrefrigerated tissue by storing it in 50% glycerol at room temperature or in pure glycerol at 4°C. Preservation can also be enhanced if a 20% suspension of infected tissue or virus culture is made with a solution that is high in protein or amino acids. Storage at ultra-low temperatures ($-30°$ to $-80°C$) prolongs virus survival for years in untreated fresh-frozen tissue. However, freezing samples in a household freezer with subsequent thawing will damage the tissue and destroy the virus for subsequent detection.

EPIDEMIOLOGY

Susceptibility

All warm-blooded animals are vulnerable to infection with rabies virus; however, the degree of species susceptibility varies considerably. Foxes, coyotes, jackals, wolves, and certain rodents are among the most susceptible animal groups. Skunks, raccoons, bats, rabbits, cattle, and some members of the families Felidae and Viverridae have a high susceptibility. Groups with only moderate susceptibility include domestic dogs, sheep, goats, horses, and nonhuman primates. All birds and primitive mammals such as the opossum have low susceptibility. Cats are actually more resistant than dogs to experimental infection with naturally occurring rabies virus but are much more prone to develop infection with vaccine virus. Younger animals are usually more susceptible to rabies infection than older ones.

Transmission

The source of rabies infection is nearly always due to the bite of an infected animal that has rabies virus in its saliva. Other modes of transmission to be described are infrequently involved in infections of the dog and cat but may serve to maintain infection in wildlife. Transmission from exhaled or excreted virus has been suggested in large colonies of cave-dwelling bats[4] and in a laboratory outbreak among terrestrial animals.[5] Such airborne infections are probably only important among highly susceptible animals that live in high-density populations. Rabies can occasionally result from the ingestion of infected tissue or secretions.[6] Transplacental rabies infections in skunks, bats, and a cow also have been reported;[7] however, the ability of such in utero infections to be transmitted in later life is unclear. Environmental transmission by fomites is rarely, if ever, involved. Human rabies has been acquired by corneal transplantation, and the disturbing number of human rabies cases in which no obvious source of exposure can be determined argues against complacency when considering the routes of rabies virus transmission. Latent rabies infections with prolonged salivary shedding of virus do exist among some animal species, so that the absence of neurologic abnormalities cannot be used to rule out the possibility of rabies infection.

Hosts and Range

There are over 27,000 cases of animal rabies reported yearly in the world with the estimated actual number of cases being many times greater. Approximately 500 human cases of rabies are reported yearly, whereas the estimated number is thought to be well over 20,000. Recent reports suggest that over 20,000 human rabies deaths may occur in South Asian countries alone. This discrepancy probably is due to inaccurate diagnosis and reporting.[8] Antarctica, Australia, New Zealand, Taiwan, some of the Caribbean islands, England, Ireland, Spain, Norway, Sweden, Iceland, and Japan are presently free of rabies.

Throughout the world, in most of the Northern Hemisphere rabies is primarily a disease of wildlife, whereas in the Southern Hemisphere, the dog is the major species infected (Fig. 31–2).[9] Despite the fact that all warm-blooded animals are susceptible, rabies virus in a given enzootic area usually restricts itself to a single dominant reservoir species. For example, wildlife reservoir species are skunks, insectivorous bats, raccoons, and foxes in various geographic areas of the United States, foxes in Europe, and mongooses in South Africa and certain Caribbean islands. Rabies in enzootic areas appears to be cyclic. It spreads into unexposed, susceptible wildlife populations in the region, with subsequent decreases and increases in the incidence of disease caused by population mortality and immunity that cycle in the wildlife population. These wild animals serve as reservoirs for disease transmission to dogs, cats, cattle, and horses, the main domestic animals that expose people to the virus.

Dogs and Cats. The highest incidence of dog and cat rabies in the United States generally occurs in areas where wildlife rabies is epizootic (Figs. 31–3 and 31–4).[10] While the incidence of wildlife rabies in recent years has been on the increase, cases of human, canine, and farm animal rabies have been decreasing (Fig. 31–5).[10] Vaccination of dogs has been the main factor responsible for this decline. Although the incidence of dog rabies has declined, dogs account for the majority of animal bites in the United States, and for this reason people often seek antirabies prophylaxis. In underdeveloped nations, where dog rabies has not been controlled, the incidence of canine and human rabies is quite high. Although not yet achieved in these regions, adequate vaccination of at least 70% of dogs in a given population has been shown to block the occurrence of epizootics.

As in dogs, an increase in feline rabies usually relates to spillover of infection from wildlife. Since 1979, cat rabies cases in the United States have shown a slight increase over the previous 7-year period, and begin-

ning in 1981, more cases of rabies in cats than in dogs have been reported annually.[11] This increase probably reflects the low numbers of cats vaccinated for rabies and recent outbreaks of wildlife rabies in the mid-Atlantic region of the United States. The frequency of human rabies exposures attributed to rabid cats is now increasing at a greater rate than that associated with dogs. Rabid cats, which usually are reclusive, may attack humans and other animals when disturbed.

Skunks. The striped skunk (*Mephitis mephitis*), the most common skunk in the United States, is presently responsible for more reported animal rabies cases than any other single species and probably has the most important role in perpetuating wildlife rabies in this country. Although the spotted skunk (*Spilogale* sp.) was a serious rabies threat in the western United States during the 1800s, the involvement of this small, secretive animal is relatively minor at the present time. The incidence of skunk rabies in the United States is highest in California, the Midwest, and parts of the Middle Atlantic states (Fig. 31–6). Skunk and fox rabies became established in Ontario, Canada in the 1940s, and epizootics periodically affect the animal populations of this region.

The threat to people from rabid skunks is based upon the skunk's increased susceptibility to the virus, the high prevalence of rabies infection in the population, skunks' ability to live in proximity to humans, and the excretion of large quantities of virus in their saliva during the prolonged (4- to 18-day) period of clinical illness. Rabid skunks often attack anything that moves with extreme fury and frequently roam during daylight hours, unusual behavior for this nocturnal animal.

Long-term, subclinical rabies in skunks is a major concern with respect to maintenance of the infection in nature. Rabies antibodies have been found in clinically normal skunks. Skunks raised in extended periods of confinement have been found to be clinically infected with rabies.[12] This may have resulted from prior infection with latency or from congenital infection combined with a prolonged incubation period.

Foxes. Foxes are important reservoirs in the ecology of wildlife rabies throughout the Northern Hemisphere. Fox rabies epizootics

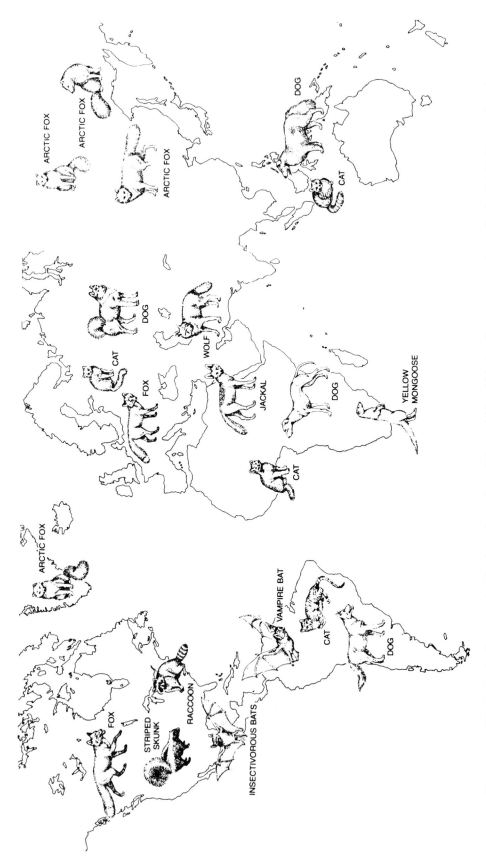

Figure 31–2. Principal animal vectors of rabies for major regions of the world in which the disease appears. Australia, the British Isles, and much of Scandinavia are free of rabies. (From Kaplan MM, Koprowski H: Rabies. *Sci Am* 242:120–234, 1980. Reprinted with permission. Copyright © 1980 by Scientific American, Inc. All rights reserved.)

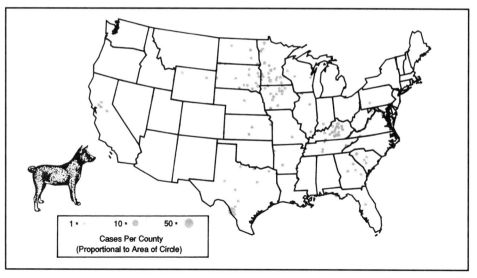

Figure 31–3. Location of counties in the United States reporting dog rabies in 1988. (From Centers for Disease Control: *MMWR* 34[SS–4], 1988.)

may be due to stress and increased contact resulting from periodic overpopulation of this species. The prevalence of the disease seems to decline when fox populations are reduced to levels in balance with available resources through either natural mortality or fox population reduction programs. Oral vaccination programs, using modified-live vaccine placed in food bait, have been used with some success to control red fox (*Vulpes vulpes*) rabies in Europe.[13]

In North America, fox rabies occurs throughout the range of the red fox, the gray fox (*Urocyon cinereoargenteus*), and the arctic fox (*Alopex lagopus*), with greatest prevalence in the province of Ontario in Canada. The outbreak occurring in upstate New York is an extension of the Canadian fox epidemic. Rabies among arctic foxes is a threat to humans and sled dogs throughout the arctic tundra.

Rabid foxes may exhibit furious or paralytic manifestations of the disease; however, the disease is invariably fatal; latency does not develop. Despite the shorter course of clinical illness, foxes can effectively trans-

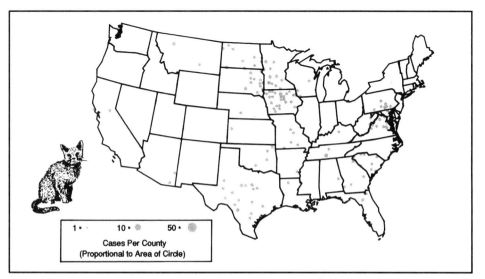

Figure 31–4. Location of counties in the United States reporting cat rabies in 1988. (From Centers for Disease Control: *MMWR* 34[SS–4], 1988.)

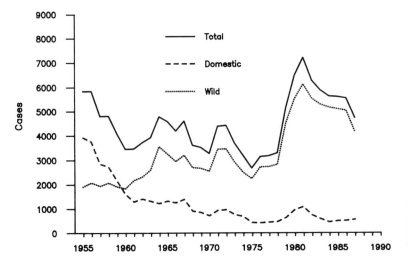

Figure 31–5. Cases of rabies in wild and domestic animals by year, United States, 1955–1987. (From Centers for Disease Control: *MMWR* 34[SS–4], 1988.)

mit the virus to other species, but human postexposure prophylaxis from direct exposure to rabid foxes is extremely low.

Raccoons. Prior to the early 1960s, rabies was not a serious problem among raccoons in the United States. However, during the 1950s the occurrence of rabid raccoons began to rise dramatically in Florida and soon spread to Georgia. By the 1970s rabies became enzootic in these states. Raccoon rabies advanced northward steadily and by 1980 included portions of Alabama and South Carolina. Virginia, West Virginia, Maryland, and Pennsylvania have reported a major raccoon rabies epizootic beginning in 1981,

owing to the translocation of infected animals from the Southeast (Fig. 31–7).[14, 15] From 1982 to 1984, the percentage of rabid raccoons of those submitted to the Department of Health of the State of Maryland increased from 8.0 to 57%.[16] Raccoons represented 77% of the total rabid animals in 1986 in the Middle Atlantic states.[11]

The danger of human exposure to rabid raccoons has increased in recent years, although to date there have been no confirmed human deaths associated with rabid raccoons. However, urban raccoon rabies is a constant threat in the United States owing to the large number of rabid raccoons in residential areas. Raccoons have adapted

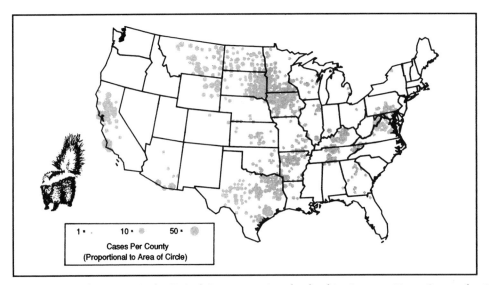

Figure 31–6. Location of counties in the United States reporting skunk rabies in 1988. (From Centers for Disease Control: *MMWR* 34[SS–4], 1988.)

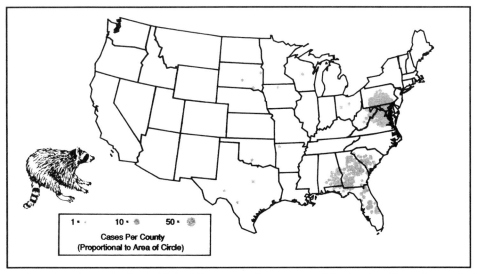

Figure 31–7. Location of counties in the United States reporting raccoon rabies in 1988. (From Centers for Disease Control: *MMWR* 34[SS–4], 1988.)

well to suburban and semiurban environments. At high population densities, the stresses of intraspecific crowding and competition for limited resources may allow for easy transmission of the virus.

Bats. Rabies in North American bats was first recognized in the early 1950s, but studies suggest that rabid bats were in this region much earlier. The ability of bats to disseminate rabies is based on a protracted clinical course rather than a subclinical carrier state. Subclinical infections could progress to more advanced clinical disease during times of stress, changes in metabolic rate, as with the cessation of hibernation, or changes in ambient temperature.

Rabid insectivorous bats in the United States rarely have attacked people. Most people are bitten by handling a rabid bat that has fallen to the ground or has been found in a building. Rabies has been transmitted to people working in a cave occupied by large numbers of insectivorous bats. Insectivorous bats might be considered a source of infection for terrestrial animals that inadvertently come into contact with them. However, there are few authenticated cases of rabies transmission to dogs and cats by insectivorous bats,[17] and studies using monoclonal antibodies indicate that bat rabies in a geographic region is independent of the persistent enzootic foci of rabies in terrestrial animals.[1, 14, 18]

Vampire bats, which feed exclusively on blood, are a major rabies threat to people and animals in Mexico, Central America, and parts of South America. Over 500,000 cases of cattle rabies attributed to vampire bats occur annually in Latin America. Their biting during routine nightly feeding makes them extremely effective in transmitting rabies virus, and the presence of rabies in vampire bats parallels that seen in insectivorous bats and terrestrial animals. Although the vampire bat is not found in North America except for Mexico, the use of the same cave by rabies-infected vampire bats and North American insectivorous bats on their southward migration may be a major source of infection for bats in the United States.

Rodents and Lagomorphs. The incidence of clinical rabies among rats, mice, squirrels, and rabbits and hares is extremely low. An increased incidence of rabies in woodchucks in the Middle Atlantic states since 1981 has been confirmed by monoclonal antibody studies to be caused by the same viral variant associated with the outbreak in raccoons in that area.[19] Isolated cases of unprovoked attacks on people by rabid rodents and rabbits have occurred.[20] Rodents and rabbits account for a high percentage of animal bites to people, but no cases of human rabies have ever been associated with these species.[21] Rodents are extremely susceptible to experimental infection with rabies virus but are rarely determined to be infected under natural circumstances. They may not survive the attack by a rabid carnivore. Generally, these species are not routinely examined for rabies in public health laboratories.

PATHOGENESIS

The incubation period of rabies is variable and depends upon such factors as the site of the bite, the amount of virus introduced, and the species that is bitten. Rabies is unique in that the incubation period, which is relatively prolonged compared with other infectious diseases, is primarily a result of the route of virus entry into and spread within the CNS (Fig. 31–8).

Entry of Virus

Following IM inoculation, virus replicates locally in myocytes that serve as amplifying sources and spreads to neuromuscular junctions and neurotendinal spindles after a variable period of days or weeks. There is no detectable viremia. Virus spreads by retrograde (centripetal) intra-axonal flow in peripheral nerves. The transport period up the

peripheral system in infected dogs and people usually requires a minimum of 21 days, but this depends upon the age of the bitten individual, the degree of innervation of the bite site, the distance from the point of inoculation to the spinal cord or brain, the strain and amount of virus introduced, post-exposure treatment, and other factors. The greater the degree of innervation at the site of the bite, the shorter the incubation period.

Although uncommon, infection by other routes is possible. Following intranasal exposure, virus enters the trigeminal nerves and ganglia in its course to the CNS. The cribriform plate and olfactory bulbs have been suggested as a route of spread, but this is not well documented. After being ingested, the virus has been shown to infect cells of the oral mucosa, taste buds, and pulmonary system (by aspiration), and intestinal mucosa. From these sites, it migrates up branches of the cranial nerves and spreads to the brain stem.

In naturally occurring cases of rabies, ranges of incubation periods before CNS signs are seen have been reported to be 3 weeks to 6 months (average, 3 to 8 weeks) in dogs, 2 to 6 weeks in cats, and 3 weeks to 12 months (average 3 to 6 weeks) in people.

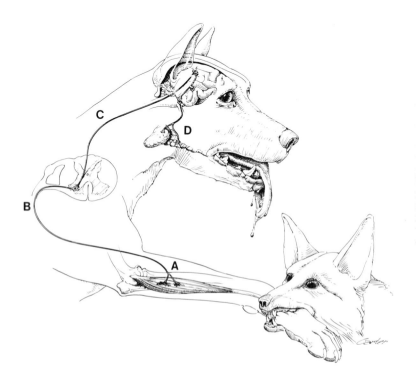

Figure 31–8. Pathogenesis of rabies virus infection. Rabies virus replicates in myocytes and spreads to motor nerve endings (A). Retrograde intra-axonal (centripetal) spread to the CNS occurs in peripheral nerves (B). Virus replicates in spinal cord neurons and spreads rapidly (probably by CSF flow) throughout the nervous system, causing progressive lower motor neuron paralysis (C). Virus enters the brain, causing cranial nerve deficits and behavioral changes. Virus spreads centrifugally in peripheral and cranial nerves, from which it enters the saliva (D) and other tissues.

Spread in CNS

After the virus begins its progression in the CNS, usually in the spinal cord, movement to the brain is rapid. Interneuronal spread of virus corresponds to the progression of clinical signs that are noted. The virus enters the spinal cord or brain stem ipsilateral to the site of initial virus inoculation. The infection then spreads to involve the contralateral neurons and ascends bilaterally in the spinal cord or brain stem to the forebrain, presumably by CSF pathways. Damage to the motor neurons causes progressive lower motor neuron (LMN) disease that in turn produces the typical flaccid paralysis of rabies infection and an ascending paralysis. Damage to the CNS caused by rabies virus has been attributed to direct viral invasion of the nervous system. Host immune responses to rabies virus may accentuate the inflammation and degeneration of nervous tissue.[21a]

Spread from CNS

Following replication within the CNS, the virus moves to other body tissues via the peripheral, sensory, and motor nerves. Both visceral and somatic portions of cranial and spinal cord nerves become involved, including the autonomic nervous system. Virus also spreads via cranial nerves to the salivary glands at this time. The spread of virus into saliva indicates that the brain has already been infected.[22] Although virtually every body tissue may be infected, centrifugal spread in the peripheral nervous system does not occur in all cases. Death may occur prior to salivary involvement. The rate (from 20% to 88% positive) of salivary gland infection also varies, depending on the species infected.

Chronic or Latent Infections

It is now recognized that in rare instances rabies can be prolonged and subclinical in nature and that recovery in dogs and in cats is possible.[23, 24] Recovery in people has been exceedingly rare.[25] In many instances, it may be difficult to demonstrate virus and to determine whether prolonged incubation, chronic infection, or complete recovery has occurred. Recovery or chronic disease following infection has been associated with high titers of antirabies virus antibody in the CSF and CNS tissue. The final outcome in rabies infections—death or recovery—is determined by host immunity and virus factors. Adequate serum titers of antirabies virus antibody, acquired by active or passive immunization, have been correlated with protection against infection and restricted viral replication.[26] However, humoral immunity is not as important as cell-mediated immunity in the eventual elimination of rabies virus.[27] Immunosuppression caused by stress or chemotherapy has worsened the clinical illness in rabies-infected animals.[26]

Excretion of Rabies Virus

Typically, virus excretion occurs for a brief period prior to the onset of neurologic signs and continues until the animal dies in 20 days or less. Most public health laws require a 10-day observation period following a bite from a suspected dog or cat because the period of virus shedding prior to neurologic signs was thought to be 1 to 5 days. Experimentally, rabies-infected dogs have been shown to shed virus in their saliva up to 13 days prior to the onset of neurologic signs, so that the 10-day observation period may have to be changed to 3 weeks. Dogs that develop neurologic signs and die suddenly actually may have lower concentrations of virus in their brains and salivary glands than those that live longer. At times, experimentally infected dogs have recovered completely from neurologic deficits but have excreted the virus in their saliva for 2 to 6 months thereafter.[23, 28] However, the amount of virus shed is exceedingly small, and the public health implication of the observation has not been determined and may, in fact, be nonexistent.[29]

CLINICAL FINDINGS

Rabies virus infection has classically been divided into three major stages: **prodromal**, **furious**, and **paralytic**. The classification and progression of infection is artificial, since rabies can be quite variable in its presentation and **atypical** signs are commonly seen. Not all animals progress through all the clinical stages, and subclinical, chronic, and recovered infections have been described.

Dogs and Cats

The **prodromal** phase in dogs usually lasts for 2 to 3 days, and apprehension, nervousness, anxiety, solitude, and variable fever may be noted. Friendly animals become shy or irritable and may snap, whereas fractious ones may become more docile and affectionate. Pupillary dilation with or without sluggish palpebral or corneal reflexes may become apparent. Most animals will constantly lick the site of viral inoculation. Some dogs may develop pruritus at the site of exposure and claw and chew at the area until it is ulcerated. The behavior of cats during the prodromal period is similar to that of dogs; however, cats more typically show unusual or erratic behavior for only a day or two.

The **furious** stage of the disease in dogs usually lasts for 1 to 7 days. Animals become restless and irritable and have increased responses to auditory and visual stimuli. They frequently become excitable, photophobic, and hyperesthetic and bark or snap at imaginary objects. As they become more restless, they begin to roam, usually becoming more irritable and vicious (Fig. 31–9). Dogs may eat unusual objects, especially wood (pica), which become gastrointestinal foreign bodies. Also, they may avoid contact with people or prefer to hide in dark or quiet places. When caged or confined, the dog often tries to bite or attack its enclosure. They usually develop muscular incoordination, disorientation, or generalized grand mal seizures during this phase. If they do not die during a seizure, they may progress to a short paralytic stage and then succumb.

Cats more consistently develop the furious phase of the disease, showing erratic and unusual behavior. When confined in cages, they may make vicious striking movements and attempt to bite or scratch at moving objects. In addition, they may have muscular tremors and weakness or incoordination. Some cats may run continuously until they die of exhaustion.

The **dumb** or **paralytic** phase of rabies usually develops within 2 to 4 days (range 1 to 10) after the first clinical signs are noted. LMN paralysis usually progresses from the site of injury until the entire CNS is involved. Cranial nerve paralysis may be the first recognizable clinical syndrome if the bite occurs on the face. When the brain stem becomes affected, a change in the tone of the bark, resulting from laryngeal paralysis, may be observed. Dogs may begin to salivate or froth excessively as a result of their inability to swallow and the deep labored respiration that occurs. A "dropped jaw" develops as a result of paralysis of the masticatory muscles. Dogs may make a choking sound, which makes an owner think that something is caught in the animal's throat. Owners or veterinarians may then become exposed to the virus in the saliva in attempting to remove a suspected foreign object. The course of the paralytic phase usually lasts 2 to 4 days. The animal often goes into a coma and dies of respiratory failure.

The paralytic disease in cats often follows the furious form of the disease and begins around the fifth day of clinical illness. As in dogs, initial paralysis of the bitten extremity can progress to paraparesis, incoordination, and ascending or generalized paralysis, terminating in coma and death. Mandibular and laryngeal paralysis is less common in cats. Cats occasionally develop the paralytic form directly after the prodromal phase with little or no signs of excitement.

Atypical, abortive forms of rabies virus infection may possibly be more common than previously realized but still are considered rare phenomena. Experimentally infected dogs that developed acute progressive LMN paralysis have shown clinical improve-

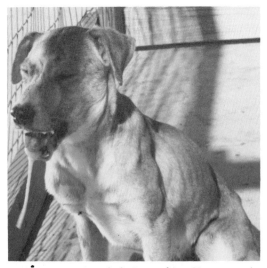

Figure 31–9. Dog with furious rabies. Note excessive salivary secretions resulting from the inability to swallow.

ment a few days to months later.[27] Survival with chronic infection has been reported to occur following experimental rabies infection in cats, but clinical recovery from paralysis has not been observed.[24]

People

The clinical syndrome of rabies in people is similar in duration and variability to that in the dog and cat. Fever, headache, anxiety, nervousness, and hyperesthesia at the bite site have been reported. As the syndrome progresses to the excitable phase, clinical signs consist of excitability, restlessness, hyperkinesis, and violent behavior. Humans salivate incessantly and refuse to drink water. They experience painful pharyngeal spasms when attempting to swallow fluids, which gives rise to the term *hydrophobia*. As disorientation and excitability continue, some patients die in convulsive episodes, whereas others develop generalized LMN paralysis and respiratory arrest. Although the rare instance of recovery has been reported following extraordinary efforts,[25] the disease is considered to be invariably fatal following the onset of clinical signs.

DIAGNOSIS

Rabies is often suspected because of the neurologic abnormalities that are present in an affected animal. However, because of the atypical nature of the clinical signs that are now recognized, rabies should be considered in any animal that suddenly develops profound behavioral changes or features of LMN paralysis or both.

No hematologic or serum biochemical changes are characteristic or specific for rabies. Biochemical changes in CSF have been minimal in experimentally infected dogs and have been rarely reported in natural infections. Increased CSF protein (110 to 150 mg/dl) and leukocytes (120 to 240/μl) with small lymphocytes predominating have been reported in dogs with postvaccinal rabies encephalomyelitis. Cats with postvaccinal rabies also have had increased CSF protein (55 to 80 mg/dl) and an increased CSF lymphocyte count (5 to 17/μl).[30]

Submission of Specimens

Selection and submission of proper specimens are critical for accurate rabies diagnosis. Handling live, suspected rabid animals must be done with extreme care. Heavy, protective gloves must be worn and use of catch-poles, cages, and other equipment often facilitates capture and transport of such animals. The animal must be euthanatized by a humane method, and the brain must be protected from damage since rabies is a neurotropic virus. The use of an ax or power saw should be discouraged when opening the skull, as these may create hazardous aerosols. A procedure to remove the brain of a suspected rabid animal has been published.[31] Small specimens such as mice and kittens may be submitted whole.

The head (or body) of an animal suspected of having rabies that has died or been euthanatized should be cooled immediately and maintained chilled (wet ice) or refrigerated until examined. The head or brain *must not be frozen*, as this delays examination and the thawing process causes brain tissue damage. A complete history should accompany each specimen. Various approved shipping containers are available and must protect the specimen as well as those handling the container.

Specimens must be sent to the laboratory as quickly as possible. Postexposure treatment is often delayed while awaiting laboratory results. It is recommended that specimens be delivered personally or by courier whenever possible to minimize delay or potential loss. Whatever method of specimen shipment is used, always mark the container to indicate that hazardous laboratory specimens are enclosed.

Direct Immunofluorescent Antibody (DFA) Testing of Nervous Tissue

This is both rapid and sensitive and presently is the most widely used method of diagnosing potential rabies infection. Unless it is completely decomposed, the head should be submitted, since specific fluorescence may still be detected. Rabies viral antigen has also been found using trypsin digestion of formalin-fixed and paraffin-embedded tissue.[32, 33, 33a] It is not necessary that animals show neurologic signs at the time of examination, and all animals excreting virus in their saliva will have detectable virus in the CNS by DFA examination.

DFA Testing of Dermal Tissues

Since virus enters extraneural tissues via centrifugal spread from the CNS, it arrives at nerve endings in the skin and at the salivary glands simultaneously. Because of the heavy sensory innervation, the skin at the nape of the neck (people) or the sensory vibrissae on the maxillary areas (animals) are most specific for DFA testing. DFA testing of a skin biopsy has a 25% to 50% probability of being positive around the time that clinical rabies develops, with an increased accuracy as the course of disease progresses.[34, 35] Rabies vaccines commonly used in dogs and cats do not give false-positive results.[34]

The skin biopsy technique shows promise in detecting infections in living animals and has already been used to detect natural infections in people, dogs, cats, skunks, cattle, and horses.[36, 37] Biopsies must include the deeper subcutaneous tissue to ensure that tactile hair follicles have been removed. Specimens are best preserved for shipment if they are fresh frozen in dry ice or refrigerated and protected from desiccation to prevent autolysis at ambient temperatures. The skin biopsy procedure has important application in testing pet animals that have bitten someone but that have a current vaccination history and normal behavioral and neurologic status. This test appears to be accurate if the virus is present; however, a negative test result does not rule out the possibility that the animal is infected. Its application is restricted at present to a few diagnostic laboratories (see Appendix 8) and has not been approved for routine laboratory diagnosis of rabies. DFA procedures have also been used on corneal impression and buccal cavity smears, but sensitivity is rather poor.[37–39]

A direct immunoperoxidase method also has been developed to detect the presence of rabies virus in skin.[40] With this procedure, conventional bright field or electron microscopy rather than fluorescent microscopy can be used to interpret the test.

Intracellular Inclusions

A classic test for the presence of rabies is to examine the brain for the presence of intracytoplasmic inclusions, known as Negri bodies, in larger neurons. They are most commonly found in the thalamus, hypothalamus, pons, cerebral cortex, and dorsal horns of the spinal cord. They are most common in neurons of the hippocampus in carnivores and in Purkinje's cells of herbivores. Negri bodies in tissue sections or impression smears of brain tissue are best demonstrated with Seller's or Van Gieson's stains, in which they stain magenta. Unfortunately, Negri bodies take time to develop and cannot be found during all stages of infection or in all infected cats. They usually cannot be detected until neurologic signs are apparent, so premature killing of the animal may reduce the chances of finding these inclusions. This test is no longer used in most developed nations for routine diagnosis.

Mouse Inoculation

Intracerebral inoculation of laboratory mice with fresh or fresh-frozen homogenized tissue is a confirmatory test for rabies and is not conducted for routine diagnosis of suspected rabies cases. Specific neutralizing antibody is incubated with extracted tissue prior to its inoculation to confirm that rabies virus is responsible for the observed neurologic signs. Brains and salivary tissues from proposed infected mice are examined for virus by DFA. This test does not distinguish between virulent and vaccine viruses because regardless of attenuation, many of the virus strains produce a similar illness in mice. Replacement of mouse inoculation by viral inoculation into tissue culture (TC) is now feasible because virulent virus can now be grown in various cell lines.[39]

Serologic Testing

Indirect immunofluorescent antibody (IFA) testing has become a rapid, sensitive, and reproducible means of quantifying rabies virus antibody. A modification of the standard IFA procedure, the rapid fluorescent-focus inhibition test (RFFIT), is used to quantify concentrations of specific rabies virus antibody in serum. A constant amount of challenge virus is added to serial dilutions of test sera. Following incubation, this mixture is inoculated onto confluent cell monolayers. After 24 hours, the cells are stained for immunofluorescence, using conjugated specific rabies virus antiglobulin. A reduction of 50% or more of the immunofluorescence indicates a significant concentration of neutralizing antibody in the serum. Disadvantages of performing the RFFIT are that it is time consuming, uses difficult-to-maintain reagents, and necessitates working with live rabies virus. Newly accepted tests for rabies virus antibodies, based on enzyme immunoassays,[41, 41a] or immune adherence hemagglutination[41b] will probably soon replace the RFFIT for serodiagnosis.

Testing for serum antibodies to rabies virus to determine recent exposure to rabies can be ambiguous unless specific IgM titers are determined. Elevated rabies antibody titers in serum can result from vaccination or from past or recent exposure to virulent virus. IgM titers increase within 3 to 4 days after vaccination and begin to decline 41 days later, while IgG titers increase 10 days after CNS infection and generally start to decline about day 225.

Testing for rabies antibody in CSF is a more accurate documentation of rabies infection since antibody is locally produced. CSF IgM titers increase two to three weeks or more after the onset of clinical rabies.[24, 41c] Because of this delay, a negative titer result does not eliminate rabies infection as a possibility. Titers in CSF usually do not increase after vaccination unless postvaccinal, vaccine virus–induced encephalomyelitis develops. In virulent or vaccine virus–induced neurologic rabies, antibody titer is usually higher in the CSF than in serum. Serum and CSF titers must be compared to eliminate the possibility that nonspecific leakage of protein has occurred from the procedure or from inflammatory processes.

Monoclonal Antibody

Monoclonal immunoglobulins produced against specific rabies virus nucleocapsid and glycoprotein moieties are able to distinguish the various antigenic variants of rabies virus. Strains of virus to be tested are grown in tissue culture and are subsequently stained to determine the antigenic composition of the virus. The pattern of staining is compared with that of reference strains of virus. This technique is extremely valuable in distinguishing between vaccine and virulent strains of rabies virus, especially in cases of human exposure to animals with postvaccinal neurologic disease.[17]

PATHOLOGIC FINDINGS

No gross lesions are detectable in the CNS with rabies infection. Despite the dramatic neurologic signs and high mortality, neuropathologic changes are mild. Pathologic changes depend on the severity and duration of infection at the time of examination. Acute polioencephalitis characterized by minimal neuronophagia, neuronal degeneration, and nonsuppurative inflammation is seen very early in the course of the disease. Necrotizing encephalitis is seen in the next phase of infection and corresponds to a gradually increasing titer in the serum and CSF. Chronic infections are characterized by focal or widespread lymphocytic and plasmacytic perivascular cuffing and focal mononuclear cell infiltrates in the CNS. A ganglioneuritis is usually present. The longer the course of illness, the more pronounced is the nonsuppurative inflammatory response in the brain and spinal cord.

THERAPY

Supportive care for rabies-infected animals is not recommended because recovered animals have been shown to excrete the virus in their saliva for extended periods. A dog or cat suspected of having rabies should be quarantined as recommended (see Compendium of Animal Rabies Vaccines, Appendix 6) or as for all other species, destroyed and the brain submitted for examination. When brain tissue has been inadvertently damaged or destroyed, spinal cord is an alternative but less desirable substitute.[42] In rare instances, a skin biopsy may be obtained for diagnosis; however, results are not confirmatory unless the test result is positive for the virus.

PREVENTION

Vaccine Types

No measure has helped reduce the incidence of human rabies as effectively as the widespread vaccination of the domestic dog population. Early vaccines were developed from virus grown in nervous tissue and later in avian embryos. Low egg passage (LEP) vaccine virus was produced by approximately 50 serial passages of the virus in chicken embryos (CEO). The virus lost its viscerotropic properties but retained some of its neurotropic traits. Vaccine-induced rabies was common if the product was used in cats. High egg passage (HEP) CEO vaccine was produced by approximately 180 passages of the virus. It no longer caused neurologic signs in laboratory mice, except when neonates had been injected intracerebrally. The vaccine was safe for dogs and for more susceptible species such as cats and cattle. For this reason, any vaccine used in cats must state that it is licensed for such use. Newer MLV vaccines were produced in TC. These products produced fewer allergic reactions, compared to CEO vaccines. Despite better immunity produced by MLV as compared with inactivated vaccines, postvaccinal rabies is a distinct disadvantage. Only one commercial MLV rabies vaccine is currently recommended for use in the United States (see Appendix 6).

To develop effective inactivated rabies virus vaccines, the virus had to be produced in high concentration, which was initially done by growing it in the nervous system of suckling mice. Neonatal mice were chosen because they lacked the antigenic myelin responsible for allergic encephalomyelitis produced by early nervous tissue origin vaccines.

An advance in the development of inactivated rabies vaccines has been the production of less allergenic and more immunogenic products. This has resulted from additional adaptation of rabies virus strains to TC cells so that large quantities of virus can be produced. Newer adjuvants, such as aluminum hydroxide, increased the immune response to the antigen in these products.[43]

Purified subunit rabies vaccines may be the recommended vaccines in the future. With purified glycoprotein vaccines, 5 to 50 times the quantity of purified glycoprotein alone is required to produce an immune response compared with intact virion vaccines. It has been suggested that the glycoprotein is absorbed on lipid complexes, which if true would greatly increase the potency of subunit vaccines.[44]

Vaccine Recommendations

Many vaccines are currently marketed in the United States for preexposure rabies prophylaxis in dogs and cats. All currently licensed products must protect 88% of vaccinates against challenge with virulent virus, while at least 80% of those challenged but not vaccinated develop rabies. Currently available MLV and inactivated vaccines have been shown to be relatively safe and effective when used in neonatal puppies and kittens. However, because of maternal antibody blockade and a relatively poor immune response in the young, the first rabies vaccination is given at a minimum of 3 months of age and then repeated 1 year later. Subsequent vaccinations are repeated every 1 or 3 years later, depending on the product and local public helath regulations. The current Compendium of Animal Rabies Vaccines (Appendix 6) and Appendices 1 and 2 should be consulted for canine and feline rabies vaccination protocols.

MLV rabies vaccines have been known to be more effective when given by the IM rather than the SC route. Presumably, like the street virus, vaccine virus must attach to nervous tissue to replicate effectively. Muscular tissue is more heavily innervated with neuromuscular end-plates and muscle spindles than are SC tissues. The advantages of SC vaccination are that it is less painful and easier to give, and it avoids the direct injury of deeper nerves or tissues. Newer inactivated TC products still generally seem to be more effective when given IM.[44a] Serum antibody titers can be misleading as a measure of protection, since previously vaccinated dogs usually show an anamnestic response to boosters, even when antibodies have already declined in their sera.[45]

Postvaccinal Reactions

The most frequent non-neurologic complications associated with rabies virus vaccine are local soreness, lameness, and regional lymphadenopathy in the injected limb. Fever and systemic signs are sometimes noted. These signs have been more frequently noted with the newer inactivated TC rabies vaccines because of the need for higher antigenic mass and adjuvants to produce an immune response equal to that produced by the older attenuated products.

Focal cutaneous vasculitis, a localized hyperpigmented alopecic macule, developed at the site of inoculation in dogs 3 to 6 months following inoculation.[46] This reaction has been primarily noted in the poodle breed, presumably because of their characteristic hair coat. Rabies virus and immunoglobulins were detected in the tissues. One dog died from presumed anaphylaxis after subsequent vaccination. These reactions, which can also produce acute painful subcutaneous swellings, are a reflection of the allergenicity of the newer TC inactivated

Table 31–1. Recommendations for Rabies Vaccination of Animals and People, Pre- and Postexposure.

ANIMAL EXPOSED	RECOMMENDATION
Preexposure	
Dogs and cats	Vaccinate at 3 months of age; revaccinate 1 year later and every 1 or 3 years thereafter depending on product recommendations
Wildlife	Discourage ownership or vaccination; none approved
People	Three doses of HDCV, 1.0 ml IM in deltoid on days 0, 7, and 28; booster based on risk group[a]
Postexposure	
Dogs and cats	Previously unimmunized: destroy immediately; if impossible or owner refuses, isolate for 6 months and vaccinate 1 month prior to release
	Previously immunized: revaccinate immediately; leash and confine at home for 3 months
Wildlife	Regard as rabid and euthanatize for examination
People	Previously unimmunized: HRIG, 20 U/kg, given half at bite site and remainder IM in gluteal muscle, and five doses HDCV, 1.0 ml IM in deltoid muscle, on days 0, 3, 7, 14, and 28
	Previously immunized: two doses HDCV, 1.0 ml IM in deltoid muscle on days 0 and 3; do not give HRIG

[a]Risk groups: Rabies vaccine production and laboratory workers have titers run every 6 months and receive boosters when the titer is low. Spelunkers, veterinarians, and wildlife control officers have titers run every 2 years and receive boosters when the titer is less than adequate. Veterinarians and veterinary students in nonenzootic areas should be vaccinated at least once with no serology or boosters until exposure. The United States population at large remains unvaccinated. HDCV = human diploid cell vaccine; HRIG = human rabies immune globulin.

rabies vaccines given in a SC site. IM inoculation results in fewer local subcutaneous reactions but because of more rapid absorption may be associated with a higher frequency of systemic allergic reactions.

Autoimmune polyradiculoneuritis has especially been observed with the use of inactivated suckling mouse brain (SMB)–origin products. Myelination of the nervous system is delayed in neonatal mice; thus, vaccines prepared from these tissues are not usually associated with neurologic complications. Some lots of SMB vaccines may have contained either older, myelinated brains or peripheral myelin from cranial nerves. A small proportion of dogs that were vaccinated with these products developed acute diffuse LMN paralysis.[47] Pain sensation remained intact, and dogs were hypersensitive to muscle palpation. Electromyographic studies showed fibrillation activity characteristic of LMN denervation. Cranial nerve abnormalities such as facial paralysis occasionally were noted. Clinical improvement began within 2 weeks following paralysis, but total recovery was delayed in some dogs for several months. Similar postvaccinal complications have been reported with the use of SMB vaccine in people.

Neurologic complications caused by MLV rabies vaccine virus–induced encephalomyelitis have been commonly observed in the past in dogs and cats.[48–51] Affected animals typically developed LMN paralysis in the pelvic limb on the side of the injection within 12 to 21 days postinoculation, which progressed to involve the opposite pelvic limb with ascending paraplegia. Progression to forelimb and intracranial involvement was more common in affected cats, whereas dogs usually recovered completely from the affliction within 17 days to 2.5 months. Injection in the cervical musculature, closer to the brain, has been associated with a much greater prevalence of neurologic complications. A peculiar feature of the paralysis in some cats is signs of hyperextended limbs rather than flaccid paralysis.

Control of Epizootic Rabies in Dogs and Cats

Where rabies epizootics have occurred, vaccination programs have been shown to greatly reduce the spread of an outbreak.[52] Management of stray and unwanted cats and dogs is essential, and unclaimed animals should be humanely destroyed. Leash laws must be enforced. Reduction in the population of wildlife vectors has been used on a limited scale when epizootics of rabies in dogs and cats have been traced to a particular wildlife reservoir species. Control through trapping and poison baits is not only difficult but may cause public resentment. As previously described, oral vaccination of wild carnivores has worked on a limited basis worldwide[52a, 52b, 52c] and will be expanded in the near future if current field trials prove successful.

Postexposure Management of Dogs and Cats

Management of a dog or cat that has been bitten or scratched by a potentially rabid mammal is difficult when the biting animal is not available for testing, because the dog or cat must be considered as having been exposed to a rabid animal (Table 31–1: Postexposure, Dogs and Cats). Differences in management depend on whether or not the exposed animal has been previously immunized. The final decision concerning the management of exposed animals generally is made by local or state public health authorities. The current Compendium of Animal Rabies Vaccines (Appendix 6) and local public health officials should be consulted when such circumstances arise.

Disposition of Animals That Bite Humans

Dogs and cats with current rabies vaccinations are of less concern as a transmission risk, although current vaccination status does not remove the need for follow-up (Table 31–2). Any illness or neurologic disease in quarantine animals must be immediately reported to local public health authorities. Stray or unwanted domestic pets or wild carnivores or bats that bite people should be sacrificed immediately, and the brain should be submitted for DFA testing or rabies virus isolation.

PUBLIC HEALTH CONSIDERATIONS

Postexposure Prophylaxis

Nearly all cases of human rabies have been acquired by exposure to saliva in bite wounds or, rarely, on abraded or scratched skin. Therapy of bite wounds should be aggressive, since immediate, thorough washing of the wound has been shown to be effective in reducing the chance of infection. Ethanol (43% or stronger) can be applied locally to open wounds. Bites should also be irrigated with large quantities of a 20% aqueous soap solution or quaternary ammonium compound (QUAT) under pressure. The optimal concentration of benzalkonium chloride, a QUAT, has been shown to be 1% to 4%; however, most commercial hospital disinfectants have a 0.13% concentration. Deep puncture wounds can be effectively cleaned by irrigation; use a 15-ml syringe fitted with a blunted 19-gauge needle that is filled with a sterile saline solution. This provides 20 pounds per square inch of pressure, sufficient for cleaning but not so excessive as to cause further tissue damage.

Approximately 20,000 people annually are given antirabies prophylaxis in the United States.[29] Specific antirabies therapy for humans has been most successful in reducing the number of deaths due to rabies when active immunization is combined with passively administered immunoglobulin (Table 31–1: Postexposure, People). Human rabies immune globulin (HRIG) is preferable to unpurified gamma globulin because of its greater immunopotency and lesser allergenicity. HRIG is given simultaneously with the initial vaccination and is not repeated because it interferes with the active immune response to subsequent vaccinations.

Rabies human diploid cell vaccine (HDCV, Rhone Merieux, Lyon, France) is highly effective and safe for pre- and postexposure immunizations. The newly licensed rabies vaccine, Rabies Vaccine Adsorbed (RVA, Michigan Department of Public Health), a rhesus monkey cell culture rabies vaccine, which is in very limited supply, and HDCV are the only commercial rabies vaccines currently available in the United States. They are more immunogenic and less allergenic than previously available human rabies vaccines. Postexposure therapy with HDCV or RVA and HRIG must begin as soon as possible, preferably within 24 hours or less (Table 31–1: Postexposure, People). Postexposure treatment failures have been noted when the vaccine has been given in the gluteal rather than the deltoid muscle.[53] A vaccine composed of live vaccinia virus with inserted genetic material for rabies glycopro-

Table 31–2. Postexposure Recommendations for Rabies Exposure of People

SOURCE OF INFECTION	SITUATION	ANIMAL DISPOSITION	POSTEXPOSURE PROPHYLAXIS FOR PEOPLE
Rodents[a]	Any episode	Usually not examined	None, but consult public health officials
Dog or cat[b]	Healthy, owned	Confine; observe for at least 10 days, especially if unprovoked attack	None or consider, if unprovoked; yes, if CNS signs develop
	Healthy, stray available or escaped	Euthanatize immediately; submit head for examination	Yes
	CNS signs or illness	Euthanatize immediately; submit head for examination	Yes, if negative FA[d] result, stop
Wild carnivore	Any episode	If captured, euthanatize immediately; submit head for examination	Yes, if positive or animal at large; if negative FA result, stop
Attenuated vaccine[c]	Any episode	Not applicable	None

[a]Squirrels, hamsters, guinea pigs, gerbils, chipmunks, rats, and mice. Lagomorphs are also included.
[b]Vaccination status of animal should not be used to make a decision on outcome for prophylaxis.
[c]Accidental inoculation. [d]FA = fluorescent antibodies.

tein has shown benefit in experimental trials of postexposure prophylaxis in animals.[54]

The decision to administer postexposure prophylaxis in people must be made immediately and is based upon a number of factors concerning the bite incident. The species of animal that inflicts the bite wound is important, because dogs, cats, and especially wild carnivores are more likely to transmit the virus. Many people might have been spared the concern and inconvenience of prophylactic therapy had cats been routinely vaccinated. Unfortunately, most public health laws that have attempted to include cats in required rabies vaccination programs have failed. Bites of rodents such as squirrels, chipmunks, rats, mice, and lagomorphs seldom if ever result in prophylactic vaccination of people (Table 31–2: Rodents). Despite that fact, postexposure prophylaxis has often been performed unnecessarily.

The circumstances behind the biting incident are also important in determining the need to initiate prophylaxis prior to laboratory confirmation (Table 31–2). Bites from rabies-infected animals usually occur without provocation. Animals that show neurologic signs at the time of the bite or soon after should be considered rabid. Bite exposures are much more likely to result in rabies infection than scratches, unless the scratches were contaminated by the animal's saliva. The prevalence of rabies in the geographic area is also important. People accidentally injected with animal rabies vaccines do not require postexposure prophylaxis.

Preexposure Prophylaxis

Preexposure prophylaxis is warranted in people with a high vocational or recreational risk of contacting rabid animals (Table 31–1: Pre- and Postexposure, People). Veterinarians, animal health technicians and caretakers, animal control officers, wildlife biologists, laboratory workers, spelunkers, and children in highly enzootic rabies areas should receive preexposure protection. Substitution of 0.1 ml of intradermal HDCV is also effective for primary immunization.[55, 56] Hypersensitivity reactions have been the main side effects noted in 1% to 6% of those receiving booster vaccinations.[57] Local and systemic immune complex–mediated allergic reaction have developed with the use of HDCV, although those reactions are less than with previously available products. Hives, urticaria, arthralgia, fever, nausea, and vomiting can develop within 1 week of booster vaccinations.[58]

The risk of veterinarians being exposed to rabid animals is over 300 times greater than that of the general population. In one study, most (230) of the 380 exposures occurred to veterinarians during nonbite contact while they examined rabid animals. Seventy-nine of the cases resulted from an animal bite, and 17 were due to exposure at necropsy. Many of these potential exposures resulted from contact with infected cattle, although a summary claimed only 13 known confirmed instances of rabies transmission from cattle to people worldwide.[59]

References

1. Smith JS, Reid-Sanden FL, Roumillat LF, et al: Demonstration of antigenic variation among rabies virus isolates by using monoclonal antibodies to nucleocapsid proteins. *J Clin Microbiol* 24:573–580, 1986.
2. Dietzschold B, Wiktor TJ, Trojanowski JQ, et al: Differences in cell-to-cell spread of pathogenic and apathogenic rabies virus in vivo and in vitro. *J Virol* 56:12–18, 1985.
3. Seif I, Coulon P, Rollin PE, et al: Rabies virulence: effect on pathogenicity and sequence characterization of rabies virus mutations affecting antigenic site III of the glycoprotein. *J Virol* 53:926–934, 1985.
4. Winkler WG: Airborne rabies virus isolation. *Bull Wildl Dis Assoc* 4:37–40, 1968.
5. Winkler WG, Baker EF, Hopkins CC: An outbreak of nonbite transmitted rabies in a laboratory animal colony. *Am J Epidemiol* 95:267–277, 1972.
6. Bell JF, Moore GJ: Susceptibility of Carnivora to rabies virus administered orally. *Am J Epidemiol* 93:176–182, 1971.
7. Howard DR: Transplacental transmission of rabies virus from a naturally infected skunk. *Am J Vet Res* 42:691–692, 1981.
8. Torres-Anjel MJ, Blenden DC, Hamory B: International aspects of rabies. (Letter.) *J Am Vet Med Assoc* 186:5–27, 1985.
9. Kaplan MM, Kaprowski H: Rabies. *Sci Am* 242:120–234, 1980.
10. Centers for Disease Control: CDC surveillance summaries, September 1988. *MMWR* 34(SS–4), 1988.
11. Centers for Disease Control: Rabies Surveillance. *Annual Summary 1986*. Issued August 28, 1987.
12. Centers for Disease Control: Rabies in pet skunks—Oregon. *MMWR* 28:481–482, 1979.
13. Beran GW, Crowley AJ: Toward worldwide rabies control. *WHO Chron* 37:192–196, 1983.
14. Smith JS, Sumner JW, Roumillat LF, et al: Antigenic characteristics of isolates associated with a new epizootic of raccoon rabies in the United States. *J Infect Dis* 149:769–774, 1984.
15. Jenkins SR: Investigation into the raccoon rabies outbreak in the mid Atlantic states. Proc North Am Symp on Rabies in Wildlife, November 7–8, 1983. Baltimore, 1986.
16. Beck AM, Felser SR, Glickman LT: An epizootic of rabies in Maryland, 1982–1984. *Am J Public Health* 77:42–44, 1987.
17. Whetstone CA, Bunn TO, Emmons RW, et al: Use of monoclonal antibodies to confirm vaccine-induced rabies in ten dogs, two cats, and one fox. *J Am Vet Med Assoc* 185:285–288, 1984.
18. Webster WA, Casey GA, Charlton KM, et al: Antigenic variants of rabies virus in isolates from eastern, central and northern Canada. *Can J Comp Med* 49:186–188, 1985.
19. Centers for Disease Control: Rabies Surveillance. *Annual Summary 1984*. Issued December 1985.
20. Centers for Disease Control: Rabid rabbit bites 4-year-old girl—Iowa. *Vet Public Health Notes* Mar:23–24, 1981.
21. Centers for Disease Control: Rabies in the United States and Canada, 1983. *In* CDC Surveillance Summaries 34(1SS):11SS–27SS, 1985.
21a. Hemachuda T, Phanuphak P, Busarawan S, et al: Immunologic studies of human encephalitic and paralytic rabies. *Am J Med* 84:673–677, 1988.
22. Charlton KM, Casey GA, Campbell JB: Experimental rabies in skunks: mechanisms of infection of the salivary glands. *Can J Comp Med* 47:363–369, 1983.
23. Fekadu M, Shaddock JH, Baer GM: Intermittent excretion of rabies virus in the saliva of a dog two and six months after it had recovered from experimental rabies. *Am J Trop Med Hyg* 30:1113–1115, 1981.
24. Murphy FA, Bell JF, Bauer SP, et al: Experimental chronic rabies in the cat. *Lab Invest* 43:231–241, 1980.
25. Hattwick MA, Weis TT, Stechschulte CJ, et al: Recovery from rabies. A case report. *Ann Intern Med* 76:931–942, 1972.
26. Lodmell DL, Ewalt LC: Pathogenesis of street rabies virus infections in resistant and susceptible strains of mice. *J Virol* 55:788–795, 1985.
27. Wiktor TJ: Triggering the immune response: how postexposure immunization works. *Rabies Report: Mounting a Strong Defense*. Lorena, KS, Veterinary Medicine Publ Co, 1986, pp 18–19.
28. Blenden DC, Breitschwerdt EB: Recovery of a dog from an experimental rabies infection. *In* Baer GM (ed): *Rabies Information Exchange* 2:9–11, 1980.
29. Baer G: Personal communication. Centers for Disease Control, Rabies Laboratory, Atlanta, GA, 1988.
30. Esh JB, Cunningham JG, Wiktor TJ: Vaccine-induced rabies in four cats. *J Am Vet Med Assoc* 180:1336–1339, 1982.
31. Tierkel ES: Shipment of specimens and techniques for preparation of animal tissues. *In* Kaplan MM, Kaprowski H (ed): *Laboratory Techniques in Rabies*. Geneva, World Health Organization, Monograph Series No 23, 1973.
32. Palmer DG, Ossent P, Suter MM, et al: Demonstration of rabies viral antigen in paraffin tissue sections: comparison of the immunofluorescence technique with the unlabeled antibody enzyme method. *Am J Vet Res* 46:283–286, 1985.
33. Anjaria JM, Jhala CI: Immunoperoxidase reaction in diagnosis of rabies. *Int J Zoon* 12:267–275, 1985.
33a. Bourgon AR, Charlton KM: The demonstration of rabies antigen in paraffin-embedded tissues using the peroxidase-antiperoxidase method: a comparative study. *Can J Vet Res* 51:117–120, 1987.
34. Blenden DC, Bell JF, Tsao AT, et al: Immunofluorescent examination of the skin of rabies-infected animals as a means of early detection of rabies virus antigen. *J Clin Microbiol* 18:631–636, 1983.
35. Blenden DC, Torres-Anjel MJ, Statlowich FT: Improve your service to clients with antemortem rabies diagnostics. *Rabies Report: Mounting a Strong Defense*. Lexena, KS, Vet Med Publ Co, 1986, pp 10–14.
36. Howard DR: Skin biopsy provides accurate rabies diagnosis. *Norden News* 56:32, 1981.
37. Anderson LJ, Nicholson KG, Tauxe RV, et al: Human rabies in the United States 1960–1979: epidemiology, diagnosis, and prevention. *Ann Intern Med* 100:728–735, 1984.
38. Rajan TSS, Padmanaban VD: Clinical diagnosis of rabies in herbivores—examination of corneal impression smears by fluorescent antibody technique. *Indian Vet J* 63:882–885, 1986.
39. Charlton KM, Webster WA, Casey GA, et al: Recent advances in rabies diagnosis and research. *Can Vet J* 27:85–96, 1986.
39a. Webster WA: A tissue culture infection test in

routine rabies diagnosis. *Can J Vet Res* 51:367–369, 1987.

40. Tsao AT, Blenden DC: Detection of rabies virus in the skin by immunofluorescence and immunoperoxidase staining and virus isolation: a blind study. *In* Baer GM (ed): *Rabies Information Exchange* 4:23–24, 1981.

41. Mammen K, Mifune K, Reid FL, et al: Microneutralization test for rabies virus based on enzyme immunoassay. *J Clin Microbiol* 25:2440–2442, 1987.

41a. Bovrhy H, Rollin PE, Vincent J, et al: Comparative field evaluation of the fluorescent-antibody test, virus isolation from tissue culture, and enzyme immunoassay for rapid laboratory diagnosis of rabies. *J Clin Microbiol* 27:519–523, 1989.

41b. Bota CN, Anderson PK, Goyal SM, et al: Comparative prevalence of rabies antibodies among household and unclaimed stray dogs as determined by immune adherence hemagglutination assay. *Int J Epidemiol* 16:472–476, 1987.

41c. Tingpalapong M, Hoke CH, Ward GS, et al: Antirabies virus IgM in serum and cerebrospinal fluid from rabid dogs. *Southeast Asian J Trop Med Public Health* 17:550–557, 1986.

42. Ito FH, Vasconcellos SA, Erbolato EB, et al: Rabies virus in different segments of brain and spinal cord of naturally and experimentally infected dogs. *Int J Zoon* 12:98–104, 1985.

43. Koutchoukali MA, Blancou J, Chappuis G, et al: Réponse sérologique du chien après primovaccination antirabique à l'aide de vaccins adjuvés ou non. *Ann Rech Vet* 16:345–349, 1985.

44. Perrin P, Portnoi D, Sureau P: Enhancement of immunogenic and protective activity of rabies glycoprotein by anchorage in liposomes. *In* Baer GM (ed): *Rabies Information Exchange* 7:16–17, 1983.

44a. Centers for Disease Control: Withdrawal of approval for subcutaneous administration of Norden rabies vaccine for dogs and cats. *MMWR* 36:628–629, 1987.

45. Derbyshire JB, Mathews KA: Rabies antibody titres in vaccinated dogs. *Can Vet J* 25:383–385, 1984.

46. Wilcock BP, Yager JA: Focal cutaneous vasculitis and alopecia at sites of rabies vaccination in dogs. *J Am Vet Med Assoc* 188:1174–1177, 1986.

47. Greene CE: Unpublished observations. Auburn University, Auburn, AL, 1975.

48. Bellinger DA, Chang J, Bunn TO, et al: Rabies induced in a cat by high-egg passage Flury strain vaccine. *J Am Vet Med Assoc* 183:997–998, 1983.

49. Bellinger DA, Chang J, Bunn TO, et al: Vaccine-induced rabies in a cat. (Letter.) *J Am Vet Med Assoc* 184:382–406, 1984.

50. Sharpee RL, Bechenhauer WH: Vaccine-induced rabies in a cat. (Letter.) *J Am Vet Med Assoc* 184:380–382, 1984.

51. Cran HR: Some clinical observations on rabies. *Vet Rec* 118:23–24, 1986.

52. Kelly VP, Gonzales JL, Nettles WD, et al: Control of 2 rabies epizootics. *Mod Vet Pract* 64:380–384, 1983.

52a. Lawson KF, Johnston DH, Patterson JM, et al: Immunization of foxes by the intestinal route using an inactivated rabies vaccine. *Can J Vet Res* 53:56–61, 1989.

52b. Brochier B, Thomas I, Iokem A, et al: A field trial in Belgium to control fox rabies by oral administration. *Vet Rec* 123:618–621, 1988.

52c. Vaccination program begun to halt spread of raccoon rabies epizootics. *J Am Vet Med Assoc* 191:394, 1987.

53. Shill M, Baynes RD, Miller SD: Fatal rabies encephalitis despite appropriate post-exposure prophylaxis. *N Engl J Med* 316:1257–1258, 1987.

54. Wiktor TJ, MacFarlan RI, Reagan KJ, et al: Protection from rabies by a vaccinia virus recombinant containing the rabies virus glycoprotein gene. *Proc Natl Acad Sci* 81:7194–7198, 1984.

55. Bernard KW, Mallonee J, Wright JC, et al: Preexposure immunization with intradermal human diploid cell rabies vaccine. *JAMA* 257:1059–1063, 1987.

56. Dreesen DW, Brown WJ, Kemp DT, et al: Preexposure rabies prophylaxis: efficacy of a new packaging and delivery system for intradermal administration of human diploid cell vaccine. *Vaccine* 2:185–188, 1984.

57. Centers for Disease Control: Systemic allergic reaction following immunization with human diploid cell rabies vaccine. *MMWR* 33:185–187, 1984.

58. Dressen DW, Bernard KW, Parker RA, et al: Immune complex–like disease in 23 persons following a booster dose of rabies human diploid cell vaccine. *Vaccine* 4:45–49, 1986.

59. US Dept. of Health and Human Services, CDC Veterinary Public Health Notes: Human rabies after exposure to rabid cattle. August:2–4, 1980.

32

PSEUDORABIES

Marc Vandevelde

ETIOLOGY

Pseudorabies virus (PRV) is an enveloped DNA virus (Fig. 32–1A and B) belonging to the α-herpesviruses. As with other herpesviruses, PRV can cause latent infection, viral DNA being incorporated in the host cell genome. The virus is relatively resistant to environmental factors and can survive outside the host for several months under favorable climatic conditions. Survival of PRV depends on temperature (10 days at 37°C, 40 days at 25°C) and pH (optimum, 7), and it is quickly inactivated by drying and exposure to UV light.[1]

EPIDEMIOLOGY

PRV infection (Aujeszky's disease, mad itch, infectious bulbar paralysis) occurs in most countries of the world with the exception of Australia and has been responsible for massive economic losses in recent years. Although many mammalian species are susceptible to infection with PRV, it is predominantly a problem in pigs, the main reservoir of the virus. However, cattle, fur-bearing animals, dogs, and cats are sporadically affected.[2, 3] It does not appear to affect people, since most reports have been circumstantial and not documented. Infection frequently is subclinical in pigs because they have become well adapted to the virus. The disease is spread by commercial movement of infected pigs or contaminated pork products. Venereal transmission occurs because infected boars may shed PRV in semen. Wild animals, such as raccoons and rats, may act as transient reservoirs; they are not important in maintaining the disease in nature.

Their role is limited to temporary local spread of virus within enzootic areas. Similarly, PRV infection in dogs and cats only occurs in areas where the disease is enzootic in pigs. In fact, the occurrence of typical pseudorabies signs in pets can be the first indication that the disease is enzootic in the local pig population. Pets almost invariably are infected as a result of consuming contaminated raw pork. Dogs also have developed pseudorabies after biting infected pigs.[4] Direct spread from dog to dog has not been shown to occur.[5]

PATHOGENESIS

Naturally acquired infection in dogs and cats occurs following ingestion of the virus, although a similar sequence of events follows parenteral inoculation of virus. PRV enters the nerve endings at the inoculation site and travels in retrograde fashion via the axoplasm of the nerve fibers to the brain. The incubation time in dogs and cats, regardless of inoculation sites, is 3 to 6 days. Experimental studies in orally infected cats have shown that PRV replicates in the tonsils and travels from the oral mucosa via the sensory branches of the ninth and tenth cranial nerves to the nucleus, tractus solitarius, and area postrema in the medulla oblongata.[6] The fifth cranial nerve has been less frequently involved. Apart from visible damage to the brain tissue associated with inflammatory changes, the virus can cause considerable functional alterations of the nerve cells.[7]

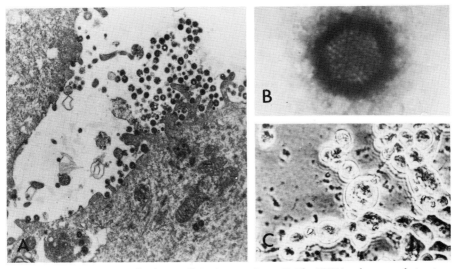

Figure 32–1. *A*, Release of PRV particles from cell in tissue culture. *B*, The PRV is a hexagonal structure composed of capsomers surrounded by an envelope. *C*, The cytopathic effect of PRV in tissue culture is characterized by syncytia formation. (Courtesy of Prof. F. Steck, Department of Veterinary Virology, University of Berne, Berne, Switzerland.)

CLINICAL FINDINGS

The majority of dogs and cats that become infected develop severe clinical signs. The onset of clinical illness is hyperacute, and signs progress rapidly until death occurs, with the total course rarely lasting longer than 48 hours. With very few exceptions, pseudorabies is always fatal in dogs. Cats may be somewhat more resistant but have rarely recovered from the disease.

The initial sign often noted by the owner is a change in behavior, such as inactivity, lethargy, and indifference, although some animals become aggressive or restless. Dyspnea, diarrhea, and vomiting are occasionally seen. Body temperature may be normal or abnormal, and hypersalivation is a common finding. The most characteristic sign, however, is intense pruritus, which usually occurs in the head region and rarely in other areas, such as the neck and shoulders. The animals violently scratch their faces and ears and rub their heads against the floor or walls. One side of the head and neck may become swollen. Self-mutilation results in erythema, excoriation, and ulceration of the skin and underlying tissues. The scratching becomes increasingly more frantic and may end in a generalized convulsion. An atypical course of the disease has also been observed. Cats may die suddenly without developing neurologic signs.[8] Pruritus has been absent in some cases of spontaneous PRV infection in dogs[9] and in experimental oral infection in cats.[6] GI signs have been the predominant feature of some infected dogs.[10] Most of the other neurologic signs that are observed in PRV infection refer to lesions in the lower brain stem and consist of one or several deficits in cranial nerve function. These deficits are usually unilateral and include anisocoria, mydriasis, lack of direct or consensual pupillary light reflexes, trismus, paresis and paralysis of the facial muscles, head tilt, inability to swallow, and vocal changes. Anisocoria and a hoarse voice are considered to be highly consistent signs in the cat.[11] Less commonly observed neurologic signs include behavioral abnormalities such as aggressiveness, generalized hyperesthesia, head pressing, and generalized convulsions. The latter often occur as a sequela to frantic scratching. Paresis and paralysis of the limbs are sometimes noted shortly before death.

DIAGNOSIS

Hematologic or biochemical abnormalities are not found in pseudorabies. The CSF may show increased protein concentration and mononuclear pleocytosis. This finding is strongly indicative of viral encephalitis but is not specific for pseudorabies. Electrocardiographic findings may include cardiac arrhythmias.[12]

Traditionally, the diagnosis of pseudorabies consisted of cutaneous inoculation of infected tissue (usually brain) into a rabbit. Scratching and automutilation of the inoculation site occurred after an incubation time of 5 to 6 days, followed by the rapid death of the animal. Virus can also be propagated in the brains of mice following intracranial inoculation.[13] Pruritus can occur in some mice at the site of inoculation. Newer diagnostic methods, such as direct immunofluorescent examination for virus, have made animal inoculation studies obsolete. This procedure can be used to detect virus in smears or frozen sections of various tissues. The brain and tonsils are the tissues of choice in such studies.

Virus can be isolated in tissue culture from lung and spleen and especially from brains and tonsils of animals with pseudorabies. Although many cell lines have been used, most laboratories employ pig kidney epithelial cells. A definite cytopathic effect consisting of syncytia formation is visible after 12 to 24 hours (see Fig. 32–1C). Virus isolation is not always easy in dogs, even in well-substantiated cases.[14] Pharyngeal washings, tonsillar swabs, and saliva are unsuitable for viral isolation in dogs.[15]

Virus neutralization, immunodiffusion, and ELISA methods commonly are used to detect serum antibody to PRV in pigs.[16] Serologic studies have been valuable in determining the prevalence of disease in pig populations from an epizootiologic and disease prevention point of view. Unfortunately, healthy virus carriers do not always develop detectable serum neutralizing antibody. However, virus neutralizing antibodies have not been found in sera from dogs tested during an outbreak of PRV infection.[15] See Appendix 8 for a list of laboratories that perform various diagnostic tests for pseudorabies.

PATHOLOGIC FINDINGS

There are no gross lesions diagnostic of pseudorabies, with the exception of skin lesions that result from intense pruritus. In some cases, an abnormal stomach content such as straw has been noted because of pica. Pulmonary edema and congestion have been consistent findings. Focal myocarditis has been found in both dogs and cats. Lesions in the CNS are almost exclusively located in the brain stem and primarily involve cranial nerve nuclei.[17] They may be unilateral and consist of perivascular cuffing with mononuclear cells and pronounced proliferation of astrocytes and microglial cells (Fig. 32–2A). The areas of focal gliosis often show degeneration (karyorrhexis) in the center and may progress to the formation of microabscesses (Fig. 32–2B and C). Severe changes occur in neurons, with chromatolysis and disintegration of the nucleus. A most significant finding is the presence of weak eosinophilic viral inclusion bodies in the nuclei of astrocytes and neurons (Fig. 32–2D). Viral antigen can be specifically demonstrated in formalin-fixed paraffin-embedded tissues with immunocytochemical methods.[18] Inflammatory changes can also be found in the nerves and ganglia associated with the site of viral entry. Severe inflammation of the myenteric plexus in the alimentary canal of dogs naturally infected with PRV has also been reported.[10,19] Experimentally infected dogs had ganglioneuritis of autonomic nerves of the heart.[12]

THERAPY

Treatment of pseudorabies is generally futile since the disease is almost always fatal. Heavy sedation and anesthesia may lessen or relieve the itching and convulsions; however, nothing can alter the outcome of the disease. Treatment with anti-PRV serum did not improve the condition of a dog with Aujeszky's disease[20] and is considered to be ineffective in the prevention of infection.[5]

PREVENTION

Prevention is the most important means of control of PRV infection in dogs and cats. Contact with pigs and, especially, feeding animals raw pork from endemic areas should be avoided. It is possible to vaccinate small animals against PRV, although this is indicated only in endemic areas, where exposure to infected pigs may occur. Natural infection with PRV has not been observed in vaccinated dogs and cats.[21] However, experimental vaccination challenge studies showed that it may be difficult to protect dogs with an inactivated vaccine, although most animals develop serum neutralizing antibodies to PRV.[5] Attenuated PRV vaccines may cause postvaccinal reactions that may be as lethal

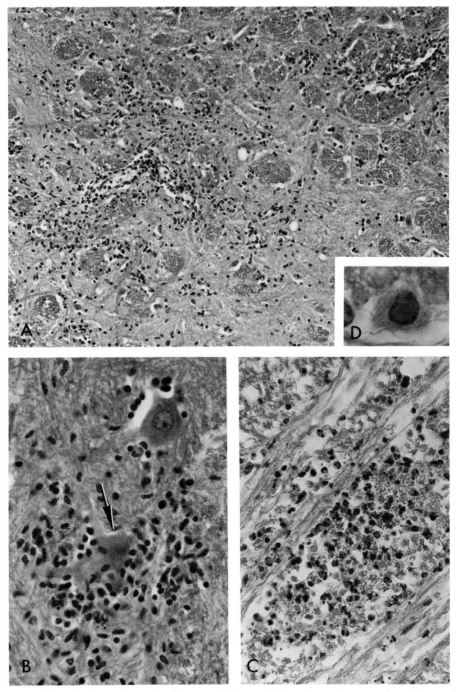

Figure 32–2. Histologic findings of pseudorabies encephalitis. *A*, Disseminated perivascular cuffing and gliosis in the medulla oblongata (H and E; × 100). *B*, Neuronal degeneration *(arrow)* with nodular gliosis (H and E; × 250). *C*, Microabscess (H and E; × 250). *D*, PRV inclusion body in glial cell nucleus (H and E; × 400).

as the natural infection. Newer subunit vaccines being developed for use in swine may be of benefit for vaccinating high risk pets in the future.[22]

References

1. Davies EB, Beran GW: Influence of environmental factors upon the survival of Aujeszky's disease virus. Res Vet Sci 31:32–36, 1981.
2. Hara M, Shimizu T, Fukuyama M, et al: A natural case of Aujeszky's disease in the dog in Japan. Jpn J Vet Sci 49:645–649, 1987.
3. Matsuoka T, Iijima Y, Sakurai K, et al: Aujeszky's disease in a dog. Jpn J Vet Sci 50:277–278, 1988.
4. Huck RA, Evans DH, Hooper RS, et al: The isolation of Aujeszky's disease virus from dogs. Vet Rec 81:172, 1969.
5. Pensaert MB, Commeyne S, Andries K: Vaccination of dogs against pseudorabies (Aujeszky's disease), using an inactivated-virus vaccine. Am J Vet Res 41:2016–2019, 1980.
6. Hagemoser WA, Kluge JP, Hill HT: Studies on the pathogenesis of pseudorabies in domestic cats following oral inoculation. Can J Comp Med 44:192–202, 1980.
7. Dolivo M, Beretta E, Bonifas V, et al: Ultrastructure and function in sympathetic ganglia isolated from rats infected with pseudorabies virus. Brain Res 140:111–123, 1978.
8. Howard DR: Pseudorabies in dogs and cats. In Kirk RW (ed): Current Veterinary Therapy IX. Philadelphia, WB Saunders Co, 1986, pp 1071–1072.
9. Whitley RD, Nelson SL: Pseudorabies (Aujeszky's disease) in the canine: two atypical cases. J Am Anim Hosp Assoc 16:69–72, 1980.
10. Frese K: Atypical Aujeszky's disease in the dog. Proceedings I. Congress European Society of Veterinary Neurology, Paris, 1987.
11. Papp L: Personal communication. University of Budapest, Budapest, Hungary, 1987.
12. Olson GR, Miller LD: Studies on the pathogenesis of heart lesion in dogs infected with pseudorabies virus. Can J Vet Res 50:245–250, 1986.
13. Steinhagen P: Contribution to the diagnosis of Aujeszky's disease in a dog. Dtsch Tierärztl Wochenschr 83:100–103, 1976.
14. Akkermans JPW: Aujeszky's disease and related problems. Tijdschr Diergeneeskd 106:332–336, 1981.
15. Hugoson G, Rockborn G: On the occurrence of pseudorabies in Sweden. II. An outbreak in dogs caused by feeding abattoir offal. Zentralbl Veterinarmed (B) 19:641–645, 1972.
16. vanDirschot JT, deWoal CAH: An ELISA to distinguish between Aujeszky's disease vaccinated and infected pig. Vet Rec 121:305–306, 1987.
17. Fankhauser R, Fatzer R, Steck F, et al: Aujeszky's disease in dogs and cats in Switzerland. Schweiz Arch Tierheilkd 111:623–629, 1975.
18. Ducatelle R, Coussement W, Hoorens J: Demonstration of pseudorabies viral antigen in thick and ultrathin tissue sections of young pigs using an immunogold method. Am J Vet Res 45:1913–1917, 1984.
19. Gore R, Osborne AD, Darke PGG, et al: Aujeszky's disease in a pack of hounds. Vet Rec 101:93–95, 1977.
20. Richter JHM, Van der Vijver JW, Fischer RF, et al: An atypical form of Aujeszky's disease in a dog. Tijdschr Diergeneeskd 100:330–334, 1975.
21. Akkermans JPW: Vaccination of "non-pigs" against Aujeszky's disease. Tijdschr Diergeneeskd 105:1084–1085, 1980.
22. Marchioli CC, Yancey RJ, Petrovskis EA, et al: Evaluation of pseudorabies virus glycoprotein gp50 as a vaccine for Aujeszky's disease in mice and swine: expression by vaccinia virus and Chinese hamster ovary cells. J Virol 61:3977–3982, 1987.

33 ENTEROVIRUS INFECTIONS

Craig E. Greene

Picornaviridae, the family of smallest RNA viruses, contains the genus *Enterovirus*. Species in this genus commonly infect humans and have classically been separated into polioviruses, coxsackieviruses, and enteric cytopathogenic human orphan (echo)viruses, and as yet unclassified enteroviruses. Newer members of the genus are called enteroviruses and are designated by a sequential numbering system. Enteroviruses, being environmentally resistant, infect people primarily via the fecal-oral route. Following replication in submucosal lymphatic tissues, the viruses may spread systemically to various other tissues.

Dogs have been tested to see if they harbor a variety of human enteroviruses because of the possible zoonotic potential (Table 33–1). Similar information is not available for cats. Dogs have been shown to be exposed to and to chronically shed human enteroviruses; however, serologic evidence of infection does not always correlate with shedding of the viruses. Although dogs appear to become infected with these viruses, clinical signs have not been apparent. The viruses can be found in their stools for a period of months, but whether the extended shedding represents reexposure is uncertain. Enteroviruses recovered from nasopharyngeal or fecal cultures of dogs have been grown and cause cytopathogenic effects, primarily in monkey kidney and not canine cell lines, supporting the fact that they are human viruses. Furthermore, neutralization tests have shown them to be indistinguishable from the human isolates.[7] In some instances, enteroviruses were found in canine feces that were "just passing through," not causing infection. These viruses could have been obtained from sources contaminated by human feces. Alternatively, they could be enteroviruses antigenically related to human enteroviruses or other viruses neutralized by nonspecific substances in the testing sera.

Table 33–1. Human Enteroviruses Recovered from Nonsymptomatic Dogs

VIRUS	SPECIMEN SOURCE	GEOGRAPHIC LOCATION
Poliovirus 1	Feces	West Bengal[1]
	Feces	Costa Rica[2]
Echovirus 6	Feces	California[3]
	Nasopharynx, feces	New Mexico[3-5]
Echovirus 7	Feces	West Bengal[1]
Coxsackievirus A9, A20	Feces	Costa Rica[2]
Coxsackievirus B₁	Nasopharynx, feces	Texas, New Mexico[3, 4]
Coxsackievirus B₃	Nasopharynx, feces	New Mexico[4]
Coxsackievirus B₅	Nasopharynx, feces	New Mexico[4]
Unclassified enteroviruses	Feces	Philippines[6]

Newer techniques to determine viral homogeneity by genetic analysis must be performed on isolates to resolve this issue.

Feeding of echovirus 6 or coxsackievirus B1 to dogs produced minimal signs suggestive of enteric disease, and although the virus could be isolated from the feces, seroconversion could not be demonstrated.[8, 9] Infection seems to be limited to the alimentary tract of dogs and does not spread systemically as such infections do in people. Although dogs shed these viruses in low amounts, viral spread to susceptible dogs has resulted in infection.[9] Whether infected dogs can be a source of human infection is uncertain.

References

1. Graves IL, Oppenheimer JR: Human viruses in animals in West Bengal: an ecological analysis. *Hum Ecol* 3:105–130, 1975.
2. Grew N, Gohd RS, Arguedas J, et al: Enteroviruses in rural families and their domestic animals. *Am J Epidemiol* 91:518–526, 1970.

3. Clapper WE: Comments on viruses recovered from dogs. J Am Vet Med Assoc 156:1678–1680, 1970.

4. Lundgren DL, Clapper WE, Sanchez A: Isolation of human enteroviruses from beagle dogs. Soc Exp Biol Med 128:463–466, 1968.

5. Pindak FF, Clapper WE: Isolation of enteric cytopathogenic human orphan virus type 6 from dogs. Am J Vet Res 25:52–54, 1964.

6. Steele JH, Arambulo PV, Beran GW: The epidemiology of zoonosis in the Philippines. Arch Environ Health 26:330–338, 1973.

7. Lundgren DL, Meade GH, Clapper WE: Cross neu-

tralization and gel double diffusion studies of enteroviruses isolated from beagle dogs. Texas Rep Biol Med 28:48–58, 1970.

8. Lundgren DL, Sanchez A, Magnuson MG, et al: A survey for human enteroviruses in dogs and man. Arch Gesamte Virusforsch 32:229–235, 1970.

9. Pindak FF, Clapper WE: Experimental infection of beagle with ECHO virus type 6. Texas Rep Biol Med 24:466–472, 1966.

10. Lundgren DL, Hobbs CH, Clapper WE: Experimental infection of beagle dogs with Coxsackievirus type B1. Am J Vet Res 32:609–613, 1971.

34 MUMPS AND INFLUENZA VIRUS INFECTIONS

Craig E. Greene

MUMPS

Mumps virus is a member of the family Paramyxoviridae and genus *Paramyxovirus*. The virus causes illness in humans, its primary natural hosts; however, nonhuman primates and other laboratory animals have been experimentally infected. Clinical signs in affected people include fever, anorexia, and progressive, independent enlargement of the parotid salivary glands. Meningitis, the main complication of infection that sometimes develops, results in headache and nuchal rigidity. Encephalitis, polyarthritis, and pancreatitis may uncommonly develop. Vaccination programs have greatly reduced the prevalence and severity of this infectious disease throughout the world.

Mumps viral antibodies have been identified in the sera of healthy dogs; however, dogs can be infected with canine parainfluenza virus (CPiV; similar to but distinct from SV-5 of nonhuman primates; see Chapters 19 and 20), which may cross-react with some mumps viral antigens. Interpretation of prior serologic studies may be misleading for this reason. Nevertheless, there are several reports of parotid salivary gland enlargement in dogs from households where children in the family have had concurrent or recent mumps-like infections.[1–4] Antibody to mumps viral antigen was detected in the serum of some affected dogs[2, 4] and a virus, neutralized by mumps viral antisera, was found in one dog.[2] Early experimental attempts to produce mumps in dogs or cats by inoculation of virus directly into the gland were inconclusive.[2, 5] Although in vivo transmission studies are inconclusive, mumps virus does grow well in primary dog kidney cell culture; this has been a source of producing attenuated vaccine for human use.[3, 6, 7] Veterinarians in practice should be aware of the possible association between mumps in children and pets, although definitive evidence for animal infection is lacking.

INFLUENZA

Influenza viruses are in the family Orthomyxoviridae. Two genera, types A and B, produce an acute self-limiting febrile illness in susceptible people as episodic outbreaks almost every winter. Type C influenza viruses are less closely related and produce similar disease. Fever, myalgia, and signs of upper or lower respiratory infections are the most common manifestations. Mortality develops from pulmonary complications. Pandemic spread of influenza may result periodically when as a result of genetic alteration of surface glycoproteins, a new virus strain, to which the world population has no immunity, emerges.

Influenza virus spreads from transfer of virus-containing respiratory secretions from an infected to a susceptible person. Small (<10 μm) aerosols are the important means of spread.

Because of the close association of pets with people there has been concern that dogs and cats may be important in the spread or maintenance of influenza infection. Many reports exist of serologic evidence of infection of dogs and cats with influenza virus. Experimental intranasal or IV infection of dogs[8–11] and cats[8, 11] with influenza virus A strains, of dogs[10] and cats[8] with B strains, and of dogs[12] with type C strains has provided convincing evidence that they do become infected. Clinical signs in infected animals were either absent or consisted of a mild conjunctivitis, serous nasal discharge,

391

or variable fever. Serologic responses to infection have been inconsistent, although viruses could be recovered from their respiratory secretions. Cats and dogs were also infected in some instances by contact with infected animals.

Spontaneous influenza viral infections of dogs and cats have been associated with human populations that are suffering from epidemics of the disease.[11, 13] There is no evidence to suggest that the virus spreads from infected pets back to people.

References

1. Chandler EA: Mumps in the dog. Vet Rec 96:365–366, 1975.
2. Noice F, Bolin FM, Eveleth DF: Incidence of viral parotitis in the domestic dog. Am J Dis Child 98:350–352, 1959.
3. Izbicky A, Frohlichova S: Influence of preincubation of primary dog kidney cell cultures on the multiplication of attenuated mumps virus. Acta Virol 23:473–480, 1979.
4. Smith RE: Mumps in the dog. Vet Rec 96:296, 1975.
5. Morris JA, BLount RE, McCown JM: Natural occurrence in dog serum of antibodies against mumps virus. Cornell Vet 46:525–531, 1956.
6. Starke G, Hlinak P: Requirements for the control of a dog kidney cell–adapted live mumps virus vaccine. J Biol Stand 2:143–150, 1974.
7. Nöbel B, Glathe H: Biological particularities of the mumps virus—its behavior in the RCT-marker. J Hyg Epidemiol Microbiol Immunol 22:203–207, 1978.
8. Paniker CK, Nair CM: Experimental infection of animals with influenza virus types A and B. Bull WHO 47:461–463, 1972.
9. Nikitin T, Cohen D, Todd JD, et al: Epidemiological studies of A/Hong Kong/68 virus infection in dogs. Bull WHO 47:471–479, 1972.
10. Todd JD, Cohen D: Studies of influenza in dogs 1. Susceptibility of dogs to natural and experimental infection with human A2 and B strains of influenza virus. Am J Epidemiol 87:426–438, 1968.
11. Romváry J, Rózsa J, Farkas E: Infection of dogs and cats with the Hong Kong influenza A (H3N2) virus during an epidemic period in Hungary. Acta Vet Acad Sci Hung 25:255–259, 1975.
12. Ohwada K, Kitame F, Homma M: Experimental infection of dogs with type C influenza virus. Sixth Int Congr Virol, Sendai, Japan, Sept 1–7, 1984.
13. Chang CP, New AG, Taylor JF, et al: Influenza virus isolations from dogs during a human epidemic in Taiwan. Int J Zoon 3:61–64, 1976.

35   ARBOVIRAL INFECTIONS

Arthropod-Borne Encephalomyelitis

Craig E. Greene

All arthropod-borne viruses known to infect dogs and cats belong to the families of Togaviridae, Flaviviridae, Bunyaviridae, or Orbiviridae (Table 35–1). These RNA viruses are usually maintained in nature by a sylvan cycle involving an arthropod vector and a vertebrate reservoir host (Fig. 35–1). Domesticated animals are usually incidental hosts, but in some cases, they act as reservoirs. As unnatural hosts, domesticated animals may be subclinically affected or show signs of disease (usually nonsuppurative, neurotropic encephalitis). The clinical susceptibility of people, dogs, and cats for each disease also varies. Since serologic cross-reactivity between certain viruses can occur and because dogs and cats can be subclinically infected, the following discussion emphasizes those cases in which virus isolation and consistent pathologic findings have been present or where experimental inoculation of dogs or cats has been performed. Serologic testing indicates a large number of these viruses may infect dogs and cats.

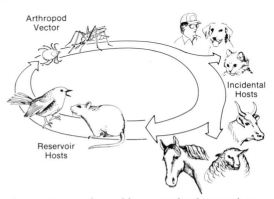

Figure 35–1. Arthropod-borne viral infections have a sylvan cycle involving arthropod vectors that feed on reservoir hosts. Domestic animals and people are usually incidental hosts, but they may serve as reservoirs in some instances (see Table 35–1).

Togaviridae

Natural and experimental susceptibility of dogs to Venezuelan equine encephalitis (VEE) virus has been well described. In both natural and experimental infections using mosquitos, viremia and seroconversion occur without clinical illness.[6] For this reason, dogs have been considered good sentinel hosts for human VEE infection and have been used to monitor the spread of infection into geographic areas. Parenteral inoculation of VEE in dogs has produced fever, leukopenia, and neurologic deficits at the peak of the febrile response.[4,5] Cerebrovascular hemorrhage and infarction were detected.[5] Nat-

urally occurring VEE was also suspected as causing encephalitis in a puppy.[20] Eastern equine encephalitis was diagnosed in three naturally infected dogs from south central Georgia.[1] All were in dogs less than 6 weeks of age with signs of diffuse encephalitis. The virus was confirmed by IFA in one case. Experimentally, dogs have developed diffuse encephalitis following intracerebral or parenteral inoculation of Western equine encephalitis virus.[3]

Flaviviridae

Dogs and cats have been more resistant to St. Louis encephalitis,[2] although serosurveys have demonstrated them to develop titers in human epidemics. Parenteral inoculation of Japanese encephalitis virus has resulted in subclinical infection, but intracranial inoculation resulted in encephalitis with corresponding neurologic deficits.[7] Louping-ill is described in a separate section of this chap-

Table 35–1. Arthropod-Borne Viral Infections Affecting Dogs and Cats[a]

DISEASE	GEOGRAPHIC DISTRIBUTION	ARTHROPOD VECTOR	USUAL HOSTS Reservoir (Domestic)	SUSCEPTIBILITY OF PEOPLE, DOGS AND CATS
Togaviridae				
Eastern equine encephalitis[1]	Eastern USA, Central America, Caribbean islands, Brazil, Guyana, Argentina	*Culiseta melanura, Aedes* spp, *Culex* spp	Birds (horses, quail, pheasants, cows, sheep)	H,D
Western equine encephalitis[2,3]	USA, Canada, Central America, Guyana, Brazil, Argentina	*Culiseta melanura, Culex* spp	Birds, small mammals, snakes (horses)	H,D
Venezuelan equine encephalitis[4-6]	Florida, Texas, northern South America, Central America	*Psorophora confinnis, Aedes* spp, *Culex* spp	Rodents (horses)	H,D,C
Flaviviridae				
St. Louis encephalitis[2]	USA, Canada, Central America, Caribbean islands, Colombia, Brazil, Argentina	*Culex* spp	Birds (usually inapparent)	H,D,[b]C[b]
Japanese encephalitis[7]	Siberia, Japan, China, many Far East countries	*Culex* spp	Birds (pigs, horses)	H,D,C[b]
Louping-Ill[8]	Scotland, Ireland	*Ixodes ricinus*	Sheep?, red grouse (sheep, cattle)	H,D
Powassan[2]	USA, Canada	*Ixodes cookei, I. marxi*	Rodents (sheep)	H,D[b]
Tick-borne encephalitis[9,10]	Europe, USSR	*Ixodes* spp, *Dermacentor* spp	Rodents, birds (sheep, goats, cattle)	H,D[b,c]
Wesselsbron disease[11]	South Africa	*Aedes* spp	Ungulates, sheep (sheep)	D
Yellow fever[12]	South America, Africa	*Aedes* spp	Nonhuman primates, humans (none)	H,C[b]
Bunyaviridae				
Tenshaw[13]	Southeastern USA	*Anopheles* spp	Rodents (cattle, dogs)	D,C
Rift Valley[14-17] fever	East Africa	*Culex theileri, Aedes caballus*	Ungulates (sheep, cattle)	H,D,[c]C[d]
Orbiviridae				
African horse sickness[18,19]	Africa	*Culicoides* spp	Equidae (horse)	D[e]

[a]H = human, D = dog, C = cat; [b]Subclinical; [c]puppies; [d]kittens; [e]subclinical, carnivorism.

ter. Dogs have developed fever, viremia, and a serologic response to Powassan virus.[2] Tick-borne encephalitis virus inoculated into puppies produced a low-titer viremia and no clinical illness, although naive ticks feeding on the dogs became infected.[10] Wesselsbron virus was isolated from the CNS of a dog with encephalitis. Material from this case was subsequently inoculated into dogs that seroconverted; a viremia developed and one dog manifested transient paralysis.[11] Yellow fever virus has produced a transient viremia in cats following inoculation[12]; however, puppies, even when splenectomized, could not be infected.[21]

Bunyaviridae

Tensaw virus inoculated into dogs and cats produced nonsymptomatic viremia.[13] Mosquito transmission from infected dogs was also demonstrated. Rift Valley fever vi-

rus has produced viremia, severe hepatic necrosis, myocarditis, splenic congestion, meningitis, diffuse petechiation, and death in puppies and kittens less than 3 weeks of age.[14-17] Virus can also be transmitted from puppies to their mother and to other puppies. Older puppies do not succumb to infection but develop viremias. The virus can cause abortion and stillbirth in pregnant bitches. Inhalation or ingestion of the virus from infected carcasses may occur under natural circumstances.[17]

Orbiviridae

Dogs can be infected subclinically with African horse sickness virus; they develop a serologic response and a viremia enabling them to transmit the infection.[18, 19] They are thought to acquire infection naturally by eating dead infected ungulate carcasses.

Louping-Ill *Hugh W. Reid*

ETIOLOGY

Louping-ill is an acute viral encephalomyelitis transmitted by the sheep tick *Ixodes ricinus*. Although it occurs most frequently in sheep, louping-ill has been reported in people, horses, pigs, goats, farmed deer, and dogs, but not in cats.

The causal virus is a member of an antigenically closely related complex of arboviruses (family Flaviviridae) that cause tick-borne encephalitis. These viruses, present throughout the northern temperate latitudes, are primarily associated with disease in people. Infection in domestic animals has been recognized regularly only in the British Isles in areas of rough pastures where sheep ticks are prevalent. However, encephalomyelitis in sheep due to infection by either louping-ill virus or closely related viruses has occurred also in Bulgaria, Turkey, Spain, and Norway, suggesting that the disease may be more widespread.[22]

Risk of infection is generally restricted to the periods of tick activity, mainly in the spring and early summer, with a recrudescence in some areas in the fall. However, the precise periods of tick activity vary with latitude and altitude. In dogs, infection has been diagnosed most frequently in working sheepdogs and gun dogs,[15, 23, 24] but any animal visiting enzootic areas during periods of tick activity may become affected. Infection is assumed to be through the bite of the tick. Alternative routes of transmission should not be overlooked, since disease in people is commonly encountered in abattoir workers. Young goats and pigs can become infected by the ingestion of virus-infected milk and carcasses, respectively.

CLINICAL FINDINGS

The initial systemic phase following infection generally is not associated with clinical signs, but during this period the animal is viremic, and virus invades the central nervous tissue. The subsequent course of disease is variable. Many infections are not recognized clinically because virus is eliminated by the immune response that subsequently maintains protection and detectable serum antibody titers, probably for the life of the animal. In animals that do develop clinical disease, initial signs, primarily due to cerebellar dysfunction, are mild paresis, ataxia, and tremors that sometimes are associated with difficulty in eating. Within 24 hours, severe incoordination develops. The affected animal is usually in lateral recumbency, paddling its limbs, but this may progress to complete tetraplegia or opisthotonos. Death may occur at any time, but in dogs that survive, recovery is slow, and locomotor dysfunction may persist for months. On recovery, temperamental and physical changes may be present, the animal being nervous, exercise-intolerant, and less tractable.

DIAGNOSIS

Diagnosis relies on the detection of a rising serum antibody response to louping-ill virus during the course of the infection. In fatal cases, histologic examination of the brain accompanied with virus isolation can confirm the disease. Histologic changes include neuronal necrosis and perivascular lymphoid cell accumulations that are particularly prominent in the spinal cord and cerebellum (Fig. 35–2). Virus may be isolated from a homogenate of brain tissue by intracerebral inoculation of 3-week-old mice or in tissue culture cells.

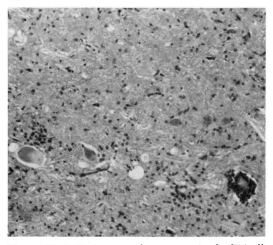

Figure 35–2. Brain stem from an animal clinically affected with louping-ill, showing neurononecrosis, gliosis, and lymphocytic perivascular cuffing (H and E, × 50) (Courtesy Dr. D. Buxton, Moredun Research Institute, Edinburgh, Scotland).

THERAPY AND PREVENTION

Supportive therapy during the acute phase is beneficial, but no specific treatment is available. An inactivated, tissue culture–propagated vaccine incorporated in an oil adjuvant is available for protection of cattle, sheep, and goats and has been used in dogs. However, dogs appear to require at least two injections to elicit a detectable serum antibody response, and a proportion of them develop painless, fluid-filled swellings at the site of injection that may require surgical drainage.[25]

The ecology of louping-ill virus is largely dependent on a sheep-tick cycle with little involvement of the native fauna. Systematic vaccination of sheep may reduce the prevalence of virus and may therefore reduce the risk of infecting other incidental hosts such as dogs.

References

1. Hall RF: Eastern encephalomyelitis in canines. *Vet Newslett* Sept:2–3, 1982.
2. Furimoto HH: Susceptibility of dogs to St. Louis encephalitis and other selected arthropod-borne viruses. *Am J Vet Res* 30:1371–1380, 1969.
3. Schlotthauer CF: The susceptibility of dogs to viruses of equine encephalomyelitis (western). *J Am Vet Med Assoc* 99:388–390, 1941.
4. Taber LE, Hogge AL, McKinney RW: Experimental infection of dogs with two strains of Venezuelan equine encephalomyelitis virus. *Am J Trop Med Hyg* 14:647–651, 1965.
5. Davis MH, Hogge AL, Corristan EC, et al: Mosquito transmission of Venezuelan equine encephalomyelitis virus from experimentally infected dogs. *Am J Trop Med Hyg* 15:227–230, 1966.
6. Bivin WS, Barry C, Hogge AL, et al: Mosquito-induced infection with equine encephalomyelitis virus in dogs. *Am J Trop Med Hyg* 16:544–547, 1967.
7. Hotta S, Kuromaru S, Funasaka K, et al: Experimental infection of dogs with Japaneses B encephalitis virus. *Acta Neuropathol* 3:494–510, 1964.
8. Mackenzie CP, Lewis WD, Smith ST, et al: Louping-ill in a working collie. *Vet Rec* 92:354–356, 1973.
9. Wandeler A, Steck F, Fankhauser R, et al: Isolierung des Virus der zentraleuropäischen Zeckencephalitis in der Schweiz. *Pathol Microbiol* 38:258, 1972.
10. Gresikova M, Weidnerova K, Nose KJ, et al: Experimental pathogenicity of tick-borne encephalitis virus for dogs. *Acta Virol* 16:336–340, 1972.
11. Simpson VR, Keubart G, Barnard B: A fatal case of Wesselsbron disease in a dog. *Vet Rec* 105:329, 1979.
12. Findley GM: Rift Valley fever or enzootic hepatitis. *Trans Roy Soc Trop Med Hyg* 25:229–262, 1931.
13. Sudia WD, Coleman PH, Chamberlain RW: Experimental vector-host studies with Tensaw virus, a newly recognized member of the Bunyamwera arbovirus group. *Am J Trop Med Hyg* 18:98–102, 1969.
14. Mitten JQ, Remmele NS, Walker JS, et al: The clinical aspects of Rift Valley fever in housepets III. Pathologic changes in the dog and cat. *J Infect Dis* 121:25–31, 1970.
15. Walker JS, Remmele NS, Carter RC, et al: The clinical aspects of Rift Valley fever in household pets I. Susceptibility of the dog. *J Infect Dis* 121:9–18, 1970.
16. Walker JS, Stephen EL, Remmele NS, et al: The clinical aspects of Rift Valley fever in household pets II. Susceptibility of the cat. *J Infect Dis* 121:19–24, 1970.
17. Keefer GV, Zebarth GL, Allen WP: Susceptibility of dogs and cats to Rift Valley fever by inhalation or ingestion of virus. *J Infect Dis* 125:307–309, 1972.
18. Dardiri AH, Ozawa Y: Immune and serologic response of dogs to neurotropic and viscerotropic African sickness viruses. *J Am Vet Med Assoc* 155:400–407, 1969
19. Salama SA, Dardiri AH, Awad FI, et al: Isolation and identification of African horsesickness virus from naturally infected dogs in Upper Egypt. *Can J Comp Med* 45:392–396, 1981.
20. Habluetzel JE, Grimes JE, Pigott MB: Serologic evidence of naturally occurring Venezuelan equine encephalomyelitis virus infection in a dog. *J Am Vet Med Assoc* 162:461–462, 1973.
21. Stokes A, Bauer JH, Hudson NP: Experimental transmission of yellow fever virus to laboratory animals. *Am J Trop Med Hyg* 8:103–164, 1928.
22. Reid HW: Louping-ill. *In* Monath T (ed): *The Arboviruses: Epidemiology and Ecology*, Vol III. Boca Raton, FL, CRC Press, 1988, pp 117–135.
23. Hobson G: Louping-ill in a working collie. *Vet Rec* 92:436, 1973.
24. Mackenzie CP: Recovery of a dog from louping-ill. *J Small Anim Pract* 23: 233–236, 1982.
25. Thomson JR, Reid HW, Pow I: Louping-ill vaccination of dogs. *Vet Rec* 120:94, 1987.

36

SALMON POISONING DISEASE

John R. Gorham
William J. Foreyt

ETIOLOGY

Salmon poisoning disease (SPD) or salmon disease, a highly fatal helminth-transmitted disease of domestic and wild Canidae, occurs on the western slopes of the Cascade Mountains from northern California to central Washington (Fig. 36–1). Occasionally, cases of SPD occur outside the indigenous range of the disease in areas where infected fish migrate or are transported. Cases in Vancouver, British Columbia, may indicate that the indigenous range of the disease is greater than previously reported.[1] The disease is caused by two rickettsiae that are antigenically distinct from other pathogenic species infecting dogs.

Salmon Disease Agent

The etiologic agent of SPD is *Neorickettsia helminthoeca*, a coccoid or coccobacillary rickettsia that is approximately 0.3 μm in size. Pleomorphic rods, up to 2 μm in length, sometimes bent in rings or crescents, have been observed. The gram-negative rickettsial organisms appear purple with Giemsa stain, red with Macchiavello's stain, black or dark brown with Levaditi's method, and pale blue with H and E. The rickettsiae almost fill the cytoplasm of cells of the mononuclear phagocyte system (MPS) that they primarily infect (Fig. 36–2). Initial attempts to grow the organism in embryonated chicken eggs, bacteriologic media, and duck embryo tissue cultures have been unsuccessful, but rickettsiae have been grown in canine monocytes,[2]

in canine leukocytes and sarcoma cells, and in mouse lymphoblasts.[3]

In dead fish, rickettsiae in metacercariae (encysted trematode larvae) do not survive 30 days at 4°C.[4] In lymph nodes, organisms resist freezing at −20°C for 31 to 158 days[5]; they remain viable in leukocytes at 4.5°C and 52.5°C for 48 hours and 2 minutes, respectively, but not at 60°C for 5 minutes.[6] At −80°C, the agent can be maintained in cell culture fluid for up to 3 months.[7]

Elokomin Fluke Fever Agent

The Elokomin fluke fever (EFF) agent[8] probably is another strain of *N. helminthoeca*.[2, 9] The disease in dogs associated with the EFF agent results in high morbidity but a lower mortality than SPD. It appears that metacercariae can harbor both EFF and SPD agents simultaneously. EFF is rarely recognized as a distinct entity in naturally occurring disease. Histologically, EFF infections in dogs are similar to but less severe than those seen with SPD.

EPIDEMIOLOGY

The vector of SPD is a trematode, *Nanophyetus salmincola*, which harbors the rickettsiae throughout its life cycle stages from egg to adult.[10] Three different hosts are required for the completion of the trematode life cycle—snails, fish, and mammals or birds (Fig. 36–3). Lists of intermediate and definitive hosts of the fluke can be found

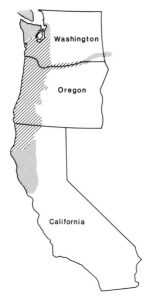

Figure 36–1. Distribution of indigenous salmon poisoning disease. Area indicated by slashed lines represents the distribution of *Oxytrema silicula* and the usual distribution of salmon poisoning disease. Area indicated by dots represents occasional cases of salmon poisoning disease usually resulting from infected migrating fish.

elsewhere.[10] The snail intermediate host, *Oxytrema silicula*, is a pleurocerid that inhabits fresh or brackish stream water in coastal areas of Washington, Oregon, and northern California. Areas of trematode infection therefore depend on the distribution of *O.*

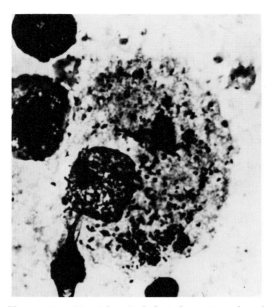

Figure 36–2. *Neorickettsia helminthoeca* in a lymph node smear (Giemsa stain; × 1000).

silicula. Cercariae (free-swimming trematode larvae) leave the snail and penetrate the second intermediate host, which is usually a salmonid fish, certain species of nonsalmonid fish, or the Pacific giant salamander (*Dicamptodon ensatus*). The metacercariae usually localize in the kidneys of fish (Fig. 36–4) but can be found in any tissue. Fish are infected in fresh water and retain the trematode and the rickettsial infection throughout their ocean migration before returning to fresh water up to 3 years later.[11]

Adult trematodes develop in the intestine approximately 6 days after the ingestion of metacercariae-infected fish by dogs and certain other fish-eating mammals, such as bears and raccoons, and birds, that serve as definitive hosts. Clinical signs of rickettsial disease occur in Canidae, primarily dogs and coyotes. However, two captive polar bears receiving long-term glucocorticoid therapy for skin conditions succumbed to an SPD-like disease after eating inadequately frozen salmon.[12] Cats are not susceptible to SPD, but trematodes will develop when infected fish are ingested.[10]

SPD also has been transmitted by parenteral injection of infected blood, spleen and lymph suspensions, adult flukes, helminth-infected snail livers, and helminth eggs. Partial transmission success was obtained by allowing ticks (*Haemaphysalis leachi* and *Rhipicephalus sanguineus*) that had fed on infected dogs to subsequently feed on susceptible dogs and by parenteral injection of suspensions of *R. sanguineus* into dogs.[13] Susceptible dogs also have been experimentally infected with aerosolized lymph node suspensions from infected dogs, and on rare occasions, direct transmission of infection between dogs has been suspected.[14]

PATHOGENESIS

After ingestion of raw, metacercariae-infected salmonid fish by a susceptible dog, the fluke matures, and the adult stage attaches to the mucosa of the intestine and by some unknown mechanism inoculates the rickettsiae (Fig. 36–5). Initial replication of rickettsiae probably takes place in the epithelial cells of the villi or in the intestinal lymphoid tissue. Inflammation of the solitary lymphoid follicles and Peyer's patches along the intestinal tract contributes to en-

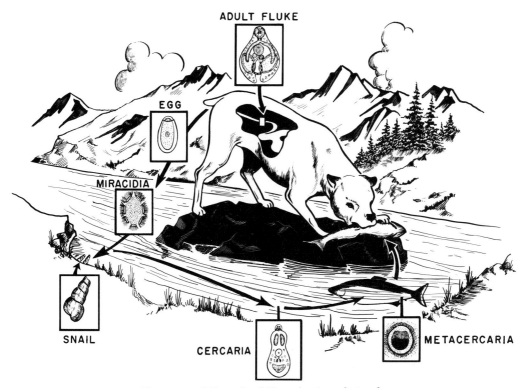

Figure 36–3. Life cycle of *Nanophyetus salmincola*.

teritis. Mild enteritis may be observed in dogs infected only with the flukes, without rickettsiae.

Rickettsiae enter the blood early in the course of the disease and spread to the lymph nodes, spleen, tonsils, thymus, liver, lungs, and brain.[9] Although secondary bacterial infections often occur, the exact cause of death in SPD is unknown. Investigations to demonstrate a toxin have been limited.

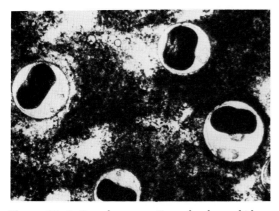

Figure 36–4. Squash preparation of salmon kidney containing numerous metacercariae of *Nanophyetus salmincola* (× 200).

CLINICAL FINDINGS

Salmon Poisoning Disease

The signs of infection are consistent in all Canidae with SPD. The usual incubation period following the ingestion of parasitized fish is 5 to 7 days, although some dogs have incubation periods as long as 19 to 33 days. The first sign usually is a sudden febrile response, which typically reaches a peak of 40° to 42°C (104° to 107.6°F) (Fig. 36–6). The temperature gradually decreases to normal or below normal over the next 4 to 8 days. Dogs are frequently hypothermic when death occurs 7 to 10 days after the initial clinical evidence of infection. Some animals show only a slight increase in temperature or a shortened febrile period; however, they may still die if left untreated.

Anorexia frequently accompanies or follows the onset of fever and may be marked and complete. Affected animals often continue to have inappetence throughout the course of the disease. Marked weight loss, weakness, and depression usually follow. Within 14 days of eating infected fish, coyotes on a controlled experiment lost approx-

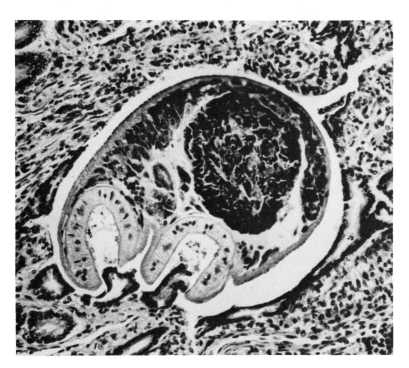

Figure 36–5. *Nanophyetus salmincola* ingesting intestinal mucosa and initiating *N. helminthoeca* infection in a dog (H and E; × 300).

imately 58% of their body weight when compared with uninfected coyotes.[4] Diarrhea and vomiting may occur, the diarrhea becoming progressively worse and often consisting primarily of blood at the time of death. The animal will occasionally exhibit extreme thirst and will drink copious quantities of water. A serous nasal discharge may be recorded early in the febrile period. Later, a mucopurulent conjunctival exudate may be seen. Enlarged cervical and prescapular lymph nodes can be palpated as early as 5 days PI.

SPD-infected dogs may show severe GI signs that are often clinically indistinguishable from canine parvovirus enteritis. Distemper and SPD can also occur concurrently, and appropriate laboratory tests can be conducted to determine which agent is involved in a particular animal.

Elokomin Fluke Fever

The incubation period is generally 5 to 12 days. The febrile period, which differs from that of SPD, is marked by a plateau of elevated temperature lasting 4 to 7 days, followed by a decline, usually to subnormal temperature.[8] Other signs are similar to those of SPD.

DIAGNOSIS

Operculated trematode eggs appear in dog feces 5 to 8 days following the ingestion of infected fish. The light brown egg is approximately 87 to 97 μm x 35 to 55 μm, with a small, blunt point on the end opposite the indistinct operculum (Fig. 36–7). Eggs can be detected on direct smears or by a washing-sedimentation technique.[15] In addition, the authors have routinely recovered *Nanophyetus salmincola* eggs with the Sheather's sugar flotation technique (specific gravity, 1.27). Eggs recovered by this latter method are somewhat deformed but recognizable. See Appendix 12 for a discussion of these procedures. Diagnosis of the rickettsial disease cannot be made entirely on the presence of trematode eggs in feces, because trematode infection does not necessarily indicate rickettsial infection. In addition, animals that have recovered from the rickettsial disease may be reinfected with the trematode. The trematode infection can remain patent for 60 to 250 days.[4]

Fluid aspirated from enlarged lymph

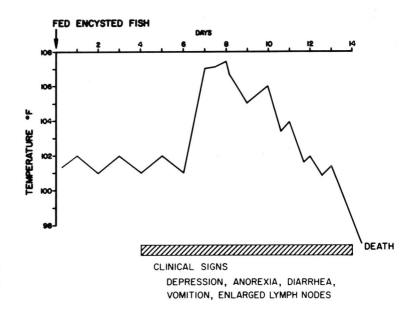

Figure 36–6. Clinical course of salmon poisoning disease in a dog.

FED ENCYSTED FISH

CLINICAL SIGNS
DEPRESSION, ANOREXIA, DIARRHEA,
VOMITION, ENLARGED LYMPH NODES

nodes can be air dried on a microscope slide, fixed, defatted for 1 minute with a mixture of equal parts of ether and absolute alcohol, and then stained by Giemsa or Macchiavello's stain. In addition, a rapid-staining Giemsa technique that involves staining the fixed smears for 2 minutes with equal parts of stock Giemsa and buffered water at pH 7.2 and then washing the slides can be used.[15] Typical intracytoplasmic rickettsial bodies are characteristically seen in MPS cells (see Fig. 36–2). Extracellular organisms are not easily separated from artifacts and should not be considered diagnostic for SPD.

Hematologic and biochemical findings of SPD are relatively nonspecific. Total leukocyte counts in naturally infected dogs range from leukopenia to leukocytosis.[16] Coyotes that had been experimentally infected with SPD rickettsiae had significantly higher numbers of band cells, lower numbers of eosinophils and lower concentrations of creatinine, glucose, calcium, inorganic phosphorus, albumin, and activity of alkaline phosphatase than did control coyotes.[4]

PATHOLOGIC FINDINGS

The principal gross findings at necropsy are changes in lymphoid tissues. The tonsils, thymus, and visceral and somatic nodes are markedly enlarged. The most pronounced swelling occurs in the ileocecal, colic, mesenteric, portal and lumbar nodes. The nodes are usually yellowish, with prominent white foci representing the cortical follicles. Occasionally, nodes show diffuse petechiae, and edema is often observed.

The spleen frequently ranges from slightly swollen to nearly twice the normal size. Splenic follicles, which often appear as grayish-white nodules in foxes, are unaffected in dogs. The spleens of animals that die of SPD are typically a dark bluish red, smooth, soft, and blood filled. Livers of dogs are usually normal, although those of foxes are usually soft and a pale yellowish brown. Hemorrhages may appear in the gallbladder wall. Petechiae may be the only change in the

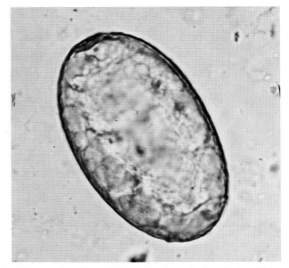

Figure 36–7. Egg of *Nanophyetus salmincola* (× 480).

pancreas. The kidneys of dogs are grossly normal, whereas those of foxes may have a slight color change toward a pale yellowish brown. The mucosa of the urinary bladder may show petechiae.

Along the intestinal tract, petechiae may be apparent in the mucosae of the lower esophagus, large intestine, ileocolic valve, distal colon, rectum, and gastric serosa. There may be bleeding ulcers in the pylorus. Intussusception of the ileum into the colon may also occur. The intestinal contents frequently contain free blood. Some blood may also appear in the colon and rectum. The intestines are typically empty except for some bile-stained mucus. Flukes in the intestinal tissue, primarily found in the duodenum, cause some tissue damage.

Microscopically, a characteristic pattern is observed in lymphocytic tissues. The lymph nodes show a marked and consistent depletion in the number of mature lymphocytes, with hyperplasia of the MPS cells in the cortex and medulla. In most foxes and dogs, there are foci of necrosis in the MPS cells. The CNS is usually involved with nonsuppurative meningitis or meningoencephalitis.[17]

THERAPY

All patients should be hospitalized so that they receive adequate monitoring and nursing care. Control of the infectious agent, N. helminthoeca, can be achieved with oral or parenteral sulfonamides, penicillin, chlortetracycline, chloramphenicol, or oxytetracycline. Aminoglycosides are ineffective. The preferred treatment schedule is oxytetracycline given for at least 3 days (Table 36–1). Oral tetracycline therapy, used for most rickettsial disease, may be difficult and may not be indicated because of the severe vomiting and diarrhea that is usually present.

Relief of dehydration, emesis, and diarrhea is also important. Fluid therapy with appropriate electrolytes should be administered IV. In cases of hemorrhagic diarrhea, transfusion of whole blood may be necessary. Other antidiarrheal treatments include fasting followed by gradual introduction of a bland, high-calorie diet. In addition, the most supportive treatment consists of keeping the dog dry, clean, and warm.

Praziquantel, when given as one dose at appropriate dosages (see Table 36–1), is highly effective against N. salmincola in coyotes and dogs.[18] Elimination of N. salmincola from infected animals will minimize the diarrhea associated from fluke infections alone and will minimize or eliminate fluke eggs from feces.

PREVENTION

Vaccines have not been developed against SPD, and therefore, keeping dogs from feeding on infected fish is the best means of preventing infection. Because metacercariae can remain viable for months in rotting fish carcasses, dogs will become infected with the fluke if they eat decomposed fish; however, they may not develop SPD. Also, in many areas, metacercariae apparently contain nonpathogenic rickettsiae.[19] Freezing fish at −20°C for 24 hours or thoroughly cooking infected fish will kill both the metacercariae and rickettsiae.[20] Supplemental prevention methods include isolation of dogs with SPD and sterilization of equipment used around infected dogs.

Infection of fish in hatcheries can be prevented by destruction of free-living cercariae by passing incoming water through an electrically charged grid or past an ultrasonic generator.[21] These methods have not been utilized on a large scale. Other control tech-

Table 36–1. Therapy for Salmon Poisoning Disease[a]

DRUG	DOSE[b] (mg/kg)	ROUTE	INTERVAL (hours)	DURATION (days)
Oxytetracycline[c]	7	IV[d]	8	3–5
Tetracycline[c]	22	PO	8	3–5
Praziquantel[e]	10–30	PO, SC	Once	

[a]IV = intravenous, PO = oral, SC = subcutaneous.
[b]Dose per administration at specified interval, expressed as mg/kg unless otherwise stated.
[c]For rickettsial infection.
[d]Parenteral therapy preferred because of GI signs.
[e]For fluke infection.

niques such as snail elimination are impractical.

References

1. Booth AJ, Stogdale L, Grigor JA: Salmon poisoning disease in dogs on southern Vancouver Island. *Can Vet J* 25:2–6, 1984.
2. Frank DW, McGuire TC, Gorham JR, et al: Cultivation of two species of *Neorickettsia* in canine monocytes. *J Infect Dis* 129:257–262, 1974.
3. Noonan WE: *Neorickettsia helminthoeca* in cell culture. PhD diss, Oregon State University, Corvallis, OR, 1973.
4. Foreyt WJ, Gorham JR, Green JS, et al: Salmon poisoning disease in juvenile coyotes: clinical evaluation and infectivity of metacercariae and rickettsiae. *J Wildl Dis* 23: 412–417, 1987.
5. Philip C, Hadlow WJ, Hughes LE: Studies on salmon poisoning disease of canines. 1. The rickettsial relationships and pathogenicity of *Neorickettsia helminthoeca*. *Exp Parasitol* 3:336–350, 1954.
6. Sims BT, Muth OH: Salmon poisoning: transmission and immunization studies. *In* Proceedings. 5th Pacific Sci Cong (1933), pp 2949–2960, 1934.
7. Brown JL, Huxsoll DL, Ristic M, et al: In vitro cultivation of *Neorickettsia helminthoeca*, the causative agent of salmon poisoning disease. *Am J Vet Res* 33:1695–1700, 1972.
8. Farrell RK: Canine rickettsiosis. *In* Kirk RW (ed): *Current Veterinary Therapy V.* Philadelphia, WB Saunders Co, 1974, pp 985–987.
9. Frank DW, McGuire TC, Gorham JR, et al: Lymphoreticular lesions of canine rickettsiosis. *J Infect Dis* 129:163–171, 1974.
10. Knapp SE, Millemann RE: Salmon poisoning disease. *In* Davis JW (ed): *Infectious Diseases of Wild Mammals.* Ames, Iowa State University Press, 1981, pp 376–387.
11. Weiseth PR, Farrell RK, Johnston SD: Prevalence of *Nanophyetus salmincola* in ocean-caught salmon. *J Am Vet Med Assoc* 165:849–850, 1974.
12. Schmidt M: Personal communication. Portland, OR, 1982.
13. Philip CB: There's always something new under the "parasitological sun" (the unique story of helminth-borne salmon poisoning disease. *J Parasitol* 41:125–148, 1955.
14. Bosman DD, Farrell RK, Gorham JR: Non-endoparasite transmission of salmon poisoning disease of dogs. *J Am Vet Med Assoc* 156:1907–1910, 1970.
15. Farrell RK, Ott RL, Gorham JR: The clinical laboratory diagnosis of salmon poisoning. *J Am Vet Med Assoc* 127:241–244, 1955.
16. Schalm OW: Leukocyte counts and lymph node cytology in salmon poisoning of dogs. *Canine Pract* 5:59–63, 1978.
17. Hadlow WJ: Neuropathology of experimental salmon poisoning in dogs. *Am J Vet Res* 18:898–908, 1957.
18. Foreyt WJ, Gorham JR: Evaluation of praziquantel against induced *Nanophyetus salmincola* infections in coyotes and dogs. *Am J Vet Res* 48: 563–565, 1987.
19. Green JS, LeaMaster BR, Foreyt WJ, et al: Salmon poisoning disease: research on a potential method of lethal control for coyotes. *In* Proceedings. Twelfth Vertebrate Pest Conference, University of California, Davis, CA, 1986, pp 312–317.
20. Farrell RK, Soave OA, Johnston SD: *Nanophyetus salmincola* infections in kippered salmon. *Am J Public Health* 64:808–809, 1974.
21. Farrell RK, Watson RE, Lloyd M: Effect of ultrasound on trematode cercariae. *J Parasitol* 59:747–748, 1973.

37

CANINE EHRLICHIOSIS

Ehrlichia canis, E. equi, *and* E. risticii *Infections*

Gregory C. Troy
S. Dru Forrester

ETIOLOGY AND EPIDEMIOLOGY

Canine ehrlichiosis is a tick-borne disease caused by the obligate intracellular parasite, *Ehrlichia canis* (Fig. 37–1). This organism is a member of the family Rickettsiaceae. The organism is located intracytoplasmically within a plasma-lined membrane, and reproduces by binary fission.[1, 2] A disease clinically resembling acute canine ehrlichiosis, caused by an organism that serologically resembles *E. canis*, has been identified recently in humans in southern regions of the United States[3–8, 8a] and in reservists at an army field station in New Jersey.[8b] Other antigenically distinguishable ehrlichial species isolated naturally in dogs include *E. platys* and *E. equi* (Table 37–1). Dogs develop subclinical infection, rickettsemia, and seropositivity for periods from 100 to 200 days after experimental inoculation of

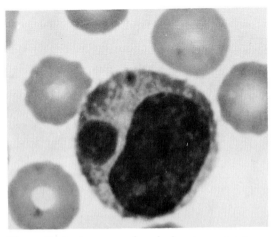

Figure 37–1. A mononuclear leukocyte containing a compact *E. canis* morula in the cytoplasm (Giemsa stain; × 2400). (Courtesy of Dr. C. F. Simpson, University of Florida, Gainesville, FL).

E. risticii, the agent of equine monocytic ehrlichiosis (EME, Potomac horse fever).[9] Cats, more commonly than dogs, have been found to be seropositive under natural conditions.[10, 11] Cats also are susceptible to experimental infection with *E. risticii* and develop rickettsemia and transient diarrhea, lymphadenomegaly, anorexia, and depression.[10, 11a] The role of dogs or cats as reservoirs and the precise insect vectors for EME are still uncertain. Except when otherwise stated, the information presented below refers to infection of dogs with *E. canis*.

The arthropod vector and primary reservoir for *E. canis* is the brown dog tick, *Rhipicephalus sanguineus*. This vector is found throughout the southern United States primarily below the forty-second parallel. Seropositive dogs have been found in most states within the continental United States (Fig. 37–2). Once infected, this three-host tick (Fig. 37–3) can transmit the disease for at least 155 days after detaching from the host. Transovarian transmission does not occur in the arthropod host. Because *R. sanguineus* carries other organisms, dogs with ehrlichiosis can be concurrently infected with *Babesia* and *Hepatozoon*.[12, 13]

PATHOGENESIS

Infection of the vertebrate host occurs when the tick ingests a blood meal and salivary secretions contaminate the feeding site. Following an incubation period of 8 to 20 days, three stages of the disease may occur in both experimental and natural infections.

The **acute phase** of ehrlichiosis lasts from

Table 37–1. Differentiating Characteristics of Ehrlichial Species Infecting Dogs, Cats, Horses, or Humans[a]

SPECIES (DISEASE)	GEOGRAPHIC DISTRIBUTION	VECTOR	LEUKOCYTES INFECTED	NATURAL HOST	EXPERIMENTAL HOST
E. canis (Canine ehrlichiosis)	Worldwide, tropical and temperate	Rhipicephalus sanguineus	Mononuclear cells, lymphocytes, rarely neutrophils	Canidae	None
E. canis-like (Human ehrlichiosis)	Worldwide, tropical	?	Mononuclear cells, granulocytes	Humans, other?	None (yet)
E. equi (Equine ehrlichiosis)	United States	?	Neutrophils, eosinophils	Horses, dogs[b]	Burros, sheep, dogs, goats, cats, nonhuman primates
E. sennetsu (Sennetsu fever)	Western Japan, Malaysia	?	Mononuclear cells	Humans	Mice, dogs, nonhuman primates
E. platys (Infectious canine thrombo-cytopenia)	Southern United States	R. sanguineus	Platelets	Dogs	Dogs
E. risticii (Equine monocytic ehrlichiosis)	United States, Canada	?	Monocytes	Horses, cats?, foxes?, wild rabbits?	Dogs, cats, mice, nonhuman primates

[a]Information from the bibliography and from unpublished information courtesy of Dr. Cynthia J. Holland, University of Illinois, Urbana, IL, and Dr. Dan B. Fishbein, The Centers for Disease Control, Atlanta, GA.

[b]Although dogs can be experimentally infected with E. equi, the presence of organisms in neutrophils of naturally infected dogs may represent infection with a particular strain of E. canis rather than infection with E. equi.

2 to 4 weeks. Replication of the organism occurs within infected mononuclear cells; then organisms spread to organs containing mononuclear phagocytes (Fig. 37–4). These target organs include the spleen, liver, and lymph nodes. The resultant lymphoreticular hyperplasia may cause organ enlargement. Infected cells apparently attach to the microvasculature or migrate to subendothelial surfaces in target organs producing vasculitis or inciting inflammation.

Decreased platelet survival, not decreased platelet production, is responsible for the thrombocytopenia.[14] Platelet destruction or utilization results from vasculitis and inflammatory responses, or the host's immunologic or coagulatory responses cause the thrombocytopenia. Platelet dysfunction can occur directly from infection or from interference by hyperglobulinemia.[15]

Leukocyte numbers vary during the acute phase. However, increased sequestration induced by immunologic mechanisms or inflammatory utilization of circulating leukocytes may lower their counts. Decreased red cell production may also become apparent as a result of the inflammatory response.

The **subclinical phase** of ehrlichiosis is associated with persistence of the organism and increased antibody response. Antibody responses reflect the host's ineffectiveness in eliminating the intracellular organism. Similar hematologic findings as in the acute phase may persist during this stage of the disease, even in the absence of clinical signs.[16]

An ineffective immune response by the host is responsible for development of the **chronic phase** of the disease. The severity of the disease has been related to the strain of the infecting organism, concomitant diseases, breed susceptibility, and the age of the animal.[1] Impaired bone marrow production of blood elements is the main feature of this phase.

CLINICAL FINDINGS

Although once considered most common during the summer months, ehrlichiosis occurs throughout the year in a variety of climatic conditions.[17–19] Because the disease is usually insidious, the duration of clinical signs from the initial acute illness until presentation is variable and may range from 3 days to 3 years, generally existing more than

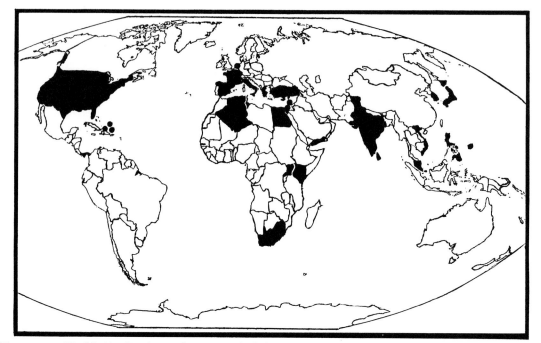

Figure 37–2. Worldwide distribution by nation (shaded areas) of reported seropositivity to *E. canis* in dogs. The actual distribution of disease is probably much greater. (Data from Dr. TJ Keefe. Personal communication, Animal Disease Diagnostic Laboratory, Kissimmee, FL, 1983.)

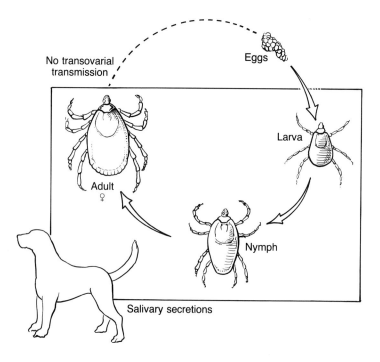

Figure 37–3. Life cycle of R. sanguineus. All three stages of this tick, including males (not shown), can feed on dogs and transmit ehrlichiosis.

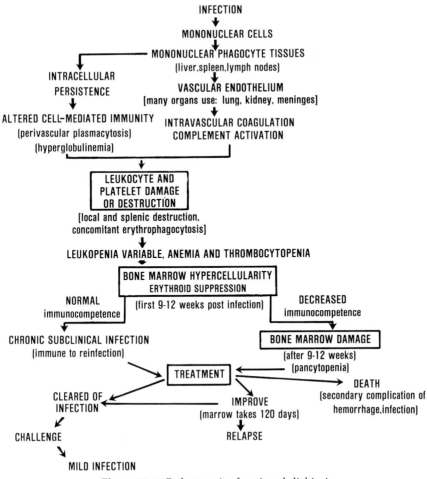

Figure 37–4. Pathogenesis of canine ehrlichiosis.

2 months.[17, 20] Of reported cases, the average age of animals at presentation is 5.22 years, with a range of 2 months to 14 years.[16, 21] The reported male to female ratio is approximately 1.5 to 1.00.[20, 22, 23]

Acute Phase

The clinical signs of the acute phase begin 1 to 3 weeks postinfection and are usually mild or inapparent. In most instances, signs are transient, often disappearing within 2 to 4 weeks. The most common historic findings have been depression and lethargy, anorexia, weight loss, and fever (Table 37–2). Hemorrhagic diatheses usually do not often occur during the acute phase, even with significant thrombocytopenia.

Respiratory signs, including increased bronchovesicular sounds, dyspnea, and cy-anosis, have been observed in some cases of ehrlichiosis as a result of hemorrhage and inflammatory changes within the lungs.[24, 25] Findings on thoracic radiographs are consistent with interstitial lung disease.[25]

Ticks are found on approximately 40% of dogs during the acute phase.[17, 19] Clinical signs of acute ehrlichiosis usually resolve without treatment. However, these dogs may remain infected and may enter the subclinical phase of illness.

Subclinical and Chronic Phase

The subclinical phase lasts from 6 to 9 weeks and may end with development of the chronic phase of ehrlichiosis. A high percentage of dogs in enzootic areas may develop subclinical disease lasting for a period of months to years.[25] Some dogs are

Table 37–2. Summary of Clinical Signs and Physical Findings in Canine Ehrlichiosis[a]

CLINICAL SIGN/ PHYSICAL FINDING	DOGS WITH ABNORMALITY (%)/ DOGS EXAMINED FOR ABNORMALITY (NO.)
Depression/lethargy	64/390
Anorexia	56/345
Weight loss	53/371
Fever (>102.5°F)	45/366
Pale mucous membranes	45/204
Bleeding tendencies	42/380
Lymphadenomegaly	36/330
Splenomegaly	20/345
Vomiting	11/265
Anterior uveitis	8/265

[a]Data summarized from references 16, 17, 19–22, 24, and 24a.

affected mildly during the chronic phase, whereas others manifest severe complications, including depression, weight loss, pale mucous membranes, abdominal tenderness, bleeding episodes, secondary infections, and scrotal and limb edema. Lymphadenopathy and splenomegaly are not usually evident, and ticks are not a common finding on physical examination during the chronic phase of infection.

Hemorrhage occurs in less than 50% of dogs with ehrlichiosis. When they develop, petechial and ecchymotic hemorrhages may be present on the abdomen and mucous membranes (e.g., vulva, prepuce, conjunctiva, and buccal cavity). Prolonged bleeding from venipuncture sites may be observed.[17] Internal hemorrhage may produce weakness, mucous membrane pallor, hyphema, epistaxis, and melena. Profound hypotension and shock secondary to severe hemorrhage and anemia may be extreme clinical manifestations.[1] Icterus rarely occurs with *E. canis* infections and is reported more frequently in dogs with concurrent *Babesia canis* infection.

Ocular abnormalities can involve the anterior and posterior segments of the eye. Initially, as a result of vasculitis, engorgement of retinal vessels occurs; however, this regresses, and perivascular lesions develop concurrently. With time, these lesions appear as dark gray spots in the tapetum and may be surrounded by areas of hyperreflectivity. Ocular lesions that occur secondary to thrombocytopenia include hyphema, subretinal hemorrhages, and retinal detachment with subsequent blindness. Anterior uveitis

characterized by conjunctivitis, corneal edema, aqueous flare, keratitic precipitates, and miosis occur in dogs with naturally occurring *E. canis* infection (see also Rickettsial Infections, Chapter 13).[26]

Neurologic signs compatible with meningitis can result from bleeding and inflammation within the meninges. The neurologic signs of ehrlichiosis are similar to those of Rocky Mountain spotted fever and can include ataxia with upper motor neuron dysfunction, acute central or peripheral vestibular dysfunction, and generalized or localized hyperesthesia.[1, 19]

Other abnormalities include anisocoria, cerebellar dysfunction, and intention tremors.[17, 19] The anisocoria may result from primary ocular or neurologic involvement.

Seizures have been observed as the primary manifestation in an infected dog.[27] All identifiable causes of seizures were eliminated, and the problem resolved with therapy with tetracycline.

Monoarthritis or polyarthritis has been associated with *E. canis* infections.[23, 28, 29] Joint effusion and soft tissue swelling can be evident radiographically. Polyarthritis may be more commonly observed in dogs infected with granulocytic cell strains of *Ehrlichia*.[30]

DIAGNOSIS

Ehrlichiosis should be suspected from the clinical history and physical examination findings. Since only 50% of infected dogs show increased bleeding tendencies, absence of hemorrhagic signs does not eliminate the possibility of ehrlichiosis. Many atypical features have been noted in spontaneously affected dogs. Clinical findings should be considered, along with results of hematology, biochemistry, and serology, in establishing a definitive antemortem diagnosis of ehrlichiosis.

Hematology

The acute stage of ehrlichiosis may not be apparent because clinical signs may be mild and transient. Thrombocytopenia occurs 10 to 20 days postinfection, and large, regenerative platelets may increase concurrently. Thrombocytopenia occurs in a high percentage of dogs with ehrlichiosis (Table 37–3) and usually persists through all phases of the disease. However, if clinical findings suggest ehrlichiosis, it should not be excluded from the differential diagnosis in the absence of thrombocytopenia.[1] The absolute platelet count does not always correlate with the severity of bleeding, and platelet numbers often fluctuate from day to day.[1, 17] Mild leukopenia occurs 3 to 4 weeks postinfection, followed by leukocytosis and monocytosis. Anemia is commonly present in dogs with ehrlichiosis and is usually nonregenerative unless concurrent B. canis infection or recent hemorrhage has occurred. Lymphocytosis has been reported infrequently during the acute phase of illness.[1] Rarely, undifferentiated or abnormal cells have been found in the circulation of some infected dogs, confusing the diagnosis with that of myeloproliferative disorders.[29] These cells disappear with appropriate therapy for ehrlichiosis. Coombs'-positive anemia may be present and can confuse the diagnosis in dogs with regenerative anemias.[1, 19, 32] These may become negative after successful treatment with antibiotics.

Bone marrow in dogs with ehrlichiosis shows marked hypercellularity of the megakaryocytic and myeloid series in the acute and subclinical phases.[2] Erythroid hypoplasia with increased M:E ratios and plasmacytosis is often noted in the chronic phase. Generalized marrow aplasia may occur in a low percentage of severely affected dogs.

Table 37–3. Summary of Hematologic and Biochemical Findings in Canine Ehrlichiosis[a]

LABORATORY ABNORMALITY	DOGS WITH ABNORMALITY (%)/ DOGS EXAMINED FOR ABNORMALITY (NO.)
Thrombocytopenia	86/327
Anemia	70/327
Eosinopenia	56/120
Lymphopenia	46/74
Increased serum ALT activity	41/271
Hypoalbuminemia	40/295
Leukopenia	31/300
Hyperproteinemia	26/299
Increased serum ALP	22/271
Elevated BUN	19/259
Elevated serum creatinine	11/238
Leukocytosis	11/300
Elevated total serum bilirubin	10/212

[a]Data summarized from references 16, 17, 19–24, and 31.

Morulae, intracellular inclusions, occur most commonly in the cytoplasm of leukocytes during the acute phase of ehrlichiosis but are transient and low in number. Inclusions are usually present in monocytes but may appear in neutrophils, lymphocytes, or eosinophils, depending on the strain or species of Ehrlichia. E. equi is the proposed agent found in neutrophils. Dogs with some granulocytic strains show positive titers to E. canis. Because of serologic cross reactivity, these infections may represent either infection with E. equi or a granulocytic strain of E. canis. Morulae consist of tightly packed organisms that stain purplish red with Wright's stain and bluish with Giemsa stain.[1, 2] Cells with morulae are most easily observed in blood from peripheral vasculature, such as ear margins, and are more likely to be detected at the feathered edge of a blood film. Examination of buffy coat smears, especially in leukopenic dogs, increases the chance of identifying morulae within cells. In addition, intracytoplasmic morulae may be identified on cytologic evaluation of bone marrow, lung, lymph node, and splenic aspirates. Because of their rarity in clinical samples, the absence of detectable morulae does not eliminate the diagnosis of ehrlichiosis.

Although clinical signs of illness are absent during subclinical phase, abnormal hematologic parameters may include thrombocytopenia, leukopenia, or anemia.[16, 21, 33] Pancytopenia is an inconsistent feature of this phase.

Pancytopenia is a typical laboratory finding in the chronic phase of ehrlichiosis. Monocytosis and lymphocytosis may be present. Eosinopenia and lymphopenia are probably secondary responses to endogenous or exogenous glucocorticoids.[20] Bone marrow during the chronic stage is usually hypoplastic, including all cell lines. However, bone marrow hypercellularity has been an inconsistent finding in one report.[22] Plasmacytosis in the bone marrow occurs regularly.[17, 20] Increased numbers of mast cells may be observed on marrow smears, but the cause is unknown.[22]

Biochemistry

The major abnormal findings are summarized in Table 37–2. ALT (formerly SGPT) and serum ALP activities may increase in dogs with ehrlichiosis, especially during the acute phase. Increased serum total bilirubin and mild icterus have been reported in a low percentage of dogs with ehrlichiosis.

Elevations in BUN and creatinine have been reported. Azotemia may be prerenal in origin (e.g., dehydration) or it may occur secondary to primary renal disease. Primary renal azotemia has been associated with glomerulonephritis and renal interstitial plasmacytosis in dogs with ehrlichiosis.[17, 20]

Hyperproteinemia, hyperglobulinemia, and hypoalbuminemia are frequently observed in ehrlichiosis. Hypoalbuminemia occurs during the acute phase and usually resolves by the subclinical phase.[34] Serum globulin levels increase progressively during the course of illness and are often apparent 1 to 3 weeks postinfection.[1, 33] The magnitude of globulin increase usually correlates directly with duration of illness. Serum protein electrophoresis usually reveals hypoalbuminemia and a polyclonal gammopathy with increased α2-, β-, and γ-globulins, typical of chronic disease.[22] A monoclonal gammopathy, characterized by increased immunoglobulin class IgG, occurs infrequently in dogs with ehrlichiosis.[16, 20, 35] For prognostic and therapeutic reasons, other causes of monoclonal gammopathy (e.g., multiple myeloma, lymphocytic leukemia) must be investigated. Hyperglobulinemia may persist for 6 to 18 months after elimination of the organism by antibiotic therapy.[1]

Tests for antinuclear or antiplatelet antibodies can have positive results.[1, 21] Autoantibodies, produced perhaps in response to persistence of the organism, may be important in the pathogenesis of chronic infections.

Proteinuria, with or without azotemia, has occurred in almost half of the dogs with ehrlichiosis. There has been an inverse relationship between the serum albumin and the quantity of urinary protein in acute, experimental ehrlichiosis.[34] Urinary protein loss has reached its maximum 3 to 4 weeks following acute, experimental infection.[34] During the subclinical phase, urinary protein values have returned to preinfection levels. Quantitation of urine protein loss, either by collecting all urine for a 24-hour period or by calculating the urine microprotein to creatinine ratio in a single sample, will aid in determining the significance of proteinuria in an affected dog. In most cases,

urinary protein losses have been consistent with glomerulonephritis. The average urine microprotein to creatinine ratio was 2.06 in four proteinuric dogs with ehrlichiosis.[23] Two dogs with monoclonal gammopathy lost 2.69 and 1.29 grams of protein per day in the urine.[20] Urine protein electrophoresis parallels that of serum, with increased IgG.[20]

Results of coagulation tests (e.g., prothrombin time, activated partial thromboplastin time, fibrin degradation products) have been normal in dogs with ehrlichiosis, unless DIC exists.[1,2] Bleeding time and clot retraction have often been abnormal owing to thrombocytopenia and platelet dysfunction.[2]

CSF analysis in dogs with signs of CNS disease has revealed increased protein levels and mononuclear pleocytosis similar to that found in viral infections.[1, 19]

Synovial fluid in dogs with arthritis is straw-colored and contains a high protein concentration with elevation in the cell count, consisting predominantly ($\geq$75%) of mature neutrophils and some macrophages and lymphocytes. Intracytoplasmic morulae may be found in a low percentage of synovial fluid neutrophils.

Serology

Serologic testing is probably the most clinically useful and reliable method to detect animals infected with ehrlichiosis, and the IFA test is the most reliable for detection of *E. canis* infection. The technique utilizes infected cell culture systems as the antigen. The test is highly sensitive and specific for *E. canis*.[36] Some cross-reaction between the various *Ehrlichia* species does exist, but IgG titers are generally highest to the agent causing infection (Table 37–4). Positive immunofluorescence at the lowest (1:10) serum dilution that is usually evaluated in dogs is considered to indicate infection, because infection and antibody titers persist unless treatment has begun.[1, 33] Little, if any, cross-reactivity occurs between *E. canis* and *Rickettsia rickettsii*, the etiologic agent of Rocky Mountain spotted fever (RMSF).[19] Because the clinical presentation of these two diseases is similar, dogs with clinical signs of ehrlichiosis in the absence of a titer to *E. canis* should be tested for RMSF by collecting serum, either a single IgM/IgG titer or

Table 37–4. Comparison of Serologic Cross-Reactivity of Ehrlichia of Humans, Horses, Dogs, and Cats

	E. canis	E. platys	E. equi	E. risticii	E. sennetsu
E. canis	+ + +	—	+ +	+	+ +
E. platys		+ + +	—	—	—
E. equi			+ + +	—	+
E. risticii				+ + +	+ +
E. sennetsu					+ + +

Information courtesy of Dr. Cynthia J. Holland, University of Illinois, Urbana, IL, and Dr. Dan B. Fishbein, The Centers for Disease Control, Atlanta, GA.

Cross-reactivity: − = none, + = low, + + = intermediate, + + + = high.

comparison of paired IgG titers to R. rickettsii, at least 2 weeks apart (see Chapter 38).[1] If IgG titers to E. canis are low (≤1:40), they can also be repeated, since demonstrating a rising titer would be more definitive. Serologic cross-reaction between E. canis and E. platys, the etiologic agent of infectious canine thrombocytopenia, does not appear to be a significant clinical problem.[1]

The first increase in detectable antibody titer occurs 7 days postinoculation (PI) and consists of IgA and IgM. IgG titers are not detected until 21 days PI.[33] All dogs become seropositive 20 days PI, with titers peaking at 80 days PI in untreated animals.[33] Antibody titers continue to rise during the course of illness, falling suddenly in some dogs just prior to death.[1, 33] There is no absolute correlation between the elevation in serum globulins and the rise in serum antibody titer.[1] Neither the hyperglobulinemia nor the increased antibody titer is protective against infection with E. canis. Serum IFA-IgG titer and elevated serum globulins decrease gradually within 3 to 9 months following elimination of the organism by treatment.[33] However, the serum IFA-IgG titer may persist following successful treatment, whereas increased γ-globulin levels do not.[1] Therefore, seropositive chronic carriers can be distinguished from seropositive dogs cleared of infection by the additional presence of persistently elevated globulin levels or thrombocytopenia.[33] See Appendix 8 for a listing of diagnostic laboratories that perform these tests.

A new plate latex agglutination test for rapid diagnosis of ehrlichial infections has been developed.[10, 37] It may assist in more rapid screening for ehrlichiosis, although subsequent confirmation may still require the IFA procedure. It primarily appears to detect earlier developing IgM reactive antibodies; however, its use in canine ehrlichial infections is limited.

PATHOLOGIC FINDINGS

Necropsy findings in dogs with ehrlichiosis depend on the stage of infection. Petechial and ecchymotic hemorrhages are present on serosal and mucosal surfaces of most organs, including the nasal cavity, lungs, kidneys, urinary bladder, and the GI tract (stomach, small and large intestines), and in subcutaneous tissues.[17] Generalized lymphadenopathy, splenomegaly, and hepatomegaly are present most often during the acute phase.[1] All lymph nodes, including the mesenteric nodes, are enlarged and have a brownish discoloration. Emaciation with loss of overall body condition is a common finding in chronic cases. Brownish mottling of the lungs may be evident. During the acute stage, the bone marrow is hypercellular and red in color. With chronic disease, the marrow becomes hypoplastic and pale owing to fatty discoloration.[2] Edema of subcutaneous tissues is often noted in dependent areas of the body.

The most characteristic finding is a perivascular plasma cell infiltrate in numerous organs, including the lungs, brain, meninges, kidneys, lymph nodes, and spleen. Therefore, tissues from these organs should be selected for histologic examination.

In the CNS, there is a multifocal, nonsuppurative meningoencephalitis involving the brain stem, midbrain, and cerebral cortex. Most lesions are located ventrally in the brain stem and around the periventricular gray and white matter. Only a very mild encephalitis of the cerebellum occurs. There is a marked lymphoplasmacytic cell infiltrate into the meninges, especially around veins.[17] Microscopic meningeal lesions are present in nearly all dogs at necropsy, yet few dogs demonstrate clinical signs of meningitis.

Lymph node and splenic architecture are altered by marked plasmacytosis and follicular hyperplasia (Fig. 37–5). During the early stages of disease, there is lymphoreticular hyperplasia in paracortical areas of lymph nodes and splenic red pulp. Splenomegaly, which usually occurs during the acute phase, is associated with congestive enlargement and diffuse proliferation of the white pulp. The activity of germinal centers increases initially and then diminishes. With time, the concentration of plasma cells progressively increases from the lymph node cortex to the outer medullary cords, where nearly all cells are plasma cells. Lymphoid follicles blend with surrounding tissue as small lymphocytes are replaced by larger lymphocytes and plasma cells. Splenic plasma cell population is usually extensive in chronically affected dogs.

Pulmonary changes in ehrlichiosis are consistent with interstitial pneumonia. Initially, there is subendothelial accumulation of mononuclear cells. Interstitial and alveolar hemorrhages may be present. *E. canis* organisms may be found in septal mononuclear cells and macrophages of the pulmonary vascular endothelium. During the chronic phase, alveolar septal wall thickening occurs owing to hypertrophy and hyperplasia of septal cells. In addition, there are increased numbers of immature reticuloendothelial cells present in the interstitium, and pulmonary vessels are surrounded by cuffs of plasma cells.

Renal lesions include a vasculitis with plasma cell infiltrate concentrated around vessels in the corticomedullary junction (Fig. 37–6). Focal areas of hemorrhage may

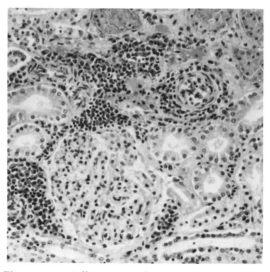

Figure 37–6. Diffuse accumulation of plasma cells in the periglomerular area of the kidney of a dog that died of ehrlichiosis (H and E; × 160).

be found in the corticomedullary area. Glomerulonephritis and interstitial plasmacytosis may occur in dogs with ehrlichiosis.[17, 20]

Centrilobular necrosis is evident in the liver during the acute phase. There is dilation of centrilobular sinusoids and occasional infiltration of plasma cells around centrilobular veins and in the portal triads.

Other organs that may be affected by gross and microscopic hemorrhages include the eyes, heart, GI tract, urinary bladder, and testicles. Plasmacytosis also occurs in the third eyelid, retina, urinary bladder, and testicles.

Ehrlichia organisms are difficult to detect histologically in tissues fixed in either formalin or Bouin's solution. Morulae are infrequently observed in mononuclear phagocytic cells of tissues stained with H and E.[1] The difficulty with which the organism is identified histologically may explain why the disease is not frequently diagnosed at necropsy.[1]

Ultrastructurally, morulae in blood monocytes are intracytoplasmic, limited by a single trilaminar membrane and contain numerous organisms called elementary bodies. The organisms are either round, ovoid, or elongated and are surrounded by a double membrane. The cytoplasm of *E. canis* contains fine fibrils and granules and is similar in appearance to other rickettsiae (*Anaplasma* spp. and *Haemobartonella* spp.).

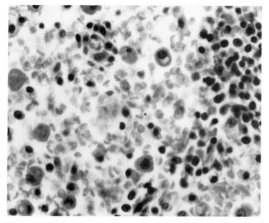

Figure 37–5. Congestion, erythrophagocytosis, and plasma cell accumulation in the spleen of a dog that died of ehrlichiosis (H and E; × 460).

THERAPY

The treatment of canine ehrlichiosis consists of antirickettsial agents and supportive therapy. Drugs used successfully include the tetracyclines, chloramphenicol, imidocarb dipropionate, or amicarbalide (Table 37–5). Generally, the earlier treatment is initiated in the disease process the more favorable the prognosis and outcome.

Tetracycline or oxytetracycline is considered the initial drug of choice.[38] In dogs with acute illness, mild clinical signs, or normal leukocyte counts, the clinical response to therapy is usually rapid and dramatic, often within 24 to 48 hours. Dogs with pancytopenia, characteristic of chronic disease, have guarded prognoses and show gradual or no improvement following treatment.[1] Hemorrhage due to thrombocytopenia and infections secondary to neutropenia often cause death in these dogs. Improvement in clinical signs usually precedes return of hematologic parameters to normal. A period of 120 days may elapse following treatment and clearance of infection before bone marrow regeneration occurs.[1]

Doxycycline and minocycline are semisynthetic, lipid-soluble tetracyclines that are readily absorbed to produce high blood and tissue concentrations (see Chapter 43). These drugs readily penetrate most cells and are apparently as effective in patients with ehrlichiosis that are refractory to tetracycline therapy. Doxycycline, given orally at lower doses in acute cases and higher doses in chronic cases, has been effective in a higher percentage of infected dogs than oxytetracycline. Also, doxycycline can be given IV in dogs that are vomiting. The IV dose is usually given for 5 days. In addition, dogs treated with oral doxycycline have had a lower incidence of relapse or reinfection than have dogs treated with oxytetracycline.[21]

Chloramphenicol has been recommended for use in puppies less than 5 months of age in order to avoid yellow discoloration of erupting teeth. Chloramphenicol may be more effective than tetracycline in eliminating infection.[29] It should be used in dogs that have persistent infections despite therapy with tetracyclines. However, because of the associated public health risks associated with use of chloramphenicol, and because it directly interferes with heme and bone marrow synthesis, its use in anemic or pancytopenic dogs should be avoided when possible. The quinolones have known antirickettsial activity, but their use in treatment of this disease has not been evaluated.

Although not available in the United States, imidocarb dipropionate has been used successfully in the treatment of ehrlichiosis.[39] When given as a single IM injection, 83.9% of dogs with ehrlichiosis have recovered. Dogs receiving this drug have had fewer relapses than those treated with tetracycline.[40] However, 10% of apparently recovered dogs may relapse.[40] Imidocarb has also been effective in 95.8% of dogs with babesiosis and in 60% of dogs with concurrent babesiosis and ehrlichiosis. Concurrent infections may be treated successfully by giving two injections at 14-day intervals. Amicarbalide may be used at this same dosage schedule (see Table 37–3). Transient, dose-dependent side effects of imidocarb dipropionate include excessive salivation, serous nasal discharge, diarrhea, and dyspnea. These signs may be the result of an anticholinesterase effect.[39]

In addition to antimicrobial therapy, supportive therapy may be needed, especially in dogs with chronic disease. Dehydration is corrected by administering balanced elec-

Table 37–5. Therapy for Canine Ehrlichiosis[a]

DRUG	DOSE[b] (mg/kg)	ROUTE	INTERVAL[c] (hours)	DURATION (days)
Tetracycline	22	PO (IV)	8	14–21
Doxycycline or minocycline	5–10	PO (IV)	12–24	7–10
Chloramphenicol	15–20	PO (IV,SC)	8	14
Imidocarb dipropionate	5	IM	24	1[d]
Amicarbalide	5–6	IM	every 2 wks	14

[a]PO = oral, IV = intravenous, SC = subcutaneous, IM = intramuscular.
[b]Dose per administration at specified interval, expressed as mg/kg unless otherwise stated.
[c]Expressed in hours, unless otherwise stated.
[d]Concurrent infections with *Babesia* require a second injection 14 days later.

trolyte solutions. Blood transfusions may be necessary in dogs that are severely anemic. Fresh blood or platelet-rich plasma should be used because platelets are inactivated by refrigeration or freezing. Intranasal epinephrine or phenylephrine may help to control severe epistaxis in emergency situations.[1] Bone marrow stimulation with androgenic steroids may be beneficial in dogs with depressed bone marrow production and pancytopenia. Oxymetholone may be given orally once a day or nandrolone decanoate (Deca-durabolin, Organon, West Orange, NJ) may be administered IM once weekly.

Short-term (i.e., 2 to 7 days) therapy with glucocorticoids may be of value early in the treatment when severe or life-threatening thrombocytopenia is present. An immune-mediated mechanism may be partially responsible for thrombocytopenia and decreased platelet function. Therefore, anti-inflammatory to immunosuppressive dosages of either dexamethasone or prednisolone have been used. Some clinicians prefer to use glucocorticoids and tetracycline in combination initially, because of the difficulty in distinguishing between canine ehrlichiosis and immune-mediated thrombocytopenia (ITP) and because of the lag time until serologic test results are available. However, these two diseases can often be differentiated on the basis of history and physical examination findings.[1] In contrast to dogs with ehrlichiosis, dogs with ITP are usually afebrile and lack constitutional signs. Usually, the presenting complaint with ITP is hemorrhage (e.g., petechiae and ecchymoses). In both diseases, clinical bleeding and hemorrhage often decrease prior to an increase in the platelet count. Since many dogs with ehrlichiosis are already immunosuppressed and leukopenic, glucocorticoids at immunosuppressive dosages for prolonged periods of time should be avoided. In addition, glucocorticoid immunosuppression may interfere with clearance and elimination of the organism following tetracycline therapy.[1]

Glucocorticoids may have to be given to dogs that develop chronic progressive polyarthritis if antimicrobial therapy is not suf-ficient in eliminating the clinical signs of fever, lameness, and joint swelling.

PUBLIC HEALTH CONSIDERATIONS

Prior to 1986, the only *Ehrlichia* species recognized as infecting people was *E. sennetsu*. This agent was isolated in Japan and is responsible for a mild mononucleosis-like syndrome. *E. canis* or more likely a closely related species has been identified as causing disease in people.[3, 5–8, 8a, 8b] Most cases were reported from the southern and south central portions of the United States and were diagnosed based on serologic evidence of infection with *E. canis*. One additional case also demonstrated intracytoplasmic inclusions in leukocytes.[3] Isolation of the suspected organism from clinical cases in people has not been accomplished at this time. Some people with serologic evidence of infection have been clinically nonsymptomatic.

Recent tick exposure has been a common denominator. People probably do not acquire the infection directly from dogs. *Rhipicephalus sanguineus* is probably not the vector of human ehrlichiosis, since unlike the canine infection most cases are seasonal (March to September) and have been associated with outdoor tick exposure 4 weeks prior to infection but independent of exposure to dogs.[40a] The major clinical findings in people include fever, headache, rigors, myalgia, ocular pain, and GI symptoms.[3, 5, 6] A petechial rash similar to RMSF was noted in only 20% of affected people.[7] Laboratory findings have included anemia, leukopenia (usually lymphopenia), and thrombocytopenia. Mildly elevated liver enzyme activities and mildly abnormal renal function test results have been observed also. A fourfold rise in IFA titer to at least 1:80 has been used to confirm a diagnosis. Treatment with tetracyclines usually leads to a rapid and complete recovery.

Although this disease should be suspected in people with pancytopenia and unexplained fever after exposure to ticks, its true prevalence in humans will be known only after further study.

Ehrlichia platys *Infection* (Infectious Cyclic Thrombocytopenia of Dogs)

John W. Harvey

ETIOLOGY

Infectious cyclic thrombocytopenia (ICT) of dogs is caused by a small rickettsial parasite classified as *Ehrlichia platys*.[41, 42] Organisms appear as blue inclusions in platelets when blood films are stained with Giemsa or new methylene blue (Fig. 37–7). *E. platys* appears to be similar to *E. canis*, but it infects platelets rather than leukocytes and is serologically distinct from other Ehrlichiae (see Table 37–4).

Ultrastructurally, organisms range from 350 to 1250 nm in diameter; are round, oval, or bean shaped; and are surrounded by a double membrane. Infected platelets may contain from one to three single membrane-lined vacuoles with one to eight organisms per vacuole (Fig. 37–8).[41]

Megakaryocytes in bone marrow have not been observed to contain organisms either prior to or during parasitemia. Organisms appear to enter platelets by endocytosis following adherence. Therefore, the vacuolar membrane probably is derived from the external platelet membrane. Repetitive binary

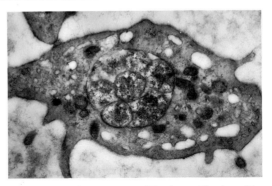

Figure 37–8. Ultrastructure of *E. platys*. Platelet with a membrane-lined vacuole containing seven visible organisms. (From Harvey JW et al: *J Infect Dis* 137:182–188, 1978. Reprinted with permission.)

fission of organisms within the vacuole results in the formation of a morula.

Attempts to culture the organism have been unsuccessful. An attempt to infect a cat by IV inoculation was also unsuccessful.

PATHOGENESIS

The incubation period following experimental IV infection in dogs is 8 to 15 days. The natural mode of transmission has not been verified experimentally, but it probably involves ticks. The highest percentage of parasitized platelets occurs during the initial parasitemic episode (Fig. 37–9).[41] Within a few days after the appearance of parasitized platelets, there is a precipitous decrease in platelet count (generally 20,000 cells/μl or less), and organisms are usually no longer seen. After the disappearance of microorganisms, platelet counts increase rapidly, reaching normal values within 3 to 4 days.

Parasitemias and subsequent thrombocytopenias recur at 1- to 2-week intervals (Fig. 37–9). Although the percentage of infected platelets decreases to as low as 1% or less with subsequent parasitemias, thrombocytopenic episodes are as severe as those following the initial parasitemia. Whereas initial thrombocytopenias may develop primarily as a consequence of direct injury to platelets by replicating organisms, immune-mediated mechanisms of platelet removal

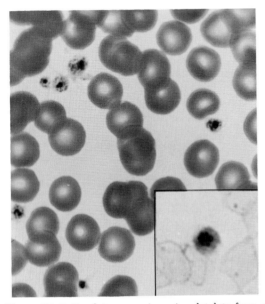

Figure 37–7. *E. platys* organisms in platelets from a dog with infectious cyclic thrombocytopenia (Giemsa stain; × 1400) *Inset:* Platelet containing morula of *E. platys* (new methylene blue; × 1500).

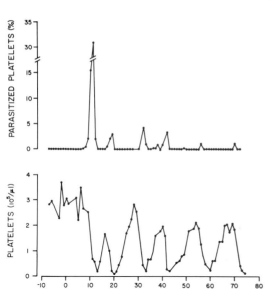

Figure 37–9. Percentage of parasitized platelets and platelet counts from a dog inoculated IV with *E. platys;* 0 on the abscissa represents the day of inoculation. (From Harvey JW et al: *J Infect Dis* 137:182–188, 1978. Reprinted with permission.)

may be more important in subsequent thrombocytopenic episodes.[43] The cyclic nature of the parasitemias and thrombocytopenias diminishes with time, resulting in mild, slowly resolving thrombocytopenias in association with sporadically occurring organisms in the blood.

In some instances, transient decreases in total leukocyte counts have occurred concomitantly with parasitemia, but values are usually not below the reference range for dogs. Mild normocytic normochromic anemias may occur during the first month of infection. Based on serum iron and bone marrow studies, decreases in PCV may be attributed to the syndrome of anemia of inflammation.[44]

CLINICAL FINDINGS

A slight increase in rectal temperature has sometimes been noted during initial parasitemias. On several occasions, a small amount of fresh blood has been observed in the feces of thrombocytopenic dogs. Splenectomy prior to infection results in higher initial platelet counts but does not alter the periodicity of the parasitemias or the severity of disease.[41] Uveitis that was present in a natural case of *E. platys* infection[45] has not been recognized in experimental animals. Conse-

quently, a cause-and-effect relationship remains to be proved.

Even though the *E. platys* isolates studied thus far in the United States do not cause clinical disease, this agent is still considered to have potential significance for several reasons. More pathogenic strains may exist in nature; preliminary studies indicate that a morphologically and serologically related organism causes illness (fever, depression, and weight loss) in dogs in Greece.[46] The occurrence of *E. platys* with other infectious agents (e.g., *E. canis* or *Babesia canis*) may potentiate the clinical disease produced by either of these agents. As with *E. canis*, certain breeds of dogs or individual animals may be more severely affected than the dogs studied experimentally. Dogs with thrombocytopenias may bleed following trauma or surgery. Finally, even if *E. platys* does not produce clinical illness, it must be considered in the differential diagnosis of thrombocytopenia in dogs.

DIAGNOSIS

A diagnosis of ICT may be made by finding organisms within platelets on stained blood films. In most instances, this method of diagnosis is not reliable because the parasites are either absent or are present in very low numbers.

An IFA test for detection of serum antibodies to *E. platys* has been developed.[42] Sera of dogs experimentally infected with *E. platys* change from negative to positive coincident with or shortly after the peak of the first parasitemia. Based on serologic studies, it appears that *E. platys* infection is widely distributed in the United States. As many as 33% of thrombocytopenic dogs in Florida and Louisiana have positive titers, and over 50% of dogs seropositive for *E. canis* also have positive titers to *E. platys*.[42,47] Evidence for positive serologic reactions to both organisms in serum samples from some dogs probably represents combined infections, inasmuch as other dogs have positive titers to either agent alone. See Appendix 8 for a listing of diagnostic laboratories that perform this test.

PATHOLOGIC FINDINGS

Generalized lymph node enlargement has been the only gross finding at necropsy in an experimental study of dogs euthanatized during the early weeks of infection.[48] Histologic lesions were generally mild and included lymphoid hyperplasia and plasmacytosis in lymph nodes and spleen, crescent-shaped perifollicular hemorrhages in the spleen, and multifocal Kupffer cell hyperplasia in the liver.

THERAPY AND PREVENTION

Based on preliminary studies, it appears that tetracyclines at dosages recommended for E. canis infections are effective against this agent (see Table 37–3).[45,46] Inasmuch as ticks, and possibly other arthropods, are probably responsible for natural transmission of the disease, adequate vector control is recommended to prevent its spread.

References

1. Greene CE, Harvey JW: Canine ehrlichiosis. In Greene CE (ed): Clinical Microbiology and Infectious Diseases of the Dog and Cat. Philadelphia, WB Saunders Co, 1984, pp 545–561.
2. Hibler SC, Hoskins JD, Greene CE: Rickettsial infections in dogs. Part II. Ehrlichiosis and infectious cyclic thrombocytopenia. Compend Cont Educ Pract Vet 8:106–115, 1986.
3. Maeda K, Markowitz N, Hawley RC, et al: Human infection with Ehrlichia canis, a leukocytic rickettsia. N Engl J Med 316:853–856, 1987.
4. Ewing SA, Johnson EM, Kocan KM, et al: Human infection with Ehrlichia canis. N Engl J Med 317:899–900, 1987.
5. Fishbein DB, Sawyer LA, Holland CJ, et al: Unexplained febrile illnesses after exposure to ticks. Infection with an Ehrlichia? JAMA 257:3100–3104, 1987.
6. Fishbein DB, Sawyer LA, McDade JE, et al: Ehrlichia canis infection in humans: a new zoonosis. J Am Vet Med Assoc 190:12, 1987.
7. Edwards MS, Jones JE, Leass DL, et al: Childhood infection caused by Ehrlichia canis or a closely related organism. Pediatr Infect Dis J 7:651–654, 1988.
8. Taylor JP, Betz TG, Fishbein DB, et al: Serological evidence of possible human infection with Ehrlichia in Texas. J Infect Dis 158:217–220, 1988.
8a. Harkness JR, Ewing SA, Crutcher JM, et al: Human ehrlichiosis in Oklahoma. J Infect Dis 159:576–579, 1989.
8b. Petersen LR, Sawyer LA, Fishbein DB, et al: An outbreak of ehrlichiosis in members of an army reserve unit exposed to ticks. J Infect Dis 159:562–568, 1989.
9. Ristic M, Dawson J, Holland CJ, et al: Susceptibility of dogs to infection with Ehrlichia risticii, causative agent of equine monocytic ehrlichiosis (Potomac horse fever). Am J Vet Res 49:1497–1500, 1988.
10. Collins DR, Practitioner's Update. Morris Animal Foundation Newsletter, February 1988.
11. Dawson JE, Holland CJ, Ristic M: Susceptibility of dogs and cats to infection with Ehrlichia risticii, causative agent of Potomac horse fever. In Proceedings, 67th Annu Mtg Conf Res Work Anim Dis, 349, 1986.
11a. Dawson JE, Abeygunawardena I, Holland CJ, et al: Susceptibility of cats to infection with Ehrlichia risticii, causative agent of equine monocytic ehrlichiosis. Am J Vet Res 49:2096–2100, 1988.
12. Gossett KA, Gaunt SD, Aja DS: Hepatozoonosis and ehrlichiosis in a dog. J Am Anim Hosp Assoc 21:265–267, 1985.
13. Van Heerden J, Reyers F, Stewart CG: Treatment and thrombocyte levels in experimentally induced canine ehrlichiosis and canine babesiosis. Onderstepoort J Vet Res 50:267–270, 1983.
14. Smith RD, Ristic M, Huxsoll DL, et al: Platelet kinetics in canine ehrlichiosis: evidence for increased platelet destruction as the cause of thrombocytopenia. Infect Immun 11:1216–1221, 1975.
15. Matus RE, Leifer CE, Hurvitz AI: Use of plasmapheresis and chemotherapy for treatment of monoclonal gammopathy associated with Ehrlichia canis infection in a dog. J Am Vet Med Assoc 190:1302–1304, 1987.
16. Codner EC, Farris-Smith LL: Characterization of the subclinical phase of ehrlichiosis in dogs. J Am Vet Med Assoc 189:47–50, 1986.
17. Troy GC, Vulgamott JC, Turnwald GH: Canine ehrlichiosis: a retrospective study of 30 naturally occurring cases. J Am Anim Hosp Assoc 16:181–187, 1980.
18. Price JE, Sayer PD, Dolan TT: Improved clinical approach to the diagnosis of canine ehrlichiosis. Trop Anim Health Prod 19:1–8, 1987.
19. Greene CE, Burgdorfer W, Cavagnolo R, et al: Rocky Mountain spotted fever in dogs and its differentiation from canine ehrlichiosis. J Am Vet Med Assoc 186:465–472, 1985.
20. Breitschwerdt EB, Woody BJ, Zerbe CA, et al: Monoclonal gammopathy associated with naturally occurring canine ehrlichiosis. J Vet Intern Med 1:2–9, 1987.
21. Codner EC: The subclinical phase of naturally occurring canine ehrlichiosis. In Proceedings, ACVIM, Section 13, pp 21–23, 1986.
22. Kuehn NF, Gaunt SD: Clinical and hematologic findings in canine ehrlichiosis. J Am Vet Med Assoc 186:355–358, 1985.
23. Troy GC: Unpublished data on 50 new cases of canine ehrlichiosis. Virginia-Maryland Regional College of Veterinary Medicine, Blacksburg, VA, 1987.
24. Woody BJ, McDonald RK: Canine ehrlichiosis. Miss Vet J 7:2–5, 1985.
24a. Waddle JR, Littman MP: A retrospective study of 27 cases of naturally occurring canine ehrlichiosis. J Am Anim Hosp Assoc 24:615–620, 1988.
25. Codner EC, Roberts RE, Ainsworth AG: Atypical findings in 16 cases of canine ehrlichiosis. J Am Vet Med Assoc 186:166–169, 1985.
26. Swanson JF: Uveitis associated with Ehrlichia canis infection. Proc Am Coll Vet Ophthalmol 13:103–115, 1982.
27. Hall CL: Personal communication. Texas A & M University, College Station, TX, 1987.
28. Bellah JR, Shull RM, Shull-Selcer EV: Ehrlichia canis–related polyarthritis in a dog. J Am Vet Med Assoc 189:922–923, 1986.

29. Madigan JE: Questions diagnosis of ehrlichiosis (letter). *J Am Vet Med Assoc* 190:244–245, 1987.

30. Stockham SL, Tyler JW, Schmidt DA, et al: Ehrlichiosis (granulocytic form) associated with arthritis in the dog. Workshop on Diseases Caused by Leukocytic Rickettsiae of Man and Animals, Abstract 032. University of Illinois, Urbana, IL, 1985.

31. Waddle JR, Littman MP: A retrospective study of 27 cases of *Ehrlichia canis* infection. *In* Proceedings, ACVIM (Research Report No. 36), 1986.

32. Heald RD: *Ehrlichia*-associated Coombs'-positive anemia in a dog. *Canine Pract* 11:34–36, 1984.

33. Buhles WC, Huxsoll DL, Ristic M: Tropical canine pancytopenia: clinical, hematologic, and serologic response of dogs to *Ehrlichia canis* infection, tetracycline therapy, and challenge inoculation. *J Infect Dis* 130:357–367, 1974.

34. Codner EC: Proteinuria associated with acute experimental canine ehrlichiosis. *In* Proceedings, ACVIM (Research Reports No. 83), 14–57, 1986.

35. Hoskins JD, Barta O, Rothschmitt J: Serum hyperviscosity syndrome associated with *Ehrlichia canis* infection in a dog. *J Am Vet Med Assoc* 183:1011–1012, 1983.

36. Ristic M, Huxsoll DL, Weisiger RM, et al: Serological diagnosis of tropical canine pancytopenia by indirect immunofluorescence. *Infect Immun* 6:226–231, 1972.

37. Ristic M, Boothe D: Diagnosis of infections with *Ehrlichia* agents with emphasis on canine ehrlichiosis. *J Am Vet Med Assoc* 190:1604, 1987.

38. Amyx HL, Huxsoll DL, Zeiler DC, et al: Therapeutic and prophylactic value of tetracycline in dogs infected with the agent of tropical canine pancytopenia. *J Am Vet Med Assoc* 59:1428–1432, 1972.

39. Adeyanju BJ, Aliu YO: Chemotherapy of canine ehrlichiosis and babesiosis with imidocarb dipropionate. *J Am Anim Hosp Assoc* 18:827–830, 1982.

40. Greene CE: RMSF and ehrlichiosis. *In* Kirk RW (ed): *Current Veterinary Therapy IX.* Philadelphia, WB Saunders Co, 1986, pp 1080–1084.

40a. Human ehrlichiosis—United States. *MMWR* 37:270–271, 1988.

41. Harvey JW, Simpson CF, Gaskin JM: Cyclic thrombocytopenia induced by a rickettsia-like agent in dogs. *J Infect Dis* 137:182–188, 1978.

42. French TW, Harvey JW: Serologic diagnosis of infectious cyclic thrombocytopenia in dogs using an indirect fluorescent antibody test. *Am J Vet Res* 44:2407–2411, 1983.

43. French TW, Shelly SM, Harvey JW: Investigation of the mechanism of thrombocytopenia in dogs with acute *Ehrlichia platys* infection (abstract). *In* Proceedings, 38th Annu Meeting Am Coll Vet Pathol, p 25, 1987.

44. Baker DC, Gaunt SD, Babin SS: Anemia of inflammation in dogs infected with *Ehrlichia platys.* *Am J Vet Res* 49:1014–1016, 1988.

45. Glaze MB, Gaunt SD: Uveitis associated with *Ehrlichia platys* infection in a dog. *J Am Vet Med Assoc* 188:916–917, 1986.

46. French TW, Papadopoulos O: Personal communication, Cornell University, Ithaca, NY, and Aristotelian University, Thessalonica, Greece, 1986.

47. Hoskins JD, Breitschwerdt EB, Gaunt SD, et al: Antibodies to *Ehrlichia canis*, *Ehrlichia platys*, and spotted fever group rickettsiae in Louisiana dogs. *J Vet Intern Med* 2:55–59, 1988.

48. Baker DC, Simpson M, Gaunt SD, et al: Acute *Ehrlichia platys* infection in the dog. *Vet Pathol* 24:449–453, 1987.

38 ROCKY MOUNTAIN SPOTTED FEVER AND Q FEVER

Craig E. Greene
Edward B. Breitschwerdt

Rocky Mountain Spotted Fever

ETIOLOGY AND EPIDEMIOLOGY

Rocky Mountain spotted fever (RMSF) is a tick-borne, rickettsial disease of the Americas that affects dogs and people. Although cats and other domestic animals can have a seropositive test result for the organism, knowledge concerning the seroprevalence of clinical disease in these animals is minimal. RMSF was recognized primarily in the western United States prior to 1930. Overall, the reported prevalence of the human disease appears to have increased since its discovery, with the highest yearly prevalence now being reported from the eastern United States (Fig. 38–1). Presumably, this increase reflects increased recognition and reporting rather than geographic spread of the disease.[1] Deciduous forests, increased humidity, and warmer temperatures are factors associated with the high prevalence of this tick-transmitted disease in these areas. RMSF is known to occur throughout the contiguous United States with the exception of Maine. It has been reported in western Canada, Mexico, Panama, Costa Rica, Honduras, Nicaragua, Colombia, and Brazil.

Rickettsia rickettsii, the etiologic agent of RMSF, is an obligate intracellular parasite in the family Rickettsiaceae (Fig. 38–2). Members of the spotted fever group (SFG), such as *R. rickettsii*, are related to the typhus group of rickettsiae (Table 38–1) but are distinct from other genera. Serologically and pathogenically distinct strains of SFG rickettsiae have been described throughout the world.[2, 2a, 2b] Four main SFG species, *R. rickettsii*, *R. montana*, *R. rhipicephali*, and *R. belli*, are isolated from ticks in the United States. *R. rickettsii* is the only SFG rickettsia in the Western Hemisphere known to be pathogenic for people and animals. The natural history and distribution of RMSF in the United States appears to center primarily on the distribution of two ticks, *Dermacentor andersoni* and *D. variabilis*, which serve as natural hosts, reservoirs, and vectors for *R. rickettsii* (Fig. 38–3).

D. andersoni (the wood tick) is a three-host tick that is found from the Cascades to the Rocky Mountains (Fig. 38–4).[2c] It is the principal vector of RMSF in the western United States and is also present in Canada in the provinces of southern British Columbia, Alberta, and Saskatchewan.

D. variabilis (American dog tick) is a three-host tick found from the Great Plains region eastward to the Atlantic Coast of the United States and southern Canada. It has also been reported in California, southwest Oregon, southern Washington, and Idaho.

Three other ticks have been incriminated in the transmission of RMSF to animals and people, but their significance is uncertain. The Lone Star tick (*Amblyomma americanum*) occurs in the United States from Texas eastward to the Atlantic coast. The brown dog tick, *Rhipicephalus sanguineus*,

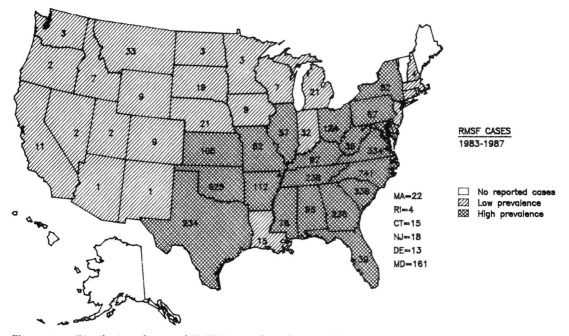

RMSF CASES
1983-1987

MA=22
RI=4
CT=15
NJ=18
DE=13
MD=161

☐ No reported cases
▨ Low prevalence
▩ High prevalence

Figure 38–1. Distribution of cases of RMSF in people in the United States for 1983 to 1987. (Data compiled from *Morbidity and Mortality Weekly Reports* by Dr. Tom Schwan, Rocky Mountain Laboratories, Hamilton, MT.)

is found throughout the United States, southern Canada, Mexico, and South America. Unlike the other vector ticks, *R. sanguineus* feeds on dogs during all three stages. *Haemaphysalis leporispalustris*, the rabbit tick, resides throughout the Western Hemisphere. Although rickettsiae recovered from this tick are antigenically similar to *R. rick-*

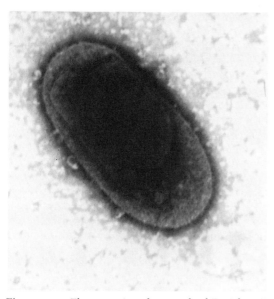

Figure 38–2. Electron microphotograph of *R. rickettsii* in yolk sac culture (× 15,000).

ettsii, they do not produce disease in laboratory animals.

Ticks become infected by two means. First, horizontal transmission can occur during feeding of noninfected ticks on small mammals, including chipmunks, voles, and ground squirrels, that have developed sufficient rickettsemia during acute infection. The primary sylvan cycle, which maintains the transmission cycle in nature, occurs between these small rodents and immature (larval and nymphal) tick stages, and it is possible that medium-sized mammals such as raccoons, opossums, and foxes are additional sources for infecting ticks. Although of minor importance, birds are a means by which infected ticks can be transported into new areas.

Second, ticks can be infected transstadially and also vertically by transovarial passage between generations. *R. rickettsii* initially replicates in the epithelial cells of the tick midgut, enters the hemocoel, and from there spreads to and multiplies in other tick tissues, including the salivary glands and ovaries. Ticks must ingest numerous rickettsiae for successful transovarial transmission.

Several restrictions may explain why RMSF is limited to geographic islands in the Americas. The overall low prevalence of infection in ticks, less than 2% even in areas

Table 38–1. Comparison of Some Pathogenic Rickettsiae Affecting Dogs and Cats[a]

DISEASE (AGENT)	GEOGRAPHIC LOCATION	INSECT VECTOR	INCIDENTAL HOST	RESERVOIR HOST
Spotted Fever Group[b]				
Rocky Mountain spotted fever (Rickettsia rickettsii)	Western hemisphere	Tick	People, dogs, cats	Rodents, dogs
Boutonneuse fever (R. conorii)	Africa, India, Mediterranean	Tick	People	Rodents, dogs
Typhus Group				
Epidemic typhus (R. prowazekii)	South America, USA? Africa, Asia	Body louse	Domestic animals	People, flying squirrels
Murine (endemic) typhus (R. typhi)	Foci worldwide	Flea	People	Rats, cats
Others				
Scrub typhus (R. tsutsugamushi)	SE Asia	Mite	People, dogs (subclinical)	Rats, birds
Q fever (Coxiella burnetii)	Worldwide	Aerosols, tick?	People, dogs	Cattle, sheep, goats, cats
Salmon poisoning (Neorickettsia helminthoeca)	Pacific NW of USA	Fluke	People (rare)	Dogs, foxes

[a]For Ehrlichiosis, see Table 37–1.

[b]Also includes Queensland tick typhus (R. australis), North Asian tick typhus (R. siberica), rickettsialpox (R. akari), and Shikoku Japan fever (R. montana–like agent).

with a high prevalence of RMSF, suggests that most mammalian hosts of adult ticks, such as dogs, rarely develop rickettsemias of sufficient magnitude and duration to infect large numbers of ticks.[3] Sampling errors also may explain why focal ecologic pockets of infected ticks have been found.

Spread of infection within tick and host populations also appears to be limited by other factors. Transmission of infection from male to female ticks during mating does not occur.[1] Immature ticks do not usually feed more than once between each stage before moulting. Adult female ticks feed only once; following a blood meal, they drop from the dog, deposit eggs, and die. Females with ovarian infection may transmit rickettsiae to as many as 100% of progeny. Adult male ticks may have some importance in spread of RMSF to mammals because they feed intermittently on a succession of hosts in search of female ticks. However, rickettsial infection of ticks is not an ideal symbiotic relationship. Since transstadial transmission may be incomplete, reproduction may be impaired, or death may occur.[1]

Figure 38–3. Distribution of D. andersoni and D. variabilis in the United States. (Modified from Bishopp FC, Trembley HL: Parasitol 31:1–54, 1945, with permission.)

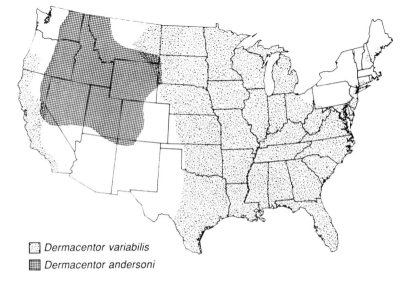

☐ Dermacentor variabilis
▦ Dermacentor andersoni

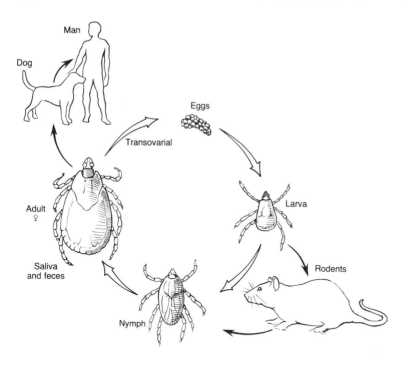

Figure 38–4. Relationship of ticks and their hosts in transmission of RMSF.

Tick immobility and restricted territorial movement of small rodents may be additional factors in limiting the uniform spread of *R. rickettsii* through tick populations. Environmental factors such as low (<50%) humidity, colder temperatures, and decreased vegetation further inhibit survival of infected ticks. Resistance to infection with *R. rickettsii* develops in ticks and possibly mammalian hosts as a result of infection with the three other common nonpathogenic SFG rickettsiae.

For reasons that are not completely understood, ticks do not usually infect a new host until they have been attached for a minimum of 5 to 20 hours. A reactivation period within the tick with an apparent increased rickettsial virulence is thought to occur after ticks reattach and take their first blood meal of the season. A period of feeding also may be needed for the production of infective organisms in the salivary glands. It may also relate to the need of the ticks to produce a cement collar around their mouth parts before they begin feeding. Although infections that people acquire from being bitten by ticks require extended attachment, those acquired from contact of mucous membranes with feces or hemolymph from ticks preengorged on animals do not appear to involve extended contact periods.

PATHOGENESIS

R. rickettsii usually enter the body through the bite of infected ticks (Fig. 38–5). Via the circulatory system, rickettsiae invade and replicate in endothelial cells of smaller blood vessels. Endothelial cell damage initiates platelet activation and activation of the coagulation system.[4, 4a] Decreased plasma levels of antithrombin III and plasminogen and increased fibrinogen degradation products are consistent with simultaneous activation of the fibrinolytic and coagulation systems. Results of coagulation factor analysis suggest activation of both the extrinsic and intrinsic pathways.[4] Progressive necrotizing vasculitis may be caused sequentially by complement activation, cellular chemotaxis, and subsequent vascular necrosis and extravasation of blood. Organs with endarterial circulation, such as the skin, brain, heart, and kidneys, are frequently affected.

Significantly increased plasma and extracellular fluid volume have been described in experimental infections of nonhuman primates.[5] Accumulation of extracellular volume and electrolytes, renal water retention, and edema were correlated with increased concentrations of aldosterone and antidiuretic hormone in people.[6] Fluid overload in the circulation and edema of the medulla

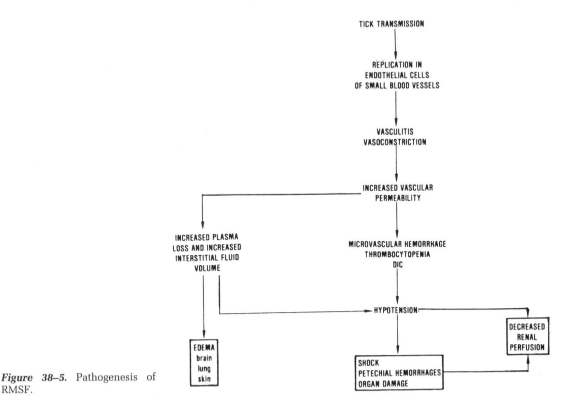

Figure 38–5. Pathogenesis of RMSF.

oblongata in experimental animals[5] suggest that IV fluid therapy be used sparingly in the management of dogs with RMSF. CNS signs and death may relate to cardiorespiratory depression through edema of medullary centers. Fulminant infection may result in peripheral vascular collapse and death in the first week of infection, before proliferative and thrombotic lesions occur. Acute renal failure, a fatal complication of RMSF

in people, has not frequently developed in dogs.

CLINICAL FINDINGS

Both clinical and subclinical illnesses have been reported in dogs with naturally occurring and experimentally produced RMSF. Most dogs are presented for examination for illness during the months of March to October. Purebred dogs appear to be more prone to develop clinical illness as compared with mixed breed dogs, and the German shepherd dog has a particularly high prevalence of disease.[7] Clinical signs of illness in dogs are similar to those in cases of naturally infected people and are summarized in Table 38–2.[7a, 7b, 7c]

Fever, one of the earliest and most consistent findings, can occur within 2 to 3 days following tick attachment. Early cutaneous lesions in some dogs consist of edema and hyperemia of the lips, penile sheath, scrotum, pinna, other extremities, and rarely on the ventral abdomen (Fig. 38–6). Discrete clear vesicles and focal erythematous macules were observed on the buccal mucosa.[8] Male dogs that develop scrotal edema or

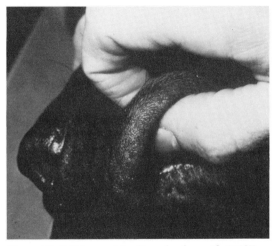

Figure 38–6. Edema of the lips of a dog with RMSF.

Table 38–2. Frequency of Clinical Findings in People and Dogs with RMSF[a]

CLINICAL FINDINGS	PEOPLE (n = 262)	DOGS (n = 79)
Low fever	99 (>37.8°C)	67 (>39.2°C)
High fever	90 (>38.9°C)	54 (>40°C)
Headache	91	NR
Rash/petechiae	88	19
Myalgia/arthralgia	83	49
Anorexia	NR	51
Known tick exposure	67	52
Nausea/vomiting	60	18
Abdominal/lumbar pain	52	30
Conjunctivitis/scleral congestion	30	34
Lymphadenomegaly	27	43
Stupor/depression/altered mental status	26	83
Vestibular deficits[b]	18	41
Cervical pain/nuchal rigidity	18	8
Coma/unconsciousness	9	4
Seizures	8	10
Diarrhea	19	16
Edema of face/extremities	18	25
Polydipsia/polyuria	NR	5
Splenomegaly	16	3
Hepatomegaly	12	3
Pneumonitis/dyspnea/cough	12	39
Jaundice	9	4
Cardiac arrhythmias	7	8
Death	4	3

Data from Helmick CG et al: *J Infect Dis* 150:480–488, 1984; Greene CE: *J Am Vet Med Assoc* 19:666–671, 1987; and Greene CE, University of Georgia, unpublished observations, 1989.

[a]NR = not reported.

[b]Deficits include vestibular signs of nystagmus, head tilt, circling, and incoordination.

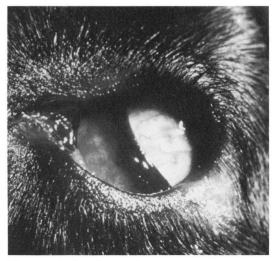

Figure 38–7. Petechiae and vascular congestion of the sclera of a dog with RMSF.

apy. Permanent organ damage may occur within 1 to 2 weeks of onset of clinical signs in severely affected dogs that survive the acute stages of illness. Necrosis of the extremities and previously hyperemic or edematous portions of the body may occur at this time (Figs. 38–9 and 38–10).[13] Dogs may die in the acute stages of illness as a result of hemorrhagic diathesis or from thrombosis of vital organs. Cardiovascular, neurologic, and renal damage are the most consistent cause of death or permanent organ injury. Death in some severely affected dogs has been caused by disseminated,

ependymal swelling often have a stiff gait and show reluctance to walk.

Petechial and ecchymotic hemorrhages may develop subsequent to the acute illness in some dogs and if present, occur on ocular, oral, and genital mucous membranes (Fig. 38–7) rather than involving the skin. Funduscopic examination provides a more sensitive means of detecting these hemorrhagic lesions (Fig. 38–8; also see Chapter 13).[9, 10] Epistaxis, melena, and hematuria may be noted in severely affected animals.

Neurologic signs of generalized cerebral and spinal cord involvement have been found (see Table 38–2). Focal or localizing neurologic signs, such as vestibular disease, are common.[7, 11, 12]

Infected dogs may make a rapid complete recovery if they are mildly affected or with the early institution of antimicrobial ther-

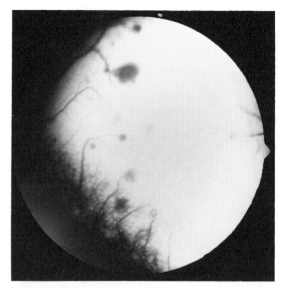

Figure 38–8. Retinal hemorrhages seen on the fundus of a dog with RMSF. (Courtesy of Dr. Renee Kaswan, University of Georgia, Athens, GA.)

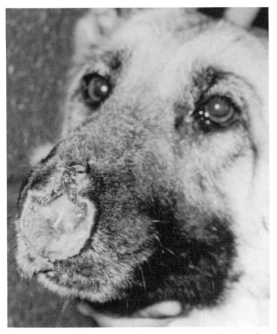

Figure 38–9. Necrosis of the planum nasale of a dog with RMSF. (Courtesy of Dr. Craig Greene.)

rapidly progressing meningoencephalitis. Shock, cardiovascular collapse, and oliguria become apparent in the terminal stages of illness.

DIAGNOSIS

Clinical Laboratory Findings

Mild leukopenia, which may develop early in the course of illness, is followed by a moderate leukocytosis with a left shift on stress hemogram. The longer the duration of clinical signs prior to diagnosis, the more pronounced is the leukocytosis. A normocytic normochromic anemia and elevated erythrocyte sedimentation rate are nonspecific hematologic changes. Fibrinogen concentration, which increases as a result of an acute phase reaction, may be decreased in severely affected dogs developing DIC.

Thrombocytopenia has been one of the most consistent hematologic abnormalities in infected dogs. Platelet counts have ranged from 23,000 to 220,000/μl. Megathrombocytosis is usually detectable in a majority of cases by examining blood smears. Platelet counting is preferable to examination of blood smears because the thrombocytopenia in RMSF is often not markedly decreased (<75,000). Rarely, DIC characterized by pro-

longation of the activated coagulation time, prothrombin time, activated partial thromboplastin time, and thrombin time with elevated fibrin (fibrinogen) degradation products occurs as a terminal event in dogs.

Biochemical abnormalities may include mildly increased serum glucose concentration and elevated serum ALP, ALT (formerly SGPT), and AST (formerly SGOT) activities. Hypercholesterolemia has been one of the more consistent findings in affected dogs. Hypoalbuminemia is often observed and probably is caused by the generalized vascular endothelial damage. Hyponatremia, hypochloremia, and metabolic acidosis are variable findings. The BUN increases in terminal stages of the disease and corresponds with oliguria and renal failure. Proteinuria and hematuria occur as results of incoagulability or glomerular and tubular injury. Bilirubinuria and hyperbilirubinemia occur in some dogs. Serum creatine phosphokinase has been mildly to moderately increased in some dogs. CSF analysis is frequently normal; however, mildly increased protein (>25 but <100 mg/μl) and polymorphonuclear or mononuclear cells have also been found.[7, 14] Analysis of synovial fluid in dogs developing polyarthritis has shown inflammatory changes, with a predominant increase in neutrophils. Results of lupus erythematosus cell, rheumatoid factor, antinuclear antibody, platelet autoantibody, and Coombs' testing and of bacterial blood culture are usually negative.

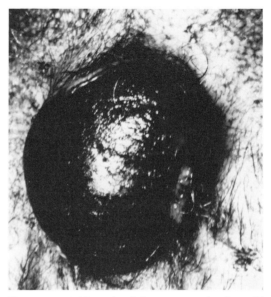

Figure 38–10. Necrosis of the scrotum of a dog with RMSF.

Electrocardiographic abnormalities, if present, consist of sinoatrial node dysfunction, ST segment and T wave depressions, and premature ventricular contractions. Thoracic radiography reveals diffuse increased interstitial density, especially in dogs presented for dyspnea and coughing.

Serologic Testing

A wide variety of mammals have detectable antibodies to SFG rickettsiae. The high prevalence of serologic reactivity in these animals as compared with the low prevalence of disease may reflect infection by antigenically related avirulent rickettsiae. Mammalian hosts differ in regard to the specificity of their immune response to rickettsiae. Well-adapted hosts, such as mice, develop highly specific antibody titers against each species of organism. Human serologic responses generally react strongly with group-reactive antibody but do not consistently distinguish between typhus-group and SFG rickettsiae. Seroreactivity of dogs appears to be intermediate between that of rodents and people. Cross-reactions in dog sera develop between SFG-antigens; however, the titer is generally highest to the specific rickettsial species causing infection. There is generally minimal reaction to typhus-group or other rickettsia. Dogs on the Atlantic seaboard have between 5% to 15% seropositivity to SFG rickettsiae.[12] The prevalence of clinical illness due to RMSF is lower than seropositivity suggests, presumably because some of the positive titers to R. rickettsii are from exposure to nonpathogenic SFG rickettsiae.[12, 15] Furthermore, subclinical or mild infections with R. rickettsii seem to be more common in dogs, which appear to be more frequently exposed and better adapted than people to the organism.

Several serologic tests have been developed to detect antibodies to RMSF in humans, including Weil-Felix, complement fixation, microscopic immunofluorescence (Micro-IF), microagglutination, indirect hemagglutination, ELISA, and latex agglutination (LA). The Micro-IF, ELISA, and LA tests appear to be the best suited to examine canine sera.

The Micro-IF test, an IFA test, and the ELISA have the advantages of requiring small amounts of sera and reagents, having high sensitivity, and classifying antibodies to R. rickettsii as IgM or IgG. Measurement of IgG antibodies to R. rickettsii using the Micro-IF method is used by most diagnostic laboratories that test canine sera (see Appendix 8). Acute and convalescent IgG titers have been generally <1:64 in uninfected dogs or those with ehrlichiosis, although titers will vary between laboratories. Actively infected dogs may have increased titers (≥1:64) by the time clinical signs are apparent and the first sample is taken. IgG titers in experimentally infected dogs have not increased until 2 to 3 weeks after infection.[16] Therefore, seronegative results do not discount the possibility of RMSF, and a second sample should be tested at a later date. An IgG titer increase of fourfold or greater is required to definitively document active infection. Dogs infected in the eastern United States usually develop higher titers than those from the western regions, which may reflect strain differences, since those in the East also appear more virulent in dogs.[17] High IgG titers that develop in actively infected dogs generally decrease after 3 to 5 months, although they may remain increased (≥1:128) for at least 10 months.[7, 16] Thus, unless single titers are markedly increased (≥1:1024 in East, ≥1:256 in West) active infection cannot be absolutely ascertained, and paired samples must be obtained. Differences can be found between laboratories performing the test and within laboratories performing the same test at a later date. Therefore, it is recommended that acute and convalescent serum samples be submitted together. Simultaneous assessment of IgM and IgG titers provides more accurate information as to the time course of infection when evaluating a single serum sample.

A modification of the test that allows for measurement of IgM has advantages in permitting more specific diagnosis of recent infection with a single convalescent titer, and IgM titers can be increased prior to increases in IgG titers. The IgM titers in naturally and experimentally infected dogs only increase (≥1:8) during the first week following infection and decrease after 4 weeks to become ≤1:8.[18–20] The maximum measured IgM titers are generally of two to four dilutions lower in magnitude than the corresponding IgG titers in the same animal.

The LA test appears to be a rapid and specific assay for recent R. rickettsii infection in dogs.[19, 20] Because the sensitivity is lower than the micro-IF test, false-negative results occur, although a single increased titer ($\geq$1:32) appears indicative of active RMSF in dogs.

Direct Immunofluorescence

Direct fluorescent antibody (FA) staining of infected tissues is a valuable test for rapid clinical or postmortem diagnosis of RMSF. Direct FA procedures have been used to detect organisms in embryonated eggs or tissue culture, tissues at necropsy, ticks, and skin biopsies from acutely infected people and dogs.[7, 8, 21, 22] Full-thickness skin biopsies should be surgically removed from visible lesions on the skin or mucosae and placed in isotonic saline, on melting ice, or in formalin at room temperature until they are processed. Rickettsiae can be found in approximately 75% of specimens taken from affected lesions and are rarely found in unaffected skin.[8] Formalin fixation causes some decrease in sensitivity of rickettsial detection.[21] Trypsin digestion and deparaffinization is needed to examine specimens that have been processed for light microscopy. Tissue sections are stained by anti–R. rickettsii fluorescent antibody for the presence of coccobacillary organisms in endothelial cells and vascular walls of the dermis.

The advantage of the direct FA procedure on tissue is that it potentially can confirm the diagnosis as early as the third or fourth day of disease on a single sample. Direct FA procedures can be performed by veterinary or human laboratories without regard to host species differences. Few false-positive results are found with the direct FA test, but many (30% to 40%) false-negative reactions can occur and are usually due to prior therapy with chloramphenicol or tetracycline or failure to obtain a sample through an area of vasculitis. Specimens should be obtained early in the course of infection because organisms are eliminated from the tissue within a few days, especially after antimicrobial therapy.[23] Owing to the usual absence of cutaneous petechiae in dogs, biopsy specimens could be obtained from mucosal hemorrhages or from vesicles that may develop in the buccal mucosa.

Rickettsial Isolation

Bioassays involving isolation of R. rickettsii in susceptible species of laboratory animals have been a research laboratory means of diagnosing RMSF. Fresh or deep frozen ($-80°C$) tissue such as liver, spleen, or brain, or clotted blood from biopsy or necropsy specimens can be inoculated into meadow voles or guinea pigs. Their serum may be tested for the presence of antibody to R. rickettsii. Tissues or blood of the affected or laboratory animal may be inoculated into embryonated chicken eggs or tissue culture to isolate and purify the agent. A staining technique using carbol basic fuchsin is widely used for the identification of SFG and typhus-group rickettsiae (Appendix 12).[24] Rickettsiae may replicate sufficiently within several days with in vitro isolation procedures, whereas bioassays often require a month to complete.

PATHOLOGIC FINDINGS

Gross lesions, if present, consist of widespread petechial and ecchymotic hemorrhages in all tissues. Generalized hemorrhagic lymphadenomegaly and splenic enlargement are usually found.

Microscopic findings consist of necrotizing vasculitis with perivascular polymorphonuclear and lymphoreticular cell infiltrations. Vascular lesions are most prominent in the skin, epididymis, testicle, GI tract, pancreas, kidneys, urinary bladder, myocardium, meninges, retina, and skeletal muscle. Acute meningoencephalitis with small focal nodular gliosis is found in brain parenchyma of dogs with acute infections (Fig. 38–11). Focal myocardial and hepatic necrosis and acute interstitial pneumonia are common lesions. Rickettsiae can be detected in many tissues by previously described staining and isolation procedures, but not by routine histologic methods.

THERAPY

Mortality in dogs with RMSF usually relates to incorrect diagnosis and treatment or to rapidly progressive shock or severe CNS infections. Antibody titers are not always available at the time the dog is admitted, and even then, results from the first sample may not be diagnostic, because it may take 1 to 3 weeks for maximal IgG response. For this reason, a response to therapy is used to increase the index of suspicion. It is judi-

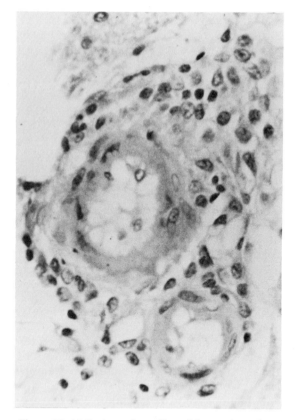

Figure 38–11. Perivascular cuffing of the meninges from a dog that died of rapidly progressive RMSF associated with meningoencephalitis.

cious to begin treatment before the return of laboratory test results. Presumptive diagnosis of RMSF can be made based upon the seasonal occurrence and clinical and laboratory abnormalities. The antibiotics used to treat RMSF are considered to be rickettsiostatic (Table 38–3).[25] Eventual eradication from the host requires adequate immune responses; the immunodeficient patient may require prolonged therapy of up to 2 weeks' duration. Tetracycline or oxytetracycline should be given for at least 7 days. Lipid-soluble tetracyclines, such as minocycline or doxycycline, have been shown to be as effective in treating rickettsial infections in people when they have been used for peri-

ods of less than 7 days.[26, 27] Chloramphenicol is equally effective and is indicated in young (<6 months old) puppies to avoid dental staining. Parenteral administration of these drugs may be required in patients that are semicomatose or have nausea or vomiting. Dogs treated early in the course of illness show clinical rapid improvement, generally within 36 to 48 hours after therapy is instituted. Delayed or incomplete recovery is associated with organ failure or with CNS damage. Some dogs treated with chloramphenicol and less commonly, with tetracycline develop depression, nausea, and vomiting, which can appear to delay their clinical recovery. Antibiotics are effective in reducing the severity of the illness only if they are given prior to the development of advanced pathologic changes, such as thrombosis and tissue necrosis. Animals that develop acryl gangrene will have eventual healing of their extremities with permanent scarring or disfigurement.

In people, use of tetracycline early in the course of illness is thought to reduce the magnitude of the serologic response that would otherwise develop. Some reduction in the intensity of antibody response in dogs has been noted following the use of tetracycline, but the clinical relevance of this finding needs to be clarified.[16] Chloramphenicol appears to reduce serologic titers to R. rickettsii in dogs to a greater extent than tetracycline. When serologic confirmation of infection is desired, chloramphenicol should not be used as the drug of first choice or prior to collecting serum for testing.[19] However, chloramphenicol appears to be more effective in clearing resistant infections in dogs that have persistent thrombocytopenia following tetracycline therapy. In addition to the previously discussed drugs, josamycin, rifampin, and ciprofloxacin have been found to be somewhat effective in vitro against R. rickettsii,[28, 29] but their clinical use has not been investigated. Ciprofloxacin has been shown to be effective in treating

Table 38–3. Therapy for Rocky Mountain Spotted Fever[a]

DRUG	DOSE[b] (mg/kg)	ROUTE PREFERRED (ALTERNATE)	INTERVAL (hours)	DURATION (weeks)
Tetracycline	22	PO (IV)	8	1–2
Chloramphenicol	15–25	PO (IV, SC, IM)	8	1–2
Doxycycline	10–20	PO (IV)	12	1

[a]PO = oral, IV = intravenous, SC = subcutaneous, IM = intramuscular.
[b]Dose per administration at specified interval, expressed as mg/kg unless otherwise stated.

R. tsutsugamushi infection (murine scrub typhus) in mice.[30]

Supportive care must be used in dogs with shock, coagulation disorders, and clinical or laboratory evidence of organ failure. IV fluid therapy must be used with caution because increased vascular permeability and expanded extracellular fluid volume can give rise to pulmonary and cerebral edema.

PREVENTION

Dogs recovering from infection with *R. rickettsii* have been immune to reinfection when challenged 6 to 12 months later.[16, 31] Infection with nonpathogenic rickettsiae such as *R. montana* does not seem to protect dogs to infection with the more virulent *R. rickettsii*.[16] Naturally infected dogs that recover from RMSF have never been shown to be reinfected. There are no vaccines available for use in dogs or people. Challenge infection in people following vaccination with inactivated products has been associated with a prolonged incubation period, a shorter and milder course of illness, and reduced prevalence of relapses, but reinfection is not prevented. Experimental, inactivated, tissue culture–origin vaccines appear to offer protection against infection in experimental animals.[32] Specific antigenic components of *R. rickettsii* responsible for producing protective antibody response were identified.[33] Inactivated vaccine containing purified surface antigens of *R. rickettsii* produced by recombinant DNA technology was used successfully to protect mice from lethal RMSF.[34, 35]

The best means of prevention of RMSF in dogs is avoidance of tick-infested areas and rapid, safe removal of attached ticks. Pets should be dipped repeatedly if they frequent areas inhabited by ticks. Tick eradication in the environment is impossible because of the maintenance of the life cycle by rodents and other reservoir hosts. Elimination of small ground rodents is difficult if not impossible to achieve. Some reduction in tick numbers has been achieved locally in the eastern and southern United States by application of insecticides in the form of aqueous suspension or dust to surrounding vegetation.

PUBLIC HEALTH CONSIDERATIONS

Of the more than 1000 cases of rickettsial diseases reported each year in the United States, approximately 90% are RMSF.[36] Mortality remains at approximately 4% to 7% of affected people. The increased incidence of infection in people in recent years may relate to population shifts into previously undeveloped localities and increased exposure to infected ticks, although increased prevalence of disease has been somewhat independent of population growth in many areas. The increase may relate to a summation of factors, including encroachment of people on undeveloped wooded areas, improved recognition and reporting of disease, and a periodic cyclicity of infection. The prevalence of seropositive reactions in dogs within a given area usually parallels human risk of infection.[22]

The seasonal occurrence of RMSF in people parallels that in dogs. The rate of infection is highest in children and young adults and is higher in males. Patients from rural areas have a greater proportion of confirmed diagnoses compared with those from suburban and urban areas.[37–39] Approximately 60% of infected people have reported a tick bite and 30% more said that they were in a wooded area just before clinical illness. The lack of known exposure does not eliminate tick involvement in infection, especially because small larval and nymphal stages can feed transiently and remain undetected. Most exposures occur at the place of residence, but a number have been related to an outdoor recreational activity. Approximately 10% of reported human cases follow only known exposure to dogs or their ticks, but this should not imply an absolute association, because common exposure to the same tick population is more likely.[40]

Dogs are a potenital source for human infections because they carry infected ticks into closer proximity to people, who become exposed by transfer of ticks from dogs to themselves or by their contact with the engorged tick's hemolymph during tick removal or by contact with tick excreta with the person's abraded skin or conjunctivae. It is not the secretions from infected dogs but the effluents from engorged, infected ticks that pose the greatest danger. Aerosol exposure from an infected dog's secretions is unlikely under natural conditions, as the organism does not survive outside host or tick cells. Aerosol exposure has occurred only in the laboratory, where inadvertent inoculation of infected tissues may also occur.

The clinical manifestations in affected people closely parallel those signs seen in dogs (see Table 38–2). Early signs in people are vague and may mimic an upper respiratory infection. Although the rash is considered typical of RMSF, it never develops in up to 12% of people, and when it does develop, it is seen in less than 50% of the cases within the first 3 days.[7b] Not all people develop all manifestations of RMSF, although fever and headache are most consistent. Neurologic signs usually develop later in the course of illness. Death appears to be more of a problem in people who develop severe hepatomegaly, jaundice, stupor, and azotemia (>25 mg/dl).[41] Cardiac arrhythmias from myocarditis, meningoencephalitis, and DIC often are detected in terminal patients. Subclinical infections in people have been suspected, but the role of nonpathogenic rickettsiae in causing the observed serologic responses has not been determined.[7b, 42]

Ticks should be removed by applying constant traction with curved forceps or less desirably with tweezers or fingers protected with facial tissue placed as close as possible to the point of insertion.[43] Ticks should not be squeezed or crushed with bare fingers since the organism can be transmitted via tick feces or hemolymph. Hands should be washed thoroughly with soap and water after removal of the tick.

Q Fever

ETIOLOGY AND EPIDEMIOLOGY

Q (query) fever, caused by the rickettsia *Coxiella burnetii* (see Table 38–1) is a zoonosis worldwide except for rare reports from Sweden, Norway, Iceland, and New Zealand. Reservoir hosts vary, depending on the geographic location, and include domestic and wild animals and their ectoparasites. Approximately 40 species of ticks and many other arthropods are naturally infected with *C. burnetii*. The tick facilitates a sylvatic cycle with the reservoir animal. Resultant infection of humans and domestic animals may occur when infected ticks feed on them. However, domestic animals and people are more commonly infected by inhalation or ingestion of environmentally resistant organisms. Cattle, sheep, and goats are the most common domestic animal reservoirs for human infection. Typically, they are subclinically infected and shed environmentally resistant organisms in their urine, feces, milk, and parturient discharges. The placenta in late gestation may contain the greatest concentration of organisms (10^9) per gram of tissue. Within the herd, infection is probably maintained by inhalation of infected dusts and aerosols or by fomites.

Serologic studies and organism isolation indicate that dogs and cats can be infected.[44, 45] Dogs and cats may acquire infection under natural circumstances by ingestion or inhalation of organisms while feeding on infected body tissues or carcasses. *C. burnetii* has been found in the blood of experimentally infected cats for 1 month and in their urine for 2 months.[46] It has been isolated from the uteri of postpartum cats.[47] Infected dogs and cats may be a source of infection for people. The organism was isolated from dogs and from *Rhipicephalus sanguineus* ticks, which were feeding upon them, on farms where human outbreaks of Q fever occurred.[48] People became infected following exposure of aerosols from contaminated environment or fomites with parturient or aborted tissues from infected cats.[47, 49–51]

PATHOGENESIS

In people, the lungs appear to be the main portal of entry of the organism to the systemic circulation. The incubation period is shorter and severity of disease greater with increased amounts of rickettsiae and increased virulence of the infecting strain and when the organism is inhaled rather than ingested. The organism has a predilection for replication in the vascular endothelium and respiratory, renal tubular, and serosal epithelia. Widespread vasculitis results in focal necrotizing hemorrhagic pneumonitis and necrosis and hemorrhage of many other organs, including the liver, CNS, and mononuclear phagocyte system. Following recovery, infection with *C. burnetii* can become latent for extended periods. During chronic infection, immune-complex phenomena develop. In chronically infected people and in subclinically infected animals, the organism remains latent until parturition, during which large numbers enter the placenta, parturient fluids, feces, urine, and milk.

CLINICAL FINDINGS

Infections in dogs and cats are usually subclinical. Splenomegaly was the only clinical finding in an infected dog.[48] Fever, anorexia, and lethargy beginning 2 days after inoculation and lasting for 3 days has been seen in experimentally infected cats.[46] Abortion has occurred in some of the cats and has been associated with human outbreaks,[46a] but the organism has also been found in cats having normal parturition. For clinical signs in people, see Public Health Considerations.

DIAGNOSIS

Lymphocytosis and thrombocytopenia are the main nonspecific hematologic changes seen in infected people. Definitive diagnosis of Q fever is made by serologic evaluation or isolation of the organism. Although information concerning human exposure can be obtained on examination of a single serum sample, it is recommended that a second sample be submitted 4 weeks later. A four-fold increase in IgG titer is diagnostic.

Three seperate serologic antigens are used in detecting antibodies. Phase-1 antigens are isolated from organisms taken directly from animals or their parasites. Phase-2 antigens are found in organisms that have been passed serially in embryonated eggs. Phase-1 antigens are extracted for lipopolysaccharide (LPS) to create the third antigen. During acute illness, antibody to phase-2 antigen increases, whereas that to phase-1 antigen is low. In convalescent infections, antibodies to phase-1 and phase-2 antigens are moderately high while those to phase-1 LPS are low. In chronic infections, antibody to phase-1 antigen equals or is greater than that

of the phase-2 type, and phase-1 LPS antibody is also high. Titers from cats involved in outbreaks have shown a similar pattern of increase. Newer diagnostic tests which can provide a convincing diagnosis on a single sample involve measurement of specific IgM to phase-2 antigen[52] or of IgA to phase-1 antigen[53] using immunofluorescent or ELISA methods.[52] Organism isolation is usually performed by inoculation of tissue samples into laboratory rodents whose serum and lymphoid tissues are examined for evidence of infection. Direct FA procedures can be used to detect the organism in tissues. See Appendix 8 for the laboratory that performs this test.

THERAPY

Rickettsiostatic drugs, such as tetracyclines and chloramphenicol, are as effective as when treating RMSF (see Table 38–3). Use of erythromycin and trimethoprim-sulfonamide has been variably successful in treating infected people. Since many affected people recover spontaneously from their acute illness, interpretation of recovery is difficult without an untreated control population. The most successful in vitro combinations have included rifampin combined with doxycycline or trimethoprim. Quinolones are active against this organism as with other rickettsiae.[54, 55]

PUBLIC HEALTH CONSIDERATIONS

Human Q fever is usually contracted by inhalation of infected aerosols such as occurs following parturition. This has been the suspected means of infection in outbreaks associated with parturient cats. Because of occupational exposure, abattoir workers, wool sorters, tanners, farm workers (shepherds, dairymen), and veterinary and laboratory personnel are particularly susceptible to infection from livestock. Investigational inactivated vaccines are available in the United States for such high-risk exposure groups. Children, who are commonly infected from ingestion of raw milk, are usually nonsymptomatic, regardless of the source of infection.

Some of the previously reported outbreaks of Q fever in urban settings may have been related to exposure to environments contaminated by infected cats. Poker players[50] and truckers[51] have been affected in this manner. In cat-associated Q fever, the incubation period, from time of contact until the first signs of illness, ranges from 4 to 30 days. Common source exposure is likely under such circumstances since the organism can be spread on clothing, dust, and other fomites to other people. Direct person-to-person transmission is uncommon but can occur since the organism is present in the body secretions of infected people.

After a prolonged (14- to 39-day) incubation period, acute systemic manifestations consist of headache, fever ($\geq 40°C$ [$104°F$]), chills, and myalgia. Less commonly, nausea, vomiting, diarrhea, arthralgia, and erythematous macules are noted. While the respiratory tract is the usual source of infection and clinical or radiographic findings of interstitial pneumonitis may develop, respiratory signs are not often found. Signs of acute hepatitis may also occur. The acute illness generally lasts 15 days and mortality rates are low, except in older or immunosuppressed individuals.

Chronic Q fever is a potentially fatal, multisystemic disorder that may develop up to 20 years after an acute episode. Signs of chronic endocarditis or hepatitis, such as fever, lethargy, dyspnea, cardiac murmurs, hepatomegaly, thrombocytopenia, and occasional thromboembolism or jaundice, occur.

References

1. McDade JE, Newhouse VF: Natural history of *Rickettsia rickettsii*. Ann Rev Microbiol 40:287–309, 1986.
2. Uchida T, Tashiro F, Funato T, et al: Isolation of a spotted fever group rickettsia from a patient with febrile exanthematous illness in Shikoku, Japan. Microbiol Immunol 30:1323–1326, 1986.
2a. Uchida T, Uchiyama T, Koyama AH: Isolation of spotted fever group rickettsiae from humans in Japan. J Infect Dis 158:664–665, 1988.
2b. Wolach B, Franco S, Bogger-Goren S, et al: Clinical and laboratory findings of spotted fever in Israeli children. Pediatr Infect Dis J 8:152–155, 1989.
2c. Bishopp FC, Trembley HL: Distribution of certain North American ticks. J Parasitol 31:1–54, 1945.
3. Norment BR, Burgdorfer W: Susceptibility and reservoir potential of the dog to spotted fever-group rickettsiae. Am J Vet Res 45:1706–1710, 1984.
4. Rao AK, Schapira M, Clements ML, et al: A prospective study of platelets and plasma proteolytic systems during the early stages of Rocky Mountain spotted fever. N Engl J Med 318:1021–1032, 1988.
4a. Herrero-Herrero JI, Ruiz-Beltran R, Battle-Forondona J: The complement system in Mediterranean spotted fever. J Infect Dis 17:1093–1095, 1988.
5. Liu CT, Hilmas DE, Griffin MJ, et al: Alterations of body fluid compartments and distribution of tissue water and electrolytes in rhesus monkeys with Rocky Mountain spotted fever. J Infect Dis 138:42–48, 1978.
6. Kaplowitz LG, Robertson GL: Hyponatremia in Rocky Mountain spotted fever: role of antidiuretic hormone. Ann Intern Med 98:334–335, 1983.
7. Greene CE, Burgdorfer W, Cavagnolo R, et al: Rocky Mountain spotted fever in dogs and its differentiation from canine ehrlichiosis. J Am Vet Med Assoc 186:465–472, 1985.
7a. Helmick CG, Bernard KW, D'Angelo LJ: Rocky Mountain spotted fever: clinical, laboratory, and epidemiological features of 262 cases. J Infect Dis 150:480–488, 1984.
7b. Greene CE: Rocky Mountain spotted fever. J Am Vet Med Assoc 191:666–671, 1987.
7c. Greene CE: Unpublished observations. University of Georgia, Athens, GA, 1989.
8. Davidson MG, Breitschwerdt EB, Walker DH, et al: Identification of rickettsiae in cutaneous biopsies from dogs with experimental Rocky Mountain spotted fever. J Vet Intern Med 3:8–11, 1989.
9. Davidson MG, Nasisse MP, Breitschwerdt EB, et al: Ocular manifestations of Rocky Mountain spotted fever in dogs. Am Col Vet Ophthalmol transcript 17, 1986.
10. Davidson MG, Breitschwerdt EB, Walker DH, et al: Experimental *Rickettsia rickettsii* vasculitis in the canine eye. Proc Int Cong Rickettsiol, 1987, p 137.
11. Keenan KP, Buhles WC, Huxsoll DL, et al: Studies on the pathogenesis of *Rickettsia rickettsii* in the dog: clinical and clinicopathologic changes of experimental infection. Am J Vet Res 38:851–856, 1977.
12. Breitschwerdt EB, Moncol DJ, Corbett WT, et al: Antibodies to spotted fever-group rickettsiae in dogs in North Carolina. Am J Vet Res 48:1436–1440, 1987.
13. Weiser I, Greene CE: Dermal necrosis associated with Rocky Mountain spotted fever in four dogs. J Am Vet Med Assoc. In press, 1990.
14. Breitschwerdt EB, Meuten DJ, Walker DH, et al: Canine Rocky Mountain spotted fever: a kennel epizootic. Am J Vet Res 46:2124–2128, 1985.
15. Hoskins JD, Breitschwerdt EB, Gaunt SD, et al: Antibodies to *Ehrlichia canis*, *Ehrlichia platys* and spotted fever group rickettsiae in Louisiana dogs. J Vet Intern Med 2:55–59, 1988.
16. Breitschwerdt EB, Walker DH, Levy MG, et al: Clinical, hematologic, and humoral immune response in female dogs inoculated with *Rickettsia rickettsii* and *Rickettsia montana*. Am J Vet Res 49:70–76, 1988.
17. Anaker RL, Mann RE, Gonzales C: Reactivity of monoclonal antibodies to *Rickettsia rickettsii* with spotted fever and typhus group rickettsiae. J Clin Microbiol 25:167–171, 1987.
18. Breitschwerdt EB: Personal communication. North Carolina State University, Raleigh, NC, 1988.
19. Greene CE: Update on neurologic and serologic findings on RMSF in dogs. Abstr Proceedings. 5th Annu Vet Med Forum, ACVIM, 1987.
20. Greene CE, Breitschwerdt EB, Marks AM, et al: Comparison of latex agglutination and microimmunofluorescence tests in the diagnosis of Rocky

Mountain spotted fever in dogs. *Am J Vet Res*, submitted, 1990.

21. Walker DH, Cain BG, Olmstead PM: Laboratory diagnosis of Rocky Mountain spotted fever by immunofluorescent demonstration of *Rickettsia rickettsii* in cutaneous lesions. *Am J Clin Pathol* 69:619–623, 1978.

22. Walker DH: Rocky Mountain spotted fever: a disease in need of microbiological concern. *Clin Microbiol Rev* 2:227–240, 1989.

23. Woodward TE: Rocky Mountain spotted fever: epidemiological and early clinical signs are keys to treatment and reduced mortality. *J Infect Dis* 150:465–468, 1984.

24. Gimenez DF: Staining rickettsiae in yolk sac cultures. *Stain Technol* 39:135–140, 1964.

25. Wisseman CL, Ordonez SV: Actions of antibiotics on *Rickettsia rickettsii*. *J Infect Dis* 153:626–628, 1986.

26. Bella-Cueto F, Font-Creus B, Segura-Porta F, et al: Comparative, randomized trial of one-day doxycycline versus 10-day tetracycline therapy for Mediterranean spotted fever. *J Infect Dis* 155:1056–1058, 1987.

27. Yagupsky P, Gross EM, Alkan M, et al: Comparison of two dosage schedules of doxycycline in children with rickettsial spotted fever. *J Infect Dis* 155:1215–1219, 1987.

28. Raoult D, Rousselier R, Vestris G, et al: In vitro antibiotic susceptibility of *Rickettsia rickettsii* and *Rickettsia conorii*: plaque assay and microplaque colorimetirc assay. *J Infect Dis* 155:1059–1061, 1987.

29. Raoult D, Rousselier P, Tamalet J: In vitro evaluation of josamycin, spiramycin, and erythromycin against *Rickettsia rickettsii* and *R. conorii*. *Antimicrob Agents Chemother* 32:255–256, 1988.

30. McClain JB, Joshi B, Rice R: Chloramphenicol, gentamicin and ciprofloxacin against murine scrub typhus. *Antimicrob Agents Chemother* 32:285–286, 1988.

31. Keenan KP, Buhles WC, Huxsoll DL, et al: Pathogenesis of infection with *Rickettsia rickettsii* in the dog: a disease model for Rocky Mountain spotted fever. *J Infect Dis* 135:911–917, 1977.

32. Ascher MS, Oster CN, Harber PI, et al: Initial clinical evaluation of a new Rocky Mountain spotted fever vaccine of tissue culture origin. *J Infect Dis* 138:217–221, 1978.

33. Feng HM, Kirkman C, Walker DH: Radioimmunoprecipitation of [³⁵S] methionine-radiolabeled proteins of *Rickettsia conorii* and *Rickettsia rickettsii*. *J Infect Dis* 154:717–721, 1986.

34. Anacker RL, List RH, Mann RE, et al: Characterization of monoclonal antibodies protecting mice against *Rickettsia rickettsii*. *J Infect Dis* 151:1052–1060, 1985.

35. McDonald GA, Anacker RL, Garjian K: Cloned gene of *Rickettsia rickettsii* surface antigen: candidate vaccine for Rocky Mountain spotted fever. *Science* 235:83–85, 1987.

36. Rocky Mountain spotted fever—United States. *MMWR* 35:247–249, 1986.

37. Smith RC, Gordon JC, Gordon SW, et al: Rocky Mountain spotted fever in an urban canine population. *J Am Vet Med Assoc* 183:1451–1453, 1983.

38. Salgo MP, Telzak EE, Currie B, et al: A focus of Rocky Mountain spotted fever within New York City. *N Engl J Med* 318:1345–1348, 1988.

39. Durack DT: Rus in Urbe, spotted fever comes to town. *N Engl J Med* 318:1388–1390, 1988.

40. Gordon JC, Gordon SW, Peterson E, et al: Rocky Mountain spotted fever in an urban canine population. *Am J Trop Med Hyg* 33:1026–1031, 1984.

41. Walker DH, Lesesne HR, Varma VA, et al: Rocky Mountain spotted fever mimicking acute cholecystitis. *Arch Intern Med* 145:2194–2196, 1985.

42. Taylor JP, Tanner WB, Rawlings JA, et al: Serological evidence of subclinical Rocky Mountain spotted fever infections in Texas. *J Infect Dis* 151:367–369, 1985.

43. Needham GR: Evaluation of five popular methods for tick removal. *Pediatrics* 75:997–1002, 1985.

44. Marrie TJ, Van Buren J, Fraser J, et al: Seroepidemiology of Q fever among domestic animals in Nova Scotia. *Am J Public Health* 75:763–766, 1985.

45. Randhawa AS, Jolley WB, Dietrich WH, et al: Coxiellosis in pound cats. *Feline Pract* 4:37–38, 1974.

46. Gillespie JH, Baker JA: Experimental Q fever in cats. *Am J Vet Res* 13:91–94, 1952.

46a. Daoust P-Y: Coxiellosis in a kitten. *Can Vet J* 30:434, 1989.

47. Marrie TJ, Durant H, Williams JC, et al: Exposure to parturient cats: a risk factor for acquisition of Q fever in maritime Canada. *J Infect Dis* 158:101–108, 1988.

48. Mantovani A, Benazzi P: The isolation of *Coxiella burnetii* from *Rhipicephalus sanguineus* on naturally infected dogs. *J Am Vet Med Assoc* 122:117–118, 1953.

49. Kosatsky T: Household outbreak of Q-fever pneumonia related to a parturient cat. *Lancet* 2:1447–1449, 1984.

50. Langley JM, Marrie TJ, Covert A, et al: Poker players' pneumonia. An urban outbreak following exposure to a parturient cat. *N Engl J Med* 319:354–356, 1988.

51. Marrie TJ, Langille D, Papukna V, et al: Truckin' pneumonia—an outbreak of Q fever in a truck repair plant probably due to aerosols from clothing contaminated by contact with newborn kittens. *Epidemiol Infect* 102:119–127, 1989.

52. Field PR, Hunt JG, Murphy AM: Detection and persistence of specific IgM antibody to *Coxiella burnetii* by enzyme-linked immunosorbent assay: a comparison with immunofluorescence and complement fixation tests. *J Infect Dis* 148:477–487, 1983.

53. Peacock MG, Philip RN, Williams JC, et al: Serological evaluation of Q fever in humans: enhanced phase I titers of immunoglobulins G and A are diagnostic for Q fever endocarditis. *Infect Immun* 41:1089–1098, 1983.

54. Sawyer LA, Fishbein DB, McDade JE: Q fever: current concepts. *Rev Infect Dis* 9:935–946, 1987.

55. Leroy D, Sivery B, Beuscart C, et al: Efficacy of ofloxacin as therapy for pneumonia due to *Legionella* sp., *Mycoplasma pneumoniae*, *Chlamydia psittaci*, or *Coxiella burnetii*. Abstr 29th Intersci Conf Antimicrob Agents Chemother, Houston, Sept. 1989, p 193.

HAEMOBARTONELLOSIS

John W. Harvey

ETIOLOGY

Haemobartonella is a genus of gram-negative, nonacid-fast, epicellular rickettsial parasites of erythrocytes, currently classified in the family Anaplasmataceae.[1] The host range of *H. felis* and *H. canis* appears to be restricted to cats and dogs, respectively, although experimental subclinical infections of cats with *H. canis* have been reported.[2] *Haemobartonella* organisms appear to contain both DNA and RNA and replicate by binary fission. Organisms have not been cultivated outside the hosts.

Haemobartonella felis

In polychrome-stained blood films, *H. felis* organisms appear as small, blue-staining cocci, rings, and rods that are usually attached to erythrocytes (Fig. 39–1). In thick blood films or thick areas of thin films, nearly all organisms appear as cocci. Ring and rod-shaped organisms are seen more readily in thin blood films or in the feathered edges of thick blood films.

The epicellular nature of *H. felis* on erythrocytes is readily apparent by scanning electron microscopic (EM) examination (Fig. 39–2). Organisms are approximately 0.5 μm in diameter and appear to be partially buried in indented foci on the surface of the erythrocytes. Discoid, conical, coccoid, rod-shaped, and doughnut-shaped organisms have been observed by using scanning EM.[4] Parasitized erythrocytes, for the most part, lose the normal biconcave shape and become spherocytes or stomatospherocytes.

The epicellular nature of *H. felis* parasites is also readily apparent by transmission EM (Fig. 39–3). A single membrane surrounds the organisms. The cytoplasm of organisms is composed of granules of varying size and density. No cytoplasmic organelles have

been recognized. Electron-lucent areas (vacuoles) appear to be present in some organisms. Organisms appear to adhere to the erythrocytic membrane by intermittent contact points.[4, 5] Although smudging of the erythrocytic membrane in association with organisms has been reported, complete erosion of the membrane has not been documented.

Haemobartonella canis

H. canis differs from *H. felis* in that it more commonly forms chains that extend across the surface of affected erythrocytes (Fig. 39–4). However, individual organisms may also appear as small dots, rods, and rings.

Results of scanning and transmission EM studies of *H. canis* indicate that it is ultrastructurally similar to *H. felis*. Although single organisms dimple the surface of the host erythrocytes in a manner similar to that

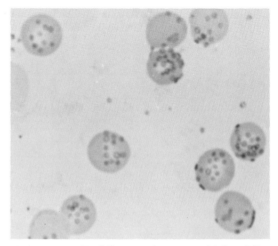

Figure 39–1. *H. felis* organisms parasitizing feline erythrocytes. Some free organisms displaced during blood film preparation are also present. (Wright-Giemsa stain, × 1600).

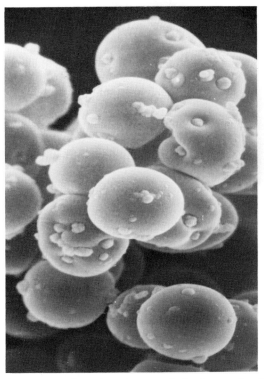

Figure 39–2. Scanning electron photomicrograph of erythrocytes from a cat infected with *H. felis* (× 6500). (Courtesy of Dr. Dallas Hyde, University of California, Davis, Davis, CA.)

described previously for *H. felis*, chains of organisms frequently occur in grooves or deep infoldings that can markedly distort the erythrocyte shape.[4]

PATHOGENESIS

Cat

Experimentally, *H. felis* infection has been transmitted by the IP and IV injections and oral administration of infected blood. Saliva and urine are not believed to be infective. Dissemination of infection by blood-sucking arthropods, such as fleas, is considered by many to be the primary mode of transmission, although such transmission has not been established experimentally in cats. *H. felis* can be transmitted from female cats with clinical disease to their newborn offspring in the absence of arthropod vectors.[6] It is not known whether transmission occurs in utero, during parturition, or via nursing. Iatrogenic transmission of *H. felis* can occur by the transfusion of blood from normal-appearing carrier cats.

The severity of disease produced by *H. felis* varies from cats that are mildly anemic and without clinical signs to cats that are markedly depressed and die as a result of severe anemia. To facilitate the understanding of feline haemobartonellosis, the disease has been divided into preparasitemic, acute, recovery, and carrier phases, or stages (Fig. 39–5). The preparasitemic phase is generally about 1 to 3 weeks after IV injection and 22 to 51 days after splenectomized cats have been given infected blood orally.[6]

The acute phase of disease represents the time from the first to last major parasitemia. This phase often lasts a month or more, but occasionally cats die quickly following the occurrence of massive parasitemias and precipitous decreases in PCV early in the course of the disease. Parasites generally appear in the blood in a cyclical manner within discrete parasitemic episodes (see Fig. 39–5). The number of parasites generally increases to a peak value over 1 to 5 days, followed by a rapid decline. The synchronized disappearance of organisms from the blood can occur in 2 hours or less.[6] Few, if any, parasites are seen in blood films for several days following parasitemic episodes.

In many instances, a rapid decrease followed by a rapid increase in PCV occurs in association with the appearance and disappearance of organisms from the blood.[6] These fluctuations in PCV appear to be associated with splenic sequestration of parasitized erythrocytes and with later release of nonparasitized erythrocytes.[7] In other instances, the PCV remains decreased or continues to decline for 1 or more days after a parasitemic episode, probably as a result of erythrocyte destruction.

Repetitive parasitemic episodes appear to result in progressive erythrocyte damage and shortened erythrocyte life spans. Some damage to erythrocytes may be caused directly by the parasite, but immune-mediated injury appears to be more important. Direct Coombs' tests may have positive results within a week following the first parasitemia. Coombs' test results remain positive during the acute stage of disease whether or not parasites are present.[8] It is postulated that the attachment of organisms to erythrocytes either exposes hidden erythrocyte antigens or results in altered erythrocyte antigens, to which the host responds by producing antierythrocyte antibodies. Inasmuch as antibodies are made against *H. felis*

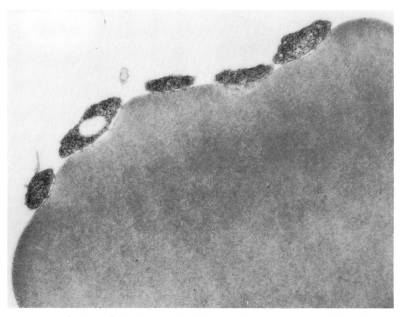

Figure 39–3. Transmission electron photomicrograph of five *H. felis* organisms in intermittent contact with the plasmalemma of a parasitized erythrocyte (× 23,000). (From Simpson CF et al: *J Parasitol* 64:504–511, 1978, with permission.)

organisms,[8] another possible mechanism of immune-mediated injury should also be considered: if complement-fixation occurs, the erythrocytic membrane may be damaged as an "innocent bystander." Minimal intravascular hemolysis occurs in this disorder. The

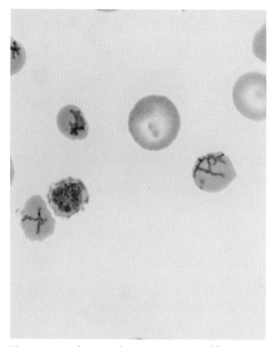

Figure 39–4. Three erythrocytes parasitized by *H. canis* organisms (Wright-Giemsa stain; × 1500).

anemia occurs primarily as a result of extravascular erythrophagocytosis by macrophages in the spleen, liver, lungs, and bone marrow.

As a lymphocyte- and macrophage-rich blood filter, the spleen is of primary importance in the clearance of bloodborne particulate antigens and the elaboration of specific immune responses to these antigens. In animals other than the cat, splenectomy is generally required before clinical disease is produced by the various species-specific *Haemobartonella* organisms.[2] *Haemobartonella* organisms are removed less readily in splenectomized cats, resulting in parasitemias lasting about twice as long as those in intact cats,[7] but splenectomy performed prior to infection does not appear to affect the incubation period or severity of disease in cats. Splenectomy after cats have recovered results in the transient reappearance of blood parasites, but in most cases the PCV does not drop to a clinically significant level.[9]

Without therapy, approximately one third of cats with uncomplicated acute haemobartonellosis die as a result of severe anemia. Cats that mount both a sufficient immune response to the organism and a regenerative bone marrow response in excess of the rate of erythrocyte destruction will recover from the disease. The recovery phase, the time

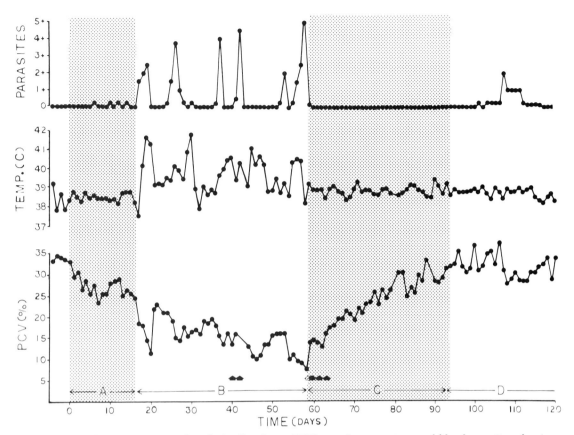

Figure 39–5. Daily measurements of packed cell volume (PCV), rectal temperature, and blood parasite value in a cat following IV inoculation with *H. felis*–infected blood on day 0. Closed arrows indicate intravenous administration of thiacetarsamide sodium (1 mg/kg). Open arrow at day 60 indicates a 25 ml IV whole blood transfusion. Phases of disease are indicated by letter and shading, with A being the preparasitemic phase, B the acute phase, C the recovery phase, and D the carrier phase. (From Harvey JW, Gaskin JM: *J Am Anim Hosp Assoc* 13:28–38, 1977, with permission.)

from the last major parasitemia until the PCV has stabilized within or close to the reference range, often takes a month or more.[6] In untreated cats, organisms are commonly observed in low numbers in the blood during the recovery phase but do not usually occur as discrete parasitemic episodes.

Cats that recover from acute infections with *H. felis* remain chronically infected for months to years, if not for life.[9] Although an extracellular parasite should be eliminated by immune mechanisms, intact organisms have been reported within phagocytic vacuoles of spleen and lung macrophages.[5] Possibly some organisms survive within the cells and account for the indefinite, chronically infected state. Chronically infected "carrier" cats appear clinically normal. They may have normal PCV or mild regenerative anemias. Low numbers of organisms are regularly observed in some cats, but in others no organisms may be visible in blood films

for weeks.[9] Carrier cats appear to be in a balanced state in which replication of organisms is balanced by phagocytosis and removal.

H. felis may be an opportunistic agent that exists commonly in healthy cats and produces disease when the cat is stressed by other diseases or surgical procedures. Many cats, however, do not appear to have identifiable predisposing disease or stress conditions.[10] Cat-bite abscesses appear to be the most frequent disorder recognized to precede haemobartonellosis by a few weeks. Although an abscess is undoubtedly stressful, the possibility of transmission of the disease through a bite has not been ruled out.

Of particular interest is the possible interrelationship between *H. felis* and feline leukemia virus (FeLV)–produced disease.[11] In one small study, 41% of cats with clinical haemobartonellosis were viremic.[12] Inasmuch as FeLV can suppress the normal immune response to unrelated antigens, it was considered likely that this virus would increase the susceptibility of cats to haemobartonellosis. Because some FeLV strains can induce anemias directly, concurrent FeLV and *H. felis* infections may produce severe anemia in an additive manner.

Dog

Transmission of *H. canis* by the brown dog tick (*Rhipicephalus sanguineus*) has been demonstrated experimentally.[13] Transstadial and transovarial transmission in ticks has also been described, indicating that the tick may be an important reservoir as well as a vector of infection. Iatrogenic transmission of *Haemobartonella* organisms by blood transfusion from clinically normal carrier dogs can also occur but is of less concern than it is in cats because the recipient dog generally must have been splenectomized before clinically significant disease occurs.[4] Haemobartonellosis resulting in the death of two animals has been recognized in a litter of 4-week-old pups.[8] Experimental studies to demonstrate transmission to puppies in utero or through nursing have not been successful,[14] but indirect evidence for in utero transmission has been given.[15] Transmission by oral administration of infected blood has also been reported.[14]

In contrast to haemobartonellosis in cats, the majority of nonsplenectomized dogs infected with *H. canis* do not develop clinical evidence of disease and probably do not become anemic or have sufficient numbers of organisms present in the blood to be recognized on routine blood film examination.[14]

The prepatent period following IV injection of infected blood into splenectomized dogs has been reported to range from 1 or 2 days[14] to 2 weeks or more.[15] Some cases have been characterized by a rapidly developing anemia associated with nearly constant parasitemia. Death generally occurs in these dogs within a month following inoculation.[14] In other dogs, the development of anemia is more gradual, occurring as a result of repetitive parasitemic episodes. Parasites are generally observed in large numbers in the blood for a week or more, with a few intervening days when organisms are not observed. From 1 to 2 months are generally

required for the PCV and hemogloblin concentration to drop to minimum values and an equal time for them to return to noral.[14, 15] Although immunologic evaluation of infected dogs has been limited, it appears that antibodies are produced against erythrocytes.[8, 16]

Although splenectomy is generally required before clinically significant haemobartonellosis occurs in dogs, cases have been described in nonsplenectomized dogs with concurrent *Ehrlichia*, *Babesia*, bacterial, and viral infections.[4, 15] Haemobartonellosis has also occurred in dogs given immunosuppressive drugs and in dogs with splenic pathology.[4] Rare cases have occurred in spleen-intact dogs when no evidence for immunosuppression was found.[8]

CLINICAL FINDINGS

Cat

Acute haemobartonellosis occurs in cats of all ages and primarily in males. The increased incidence in adult male cats has been attributed to their increased roaming and fighting behavior, with greater exposure to cats infected with *H. felis*.[12]

The most common clinical signs in cats are depression, weakness, anorexia, weight loss, paleness of mucous membranes, and at times, splenomegaly. Icteric mucous membranes are occasionally noted. Clinical signs depend on the stage of disease and the rapidity with which anemia develops. If anemia develops gradually, a cat may exhibit weight loss but remain bright and alert. In contrast, a precipitous drop in PCV early in the disease in association with a severe parasitemia causes little weight loss, but marked mental depression occurs.

The rectal temperature generally is normal except during the acute phase of disease, when it is increased approximately 50% of the time.[6] Subnormal temperatures may be present in moribund cats.

Dog

Unless other diseases are also present, clinical signs are rarely apparent in nonsplenectomized dogs infected with *H. canis*. Splenectomized experimental dogs become listless and have pale mucous membranes as the anemia develops but generally have normal rectal temperatures and appetites.[14]

DIAGNOSIS

Cat

H. felis organisms are present in sufficient numbers to be easily recognized in stained blood films only about 50% of the time during the acute phase of disease.[10] The PCV is usually below 20% and frequently below 10% before clinical signs of disease are apparent to the client.[5] The PCV is not always a good indicator of total erythrocyte mass in cats with haemobartonellosis. Parasitized erythrocytes that are primarily sequestered in the spleen and other organs may return to the general circulation following the removal of organisms.[6]

If the PCV decreases rapidly, the mean corpuscular volume (MCV) may be normal with little polychromasia and few reticulocytes present. In most instances, by the time clinical signs of disease are apparent, there is a regenerative anemia with polychromasia and reticulocytosis. Erythrocytes are usually macrocytic, with a MCV greater than 50 fl, and frequently hypochromic, with a MCHC less than 32%.[4] Although anisocytosis, nucleated erythrocytes, and increased number of Howell-Jolly bodies are consistently observed in the circulation during the acute phase of feline haemobartonellosis, these findings are not reliable indicators of regenerative response in the cat. Howell-Jolly bodies are often observed in normal cats, nucleated erythrocytes may appear in a wide variety of feline diseases, and marked anisocytosis without polychromasia has been reported in cats with myeloproliferative disease.[4] Cats with latent infections (carriers) occasionally have low numbers of parasites visible in the blood. The PCV fluctuates over time and may be normal or slightly to moderately decreased (never below 20%). Slight polychromasia and reticulocytosis and increased MCV are present at times.[9]

Since two morphologic forms of reticulocytes have been described in cats, it is important to know what criteria a reference laboratory uses to count reticulocytes. Aggregate reticulocytes occur in a low proportion (0% to 0.4%) of the erythrocytes in blood from normal cats. The percentage of this form correlates well with the percentage of polychromatophilic erythrocytes. A greater proportion (up to 10%) of circulating erythrocytes in normal cats contains punctate reticulocytes, which consist of precipitated ribosomes. Punctate reticulocyte counts are not valid in blood heavily parasitized with H. felis, because organisms also stain as punctate blue inclusions.

Total and differential leukocyte counts are quite variable and of limited diagnostic assistance. Absolute monocyte counts are however frequently increased, and erythrophagocytosis by monocytes or macrophages may be observed if blood films are scanned at low magnification.[4, 6]

Phagocytosis of erythrocytes by mononuclear cells in the circulation appears to occur as a result of antibodies and complement on the erythrocyte surface. Autoagglutination is frequently observed in blood collection vials during early stages of acute haemobartonellosis.[8] The direct Coombs' test result is generally positive by the time a patient is presented for diagnostic evaluation. Only Coombs' reagents made specifically for cats can be used in this test.

Bone marrow myeloid to erythroid (M:E) ratios are normal in the early stages of disease but are generally decreased later in the disease. Erythroid hyperplasia is evident not only by an increase in the total number of erythroid cells but also by an increased proportion of immature stages. Slight to marked erythrophagocytosis by macrophages is often present.

Icteric plasma is not consistently observed in feline haemobartonellosis but may be present within 1 to 2 days after a rapid decrease in PCV. The fact that icterus index values and bilirubin content are not always increased subsequent to rapid decreases in PCV is probably due to the fact that erythrocytes can be sequestered in capillaries and vascular spaces within the spleen without being destroyed.[6] Plasma protein concentrations are usually in the reference range (6 to 8 g/dl) but may be increased in some cats. Moribund cats may be markedly hypoglycemic.

Presently, the only readily available method for the diagnosis of H. felis infections is the demonstration of organisms in the blood. Thin, well-stained blood films, without artifacts caused by improper drying or fixation or by precipitated stain, are required (see also Preparation of Blood Films, Chapter 76 and Appendix 12 for additional information). Blood films must be examined before therapy is begun, since organisms are absent while cats are being treated with tetracyclines. One must be able to differentiate H. felis organisms from Howell-Jolly bodies, basophilic stippling, and Cytauxzoon parasites, which are small protozoa with both a nucleus and cytoplasm. New methylene blue wet preparations are not recommended for demonstration of H. felis organisms, because organisms are difficult to discern unless massive numbers are present.

Owing to the cyclic nature of the parasitemias, the absence of H. felis organisms from blood does not rule out a diagnosis of haemobartonellosis. A regenerative anemia with a positive Coombs' test result, the presence of autoagglutination, or erythrophagocytosis by blood monocytes is suggestive of haemobartonellosis, but other diseases such as primary autoimmune hemolytic anemias or FeLV-induced hemolytic anemia should also be considered.

The mere presence of H. felis organisms in the blood does not necessarily indicate that the clinical illness present was produced by this agent, because parasites may be incidentally observed in carrier cats with other diseases. On the other hand, one should not automatically discount the significance of organisms in cats because the anemia appears nonregenerative. If the PCV drops precipitously after infection, a cat can be depressed and anemic for several days before a substantial regenerative bone marrow response is evident in the peripheral blood.[6] However, a persistent nonregenerative anemia should make one pursue other causes of anemia, such as FeLV infection.

Acridine orange and direct immunofluorescent staining techniques are reported to be more sensitive than standard Romanowsky-type stains for demonstrating H. felis.[15a] These procedures are not generally available and have definite limitations. Diagnosis using these staining techniques is limited by the presence of organisms in the blood. Both procedures require a fluorescent microscope (not available to most practicing veterinarians) and a person trained in fluorescent microscopy (staining techniques are more difficult than routine blood stains and nonspecific fluorescence might give false-positive results).

Dog

Haemobartonella organisms are usually present when clinical evidence of anemia is recognized in dogs. Although the anemia has varied from mild to severe in studies of splenectomized experimental dogs, the PCV has generally been below 20% before clinical signs of haemobartonellosis were observed.[16] Organisms may be found incidentally on hematologic screening when an animal is examined early in the disease because of clinical signs attributable to other concurrent disorders.

In most cases, sufficient time has elapsed between the development of anemia and initial recognition of the disease for there to be peripheral blood evidence of a regenerative bone marrow response. Hematologic findings include reticulocytosis, increased polychromasia and anisocytosis, circulating nucleated erythrocytes, and frequent Howell-Jolly bodies. Macrocytosis takes more time to develop and may therefore not be present when cases are initially presented.

No consistent leukogram abnormalities are recognized in canine haemobartonellosis. Neither icteric plasma nor hemoglobinemia is generally recognized in uncomplicated cases, but substantial bilirubinuria may occur. Spherocytosis and positive direct Coombs' test results occur in some cases.[8, 16] Dogs with latent infections generally have normal hemograms.

The diagnosis of canine haemobartonellosis depends on the recognition of organisms in the blood. One must be able to differentiate between organisms and staining artifacts, basophilic stippling, and Howell-Jolly bodies. The most useful criterion is the tendency of H. canis to form chains of organisms across the erythrocyte surface. Blood films should be inspected closely if an anemia develops or becomes worse in a dog after splenectomy.

PATHOLOGIC FINDINGS

Gross necropsy findings in cats include pale-appearing tissues in all cases, emaciation in approximately 75% of the cats, slight-to-marked splenomegaly in approximately 50%, and slight-to-moderate icterus in some instances.

Abnormal histologic findings are variable

and include erythroid and at times myeloid hyperplasia of bone marrow and passive congestion, extramedullary hematopoiesis, follicular hyperplasia, erythrophagocytosis, and increased hemosiderin in the spleen. In some cases, fatty degeneration and centrilobular necrosis of the liver is recognized.

Necropsy findings in canine haemobartonellosis have not been thoroughly reported. The blood appears thin and tissues pale. The bone marrow is red and gelatinous. Hyperplasia of the mononuclear phagocyte system has been mentioned.

THERAPY

Cat

Blood transfusions are probably not needed in cats if the PCV is 15% or greater. The necessity of a blood transfusion is related to the rapidity of onset of the hemolytic crisis. The physical appearance of the patient is an important consideration when one must decide whether a transfusion is needed. If the cat is comatose, parenteral glucose may be indicated.[6]

Cats should be treated orally for 3 weeks with oxytetracycline (Table 39–1). Some tetracycline products appear to produce a fever and evidence of illness as adverse side effects in some cats.[8] A lower dosage or a different tetracycline product may be used, or the drug may be discontinued altogether. Tetracycline antibiotics do not appear to totally eliminate organisms from infected cats; consequently, "recovered" animals remain chronically infected.[6]

In addition to tetracycline therapy, treatment with an orally administered glucocorticoid such as prednisolone (see Table 39–1) is indicated in severely anemic cats. The immediate benefit of prednisolone is to inhibit erythrophagocytosis. The glucocorticoid dosage should be decreased gradually as desired increases in PCV are measured. Unless parasites are present in the circulation, it is impossible to differentiate haemobartonellosis from autoimmune hemolytic anemia. Consequently, the same therapeutic approach to both diseases is indicated.

Thiacetarsamide sodium IV has been recommended in the past, but recent studies indicate a lack of effectiveness of this drug.[6, 17] Chloramphenicol has also been recommended for the treatment of haemobartonellosis. Unfortunately, this drug produces significant (albeit reversible) erythroid hypoplasia and clinical signs of illness at therapeutic dosages recommended for cats, and its efficacy has been questioned.[17]

The long-term prognosis of cats following recovery from uncomplicated haemobartonellosis appears to be good. Although carrier cats are believed to be prone to relapse into clinical disease following periods of "stress," when body defenses are weakened, experimental studies thus far have not been able to verify this phenomenon.[9]

Dog

Experimental studies evaluating therapy for canine haemobartonellosis have been limited. Blood transfusions should be administered when the anemia is considered to be life-threatening. Oxytetracycline, administered orally, is reported to be effective in treating *H. canis* infections (see Table 39–1).[18, 19] If an animal relapses after therapy, it may be advantageous to follow a second course of therapy with a lower dose of oxy-

Table 39–1. Drug Dosages for Canine and Feline Haemobartonellosis[a]

DRUG	SPECIES	DOSE[b] (mg/kg)	ROUTE	INTERVAL (hours)	DURATION (days)
Tetracyclines	C	20	PO (IV)	8	21
	D[c]	40	PO (IV)	8	14
Chloramphenicol	D[d]	22	PO (IV)	12	9
Thiacetarsamide	D[e]	2.2	IV	24	9
Prednisolone	B	1–2	PO	12	prn

[a]C = cat, D = dog, B = dog and cat, PO = oral, IV = intravenous, prn = as needed.
[b]Dose per administration at specified interval, expressed as mg/kg unless otherwise stated.
[c]If relapse occurs, use 40 mg/kg, PO, every 24 hours for at least 30 days.
[d]Can cause bone marrow suppression, more noticeable in cats, so reserved for use in dogs.
[e]Apparent lack of effectiveness for cats, see text.

tetracycline for a month or more to prevent recurrence.[20]

Successful treatment has been reported in three experimentally infected dogs with thiacetarsamide sodium IV and in one experimentally infected dog with chloramphenicol IV (see Table 39–1).[18] Dogs that recover from haemobartonellosis probably have latent infections.

PREVENTION

Elimination of blood-sucking arthropods from dogs and cats is recommended, because they may transmit infectious diseases, including haemobartonellosis. Iatrogenic transmission of canine haemobartonellosis is usually of concern only if the recipient has had a splenectomy. Iatrogenic transmission can be prevented in both cats and dogs by splenectomizing blood donor animals and examining blood films for organisms for 10 days thereafter to make sure they do not have latent infections.[9, 14]

References

1. Kreier JP, Ristic M: Haemobartonella. In Krieg NR, Holt JG (ed): Bergy's Manual of Systemic Bacteriology, vol 1. Baltimore, Williams & Wilkins, 1984, pp 724–726.
2. Kreier JP, Ristic M: Haemobartonellosis, eperythrozoonosis, grahamellosis and ehrlichiosis. In Weinman D, Ristic M (ed): Infectious Blood Diseases of Man and Animals, vol 2. New York, Academic Press, 1968, pp 387–472.
3. Harvey JW: Feline hemobartonellosis. In Kirk RW (ed): Current Veterinary Therapy VII. Small Animal Practice. Philadelphia, WB Saunders Co, 1980, pp 410–413.
4. Jain NC: Schalm's Veterinary Hematology, ed 4. Philadelphia, Lea & Febiger, 1986, pp 602–608.
5. Simpson CF, Gaskin JM, Harvey JW: Ultrastructure of erythrocytes parasitized by Haemobartonella felis. J Parasitol 64:504–511, 1978.
6. Harvey JW, Gaskin JM: Experimental feline hae-
mobartonellosis. J Am Anim Hosp Assoc 13:28–38, 1977.
7. Maede Y: Studies on feline haemobartonellosis. V. Role of the spleen in cats infected wtih Haemobartonella felis. Jpn J Vet Sci 40:141–146, 1978.
8. Harvey JW: Unpublished observations. University of Florida, Gainesville, FL, 1987.
9. Harvey JW, Gaskin JM: Feline haemobartonellosis: attempts to induce relapses of clinical disease in chronically infected cats. J Am Anim Hosp Assoc 14:453–456, 1978.
10. Hayes HM, Priester WA: Feline infectious anemia. Risk by age, sex and breed; prior disease; seasonal occurrence; mortality. J Small Anim Pract 14:797–804, 1973.
11. Bobade PA, Nash AS, Rogerson P: Feline haemobartonellosis: clinical, haematological and pathological studies in natural infections and the relationship to infection with feline leukaemia virus. Vet Rec 122:32–36, 1988.
12. Cotter SM, Hardy WD, Essex M: Association of feline leukemia virus with lymphosarcoma and other disorders in the cat. J Am Vet Med Assoc 166:449–454, 1975.
13. Seneviratna P, Weerasinghe N, Ariyadasa S: Transmission of Haemobartonella canis by the dog tick Rhipicephalus sanguineus. Res Vet Sci 14:112–114, 1973.
14. Lumb WV: Haemobartonellosis in the dog. In Proceedings. 8th Gaines Veterinary Symposium, 15–16, 1958.
15. Krakowka S: Transplacentally acquired microbial and parasitic diseases of dogs. J Am Vet Med Assoc 171:750–753, 1977.
15a. Bobade PA, Nash AS: A comparison of the efficiency of acridine orange and some Romanowsky staining procedures in the demonstration of Haemobartonella felis in feline blood. Vet Parasitol 26:169–172, 1987.
16. Bundza A, Lumsden JH, McSherry BJ, et al: Haemobartonellosis in a dog in association with a Coombs' positive anemia. Can Vet J 17:267–270, 1976.
17. Watson ADJ, Farrow BRH, Haskins LP: Some observations on treating cats infected with Haemobartonella felis. Aust Vet Pract 8:129–132, 1978.
18. Pryor WH, Bradbury RP: Haemobartonella canis infection in research dogs. Lab Anim Sci 25:566–569, 1975.
19. Middleton DJ, Moore AS, Medhurst CL: Haemobartonellosis in a dog. Aust Vet J 59:29–31, 1982.
20. Kuehn NF, Gaunt SD: Hypocellular marrow and extramedullary hematopoiesis in a dog: hematologic recovery after splenectomy. J Am Vet Med Assoc 188:1313–1315, 1986.

40 CHLAMYDIAL INFECTIONS

Craig E. Greene

ETIOLOGY

The genus *Chlamydia* is a member of the class Microtatobiotes, order Chlamydiales, and family Chlamydiaceae. Chlamydiae are obligate intracellular parasites that, like bacteria, have a cell wall, DNA, and RNA but lack the metabolic machinery required for autonomous survival and replication. They have an unusual developmental cycle that involves both extracellular and intracellular forms (Fig. 40–1).

Elementary bodies are small (0.3 μm), resistant particles with rigid cell walls. They undergo a transient extracellular migration to infect new cells, where they subsequently grow into larger (0.5 to 1 μm) initial bodies

that lack cell walls and are noninfectious. The initial bodies proliferate by means of budding and fission within a cytoplasmic vesicle, or phagosome, of the host cell. This proliferation is followed by a phase of rapid division, in which the initial bodies divide to become a large, membrane-bound population of elementary bodies. These are released from the cell following lysis, and free elementary bodies are able to infect new host cells.

Chlamydiae persist as commensal flora on the ocular, respiratory, GI, and genitourinary mucosae. They produce inapparent to overt infections in a variety of hosts. Their tendency to cause chronic, relapsing, or latent infections indicates that only a partial host immune response is evoked. *C. trachomatis* and *C. psittaci*, are the two recognized species within this genus. *C. trachomatis* is a parasite of people that produces ocular, urogenital, and pulmonary infections. *C. trachomatis* forms compact rigid cell wall inclusions, containing glycogen, that stain with iodine, a characteristic distinguishing it from *C. psittaci*. *C. psittaci* has many host-adapted strains that can infect other animals. In this regard, it has little host or tissue specificity. The discussion below concentrates on those infections in dogs and cats.

CLINICAL FINDINGS

Dogs

Serologic surveys have detected antibodies to chlamydiae in up to 50% of healthy dogs.[1, 2] Chlamydiae have been suggested as a cause of chronic superficial keratitis in dogs[3]; however, they can be found as ocular

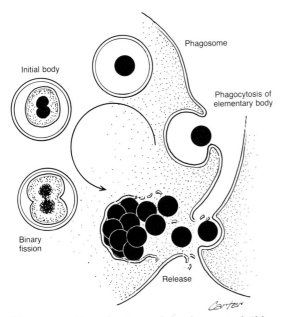

Figure 40–1. Reproduction and development of *Chlamydia*.

Phagosome

Initial body

Phagocytosis of elementary body

Binary fission

Release

Carter

flora in clinically healthy animals. Although never established as the cause, chlamydiae were isolated from dogs with encephalitis and systemic illness.[4, 5] A chlamydia isolated from a sheep with polyarthritis produced fever, anorexia, depression, pneumonia, joint pain, and diarrhea in experimentally inoculated dogs.[6] Although chlamydiosis was a presumptive diagnosis, a dog developed coughing and a radiographically consolidated lung lobe after being exposed to an aviary of budgerigars suffering from an epidemic of psittacosis.[7]

Cats

Positive antibody titers to chlamydiae have been detected in as high as 9% of healthy, laboratory-reared cats[2] and 45% of farm cats.[8, 9] Despite this high prevalence of seropositivity, chlamydiae were only isolated from conjunctival or rectal swabs from 6% and 4%, respectively, of clinically healthy cats.[9] Isolation rates of up to 30% of household cats with conjunctivitis were reported.[8] Chlamydiae have been well recognized as a cause of ocular, nasal, and lower respiratory infections of cats (see Chapter 27). They also colonize the gastrointestinal and genital mucosae.

Chlamydiae were isolated from the superficial mucus-producing cells of the gastric mucosa.[10, 11] There has been no consistent association of infected cats with GI or respiratory disease, and this may represent latent infection. Experimental inoculation of the gastric chlamydiae into the respiratory tract produced upper respiratory infection similar to that caused by the feline pneumonitis agent.[10] Inoculation of the feline conjunctivitis agent directly into feline oviducts produced chronic salpingitis, and the organism was isolated for up to 2 months after inoculation.[12] This infection was similar to that produced by C. trachomatis in people, although anatomic differences would limit the spread of genital chlamydiae up the oviducts. Peritonitis also was attributed to chlamydial infection in cats.[13]

Experimental ocular infection of specific pathogen-free cats with the feline pneumonitis strain of C. psittaci produced acute conjunctivitis and persistent genital and GI infection in some cats.[14] Whether chlamydiae are responsible for reproductive disorders in cats is uncertain. Genital infections

may be a means by which infection is spread from queens to their kittens.[15]

DIAGNOSIS

Swab specimens of surface tissues or aspirations or washings from deeper tissues are inoculated in McCoy cell tissue culture in the laboratory.[16] Vigorous swabbing is essential to obtain enough epithelial cells that contain the organism. Cotton swabs are best; dacron swabs or those with wooden sticks should not be used. Swabs should be placed immediately in a chlamydial transport medium such as 2SP (0.2 M sucrose and 0.02 M phosphate).[17] Routine viral transport media contains antibiotics that will inactivate the organisms. The sample should be refrigerated (4°C) if it is not immediately sent to the laboratory; however, the specimens ideally should be frozen at $-70°C$. Examining the amino acid nutritional requirements can differentiate the strains of C. psittaci.[18]

Giemsa is the traditional stain for demonstrating chlamydiae, but artifacts in the cytoplasm may stain similarly. FA techniques using monoclonal antibodies make identification highly specific. ELISA methodology can be used to detect antigen directly in patient specimens.[19] Cross-reaction with all the members of the genus occurs with these tests as presently employed commercially (Chlamydiazyme, Abbott Labs, Chicago IL; IDEIA Chlamydia Test, Boots-Celltech Diagnostics Inc, East Hanover, NJ; see Appendix 8). ELISA methods are relatively specific but less sensitive than cell culture in detecting feline infections.[19] Serologic testing for antibodies to chlamydiae is of limited diagnostic benefit in determining active infection, since the IgG antibody titer increase is variable or prolonged and IgM antibody titers are inconsistently elevated. However, highest antibody titers are generally associated with symptomatic cats.[8] Chlamydial infections persist in the presence of high serum antibody levels; therefore, serologic testing only documents exposure and cannot be used to evaluate protection afforded by vaccines.

THERAPY

Treatment of chlamydial infections primarily involves the use of tetracyclines. Oral administration is usually preferred at a dosage of 22 mg/kg, given three times daily for 3 to 4 weeks. Ocular infections respond best to tetracycline eye ointment applied three times daily. In cat colonies with chlamydial infection, treatment may have to be continued for up to 6 weeks, and the entire population may have to be treated simultaneously.

PREVENTION

Both inactivated and modified live vaccines have been available for the protection against chlamydial respiratory disease in cats (see Prevention, Chapter 27, and Feline Respiratory Disease, Chapter 2). Even modified live vaccines, which provide the best protection, do not entirely prevent colonization of mucosae and shedding of chlamydiae following challenge.[14, 20] They minimize the replication of the organism and hence reduce the clinical signs in subsequently infected cats.

PUBLIC HEALTH CONSIDERATIONS

Chlamydia of feline origin have been suspected as the cause of human conjunctivitis on several occasions.[21–23] In one instance, chlamydiae isolated from an infected person were inoculated into experimental cats and produced acute conjunctivitis and persistent chlamydial infection, attesting to their potential feline origin.[21] Although these associations are difficult to document, people should take precautions in medicating cats with conjunctivitis, and infected cats may have to be treated simultaneously in households where people develop chlamydial conjunctivitis.

References

1. Weber A, Kraus H, Schmatz HD: Serum epidemiological studies on the occurrence of chlamydial infections in beagles from experimental kennels. A Versuchstierk 19:270–275, 1977.
2. Fukushi H, Ogawa H, Minamoto N, et al: Seroepidemiological surveillance of Chlamydia psittaci in cats and dogs in Japan. Vet Rec 117:503–504, 1985.
3. Voigt A, Dietz O, Schmidt V: Klinische und experimentelle Untersuchungen zur Atiologie der Keratitis superficialis chronica (uberretier). Arch Exp Vet Med 20:259–274, 1966.
4. Contini S: Su di un caso della nalatti di Giroud et Groulade del can. Atti Soc Ital Sci 10:736–740, 1956.
5. Groulade P, Roger F, Dortois N: Contribution a l'étude d'un syndrome infectieux du chien répondant sérologiquement à une souche do Rickettsia psittaci. Rev Pathol Comp Med Exp 54:1426–1432, 1954.
6. Young S, Storz J, Maierhofer CA: Pathologic features of experimentally induced chlamydial infection in dogs. Am J Vet Res 33:377–383, 1972.
7. Fraser G, Norval J, Withers AR, et al: A case history of psittacosis in the dog. Vet Rec 85:54–58, 1969.
8. Wills JM, Howard PE, Gruffydd-Jones TJ, et al: Prevalence of Chlamydia psittaci in different cat populations in Britain. J Small Anim Pract 29:327–339, 1988.
9. Gethings PM, Stephens Gl, Wills JM, et al: Prevalence of Chlamydia, Toxoplasma, Toxocara and ringworm in farm cats in south-west England. Vet Rec 128:213–216, 1987.
10. Gaillard ET, Hargis AM, Prieur DJ, et al: Pathogenesis of feline gastric chlamydial infection. Am J Vet Res 45:2314–2321, 1984.
11. Hargis AM, Prieur DJ, Gaillard ET: Chlamydial infection of the gastric mucosa in twelve cats. Vet Pathol 20:170–178, 1983.
12. Kane J: Chlamydial pelvic infection in cats: a model for the study of human pelvic inflammatory disease. Genitourin Med 61:311–318, 1985.
13. Dickie CW, Shiff ES: Chlamydia infection associated with peritonitis in a cat. J Am Vet Med Assoc 176:1256–1259, 1987.
14. Wills JM, Gruffydd-Jones TJ, Richmond SJ: Effect of vaccination on feline Chlamydia psittaci infection. Infect Immun 55:2653–2657, 1987.
15. Wills J, Gruffydd-Jones TJ, Richmond S, et al: Isolation of Chlamydia psittaci from cases of conjunctivitis in a colony of cats. Vet Rec 114:344–346, 1984.
16. Richmond SJ, Stirling P: Localization of chlamydial group antigen in McCoy cell monolayers infected with Chlamydia trachomatis or Chlamydia psittaci. Infect Immun 34:561–570, 1981.
17. Spencer WN, Johnson FW: Simple transport medium for the isolation of Chlamydia psittaci from clinical material. Vet Rec 113:535–536, 1983.
18. Johnson FW: Isolation of Chlamydia psittaci from nasal and conjunctival exudate of a domestic cat. Vet Rec 114:342–344, 1984.
19. Wills JM, Millard WG, Howard PE: Evaluation of a monoclonal antibody based ELISA for detection of feline Chlamydia psittaci. Vet Rec 119:418–420, 1986.
20. Shewen PE, Povey RC, Wilson MR: A comparison of the efficacy of a live and four inactivated vaccine preparations for the protection of cats against experimental challenge with Chlamydia psittaci. Can J Comp Med 44:244–251, 1980.
21. Ostler HB, Schacter J, Dawson R: Acute follicular conjunctivitis of epizootic origin. Arch Ophthalmol 82:587–591, 1969.
22. Bialasiewicz AA, Jahn GJ: Ocular findings in Chlamydia psittaci–induced keratoconjunctivitis in the human. Fortschr Ophthalmol 83:629–631, 1986.
23. Schmeer N, Jahn GJ, Bialasiewicz AA, et al: The cat as a possible source for Chlamydia psittaci–induced keratoconjunctivitis in the human. Tierarztl Prax 15:201–204, 1987.

MYCOPLASMAL INFECTIONS

S. Rosendal

ETIOLOGY

Mycoplasmas, the smallest free-living microorganisms, are prokaryotes, with replicating cells as small as 300 nm and a DNA molecule expressing as few as 700 genes (Fig. 41–1). Although this is enough for an extracellular existence, it restricts their metabolic and synthetic capacity. Therefore, mycoplasmas depend on nourishment from a rich environment, which they find on mucosal membranes of the respiratory and urogenital tracts of their warm-blooded hosts. The lack of a rigid protective cell wall makes mycoplasmas rather fragile outside the host but resistant to lysozyme and cell wall–inhibiting antibiotics, such as penicillins, cephalosporins, and bacitracin.

Mycoplasmas of the genera *Mycoplasma*, *Ureaplasma*, and *Acholeplasma* are represented in the natural flora of dogs and cats. Many species may have a role in diseases by virtue of being isolated from disease processes, but few have been conclusively proved to be pathogenic. Table 41–1 contains a list of diseases of dogs and cats in which mycoplasmas may be a causal factor.

CLINICAL FINDINGS

Ocular

It is fairly well established that *M. felis* is a significant pathogen in conjunctivitis of cats.[1, 2] The clinical signs for mycoplasmal conjunctivitis have been described as serous discharge followed by mucoid and sticky exudate. The conjunctiva is initially hyperemic and edematous and later becomes indurated. Untreated cats may show signs for

as long as 60 days, but the cornea is usually not involved.

Respiratory

Most of the mycoplasma species normally present in the upper respiratory tract have also been isolated at necropsy from lungs of dogs and cats with various types of pneumonia but are not generally present in the lungs of normal animals.[3–7] In animals with impaired pulmonary clearance due to viral infection, mycoplasmas inhaled from the upper respiratory tract may establish an infection in the lung as secondary opportunistic pathogens. When a number of mycoplasmal species isolated from lungs of dogs with distemper pneumonia were evaluated for virulence by experimental exposure of healthy puppies, only one strain of *M. cynos* induced pulmonary pathology. Although it is not likely to play a primary role, it undoubtedly contributes to the multifactorial cause of canine pneumonia.[3] It is possible that *M. felis* in the cat should be viewed in a similar manner since pneumonia has been found with experimental challenge of kittens.[1]

Genitourinary

It is not uncommon to isolate mycoplasmas in large numbers from the urine of dogs with urinary tract disease. Although in most situations they are in mixed culture with bacteria, they are also occasionally isolated alone.[8] The same conditions predisposing to bacterial infection may promote mycoplasmal infection, such as tumors and urinary

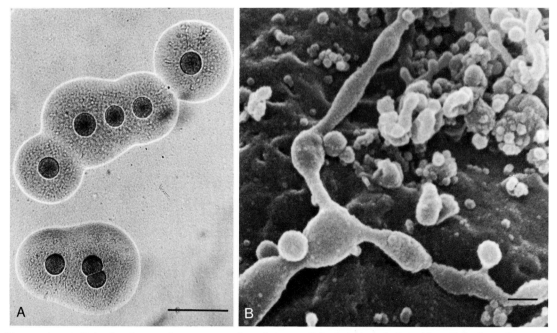

Figure 41–1. A, Colonies of mycoplasmas grown for 4 days on solid substrate and viewed in a dissecting microscope (bar = 1 mm). B, Scanning electron micrograph of mycoplasmas colonizing the surface of epithelial cells (bar = 200 nm). (Courtesy of V. Bermudez, Ontario Veterinary College, Guelph, ON.)

calculi. The source of the mycoplasmas in the urinary tract is undoubtedly the rich natural flora in the distal urogenital tract. No distinct clinical signs can predict mycoplasmal urinary tract infection.

M. canis has been isolated from dogs with endometritis.[9, 18] The assumed opportunistic role of mycoplasmas in endometritis is probably overlooked in many cases of mixed infection for which only bacteria are cultured. On the other hand, opportunistic bacterial infections may be responsible for the reproductive disorders in kennels where both mycoplasmas and bacteria are found.

Vaginal and preputial swabs and semen samples are often submitted for mycoplasmal culture in dogs with infertility problems. Very often these give positive results; however, their significance as pathogens is uncertain. It is important to weigh the cultural results in relation to other diagnostic findings and make a judgment whether antibiotic treatment for mycoplasmas will solve the infertility problem. Deep vaginal or semen cultures are the most accurate means of determining the presence of the organisms.

A survey of dogs with infertility and normal animals showed that infertile dogs had

Table 41–1. Disease Conditions in Dogs and Cats and Associated Mycoplasma Species[a]

DISEASE	HOST	MYCOPLASMA SPP. INVOLVED
Conjunctivitis	C	M. felis[1,2]
Pneumonia	D	M. cynos (M. spumans, M. gateae, M. canis, M. edwardii, M. feliminutum, Ureaplasma sp.)[b, 3–5]
	C	(M. felis, M. arginini)[b, 6, 7]
Nephritis, cystitis	D	(M. canis, M. spumans, M. cynos)[b, 8]
Reproductive diseases, infertility	D	M. canis, Ureaplasma sp. (M. maculosum, M. spumans, M. edwardii, M. cynos, M. molare, M. sp.)[b, 9, 10]
Systemic diseases, polyarthritis	D	M. spumans, (M. canis, M. edwardii, M. maculosum)[b, 11–13]
	C	M. gateae, M. felis[14]
Colitis	D	(M. canis, M. spumans, M. sp. HRC 689)[b, 15]
Abscesses	C	Unidentified M. sp.[c, 16, 17]

[a]D = dog, C = cat
[b]The evidence for the causal role of the bracketed Mycoplasma spp. is presumptive and is based on cultural association with the disease condition only.
[c]These may represent L-form infections. See also Chapter 50 under this heading.

ureaplasmas in vaginal and preputial samples more often than fertile dogs. This difference was statistically significant in male dogs, but not in female dogs.[10] Because ureaplasmas are associated with infertility in other animals, research work is urgently needed to evaluate the role of these organisms in dogs and cats.

Systemic

It is generally assumed that microorganisms from the natural flora cross the mucosal barrier with regularity, but healthy individuals eliminate these invaders by specific and nonspecific defense reactions. Mycoplasmas originating from the natural flora may, therefore, occasionally be isolated from parenchymatous organs of dogs and cats with debilitating diseases, such as malignancies or immunosuppression.[11, 12, 12a] A reported *M. gateae* case of polyarthritis in a cat should probably be viewed in this light. Cats injected IV developed polyarthritis, thus confirming the potential virulence of this organism.[14] Predisposing conditions were not identified in a young greyhound with polyarthritis caused by *M. spumans*.[13]

Mycoplasmas are occasionally isolated from rectum and colon biopsy samples of dogs with colitis, but there is no conclusive evidence for their etiologic role in the inflammatory condition.[15]

Organisms with the characteristics of mycoplasmas have been isolated from cats with abscesses, most likely introduced by bite-inflicted wounds.[16, 17] Unfortunately, the isolates have been difficult to adapt to in vitro conditions and therefore have been impossible to classify. In one report, three cats had mycoplasmal abscesses in subcutaneous and muscle tissue and another cat was diagnosed with a cervical and a pulmonary abscess. In all situations, the abscesses responded to treatment with tetracycline or tylosin (see also L-Form Infections, Chapter 50).

DIAGNOSIS AND THERAPY

The clinician should be aware of the fragile nature of mycoplasmas. Cotton swabs placed in Hayflicks broth medium or commercially available swabs with either Amies medium (without charcoal) or modified Stuart bacterial transport medium can be submitted to the diagnostic laboratory for mycoplasma culture. The specimens should be cooled and shipped with an ice pack if transport time is less than 24 hours but must be frozen and shipped on Dry Ice if longer transport time is expected. Mycoplasmas from dogs and cats grow on media prepared according to Hayflicks formula and can be identified quite easily, provided specific reference antisera are available.

Susceptibility testing to antimicrobial agents is not available for mycoplasmas on a routine basis. They are generally susceptible to the macrolides (tylosin, erythromycin), tetracyclines, chloramphenicol, lincomycin, nitrofuran, tiamulin, and aminoglycosides, but it is necessary to treat for an extended period of time (see Appendix 14 for dosages). Because tetracycline and chloramphenicol should not be used in pregnant animals,[18] erythromycin and lincomycin, although less effective, are safer to use. The newer quinolones have been shown to be effective against mycoplasmas.

PUBLIC HEALTH CONSIDERATIONS

Mycoplasmal infections of dogs and cats have not been considered as public health risks. A veterinarian developed suppurative tenosynovitis 1 week after being scratched on a finger by a cat being treated for colitis.[19] The infection was resistant to erythromycin, cloxacillin, and penicillin but was cured with doxycycline. This was the first report of mycoplasmal infection as a zoonosis and the first report that mycoplasma produced an abscess in people.

References

1. Tan RJS: Susceptibility of kittens to *Mycoplasma felis* infection. *Jpn J Exp Med* 44:235–240, 1974.
2. Campbell LH, Snyder SB, Reed C, et al: *Mycoplasma felis*–associated conjunctivitis in cats. *J Am Vet Med Assoc* 163:991–995, 1973.
3. Rosendal S: Canine and feline mycoplasmas. In Barile MF, et al (eds): *The Mycoplasmas*, vol 2. New York, Academic Press, 1979, pp 217–234.
4. Ball HJ, Bryson DG: Isolation of ureaplasmas from pneumonic dog lungs. *Vet Rec* 111:585, 1982.
5. Rosendal S: Canine mycoplasmas: their ecologic niche and role in disease. *J Am Vet Med Assoc* 180:1212–1214, 1982.
6. Spradbrow PB, Marley J, Portas B, et al: The isolation of mycoplasmas from cats with respiratory disease. *Aust Vet J* 46:109–110, 1970.

6a. Kirchner BK, Mayoc TJ, Sidor MA, et al: Isolation of three untyped *Mycoplasma* sp. from dogs with respiratory disease. *Lab Anim Sci* 33:483, 1983.

6b. Ruben Z, Port CD: Spontaneous bronchopneumonia and tracheitis in laboratory dogs infected with untyped *Mycoplasma* sp. *Lab Anim Sci* 33:483, 1983.

7. Tan RJS, Miles JAR: Incidence and significance of mycoplasmas in sick cats. *Res Vet Sci* 16:27–34, 1974.

8. Jang SS, Ling GV, Yamamoto R, et al: Mycoplasma as a cause of canine urinary tract infection. *J Am Vet Med Assoc* 185:45–47, 1984.

9. Holzmann A, Laber G, Walzl H: Experimentally induced mycoplasmal infection in the genital tract of the female dog. *Theriogenology* 12:355–370, 1979.

10. Doig PA, Ruhnke HL, Bosu WTK: The genital mycoplasma and ureaplasma flora of healthy and diseased dogs. *Can J Comp Med* 45:233–238, 1981.

11. Koshimizu K, Yamamoto K, Ogata M: Mycoplasmas isolated from dogs with malignant lymphoma. *Jpn J Vet Sci* 35:123–132, 1973.

12. Henricks PM: Isolation of two mycoplasma species from the peritoneal cavity of a dog. *Can Vet J* 28:437–438, 1987.

12a. Hooper PT, Ireland LA, Carter A: Mycoplasma polyarthritis in a cat with probable severe immune deficiency. *Aust Vet J* 62:352, 1985.

13. Barton MD, Ireland L, Kirschner JL, et al: Isolation of *Mycoplasma spumans* from polyarthritis in a greyhound. *Aust Vet J* 62:206, 1985.

14. Moise NS, Crissman JW, Fairbrother JF, et al: *Mycoplasma gateae* arthritis and tenosynovitis in cats: case report and experimental reproduction of the disease. *Am J Vet Res* 44:16–21, 1983.

15. Bowe PS, Van Kruiningen HJ, Rosendal S: Attempts to produce granulomatous colitis in boxer dogs with a mycoplasma. *Can J Comp Med* 46:430–433, 1982.

16. Keane DP: Chronic abscesses in cats associated with an organism resembling mycoplasma. *Can Vet J* 24:289–291, 1983.

17. Crisp MS, Birchard SJ, Lawrence AE, et al: Pulmonary abscess caused by a *Mycoplasma* sp. in a cat. *J Am Vet Med Assoc* 191:340–342, 1987.

18. Lein DH: Canine *Mycoplasma*, *Ureaplasma*, and bacterial infertility. *In* Kirk RW (ed): Current Veterinary Therapy IX. Philadelphia, WB Saunders Co, 1986, pp 1240–1243.

19. McCabe SJ, Murray JF, Ruhnke HL, et al: Mycoplasma infection of the hand acquired from a cat. *J Hand Surg* 12A:1085, 1987.

BACTERIAL INFECTIONS

SECTION III

42 LABORATORY DIAGNOSIS OF BACTERIAL INFECTIONS

Robert L. Jones

The purpose of clinical bacteriology is to rapidly and accurately provide information concerning the presence or absence of a bacterial agent in an infectious disease process. It usually requires at least 24 to 72 hours for bacteria to be isolated, but the clinician can seldom wait that long to institute therapy. Knowledge of the prevalence of specific pathogens responsible for defined clinical syndromes and trends in the antimicrobial susceptibility patterns can provide the basis for making rational treatment decisions and selecting the antimicrobial agent most likely to succeed.

Utilization of the microbiology laboratory is subject to unique pitfalls posed by the diversity of bacterial agents, each with unique requirements for laboratory identification; multiple and often poorly accessible sites for collection of specimens; contamination of specimens with indigenous flora; and the necessity for subjective interpretation of results. The request for a culture is an implied request to search for anything in the specimen that could contribute to the diagnosis and treatment of an infectious disease. Problems then occur in communication between the microbiology laboratory and the clinician regarding the suitability of the specimen for laboratory examination, uncertainty of the significance of bacterial isolates, wrong interpretation of reports, and the length of delay between the submission of the specimen and the production of useful information. Current kits and devices provide the microbiology laboratory with the capability of identifying and susceptibility testing bacteria with a degree of accuracy previously unavailable. However, cost constraints increasingly limit the extent of microbiologic services that can reasonably be afforded.

It is unreasonable to expect equal capabilities for isolation of all possible pathogens from all microbiology laboratories. Material should be referred to specialized laboratories when a diagnosis is suspected that cannot be established by the laboratory facilities at hand.

DIAGNOSTIC METHODS

Diagnosis and treatment of infectious diseases generally require detection and identification of the etiologic agent(s). Microbiologic studies complement clinical judgment, enhance the clinician's ability to select specific antimicrobial drugs, and ultimately improve patient care.

Direct Microscopic Examination

Direct microscopic examination of exudates or infected body fluids is the single most important and cost-effective laboratory procedure that can be used for diagnosis and management of infections. It provides immediate information on the number, morphology, and Gram-staining properties (Table 42–1) of bacteria and the host cellular response. Purulent inflammatory responses are most suggestive of bacterial infection. Microscopic examination also gives an indication of the suitability of the specimen for culture, the likelihood of the presence of infection, the likely pathogen(s), and the predominant organisms in a mixed infection. This information may be used as a basis for interpretation of the significance of subsequent culture results.

Bacteria are readily observed on a smear when present in the specimen at a concen-

Table 42–1. Microscopic Appearance of Bacteria in Clinical Specimens

MORPHOLOGY AND GRAM-STAINING REACTION	POSSIBLE MICROORGANISMS
Gram-positive cocci	*Staphylococcus, Streptococcus,* anaerobic cocci
Gram-positive rods with endospores	*Clostridium*
Gram-positive, branching filaments; may show beading	*Actinomyces, Nocardia*
Gram-negative rods	Enterics, *Pseudomonas, Pasteurella, Bordetella,* anaerobic rods

tration of about 10,000 to 100,000/ml. Therefore, examination of specimens such as blood or CSF for bacteria is usually unrewarding because even when present bacteria are too few in number to be detected. Some bacteria, such as spirochetes and mycoplasmas, do not stain well with Gram stain. Darkfield microscopy allows visualization of spirochetes, but mycoplasmas are too small for observation by light microscopy.

Isolation and Identification

Whether isolation and identification are attempted depend upon many factors, chief among them being the source of the specimen and whether or not a presumptive diagnosis can be made microscopically. There are predictable agents commonly recovered from specific sites. Liquid broth media provide enrichment of organisms present in small numbers and facilitate isolation of fastidious organisms. In some cases, selective media must be used to suppress growth of contaminants and normal microflora while allowing growth of the pathogen.

Some bacteria with specific growth conditions may be more efficiently identified by direct detection of their antigens or toxins. For diagnosis of some clostridial diseases, such as botulism (Chapter 47), tetanus (Chapter 48), and *Clostridium difficile* enterocolitis (see also Clindamycin, Chapter 43), it is imperative that the toxin be identified in the specimen rather than relying solely upon isolation. Direct or indirect fluorescent antibody stains are extremely useful for a rapid presumptive diagnosis of infection with some bacteria. Because *Yersinia pestis* (Chapter 59) and *Francisella tularensis*

(Chapter 60) are hazardous to laboratory personnel, antigen detection by fluorescent antibody staining of exudates or tissue is the best tool for their rapid and specific identification.

Specimen Collection

This is most important for assembling information required for a clinical decision. Ideally, the microbiology laboratory should provide the clinician with directions for collecting, ordering, and transporting specimens for analysis. In turn, the clinician should provide the laboratory with sufficient information for proper processing of the specimen and interpretation of results. The extra time and effort spent in collecting the best specimen is the best way to ensure quality results and to avoid the necessity of collecting a second specimen.

Specimens must be collected from the actual site of infection with a minimum of contamination from adjacent tissues, organs, or secretions (Fig. 42–1). Some specimens are likely to become contaminated with indigenous flora during the collection process. Great care should be taken to use aseptic technique when collecting specimens. Some specimens are simply inaccessible except by aspiration or biopsy of deeper tissues. Skin decontamination should be performed as for surgery for all specimens obtained by needle or aspiration. Often, by reviewing the pathogenesis of the infection and target organs, one can select the most appropriate collection site that will best verify the presence or absence of the particular pathogen. Specimens should be collected as early in the course of the disease process as possible. As the disease progresses and necrosis of tissue occurs, some microorganisms may die or be overgrown by other bacteria.

Whenever possible, obtain specimens before the administration of antimicrobials. However, their use does not necessarily preclude the recovery of bacteria from selected tissues where low antibiotic concentrations are achieved or from those cases with antimicrobial resistant bacteria. If it is not possible to collect the specimen before any antimicrobials are administered, the specimen should be taken just before the next dose is given. If antimicrobials are concentrated at the specimen site, such as urine,

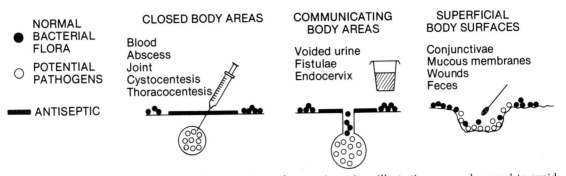

Figure 42–1. Collection of bacterial culture specimens from various sites, illustrating approaches used to avoid excessive contamination of the specimen and probable sources of contamination. (From Jones RL: In McCurnin DM (ed): *Clinical Textbook for Veterinary Technicians.* WB Saunders Co, 1985, pp 110–147. Reprinted with permission.)

then it is best to wait 48 hours after the last dose before collecting a specimen.

An adequate (several milliliters or grams) quantity of material should be obtained for appropriate laboratory tests. All too frequently, an inadequate amount of material is obtained with a swab, making it nearly impossible for the laboratory to make appropriate smears and adequate cultures. A swab should *never* be submitted in lieu of curettings, biopsy material, fluid (especially urine), or surgically removed tissue.

Multiple specimens should be submitted when lesions are present at several sites or when more than one laboratory procedure is requested. Multiple blood samples are necessary because bacteria may be shed intermittently into the blood. Multiple fecal samples are also indicated for detection of salmonellae.

In most cases of infection of unknown etiology that do not yield results after initial culturing attempts, an individual approach, including consultation between the microbiologist and clinician, is recommended. Simply repeating culture after culture is expensive and often unsuccessful.

Collection Devices and Transport. Appropriate collection devices and specimen transport systems are needed to ensure survival of the microorganism without overgrowth and for optimal isolation and identification. A variety of containers are commercially available, ranging from simple swab and plastic tube combinations to complicated specimen collection devices (Fig. 42–2). Swabs must be made of approved, noninhibitory materials and transported in a sterile container. Many bacteria are susceptible to desiccation during transport. Therefore, swabs are only acceptable for transportation

of specimens when provided with a humidified transporting chamber or placed in transport medium. Tissue, exudate, or fluid should be submitted in an appropriate closed sterile container. Glass or plastic containers, screw-capped jars, or tubes are recommended. Each tissue or specimen must be placed in a separate container. Direct aspiration into a syringe is often the most convenient and satisfactory means of collection of tissues and fluids. The needle should be plugged with a sterile stopper or removed, and the syringe should be capped.

A variety of media may be used directly for transporting specimens to the laboratory. Transport medium is usually buffered and may contain charcoal to absorb toxic metabolic products from the bacteria to ensure survival. These transport devices usually should be refrigerated or chilled during transport to the laboratory. Transport media, such as Stuart, Carey-Blair, and Amies (all from Difco, Detroit, MI), are nonnutritive and help to preserve the organisms in the specimen as well as to minimize overgrowth by those in a mixture, especially when there are low numbers or fastidious bacteria. Ordinary nutrient-type broth such as that in blood culture bottles may be used only when swabs or aspirates are collected from normally sterile body sites (e.g., CSF, synovia) and when great care has been taken to avoid any contamination. Special anaerobic transport devices must be used to prevent exposure of obligate anaerobes to lethal concentrations of oxygen (Chapter 49). Because reduced oxygen is not lethal for the aerobes and facultative anaerobes, they can be transported in the same anaerobic transport devices. Tissue in formalin, dry swabs, urine collected several hours earlier and not refrigerated, and swabs for attempted isolation

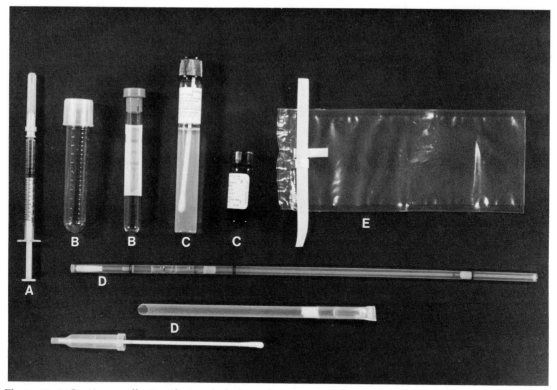

Figure 42–2. Specimen collection devices include swabs, syringes, tubes, and plastic bags. Fluid specimens can be transported in syringes (A) or tubes (B). Swabbed specimens can be transported in transport media (C) or special chambers (D). Tissues and fecal specimens can be placed in plastic bags (E).

of mycobacteria are unsuitable for bacterial culture.

Blood. Successful isolation of microorganisms from blood requires an understanding of the intermittency and low order of magnitude of most bacteremias (see Blood Culture, Chapter 7). It is most important to take several specimens for culture over a period of time. The usual recommendation is that blood cultures be drawn as the fever begins. Another suggestion is to take three or four cultures within 1 to 3 hours; if more than one culture shows growth, it is probably significant. See Chapter 7 for the appropriate technique.

Urine. The collection, transport, and storage of urine specimens are important adjuncts to the reliability of culture results. Urine is an excellent bacterial growth medium, allowing a small or insignificant number of bacteria to multiply rapidly to large numbers unless certain precautions are taken.

Culture results of a voided specimen taken without cleansing are useful only if there is no growth; any growth may be urethral con-

tamination, infection, or both. Contamination of a midstream-voided sample must be considered when less than 10^5 colony-forming units/ml are isolated, although total counts of viable bacteria may be reduced in some infections. Gram's stain of a drop (allowed to dry without spreading) of well-mixed urine will not only provide a means of determining the adequacy of its collection but will also provide the diagnosis of significant bacteriuria ($>10^5$ colony-forming units/ml) when at least two bacteria per oil immersion (1000 magnification) field are found.

Urine collection for culture by urethral catheterization is seldom indicated, except in those cases in which catheterization must otherwise be done for diagnostic or therapeutic reasons. Contamination of the urine by urethral microflora is best avoided by cystocentesis, a relatively safe and simple procedure in experienced hands (Chapter 11). This will solve the problem of equivocal counts and the risk of nosocomial urinary tract infection associated with catheterization.

The urine must be collected directly into

a sterile capped syringe or a screw-capped container or tube, not into a "clean" cup or swab. If the urine cannot be cultured within 1 to 2 hours after its collection, it must be refrigerated for a maximum of 18 to 24 hours. For longer storage or transport and storage, a urine preservation tube (Vacutainer Urine Transport Kit, Becton-Dickinson, Rutherford, NJ) allows for analysis and culture of specimens held for up to 48 hours at room temperature and for quantitative culture held for up to 72 hours refrigerated.

Transudates and Exudates. A sterile syringe and needle should be used to collect a generous quantity of liquid material from unopened abscesses and body cavities after antiseptic has been applied to the surface. After aspiration, air remaining in the syringe should be expelled and the end capped or the specimen transferred immediately to an anaerobic transport device.

When a wash solution is used to aid in collection of a specimen such as a tracheal aspirate, it is imperative to use a solution that does not contain a bacteriostatic preservative. Best results can be expected when a buffered solution such as lactated Ringer's solution is used instead of isotonic saline solutions, which tend to be acidic.

Feces. Proper collection and preservation of feces is a frequently neglected but important requirement for the isolation of microorganisms contributing to intestinal disease. Salmonellae may not survive unless the specimen can be taken immediately to the laboratory and properly handled upon delivery, because of the pH changes that occur with a drop in temperature. A small (2- to 3-g) quantity of stool is the preferred specimen; a rectal swab specimen is less satisfactory, yielding fewer positive results. It is best to choose portions of the stool that contain mucus and blood. These areas may harbor a larger number of the organisms that are involved in the disease process. Stools should be collected in clean containers that can be sealed for leakproof transport to the laboratory.

Repeated cultures are often required for screening stool specimens, as some pathogens may appear only several days after onset of diarrhea, whereas other organisms may be few or absent later in the disease. Although the number three is not inviolate, repeated cultures are indicated if the clinical picture suggests GI infection by pathogenic bacteria and the first cultures are unrewarding.

Tissue Samples. A portion of the tissue rather than a swabbed specimen should be submitted. Surgical biopsy specimens are of considerable importance for culture and may represent the entire pathologic process. They are usually obtained at considerable expense and some risk to the patient. Therefore, they should be handled carefully to avoid contamination or desiccation that would reduce their diagnostic value. When the lesion is large or when there are several lesions, multiple specimens from different sites should be collected. Samples from an abscess should include pus and a portion of the wall of the abscess.

When collecting necropsy specimens, it is best to anticipate the specimens that will be needed for microbiologic analysis before starting the necropsy and then to collect these samples first, before excessive tissue handling causes further contamination. Samples from the GI tract should be taken last in order to avoid contaminating other tissues. When collecting fluid from a body compartment (joints, CSF, pericardial fluid), use a syringe and needle, aseptically aspirating a sample of fluid rather than using a swab.

The specimen should be placed unfixed in a sealed sterile container to prevent contamination or desiccation. If there will be a delay in delivering the specimen to the laboratory, it should be refrigerated.

INTERPRETATION OF CULTURE RESULTS

Specimens that have been properly obtained from the animal, carefully transported to the laboratory, and processed for bacteriologic culture and susceptibility testing frequently yield important information about the cause of the infection and the antibiotic expected to be most effective. However, laboratory identification of a bacterium is not necessarily indisputable evidence of disease. The findings must be interpreted by evaluating (1) the clinical signs or lesion, (2) the site of collection of the specimen, (3) the presence of normal flora or other contaminants, (4) the method of handling and transporting the specimen to the laboratory, and

(5) the number of different bacteria isolated and the quantitative recovery of the agents.

Provision of a history and description of the specimen source enable the microbiologist to better assist the clinician with the recognition of significant results and their proper interpretation.

Normal Flora

All mucous membranes and external body surfaces are potentially colonized with bacteria as part of the normal microflora. These bacteria may be pathogenic if invading and causing inflammation, or they may be just colonizing the surfaces. Therefore, culture results must be correlated with clinical signs. Semiquantitation of culture results is often an aid to evaluating the significance of the results.

Quantitation of Growth

The amount of bacterial growth can aid in interpreting the significance of isolates, although the number of bacteria can be related to the vigor of swabbing to collect the specimen. The laboratory report should indicate whether growth is light, moderate, or heavy. Finding large numbers of a single microorganism in nearly pure culture is a strong indicator of significance. Light growth, including growth from broth enrichment alone, is often typical of normal flora, insignificant contaminants, or suppression of growth by antimicrobials. Culture results usually have limited significance unless the sample was taken from a normally sterile body site and there is knowledge that the specimen was properly collected. Isolation of a mixture of four or more aerobic microorganisms in light or moderate numbers is usually typical of normal microflora.

Absence of Specified Pathogens

Sometimes it is more important to know that the laboratory sought to isolate specific pathogens but was unable to find them than to receive a report identifying the microorganisms that were present. For example, a culture report on a fecal sample stating that no *Salmonella* or *Campylobacter* were isolated is much more useful than a report that

names several species of normal fecal microflora, because this indicates that a specifically directed effort was made to identify these pathogens in the specimen.

No-Growth Cultures

Failure to isolate bacteria may be a false-negative result for a number of reasons, including the following: (1) sampling and transporting mistakes, such as desiccation or failure to use transport media; (2) previous antimicrobial therapy; and (3) infections due to fastidious microorganisms for which proper culture procedures were not performed, such as *Mycoplasma*, obligate anaerobes, and spirochetes. If microscopic examination of the specimen reveals microorganisms but comparable microorganisms are not isolated, transporting and culturing procedures should be evaluated in consultation with the microbiologist.

ANTIMICROBIAL SUSCEPTIBILITY TESTS

Testing bacteria for their susceptibility to antimicrobials has become established as one of the laboratory procedures that has significant impact on the prescribing of antimicrobials. In order to improve the predictive value of susceptibility tests, the indications for these tests and their limitations must be understood.

The words *susceptible* and *resistant* are relative terms (and somewhat arbitrarily defined), since within the animal a microorganism may be susceptible in one location because of attainable antimicrobial concentrations but may be resistant in another. Susceptibility tests measure the lowest concentration of antimicrobial required to macroscopically inhibit growth of the microorganism, called the minimum inhibitory concentration (MIC). The concentration of antimicrobial that inhibits the infectious agent, either by killing it outright or by slowing its growth sufficiently so that normal body defense mechanisms can take over is assumed to be similar to the in vitro MIC. Comparison of the MIC with the concentration of antimicrobial that can be attained in various body compartments can be done to predict the susceptibility or resistance of the organism to the drug at the infection site.

Indications

Some microorganisms that can be expected in the site of involvement are predictably susceptible to certain inexpensive, relatively nontoxic antimicrobials that should always be the first choice treatment. Some are naturally resistant to common antimicrobials, whereas others are capable of developing or acquiring resistance. If the possibility exists that species with an unpredictable antimicrobial susceptibility pattern are present, it is paramount that the clinician know this as soon as possible so that antimicrobial susceptibility tests can be performed. Although broad-spectrum antimicrobials can be selected without culture, they tend to be more expensive and more toxic. Generally, isolates from normally sterile body fluids should be tested, although questions have been raised about the cost-effectiveness of routine testing of all urinary tract isolates. Susceptibility testing of multiple bacterial isolates from abscesses and wounds is meaningless. Testing the susceptibility of anaerobes remains a technical problem and an unsettled issue; most anaerobes except those that produce β-lactamases are predictably susceptible.

Test Methods

The reference method of antimicrobial susceptibility testing measures the MIC in µg/ml by incorporating serial twofold dilutions of antimicrobials in a bacteriologic growth medium (Fig. 42–3). These dilutions can be in microdilution wells, a procedure used by many larger laboratories. The clinical significance is determined by interpreting the results according to the criteria in Table 42–2.

In contrast to the MIC, the most commonly used method of antimicrobial susceptibility testing in small laboratories and veterinary practices is the agar diffusion test. This method uses antimicrobial-impregnated paper disks applied to the surface of agar that has been inoculated with pure cultures of the test organism (Fig. 42–4). The diameter of the zone of inhibition of growth around the disk correlates inversely with the MIC. The disk diffusion technique is easy to perform; however, strict guidelines must be followed in order to use the standard zone size interpretive chart worked out for each

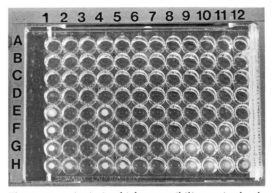

Figure 42–3. Antimicrobial susceptibility testing by the microdilution method. Each column of microwells contains serial twofold dilutions of an antimicrobial. The lowest concentration of drug that inhibits growth of the bacteria is defined as the MIC. For example, the first column contains ampicillin (32 µg/ml in well A1, decreasing to 0.25 µg/ml in well H1). The pellet of bacteria in the lower four wells (E1–H1) indicates that 4 µg/ml (well D1) is the MIC. Susceptibility to eleven other drugs has also been tested in this microwell plate.

drug. Any variation in technique changes the relationship between the zone size and the MIC, leading to misinterpretation of the test result.

Interpretations

In general, in vitro susceptibility testing is useful and reliably applied only to common, rapidly growing microorganisms such as staphylococci, enterococci, Enterobacteriaceae, and *Pseudomonas aeruginosa*. More fastidious bacteria are usually treated more reliably on the basis of published guidelines. A useful guide to empiric therapy is the tabulation of susceptibility trends that can be related to outbreaks of disease and to the use of antimicrobials in the region (see Appendix 13).

Susceptibility test results are a prediction of an expected response to therapy, not a guarantee. Most susceptibility tests use class-representative drugs rather than testing for each possible antibiotic. Furthermore, the interpretative criteria frequently applied to results are based on the average blood levels of antimicrobials that are expected to be achieved in people. Drug dosages and disposition may be significantly different in other species, ages, and body sizes. Levels of drug in tissues may significantly differ from levels in serum, such as low levels in CSF, or high concentrations in urine. Although in vitro susceptibility testing indi-

Table 42–2. Interpretation Categories for Microdilution Antimicrobial Susceptibility Tests

CATEGORY	DEFINITION
Susceptible	The microorganism is inhibited by levels of antimicrobial attained in blood or tissue with usual dosages, including oral administration
Moderately susceptible	The microorganism is inhibited only by blood levels achieved with maximum dosages, usually requiring IV administration with increased frequency (in some animals, these dosages may be toxic)
Resistant	The microorganism is resistant to achievable systemic concentrations of the antimicrobial; there still may be efficacy when the drug reaches high concentrations, such as in the urine, if the laboratory does not use the conditionally susceptible category
Conditionally susceptible	The microorganism can be inhibited only on the condition that the infection is in a site where antimicrobial concentrations that are considerably higher than blood levels, e.g., lower urinary tract infections, and topical therapy can be achieved

cates effectiveness, the drug may not be able to penetrate to the site of infection. Therefore, the predictive value of susceptibility tests for a favorable response is moderate at best. Their value in predicting failure is much better but is still not totally accurate. For example, an MIC result interpreted as resistant according to blood levels may not take into account that the organism was recovered from urine, where the drug is concentrated. Some agar diffusion tests use disks containing large amounts of antimicrobial that are applicable only to urinary tract infection.

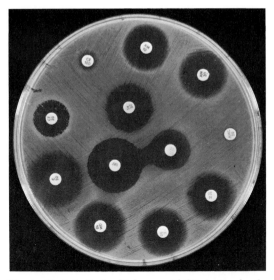

Figure 42–4. Antimicrobial susceptibility testing by the agar diffusion method, using disks containing antimicrobials. The diameter of the zone of inhibited microbial growth correlates inversely with the susceptibility of the microorganism.

SEROLOGIC TESTING

Detection of specific antibodies in the serum of an animal can be an indication of previous exposure, infection, vaccination, or passively acquired antibody. It is not always easy to discern the origin of these antibodies. Therefore, serology is most efficient as a diagnostic tool when the prevalence of antibodies in a population is low. Paired serum samples are also useful for interpreting the significance of serologic assays. The more common bacterial infections for which serologic tests are useful include leptospirosis (Chapter 45), Lyme disease (Chapter 46), and brucellosis (Chapter 52) (see also Appendix 8).

Reference

1. Jones RL: Clinical microbiology. *In* McCurnin DM (ed): *Clinical Textbook for Veterinary Technicians.* Philadelphia, WB Saunders Co, 1985, pp 110–147.

43

ANTIBACTERIAL CHEMOTHERAPY

Craig E. Greene
Duncan C. Ferguson

Antibacterials, among the most widely used drugs in veterinary practice, are commonly administered without adequate documentation that an infection exists. Although not harmful to the immediate needs of the patient, routine and irrational use of antimicrobials may cause several undesirable consequences for future use of that antibacterial. Unrestricted use encourages the selection of resistant strains of bacteria that subsequently limits the choice of effective agents. Long-term use of antimicrobials may suppress the animal's resident microflora, thereby allowing the overgrowth of more resistant microorganisms.

This chapter presents a review of the general properties of antibacterial drugs by pharmacologic groupings. It supplements the information on antibacterial drugs used in the dog and cat since the publication in 1984 of *Clinical Microbiology and Infectious Diseases of the Dog and Cat*. Because of space limitations and because that subject matter has changed marginally, discussion of general principles of antibacterial chemotherapy and reference information have been omitted here. Discussions of antibacterial resistance and prophylaxis are discussed in Chapter 1, and the use of antibacterial drugs in treating infections of various organ systems is covered in Chapters 44 through 61. Dosage charts are listed in each of these chapters, in addition to Appendix 14. Appendix 13 contains a list of appropriate antibacterial drugs for particular types and locations of infections.

PENICILLINS

Natural Penicillins

Penicillin G is a naturally occurring bactericidal antibiotic produced by the mold *Penicillium chrysogenum*. It primarily inhibits synthesis of the gram-positive bacterial cell wall, which contains peptidoglycans, and results in an osmotically fragile bacteria. Penicillin G, the parent molecule of the natural penicillins, has three significant therapeutic limitations: it is degraded by gastric acid, which reduces absorption via the oral route; it is inactivated by the enzyme β-lactamase (formerly penicillinase), which is produced by certain staphylococci and many gram-negative organisms; and at usual therapeutic dosages it is primarily used against gram-positive organisms (Table 43–1). Newer semisynthetic penicillins have been produced that have overcome the disadvantages of the parent compound.

Despite the production of newer derivatives, penicillin G is still the most active against gram-positive bacteria. Most streptococci, with the exception of enterococci, are susceptible. Many gram-positive bacilli and anaerobic bacteria with the exception of β-lactamase–producing *Bacteroides* spp. are susceptible. Staphylococci are usually resistant.

Penicillin V (phenoxymethyl penicillin) is an acid-stable derivative that is absorbed from the GI tract, although the resulting blood concentration is much lower than that

Table 43–1. Properties of Penicillins and β-Lactam Derivatives[a]

GENERIC NAME (TRADE NAME)	ROUTE OF ADMINISTRATION	ANTIMICROBIAL SPECTRUM					
		Gastric Acid Stability	β-Lactamase Resistance	Gram-Positive	Gram-Negative	Anaerobic	*Pseudomonas*
Natural Penicillins							
Penicillin G (many)	PO, IM, IV	−	−	+	−	+	−
Penicillin V (many)	PO	+	−	+	−	+	−
Phenethicillin (many)	PO	+	−	+	−	−	−
β-Lactamase-Resistant Penicillins							
Methicillin (Staphcillin, Celbenin)	IM, IV	−	+	+	−	−	−
Isoxazolyl Penicillins[b]							
Nafcillin (Unipen, Nafcil)	IM, IV	±	+	+	−	−	−
Cloxacillin (Tegopen)	PO	+	+	+	−	−	−
Dicloxacillin (Veracillin, Pathocil, Dynapen)	PO	+	+	+	−	−	−
Oxacillin (Prostaphylin, Bactocil)	PO, IM, IV	+	+	+	−	−	−
Aminopenicillins[c]							
Ampicillin (many)	PO, IM, IV	+	−	+	±	±	−
Amoxicillin (Omnipen)	PO, IM	+	−	+	±	±	−
Hetacillin (Hetacin)	PO	+	−	+	±	±	−
Extended Spectrum Carboxypenicillins[d]							
Carbenicillin (Pyopen, Geopen)	IM, IV	−	−	±	+	+	+
Ticarclllin (Ticar)	IM, IV	−	−	±	+	+	+
Ureidopenicillins[e]							
Mezlocillin (Mezlin)	IM, IV	−	−	+	+ +	±	+ +
Piperacillin (Pipracil, Pipral)	IM, IV	−	−	+	+ +	±	+ +
Amdinopenicillins							
Amdinocillin [mecillinam] (Coactin)	IM, IV	−	−	−	+ +	−	−
Pivamdinocillin[f]	PO	+	−	−	+ +	−	−
6-Methoxypenicillins							
Temocillin (TEM-30)	IM, IV	−	+	±	+ +	−	+
Other β-Lactams							
Aztreonam (Azactam)	IM, IV	−	+ +	−	+ +	−	+ +
Imipenem-cilastatin (Primaxin)	IV	−	+ +	+ +	+ +	+ +	+ +
β-Lactam Inhibitors							
Clavulanic acid [CA][f]	PO, IV	+	+ +	−	−	−	−
CA + amoxicillin (Clavulox, Clavamox, Augmentin)	PO	+	+ +	+ +	+	±	−
CA + Ticarcillin (Timentin)	IV	−	+ +	±	+	+	+
Sulbactam [SB][f]	IV	−	+ +	+	±	±	−
SB + ampicillin (Unasyn, Synergistin)	IV	−	+ +	+	+	+	+

[a]PO = oral, IM = intramuscular, IV = intravenous, − = none, + = good, + + = excellent, ± = variable. See Appendix 14 for dosages.
[b]Also includes flucloxacillin and floxacillin.
[c]Also includes bacampicillin (Spectrobid), cyclacillin (Cyclapen), epicillin, pivampicillin, and talampicillin.
[d]Also includes indamylcarbenicillin, carindacillin, and carfecillin.
[e]Also includes azlocillin (Azlin).
[f]Susceptibility studies indicate efficacy of inhibitor alone, although the drug is not available by itself.

produced following parenteral administration of the same dose of penicillin G. Therapeutic effects equivalent to those obtained with penicillin V may be achieved at less expense by giving oral penicillin G to fasting animals at four times the usual parenteral dosage.

β-Lactamase–Resistant Penicillins

Methicillin, the first semisynthetic penicillin developed, resists β-lactamase; how-ever, it is inactivated by gastric acid and has relatively low potency, both factors that limit its clinical usefulness. Newer isoxazolyl derivatives, which include nafcillin, cloxacillin, dicloxacillin, and oxacillin, are also β-lactamase resistant, and all except nafcillin can be administered orally with relatively good absorption from the GI tract.

Aminopenicillins

Ampicillin, amoxicillin, and hetacillin are susceptible to β-lactamase, but they can be given either orally or parenterally and have a wider spectrum of action against gram-negative organisms than do the previously discussed penicillin derivatives. Amoxicillin has an antibacterial spectrum identical with that of ampicillin but is absorbed better from the GI tract and has more rapid bactericidal activity and longer duration of action. Hetacillin is an inactive acetone derivative of ampicillin that is more stable in the presence of gastric acid and is broken down in the body into ampicillin. Bioavailability of orally administered ampicillin is also dependent on the dissolution and breakdown of a particular formulation prior to absorption. In cats 42% of the orally administered dose of anhydrous hard gelatin capsules is absorbed compared with 18% of the oral suspension.[1] Bacampicillin, pivampicillin, and talampicillin are similar derivatives. Cyclacillin is more β-lactamase resistant than the other compounds and produces higher serum and urine concentrations than ampicillin.

Carboxypenicillins

Newer members of the group, carbenicillin and ticarcillin, have increased activity against gram-negative bacteria, including *Pseudomonas* and some anaerobes. All carboxypenicillins are destroyed by β-lactamase and are less effective against gram-positive organisms. Ticarcillin has more activity against *Pseudomonas* than carbenicillin.[2] Because the minimum inhibitory concentrations (MICs) for these organisms are relatively high, large dosages of the drugs must be administered to be effective. The spectra and activities of these penicillins are increased synergistically when they are combined with aminoglycosides. They are not well absorbed when administered orally and so must be given parenterally.

Ureidopenicillins

Azlocillin, mezlocillin, and piperacillin have the widest antimicrobial activity in this class. Their acid instability and β-lactamase resistance is similar to that of the antipseudomonas penicillins; however, they have greater activity against gram-negative and *Pseudomonas* species, with less activity against some anaerobes. Antipseudomonal

activity of piperacillin is greater than that of any other penicillin derivative. It is also one of the few drugs that is consistently effective against *Bacteroides fragilis* and enterococci.

Amdinopenicillins

Amdinocillin (formerly mecillinam) is extremely active against gram-negative species but has poor gram-positive activity and is inactive against *Pseudomonas* and anaerobic bacteria. It acts synergistically with other penicillins but not with aminoglycosides. It is acid-unstable and cannot be given orally. However, an investigational ester, pivamdinocillin, is well absorbed and hydrolyzed, yielding active drug. It crosses the inflamed meninges better than ampicillin and is effective in treating gram-negative meningitis.

6-Methoxypenicillins

Temocillin is a 6-α-methoxy derivative of ticarcillin that is extremely resistant to β-lactamases. The drug has an increased efficacy against gram-positive and *Pseudomonas* species. Given parenterally, it has been used to treat soft tissue and urinary infections caused by susceptible gram-negative species. Studies in dogs have shown it to be safe, to have a wide distribution in body tissues, and to be primarily excreted in the urine.[2a]

Pharmacology

The absorption and the duration of activity of penicillins depend on the dosage administered, the vehicle in which the drug is contained, and the solubility of the salt formulation in which it is used. The inorganic potassium and sodium salts are soluble and can be given orally, IM, SC, IV, and topically, whereas insoluble trihydrate salts are less rapidly absorbed when administered by the oral, IM, or SC route. Soluble penicillin derivatives are absorbed from all serous and mucosal surfaces but not through unbroken skin. Food in the stomach can have a marked effect on the bioavailability of orally administered penicillins in dogs.[3] All penicillins are eliminated by the kidney through active renal tubular secretion. As a result, soluble salts of penicillin derivatives must be given at a minimum of 4-hour intervals to maintain serum concentrations at therapeutic levels. Probenecid was developed to inhibit this rapid elimination. Activity can also be prolonged by delaying release of these agents from a tissue depot by placing them in water-insoluble vehicles or combining them with organic salts. Examples are procaine penicillin and benzathine penicillin.

Penicillins are widely distributed into most body fluids and bone with the exception of the brain and CSF. Penicillins and aminopenicillins enter the CSF when the meninges are inflamed. Only the highly protein-bound isoxazolyl derivatives have difficulty in penetrating many body fluids. The dosage of penicillins may not have to be adjusted in patients with renal failure, despite their impaired excretion, because of the low toxicity of the drugs and the increased percentage of biliary secretion obtained with the semisynthetic derivatives. Potassium-containing penicillins should not be given IV to oliguric patients because of the risk of hyperkalemia.

Most aqueous solutions of penicillins are unstable, an effect that is accelerated at higher temperatures. They should be maintained at a pH between 5.5 and 7.5 and should not be added to solutions containing bicarbonate or other alkalinizing ingredients. Oral suspensions of penicillins must be kept refrigerated after reconstitution, and then they remain stable for only a week. IV solutions should be used within 24 hours of preparation. For example, aqueous sodium ampicillin for IV injections is not stable for more than 1 hour after reconstitution with water if it is not further diluted in IV fluids. If added to IV fluids for infusion, sodium ampicillin is stable for 24 hours. Therefore, portions of the reconstituted drug that are not used immediately should be discarded.

Parenteral penicillins such as carbenicillin are administered in high dosages by rapid periodic infusions of small volumes of fluid. Penicillins should never be mixed with blood, plasma, or other proteinaceous fluids or with other antibiotics prior to administration. They display in vivo antagonism with tetracycline and chloramphenicol; variable interactions with erythromycin, novobiocin, and lincomycin; no antagonism with sulfonamides; and possible synergism with aminoglycosides, cephalosporins, and polymyxins. As a matter of course, penicillins should not be mixed in the same syringe with aminoglycosides because of known inactivation of both drugs.

Toxicity

Toxic reactions are relatively rare with penicillin derivatives, which generally have a high therapeutic margin of safety. Rapid IV infusion may cause neurologic signs and convulsions.[4] Hypersensitivity reactions such as hives, fever, joint pain, and acute anaphylaxis have been noted immediately following administration to dogs and cats. Use of any penicillin derivatives should be avoided in known sensitized animals because of cross-reactivity.

Clinical bleeding, presumably caused by interference with coagulation factors, has been an important side effect in human patients treated with the antipseudomonas and extended spectrum penicillins and third generation cephalosporins.[5] Thrombocytopenia has been rare, and the bleeding has been attributed to various factors, including delayed fibrin polymerization, suppression of vitamin K–dependent procoagulants, and platelet dysfunction.

OTHER β-LACTAM DRUGS

Monobactams

Aztreonam and carumonam are the most clinically effective members of this monocyclic β-lactam group. Aztreonam is very resistant to β-lactamase and highly but exclusively effective against typically antibiotic-resistant, aerobic and facultative gram-negative bacteria, including most *P. aeruginosa*. It is not active against gram-positive or anaerobic bacteria. It is not absorbed after oral use, must be given parenterally, and is primarily excreted in the urine. It enters many body tissues and fluids of dogs, including the CSF.[5a] Adverse effects are minimal and include diarrhea and vomiting. Its primary use has been to treat serious gram-negative infections to resistant species such as *Escherichia coli, Klebsiella, Serratia,* and *Pseudomonas* in lungs, bone, blood, and urinary tract. It has been used safely and effectively in combination with clindamycin, erythromycin, metronidazole, penicillins, and vancomycin.[6] It may be indicated when a single parenteral drug is required for a urinary tract infection and resistance or toxicity to aminoglycosides is anticipated.

Carbapenems

This series of atypical β-lactams, the most important of which is a semisynthetic derivative known as N-formimidoyl thienamycin, or imipenem, has the widest spectrum of activity of any known antibiotic, partly owing to its β-lactamase resistance.[7] Imipenem has an antibacterial spectrum that includes gram-positive, gram-negative, and anaerobic bacteria. It is primarily indicated in the treatment of infections caused by cephalosporin-resistant members of the family Enterobacteriaceae. Typically resistant organisms such as P. aeruginosa, Serratia spp., Enterobacter spp., and gram-negative anaerobes are susceptible to its bactericidal activity. Little cross-resistance occurs with penicillins or cephalosporins. Emergence of resistant Pseudomonas isolates has occurred during the course of therapy. It appears to be nephrotoxic and is metabolized in the kidney, with minimal amounts appearing in the urine. Co-administration of a metabolic inhibitor of renal tubular enzymes such as cilastatin in an equal-dose ratio (imipenem-cilastatin) allows for obtaining urinary concentrations and eliminates the nephrotoxic effects. Parenteral administration is necessary since neither imipenem or cilastatin are absorbed orally. The dosage of the combination drug must be reduced in cases of renal failure. Adverse effects have included nausea, vomiting, diarrhea, phlebitis at the infusion site, fever, and seizures.

β-LACTAMASE INHIBITORS

Clavulanic Acid

Some naturally occurring β-lactam products, such as clavulanic acid, a β-lactamase inhibitor, have no antibacterial activity by themselves but irreversibly bind to and inactivate β-lactamase. Concurrent administration of drugs such as clavulanic acid increases the activity of penicillins and decreases the in vitro MIC required to inactivate many β-lactamase–producing organisms, such as staphylococci, E. coli, K. pneumoniae, some Proteus spp., Bacteroides fragilis, and Campylobacter.[8–10] Organisms

such as P. aeruginosa are still resistant. Clavulanate is rapidly absorbed, unaffected by food, and widely distributed in extravascular sites with the exception of the CNS. It is rapidly excreted, unchanged, in the urine. Uses include therapy of sinusitis; otitis media; and skin, lower respiratory tract, and soft tissue infections. The primary side effect with its use has been diarrhea, and as with amoxicillin and ampicillin, it may give a false-positive glucosuria result on screening with Clinitest (Ames Laboratories, Elkhart, IN).

An orally administered product consisting of amoxicillin combined with clavulanic acid is licensed for small animal use, as is a parenteral formulation of clavulanic acid with ticarcillin for human and equine use.[11] In vitro susceptibility testing has shown that isolates from dogs and cats that are usually sensitive to ticarcillin-clavulanic acid are Staphylococcus aureus, S. intermedius, Enterobacter aerogenes, E. agglomerans, Pasteurella multocida, Bordetella bronchiseptica, Proteus mirabilis, and Serratia spp.[11a] Following IV or IM administration to dogs, absorption and elimination of clavulanic acid is more rapid than that of ticarcillin.[11b] Dosages of 50 mg/kg of ticarcillin and 1.7 mg/kg of clavulanic acid should be effective for treating most resistant infections caused by members of the family Enterobacteriaceae, with the exception of pseudomonads. The oral formulation must be kept dry in foil wrappers because it absorbs moisture from the air and becomes inactivated. The amoxicillin-clavulanic acid combination has been shown to be effective in treating experimental E. coli cystitis[12,13] and staphylococcal skin infections[14] in dogs

Sulbactam

This drug, an irreversible β-lactamase inhibitor, resembles clavulanic acid, having weak antibacterial activity against most gram-positive and some gram-negative organisms, with best activity against Neisseria and Bacteroides. As with clavulanic acid, it acts synergistically with penicillins and cephalosporins, which are degraded by β-lactamases. It is primarily excreted in the urine. It is available as a sodium salt for parenteral use or in combination with ampicillin for oral use but is usually given parenterally because oral use has been associated with diarrhea. It has been used in conjunction with ampicillin to treat resistant bacterial meningitis in people[15] and intra-abdominal, pelvic, skin, soft tissue, bone, and joint infections.[16]

Investigational Inhibitors

Tazobactam is a triazolylmethyl penicillanic acid, β-lactamase inhibitor that is under development. The combination of tazobactam with piperacillin, in a 1:8 ratio has markedly improved the spectrum of piperacillin, and the efficacy is increased against many Enterobacteriaceae, S. aureus, and B. fragilis in vitro. TAIHO (YTR 830) is a β-lactamase inhibitor of the penicillinate-sulfone group and is one of the most potent drugs of this class. It has been shown to have similar potentiating effects on piperacillin when used in combination.

CEPHALOSPORINS

With the exception of cefoxitin, a cephamycin produced from an actinomycete, and moxalactam, a totally synthetic compound, the cephalosporins are a group of antibiotics composed of semisynthetic derivatives of 7-amino-cephalosporanic acid, which is produced by the fungus Cephalosporium acremonium. Like penicillins, cephalosporins are β-lactam antibiotics that are bactericidal, inhibiting synthesis of peptidoglycan in the bacterial cell wall. These drugs are generally more effective in penetrating the outer cell wall of gram-negative bacteria and are less susceptible to inactivation by β-lactamase–producing bacteria than are penicillins.[17]

Cephalosporins have been separated into three generations, or classes, based upon the chronology of discovery, chemical structure, and therapeutic activity. The characteristics of the classes are compared in Table 43–2 and clinically significant features of the most common cephalosporins are presented in Table 43–3.

First Generation

The first-generation cephalosporins are primarily active against gram-positive bacteria with the exception of some staphylococci and against some gram-negative bacteria, such as E. coli, Klebsiella, and P. mirabilis. This activity against both gram-positive and gram-negative bacteria exceeds that of penicillin G. They are relatively ineffective against Bacteroides. First-generation cephalosporins can be administered orally or parenterally, depending on the drug, and have variable protein binding with wide distribution into pleural, pericardial, peritoneal, and synovial fluids and most soft tissues. They enter the CSF only in the presence of meningeal inflammation. Most are excreted unchanged in the urine. Many cephalosporins interfere with glucose oxidase methods for determining urine glucose with test strips.

Two members of this group are of historic significance but are no longer used. Cephalothin is found in susceptibility disks; however, its use is limited because of pain and sterile abscesses produced on IM inoculation. Cephaloridine, initially licensed for veterinary use, produces similar complications, in addition to nephrotoxicity. It is the only first generation drug to reach high concentration in the CSF.

Cefadroxil has been marketed for veterinary use. It has a wide variety of uses in treating gram-negative urinary and gram-positive skin infections in dogs and skin and soft tissue infections in cats.[18] Both cefadroxil[19] and cephalexin[20–22] reach effective serum concentrations following oral dosing of dogs and cats. Approximately 25% less cephalexin is available when oral is compared with parenteral administration.[22]

Second Generation

Second-generation cephalosporins have a broader spectrum of antibacterial activity and greater efficacy against gram-negative bacteria and anaerobes than the first generation. They are slightly inferior to the first group but are equal to penicillin in their efficacy against gram-positive bacteria. They are more effective than the first-generation drugs against Proteus spp. other than P. mirabilis, Enterobacter, Citrobacter, and anaerobic bacteria. As with first-generation drugs, second- and third-generation cephalosporins are relatively ineffective against Bacteroides spp. Exceptions are cefoxitin, cefotetan, and moxalactam, which are effective against most obligate anaerobes. Cefoxitin is effective against Serratia and B. fra-

Table 43–2. Comparison of Antimicrobial Activity of Cephalosporins[a]

| GENERATION | BACTERIAL SUSCEPTIBILITY | | | | SELECTED SUSCEPTIBLE ORGANISMS |
	Gram-Positive	Gram-Negative	Anaerobes	β-Lactamase–Resistant	
First	+ + +	+	−	−	*Staphylococcus intermedius*
Second	+ +	+ +	+	+	*Proteus*
Third	±	+ + +	+ +	+ +	*Pseudomonas* sp. variable[b]

[a]+ + + = excellent, + + = very good, + good, ± = variable, − = poor. See Appendix 14 for dosages.
[b]See Table 43–3 for antipseudomonal efficacy of selected cephalosporins.

Table 43–3. Properties of Cephalosporins[a]

GENERIC NAME (TRADE NAME)	ROUTE OF ADMINISTRATION	COMMENTS
First Generation[b]		
Cephalexin (Keflex)	PO	Less active against staphylococci
Cefazolin (Ancef, Kefzol)	IV, IM	Achieves greatest serum concentration; longest half-life; most protein-bound; more active against *Escherichia coli, Klebsiella, Enterobacter*
Cephapirin (Cefadyl)	IV, IM	Resists β-lactamase; high dosages for serious life-threatening infections when causative organism shows susceptibility to first generation drugs
Cefadroxil (Duricef, Cefa-Tabs)	PO	Rapid and complete oral absorption even with food; enters prostate
Cephradine (Velosef, Anspor)	IV, IM, PO	Spectrum identical with that of cephalexin; less active against some gram-negative organisms
Second Generation[c]		
Cefaclor (Ceclor)	PO	Similar spectrum but more active than other oral derivatives; adequate soft tissue concentrations; minor amount excreted in urine unchanged
Cefoxitin (Mefoxin)	IV, IM	Pain on IM injection; activity against *Bacteroides fragilis* and *Serratia; Clostridium difficile* resistant; effective against anaerobes
Cefamandole (Mandol)	IV, IM	Wide distribution in tissues, bile, synovia; high activity against *E. coli, Klebsiella, Enterobacter, Hemophilus, Proteus, Salmonella, Shigella*
Third Generation[d]		
Cefotaxime (Claforan)	IV	Activity against gram-negative organisms except *Pseudomonas*; metabolized in liver to active drug
Moxalactam (Moxam)	IV, IM	Primarily renal excretion; active against many gram-negative organisms that resist aminoglycosides, i.e., *Proteus, Serratia, Enterobacter,* and some *Pseudomonas*; gram-positive organisms resistant; most active against anaerobes
Antipseudomonal Third Generation[e]		
Ceftazidime (Fortaz)	IV	Primarily active against gram-negative organisms and *Pseudomonas*
Cefoperazone (Cefobid)	IV	Less active against gram-positive and -negative organisms except *Pseudomonas*; can produce vitamin K deficiency

[a]Technically, cefoxitin and cefotetan are cephamycins, and moxalactam is an oxacephem, but they are included here. PO = oral, IV = intravenous, IM = intramuscular. See Appendix 14 for appropriate dosages.
[b]Also includes cephaloglycin, cephalothin, cephaloridine.
[c]Also includes cefotiam, cefuroxime (Zinacef, Kefurox), ceforanide, cefmetazole, cefonicid (Monocid).
[d]Also includes ceftriaxone (Rocephin), ceftizoxime (Cefizox), flomoxef, ceftibuten, cefmenoxime, cefotetan (Cefotan), cefbuperazone (Cefobid), ceftiofur (Naxcel).
[e]Also includes cefsulodin, cefpiramide.

gilis. Cefamandole, which works against Salmonella and Shigella, has been recommended as a substitute for gentamicin in treating bowel-related infections because gentamicin alone is not effective against anaerobic bacteria. Most are given parenterally, with the exception of cefaclor and a derivative, cefuroxime axetil (ceftin), an orally administered pro-drug of cefuroxime with the same spectrum of activity as the parent drug.

Third Generation

The relatively new third-generation cephalosporins have a longer duration of activity than drugs in the other two classes. Excretion in either the urine or the bile is variable, depending on the drug, although most undergo some inactivation and excretion by the liver. Up to 80% of cefoperazone is excreted in the bile. Third-generation drugs, with the exception of moxalactam, ceftriaxone, and cefotaxime, do not penetrate the CSF under most circumstances. Third-generation cephalosporins have marked activity against anaerobic and aerobic gram-negative organisms and minimal effect on aerobic gram-positive organisms. Unlike other cephalosporins, cefoperazone, moxalactam, and cefotaxime are somewhat effective against P. aeruginosa. Ceftazidime is uniquely extremely active against P. aeruginosa. However, third-generation cephalosporins are not as effective against Pseudomonas as the newer extended spectrum penicillins. Third-generation cephalosporins have been recommended for use in septicemia, bacteremia, intra-abdominal infections, and endocarditis when they are given IV. Because of the extremely broad spectrum of activity, third-generation drugs such as ceftazidime have been used alone or in combination in human patients with neutropenia and fever of unknown origin with suspected bacteremia.[23] Second- and third-generation drugs have had good efficacy against drug-resistant salmonellae isolated from people.[24] Ceftriaxone has been found to be effective in the treatment of chronic resistant meningitis or arthritis with Lyme borreliosis (see Therapy, Chapter 46). Cefotaxime has been shown to be effective as a substitute for penicillin in treating human leptospirosis.[2] Both an aqueous[25] and a slow-release oil suspension[26] of this drug have been found to be bioavailable and produce sufficient plasma concentrations in dogs. Aqueous preparations have been similarly effective in cats.[27]

Indications

The varied indications for use of cephalosporins include treatment of bacterial infections of the respiratory, urinary, and genital tracts, soft tissues, bones and joints, and skin. Cephalosporins are effective when given prophylactically for polymicrobial intra-abdominal infections following bowel surgery. In addition, they have also been recommended for both prophylactic use in biliary tract surgery and for treating biliary tract infection, because many are excreted in the bile unchanged. However, they do not enter the biliary tract when complete biliary obstruction and jaundice are present. Cefotaxime, moxalactam, and some other third-generation cephalosporins effectively enter the blood-CSF barrier and are very effective in the treatment of meningitis caused by drug-resistant bacteria.

Most orally used cephalosporins in small animal practice are first-generation drugs that are expensive when compared with other antibiotics. Second- and third-generation cephalosporins are available only for parenteral use. Presently, their cost is somewhat prohibitive for general use in veterinary practice. The newer generation of parenteral cephalosporins are reserved for treating severe infections and should be mixed with isotonic saline or dextrose for IV administration. Such formulations should be used within 24 hours after reconstitution. Continuous peritoneal lavage with moxalactam has been shown to produce effective intraperitoneal and sustained serum concentrations in dogs treated for peritonitis.[27a] Following parenteral administration, moxalactam also enters the peritoneal cavity in high concentrations in dogs with peritonitis.[27b]

Toxicity

The toxicity of cephalosporins is minimal compared with that of other antibiotics; and in this regard, the cephalosporins are similar to the penicillin derivatives. Allergic skin reactions have been reported with the use of cephalexin for skin infection in a dog.[28] Cephaloridine has been shown to be nephrotoxic, but this feature is not characteristic of the newer drugs. Because most cephalosporins are excreted by the kidney, their concentrations are increased and their half-lives are prolonged in cases of renal failure, or when probenecid, loop diuretics, or aminoglycosides are used. All parenteral formulations of cephalosporins may cause phlebitis and myositis following IV and IM administration, respectively. GI irritation may cause vomiting and diarrhea when oral formulations are used. As mentioned under penicillins, bleeding disorders in people have been associated with the use of third-generation cephalosporins, specifically moxalactam.[29,30] Cephalosporin-induced blood dyscrasias, as a result of immune-mediated destruction of blood cells and direct bone marrow toxicity, have been produced in dogs given high-dose, long-term cephalosporins.[30a] A dramatic reversal of myelosuppression occurs when therapy is withdrawn.

AMINOGLYCOSIDES

These bactericidal antibiotics interfere with the synthesis of bacterial protein. They are relatively small, primarily basic, water-soluble molecules that are active against certain gram-negative and gram-positive bacteria and mycobacteria. They are generally effective against aerobic gram-negative bacilli such as *E. coli*, *Klebsiella*, *Proteus*, and *Enterobacter*, and some are effective against *P. aeruginosa*. Aminoglycosides are not active against fungi or anaerobic bacteria and should not be used to treat abscesses or granulomatous infections. When used alone, they are relatively ineffective against streptococci but are effective against *Staphylococcus intermedius*. The properties and indications for use of various aminoglycosides are summarized in Table 43–4.

Dihydrostreptomycin, streptomycin, neomycin, and kanamycin have been extensively used for many years. However, with such frequent use, extensive bacterial resistance has developed. Amikacin and gentamicin are more effective and routinely used. Tobramycin, netilmicin, and dibekacin are newer drugs that have been used clinically to treat infections in people. Sisomicin, framycetin, isepamicin, and dactimicin are newer aminoglycosides being evaluated for clinical use. Isepamicin is a derivative of

gentamicin. Dactimicin is a new pseudodisaccharide aminoglycoside. Both of these have broad spectrum activity against gram-positive and gram-negative organisms.

Pharmacology

The pharmacokinetics of many of the aminoglycosides have been studied in dogs[31] and cats.[32–35a] Aminoglycosides are poorly absorbed from the GI tract and must be administered parenterally to achieve therapeutic serum concentrations; however, some are administered orally for the local treatment of bacterial enteritis. They are poorly absorbed through intact skin, although they may cross damaged squamous or mucosal epithelium. Topical aminoglycoside creams and solutions have been shown to be of benefit in controlling bacterial growth and facilitating the healing of open wounds.[36] They are rapidly absorbed following IM or SC administration. They are minimally bound to plasma proteins but penetrate little beyond the extracellular fluid spaces, including the synovial, peritoneal, and pleural spaces. Following IV administration, they enter surgical wounds for a time that parallels their serum concentration.[36a] Because of their lipid insolubility, they are minimally excreted in the bile and the feces, and diffuse poorly into the CNS, prostate, amniotic fluid, and the eye. Concentrations in these latter tissues remain inadequate even in the presence of inflammation. All aminoglycosides are rapidly excreted unchanged in the urine. The pH at which optimal antibacterial activity occurs is 7.5 to 8.0. Streptomycin may produce spuriously high results with measurements of urine glucose by strips, using the oxidase method. Aminoglycosides such as gentamicin have been shown to be effective in treating bronchopulmonary infections when given to dogs by the aerosol route. Concentration of drug in the airway lumen is maximal. Toxicity is minimized because of the lack of absorption from this site.

Bacteria are prone to develop resistance to aminoglycosides by one of three mechanisms. These are alteration of the receptor sites on bacterial ribosomes, decreased bacterial cell penetrability, and plasmid-associated production of enzymes that inactivate

Table 43–4. Properties of Aminoglycosides[a]

GENERIC NAME (TRADE NAME)	ROUTE OF ADMINISTRATION	COMMENTS
Streptomycin (many)	IM	PO rarely used for enteric pathogens; occasionally for bacteremias, *Brucella canis*; clears *Leptospira* carriers
Dihydrostreptomycin (many)	IM	Identical with those for streptomycin; many resistant strains
Neomycin (Biosol, Mycifradin)	PO	PO for local GI effect; topical use as irrigating preparation; spectrum similar to that of kanamycin; absorbed and toxic if bowel wall is damaged
Kanamycin (Kantrim, Kantrex, Klebcil)	PO, IM	PO for local GI effect; useful in urinary tract, superficial, and systemic infections; spectrum similar to that of gentamicin, but resistant strains much more common; effective for staphylococci
Gentamicin (Gentocin, Garamycin, Apogen, Bristagen, U-Gencin)	IM, IV, aerosol, topical	Bacteremia; respiratory (aerosol) infections caused by *E. coli*, *Pasteurella*, *Pseudomonas*, *Proteus*, staphylococci, *Enterobacter*, *Serratia*, *Klebsiella*, *Bordetella* (aerosol)
Paromomycin (Humatin)	PO	PO for local GI effect; used for susceptible staphylococci, *E. coli*, *Salmonella*, and protozoa (*Entamoeba* and *Balantidium*)
Tobramycin (Nebcin)	IM	Gram-negative spectrum similar to that of gentamicin; effective against some strains of *Pseudomonas* that are resistant to gentamicin and is less nephrotoxic
Amikacin (Amikin, Amiglyde)	IM	Widest antibacterial spectrum among currently used aminoglycosides; effective against *Pseudomonas* and many gram-negative bacilli that are resistant to gentamicin and tobramycin (e.g., *Klebsiella*)
Sisomicin (Sisomin)	IM	More active than gentamicin against many bacteria, especially *Pseudomonas* and *E. coli*; not effective against organisms resistant to gentamicin, toxicity parallels gentamicin
Netilmicin (Netromycin)	IM	Staphylococci highly susceptible; active against some organisms resistant to gentamicin; more active than sisomicin or tobramycin; slightly less active than amikacin against *Pseudomonas*; less toxic than tobramycin
Framycetin (Sulframycin, Neomycin B)	PO, topical	Gram-negative spectrum; effective in presence of pus, serum, blood, and debris
Dactinomycin[b]	SC	Intra-abdominal infections; wide activity against gram-positive and gram-negative organisms when combined with anaerobic drug, metronidazole; most active against *Acinetobacter* and staphylococci
Isepamicin[b]	IV	Exceptional activity against Enterobacteriaceae and *Pseudomonas*

[a]IM = intramuscular, PO = oral, IV = intravenous. See Appendix 14 for appropriate dosages.
[b]Not available commercially.

the drugs. Bacterial resistance to aminoglycosides is greater with the older drugs and is less with the newer compounds. Cross-resistance is not uniform among all members of the class. For example, although many *K. pneumoniae* are resistant to kanamycin and gentamicin, they are susceptible to amikacin, a semisynthetic derivative of kanamycin.[37] In general, there is a high degree of cross-resistance between gentamicin and other aminoglycosides, except for amikacin and tobramycin.[38]

Toxicity

Toxicities with aminoglycoside antibiotics are relatively common and are a result of the individual drug used, dosage, duration of therapy, state of patient hydration, presence of upper urinary tract infection, and pretreatment renal function.[39,40] In decreasing order of nephrotoxicity are neomycin, gentamicin, tobramycin, kanamycin, amikacin, and streptomycin. Nephrotoxicity has been associated with trough serum concentration greater than 2.0 μg/ml (5.0 μg/ml for amikacin).[41] Frequent administration of small doses to maintain serum aminoglycoside concentrations is more toxic than less frequent usage of larger dosages.[42-44] Frequent (three to four times daily) dosing has been recommended for treatment of systemic infections in animals, although renal function must be closely monitored with such protocols. In contrast, pulse administration of large (10 mg/kg) IM doses of gentamicin at 5-day intervals has been shown to maintain effective tissue concentrations in dogs.[45] The pulse administration should be less nephrotoxic than more frequent dosing because the serum concentrations decrease sufficiently during the longer treatment period; however, documentation of the clinical efficacy of such regimens is lacking. Use of aminoglycosides should be avoided in puppies and kittens because they are more prone to develop renal failure than older animals. Renal proximal tubular dysfunction is the most common and serious side effect of administration of most aminoglycosides. The earliest method of predicting and monitoring tubular dysfunction is to examine the urine for casts, which appear to be more sensitive indicators than BUN or creatinine concentration. Although still clinically impractical research tools, the most sensitive way to detect aminoglycoside toxicity in dogs and cats is to measure urinary concentrating ability and urinary enzyme activities.[46,47,47a] Acute renal failure typically develops several days after therapy is initiated and may develop several days after the drug is discontinued. Once it develops, the prognosis for recovery from renal failure is very poor in dogs and cats.[39]

Clinical reports from human hospitals have noted increased nephrotoxicity when the aminoglycosides are given with cephalosporins. However, studies in rats indicate that the combination may actually be protective. Similarly, combinations of piperacillin with gentamicin or cephaloridine have been shown to have reduced nephrotoxicity.[47b] Furosemide may enhance both the nephrotoxicity and the ototoxicity of aminoglycosides.[48] Toxicity is thought to result from reduced extracellular fluid volume with decreased excretion and increased serum concentration. Other diuretics may have similar adverse effects and should be avoided in combination with aminoglycosides. Cats and dogs should be well hydrated whenever aminoglycoside therapy is instituted.

Gentamicin-impregnated methymethacrylate beads have been implanted in the joints of a dog with septic arthritis.[48a] Local release of the drug into the surrounding tissues and synovial fluid allowed for long-term therapy, an effective cure, and no side effects.

Ototoxicity has been a problem with aminoglycoside therapy; both vestibular and auditory impairment from damage to the sensory end-organs have been reported. Aminoglycosides also can cause ototoxicity when they are directly instilled into the external ear canal of dogs and cats, especially if the tympanic membrane has been ruptured.[49] Table 43–5 is a summary of relative otic and renal toxicities of the aminoglycosides for dogs and cats.[49a,50] In cats the comparative ototoxicity between drugs in decreasing order was determined to be gentamicin, tobramycin, and netilmicin, with vestibular more likely than cochlear damage.[50]

Aminoglycosides may produce neuromuscular blockade by competitive antagonism of acetylcholine at the myoneural junction. In addition to their own neuromuscular-blocking effects, they enhance the actions of other neuromuscular-blocking agents and general anesthetics. Therefore, irrigation of body cavities or parenteral administration of aminoglycosides should be avoided during surgery requiring general anesthesia.

Circulatory depression, manifest by decreased systemic blood pressure and heart rate, has been found in cats, dogs, and nonhuman primates given aminoglycosides during pentobarbital anesthesia. Neomycin, streptomycin, kanamycin, gentamicin, and dihydrostreptomycin have all been shown

Table 43–5. Relative Toxicity of Aminoglycosides[a]

DRUG	KIDNEY	VESTIB-ULAR	AUDITORY
Streptomycin	−	+	−
Dihydrostreptomycin	?	−	+
Neomycin	+	+	+
Gentamicin	+	+	−
Kanamycin	+	−	+
Tobramycin	+	+	+
Amikacin	+	−	+
Netilmicin	±	±	±

Adapted from data from Conzelman GM: *J Am Vet Med Assoc* 176:1078–1080, 1980; McCormick GC et al: *Toxicol Appl Pharmacol* 77:478–489, 1985.

[a] + = lesions have been detected, ± = milder lesions than +, − = lesions have not been detected, ? = information concerning lesions is lacking.

See Appendix 14 for appropriate dosages.

to decrease cardiac output and to produce hypotension and bradycardia. Cardiac arrest has been reported in humans receiving overdoses of kanamycin. If possible, aminoglycoside administration should be avoided in pregnant animals or in those in shock or with cardiovascular insufficiency. Calcium gluconate can be given IV to reverse aminoglycoside-induced neuromuscular blockade or myocardial depression and to restore blood pressure.

Prolonged high oral dosages of neomycin or paromomycin may produce diarrhea and malabsorption owing to selective overgrowth of resistant indigenous intestinal flora. Although rare, hypersensitivity and allergic reactions have been reported in humans receiving aminoglycosides. Aminoglycosides should not be administered to pregnant animals because these drugs can cross the placenta and may produce fetal intoxication. Penicillins and aminoglycosides should never be mixed in the same solution prior to administration. Depending on the type and concentration of penicillin used, mixing can cause direct inactivation of the aminoglycoside.

SPECTINOMYCIN

Aminocyclitol antibiotics, composed of a basic cyclic structure with an amino group, include spectinomycin and the aminoglycosides. Being structurally related, spectinomycin shares many properties with the aminoglycosides, including minimal binding to plasma proteins, high water solubility, poor GI absorption, primary renal excretion, and optimal activity at a pH of 8. Spectinomycin is also similar to aminoglycosides in that it inhibits protein synthesis by bacterial ribosomes.

Spectinomycin is a broad-spectrum antibiotic effective against gram-negative bacteria such as E. coli, Klebsiella, Salmonella, Enterobacter, and Proteus and gram-positive organisms, including streptococci and staphylococci, as well as against mycoplasmas. It has low efficacy against obligate anaerobes, most pseudomonads, and chlamydiae. Parenteral administration of spectinomycin is advantageous for treatment of bacteremia associated with infectious gastroenteritis caused by susceptible enteropathogenic bacteria and for treatment of intra-abdominal sepsis (see Intra-abdominal Infections, Chapter 9). As with some of the aminoglycosides, development of resistant bacteria is a problem with spectinomycin. Its use in humans is currently limited to the treatment of Neisseria gonorrhoeae infections.

Combinations of aminocyclitols with other antibiotics may be antagonistic or synergistic. Antagonism is primarily restricted to use with chloramphenicol or tetracycline. Spectinomycin combined with lincomycin is thought to be effective against mycoplasmal infections. Penetration of spectinomycin into intraocular tissue is minimal, and it enters meningeal tissue and CSF only in the presence of inflammation.

The advantage of spectinomycin is that its toxicity is lower than that of the aminoglycosides. It is neither ototoxic nor nephrotoxic and can be used in some patients with impaired renal function. Neuromuscular blockade is a rare side effect that occurs with both spectinomycin and the aminoglycosides.

GLYCOPEPTIDES

Vancomycin

This narrow-spectrum bactericidal antibiotic acts on replicating organisms by inhibiting the biosynthesis of cell wall phospholipids and peptidoglycan polymers. It also inhibits the synthesis of RNA and alters the cytoplasmic membranes.

Vancomycin is a complex, soluble glycopeptide that is approximately 10% bound to plasma proteins. It diffuses well into body cavities and across inflamed meninges. Excretion occurs almost exclusively by the kidneys, with minimal amounts entering the bile.

Vancomycin is primarily active against gram-positive organisms and few gram-negative cocci, such as Neisseria, and against some protozoa, such as amoebae. Gram-positive cocci such as S. aureus, S. intermedius, S. epidermidis, Streptococcus pyogenes, and S. pneumoniae are highly susceptible to this antibiotic. Microaerophilic streptococci, Clostridium sp., Bacillus anthracis, Actinomyces sp., Corynebacterium diphtheriae, and N. gonorrhoeae are usually susceptible. Vancomycin is not effective against gram-negative bacilli, mycobacteria, or fungi. Resistance rarely develops during therapy, and there is no cross-resistance with other antibiotics. Vancomycin has been the drug of choice in treating people with pseudomembranous enterocolitis caused by overgrowth of enteric *Clostridium difficile* due to antimicrobial therapy.[51] It is also important in the treatment of infections caused by methicillin-resistant staphylococci.

Absorption from the GI tract is poor, so vancomycin must be given IV for systemic infections. The IM route is less desirable because the drug produces pain at the site of injection. Vancomycin may be administered orally in treating susceptible enteric pathogens. It is incompatible with many other drugs, including chloramphenicol, glucocorticoids, and methicillin, when given in IV solutions.

The most frequent side effects of vancomycin therapy in people have been fever, chills, and phlebitis at the site of injection. These can be reduced if the drug is administered slowly in a large volume of fluid. Leukopenia and eosinopenia have been reported. Nephrotoxicity, characterized by the presence of hematuria, proteinuria, urinary casts, and azotemia, has been an infrequent and usually mild complication. The most important adverse reaction is damage to auditory function. The use of vancomycin has been limited in veterinary medicine.

Teicoplanin

This complex glycopeptide under investigational use is similar in structure to vancomycin. It is primarily active against aerobic and some anaerobic gram-positive organisms. In contrast to vancomycin, teicoplanin is 90% protein-bound and lipophilic. Its half-life in plasma is much longer and may allow administration only once daily. It has a greater affinity for the microbial cell compared with albumin, which explains its relative efficacy despite its high degree of protein binding.

Orienticins

These glycopeptides are similar in activity to vancomycin. They are active against gram-positive aerobic and anaerobic organisms. Staphylococci, streptococci, and clostridia are susceptible.

POLYMYXINS

These closely related, cationic, branched decapeptides are elaborated by strains of *Bacillus polymyxa*. Of the types A through E, polymyxin B and polymyxin E (colistin) are therapeutically most important. Polymyxins appear to exert their effects as cationic detergents, disrupting the lipophilic fraction, and hence the cytoplasmic membrane, of gram-negative bacteria. This process is synergistic with complement but is inhibited by calcium. Administration of these drugs prior to infusion of gram-negative endotoxin has been effective in protecting experimental animals. Most gram-negative organisms, such as *Pasteurella*, *Shigella*, *Salmonella*, *Bordetella*, and some *Klebsiella* and *Pseudomonas*, are susceptible, whereas *Brucella* and *Proteus* are frequently resistant. Resistance is also a factor of increased usage, and although emergent strains develop during usage, they revert to being susceptible once polymyxin therapy is stopped.[52]

Polymyxins are poorly absorbed when given orally and topically. They do not produce high blood concentrations following parenteral administration, presumably because of their affinity for host cell membranes. They are primarily excreted in the urine.

These drugs are used chiefly as topical preparations for treating localized infections in the ear canal, eye, bowel, and urinary tract. Respiratory therapy may be achieved by means of nebulization. Intrathecal administration has been performed with aqueous preparations; however, they are highly irritating. Polymyxins have been combined with neomycin and bacitracin or tetracycline to broaden the antibacterial spectrum.

Polymyxins have been given systemically to treat infections that are resistant to aminoglycosides and as such have shown some synergism with trimethoprim. Methane sulfonate colistin (sodium colistimethate) is the least toxic parenteral preparation. The major side effect of the polymyxins is nephrotoxicity, although pain at the injection site, CNS signs, and neuromuscular blockade have also been noted.

CHLORAMPHENICOL

Chloramphenicol is a highly lipid-soluble, broad-spectrum antibiotic that is predominantly bacteriostatic and inhibits protein synthesis. It is effective against a variety of pathogens, including mycoplasmas, rickettsiae, *Bacteroides*, staphylococci, salmonellae, *Pasteurella*, *Bordetella*, *Hemophilus*, enteric coliforms, and *Chlamydia*. Chloramphenicol can be administered orally or parenterally, and absorption is unimpeded by food. Less than 50% of the drug is bound to plasma protein. In dogs, approximately 90% of the drug is metabolized by the liver to an inactive metabolite that is excreted in the urine. A trace amount of the metabolite is excreted in the bile, where it undergoes enterohepatic circulation. The remaining 10% of active drug is primarily excreted unchanged in the urine. In cats and neonatal dogs, metabolism differs, and approximately 25% of the active drug is excreted in the urine.[53] The concentration of active chloramphenicol in the urine is usually sufficient to be effective against susceptible bacteria. Optimal activity occurs at a pH of 7.5 to 8.0. Chloramphenicol in urine may cause a spuriously positive test result for glucose when glucose oxidase strips are used.

Administration

Chloramphenicol is available in a variety of forms, and that used depends on the route of administration selected. The drug is usually given orally in capsular form but can be bitter tasting, causing salivation and anorexia if the capsules are not swallowed intact. As an oral suspension, chloramphenicol palmitate must be flavored because of its bitter taste. Since the palmitate form of the drug requires hydrolysis by digestive enzymes before absorption can occur, therapeutic serum concentrations are reached slowly. The bioavailability of the palmitate ester is low in cats, so capsules should be used in that species.[54] Chloramphenicol sodium succinate, a water soluble ester, is recommended for parenteral use. It can be given IV, SC, or IM, but because it offers no advantage over IV or SC administration and requires frequent injection, the IM route is not routinely recommended. In contrast to conflicting reports in the human and veterinary literature, it appears to be well absorbed

after IM administration.[55] Otic, ophthalmic, and topical preparations are also available.

Pharmacology

Chloramphenicol diffuses rapidly and well into most tissues. Highest concentrations are found in the liver, kidney, bile, spleen, lung, pancreas, and urine. The drug penetrates into pleural, ascitic, and synovial fluids, saliva, aqueous and vitreous humors, milk, prostatic fluid, CSF, and amniotic fluid.[56]

Chloramphenicol ranks second only to sulfanilamide in its ability to diffuse into CSF. It takes several hours for brain tissue concentration to approximate that of blood concentrations; however, brain tissue concentration remains adequate for up to 12 hours, although blood concentration diminishes before that time. Chloramphenicol penetration into CSF is also relatively high and is not affected by inflammation or simultaneous glucocorticoid therapy.

Because it is minimally excreted by the kidneys, no change in the dosage of chloramphenicol is necessary in patients with subclinical renal failure. Chloramphenicol is considered useful in the treatment of urinary tract infections in dogs with subnormal renal function. A 10% decrease in dosage is recommended if uremia is present because of the catabolic effects of the drug on protein metabolism.

Indications

Chloramphenicol is effective against most aerobic and anaerobic bacteria as well as many respiratory pathogens in dogs and cats. It is the preferred antibiotic for treating *Salmonella* and *E. coli* infections in the GI tract and has been recommended for prophylactic use prior to intestinal surgery or dental prophylaxis. Staphylococcal infections, commonly associated with prolonged soft tissue and orthopedic surgeries, can be prevented by the prior administration of chloramphenicol (see Antimicrobial Prophylaxis, Chapter 1).

Chloramphenicol penetrates the cornea well because it is lipid soluble and has a low molecular weight. Systemic administration is required for the treatment of intraocular and orbital infections and deep corneal lesions.

Toxicity

The most frequent side effect of chloramphenicol administration in dogs and cats is GI irritation, which is manifested by depression, anorexia, dysphagia, salivation, nausea, vomiting, and sporadic diarrhea. Blood dyscrasias and severe irreversible pancytopenia have been reported in humans. The pancytopenia is idiosyncratic and not dose related. However, only reversible bone marrow suppression has been demonstrated in dogs and cats when erythropoiesis and myelopoiesis are variably suppressed.

Nonregenerative anemia has primarily been noted in dogs with pre-existing or concurrent blood loss or hemolysis at the time chloramphenicol therapy was instituted. The anemia is apparently caused by the inhibition of ferrochelatase, an enzyme important in hemoglobin synthesis. Regeneration is evident once chloramphenicol therapy is discontinued. Morphologic bone marrow effects are not routinely found in treated dogs.

Chloramphenicol is more toxic to cats than to dogs, perhaps because of the cat's inability to conjugate glucuronic acid, which is an important step in elimination of chloramphenicol in other species. Bone marrow changes in cats after 1 week of therapy, (50 mg/kg, given every 12 hours) include hypocellularity, decreased mitotic activity, erythroid maturation arrest, and vacuolation of precursor cells and lymphocytes.[57] After 3 weeks of therapy, neutropenia, lymphopenia, nonregenerative anemia, and thrombocytopenia are seen. Anorexia, mental depression, and dehydration also occur. Toxic changes do not develop if cats are given the drug on an intermittent basis or a lower dosage regimen. Clinical improvement and resolution of hematologic changes usually occur within several days after cessation of therapy. A normal hemogram does not rule out toxicosis, as bone marrow changes precede those in peripheral blood.

The public health hazard associated with inadvertent contact with small amounts of chloramphenicol has limited its use in food-producing species and may increase the veterinarian's liability to owners handling the drug intended for their pets. Thiamphenicol, an analog of chloramphenicol, has been widely used in European countries as a subsitute. It has similar antibacterial properties, enhanced renal excretion of active drug, and a low frequency of complications of aplastic anemia in people.

Because of its potent effects on cellular protein synthesis, there are many potential contraindications to the use of chloramphenicol. It should not be given to a pregnant animal because the fetus is unable to metabolize it, nor should it be used in animals with impaired liver function. The drug should not be administered to cardiac patients because of myocardial depression associated with its use. Theoretically, chloramphenicol should not be used in conjunction with active immunization or in treating extensive wounds because it interferes with immunoglobulin and protein synthesis, respectively. No interference could be found in puppies vaccinated for canine distemper when chloramphenicol was given simultaneously.[58] Because it has been shown to decrease gonadal activity, it should be avoided in breeding animals. By interfering with hepatic biotransformation, chloramphenicol can potentiate or prolong the action of drugs such as diphenylhydantoin, phenobarbital, primidone, digoxin, warfarin, cyclophosphamide, salicylates, and inhalation anesthetics.[59] This interaction has even been noted when chloramphenicol ophthalmic preparations were used.[60] As a bacterial protein synthesis inhibitor, it may also interfere with the action of the concurrently administered bactericidal drugs, penicillins and aminoglycosides.

TETRACYCLINES

Tetracycline antibiotics are bacteriostatic and interfere with protein synthesis of bacterial RNA. As a group, they have a broad spectrum of activity that includes certain aerobic and anaerobic gram-positive and gram-negative bacteria, spirochetes, mycoplasmas, rickettsiae, chlamydiae, and some protozoa (Table 43–6). The second-generation lipid-soluble tetracyclines, doxycycline and minocycline, are more active against anaerobes and several facultative intracellular bacteria like *Brucella canis* than are other tetracyclines. Minocycline is more active in vitro against *Nocardia* and staphylococci that are resistant to the other tetracyclines. Tetracycline has potential benefit for treatment of canine urinary tract infections caused by *P. aeruginosa*.[61]

Table 43–6. Properties of Tetracyclines[a]

GENERIC NAME (TRADE NAME)	ROUTE OF ADMINISTRATION	COMMENTS AND SPECIFIC INDICATIONS
Short-Acting, Water Soluble		
Tetracycline (Panmycin, Achromycin, Tetracyn)	PO, IV, IM	Therapeutic or prophylactic use for *Ehrlichia canis*; IM injections painful; do not inject intra-articularly
Oxytetracycline (Terramycin)	PO, IV, IM	Reaches high concentration in lung, liver, kidney, and mononuclear phagocyte system; better tolerated orally by cats
Chlortetracycline (Aureomycin)	PO	pH is very important for activity
Intermediate-Acting[b]		
Demeclocycline[c] (Declomycin)	PO	Photosensitivity may occur; dosage-dependent diabetes insipidus
Long-Acting, Lipid Soluble		
Minocycline (Minocin, Vectrin)	PO, IV	More effective against *E. canis*, *Babesia canis*; greater activity against *Nocardia*, *Staphylococcus aureus*, and anaerobes; wide distribution in tissues
Doxycycline (Vibramycin, Doxychel)	PO, IV	Same as for minocycline; tetracycline of choice for extrarenal infections in renal failure patients; more active against *Bacteroides fragilis*; prophylaxis for bowel surgery; used to treat chronic prostatitis

[a]PO = oral, IV = intravenous, IM = intramuscular.
[b]Also includes methacycline.
[c]Formerly demethylchlortetracycline.
See Appendix 14 for appropriate dosages.

Pharmacology

The tetracyclines vary markedly in their lipid solubility, a factor that determines their relative GI absorption; degree of protein binding; and tissue penetration. Highly lipid-soluble doxycycline and minocycline are superior to other tetracyclines in these three properties. Absorption, a passive process that occurs primarily in the duodenum, is interfered with by divalent and trivalent cations in food, milk, aluminum hydroxide gels, sodium bicarbonate, calcium and magnesium salts, and iron preparations. Because the absorption of doxycycline and minocycline is somewhat less affected by food or drugs than is absorption of the other tetracyclines,[62] these two agents are often given with meals to reduce GI irritation. However, because they undergo enterohepatic circulation, intraintestinal divalent cations can still chelate and reduce the bioavailability of parenterally administered drug.[62]

Tetracyclines enter most tissues, including the eye and CNS of dogs.[63] They even penetrate well into the paranasal sinuses and secretions, so they are good for treating bacterial sinusitis. Tetracyclines are less active in alkaline media; pH is an especially important factor if the use of chlortetracycline is being considered.

Less lipid-soluble tetracyclines are primarily excreted unchanged in the urine.

Sixty percent of the active drug is recovered in urine, whereas 40% is excreted by the liver and found in feces. In contrast, minocycline is primarily excreted by enterohepatic recirculation, and only 10% of the administered dose enters the urine. The excretion of doxycycline does not depend on hepatic or renal function; this drug is unique, being excreted directly into the GI tract. Minocycline and doxycycline do not reach high enough concentrations in the urine to be effective.

Resistance

Bacterial resistance to tetracyclines is usually mediated by plasmids, although it may occur following genetic mutation. Resistance has been a major problem with conventional tetracyclines but occurs less often with doxycycline and minocycline.

Toxicity

Numerous side effects have been associated with the use of tetracyclines. GI disturbances result from irritative diarrheas and from changes in the enteric microflora. Because doxycycline and minocycline are well absorbed in the upper GI tract, they are less likely than other tetracyclines to alter the intestinal flora. Orally administered tetracyclines in cats frequently produce fever with or without severe GI upsets from local irritation. Similarly, esophagitis has been found in people given tetracyclines[64] and probably occurs in animals. Clinical signs of GI irritation include depression, fever, anorexia, vomiting, and diarrhea. As with chloramphenicol, tetracyclines inhibit hepatic microsomal enzymes and may delay elimination of hepatically metabolized drugs. Increased hepatic enzyme activities (ALT, formerly SGPT) have been found in animals receiving tetracyclines.

Except for doxycycline, tetracyclines should be avoided in patients with renal failure because drug excretion is delayed in such cases. Dogs receiving tetracyclines have developed azotemia that was out of proportion to the renal damage, presumably because of the catabolic effect the drug had on protein synthesis.[65,65a] The use of tetracyclines in dogs has been associated with direct nephrotoxicity from acute tubular necrosis,[66] and in people use of outdated tetracyclines or the drug's breakdown products have produced a Fanconi-like syndrome with reversible renal tubular dysfunction.[67] Findings on urinalysis have included glucosuria, phosphaturia, and aminoaciduria, with or without proteinuria. The nephrotoxicity occasionally produced by methoxyflurane anesthesia is accentuated by tetracyclines given prior to surgery.[68]

Anaphylactoid reactions to parenterally administered tetracyclines or their vehicles have occasionally been noted in dogs and cats. Hypotension, shock, and urticaria developed in dogs given rapid IV doses of minocycline.[69] Phototoxic reactions in people following exposure to UV light, characterized by erythema and edema of the skin, have been associated with the use of certain tetracyclines. Demeclocycline has been shown to induce acute reversible nephrogenic diabetes insipidus in humans.

Tetracyclines become fixed in growing osseous structures. Staining of deciduous teeth of neonates may occur when tetracyclines are given to a bitch or queen during the last 2 or 3 weeks of pregnancy; the deciduous teeth of puppies or kittens may also be stained if they are given these drugs during the first months of life. In children, doxycycline and oxytetracycline are least likely to produce this effect.

Thrombophlebitis frequently occurs following IV injections of tetracycline and is seen more frequently with the lipid-insoluble tetracyclines. IM administration of tetracycline is discouraged, as it is painful and irritating. A long-acting, somewhat less painful formulation of injectable oxytetracycline has been developed for use in food-producing animals. It consists of a vehicle containing a solvent, 2-pyrrolidone, with a povidone (polyvinylpyrrolidone) base.

IV administration of minocycline in dogs has been associated with toxic side effects. Minocycline given at 10 to 20 mg/kg daily for 1 month decreased erythrocyte count, hemoglobin concentration, and hematocrit and increased ALT activity.[69a] Daily IV dosages of 40 mg/kg produced increased urine calcium and bromosulfophthalein (BSP) retention, decreased food consumption, and weight loss. None of these side effects was observed with equivalent oral dosages. Certain vehicles such as propylene glycol in the IV tetracycline preparations may be responsible for acute reactions mimicking acute anaphylaxis that occur. Sudden ataxia, shivering, dyspnea, hypotension, and arrhythmias have occurred.[70] Rapid IV infusion of doxycycline at 5 mg/kg has not produced any adverse effects in dogs.[71]

Tetracyclines may cause false-positive urine test results for glucose if copper sulfate reagents are used (Clinitest, Ames Laboratories, Elkhart, IN), and false-negative tests may occur with glucose oxidase reagents. Leukocytosis, atypical lymphocytes, toxic granulation, and immune hemolytic anemia have been reported with tetracycline use in humans. Interference of tetracycline with coagulation factors has also been noted.

Vestibular side effects have frequently been reported with the use of minocycline in humans. This complication is peculiar to humans because minocycline is appreciably biotransformed in humans but not in dogs and cats. A metabolite of minocycline may be responsible for the vestibular toxicosis. Long-acting IM oxytetracycline formulations containing polyvinylpyrrolidone have been shown to produce pain at the site of injection and generalized anaphylaxis in dogs.

ERYTHROMYCIN

This drug is the most important of the macrolides, a group of antibiotics produced by the actinomycete *Streptomyces erythreus*.

Oleandomycin and its synthetic congener, troleandomycin, are less active and more toxic than erythromycin; therefore, they are rarely used. Rosamycin is similar to erythromycin in antibacterial spectrum and usage. Josamycin, an erythromycin derivative, is better absorbed and less toxic and is less likely to develop bacterial resistance than erythromycin. Rokitamycin, an experimental macrolide, has a higher stability in the stomach and achieves higher serum concentrations after oral administration than erythromycin. Dirithromycin is a potent erythromycin derivative that has been shown to have higher and longer-lasting serum levels than erythromycin base. Because of its antiprotozoal efficacy, the macrolide spiramycin is discussed in Chapter 77.

Erythromycin, which is bacteriostatic for most organisms at commonly used dosages, inhibits RNA-dependent protein synthesis in bacterial cells. Because this mechanism of action is similar to that of chloramphenicol and lincomycin, erythromycin can compete with these two drugs for binding sites.

Formulations

Erythromycin, a weak base, is unstable in the presence of gastric acid, which inhibits its bioavailability following oral administration. Different formulations of erythromycin, made to prevent destruction of erythromycin base by digestive enzymes, have incorporated enteric coating, acid-stable salts (stearate), esters (ethylsuccinate), and salts of esters (estolate) (Table 43–7). Erythromycin base is absorbed intact, but absorption is reduced when the drug is taken with food. Absorption of stearate is also inhibited by food and is partially decreased by gastric acid. The base and stearate formulations should be given on an empty stomach. The stearate compound readily dissociates into the base following absorption. The facts that ethylsuccinate and estolate preparations are absorbed as esters and require hydrolysis within the body to form limited amounts of free (active) drug have caused considerable controversy concerning their therapeutic effectiveness. Erythromycin ethylsuccinate is nonirritating and tasteless, and is good as an oral suspension for use in puppies and kittens. Erythromycin estolate is not affected by the presence of gastric acid or food and

gives the highest and most prolonged serum activity. Erythromycin is formulated as lactobionate and gluceptate esters that can be administered parenterally, although these are relatively expensive to use. Topical preparations are also available for general use and as ophthalmic ointments.

Pharmacology

Erythromycin diffuses readily into most tissues, and extracellular fluid compartments, with the exception of CSF, and therapeutic concentrations are reached within 2 to 3 hours.[72] It is concentrated by the liver, and is excreted in the bile in high concentration or undergoes enterohepatic circulation and finally is excreted in feces. High concentrations are also found in most body fluids and secretions with the exception of urine. Only 4% of the oral and 15% of the parenteral dose is found in urine; therefore, minimal dosage adjustment is required for patients with renal failure.

Indications

Erythromycin, which has a primarily grampositive spectrum, is most effective against streptococci, staphylococci, *Erysipelothrix*, *Clostridium*, *Bacteroides*, *Borrelia*, and *Fusobacterium*. It is also effective against a few gram-negative organisms, such as *Pasteurella* and *Bordetella*, but not against aerobic enteric bacteria unless the environmental pH is alkaline. Erythromycin has exceptional activity against *Campylobacter fetus*, *Legionella pneumophila*, mycoplasmas, chlamydiae, rickettsiae, spirochetes, some atypical mycobacteria, *Leptospira*, and amebae. Resistance has developed with increasing frequency because the drug is being used more routinely. It has been combined with sulfonamides to achieve a broader spectrum of effectiveness and with neomycin as prophylaxis against peritoneal contamination during colonic surgery. Erythromycin is rarely used as a first choice drug, with the exception of treatment of *Campylobacter* or *Legionella* infections but more often as an alternative.

Toxicity

Erythromycin has relatively low toxicity; the most frequent side effect is GI irritation

Table 43–7. Comparison of Erythromycin Formulations for Oral Use[a]

GENERIC DRUG (TRADE NAMES)	ABSORBED AS FREE BASE	ABSORPTION AFFECTED BY GASTRIC ACID/FOOD	ROUTE OF ADMINISTRATION (FORMULATION/COMMENTS)
Erythromycin base (Erythromycin, Ilotycin, Robimycin, E-Mycin, Eryc)	+	+ / ±	PO (Tablets/enteric-coated)
Erythromycin stearate (Erythrocin, Ethril, Erypar, Wyamycin)	+	± / −	PO (Tablets/absorption increased by drinking large amounts of water)
Erythromycin estolate (Ilosone)	−	− / −	PO (Drops, tablets, suspension/associated with increased risks of cholestasis and hepatotoxicity)
Erythromycin ethylsuccinate (Pediamycin, Eryped, E.E.S.)	−	± / ±	PO (Drops, capsules, tablets, suspension/milk enhances absorption)

[a] + = yes, ± = variable, − = no, PO = oral.
See text for the comparative properties and indications for each product.
See Appendix 14 for appropriate dosages.

manifested as nausea, vomiting, and diarrhea. Water or dilute solutions of antacids given with the drug may decrease irritation and facilitate absorption. Erythromycin estolate and occasionally erythromycin ethylsuccinate have been associated with an increased risk of cholestasis and hepatotoxicity, which may cause increased serum bilirubin concentration and hepatic enzyme activity. All parenteral preparations are irritating at the site of injection.

TYLOSIN

This bacteriostatic macrolide antibiotic, produced by *Streptomyces fradiae*, is related to erythromycin. Oral absorption is variable, depending on the product formulation used, and the drug is metabolized by the liver and excreted in both the urine and the bile. Tylosin base is adequately absorbed when given orally. Tylosin has been recommended for use in the management of ulcerative colitis in dogs and in the treatment of feline infectious peritonitis; however, proof of its efficacy in treating either syndrome is lacking. Gram-positive bacteria, *Campylobacter*, and mycoplasmas are particularly susceptible to its effects, as are most organisms that are susceptible to erythromycin.

High dosages (200 to 400 mg/kg/day, given for a 2-year period) have been tolerated by clinically healthy dogs with no apparent side effects. Dosages as low as 5 mg/kg/day have increased the tendency of dogs to develop ventricular tachycardia following ex-

perimental myocardial ischemia. IM injections produce pain and localized swelling. Nausea and vomiting may occur with oral administration. Contact dermatitis has developed in veterinarians handling the drug.

LINCOMYCIN AND CLINDAMYCIN

Lincomycin was the first member of a new group of antibiotics isolated from *Streptomyces lincolnensis*. Although it has many similarities to erythromycin, there are distinct differences as well. Depending on the dosage employed, lincomycin is bacteriostatic to bactericidal; it works by inhibiting bacterial protein synthesis. Clindamycin, a chlorosubstituted lincomycin, has increased bactericidal activity and rate of absorption and has shown a low level of toxicity in animals when compared with lincomycin.

Pharmacology

The absorption of lincomycin from the GI tract is incomplete and variable and is further impeded by the presence of food. Most (77%) of an oral dose given on an empty stomach is excreted in the bile; only 14% appears in urine. When the drug is given with food, 38% and 49% are excreted in the bile and urine, respectively. Therefore, the dosage of lincomycin must be reduced in patients with renal failure. IM administration yields a higher serum concentration of the drug.

Clindamycin is rapidly and completely absorbed from the GI tract regardless of the presence of food. As it is predominantly (>90%) excreted in the bile with only 10% excreted in the urine, dosage adjustments are not required in cases of renal failure. However, the dosage should be reduced or the drug should be avoided in patients with hepatic insufficiency or evidence of cholestasis. Because of biliary excretion, antibacterial activity may persist in the feces for 5 or more days after therapy is discontinued.

Lincomycin and clindamycin are widely distributed in body tissues and fluids, including bile, peritoneal and pleural fluids, milk, placenta, prostatic fluid, and bone. Lincomycin will not enter the CSF or ocular structures unless inflammation is present. Little is known about CSF or ocular penetration by clindamycin, but it appears to work in treatment of infections in these tissues when inflammation is present. The drug does accumulate in neutrophils and macrophages and in abscesses, features which would seemingly make it useful in treating infections caused by anaerobic or persistent intracellular pathogens (see Therapy of Anaerobic Infections, Chapter 49, and Therapy of Toxoplasmosis, Chapter 86).

Indications

Lincomycin and clindamycin are primarily indicated for the treatment of infections caused by gram-positive aerobes and gram-positive and gram-negative anaerobes. Lincomycin has been recommended for use in a variety of respiratory, GI, soft tissue, and bone infections, especially when gram-positive organisms are involved. Clindamycin, which is generally more active than lincomycin, is known to be effective against a greater variety of organisms, including anaerobic bacteria and protozoa such as *Toxoplasma* (see Therapy, Chapter 49 and Therapy, Chapter 86). It is active against several gram-negative species, including *Klebsiella*, *Pasteurella*, *Pseudomonas*, and *Salmonella*. Clindamycin has been shown to be effective when combined with aminoglycosides in treating peritoneal infections caused by a mixture of anaerobic and gram-negative bacteria from the bowel. Clindamycin is very effective in treating anaerobic infections in

dogs[73] and could be considered over chloramphenicol or metronidazole. It has been effective in the treatment of experimental post-traumatic osteomyelitis caused by S. aureus in dogs.[74] It is of benefit in the treatment of staphylococcal pyoderma or diskospondylitis in dogs (see Therapy, Chapters 5 and 6, respectively).

Clindamycin susceptibility disks have been used to test for in vitro susceptibility to either drug. Bacterial resistance, which may develop after repeated exposure to either drug, is usually cross-reacting.

Toxicity

Toxicity of lincomycin and clindamycin has been relatively low in dogs that received supratherapeutic dosages for relatively long periods. GI irritation, vomiting, and diarrhea may be seen if the drug is given orally; IM injections cause local pain. Rapid IV administration of lincomycin causes hypotension and cardiopulmonary arrest. To avoid GI irritation, the administration of the drug can be temporarily discontinued or the dosage lowered until side effects are no longer observed.

Pseudomembranous colitis, a complicating syndrome of humans treated with either drug, is manifested clinically by abdominal pain, fever, and mucus or blood in the stools. This syndrome is thought to be caused by overgrowth of resistant, toxin-producing strains of *Clostridium difficile*. Although diarrhea develops in dogs and cats with use of clindamycin or lincomycin, it does not seem to be caused by *C. difficile* toxin.[74a] If this colitis does occur, clindamycin should be discontinued; vancomycin or metronidazole should be substituted. Although not licensed for use in cats, oral clindamycin given at daily dosages of 11 to 22 mg/kg for 10 days[74b] or 25 to 50 mg/kg for 6 weeks[75] caused minimal signs of GI or other toxicities in cats.

NOVOBIOCIN

This antibiotic, produced by *Streptomyces niveus*, has an antibacterial spectrum similar to, but not as consistent as, that of penicillin. Many gram-positive organisms, including streptococci and staphylococci, are susceptible to it. Variable effectiveness has been found against *Proteus, Pseudomonas,* and *Pasteurella multocida.* Novobiocin inhibits RNA synthesis, and antibacterial resistance to this drug does not transfer to other antibiotics.

Novobiocin is absorbed well after oral administration and is excreted in the bile, urine, and feces. It has been marketed in the United States, primarily in fixed combination with tetracyclines. In vitro studies have suggested possible inhibition reactions between these compounds. However, a subjective clinical evaluation reported more clinical improvement in upper respiratory tract infections in dogs treated with novobiocin combined with tetracycline than in dogs given either drug alone.

BACITRACIN

This antibiotic is a polypeptide produced by *Bacillus subtilis* that is relatively unstable in water-soluble formulations at room temperature. The exact mode of its action is unknown, but it appears to interfere with bacterial cell wall synthesis. Although it is not absorbed after oral or topical administration, bacitracin has been combined in a variety of ointments and solutions for use as a topical dressing or for local application by irrigation. Its activity is not impaired by blood, pus, or necrotic tissue. Bacitracin has been used to treat infectious processes in wounds, the genitourinary tract, and in the eyes and ears. It has been given orally as an antidiarrheal agent in the treatment of intestinal pathogens and is rarely, if ever, intended for systemic use.[51] Activity is greatest against gram-positive organisms such as staphylococci, streptococci, *Corynebacterium,* and anaerobes such as *Clostridium* and *Actinomyces,* and the drug is also quite effective in treating diarrhea caused by *Entamoeba.* Toxicity of bacitracin is manifested primarily as hypersensitivity associated with topical administration.

NITROFURANS

This class of antibacterial compounds includes chemical derivatives of 5-nitrofuraldehyde. Their exact mechanism of action is uncertain, although they are known to interfere with many cellular enzymes. Nitrofurans are bacteriostatic or bactericidal,

depending on the susceptibility of the organisms and the amount of drug at the site of infection. Table 43–8 summarizes the uses of these compounds in veterinary practice.

Nitrofurantoin is rapidly absorbed following oral ingestion; however, its concentration in plasma is never sufficient to treat systemic infections. Most of the administered dose is excreted in the urine, which makes the drug useful only for urinary tract infections. Nitrofurantoin in urine may cause a spuriously positive test result for glucose when glucose oxidase test strips are used. Alkalinization of the urine, which increases the amount of nitrofurantoin that is excreted, should be avoided because the drug is more effective in an acid pH. Macrodantin, a crystalline form of nitrofurantoin, was developed to decrease the rate of absorption, thereby minimizing the irritating effect on the GI mucosa. Nifuratel is an analog of nitrofurantoin with a similar pattern of absorption; however, it is unaffected by urine pH and has a wider spectrum of activity, including efficacy against *Candida.*

Furazolidone is not absorbed by the GI mucosa following oral administration and has been used for treatment of local infections caused by enteric pathogens. Nitrofurazone is a nonabsorbable, topically applied antimicrobial powder, cream, or spray solution. There is evidence that the spray preparation may be carcinogenic. It is frequently incorporated in an oil base rather than a water-soluble cream; however, this incorporation reduces its antibacterial effectiveness.

The nitrofurans as a group have a relatively broad spectrum of activity, although they are generally more effective against gram-negative organisms. *E. coli,* staphylococci, and streptococci are usually susceptible, whereas *Pseudomonas* and some *Proteus* spp. are fairly resistant. *Pseudomonas* can actually grow in many preparations of nitrofurazone, which may lead to nosocomial wound contamination. Resistance rarely develops during therapy with nitrofurans, in contrast to that which occurs with the use of other antibacterials.

Nitrofurantoin is indicated for use in urinary tract infections only when other agents fail. Nitrofurazone does not interfere with the healing of wounds, but when used as an oil-based medicament it may result in maceration of the wound, which prolongs healing. It is one of the few antibacterials that are effective in the presence of blood and pus.

Table 43–8. Comparison of Properties of Nitrofurans[a]

GENERIC NAME (TRADE NAMES)	ROUTE OF ADMINISTRATION (FORMULATION)	USES/COMMENTS
Nitrofurantoin (Furadantin, Macrodantin)	PO (tablets, suspension) IM (solution)	Urinary tract infections/avoid in renal failure; macrocrystalline is absorbed slower and is less toxic
Nifuratel (Magmilor)	PO (tablets)	Urinary tract infection, also effective against *Candida* at any urine pH
Furazolidone (Furoxone)	PO (tablets, suspension)	Orally: for enteric pathogens, not absorbed, used for *Salmonella* and coccidia
Nitrofurazone (Furacin)	Topical (ointment, powder, solution, cream, suppositories)	For skin and mucosal infections/*Pseudomonas* can contaminate
Nifuroxime (Micofur)	Topical (suppositories, cream)	Antifungal properties/used combined with other nitrofurans

[a]PO = oral, IM = intramuscular.
See Appendix 14 for appropriate dosages.

Table 43–9. Properties of Commonly Used Sulfonamides[a]

GENERIC NAME (TRADE NAMES)	ROUTE OF ADMINISTRATION	INDICATIONS AND COMMENTS
Short Acting[b]		
Sulfadiazine (Suladyne, Debenal)	PO, IM	Systemic and urinary tract infections and nocardiosis/frequently combined as triple sulfate to minimize renal tubular precipitation; sulfadiazine and sulfamethoxazole combined with trimethoprim (see below)
Sulfamerazine (Supronal)	PO, IM	As above
Sulfamethazine (Sulmet, Sulfamezathine)	PO, IM	As above
Sulfamethoxazole (Gantanol, Methoxal)	PO, IM	As above
Intermediate Acting[c]		
Sulfisoxazole (Gantrisin, Soxisol, Sulfasox)	PO	Urinary tract infections
Sulfamethoxypyridazine (Midicel, Kypnx, Quinoseptyl)	PO	Urinary tract and respiratory infections/has advantage of less frequent administration
Sulfadimethoxine (Sudine, Bactrovet, Albon, Madribon)	PO	As above
Gastrointestinal Preparations[d]		
Succinylsulfathiazole (Sulfasuxidine)	PO	Local antibacterial effects on GI tract/administer with kaolin-pectin
Phthalylsulfathiazole (Sulfathalidine)	PO	*Shigella* enteritis, preoperative prophylaxis for GI surgery/mineral oil, laxatives, and purgatives interfere with action
Special Preparations		
Salicylazosulfapyridine (Azulfidine, Sulfasalazine)	PO	Ulcerative colitis/salicylate component may help in therapy
Mafenide (Sulfamylon cream)	Topical	Burns/prophylaxis only
Trimethoprim and sulfamethoxazole (Septra, Bactrim)	PO	Systemic, respiratory, urinary tract infections, *Pneumocystis* pneumonia, brucellosis/must be given to dogs at least twice daily; effective when given once daily for treatment of urinary tract infections
Trimethoprim and sulfadiazine (Tribrissen, Di-Trim)	PO, IM	As above

[a]PO = oral, IM = intramuscular.
[b]Rapidly absorbed and rapidly excreted.
[c]Rapidly absorbed and slowly excreted.
[d]Poorly absorbed.
See Appendix 14 for appropriate dosages.

Adverse reactions to nitrofurans are not uncommon. Nitrofurantoin frequently causes nausea and emesis in dogs and cats. Acute polymyositis developed in a dog as a complication of nitrofurantoin use.[75]

SULFONAMIDES

These first effective drugs developed for treating bacterial disease have now been superceded by a variety of antimicrobial agents. They are derivatives of sulfanilamide and act primarily by interfering with bacterial synthesis of folic acid from para-aminobenzoic acid (PABA). Sulfonamides are bacteriostatic compounds and are ineffective in the presence of pus, necrotic tissue, or serum that contains PABA.

Pharmacology

Except for a few poorly absorbed compounds, most sulfonamides are readily and rapidly absorbed and reach bacteriostatic concentrations in serum. They are variably bound to plasma protein and become widely distributed to all tissues of the body, including pleural, peritoneal, synovial, and ocular fluids. They are able to cross the placenta and, because they readily enter CSF, are effective in treating meningeal infections. Sulfonamides are generally metabolized in the liver and excreted in small amounts in the bile. Most of the metabolized drug is excreted in the urine. The serum concentration is dependent upon the route of administration and the dosage.

Indications

The orally absorbed sulfonamides can be divided into three groups on the basis of their duration of action (Table 43–9). The short-acting drugs, rapidly absorbed and excreted, require doses at 8-hour intervals. They are the sulfonamides of choice for systemic and urinary tract infections. The intermediate-acting sulfonamides have a lower excretion rate, are administered every 12 to 24 hours, and are primarily used for treating urinary tract infections. Sulfisoxazole is the most frequently used member of the group. Long-acting sulfonamides such as sulfadoxine have slow excretion rates and require administration every few days. They have been used in countries other than the United States for treatment of malaria, chronic bronchitis, and urinary tract infections in humans.

Certain sulfonamides, poorly absorbed from the GI tract, are used to alter enteric microflora but do not disrupt the balance of microflora and rarely cause superinfection. Phthalylsulfathiazole has been used to reduce coliform flora, stool bulk, and gas prior to colonic surgery.

Although marketed for topical use, sulfonamides are relatively ineffective in the presence of exudates. Mafenide, the only exception, is the drug of choice for prophylaxis in burn patients because of its ability to inhibit *Pseudomonas*.

Certain sulfonamides have been used for specific diseases. Sulfapyridine, which is relatively toxic, is indicated only for the treatment of dermatitis herpetiformis. Salicylazosulfapyridine is used for the treatment of ulcerative colitis.

Organisms that are highly susceptible to sulfonamides include streptococci, *Bacillus*, *Corynebacterium*, *Nocardia*, *Brucella*, *Campylobacter*, *Pasteurella*, and *Chlamydia*. *Pseudomonas*, *Serratia*, and *Klebsiella* are generally resistant. Caution must be exercised in interpreting disk susceptibility test results, because they frequently do not correlate with in vivo susceptibility. An increasing number of organisms are becoming resistant to sulfonamides. Resistance appears to develop more commonly with long-term therapy.

Toxicity

Toxic reactions to sulfonamides are relatively uncommon in dogs and cats. Acute hemolytic complications and precipitation of sulfonamide metabolites in renal tubules, as seen in humans, have not been noted in small companion animals. That dogs do not acetylate sulfas may partly explain their relative insusceptibility to these complications. Dogs given high dosages of sulfonamides can develop sulfonamide cystic urolithiasis (see Trimethoprim-Sulfonamides, Chapter 5). However, cats may develop azotemia and renal failure during sulfonamide or trimethoprim-sulfonamide therapy.[75] Keratitis sicca has been the most common problem with long-term administration in dogs.[76,76a]

TRIMETHOPRIM-SULFONAMIDES

Sulfonamides by themselves inhibit bacterial synthesis of dihydrofolic acid. Trimethoprim interferes with dihydrofolate reductase, subsequently preventing the conversion of dihydrofolic acid (folic acid) to tetrahydrofolic acid (folinic acid), which is essential for synthesis of purines, pyrimidines, and the resulting nucleic acids. Mammals, unlike microorganisms, acquire most folic acid preformed in the diet, and this explains the selective action of these folate synthesis inhibitors. Trimethoprim has less affinity for dihydrofolate reductase in mammals than in microorganisms, which helps to explain the reduced toxicity of the drug for mammalian cells. The combination of two bacteriostatic drugs, trimethoprim and a sulfonamide in a 1:5 ratio, is synergistic and results in a bactericidal drug when an optimal in vivo ratio of 1:2 is achieved.

Pharmacology

Trimethoprim is rapidly and completely absorbed following oral administration. It is similar to the sulfonamides in having a wide distribution in many tissues that are not penetrated by most antibiotics, including the CSF and prostate. Therapeutic concentrations are achieved in the brain, eye, bone, and joints. In dogs, approximately 60% to 80% of the administered dose is excreted in the urine within 24 hours. It is not necessary to reduce the dosage unless renal failure is severe.

Sulfadiazine has been formulated for use with trimethoprim in dogs, whereas sulfamethoxazole is combined in human preparations. This difference in formulation stems from the fact that people excrete sulfamethoxazole and trimethoprim at a similar rate, making the combination effective when administered twice daily. In contrast, the half-life of trimethoprim (3 hours) in dogs is shorter than the excretion of sulfadiazine (10 hours), so that twice-daily dosing is essential to maintain therapeutic concentrations of both drugs. Once-daily dosing may be sufficient in the treatment of urinary infections or for systemic infections when or-

ganisms are particularly susceptible to sulfonamides alone.

Indications

Trimethoprim is available by itself for use in countries other than the United States; however, because it has lower activity and is no less toxic than the combined product, there is little advantage in its use. Trimethoprim-sulfonamide is available in an oral formulation for small animals, as well as in a parenteral solution used to treat severe infections and for use in comatose patients.

Trimethoprim-sulfonamide has been recommended primarily for the treatment of respiratory and urinary tract infections caused by *E. coli*, streptococci, *Proteus*, *Salmonella*, *Shigella*, and *Pasteurella*. Lesser and more variable activity is noted against staphylococci, *Klebsiella*, *Fusiformis*, *Corynebacterium*, *Clostridium*, and *Bordetella*. *Moraxella*, *Nocardia*, and *Brucella* are usually only moderately susceptible. The drug is ineffective against mycobacteria, *Leptospira*, *Pseudomonas*, *Erysipelothrix*, and *Bacteroides*. Despite its in vitro efficacy against some anaerobes,[77] the drug does not work well clinically in treatment of anaerobic infections. It has been used simultaneously with polymyxins or aminoglycosides to increase the spectrum of effectiveness against gram-negative organisms. Bacterial resistance has developed with continued usage. Because of good CNS penetrability, it is an excellent choice for gram-negative pathogens producing meningitis.[78]

Trimethoprim-sulfonamide has been especially recommended for long-term, low-dose therapy for chronic infections of the urinary tract because it is found in high concentration throughout the urinary system and does not usually cause overgrowth of resistant bowel flora during long-term usage. The drug has also been used in treatment of or prophylaxis for *Pneumocystis carinii*, *Toxoplasma gondii*, and enteric coccidial infections.

Daily dosing of trimethoprim-sulfonamide as recommended on the label should be reserved for prophylactic use and treatment of chronic urinary tract infections. One-time dosing of 30 to 90 mg/kg for urinary tract infections in dogs has not been sufficient compared with the conventional daily dosing.[79,80] For treatment of systemic infections, larger (30 to 45 mg/kg) doses, given at least twice a day, are required. Crushing the tablets and mixing them with food will have minimal effects on the absorptive process.

Toxicity

All the side effects noted previously with sulfonamide therapy can be seen with this drug combination. Trimethoprim-sulfonamide causes greater adverse reactions and has a smaller margin of safety when given to cats compared with treatment of dogs. The drug is not currently marketed for use in cats. Azotemia and renal failure may develop in some treated cats (see Toxicity, Sulfonamides). Cats given standard therapeutic dosages had anorexia, whereas much higher (300 mg/kg) dosages resulted in severe anorexia, leukopenia, and anemia. These abnormalities disappeared after therapy was discontinued. Because they cause excessive salivation and have a bitter taste, crushed tablets should not be administered to cats. Vomiting is a common complication of oral administration of trimethoprim-sulfonamide to cats.

Other toxicities have been reported to occur in dogs and cats. Ataxia has sometimes been observed in dogs and cats given higher therapeutic dosages of trimethoprim-sulfonamide. Neurologic signs usually disappear within 24 to 48 hours after the drug therapy is discontinued. Cholestatic hepatitis, causing icterus, anorexia, and vomiting, was described in people receiving the drug.[81] A similar phenomenon in the dog was described previously[82] and has been observed, especially in dogs with preexisting hepatic disease.[75] Aplastic anemia was associated with trimethoprim-sulfadiazine and fenbendazole administration in a dog.[83] The anemia resolved after withdrawal of the drug and may have been related to a drug idiosyncrasy or immune-hypersensitivity rather than to folate metabolism inhibition.

Treatment with trimethoprim-sulfadiazine combination has been associated with allergic immune-complex reactions in dogs specifically due to the sulfadiazine.[84–87] Polyarthritis, lymphadenopathy, fever, polymyositis, glomerulonephritis, urticaria, focal retinitis, anemia, leukopenia, and thrombocytopenia have been noted. These adverse drug reactions developed within 1 to 3 weeks after the first use of the drug or within 1 hour to 10 days after repeated usage.[84] Doberman pinschers have shown a predilection for developing immune-complex complications but many other large breed dogs have been affected. The immune-mediated reaction subsides within 24 to 48 hours of withdrawal of the drug and immunosuppressive doses of glucocorticoids. Immune-mediated ulcerative skin disease has occurred in a dog being treated with trimethoprim-sulfamethizole.[88] Similarly, a presumed immune-mediated meningitis was described in people being treated with trimethoprim-sulfamethoxazole.[89]

Dietary supplementation or administration of folinic acid (leucovorin) at a dosage of 0.5 to 1 mg/day can overcome the anemia and leukopenia due to interference with folic acid metabolism. Therapy with trimethoprim-sulfonamide must be discontinued, and doses of folinic acid of up to 15 g total/day may be needed to overcome existing toxicity.[90,91] Addition of folinic acid merely reduces the effect of trimethoprim-sulfonamide on enterococci. Folic acid supplementation should not be used, because its activation to folinic acid is blocked by trimethoprim.[90] Folinic acid supplementation will counteract the antibacterial or antiprotozoal effectiveness of sulfonamides unless trimethoprim or pyrimethamine is used in combination.[92] Hematologic studies should be performed at least once a month whenever dogs or cats receive trimethoprim-sulfonamide for longer than 2 weeks. Use of this drug should be restricted in animals with preexisting anemia or leukopenia.

QUINOLONES

Pharmacology

The fluoroquinolones are a diverse group of bactericidal naphthyridine derivatives that prevent bacterial DNA synthesis by partially inhibiting the bacterial enzyme, DNA gyrase. This effect is antagonized by protein synthesis inhibitors such as chloramphenicol or rifampin but is synergistic with the effects of co-administered aminoglycosides. Nalidixic and oxolinic acid are the nonfluorinated parent compounds of this group. They are well absorbed following oral administration and undergo hepatic metabolism to biologically active metabolites that are excreted in urine. Plasma concentrations are low; the only therapeutic benefit of these two parent drugs has been in treatment of intestinal or urinary tract infections. Fluoroquinolones achieve effective urinary concentrations, but those with a piperacine group at the C-7 position, such as ciprofloxacin and norfloxacin, are inactive below pH of 6.8, and their efficacy can be enhanced by raising urine pH with concurrent administration of bicarbonate. Unfortunately, alkaline urine may favor renal tubular crystalluria (see Toxicity). Newer clinically available quinolones and those under investigation are listed in Table 43–10. Compared with nalidixic and oxolinic acids, the newer commercially available quinolones such as ciprofloxacin, norfloxacin, and enrofloxacin have less toxicity, increased potency, and less bacterial resistance. Variable GI absorption occurs with fluoroquinolones, with ofloxicin, ciprofloxacin, pefloxacin, enrofloxacin, and norfloxacin being absorbed effectively in decreasing order. Food inhibits their absorption so that they should be administered on an empty stomach. Absorption is impaired by concurrent administration of magnesium or aluminum-containing preparations such as antacids by sucralfate-containing preparations.[92a] To achieve better serum concentrations in dogs and cats with some of the compounds, IM administration may be advised. When effective blood levels are achieved, the drugs have good penetration into body fluids and secretions and other harder-to-enter tissues, including the CSF, prostate, and bone.[93–98] Fluoroquinolones are partially metabolized in the liver and excreted in the bile or urine partly as active drug or metabolites. Concentrations achieved in bile and urine are 10 to 20 times higher than those of serum. Urine recovery varies from 30% to 70%, depending on the drug being considered. The dose should be reduced by at least 50% in patients with evidence of renal failure.

Indications

The fluoroquinolones are primarily active against gram-negative organisms. Although many gram-positive and other bacteria are susceptible, MIC ranges usually are higher than for gram-negative organisms. They are not very effective for treating anaerobic or streptococcal or some staphylococcal infections. Staphylococci spp. that are resistant to many other drugs may be susceptible to the quinolones. Some rickettsiae have been shown to be susceptible to treatment with quinolones. Some quinolones have also been shown to have activity against *Chlamydia*, *Mycoplasma*, and some mycobacteria. They have good activity against bacterial enteropathogens, such as *Salmonella* spp., *Shigella* spp., *Campylobacter* spp., *Yersinia enterocolitica*, and *E. coli*. Ciprofloxacin has more activity than norfloxacin.[99] They kill bacteria at concentrations that are close to inhibitory concentrations and they have marked postantibiotic inhibitory effect in vivo.[100] Recurrent urinary tract infections caused by resistant organisms such as *Pseudomonas*, *Proteus*, or *Klebsiella* are the primary indications for their use. They have also been used to treat enteropathogenic and

Table 43–10. Dosages of Fluoroquinolones Recommended for Dogs and Cats[a]

DRUG (BRAND, MFR)	SPECIES	DOSE[b] (mg/kg)	ROUTE	INTERVAL (hours)	INFECTION SITES
Norfloxacin[93] (Noroxin, Merck)	B	5–11[c]	PO	12	Urine, urinary tract
	D	11–22[d]	PO	12	Skin and soft tissues
Ciprofloxacin[94] (Cipro, Miles)	D	5–11	PO	12	Urine and urinary tract
	D	10–15	PO	12	Skin and soft tissue
Enrofloxacin[95] (Baytrill, Mobay)	B	2.5–5	PO, SC	12	Urine and urinary tract
	D	5–15	PO	12	Skin and soft tissues

[a]Under development is Enoxacin (Warner-Lambert[96]), lomefloxacin (Searle), amifloxacin (Sterling-Winthrop), ibafloxacin (Beecham), ofloxacin, pefloxacin, fleroxacin, difloxacin, Temafloxacin (Abbott), Danofloxacin (Pfizer), tosufloxacin. D = dog; B = dog and cat.

[b]Dose per administration at specified interval, expressed as mg/kg unless otherwise stated.

[c]Dose adequate for *Staphylococcus intermedius*, *Escherichia coli*, *Klebsiella pneumoniae*, and *Serratia marcescens*.

[d]Dose adequate for *Pseudomonas aeruginosa* and *Enterobacter cloacae*.

respiratory infections caused by resistant organisms. In addition, they offer the advantage of oral therapy for chronic resistant osteomyelitis. In intra-abdominal infections, when mixed flora are present, quinolones have been effective against aerobic or facultative bacteria when used in combination with drugs, such as clindamycin and metronidazole, that are effective against anaerobes.

Bacterial resistance does occur with quinolones; it has developed most commonly in treatment of infections caused by *P. aeruginosa*, *K. pneumoniae*, *Acinetobacter* spp., *S. marcescens*, enterococci, and staphylococci.[99a] Cross-resistance among the quinolones is usual but does not occur with antibiotics in other classes.

Toxicity

Eukaryotic DNA enzyme is partially affected by these compounds. Side effects following use of nalidixic and oxolinic acids have included vomiting, diarrhea, hepatotoxicity, and CNS signs. In comparison, extremely high concentrations of the newer quinolones are needed to be toxic. Rapid IV administration of 10 to 30 mg/kg of quinolones to anesthetized dogs or cats produces systemic hypotension, presumably related to histamine release.[101a] Hypotension and tachycardia have also been seen after oral administration. Abnormal electroencephalographic (EEG) changes have also been observed in dogs and cats after IV administration of 25 mg/kg or greater. Seizures have been precipitated by administration of parenteral doses of quinolones with concurrent use of nonsteroidal analgesic drugs such as fenbufen. Toxic effects were noted in the eye, kidney, and joints of juvenile animals given oral dosages.[101,101a] Dogs given high dosages have had subcapsular cataract formation in the lens and an associated inflammatory response after treatment for 8 to 12 months.[101a] Quinolones have limited solubility at alkaline pH and may crystallize. At high dosages in dogs, renal toxicity developed from crystalluria and crystal deposition in tubular lumens. Nephrotoxicity has also been an uncommon finding in people and dogs treated with usual therapeutic dosages. Cartilaginous defects occurred in growing cartilage of young dogs, and this has been accentuated with exercise and has been prevented with restriction of activity. Nevertheless, use of quinolones is contraindicated during the rapid growth phase, between 2 to 8 months in small and medium breeds, 1 year in large breeds, and 18 months in giant breeds of dogs.[101b] Cats given high doses of ciprofloxacin developed erythema of their pinnae, vomiting, and clonic muscle spasms. Dogs consistently vomited when given higher dosages of medicine and, therefore, did not show other systemic manifestations of toxicity. High IV dosages administered to anesthetized dogs or cats have produced EEG abnormalities suggestive of brain irritation. Unanesthetized dogs given ciprofloxacin and ibuprofen have had reduced seizure thresholds. Because of their effects on nucleic acid synthesis and known fetal toxicity in other species, these drugs should not be given to young (<6 months of age) or pregnant dogs or cats. Since they are excreted in milk, use in lactating animals should similarly be avoided. High dosages (100 mg/kg) for longer than 3 months have been associated with impaired spermatogenesis and testicular atrophy in dogs.[101a]

PHOSPHONOPEPTIDES

Alafosfalin, fosfomycin, and fosmidomycin are members of a new antibacterial class of phosphonic acid compounds. Fosmidomycin has been evaluated in dogs, and a majority of the drug was excreted unchanged, making it a possible alternative in management of urinary infections.[102] Alafosfalin reaches high concentration in inflammatory exudates and in most tissues except the brain after parenteral injection. It possesses little antibacterial activity and must be transported into bacteria, where it is metabolized to become effective.

URINARY ANTISEPTICS

Methenamine (hexamethylenetetramine), a highly water-soluble organic compound, decomposes at an acid pH to form formaldehyde. Reserved for chronic treatment and long-term prophylaxis of urinary tract infections, it is dispensed in an enteric-coated tablet to prevent degradation by gastric acid. Following oral administration, it is rapidly absorbed and is primarily excreted in the urine. Formulations containing organic acids (mandelic, hippuric, and sulfosalicylic salts) have been prepared in an attempt to facilitate the lowering of pH when these substances are simultaneously excreted. Antibacterial activity is primarily confined to the bladder, because urinary transit in the upper tract is brief and time is required for the generation of formaldehyde.

ANTITUBERCULOUS DRUGS

Isoniazid

This hydrazide derivative of isonicotinic acid is one of the most active compounds against *Mycobacterium tuberculosis*. It acts by interfering with the synthesis of mycolic acids found in the bacterial cell walls and is active only against replicating bacteria; slow-growing or inactive organisms are not affected. The MIC for *M. tuberculosis* is 0.025 to 0.15 µg/ml. The absorption of isoniazid from the intestine is rapid but is inhibited by antacids, and a major portion of the dose is excreted unchanged in the urine within 24 hours. It penetrates most tissues well. CSF concentration is 20% of that of serum but increases to 100% in the presence of inflammation. Most but not all strains of *M. tuberculosis* are sensitive to isoniazid. Because resistance usually develops during the course of therapy, drug susceptibility testing is recommended.

The principal side effects of isoniazid, hepatotoxicity and hepatic enzyme elevation, are reversed if therapy is discontinued immediately. Peripheral neuropathy and CNS excitability may be caused by monoamine oxidase antagonism. Seizures, tremors, and hyperexcitability were noted in dogs that have been overdosed.[103] Immune-mediated thrombocytopenia was also noted in a dog treated with isoniazid.[70] GI irritation and allergic skin reactions and vasculitis have also been reported in people.

Rifampin

This semisynthetic hydrazone derivative of rifampin B, is a complex macrocyclic antibiotic produced by *Streptomyces mediterranei*. Rifampin interferes with RNA synthesis. It is well absorbed from the GI tract, and because it is lipid-soluble, it is 75% to 90% bound to serum protein. It effectively penetrates all body tissues and exceeds serum levels in the lung, liver, bile, cholecystic wall, and urine. Therapeutic levels of rifampin are attained in pleural exudate, ascites, milk, the urinary bladder wall, soft tissues, and CSF. A major part of the administered dose is metabolized by the liver and excreted in the bile. Only 6% to 30% of the drug appears in the urine.

Rifampin has antibacterial, antichlamydial, and some antiviral activity (see also Reverse Transcriptase Inhibitors, Chapter 15). It is primarily used to treat infections caused by *M. tuberculosis*. It is one of the most active antibiotics against staphylococci and is effective against some gram-negative bacteria. It is frequently useful in combination with β-lactam drugs in the treatment of resistant staphylococcal endocarditis or osteomyelitis. Although ineffective against fungi when used alone, rifampin has been shown to enhance the effect of amphotericin B and miconazole against *Candida*. It has been combined with vancomycin and with cephalosporins to achieve increased efficacy against staphylococci. Rifampin was shown to be superior to tetracycline for treatment of experimental brucellosis in laboratory animals but was not as successful as minocycline in the treatment of canine brucellosis.

Resistance to rifampin, which may develop rapidly when it is used alone, can be prevented by combining it with another drug. Side effects of rifampin therapy include orange-colored urine, tears, saliva, and sweat. Rash, GI complaints, and asymptomatic increases in liver enzymes may be associated with long-term daily use. Many other side effects have been noted at higher dosages. Rifampin accelerates the hepatic metabolism of other drugs and thus reduces the activity of concurrently administered glucocorticoids, digoxin, quinidine, barbiturates, isoniazid, dapsone, and theophylline.

Ethambutol

This tuberculostatic drug interferes with RNA synthesis and is active only against dividing organisms. It is well absorbed from the GI tract and is widely distributed in body tissues, including the CSF. Most of the drug is excreted unmetabolized in the urine; therefore, the dosage must be reduced in patients with renal failure. Its primary toxic effects are optic and peripheral neuritis.

Miscellaneous Drugs

Para-aminosalicylic acid is an analogue of para-aminobenzoic acid that is mycobacteriostatic, interfering with folic acid synthesis. It potentiates the effect of isoniazid by delaying its metabolism. Pyrazinamide, a tuberculostatic drug with an unknown mode of action, is relatively hepatotoxic. Cycloserine inhibits bacterial cell wall synthesis and is excreted primarily by the kidneys. Ethionamide inhibits protein synthesis and has widespread tissue distribution. It is combined in therapy when resistance is found to other drugs. Viomycin, capreomycin, kanamycin, and amikacin have all been shown to be effective against mycobacteria when combined with other drugs. See Chapter 51 for a discussion of tuberculosis in dogs and cats.

AGENTS EFFECTIVE AGAINST ATYPICAL MYCOBACTERIA

Certain antituberculous drugs, such as isoniazid, rifampin, and aminoglycosides, are effective in treating some strains of atypical mycobacteria. Antibiotics, including erythromycin, tetracyclines, and trimethoprim-sulfonamide, have also been successful in some cases, as have drugs used to treat human leprosy.

Dapsone is a sulfone derivative that is bacteriostatic to bactericidal against *Mycobacterium leprae*. It is completely absorbed from the bowel, metabolized in the liver, and primarily eliminated by renal excretion. Toxic effects in dogs have consisted of hemolytic anemia, leukopenia, thrombocytopenia, and increased liver enzyme activities. Acedapsone is another derivative with a longer duration of action. Quinolones and clofazamine are two newer drugs that have been effective in treating atypical mycobacterial infections when other antibacterial agents have failed (see sections on Therapy, Chapter 51).

MUPIROCIN

The major metabolite of *Pseudomonas fluorescens* is a novel antibiotic, unrelated

Table 43–11. Improved Formula for Buffered-EDTA Solution

1. Dissolve 1.2 g of ethylenediaminetetraacetate (EDTA) in 1 L of 0.05 M (6.05 g) tromethamine (hydroxymethyl)aminomethane (TRIS) and 1.9 g/L sodium dodecyl sulfate (SDS)[a]
2. Adjust pH to 8.0 (usually requires concentrated NaOH)
3. Sterilize in autoclave (121° C for 20 min) or filter with 0.22 μm filter
4. Store in sterile bottles at room temperature

[a]SDS is added to improve efficacy.[106]

in structure and action to other antimicrobials. It inhibits bacterial protein synthesis. It has marked bactericidal action against aerobic gram-positive and some gram-negative and anaerobic organisms, especially those associated with skin infections.[104] The drug is available commercially as a topical ointment (2%) in a polyethylene glycol base.[105] The only side effect observed with its use has been a local dermal hypersensitivity reaction at the site of application in some animals.

TOPICAL BUFFERED-EDTA SOLUTION

Many gram-negative bacteria are susceptible to the action of chelating agents such as EDTA. The bactericidal effect appears to occur by means of the removal of cations from the bacterial cell wall, which results in the leakage of cell solutes. Alkaline pH appears to facilitate bactericidal activity. Experimental and clinical research has proved EDTA to be safe when applied topically to animal tissues. Appropriate pH is maintained by combining it with stable amino buffers such as tromethamine (TRIS)-HCl at a pH of 8. Use of this combination (Wooley's solution) is restricted to topical application or irrigation because of the undesirable toxicity that results from removal of blood cations such as calcium and the production of nephrocalcinosis. The buffered-EDTA solution can be made with easily obtainable ingredients (Table 43–11). Modification of the formulation to incorporate sodium dodecyl sulfate (SDS), an ionic detergent, has improved the efficacy of the solution.[106]

Buffered-EDTA solutions have been used alone and in combination with several different antimicrobial agents to treat a variety of resistant bacterial infections in dogs and cats. Therapy with buffered-EDTA solutions has primarily been directed against *Pseudomonas* organisms, which are inherently resistant to many antibacterial drugs. Buffered-EDTA solutions have been combined with lysozyme, gentamicin, and oxytetracycline in an attempt to increase the potency of these antimicrobials and to reduce the incidence of antimicrobial resistance.[107] Buffered-EDTA solutions may work synergistically to increase gram-negative bacterial cell wall permeability, thereby facilitating the penetration and resultant activity of antimicrobial drugs. Overgrowth of fungi may occur during treatment with buffered-EDTA solutions unless additional antimicrobial therapy is used against these organisms. Such overgrowth is a problem when infections are treated in regions of the body that lack a normal competitive microflora, as in the urinary bladder. Repeated catheterization and flushing of these drugs may serve to introduce resistant strains.

References

1. Baggot JD: Factors involved in choice of routes of administration of antimicrobial drugs. *J Am Vet Med Assoc* 185:1076–1082, 1984.
2. Alexander AD, Rule PL: Penicillins, cephalosporins, and tetracyclines in treatment of hamsters with fatal leptospirosis. *Antimicrob Agents Chemother* 30:835–839, 1986.
2a. Cockburn A, Mellows G, Jackson D, et al: Temocillin, summary of safety studies. *Drugs* 5:103–105, 1985.
3. Watson ADJ, Emslie DR, Martin ICA, et al: Effect of ingesta on systemic availability of penicillins administered orally in dogs. *J Vet Pharmacol Ther* 9:140–149, 1986.
4. Currie TT, Hayward NJ, Campbell PC, et al: Epilepsy in dogs caused by large doses of penicillin and concurrent brain damage. *Br J Exp Pathol* 51:492–497, 1970.
5. Fass RJ, Copelan EA, Brandt JT, et al: Platelet-mediated bleeding caused by broad-spectrum penicillins. *J Infect Dis* 155:1242–1248, 1987.
5a. Kita Y, Fugona T, Imada A: Comparative pharmakokinetics of carumonam and aztreonam in mice, rats, rabbits, and cynomologus monkeys. *Antimicrob Agents Chemother* 29:127–134, 1986.
6. Nue HC: Aztreonam: the first monobactam. *Med Clin North Am* 72:555–566, 1988.
7. Donowitz GR, Mandell GL: Drug therapy. Beta-lactam antibiotics, part II. *N Engl J Med* 318:490–500, 1988.
8. Indiveri MC, Hirsh DC: Clavulanic acid-potentiated activity of amoxicillin against *Bacteroides fragilis*. *Am J Vet Res* 46:2207–2209, 1985.
9. Corbel MJ, Ibrahim MEM, Gill KPW: Sensitivity of campylobacter isolates to clavulanate-potentiated amoxycillin. *Vet Rec* 115:465, 1984.
10. Bywater RJ, Palmer GH, Buswell JF, et al: Clavulanate-potentiated amoxycillin: activity in vitro and bioavailability in the dog. *Vet Rec* 116:33–36, 1985.
11. Woodnut G, Kernutt I, Mizen L: Pharmacokinetics and distribution of ticarcillin-clavulanic acid (Timentin) in experimental animals. *Antimicrob Agents Chemother* 31:1826–1830, 1987.
11a. Sparks SE, Jones RL, Kilgore WR: In vitro susceptibility of bacteria to a ticarcillin-clavulanic acid combination. *Am J Vet Res* 49:2038–2040, 1988.
11b. Garg RC, Keefe TJ, Vig MM: Serum levels and pharmacokinetics of ticarcillin and clavulanic acid in a dog following parenteral administration of timentin. *J Vet Pharmacol Ther* 10:324–330, 1987.
12. Senior DF, Gaskin JM, Buergelt CD, et al: Amoxicillin and clavulanic acid combination in treatment of experimentally induced bacterial cystitis in cats. *Res Vet Sci* 39:42–46, 1985.
13. Senior DF, Gaskin JM, Buergelt CD, et al: Amoxicillin and clavulanic acid combination in the treatment of experimentally induced bacterial cystitis in dogs. *J Am Anim Hosp Assoc* 22:227–233, 1986.
14. Bywater RJ, Hewett GR, Marshall AB, et al: Efficacy of clavulanate-potentiated amoxycillin in experimental and clinical skin infections. *Vet Rec* 116:177–179, 1985.
15. Foulds G, McBride TJ, Knirsch AK, et al: Penetration of sulbactam and ampicillin into cerebrospinal fluid of infants and young children with meningitis. *Antimicrob Agents Chemother* 31:1703–1705, 1987.
16. Donowitz GR, Mandell GR: Beta-lactam antibiotics, part I. *N Engl J Med* 318:419–426, 1988.
17. Thomson TD, Quay JF, Webber JA: Cephalosporin group of antimicrobial drugs. *J Am Vet Med Assoc* 185:1109–1114, 1984.
18. Barsanti JA, Chatfield RC, Shotts EB, et al: Efficacy of cefadroxil in experimental canine cystitis. *J Am Anim Hosp Assoc* 21:89–93, 1985.
19. Chatfield RC, Gingerich DA, Rourke JE, et al: Cefadroxil: a new orally effective cephalosporin antibiotic. *VM/SAC* 79:339–346, 1984.
20. Crosse R, Burt DG: Cephelexin: interpretation of sensitivity disks in veterinary practice. *Res Vet Sci* 36:259–262, 1984.
21. Crosse R, Burt DG: Antibiotic concentration in the serum of dogs and cats following a single oral dose of cephalexin. *Vet Rec* 115:106–107, 1984.
22. Silley P, Rudd AP, Symington WM, et al: Pharmacokinetics of cephalexin in dogs and cats after oral, subcutaneous and intramuscular administration. *Vet Rec* 122:15–17, 1988.
23. Pizzo PA, Hathorn JW, Hiemenz J, et al: Randomized trial comparing ceftazidime alone with combination antibiotic therapy in cancer patients with fever and neutropenia. *N Engl J Med* 315:552–558, 1986.
24. Cherubin CE, Eng RH, Smith SM, et al: Cephalosporin therapy for salmonellosis. Questions of efficacy and cross resistance with ampicillin. *Arch Intern Med* 1465:2149–2152, 1986.
25. Guerrini VH, English PB, Filippich LJ, et al: Pharmacokinetics of cefoxamine in the dog. *Vet Rec* 119:81–83, 1986.
26. Guerrini VH, English PB, Filippich LJ, et al: Pharmacokinetic evaluation of a slow-release cefotaxime suspension in the dog and in sheep. *Am J Vet Res* 47:2057–2061, 1986.

27. McElroy D, Ravis WR, Clark CH: Pharmacokinetics of cefotaxime in the domestic cat. Am J Vet Res 47:86–88, 1986.

27a. Fry DE, Trachtenberg L, Polk HC: Serum kinetics of intraperitoneal moxalactam. Arch Surg 121:282–284, 1986.

27b. Rubinstein E, Meissel D, Klein E, et al: Effect of pancreatitis on moxalactam excretion in pancreatic fluids of dogs and man. World J Surg 12:411–414, 1988.

28. Scott DW, Miller WH, Goldschmidt MH: Erythema multiforme in the dog. J Am Anim Hosp Assoc 19:453–459, 1983.

29. Brown RB, Klar J, Lemeshow S, et al: Enhanced bleeding with cefoxitin or moxalactam. Statistical analysis within a defined population of 1493 patients. Arch Intern Med 146:2159–2164, 1986.

30. Barza M, Furie B, Brown AE, et al: Defects in vitamin K dependent carboxylation associated with moxalactam treatment. J Infect Dis 153:1166–1169, 1986.

30a. Deldar A, Lewis H, Bloom J, et al: Cephalosporin-induced changes in ultrastructure of canine bone marrow. Vet Pathol 25:211–218, 1988.

31. Baggot JD: Pharmacokinetics of kanamycin in dogs. J Vet Pharmacol Therap 1:163–170, 1978.

32. Jacobson ER, Groff JM, Gronwall RR, et al: Serum concentrations of gentamicin in cats. Am J Vet Res 46:1356–1358, 1985.

33. Shille VM, Brown MP, Gronwall R, et al: Amikacin sulfate in the cat: serum, urine and uterine tissue concentrations. Theriogenology 23:829–839, 1985.

34. Jernigan AD, Hatch RC, Wilson RC: Pharmacokinetics of tobramycin in cats. Am J Vet Res 49:608–612, 1988.

35. Jernigan AD, Wilson RC, Hatch RC, et al: Pharmacokinetics of gentamicin after intravenous, intramuscular, and subcutaneous administration in cats. Am J Vet Res 49:32–35, 1988

35a. Jernigan AD, Hatch RC, Wilson RC et al: Pharmacokinetics of gentamicin in cats given Escherichia coli endotoxin. Am J Vet Res 49:603–607, 1988.

36. Lee AH, Swaim SF, Yang ST, et al: Effects of gentamicin solution and cream on the healing of open wounds. Am J Vet Res 45:1487–1492, 1984.

36a. Rosin E, Ebert S, Uphoff TS, et al: Penetration of antibiotics into the surgical wound in a canine model. Antimicrob Agents Chemother 33:700–704, 1989.

37. Baggot JD, Ling GV, Chatfield RC: Clinical pharmacokinetics of amikacin in dogs. Am J Vet Res 46:1793–1796, 1985.

38. Amikacin sulfate. Case reports and applied research. Proc Symp, Bristol Veterinary Products, April 3, 1984.

39. Brown SA, Barsanti JA, Crowell WA: Gentamicin-associated acute renal failure in the dog. J Am Vet Med Assoc 186:686–689, 1985.

40. Fraxier DL, Aucoin DP, Riviere JE: Gentamicin pharmacokinetics and nephrotoxicity in naturally acquired and experimentally induced disease in dogs. J Am Vet Med Assoc 192:57–63, 1988.

41. Brown SA, Engelhardt JA: Drug-related nephropathies. Part 1. Mechanisms, diagnosis, and management. Compend Cont Educ Pract Vet 9:148–160, 1987.

42. Jernigan AD, Hatch RC, Brown J, et al: Pharmacokinetic and pathologic evaluation of gentamicin in cats given a small intravenous dose repeatedly for five days. Can J Vet Res 52:177–180, 1988.

43. Benitz AM: Future developments in the aminoglycoside group of antimicrobial drugs. J Am Vet Med Assoc 185:1118–1123, 1984.

44. Jernigan AD, Hatch RC, Wilson RC, et al: Pathologic changes and tissue gentamicin concentrations after intravenous gentamicin administration in clinically normal and endotoxemic cats. Am J Vet Res 49:613–617, 1988.

45. Spreat SR, Van Hoose LM: Tissue concentration in dogs treated with gentamicin. VM/SAC 74:337–341, 1979.

46. Greco DS, Turnwald GH, Adams R, et al: Urinary γ-glutamyl transpeptidase activity in dogs with gentamicin-induced nephrotoxicity. Am J Vet Res 46: 2332–2335, 1985.

47. Hardy ML, Hsu R-C, Short CR: The nephrotoxic potential of gentamicin in the cat: enzymuria and alterations in urine concentrating capability. J Vet Pharmacol Therap 8:382–392, 1985.

47a. Short CR, Hardy ML, Clarke CR, et al: The nephrotoxic potential of gentamicin in the cat: a pharmacokinetic and histopathologic investigation. J Vet Pharmacol Ther 9:325–329, 1986.

47b. Hayashi T, Wantanabe Y, Kumano K, et al: Protective effect of piperacillin against nephrotoxicity of cephaloridine and gentamicin in animals. Antimicrob Agents Chemother 32:912–918, 1988.

48. Raisbeck MF, Hewitt WR, McIntyre WB: Fatal nephrotoxicosis associated with furosemide and gentamicin therapy in a dog. J Am Vet Med Assoc 183:892–893, 1983.

48a. Brown A, Bennett D: Gentamicin-impregnated polymethylmethacrylate beads for the treatment of septic arthritis. Vet Rec 123:625–626, 1988.

49. Webster JC, Carroll R, Benitez JT, et al: Ototoxicity of topical gentamicin in the cat. J Infect Dis 124 (Suppl):S138–S144, 1971.

49a. Conzelman GM: Pharmacotherapeutics of aminoglycoside antibiotics. J Am Vet Med Assoc 176:1078–1080, 1980.

50. McCormick GC, Weinberg E, Szot RJ, et al: Comparative ototoxicity of netilmicin, gentamicin, and tobramycin in cats. Toxicol Appl Pharmacol 77:479–489, 1985.

51. Dudley MN, McLaughlin JC, Carrington G, et al: Oral bacitracin vs vancomycin therapy for Clostridium difficile–induced diarrhea. A randomized double-blind trial. Arch Intern Med 146:1101–1104, 1986.

52. Sogaard H: The pharmacodynamics of polymyxin antibiotics with special reference to drug resistance liability. J Vet Pharm Therap 5:219–231, 1982.

53. Knifton A: The responsible use of chloramphenicol in small animal practice. 1. Pharmacological considerations. J Small Anim Pract 28:537–542, 1987.

54. Watson ADJ: Effect of ingesta on systemic availability of chloramphenicol from two oral preparations in cats. J Vet Pharm Therap 2:117–121,1979.

55. Shann F, Linnemann V, Mackenzie A, et al: Absorption of chloramphenicol sodium succinate after intramuscular administration in children. N Engl J Med 313:410–414, 1985.

56. Harper RC: The responsible use of chloramphenicol in small animal practice. 2. Clinical considerations. J Small Anim Pract 28:543–547, 1987.

57. Watson ADJ: Further observations on chloram-

phenicol toxicosis in cats. *Am J Vet Res* 41:293–294, 1980.

58. Nara PL, Davis LE, Laverman LH, et al: Effects of chloramphenicol on the development of immune responses to canine distemper virus in Beagle pups. *J Vet Pharmacol Therap* 5:177–185, 1982.

59. Campbell CL: Primidone intoxication associated with concurrent use of chloramphenicol. *J Am Vet Med Assoc* 182:992–993, 1983.

60. Stowe CM: Antimicrobial drug interactions. *J Am Vet Med Assoc* 185:1137–1141, 1984.

61. Ling GV, Creighton SR, Ruby AL: Tetracycline for oral treatment of canine urinary tract infection caused by *Pseudomonas aeruginosa*. *J Am Vet Med Assoc* 179:578–579, 1981.

62. Shaw DH, Rubin SI: Pharmacologic activity of doxycycline. *J Am Vet Med Assoc* 189:808–810, 1986.

63. Barza M, Brown RB, Shanks C, et al: Relation between lipophilicity and pharmacological behavior of minocycline, doxycycline, tetracycline, and oxytetracycline in dogs. *Antimicrob Agents Chemother* 8:713–720, 1975.

64. Amendola MA, Spera TD: Doxycycline-induced esophagitis. *JAMA* 253:1009–1011, 1985.

65. Sedwitz J, Bateman JC, Klopp CT: Oxytetracycline toxicity studies in dogs. *Antibiot Chemother* 3:1015–1019, 1953.

65a. English PB: Antimicrobial chemotherapy in the dog. III. Possible adverse reactions. *J Small Anim Pract* 24:423–436, 1983.

66. Stevenson S: Oxytetracycline nephrotoxicosis in two dogs. *J Am Vet Med Assoc* 176:530–531, 1980.

67. Benitz KF, Diermeier HF: Renal toxicity of tetracycline degradation products. *Proc Soc Exp Biol Med* 115:930–935, 1964.

68. Brunson DB, Stowe CM, McGrath CJ: Serum and urine inorganic fluoride concentrations and urine oxalate concentrations following methoxyflurane anesthesia in the dog. *Am J Vet Res* 40:197–203, 1979.

69. Wilson RC, Kitzman JV, Kemp DT, et al: Compartmental and noncompartmental pharmacokinetic analyses of minocycline hydrochloride in the dog. *Am J Vet Res* 46:1316–1318, 1985.

69a. Noble JF, Kanegis LA, Hallesy DW: Short-term toxicity and observations on certain aspects of the pharmacology of a unique tetracycline-minocycline. *Toxicol Appl Pharmacol* 11:128–149, 1967.

70. Davis L: Hypersensitivity reactions induced by antimicrobial drugs. *J Am Vet Med Assoc* 185:1131–1136, 1984.

71. Wilson RC, Kemp DT, Kitzman JV, et al: Pharmacokinetics of doxycycline in dogs. *Can J Vet Res* 52:12–14, 1988.

72. Wilson RC: Macrolides in veterinary practice. *In* Omura S (ed): *Macrolide Antibiotics: Chemistry, Biology, and Practice*. Orlando, Academic Press, 1984, pp 301–347.

73. Berg JN, Scanlan CM, Buening GM, et al: Clinical models for anaerobic bacterial infections in dogs and their use in testing the efficacy of clindamycin and lincomycin. *Am J Vet Res* 45:1299–1306, 1984.

74. Braden TD, Johnson CA, Gabel CL, et al: Posologic evaluation of clindamycin, using a canine model of posttraumatic osteomyelitis. *Am J Vet Res* 48:1101–1105, 1987.

74a. Jacobs G, Lappin M, Marks A, et al: Effects of clindamycin on factor VIII activity in healthy cats. *Am J Vet Res* 50:393–395, 1989.

74b. Brown SA, Dieringer JM, Hunter RP, et al: Oral clindamycin disposition after single and multiple doses in normal cats. *J Vet Pharmacol* 12:209–216, 1989.

75. Greene CE: Unpublished observations. University of Georgia, Athens, GA, 1988.

76. Morgan RV, Bachrach A: Keratoconjunctivitis sicca associated with sulfonamide therapy in dogs. *J Am Vet Med Assoc* 180:432–434, 1982.

76a. Sansom J, Barnett KC, Long RD: Keratoconjunctivitis sicca in the dog associated with the administration of salicylazosulphapyridine (sulphasalazine). *Vet Rec* 116:391–393, 1985.

77. Indiveri MC, Hirsh DC: Susceptibility of obligate anaerobes to trimethoprim-sulfamethoxazole. *J Am Vet Med Assoc* 188:46–48, 1986.

78. Levitz RE, Quintiliani R: Trimethoprim-sulfamethoxazole for bacterial meningitis. *Ann Intern Med* 100:881–890, 1984.

79. Turnwald GH, Gossett KA, Cox HU, et al: Comparison of single-dose and conventional trimethoprim-sulfadiazine therapy in experimental *Staphylococcus intermedius* cystitis in the female dog. *Am J Vet Res* 47:2621–2623, 1986.

80. Rogers KS, Lees GE, Simpson RB: Effects of single-dose and three-day trimethoprim-sulfadiazine and amikacin treatment of induced *Escherichia coli* urinary tract infection in dogs. *Am J Vet Res* 49:345–349, 1988.

81. Thies PW, Dull WL: Trimethoprim-sulfamethoxazole–induced cholestatic hepatitis. *Arch Intern Med* 144:1691–1692, 1984.

82. Anderson WI, Campbell KL, Wilson RC, et al: Hepatitis in a dog given sulfadiazine-trimethoprim and cyclophosphamide. *Mod Vet Pract* 65:115, 1984.

83. Weiss DJ, Adams LG: Aplastic anemia associated with trimethoprim-sulfadiazine and fenbendazole administration in a dog. *J Am Vet Med Assoc* 191:1119–1120, 1987.

84. Giger U, Werner LL, Millichamp NJ, et al: Sulfadiazine-induced allergy in six Doberman pinschers. *J Am Vet Med Assoc* 186:479–484, 1985.

85. Werner LL, Bright JM: Drug-induced immune hypersensitivity disorders in two dogs treated with trimethoprim-sulfadiazine: case reports and drug challenge studies. *J Am Anim Hosp Assoc* 19:783–790, 1983.

86. Whur P: Possible trimethoprim-sulphonamide–induced polyarthritis. *Vet Rec* 121:91–92, 1987.

87. Grondalen J: Trimethoprim-sulphonamide–induced polyarthritis. *Vet Rec* 121:155, 1987.

88. Scott DW, Smith FWK, Smith CA: Erythema multiforme and pemphigus-like antibodies associated with sulfamethoxazole-trimethoprim administration in a dog with polycystic kidneys. *Canine Pract* 13:35–38, 1986.

89. Derbes SJ: Trimethoprim-induced aseptic meningitis. *JAMA* 252:2865–2866, 1984.

90. Kinzie BJ, Taylor JW: Trimethoprim and folinic acid. *Ann Intern Med* 101:565, 1984.

91. Hollander H: Leukopenia, trimethoprim-sulfamethoxazole, and folinic acid. *Ann Intern Med* 102:138, 1985.

92. Luft BJ, Stemberg S, Frankel R: The effect of folic and folinic acid on the antitoxoplasma activity of pyrimethamine and sulfadiazine. Abstr 28th Intersci Conf Antimicrob Agents Chemother, 1988, p 330.

92a. Parpia SH, Nix DE, Hejmanowski LG, et al: Sucralfate reduces the gastrointestinal absorption of norfloxacin. *Antimicrob Agents Chemother* 33:99–102, 1989.

93. Walker RD, Stein GE, Budsberg SC, et al: Norfloxacin serum and tissue concentrations after oral administration in healthy dogs. *Am J Vet Res* 50:154–157, 1989.
94. Walker RD, Stein GE, Budsberg SC, et al: Serum and tissue concentrations of ciprofloxacin in the dog. Abstr 69th Conf Res Workers Anim Dis, Chicago, November 1988.
95. Bauditz R: Results of clinical studies with Baytril in dogs and cats. *Vet Med Rev* 2:137–140, 1987.
96. Tho TV, Armengavd A, Davet B: Diffusion of enoxacin into the cerebrospinal fluid in dogs with healthy meninges and with experimental meningitis. *J Antimicrob Chemother* 14(Suppl C):57–62, 1984.
97. Jensen KM, Madsen PO: Distribution of quinolone carboxylic acid derivatives in the dog prostate. *Prostate* 4:407–414, 1983.
97a. Gasser TC, Graversen PH, Madsen PO: Fleroxacin distribution in canine prostatic tissue and fluids. *Antimicrob Agents Chemother* 31:1010–1013, 1987.
97b. Gasser TC, Graversen PH, Larsen EH, et al: Quinolone penetration into canine vaginal and urethral secretions. *Scand J Urol Nephrol Suppl* 104:101–105, 1987.
98. Scheer M: Concentrations of active ingredient in the serum and in tissues after oral and parenteral administration of Baytril. *Vet Med Rev* 2:104–118, 1987.
99. Scully BE, Neu HC, Parry MF, et al: Oral ciprofloxacin therapy of infecions due to *Pseudomonas aeruginosa. Lancet* 1:819–822, 1986.
99a. Desgrandchamps D, Munzinger J: Increasing rates of in vitro resistance to ciprofloxacin and norfloxacin in isolates from urine specimens. *Antimicrob Agents Chemother* 33:595–596, 1989.
100. Neu HC: Quinolones: a new class of antimicrobial agents with wide potential uses. *Med Clin North Am* 72:623–636, 1988.
101. Schluter G: Ciprofloxacin: review of potential toxicologic effects. *Am J Med* 82 (Suppl 4A):91–93, 1987.
101a. Christ W, Lehnert T, Ulbrich B: Specific toxic aspects of the quinolones. *Rev Infect Dis* 10(Suppl):S141–S146, 1988.
101b. Baytril, Professional Services Bulletin, Mobay Corp, Animal Health Division, Shawnee, KS, 1989.
102. Murakawa T, Sakamoto H, Fukada S, et al: Pharmacokinetics of fosmidomycin, a new phosphonic acid antibiotic. *Antimicrob Agents Chemother* 21:224–230, 1982.
103. Doherty T: Isoniazid poisoning in a dog. *Vet Rec* 111:460–461, 1982.
104. Hill R, Casewell T, Ware R: Reduction in bacterial contamination of internal jugular cannulae by the local application of calcium mupirocin—a controlled trial. Conf Curr Exp Beta-Lactamase Inhibition. Taormina, Italy, May 1988.
105. Bactoderm (Mupirocin) Veterinary Ointment, Product Information, Beecham Laboratories, Bristol, TN, 1988.
106. Wooley RE, Dickerson HW, Engen WR: Treatment of otitis externa in dogs by EDTA-tris-SDS lavage. *Vet Med* 83:1088–1091, 1988.
107. Wooley RE, Jones MS, Gilbert JD, et al: In vitro action of combinations of antimicrobial agents with EDTA-tromethamine on *Proteus vulgaris* of a canine origin. *Am J Vet Res* 45:1451–1454, 1984.

44

ENDOTOXEMIA
Elizabeth M. Hardie

ETIOLOGY

Endotoxemia is the presence of endotoxin, a lipopolysaccharide released from the cell wall of gram-negative bacteria, in the blood-stream of the host. Endotoxemia occurs with gram-negative bacterial infections, particularly during surgical manipulation of infected tissue. Large amounts of endotoxin may also be released from the intestine when mucosal integrity is compromised in diseases such as gastric dilation-volvulus[1] or hemorrhagic diarrhea.[2]

Endotoxemia rapidly results in shock, owing to generalized activation of inflammatory mediators that are normally localized to the site of infection. Cytokines, products of stimulated macrophages such as tumor necrosis factor (TNF, cachectin) that are released in response to circulating endotoxin, are now thought to be central mediators of the host response to bacterial infection.[3] TNF probably mediates cellular injury through stimulation of the cyclooxygenase pathway. The dog and cat have species-specific responses to endotoxemia. The dog develops portal hypertension, resulting in GI congestion and edema. Cardiac output drops rapidly owing to lack of venous return. The cat develops pulmonary hypertension and bronchoconstriction, resulting in acute respiratory failure. As shock progresses in both species, compromised vascular integrity, myocardial failure, generalized hypotension, DIC, and hypoglycemia develop.

CLINICAL FINDINGS

Initially, endotoxemia is characterized by fever, chills, tachypnea, tachycardia, and hypotension. Mucous membranes are congested, and the pulse is usually rapid and thready. The extremities may be cool owing to peripheral vasoconstriction or warm and congested owing to vasodilation, depending on how rapidly endotoxin is being released. Dogs develop mucoid bloody diarrhea, whereas cats may show acute respiratory distress and pulmonary edema. Oliguria usually develops as shock progresses.

Signs of hemorrhagic diathesis such as excessive bleeding from venipuncture sites or petechiae may also be present as a result of DIC. Death occurs due to cardiovascular collapse.

DIAGNOSIS

Thrombocytopenia is the most consistent hematologic finding in endotoxemia. Leukopenia is present early, but leukocytosis develops later in the course of endotoxemia. Relative polycythemia, hypoglycemia, hypoalbuminemia, increased liver enzyme activities, bilirubinemia, and azotemia may be present. Urinary concentrating ability is usually impaired. Metabolic acidosis with respiratory compensation develops in dogs, whereas cats develop severe metabolic acidosis and hypoxemia. Increased clotting times and fibrin degradation products may be present.

THERAPY

A summary of the dosage recommendations for treating septic shock are listed in Table 44–1.[4–15] Guidelines for their use are discussed below.

Fluids

Maintenance of the circulating blood volume of animals in endotoxic shock is critical. Although only a few studies have been

Table 44–1. Dosages of IV Drugs used to Treat Endotoxemia in Dogs and Cats

DRUG	DOSE	FREQUENCY
Colloids		
Plasma[4]	7 ml/kg	Hourly rate for 3 hr (maximum 20 ml/kg/24 hr)
Dextran 40 (10%)[5]	0.5–1.5 ml/kg	Hourly rate for maximum 15 ml/kg/24 hr
Crystalloids		
Lactated Ringer's[6]	10–12 ml/kg	Hourly rate
Glucose-insulin-potassium solution[7]	3 g glucose, 1–2 U insulin, 0.5 mEq/kg potassium	Add to 250 ml lactated Ringer's (10% volume bolus, 90% infused over 4.5 hr)
Hypertonic saline[8]	12 ml/kg	Infused over 4.5 hr
Glucocorticoids		
Methylprednisolone succinate[9, 10]	30 mg/kg	Once, early in shock
	10 mg/kg	3–4 times every 2 hr
Dexamethasone sodium phosphate[9]	3 mg/kg	Once, early in shock
Prostaglandin Inhibitors		
Flunixin meglumine[11]	1.1 mg/kg	Twice, 3–12 hr interval
Antimicrobials		
Gentamicin	2–4 mg/kg	Every 6 hr[a], potentially nephrotoxic
Chloramphenicol	50 mg/kg	Every 8 hr[a]
Cephalothin	20–30 mg/kg	Every 6 hr[a]
Ampicillin	20 mg/kg	Every 6–8 hr[a]
Cardiovascular Support Drugs		
Naloxone[12]	2.0–2.5 mg/kg	Hourly rate for 4 hr
Sodium nitroprusside[13]	20 g/kg	Rate/minute
Phenoxybenzamine[14]	1 mg/kg	Over 2 hr
Dopamine[15]	5–10 μg/kg	Rate/minute
Dolbutamine[15]	5–20 μg/kg	Rate/minute

[a]Bolus or continuous intravenous infusion.

conducted to determine the fluids of choice, those studies indicate that colloids are preferable to crystalloids.[4,6] Plasma, 3% albumin, or 10% Dextran 40 solutions have been shown to increase survival during endotoxemia. Colloid therapy should be initiated prior to the development of profound hypoproteinemia, as this condition is extremely difficult to reverse once it develops.

Hyperosmolar glucose or saline solutions have been shown to have beneficial effects during endotoxemia.[7,8] Improved cardiovascular status and increased tissue oxygen consumption result when endotoxic dogs are resuscitated with hypertonic rather than isotonic saline solutions, but the effect on survival remains to be determined. Hypertonic glucose, potassium, and insulin mixtures have been shown to improve both cardiovascular status and survival.

Glucocorticoids

Methylprednisolone sodium succinate improves survival in specific canine shock models such as slow IV endotoxin infusion or IV infusion of *Escherichia coli* but does not improve survival when endotoxin is administered in a bolus IV injection.[9, 16] Treatment can only be delayed 15 minutes in the dog compared to 2 hours in the primate.[17]

Prostaglandin and Leukotriene Inhibitors

Abundant evidence suggests that prostaglandin inhibitors block the early cardiovascular and respiratory effects of endotoxin. Aspirin, indomethacin, or ibuprofen pretreatment improves survival in dogs,[18, 18a] but effects of treatment on survival after endotoxin administration are not well documented. Flunixin meglumine has had benefit when given early.[11] Ibuprofen has been tested in several studies and definitely does *not* improve survival in canine endotoxic shock.[10, 19] Benoxaprofen, a prostaglandin and leukotriene inhibitor, has been shown to improve survival during canine endotoxemia, and treatment could be delayed up to 2 hours.[20]

Antimicrobial Therapy

Endotoxemia in the dog and cat usually occurs secondary to severe gram-negative infection; thus antimicrobial therapy should be instituted at once. Gentamicin sulfate, the drug of choice, has beneficial effects on survival beyond its action as an antibiotic.[21] There is evidence that endotoxin liberation during therapy for gram-negative sepsis is greater with bactericidal antibiotics such as gentamicin or moxalactam as compared with antibiotics such as chloramphenicol.[21a] Nevertheless, bactericidal antibiotics may be preferred because they more rapidly kill intravascular bacteria and their extravascular source of seeding than their bacteriostatic counterparts.[21a]

Combination Therapy

Multiple drug therapy results in improved survival compared with use of single agents. Improved long-term survival in canine sepsis or endotoxemia has been achieved with methylprednisolone combined with gentamicin or ibuprofen or methylprednisolone combined with ibuprofen and naloxone.[10,16] Naloxone therapy is controversial since it only has been beneficial in canine endotoxic shock. Combinations of steroids and nonsteroidal anti-inflammatory drugs have a high risk of causing GI perforation in the dog and should be used with caution.[22] Agents such as nitroprusside or phenoxybenzamine have been used to overcome peripheral vasoconstriction, but they can cause severe hypotension when used inappropriately or without careful monitoring of blood pressure.

Other Drugs

The two major experimental approaches toward endotoxin therapy are to block the action of endotoxin with antitoxin or endotoxin analogs and to block the actions of the inflammatory mediators. Compounds under investigation include phospholipase inhibitors, platelet-activating factor inhibitors, tumor necrosis factor (TNF) inhibitors, oxygen-radical production inhibitors, oxygen-

radical trappers, antiproteases, calcium antagonists, glucagon, and anti-thrombin III. There have also been benefits in treatment of dogs with gram-negative sepsis or pyometra with antiendotoxin immunotherapy.[2, 23] Until the diverse effects of endotoxin are better characterized, firm recommendations as to therapy with these newer agents cannot be given.

References

1. Fessler JF, Bottoms GD: Plasma endotoxin concentrations in experimental and clinical equine and canine subjects. Vet Surg 17:32, 1988.
2. Wessels BC, Gaffin SL, Wells MT: Circulating plasma endotoxin (lipopolysaccharide) concentrations in healthy and hemorrhagic enteric dogs: antiendotoxin immunotherapy in hemorrhagic enteric endotoxemia. J Am Anim Hosp Assoc 23:291–295, 1987.
3. Michie HR, Manogue KR, Spriggs DR, et al: Detection of circulating tumor necrosis factor after endotoxin administration. N Engl J Med 318:1481–1486, 1988.
4. Walker RI, French JE, Walden DA, et al: Protection of dogs from lethal consequences of endotoxemia with plasma infusions. Circ Shock 6:190, 1979.
5. Donaldson LA, Williams RW, Worthington GS: Experimental pancreatitis: effect of plasma and dextran on pancreatic blood flow. Surgery 84:313–321, 1978.
6. Davidson I, Ottosson J, Reisch JS: Infusion volumes of Ringer's lactate and 3% albumin solution as they relate to survival after resuscitation of a lethal intestinal ischemic shock. Circ Shock 18:277–288, 1986.
7. Manny J, Rabinovici N, Manny N, et al: Effect of glucose-insulin-potassium on survival in experimental endotoxic shock. Surg Gynecol Obstet 147:405–409, 1978.
8. Luypaert P, Vincent J-L, Domb M, et al: Fluid resuscitation with hypertonic saline in endotoxic shock. Circ Shock 20:311–320, 1986.
9. White GL, Archer LT, Beller BK, et al: Increased survival with methylprednisolone treatment in canine endotoxin shock. J Surg Res 25: 357–364, 1978.
10. Almqvist PM, Ekstrom B, Kuenzig M, et al: Increased survival of endotoxin-injected dogs treated with methylprednisolone, naloxone, and ibuprofen. Circ Shock 14:129–136, 1984.
11. Hardie EM, Rawlings CA, Collins LG: Canine Escherichia coli peritonitis: long-term survival with fluid, gentamicin sulfate, and flunixin meglumine treatment. J Am Anim Hosp Assoc 21:691–699, 1985.
12. Cronenvett JL, Baver-Neff BS, Grekin RJ, et al: The role of endorphins and vasopressin in canine endotoxin shock. J Surg Res 41:609–619, 1986.
13. McIntosh JJ: The use of vasodilators in treatment of congestive heart failure: a review. J Am Anim Hosp Assoc 17:255–260, 1981.
14. Anderson RW, James PM, Bredenberg CE: Phenoxybenzamine in septic shock. Ann Surg 165:341–350, 1967.

15. Disesa VJ, Modge GH, Cohn LH: Hemodynamic comparison of dopamine and dolbutamine in the postoperative volume-loaded, pressure-loaded, and normal ventricle. *J Thorac Cardiovasc Surg* 83:256–263, 1982.

16. Hinshaw LB, Bellar BK, Archer LT, et al: Recovery from lethal *Escherichia coli* shock in dogs. *Surg Gynecol Obstet* 149:545–553, 1978.

17. Hinshaw LB, Bellar-Todd BK, Archer LT: Current management of the septic shock patient: experimental basis for treatment. *Circ Shock* 9:543–553, 1982.

18. Erdos EG: Effect of nonsteroidal anti-inflammatory drugs in endotoxin shock. *Biochem Pharmacol* 17(suppl):283–291, 1968.

18a. Hubbard JD, Jansen HF: Increased microvascular permeability in canine endotoxic shock: protective effects of ibuprofen. *Circ Shock* 26:169–183, 1988.

19. Beck RS, Abel FL: Effect of ibuprofen on the course of canine endotoxin shock. *Circ Shock* 23:59–70, 1987.

20. Toth PD, Hamburger SA, Hastings GH, et al: Benoxaprofen attenuation of lethal canine endotoxic shock. *Circ Shock* 15:89–103, 1985.

21. Bosson S, Kuenzig M, Schwartz S: Increased survival with calcium antagonists in antibiotic-treated bacteremia. *Circ Shock* 19:69–74, 1986.

21a. Shenep JL, Barton RP, Mogan KA: Role of antibiotic class in the rate of liberation of endotoxin during therapy for experimental gram-negative bacterial sepsis. *J Infect Dis* 151:1-12–1018, 1985.

22. Dow S: Unpublished observations. Colorado State University, Fort Collins, CO, 1987.

23. Wessels BC, Wells MT: Antiendotoxin immunotherapy for canine pyometra endotoxemia. *J Am Anim Hosp Assoc* 25:455–460, 1989.

45 LEPTOSPIROSIS

Craig E. Greene
Emmett B. Shotts

ETIOLOGY

Leptospirosis, a zoonotic disease of worldwide significance in many animals, is caused by infection with antigenically distinct serovars of *Leptospira interrogans*. They are maintained in nature by numerous wild and domestic animal reservoir hosts (Table 45–1). These hosts serve as a potential source of infection for humans and other accidental hosts.

Leptospires are thin, flexible, filamentous bacteria (0.1 to 0.2 μm wide by 6 to 12 μm long) made up of fine spirals with hook-shaped ends (Fig. 45–1). They are composed of a protoplasmic cylinder that is wound around a straight central axial filament. The outer envelope is composed of antigenic mucopeptide. They are motile, making writhing and flexing movements while rotating along their long axis.

L. icterohaemorrhagiae, *L. canicola*, and *L. grippotyphosa* are the most common serovars isolated from dogs with leptospirosis. Despite the widespread presence of increased antibody titers in the feline population, clinical reports of leptospirosis are infrequent. Cats appear to be less affected than dogs in both spontaneous and experimental infections.[2,3]

Leptospires are transmitted between animals by direct contact, venereal and placental transfer, bite wounds, or ingestion of infected meat. Spread of infection is enhanced by crowding of animals. Recovered dogs excrete organisms in urine intermittently for months to years following infection. Indirect transmission occurs through exposure of susceptible animals to contaminated vegetation and soil, food and water, bedding, and other fomites. Spirochetes survive in insects and other invertebrate hosts, but the role of these vectors in transmission is uncertain.

Stagnant or slow-moving warm water, while not essential, provides a suitable habitat for spirochetes in the environment. Disease outbreaks increase during periods of flooding. In arid areas, infections of accidental hosts are more common around water sources. Spirochetes survive only transiently in acid urine (pH, 5.0 to 5.5) or frozen water. Optimum survival in soil is favored by neutral or slightly alkaline pH. Optimal ambient temperatures for survival and replication of leptospires are between 0° to 25°C. A higher seasonal incidence of the disease is noted in summer and early fall, and more cases occur in the southern semitropical belt of the United States and similar climatic regions worldwide.

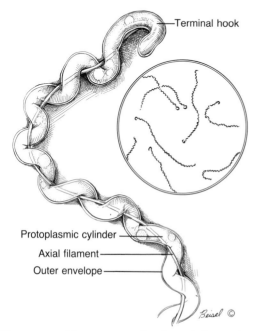

Terminal hook

Protoplasmic cylinder

Axial filament

Outer envelope

Beisel ©

Figure 45–1. Ultrastructure of pathogenic leptospires.

Table 45–1. Range for Common Serovars of Leptospira Interrogans Infecting Dogs or Cats

SEROVAR	KNOWN PRIMARY RESERVOIR HOSTS	INCIDENTAL HOSTS				
		Dog	Cat	Human	Other Domesticated Animals	Representative Wild Animals
Australis	Rat	+	–	+	Cow, horse	Mouse, raccoon, opossum, hedgehog, vole, fox, skunk, bandicoot, weasel, nutria
Autumnalis	Mouse	+	–	+	Cow	Rat, raccoon, opossum, bandicoot
Bataviae	Dog, rat, mouse	+	+	+	Cow	Hedgehog, vole, armadillo, bandicoot, shrew, leopard cat
Canicola	Dog	+	+	+	Cow, horse, pig	Rat, raccoon, hedgehog, armadillo, mongoose, bandicoot, nutria, vole, jackal, skunk
Grippotyphosa	Vole	+	+	+	Cow, pig, sheep, goat, rabbit, gerbil, cavy	Mouse, rat, raccoon, opossum, fox, bandicoot, squirrel, bobcat, skunk, shrew, hedgehog, muskrat, weasel, mole, leopard cat
Icterohaemorrhagiae	Rat	+	–	+	Cow, horse, pig, cavy	Mouse, raccoon, opossum, hedgehog, fox, woodchuck, nutria, ape, skunk, civet, muskrat, mongoose
Pomona	Cow, pig	+	+	+	Horse, sheep, goat, rabbit, cavy	Mouse, raccoon, opossum, hedgehog, wolf, fox, woodchuck, vole, sea lion, deer, civet

Modified from Alexander AD: Leptospira. In Braude AL (ed): *Microbiology*, ed 2. Philadelphia, WB Saunders Co, 1986, p 384.

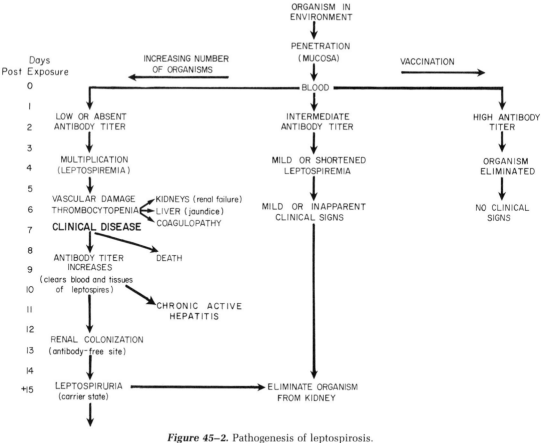

Figure 45–2. Pathogenesis of leptospirosis.

PATHOGENESIS

Leptospires penetrate mucous membranes or abraded skin and multiply rapidly upon entering the blood vascular space (Fig.45–2). The extent of damage to internal organs is variable, depending on the virulence of the organism and host susceptibility. Certain serovars are more pathogenic for particular hosts. For example in dogs, *L. canicola* and *L. icterohaemorrhagiae* produce illness, whereas *L. pomona* causes subclinical disease. Eventual recovery is dependent on increased specific antibody in the circulation within 7 to 8 days following infection.

Renal colonization occurs in most infected animals because the organism replicates and persists in renal tubular epithelial cells, even in the presence of serum-neutralizing antibodies (Fig. 45–3). Acute impairment of renal function may result from decreased glomerular filtration caused by interstitial swelling and decreased renal perfusion (Fig. 45–4). Those animals with adequate functional kidney tissue remaining will recover.

Pathologic changes will persist in the severely affected kidney despite clinical improvement (Fig. 45–5). In surviving reservoir hosts, renal colonization will be long-term, with shedding in urine.

The liver is the second major parenchymatous organ damaged during leptospiremia. Profound hepatic dysfunction may occur without major histologic changes because of subcellular damage produced by leptospiral toxins. The degree of icterus in both canine and human leptospirosis usually corresponds to the severity of hepatic necrosis. In contrast, icterus, hemoglobinemia, and hemoglobinuria that develop in cattle with leptospirosis result from a serovar-specific hemolytic toxin produced by *L. pomona*.

Chronic active hepatitis has been a sequela to *L. grippotyphosa* infection in dogs.[4] Presumably, initial hepatocellular injury and persistence of the organism in the liver result in altered hepatic circulation, fibrosis, and immunologic disturbances that perpetuate the chronic inflammatory response. Exten-

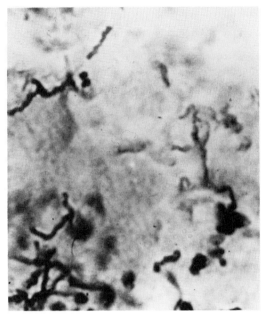

Figure 45–3. Leptospires in renal tubular epithelium from an infected dog (silver stain; × 1800).

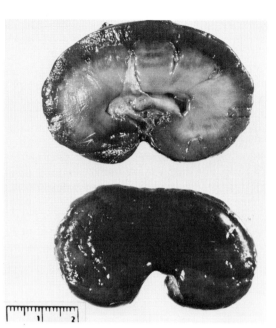

Figure 45–5. Shrunken and fibrotic kidneys from an 8-month-old puppy that had acute icterus and renal failure; the illness had been diagnosed as leptospirosis by serologic testing 5 months previously. The dog was clinically normal until the time of death.

sive hepatic fibrosis and failure may result from this process.

Other body systems are damaged during the acute phase of infection. A benign meningitis is produced when leptospires invade the nervous system. Uveitis occasionally occurs in clinical and experimental leptospirosis and results from an immunologic reaction in the eye (see Chapter 13). Abortion or infertility due to transplacental transmission of leptospires has occurred in a dog associated with *L. bataviae* infection.[5]

CLINICAL FINDINGS

Clinical signs in canine leptospirosis depend on age and immunity of the host,

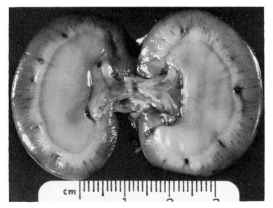

Figure 45–4. Swollen kidney from a dog that died of acute leptospirosis.

environmental factors affecting the organisms, and virulence of the infecting serovar. Peracute leptospiral infections are manifested by massive leptospiremia and death. Pyrexia (39.5° to 40°C [103° to 104°F]), shivering, and generalized muscle tenderness are the first clinical signs. Subsequently, vomiting, rapid dehydration, and peripheral vascular collapse occur. Tachypnea, rapid and irregular pulse, and poor capillary perfusion have been noted. Coagulation defects and vascular injury are apparent with hematemesis, hematochezia, melena, epistaxis, and widespread petechiae. Terminally ill dogs become depressed and hypothermic, and renal and hepatic failure do not have time to develop.

Subacute infections are characterized by fever, anorexia, vomiting, dehydration, and increased thirst. Reluctance to move and paraspinal hyperesthesia in dogs may result from muscular, meningeal, or renal inflammation. Mucous membranes appear injected, and petechial and ecchymotic hemorrhages are widespread. Conjunctivitis, rhinitis, and tonsillitis are usually accompanied by coughing and dyspnea. Progressive deterioration in renal function is manifested by oliguria or anuria. Renal function in dogs surviving subacute infections may return to normal within 2 to 3 weeks or chronic compensated polyuric renal failure may develop.

Icterus is more common in dogs affected with the subacute form of the disease. Intrahepatic cholestasis from hepatic inflammation may be so complete that fecal color changes from brown to gray. Dogs with chronic active hepatitis or chronic hepatic fibrosis as a sequela to leptospirosis may demonstrate overt signs of liver failure, including chronic inappetence, weight loss, ascites, icterus, or hepatoencephalopathy.

Intestinal intussusceptions occur with some frequency in dogs with subacute infections. Careful abdominal palpation should be performed in dogs that develop persistent vomiting and diarrhea. Feces becomes scanty in such cases, and hematochezia or melena will be apparent.

A majority of leptospiral infections in dogs are chronic or subclinical. Serologic and microbiologic evaluation for leptospirosis should be performed on dogs with fever of unknown origin or unexplained anterior uveitis. Clinical signs are usually mild or inapparent in feline leptospirosis despite the presence of leptospiremia and leptospiruria and histologic evidence of renal and hepatic inflammation.[2]

DIAGNOSIS

Clinical Laboratory Findings

Hematologic findings in typical cases of canine leptospirosis include leukocytosis and thrombocytopenia. Leukocyte counts fluctuate, depending on the stage and severity of infection. Leukopenia, common in the leptospiremic phase, develops into leukocytosis with a left shift. Marked increases in erythrocyte sedimentation rate correspond with hyperfibrinogenemia and hyperglobulinemia.

BUN and creatinine increases are found in dogs with varying severity of renal failure. Electrolyte alterations usually parallel the degree of renal and gastrointestinal dysfunction.[6] Hyponatremia, hypochloremia, hypokalemia, and hyperphosphatemia are present in most cases, whereas hyperkalemia and hyperglycemia develop in those with terminal renal failure. Mild hypocalcemia relates to hypoalbuminemia and decreased concentration of the protein-bound calcium fraction. Blood pH and serum bicarbonate con-

centration are reduced in severely affected animals, reflecting metabolic acidosis. Hypoglycemia is occasionally present with severe hepatic failure. Liver damage is demonstrated by increased serum ALT (formerly SGPT), AST (formerly SGOT), serum lactic dehydrogenase, and serum ALP activities and bilirubin concentration. Marked bilirubinuria usually precedes hyperbilirubinemia. Bilirubin in serum is primarily conjugated and peaks by days 6 to 8 following the onset of disease. Increased sulfobromophthalein retention (>5%) can be found in acute leptospirosis prior to the onset of icterus[7] and in dogs that later develop chronic active hepatitis.[4] Increased serum amylase concentration without corresponding changes in serum lipase reflects release from hepatic and small intestinal sources and decreased renal function. Dogs with intussusception have the highest serum amylase concentrations. Serum creatine phosphokinase activity is increased when skeletal muscle inflammation occurs. Urinalysis is characterized by proteinuria and bilirubinuria by increased numbers of granular casts, leukocytes, and erythrocytes in the sediment.

Thrombocytopenia and increased fibrin(ogen) degradation products recently have been found in dogs experimentally infected with *L. icterohaemorrhagiae*.[8] In a majority of dogs, other clotting parameters are normal, suggesting compensated hemostatic mechanisms. Severely affected dogs frequently have vascular endothelial damage with hypofibrinogenemia and thrombocytopenia resulting from DIC.

Although meningitis occurs subclinically in many dogs, increased protein concentration and cell count can be detected by CSF analysis.

Serologic Testing

The microscopic agglutination (MA) test, the standard serologic means to diagnose leptospirosis, requires darkfield microscopy. It is relatively nonspecific, so that numerous antigens must be used to identify the serovar causing disease. Organisms grown in liquid media are exposed to serial dilutions of patient's sera. The endpoint is the highest serum dilution that causes 50% of the organisms to agglutinate. Positive reactions are not necessarily serovar-specific. Further dilutions are done against positive-reacting antigens to determine which antibody is present in highest concentration.[9]

Demonstration of a fourfold rise in MA titer is often required for serologic confirmation of disease. Because titers are often negative in the first week of illness, a second and sometimes a third serum sample should be obtained within 2- to 4-week intervals.

An ELISA has been developed for use in dogs that detects IgG or IgM antibodies to leptospires.[10] In comparison, the MA titer appears to parallel the IgM titer more than it does the IgG titer. The IgM-ELISA becomes increased within 1 week after initial infection, and the maximum titer develops within 14 days, with a subsequent decrease thereafter.[11] The IgM-ELISA appears to be more sensitive in detecting antibody and more serovar-specific than the MA test for determining infection in dogs.[11] Dogs that have died within the first week of illness have had high IgM titers, whereas the MA titer had not had time to increase.[12]

Increased IgG-ELISA titers develop after 2 to 3 weeks following infection, with a maximum titer being found after 1 month. IgG-ELISA titers better parallel protection against infection than do MA titers. Using combined IgG and IgM measurements, the ELISA is better suited to distinguish between natural infection or vaccine-induced immunity than is the MA test. ELISA testing in dogs that have received more than one vaccination demonstrates a high IgG titer accompanied by a low or negative IgM titer, even within the first few weeks after vaccination. In contrast, the MA titers are increased both following natural and vaccine exposures, although titers greater than 1:300 that persist may indicate infection.[13] See Appendix 8 for a listing of diagnostic laboratories that perform these tests.

A microscopic microcapsular agglutination test (MCAT) using a synthetic polymer to carry leptospiral antigens has been developed.[13a] Serum titers with the MCAT in infected dogs are increased for a short period of time after inoculation. The MCAT titers correlate with IgM antibody and appear to detect recent infections.

Isolation

Proper timing and technique are essential for the recovery of leptospires because of their fastidious growth requirements and susceptibility to adverse environmental conditions. Samples should be taken prior to initiation of antibiotic therapy. Dogs are leptospiremic during the first week of infection, but the numbers of circulating organisms subsequently decrease as serum antibody titer increases. Occurrence of leptospires in CSF parallels that in blood. Urine is the ideal fluid to be cultured thereafter; however, multiple sampling is required because of intermittent shedding of organisms.

Premortem isolation is preferred, because postmortem tissue contaminants will overgrow fastidious leptospires unless selective media are used. A small volume of tissue (preferably liver or kidney) or body fluid for culture should be collected aseptically in a clean sterile glass container. Catheterized or voided urine is frequently contaminated by normal flora that interfere with the growth of leptospires; therefore, cystocentesis is preferred. Inhibiting substances such as antibody in host tissues and fluids require dilution of the sample by at least 1:10 (v/v) with buffered saline, 1% bovine serum albumin, or culture media. As an alternative, 0.25 to 0.5 ml of blood, urine, or CSF taken at the appropriate stage of infection can be directly inoculated into 7 to 10 ml of transport media. Blood should be anticoagulated with heparin or sodium polyethylene sulfonate for transport to the laboratory if it cannot be diluted immediately. Citrate anticoagulants should be avoided, since they inhibit leptospires. Diluted urine can be alkalinized during transport to enhance recovery. Tissue or fluid samples, if shipped, should be kept in transport medium or on ice but not frozen. For research purposes, organisms can be frozen in semisolid or transport media and stored at temperatures of $-60°C$ to $-70°C$ for up to 6 years prior to culture.

Media for isolation of leptospires are liquid, semisolid, or solid in nature. EMJH is a liquid or semisolid media containing polysorbate-80 and fetal calf serum or bovine serum albumin.[14,15] Modification of standard medium by adding antibiotics or 5-fluorouracil has produced improved results in isolation of certain leptospiral serovars.[16] Leptospires commonly lose their virulence on culture in artificial media, but this can be reversed by passage in susceptible animals.

Organism Identification

Darkfield examination is necessary for rapid identification of viable leptospires, because they cannot be stained by simple methods using aniline dyes. Wet mount preparations are also necessary to help characterize their writhing and flexing movements. A variety of bacteria that can be confused with leptospires produce more random movement in wet-mount preparations. Cellular fibrils or extrusions and fibrin strands, which can be mistaken for organisms, can be removed by centrifugation. Because of the inaccuracies of darkfield examination, it should always be followed by cultural or serologic procedures.

Leptospires can be seen by light microscopy in tissue sections or on air-dried smears with Giemsa stain or silver impregnation (see Fig. 45–3).

Fluorescent antibody (FA) techniques have been adapted to identify leptospiral serovars in tissues and body fluids. FA testing can be used as a screening method to identify animals shedding organisms in urine when culture is impossible or too time consuming. Leptospires have been detected in biologic fluids by the very sensitive method of DNA hybridization.[17]

Agglutination-adsorption techniques have been used in specialized laboratories to serotype isolates. Restriction endonuclease analysis has been shown to be a sensitive and accurate taxonomic means compared with serotyping.[18] Genetic probes have been used to detect urinary shedding of leptospires.[18a]

PATHOLOGIC FINDINGS

External gross lesions include injected and icteric mucous membranes with diffuse petechiation. Focal ulcerations are seen on the tongue and in the buccal cavity, and tonsillar enlargement is usually present. The entire respiratory tract may be edematous. The lungs are frequently congested, and there may be spotty, diffuse, pneumonic infiltrates present. Petechial and ecchymotic hemorrhages are commonly found on the pleural surface (Fig. 45–6). The liver is enlarged and friable, with pronounced interlobar markings and yellow-brown discoloration. Petechiae and ecchymoses are found throughout the leptomeninges.

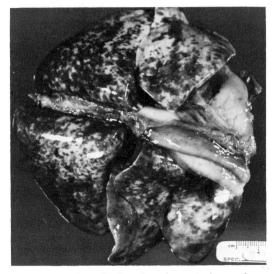

Figure 45–6. Petechial and ecchymotic hemorrhages on the serosal surfaces of the lungs from the dog in Figure 45–4.

Necrosis and hemorrhage are occasionally present in the bowel with intestinal intussusceptions. Frequently, free blood or acholic feces can be found in the colon and rectum of some animals. The spleen is pale and shrunken.

Kidneys are enlarged in animals that die of acute infection. They are pale and yellow-gray in color and bulge on the cut surface (see Fig. 45–4). The renal capsule may be adherent to the surface of the kidneys, and subcapsular hemorrhages are common. Swelling and focal, white spotting may be seen in the renal cortex on cut sections. Leptospires can be cultured from macerated kidney tissue.

Histologic changes in the lung consist of fibrinoid necrosis of blood vessels, and perivascular, intra-alveolar, and subpleural hemorrhages. Mononuclear cell infiltrates surround thrombosed pulmonary vessels. Focal necrosis of hepatic parenchyma is present. Hepatocytes are rounded, with pyknotic nuclei, and contain an eosinophilic granular cytoplasm. Intrahepatic bile stasis and severe hepatocellular injury are usually evident in icteric animals. The clinical severity of hepatic disease and histologic changes in the liver correlate well with leptospirosis. Subclinical cases usually have mild fatty changes in hepatocytes, whereas moderately ill dogs have fragmented hepatic cords, with lymphocytic infiltrates in areas of necrosis, and severely affected dogs have widespread necrosis of hepatic parenchyma and disintegration of nuclei. Chronically infected dogs develop chronic active hepatitis and hepatic fibrosis. Organisms may be demonstrated in intercellular locations within hepatic cords.

Neurologic damage includes perivascular hemorrhage (uncommon in the cat), mononuclear cell infiltrates, and occasionally, vascular thrombosis. When a silver stain is used, leptospires can be found in pericapillary areas.

Although gross lesions are absent in the heart, focal lymphocytic myocarditis is evident on histologic examination. Histologic changes seen in renal tissue include desquamation of degenerate renal tubular epithelium and swollen glomeruli, necrosis being associated with mononuclear cell infiltrates. Renal function abnormalities do not always correlate with histologic changes. Kidneys of chronically affected animals have mild-to-diffuse lymphocytic infiltration, with randomly scattered macrophages. Large numbers of atrophied tubules contain eosinophilic tubular casts. Glomeruli of some animals are swollen and have proteinaceous accumulations in Bowman's space.

THERAPY

Supportive therapy for animals with leptospirosis depends upon the severity of infection and the presence of renal or hepatic dysfunction and other complicating factors. Dehydration and shock occur in severely affected animals. Fluid loss results from vomiting and diarrhea, and balanced polyionic IV fluids should be used to correct the deficits. Petechial and ecchymotic hemorrhages indicate thrombocytopenia and can be corrected with fresh whole blood transfusions in severely affected animals. However, transfusions should be given with caution and only with concurrent low-dose heparin for ongoing DIC.

Oliguria and anuria are treated initially with rehydration. Osmotic diuretics, such as 10% glucose (5 ml/kg) or mannitol, should be given IV when impaired renal function persists following rehydration. If treatment with these diuretics fails, dopamine (10 µg/kg/min) or dobutamine may be administered by IV infusion. Tubular diuretics such as furosemide can be used as a last resort to increase urine flow; however, the effect on

improving glomerular filtration is debated. Adequate fluids should be given once polyuric renal failure ensues. Peritoneal dialysis can be considered if oliguria persists, since renal function is potentially reversible.

Antibiotics usually reduce fever within a few hours following administration. They immediately inhibit multiplication of the organism and rapidly reduce fatal complications of infection such as hepatic and renal failure. Penicillin is the antibiotic of choice for terminating leptospiremia (Table 45–2). Tetracycline and chloramphenicol are less effective. Dihydrostreptomycin is the drug of choice for eliminating the organism from the kidney and suppressing the carrier state, but it should not be used until renal function tests have returned to normal. Tetracycline also eliminates leptospires from the kidney. Ampicillin and doxycycline have been effective in the treatment of people with leptospirosis.[19, 20] In experimental studies, cephalosporins and erythromycin are also effective. Ciprofloxacin is effective in vitro and in vivo against virulent strains of leptospires, but its clinical use has been limited.[20a]

PREVENTION

Prevention of leptospirosis involves elimination of the carrier state. Unfortunately, wild animal reservoirs and subclinically affected domestic animals continue to harbor and shed organisms. Therefore, control of rodents in kennels, maintenance of environmental conditions to discourage bacterial survival, and isolation of infected animals are important to prevent spread of the disease. Doxycycline has been given at a low (200 mg once weekly) dosage to humans in endemic areas for prophylaxis when vaccination with appropriate serovars is unavailable.[21, 22]

Bivalent bacterins that contain two main serovars, *L. canicola* and *L. icterohaemorrhagiae*, have been produced for dogs. Ideally, vaccines should contain serovars that have a broad immunogenic spectrum since cross-protection is limited. Currently marketed vaccines are chemically inactivated whole cultures, which makes them relatively allergenic in comparison with the tissue culture lines of virus vaccines (see Postvaccinal Complications, Chapter 2).

Table 45–2. Recommended Therapy for Leptospirosis[a]

DRUG	SPECIES	DOSE[b] (mg/kg)	ROUTE	INTERVAL (hours)	DURATION (weeks)
Penicillin G	B	25,000–40,000 units	IM, IV	12	2
Ampicillin	B	10–20	PO, SC, IV	8–12	2
Amoxicillin	D	10	PO	12	2
Dihydrostreptomycin[c]	B	15	IM	12	2
	B	10	IM	8	2
Tetracycline[c]	B	22	PO	8	10
Doxycycline[c, d, e]	H	2.5–5	PO, IV	12–24	1–2

[a]B = dog and cat, D = dog, H = human, IM = intramuscular, IV = intravenous, SC = subcutaneous.
[b]Dose per administration at specified interval, expressed as mg/kg unless otherwise stated.
[c]Use following penicillin to clear the renal carrier state when azotemia has resolved.
[d]Will also treat the renal carrier state but not affected by azotemia.
[e]Can be given at 200 mg once weekly as prophylaxis. See text.

Immunization has been effective in reducing the prevalence and severity of canine leptospirosis, but it does not prevent the carrier state. Adequate initial immunization, using many of the available products, takes three to four injections 2 to 3 weeks apart to produce immunity to challenge infection that will last 6 to 8 months. Newer vaccines, produced by growing leptospires in synthetic protein-free media, protected against postinfection shedding when dogs were challenged 2 to 4 weeks after two doses of vaccine.[23]

Experimental vaccines have been produced from the outer envelope (membrane complex) of leptospires,[24–26] which is the site of leptospirocidal activity of antibody and complement. Antigenic material has been reduced by culture in a protein-free media, adjuvants have been removed, and up to five *Leptospira* serovars have been included in such vaccines. Maximal antibody titers have been produced in dogs within 2 weeks after a single vaccination, and dogs have been protected against infection and urinary shedding following challenge. A vaccine (Duramune, Puppyshot, Fort Dodge Labs, Fort Dodge, IA) incorporates the outer envelope fraction of the organism. Initially, the product was developed to reduce allergic reactions associated with combining leptospiral antigens with coronaviral vaccine adjuvants.

IgG titers, which are primarily responsible for protection, are produced for at least 1 year following the third vaccination in dogs.[10] Since highest titers are produced by multiple injections, frequent vaccinations should be given to dogs in endemic areas and all dogs should receive *at least three* injections in their primary vaccination series.

PUBLIC HEALTH CONSIDERATIONS

The majority of infections in people are among those who engage in water sports activities or who have occupational exposure to wildlife or domestic animal hosts. Contaminated urine is highly infectious for people and for susceptible animal species; therefore, contact with it on mucous membranes or skin abrasions should be avoided. Canine infection and leptospiruria has been found in healthy vaccinated dogs with resultant development of the disease in people.[27] All known or suspected shedders should be treated with dihydrostreptomycin or streptomycin. Areas contaminated by infected urine should be washed with detergent and then treated with iodine-based disinfectants to which the organism is very susceptible.

References

1. Alexander AD: Leptospira. In Braude AI (ed): *Microbiology*, ed 2. Philadelphia, WB Saunders Co, 1986, pp 381–385.
2. Fessler JF, Morter RL: Experimental feline leptospirosis. *Cornell Vet* 54:176–190, 1964.
3. Bryson DG, Ellis WA: Leptospirosis in a British domestic cat. *J Small Anim Pract* 17:459–465, 1976.
4. Bishop L, Strandberg JD, Adams RJ, et al: Chronic active hepatitis in dogs associated with leptospires. *Am J Vet Res* 40:839–844, 1979.
5. Ellis WA: Leptospirosis. *J Small Anim Pract* 27:683–692, 1986.
6. Finco DR, Low DG: Water, electrolyte and acid-base alterations in experimental canine leptospirosis. *Am J Vet Res* 29:1799–1807, 1968.
7. Finco DR, Low DG: Fibrinogen content and fibrinolytic activity of plasma from dogs infected with

Leptospira canicola. Am J Vet Res 29:2037–2040, 1968.

8. Navarro CEK, Kociba GJ: Hemostatic changes in dogs with experimental *Leptospira interrogans* serovar *icterohaemorrhagiae* infection. *Am J Vet Res* 43:904–906, 1982.

9. Shotts EB: Laboratory diagnosis of Leptospirosis. In Johnson RC (ed): *The Biology of Parasitic Spirochetes.* New York, Academic Press, 1976, pp 209–224.

10. Hartman EG, van Houten M, van der Donk JA, et al: Determination of specific anti-leptospiral immunoglobulins M and G in sera of experimentally infected dogs by solid-phase enzyme-linked immunosorbent assay. *Vet Immunol Immunopathol* 7:43–51, 1984.

11. Hartman EG, van Houten M, van der Donk JA, et al: Serodiagnosis of canine leptospirosis by solid-phase enzyme-linked immunosorbent assay. *Vet Immunol Immunopathol* 7:33–42, 1984.

12. Hartman EG, van den Ingh TSGAM, Rothuizen J: Clinical, pathological and serological features of spontaneous canine leptospirosis. An evaluation of the IgM- and IgG-specific ELISA. *Vet Immunol Immunopathol* 13:261–271, 1986.

13. Weaver AD: Leptospirosis in greyhounds. *Vet Rec* 74:1457–1463, 1962.

13a. Arimitsu Y, Haritan K, Ishiguro N, et al: Detection of antibodies to leptospirosis in experimentally infected dogs using the microcapsule agglutination test. *Br Vet J* 145:356–361, 1989.

14. Ellinghauser HC, McCullough WG: Nutrition of *Leptospira pomona* and growth of 13 serotypes: fractionation of oleic acid albumin complex and a medium of bovine albumin and polysorbate 80. *Am J Vet Res* 26:45–51, 1965.

15. Johnson RC, Harris VG: Differentiation of pathogenic and saprophytic leptospires. *J Bacteriol* 44:27–31, 1967.

16. Adler B, Faine S, Christopher WL, et al: Development of an improved selective medium for isolation of leptospires from clinical material. *Vet Microbiol* 12:377–381, 1986.

17. Millar BD, Chappel RJ, Adler B: Detection of leptospires in biological fluids using DNA hybridization. *Vet Microbiol* 15:71–78, 1987.

18. Thiermann AB, Handsaker AL, Foley JW, et al: Reclassification of North American leptospiral isolates belonging to serogroups Mini and Sejroe by restriction endonuclease analysis. *Am J Vet Res* 47:61–66, 1986.

18a. Zuerner RL, Bolin CA: Repetitive sequence element cloned from *Leptospira interrogans* serovar hardjo type hardjo-bovis provides a sensitive diagnostic probe for bovine leptospires. *J Clin Microbiol* 26:2495–2500, 1988.

19. Munnich D, Lakatos M: Treatment of human leptospira infections with ampicillin or amoxicillin. *Chemother* 22:372, 1976.

20. McClain JB, et al: Doxycycline therapy for leptospirosis. *Ann Intern Med* 100:696–698, 1984.

20a. Shalit I, Barnea A, Shahar A: Efficacy of ciprofloxacin against *Leptospira interrogans* serogroup Icterohaemorrhagiae. *Antimicrob Agents Chemother* 33:788–789, 1989.

21. Takafuji ET, Kirkpatrick JJ, Miller RN: Prophylaxis against leptospirosis with doxycycline. *N Engl J Med* 311:54, 1984.

22. Takafuji ET, Kirkpatrick JW, Miller RN, et al: An efficacy trial of doxycycline chemoprophylaxis against leptospirosis. *N Engl J Med* 310:497–500, 1984.

23. Broughton ES, Scarnell J: Prevention of renal carriage of leptospirosis in dogs by vaccination. *Vet Rec* 117:307–311, 1985.

24. Bey RF, Johnson RC: Humoral immune response of dogs vaccinated with leptospiral pentavalent outer envelope and whole culture vaccines. *Am J Vet Res* 39:831–836, 1978.

25. Bey RF, Johnson RC: Immunogenicity and humoral and cell-mediated immune responses to leptospiral whole cell, outer envelope, and protoplasmic cylinder vaccines in hamsters and dogs. *Am J Vet Res* 43:835–840, 1982.

26. Bey RF, Johnson RC: Leptospiral vaccines in dogs: immunogenicity of whole cell and outer envelope vaccines prepared in protein-free medium. *Am J Vet Res* 43:831–834, 1982.

27. Feigin RD, Lobes LA, Anderson D, et al: Human leptospirosis from immunized dogs. *Ann Intern Med* 79:777–785, 1973.

46 LYME BORRELIOSIS
Russell T. Greene

ETIOLOGY

Lyme borreliosis, a complex multiorgan disorder, in recent years has been one of the more commonly reported human tick-borne illnesses in the United States.[1] A similar disease syndrome has been reported in dogs.[2-5] The disease in cats is poorly documented.[6] *Borrelia burgdorferi* is the causative spirochete. Several strains have been isolated; however, the clinical importance of strain differences is still uncertain. Like most spirochetes, *B. burgdorferi* is small (0.2 μm × 30 μm) and darkfield or phase microscopy is necessary for proper visualization (Fig. 46–1).

The primary vectors are various species of hard ticks. Disease prevalence follows the distribution of these ticks worldwide (Fig. 46–2). *Ixodes ricinus* is the primary vector in Europe, whereas in the United States the important vectors are *I. dammini* in the Northeast and Midwest, *I. pacificus* in the West, and most likely *I. scapularis* in the Southeast.[7,8] *I. dammini* is a three-host tick with a 2- to 3-year life cycle (Fig. 46–3). Larvae and nymphs (which measure only 0.5 to 1.0 mm long) primarily feed on rodents and small mammals, whereas adult ticks (2.5 to 3.0 mm long) feed on deer or larger mammals (Fig. 46–4). Unlike many other tick species, the nymphal stage is active earlier in the year than the larval stage.[9] This "reversed" pattern of seasonal activity of larvae and nymphs is essential to the effective yearly transmission since transovarial transmission of this pathogen is minimal. Larvae acquire infections that had been transmitted to a reservoir host by nymphs feeding earlier in the season. The nymphal stage is considered most responsible for transmission of spirochetes to people and dogs.

Other tick species, deerflies, horseflies, botflies, mosquitoes, and fleas also have been found to harbor *B. burgdorferi*.[10, 10a] The significance of these various arthropods as vectors is questionable. The wide variety of competent and incidental hosts may be one reason for the global dispersion of the organism.

PATHOGENESIS

The pathogenesis of the clinical syndrome is poorly understood. Spirochetes are able

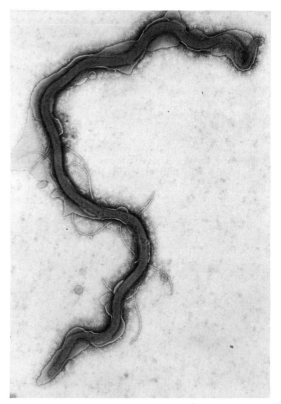

Figure 46–1. Transmission electron micrograph of *B. burgdorferi* showing periplasmic flagella that have been released from the confines of the outer membrane secondary to specimen preparation (phosphotungstic acid, × 7100).

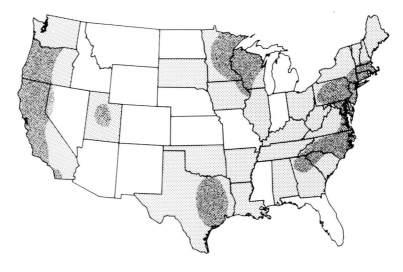

Figure 46–2. In the United States, Lyme borreliosis has been reported to occur in people in at least 43 states. Lighter shading indicates states where indigenous cases have been reported. Less is known of the seroprevalence and frequency of canine infections with *B. burgdorferi*. The darker shaded areas are regions where the highest prevalence of seropositivity has been reported. (Information courtesy of Dr. Willy Burgdorfer and Dr. Tom Schwan, Rocky Mountain Laboratories, Hamilton, MT.)

to survive within a host and may be detected within organs that are not inflamed, despite elevated specific antibody titers. When clinical signs occur, an inflammatory process, thought to be related to the persistence of the organism and possibly immune complex

deposition, is often present. Although controversial, it is theorized that a lipopolysaccharide-like component in the cell wall of *B. burgdorferi* causes the release from monocytes, of interleukin-1 which is directly responsible for tissue damage that leads to clinical illness (Fig. 46–5).[11, 12, 12a] The fact that human patients with certain B cell alloantigens tend to have severe and prolonged illnesses suggests that host factors may also play a role in the disease pathogenesis.[13]

CLINICAL FINDINGS

Canine manifestations are categorized as either acute or chronic.[14] Fever, inappetence, lethargy, lymphadenomegaly, and acute onset of stiffness, lameness, or pain are variably observed in acute infections. Acutely affected dogs often do not have swollen joints, and it is frequently difficult to localize the

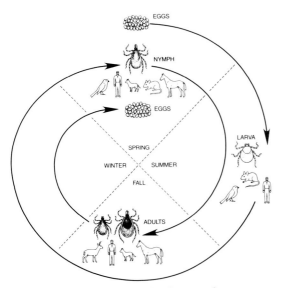

Figure 46–3. The life cycle of *I. dammini* lasts 2 years. Eggs are oviposited in the spring, and the larvae emerge approximately 1 month later. They feed once in the summer, usually on small rodents or mammals, and then overwinter. The following spring, the larvae molt into nymphs, which then feed in late spring or early summer. The nymphs feed on mice or larger mammals such as dogs, deer, or human beings and are considered the most likely source of infection for dogs and humans. Nymphs then molt into adults in the fall. The adults usually feed on larger mammals (often the white-tailed deer), where they mate. The females lay their eggs and die in the spring to repeat the 2-year cycle. (Habicht et al: *Sci Am* 257(1):78–83, 1987. Reprinted with permission.)

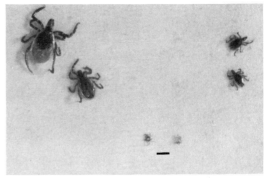

Figure 46–4. *I. dammini* is smaller than other ticks commonly found on dogs. From largest to smallest, 2 adults (male, female), 2 nymphs, 2 larvae (Bar = 1 mm). (Courtesy of Mike DeRosa, West Somerville, MA).

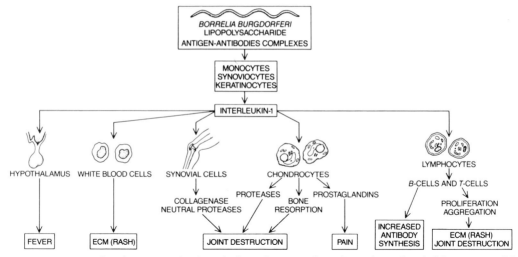

Figure 46–5. A proposed pathogenesis of *B. burgdorferi* infection is that a lipopolysaccharide-like compound from the cell wall causes the release of interleukin-1. This protein is then directly responsible for the development of the various clinical signs. (Habicht et al: *Sci Am* 257(1):78–83, 1987. Reprinted with permission.)

origin of the pain. Lameness may be intermittent and may often shift from one leg to another.

Recurrent, intermittent, nonerosive arthritis is considered the primary clinical manifestation of chronic canine Lyme borreliosis. The majority of affected dogs often have two or more joints involved.[2–5, 15] The carpus is commonly affected.

Erythema chronicum migrans (ECM, see Public Health Considerations) has not yet been documented in experimental or natural canine infections. Dermal erythema or hemorrhage has been reported in seropositive dogs; however, histology was not performed.[5] In experimental canine infections, areas of nonexpanding erythema were detectable at the site of tick attachment, but these lesions resolved after tick detachment.[16] In dogs in endemic areas, expanding lesions have been observed on the abdomen or other sparsely haired areas, but it has been difficult to definitively relate these lesions to ECM. The expanding nature of these lesions should differentiate them from localized reactions to tick bites.

Atrioventricular heart block has been documented in a dog from an endemic area that was strongly seropositive for *B. burgdorferi*.[17] Myocardial necrosis and vegetative endocarditis were found. Presence of the organism in the myocardium was suggested by immunohistochemical staining, but the organism could not be isolated from body tissues.

Neurologic manifestations have not been reported in either experimental or natural canine infections. There are suggestions that signs of meningitis or encephalitis in endemic areas may be manifestations of canine Lyme borreliosis. With time and increased awareness of these disease syndromes, these manifestations in dogs are likely to be better documented.

There is evidence that renal lesions develop secondary to *B. burgdorferi* infections in dogs.[15, 18] Glomerulonephritis and tubular damage have been observed in seropositive dogs, but it is often difficult to confirm a cause-and-effect relationship. Further epidemiologic studies are needed to determine the frequency of occurrence of these lesions in seropositive and seronegative dogs.

DIAGNOSIS

Nonspecific biochemical changes of increased erythrocyte sedimentation rates and mild increases in ALT (SGPT) and AST (SGOT) activities have been reported in affected human patients. Test results for rheumatoid factor or antinuclear antibodies are negative, but concentrations of certain complement components may be elevated. In dogs, no specific hematologic or biochemical changes have been documented. Dogs with renal localization of infection have been reported to develop azotemia, proteinuria with variable hematuria, pyuria, and tubular casts.[15, 18]

In people, synovial fluid from painful

joints has had leukocyte counts that vary from 500 to 110,000 WBC/mm³ (average 25,000/mm³), with mostly polymorphonuclear leukocytes. Total protein ranged from 3.0 to 8.0 g/dl. Examination of joint fluid from chronically lame dogs revealed a purulent exudate and, rarely, spirochetes.[3] The mean cell count was 46,300 cells/mm³.

Analysis of CSF from human patients with neurologic signs often shows moderate pleocytosis with a preponderance of lymphocytes. Protein concentration of the CSF is mildly elevated (mean 70 mg/dl), and glucose is normal. Spirochetes rarely have been isolated from the CSF of human patients. Documentation of increased intrathecal CSF antibody titers may be a useful diagnostic aid, especially when the titers are compared with serum levels early in the disease. These parameters have not been tested in dogs.

Serologic Testing

Both IFA and ELISA are used for diagnosis in people and dogs.[15, 16, 19, 20] As with other serologic testing, interlaboratory differences in the absolute titers exist.[19] In people, specific IgM titers usually peak by 14 days after the onset of initial clinical signs and sometimes remain increased throughout the illness.[21, 21a] Specific IgG titers rise slowly and are generally highest months later. IgG levels increase as neurologic and arthritic manifestations develop, such that all patients with arthritis have IgG titers.[21] If antibiotics are administered to human patients at the first sign of ECM, the serologic response may be lessened or even prevented.[21a] A specific T lymphocyte stimulation response to *B. burgdorferi* antigens may indicate infection in these seronegative patients;[21b] however, results of these studies have been questioned.[21c] ELISA procedures for IgG and IgM, using extracted flagellar antigens, improves serodiagnostic detection of early infections in people.[21d] The usefulness of these tests in dogs is uncertain.

After a single experimental IV inoculation of large quantities of *B. burgdorferi* in dogs, ELISA-IgM titers increased and remained high for approximately 2 months.[16] Specific ELISA-IgG titers increased rapidly and high titers persisted for up to 8 months. Persistence of high IgG titers makes it difficult to draw conclusions from such results on a single sample.[21e, 21f] Simultaneous measurement of IgG and IgM antibody titers in a single sample might be more meaningful than evaluation of either antibody class alone.

In naturally infected dogs, there is considerable overlap between the IgG antibody titers of those dogs with clinical and those with subclinical infections.[3, 4, 15, 16] An IFA-IgG titer greater than 1:64 has often been considered positive, although dogs in endemic areas can be asymptomatic and have an IgG titer of 1:8192.[3, 4] In serologic surveys from endemic areas, up to 53% of tested dogs had IFA-IgG titers greater than 1:64.[22] The IFA titers of the clinically affected dogs have ranged from 1:256 to 1:16,384.[2, 3, 15] The role of other cross-reacting, and presumably less pathogenic *Borrelia* species, such as *B. theileri, B. hermsii, B. parkeri, B. turicatae,* or *B. recurrentis* or potentially less pathogenic strains of *B. burgdorferi,* in producing these titers has not been fully determined.[22a] Immunoblot reactivities using sera from symptomatic and nonsymptomatic dogs are so similar that immunoblots cannot be used to determine clinical significance of high IgG titers.[23] See Appendix 8 for a list of some laboratories that perform serotesting for antibodies to *B. burgdorferi.*

Isolation

Identification or isolation of *B. burgdorferi* from the blood, CSF, urine, and joint fluid from affected human and canine patients has been difficult. This suggests that the number of circulating organisms is low or that ideal isolation methods are not being used. A special medium, Barbour-Stoenner-Kelly II, is required to grow *Borrelia.* Blood samples anticoagulated with citrate may be submitted to an appropriate laboratory for isolation. CSF or urine may also be submitted, especially if neurologic or renal disease is suspected. Positive identification of isolated organisms by using monoclonal antibodies is important, since nonpathogenic spirochetes exist, as do artifacts that mimic spirochetes.[24] Another important consideration is that isolation of *B. burgdorferi* in tissues may be an incidental finding. This organism has been isolated from tissues and body fluids of asymptomatic wildlife, laboratory animals, and seropositive dogs.[20, 25, 26] Enzyme immunoassay methods to detect an-

512 BACTERIAL DISEASES

tigen at concentrations of 10^5 organisms/ml are described.[26a, 26b]

Tissue samples can be evaluated microscopically for the presence of pathogenic spirochetes. As in culture, monoclonal antibodies are necessary for positive identification. *B. burgdorferi* has been observed in tissues of clinically healthy animals. Therefore, to be a significant finding, the spirochetes probably should be surrounded by an inflammatory process.

THERAPY

Tetracycline, ampicillin, or less desirably, erythromycin is utilized for treatment of dogs with acute infections (Table 46–1). Their use has been based on therapeutic trials in affected people and in vitro susceptibility testing.[27] In the one report of a treated dog, 500 mg ampicillin was administered orally every 8 hours for 10 days.[2] The arthritis resolved after 1 week of therapy, but long-term follow-up was not reported. *B. burgdorferi* was isolated from the blood of this dog after 3 days of the ampicillin therapy. In vitro susceptibility testing has shown that ceftriaxone is also an effective antibiotic, but it is expensive, and controlled therapeutic trials of this drug have not been performed.

In people, neurologic and arthritic manifestations are less responsive to antibiotics. Therefore, doxycycline or high doses of IV penicillin G for 10 days are recommended.[27a, 27b] Similarly, dogs with chronic Lyme borreliosis that do not respond to the initial antibiotics may benefit from IV penicillin G.[14]

Aspirin or other nonsteroidal anti-inflammatory drugs may be helpful for pain relief during episodes of synovitis, but treatment is not useful during asymptomatic periods. Treatment for the pain in acute canine cases is not usually indicated since the response to antibiotic therapy often occurs within 24 hours. Glucocorticoids may give rapid pain relief, but there is evidence that they may interfere with the response to antibiotics. Dexamethasone caused recrudescence of spirochetemia and increased antibody titers in experimentally inoculated dogs, although the dogs were not clinically ill before or after glucocorticoid treatment.[28]

PREVENTION

As the disease becomes better understood and easier to recognize, rapid diagnosis and treatment will result in fewer late-stage complications. In dogs, many aspects of the disease are probably still unrecognized. A better understanding of the serology, improved isolation, or newer antigen detection techniques will allow accurate diagnosis of the disease.

People and animals are coming into contact with the causative organism with increased frequency, especially as urban development spreads. As with other tick-borne diseases, rapid removal of the tick helps to prevent infection. There is evidence that it may take up to 24 hours of tick feeding before the organism is transmitted in the tick saliva.[29] For people who spend much time in the outdoors, 0.5% permethrin or 20% to 30% DEET has been determined to be an excellent repellent against *I. dammini*.[30]

The isolation of *B. burgdorferi* from many arthropods and mammals is cause for alarm. If vaccinations were ever needed for an endemic population, they might be successful, as hamsters have been successfully immunized passively and actively.[31, 32] In addition,

Table 46–1. Treatment of Canine Lyme Disease[a]

DRUG	DOSE[b] (mg/kg)	ROUTE	INTERVAL (hours)	DURATION (days)
Tetracycline[c]	22	PO, IV	8	10–14
Amp(amox)icillin	20	PO	8	10–14
Erythromycin	10	PO	8	10–14
Penicillin[d]	22,000 units/kg	IV	6	7
Ceftriaxone[d]	20	IV, SC	12	7–10

[a]PO = oral, IV = intravenous, SC = subcutaneous. Information is based on extrapolation from the human literature; no canine clinical trials have been reported.
[b]Dose per administration at specified interval, expressed as mg/kg, except when otherwise stated.
[c]Doxycycline may be substituted at 10 mg/kg given every 12 hours. Tetracyclines should be avoided in pups.
[d]Used for resistant cases when response to other antibiotics is not noted.

there did not seem to be major differences between Minnesota and Connecticut isolates in the ability to produce protection.

PUBLIC HEALTH CONSIDERATIONS

The clinical signs that develop in infected people are multisystemic and mimic those of many other diseases.[32] Three variable clinical stages, which encompass dermatologic, cardiac, neurologic, and arthritic manifestations, are observed in human Lyme borreliosis. The characteristic dermatologic lesion, ECM, is a nonpainful, spreading erythematous macule or papule that typically manifests in 1 to 2 weeks at the site of a tick bite. The lesion may be accompanied by fatigue, fever, headache, vomiting, myalgia, arthralgia, regional lymphadenomegaly, or splenomegaly. Several chronic dermatologic manifestations have been related to human Lyme borreliosis. Acrodermatitis chronica atrophicans and lymphadenosis benign cutis are chronic skin lesions related to preceding ECM. *B. burgdorferi* has been cultured from skin lesions of patients with these syndromes which have also been correlated with cardiac, neurologic, and arthritic manifestations of the disease. Other dermatologic lesions such as morphea, localized scleroderma, or lichen sclerosis et atrophicans have also been associated with *B. burgdorferi* infection in people.

Syncope is the most common cardiac manifestation. Rarely, signs of congestive heart failure develop. Varying degrees of atrioventricular block, occasionally with complete heart block, are the most common electrocardiographic abnormalities.

Neurologic manifestations caused by meningitis or encephalitis include headache, neck stiffness, photophobia, somnolence, lethargy, irritability, poor memory, cranial nerve defects, or concentration difficulties. Peripheral spinal neuritis with corresponding sensory and motor loss is occasionally observed.

Arthritis is the chronic clinical finding in people and develops in 60% of untreated patients. The attacks are usually mono- or oligoarticular and usually of 1 or more weeks' duration.

Whether dogs can transmit infection directly to people has not been determined. In endemic regions, high levels of serum IgG to *B. burgdorferi* were more prevalent in household dogs than in their human counterparts.[34] Dogs may be at greater risk of exposure than people owing to greater contact with the vector and delayed removal of their ticks following attachment. Spirochetemia has been found in nonsymptomatic dogs, suggesting that local dogs may act as a source for the disease.[22] The possibility must be considered that family-owned dogs or cats may bring infected ticks into the household or neighborhood.[35] Exposure of people and dogs in endemic areas to the same tick-infested environment is probably a more common means of human infection.[36] In addition, transmission of *B. burgdorferi* in the urine of dogs has been suggested, and this may pose a potential public health threat.

References

1. Centers for Disease Control: Update: Lyme disease and cases occurring during pregnancy. *MMWR* 34:376–384, 1985.
2. Lissman BA, Bossler EM, Camay H, et al: Spirochete-associated arthritis (Lyme disease) in a dog. *J Am Vet Med Assoc* 185:219–220, 1984.
3. Kornblatt AN, Urband PH, Steere AC: Arthritis caused by *Borrelia burgdorferi* in dogs. *J Am Vet Med Assoc* 186:960–963, 1985.
4. Magnarelli LA, Anderson JF, Kaufmann AF, et al: Borreliosis in dogs from southern Connecticut. *J Am Vet Med Assoc* 186:955–958, 1985.
5. Eugster AK, Angulo AB: Lyme disease. *Southwest Vet* 37:22–25, 1985.
6. Angulo AB: Lyme disease in cats. *Soutwest Vet* 37:108–109, 1986.
7. Barbour AG, Burgdorfer W, Hayes SF, et al: Isolation of a cultivable spirochete from *Ixodes ricinus* ticks of Switzerland. *Curr Microbiol* 8:123–126, 1983.
8. Steere AC, Malawista SE: Cases of Lyme disease in the United States: locations correlated with distribution of *Ixodes dammini*. *Ann Intern Med* 91:730–733, 1979.
9. Matuschka FR, Spielman A: The emergence of Lyme disease in a changing environment in North America and Central Europe. *Exp Appl Acarol* 2:337–353, 1986.
10. Magnarelli LA, Anderson JF, Barbour AG: The etiologic agent of Lyme disease in deer flies, horse flies, and mosquitoes. *J Infect Dis* 154:355–358, 1986.
10a. Magnarelli LA, Anderson AF: Ticks and biting insects infected with etiologic agent of Lyme disease, *Borrelia burgdorferi*. *J Clin Microbiol* 26:1482–1486, 1988.
11. Habicht GS, Beck G, Benach JL: Lyme disease. *Sci Am* 257(1):78–83, 1987.
12. Beck G, Habicht GS, Benach JL, et al: A role for interleukin-1 in the pathogenesis of Lyme disease. *Zentralbl Bakteriol Mikrobiol Hyg [A]* 263:133–136, 1986.

12a. Takayama K, Rothenberg RJ, Barbour AG: Absence of lipopolysaccharide in the Lyme disease spirochete, Borrelia burgdorferi. Infect Immun 55:2311–2113, 1987.

13. Steere AC, Gibofsky A, Pattarroyo ME, et al: Chronic Lyme arthritis: clinical and immunogenetic differentiation from rheumatoid arthritis. Ann Intern Med 90:896–901, 1979.

14. Burgess EC: Borreliosis (Lyme disease). In Barlough J (ed): Manual of Small Animal Infectious Diseases. New York, Churchill Livingstone, 1988, pp 153–159.

15. Magnarelli LA, Anderson JF, Schreier AB, et al: Clinical and serologic studies of canine borreliosis. J Am Vet Med Assoc 191:1089–1094, 1987.

16. Greene RT, Levine JF, Breitschwerdt, et al: Clinical and serological evaluations of induced Borrelia burgdorferi infection in dogs. Am J Vet Res 49:752–757, 1988.

17. Levy SA, Duray PH: Complete heart block in a dog seropositive for Borrelia burgdorferi. J Vet Intern Med 2:138–144, 1988.

18. Grauer GF, Burgess EC, Cooley AJ, et al: Renal lesions associated with Lyme borreliosis in a dog. J Am Vet Med Assoc 193:237–239, 1988.

19. Hedberg CW, Osterholm MT, MacDonald KL, et al: An interlaboratory study of antibody to Borrelia burgdorferi. J Infect Dis 155:1325–1327, 1987.

20. Magnarelli LA, Meegan JM, Anderson JF, et al: Comparison of an indirect fluorescent-antibody test with an enzyme-linked immunosorbent assay for serological studies of Lyme disease. J Clin Microbiol 20:181–184,1984.

21. Craft JE, Fischer DK, Shimamoto GT, et al: Antigens of Borrelia burgdorferi recognized during Lyme disease: appearance of a new immunoglobulin M response and expansion of the immunoglobulin G response late in the illness. J Clin Invest 78:934–939, 1986.

21a. Bernardi VP, Weeks KE, Steere AC: Serodiagnosis of early Lyme disease: analysis of IgM and IgG antibody responses using an antibody-capture enzyme immunoassay. J Infect Dis 158:754–760, 1988.

21b. Dattwyler RJ, Volkman DJ, Luft BJ, et al: Seronegative Lyme disease: dissociation of specific T- and B-lymphocyte responses to Borrelia burgdorferi. N Engl J Med 319:1441–1446, 1988.

21c. Nesher G, Osborn TG, Moore TL: Seronegative Lyme disease. N Engl J Med 320:1279, 1989.

21d. Hansen K, Åsbrink E: Serodiagnosis of erythema migrans and acrodermatitis chronica atrophicans by the Borrelia burgdorferi flagellum enzyme-linked immunosorbent assay. J Clin Microbiol 27:545–551, 1989.

21e. Greene RT: Lameness and asymptomatic Borrelia burgdorferi seropositivity in dogs. J Infect Dis 160:346, 1989.

21f. Frank JC: Taking a hard look at Borrelia burgdorferi. J Am Vet Med Assoc 194:1521, 1989.

22. Burgess EC: Natural exposure of Wisconsin dogs to the Lyme disease spirochete (Borrelia burgdorferi). Lab Anim Sci 36:288–290, 1986.

22a. Anderson JF, Magnarelli LA, McAninch JB: New Borrelia burgdorferi antigenic variant isolated from Ixodes dammini from upstate New York. J Clin Microbiol 26:2209–2212, 1988.

23. Greene RT, Walker RL, Nicholson WL, et al: Immunoblot analysis of the immunoglobulin G response to the Lyme disease agent (Borrelia burgdorferi) in experimentally and naturally exposed dogs. J Clin Microbiol 26:648–653, 1988.

24. Schmid GP, Steere AC, Kornblatt AN, et al: Newly recognized Leptospira species ("Leptospira inadai" serovar lyme) isolated from human skin. J Clin Microbiol 24:484–486, 1986.

25. Anderson JF, Magnarelli LA, Burgdorfer W: Spirochetes in Ixodes dammini and mammals from Connecticut. Am J Exp Med Hyg 32:818–824, 1983.

26. Johnson RC, Marek N, Kodner C: Infection of Syrian hamsters with Lyme disease spirochetes. J Clin Microbiol 20:1099–1101, 1984.

26a. Hyde FW, Johnson RC, White TJ, et al: Detection of antigens in the urine of mice and humans infected with Borrelia burgdorferi, etiologic agent of Lyme disease. J Clin Microbiol 27:58–61, 1989.

26b. Greene RT: Clinical and serologic response of dogs to the Lyme disease agent (Borrelia burgdorferi). PhD diss. North Carolina State University, Raleigh, NC, 1988.

27. Steere AC, Green J, Hutchinson GJ, et al: Treatment of Lyme disease. Zentralbl Bakteriol Mikrobiol Hyg [A] 263:352–356, 1986.

27a. Dotevall L, Hagberg L: Penetration of doxycycline into cerebrospinal fluid in patients treated for suspected Lyme borreliosis. Antimicrob Agents Chemother 33:1078–1080, 1989.

27b. Abramowicz M (ed): Treatment of Lyme disease. Med Lett 31:57–60, 1989.

28. Burgess EC: Experimental inoculation of dogs with Borrelia burgdorferi. Zentralbl Bakteriol Mikrobiol Hyg [A] 263:49–54, 1986.

29. Benach JL, Coleman JL, Skinner RA, et al: Adult Ixodes dammini on rabbits: a hypothesis for the development and transmission of Borrelia burgdorferi. J Infect Dis 155:1300–1306, 1987.

30. Schreck CE, Snoddy EL, Spielman A: Pressurized sprays of permethrin or DEET on military clothing for personal protection against Ixodes dammini (Acari: Ixodidae). J Med Entomol 23:396–399, 1986.

31. Johnson RC, Kodner C, Russell M: Passive immunization of hamsters against experimental infection with the Lyme disease spirochete. Infect Immun 53:713–714, 1986.

32. Johnson RC, Kodner C, Russell M: Active immunization of hamsters against experimental infection with Borrelia burgdorferi. Infect Immun 54:897–898, 1986.

33. Steere AC, Bartenhagen NH, Craft JE, et al: Clinical manifestations of Lyme disease. Zentralbl Bakteriol Mikrobiol Hyg [A] 263:201–205, 1986.

34. Eng TR, Wilson ML, Spielman A, et al: Greater risk of Borrelia burgdorferi infection in dogs than in people. J Infect Dis 158:1410–1411, 1988.

35. Curran KL, Fish D: Increased risk of Lyme disease for cat owners. N Engl J Med 320:183, 1989.

36. Falco RC, Fish D: Potential for exposure to tick bites in recreational parks in a Lyme disease endemic area. Am J Public Health 79:12–15, 1989.

47

BOTULISM
Jeanne A. Barsanti

ETIOLOGY

Clostridium botulinum is a gram-positive, spore-forming, saprophytic anaerobic rod that is distributed in soil worldwide. Botulism is an intoxication caused by a neurotoxin produced by the organism. In order to produce disease, either the organism or its spores must contaminate a potential food-source.

Eight types (A, B, C_1, C_2, D, E, F, and G) of *C. botulinum* have been identified, based on their antigenically distinct neurotoxins. All the toxin types are approximately the same size (molecular weight 150,000) and have the same neurotoxic effect. Types A, B, and E are associated mainly with human disease. Most cases of botulism in animals are caused by types C and D. In addition to the eight antigenic types, the organism can be subtyped on the basis of its proteolytic capacities and the species of animals usually affected. All canine cases to date have been due to type C toxin with the exception of two cases of type D reported from Sénégal.[1, 2] Natural cases in dogs have been attributed to eating carrion or raw meat.

Although the disease has been experimentally produced in cats,[3] no natural cases have yet been reported. This may be related either to the cat's more selective feeding habits or to lack of recognition of such cases. The present discussion is limited to dogs, but the disease in cats should be similar since botulinal neurotoxins cause similar signs in all species studied to date. Type C botulism has been reported in lions.[4]

The organism grows best under anaerobic conditions and warmth (30°C), although some strains can grow at temperatures as low as 6°C. Strict anaerobiosis is not essential. Mildly alkaline pH stimulates growth of some types, but pH 5.7 is optimal for type C-producing strains. Botulinal toxin is a protein released mainly from vegetative cells

following lysis of the cell or by diffusion through the cell wall. The amount of toxin in spores is only about 1% of that found in vegetative cells, but the intrasporal toxin is resistant to heat denaturation. Vegetative cells produced by germinating spores begin to produce toxin within several days after germination. In addition to *C. botulinum*, *C. barati* and *C. butyricum* have produced botulism in human infants.[5, 6]

PATHOGENESIS

Botulism is usually due to ingestion of the preformed toxin, although a variant of the disease in people, infant botulism, is due to intestinal colonization by *C. botulinum* and in vivo production of toxin.[5] Normal adults are resistant to intestinal colonization with *C. botulinum*, largely because of intestinal microflora, since colonization can be induced in adult animals or people only if they are germ free or are being treated with antibiotics.[5, 7] Persistent intestinal colonization with *C. botulinum* in adults has been rarely reported to cause clinical illness.[7a] Intestinal colonization was established experimentally in 8- to 11-day-old puppies, but no intoxication occurred.[8] Intestinal colonization has been found in a natural case of botulism in a 6-month-old dog.[9] However, the dog recovered without antibiotic therapy, even though intestinal colonization continued for several months.

Once ingested, the toxin is absorbed from the stomach and upper small bowel into lymphatics. Some toxin is denatured by digestive processes. An exception is type E toxin, which is activated and made more potent by gastric and intestinal proteolytic enzymes. Toxin can continue to be absorbed from the lower small bowel and colon, but this absorption proceeds more slowly. The toxin circulates to the neuromuscular junction of cholinergic nerves, where it exerts its effects.

Botulinal toxin is the most potent biologic poison known. The relative potency of each toxin varies with the species of animal and with the resistance of the individual. The toxin prevents presynaptic release of acetylcholine. Both the spontaneous release of acetylcholine, producing miniature endplate potentials, and its release due to a nerve action potential are inhibited.

Botulinal toxin first binds to a receptor molecule, postulated to be sialic acid, on the external surface of the nerve cell membrane. Binding occurs very quickly, is unaffected by temperature, and is independent of neural activity. During this stage the toxin is susceptible to inactivation by antitoxin, and paralysis does not result. As acetylcholine is released from the nerve ending, the toxin passes through the cell membrane. Whether this movement is due to active transport is unknown. Once inside the cell, the toxin is resistant to inactivation by antitoxin.

Intracellularly, the toxin interacts with another receptor molecule to block acetylcholine release. How the release of acetylcholine is blocked is not known. One theory is that the toxin's presence necessitates a higher concentration of calcium for exocytosis of acetylcholine to occur (Fig. 47–1).

Under light microscopy, no lesions are apparent at the neuromuscular junction. However, changes in terminal axons, synaptic clefts, and adjacent muscle fibers have been noted by electron microscopy of neuromuscular junctions from human cases. The blockage of acetylcholine release results in generalized lower motor neuron disease and parasympathetic dysfunction. Recovery is postulated to occur only by development of new terminal axons to form new neuromuscular junctions.[8]

CLINICAL FINDINGS

The reported clinical signs in canine botulism Type C have been the same whether experimentally or naturally induced.[2,10–17] The severity of the signs varies with the amount of toxin ingested and the individual susceptibility of the dog. The first signs are a progressive, symmetric, ascending weakness from the rear to the forelimbs that can result in quadriplegia, although tail wag is

maintained (Fig. 47–2). A complete neurologic examination will show hyporeflexia and hypotonia, indicating generalized lower motor neuron disease. Cranial nerves are often affected: mydriasis with sluggish pupillary responses, decreased jaw tone, decreased gag reflex with excess salivation, diminished palpebral reflexes, and weak vocalization have been found in affected dogs. Conjunctivitis and ulcerative keratitis may develop owing to the weak palpebral reflex. Bilateral keratoconjunctivitis sicca has been noted.[12] In severely affected dogs, there may be decreased abdominal muscle tone and primarily diaphragmatic respiration. The heart rate is variable (increased or decreased) and constipation and urinary retention may develop. Megaesophagus has been noted in six affected dogs.[13, 16, 18] Pain perception and an alert mental attitude are maintained (Fig. 47–3). Muscle atrophy is variable. There is no hyperesthesia. Death may result from respiratory paralysis or from secondary respiratory or urinary infections. On necropsy there are no gross or light microscopic abnormalities in the nervous system.

The progression of signs is explained by differences in muscles affected, the diaphragm being much more resistant than skeletal muscle to paralysis with progressive neuromuscular blockade.

The incubation period following ingestion of contaminated food in dogs has been from hours to 6 days and the earlier the signs appear, the more serious the disease.[10, 13] The duration of illness in dogs that recovered has ranged from 14 to 24 days. In affected people, signs generally improve within 7 days, but full recovery may take months. Cranial nerve, neck, and forelimb function tends to return first in affected dogs. If recovery occurs, it is complete (Fig. 47–4).

In cases of type D botulism, the dogs died suddenly with signs of generalized hemorrhage and without observed neurologic deficits.[1, 2]

DIAGNOSIS

All results of routine laboratory work (CBC, blood chemistry profile, urinalysis) are normal unless a secondary infection develops.[10, 13] CSF has been normal in affected dogs and people.

Electromyography (EMG) showed that lower motor neuron dysfunction in clini-

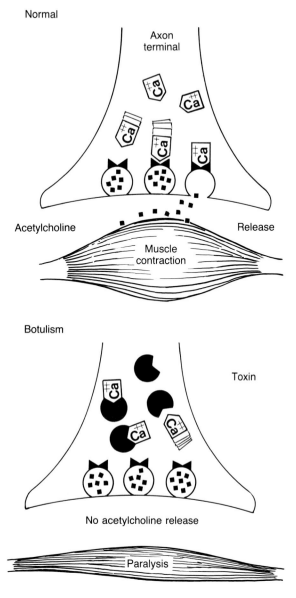

Normal

Axon
terminal

Acetylcholine

Release

Muscle
contraction

Botulism

Toxin

No acetylcholine release

Paralysis

Figure 47–1. Schematic drawing of the blockage of acetylcholine release by botulinal toxin at the neuromuscular junction. The toxin binds calcium so that it is no longer available to assist in exocytosis of acetylcholine.

Figure 47–2. Dogs with quadriplegia due to botulism.

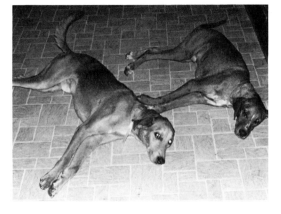

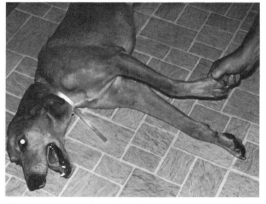

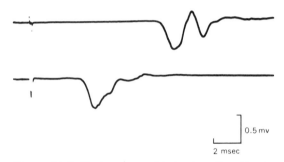

Figure 47–5. Electromyographic tracing after stimulation of the right tibial nerve of a dog with botulism. The upper tracing is the response to stimulation at the level of the femoral trochanter, and the lower tracing is the response to stimulation at the popliteal fossa. The amplitudes of the evoked potentials are markedly subnormal.

Figure 47–3. Dog with botulism showing normal pain perception but lack of a withdrawal reflex.

cally affected dogs is due to a problem at the neuromuscular junction and perhaps to peripheral nerve conduction.[10, 18] When a motor nerve was stimulated, motor unit potentials were subnormal in amplitude but not polyphasic (Fig. 47–5). Decrements in motor unit potentials were variable following repetitive stimulation. Fibrillation potentials have been noted in one study[10] but not in another,[18] which may be related to the difference in the time of performance of EMGs (mean of 16 and 12 days, respectively). Nerve conduction velocity was mildly decreased, even with correction for hypothermia.[19,39] As the dogs recovered, increased electrode insertional activity and positive sharp waves were found.

Confirmatory diagnosis of botulism is based on the finding of the toxin in serum, feces, vomitus, or samples of the food that was ingested. Serum should be collected as early in the disease course as possible and when clinical signs are maximal.[14] About 10 ml of serum or 50 g of feces, vomitus, or food is needed to conduct the test.

The preferred method of identifying the toxin is the neutralization test in mice. In this test, serum or an extract of feces, vomitus, or food is injected alone and in combination with type-specific antitoxin into the peritoneal cavity of mice. The mice are then observed for signs of botulism. Survival of one group protected with one type of antitoxin and death of the other groups with signs consistent with botulism confirm the presence of botulinal toxin. Botulinal toxin has never been found in feces of clinically normal people or in feces of people with diseases other than botulism.[19] See Appendix 8 for a listing of diagnostic laboratories that perform the mouse inoculation test.

Newer in vitro tests have been developed to identify botulinal toxin. These tests include radioimmunoassay techniques, passive hemagglutination, and ELISA. To date these tests have not replaced the mouse test because they measure antigenicity rather than toxigenicity. Antigenicity does not equal toxigenicity because of the methods of production of type-specific antitoxin.[8]

The diagnostic importance of isolation of the organism *C. botulinum* from feces is controversial. The organism can be isolated from feces of only 60% of humans with botulism.[19] Although isolation of the organism in association with clinical signs provides some evidence for the diagnosis, it is not as conclusive as toxin identification. Newer techniques combine organism isolation with toxin identification.[20] The type C organism is one of the most difficult types to culture, as it is a strict anaerobe. Often

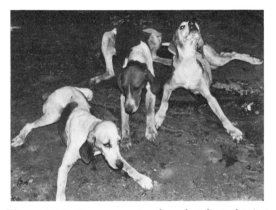

Figure 47–4. Dogs recovering from botulism, having regained the ability to resume sternal recumbency and to move the head and neck.

Table 47–1. Drug Therapy for Canine Botulism[a]

DRUG	DOSE[b] (mg/kg)	ROUTE	INTERVAL (hours)	DURATION (days)
Antitoxin[c]	10,000–15,000 U	IV, IM	4	2 doses
Antibiotics[d]				
Penicillin	20,000–40,000 U/kg	IV (IM)	6–12	10
Metronidazole	10	IV, PO	8	5

[a]IV = intravenous, IM = intramuscular, PO = oral.
[b]Dose per administration at specified interval, expressed as mg/kg unless otherwise stated.
[c]Toxin type-specific or polyvalent needed; dosage recommended is that for an average human. See text for further information.
[d]Rarely indicated; supportive care is as important or more important; see text.

the presence of toxin in an extract of cultured feces is used as evidence of the organism's presence.[19, 21]

THERAPY

Supportive Care

Supportive treatment is most important, since spontaneous recovery will occur if the amount of toxin ingested is not too large and if respiratory and urinary tract infections can be avoided. Affected animals should be assisted to eat, drink, and move about. Water beds or cage padding should be used to reduce the incidence of decubital sores. Ability to urinate should be monitored and the bladder expressed as needed. Enemas and stool softeners should be used for constipation. Parenteral fluids should be used as necessary to avoid dehydration, especially if swallowing is impaired. Antibiotics should be used if infection develops, but aminoglycosides should be avoided if possible since they also have the potential to block neuromuscular transmission. To avoid altering the intestinal microflora, which might allow *C. botulinum* to grow, antibiotics should be used only when necessary.[21] Nonmedicated or antibiotic ophthalmic ointments should be used to prevent exposure keratitis in dogs with poor palpebral function.

Antitoxin

Specific treatment for botulism is limited. Antitoxin is not effective after the toxin has penetrated the nerve endings, which occurs rapidly after the toxin enters the blood stream. Antitoxin may prevent further toxin binding if intestinal absorption and circula-

tion are still occurring. Since most cases in dogs to date have been type C, type C antitoxin should be given. The recommended dose for treating dogs (Table 47–1) is extrapolated from that used in treating people. The antitoxin will remain in circulation for 40 days following administration, so there is no need for further administration. Five ml of polyvalent antitoxin (types A, B, C, D, E, F, Statens Serum Institute, Copenhagen, Denmark) administered IV or IM has been used in dogs treated to date. Anaphylaxis is a potential risk. Intradermal skin testing can be performed with 0.1 ml of antitoxin 20 minutes prior to IV injection of antitoxin. Any immediate reaction at the test site should be advance warning that an allergic response may develop.

Antibiotics

Penicillin or metronidazole has been used in dogs and people to reduce any intestinal population of clostridia.[7, 10, 19] The efficacy of these drugs is doubted because in most cases disease is due to ingestion of preformed toxin and because neither drug is certain to eradicate *C. botulinum* from the intestine.[5,7] The possibility that these drugs could make the disease worse by releasing more toxin through bacterial lysis or by promoting intestinal infection has also been raised.[21, 22] Metronidazole predisposes to intestinal colonization in mice.[23] Dosage recommendations are listed in Table 47–1.

Neuromuscular Potentiators

Guanidine hydrochloride has been used with questionable efficacy in human cases to increase acetylcholine release. The mechanism of action is by increasing intraneuronal calcium concentration. Respiratory muscles respond to a lesser degree than limb or extraocular muscles, so the drug is less useful in severe cases in which successful therapy is crucial. Side effects of the drug include GI upsets, tremors, and twitching. Administration of guanidine hydrochloride to an affected lion resulted in seizures and pyrexia. The animal died 2 days after drug administration.[4]

Another experimental drug, 4-aminopyridine, has been able to restore neuromuscular transmission for short time periods in rats. The drug can cause convulsions and has not been clinically evaluated for treatment of botulism in people. Diaminopyridine was given to two lions, with improvement in signs for only 30 minutes.[4]

PREVENTION

Botulinal toxin is destroyed by heating to 80°C for 30 minutes or to 100°C for 10 minutes. Preventing access to carrion and thorough cooking of any food fed to dogs will prevent the disease. Foxhounds appear predisposed to the disease because they are commonly fed raw meat.

References

1. Doutre MP: Le botulisme animal de type D au Sénégal: première observation chez le chien. Rev Elev Med Vet Pays Trop 35:11–14, 1982.
2. Doutre MP: Seconde observation de botulism de type D chez le chien au Sénégal. Rev Elev Med Vet Pays Trop 36:131–132, 1983.
3. Mikhailov VV, Mikhailov VV: Effects of pathogenic action of botulinus toxin on spinal motoneurons of various types. Bull Exp Biol Med 80:1288–1290, 1975.
4. Greenwood AG: Diagnosis and treatment of botulism in lions. Vet Rec 117:58–60, 1985.
5. Arnon SS: Infant botulism: anticipating the second decade. J Infect Dis 154:201–206, 1986.
6. Aureli P, Fenicia L, Pasolini B et al: Two cases of type E infant botulism caused by neurotoxigenic Clostridium butyricum in Italy. J Infect Dis 154:207–211, 1986.
7. Chia JK, Clark JB, Ryan CA, et al: Botulism in an adult associated with food-borne intestinal infection with Clostridium botulinum. N Engl J Med 315:239–240, 1986.
7a. McCroskey LM, Hatheway CL: Laboratory findings in four cases of adult botulism suggesting colonization of the intestinal tract. J Clin Microbiol 26:1052–1054, 1988.
8. Sugiyama H: Clostridium botulinum neurotoxin. Microbiol Rec 44:419–448, 1980.
9. Farrow BRH, Murrell WG, Revington ML, et al: Type C botulism in young dogs. Aust Vet J 60:374–377, 1983.
10. Barsanti JA, Walser M, Hatheway CL, et al: Type C botulism in American foxhounds. J Am Vet Med Assoc 172:809–813, 1978.
11. Borst GHA, Lambers GM, Haagsma J: Botulismus type C bij de hond. Tijdschr Diergeneeskd 111:1104–1105, 1986.
12. Cornellissen JMM, Haagsma J, Van Nes JJ: Type C botulism in 5 dogs. J Am Anim Hosp Assoc 21:401–404, 1985.
13. Darke PGG, Roberts TA, Smart JL, et al: Suspected botulism in foxhounds. Vet Rec 99:98–99, 1976.
14. Marlow GR, Smart JL: Botulism in foxhounds. Vet Rec 111:242, 1982.
15. Richmond RN, Hatheway C, Kaufman AF: Type C botulism in a dog. J Am Vet Med Assoc 173:202–203, 1978.
16. Wallace V, McDowell DM: Botulism in a dog—first confirmed case in New Zealand. N Z Vet J 34:149–150, 1986.
17. Blakemore WF, Rees-Evans ET, Wheeler PEG: Botulism in foxhounds. Vet Rec 100:57–58, 1977.
18. VanNes JJ: Electrophysiological evidence of peripheral nerve dysfunction in 6 dogs with botulism type C. Res Vet Sci 40:372–376, 1986.
19. Dowell VR, McCroskey LM, Hatheway CL, et al: Coproexamination for botulinal toxin and Clostridium botulinum. JAMA 238:1829–1832, 1977.
20. Silas JC, Carpenter JA, Hamdy MK, et al: Selection and differential medium for detecting Clostridium botulinum. Appl Environ Microbiol 50:1110–1111, 1985.
21. Philip A: Infant botulism. Lab Management 19:53–58, 1981.
22. Bartlett JC: Infant botulism in adults. N Engl J Med 315:254–255, 1986.
23. Wang Y, Sugiyama H: Botulism in metronidazole-treated conventional adult mice challenged orogastrically with spores of Clostridium botulinum type A or B. Infect Immun 46:715–719, 1984.

48 TETANUS

Craig E. Greene

ETIOLOGY

Tetanus is caused by the action of a potent neurotoxin formed in the body during the vegetative growth of *Clostridium tetani*. *C. tetani* is a motile, gram-positive, nonencapsulated, anaerobic, spore-forming bacillus. Although strain differences of *C. tetani* exist throughout the world, the toxin produced in all cases is antigenically homogeneous. Resistant spores of the organism can be found in the environment, especially in the soil, where moisture, cultivation, and fertilization favor their survival. Organisms are routinely isolated from the feces of many domestic animals, including the dog and cat. Isolation from human feces occurs with greater frequency in those occupationally exposed to farm animals. Spores can survive adverse weather conditions in the absence of direct sunlight for months or years and can be found readily in dust and debris in indoor environments. Spores are resistant to boiling water, phenol, cresol, and mercury bichloride, and they resist an autoclave temperature of 120°C for 15 to 20 minutes. The vegetative phase of *C. tetani*, however, is no more resistant to chemical and physical inactivation than other microorganisms.

EPIDEMIOLOGY

Tetanus develops when spores are introduced into wounds or penetrating injuries. The spores vegetate in response to anaerobic conditions at the site of injury. The presence of a foreign body, tissue necrosis, other microorganisms, or abscess formation contributes to germination. Two toxins have been identified from *C. tetani*. Tetanolepsin causes hemolysis of erythrocytes during rapid in vitro growth of the bacteria; however, it is not considered clinically significant. In contrast, tetanospasmin (molecular weight 176,000) enters the body from the wound site and produces marked effects on neurologic function. It is not absorbed from the GI tract because it is usually destroyed by digestive juices. Its large molecular weight precludes its entry into the placenta.

The prevalence of the disease in dogs and cats is relatively low compared with that in other domestic animals, which may be related to the natural resistance of dogs and cats to this toxin (Table 48–1).

PATHOGENESIS

Many experimental studies have been performed with dogs, cats, and other laboratory animals to elucidate the mechanism by which tetanospasmin enters and affects the CNS. The site and route of administration of toxin are important in determining the type of disease that develops. Localized tetanus can be produced by IM or SC injection of toxin at a specific site. Toxin enters the

Table 48–1. Relative Susceptibility[a] of Animals to Tetanus Toxin

Horse	1	Most susceptible
Guinea pig	2	
Human	3	
Mouse	12	
Rabbit	24	
Dog	600	
Cat	7,200	
Chicken	360,000	Least susceptible

[a]The horse is assigned an arbitrary value of 1. Comparison relates to the amount of toxin required to produce clinical illness.

axons of the nearest motor nerves at the neuromuscular endplate and migrates by retrograde transport within motor axons to the neuronal cell body within the spinal cord (Fig. 48–1).

Spread of toxin within the nervous system, following local inoculation, occurs in the spinal cord in a bilateral ascending fashion until it reaches the brain (Fig. 48–2). IV administration of large amounts of toxin usually results in intracranial signs prior to development of generalized limb rigidity. Small amounts of blood-borne toxin are thought to enter the CNS through the intact blood-brain barrier. Generalized convulsions, increased facial muscle tone, and respiratory arrest may occur suddenly with hematogenous spread. Alternatively, hematogenously administered toxin is thought to localize preferentially in the neuromuscular endings of many motor nerves throughout the body, from which it may ascend by retrograde axonal transport into many areas of the nervous system. The initial involvement of facial musculature following hema-

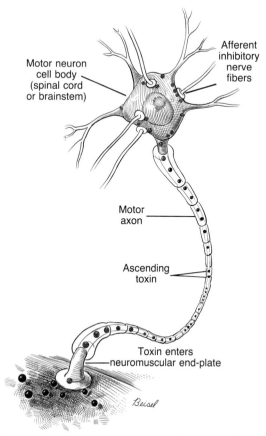

Figure 48–1. Retrograde intra-axonal transport of tetanus toxin into the CNS.

togenous spread of toxin is explained by the fact that cranial nerve motor axons (e.g., facial nerve) are shorter than those of the limbs.

The clinical signs of tetanus intoxication can be explained by the known pathophysiologic effects of tetanus toxin on the nervous system. Most experimental evidence has confirmed the effect of toxin at the spinal cord; however, brain, neuromuscular junctions, and autonomic nervous system can also be affected. In the spinal cord and brain stem, tetanus toxin has been shown to block inhibitory transmission to motor neurons. Tetanus toxin has an affinity for gangliosides within the gray matter of the CNS, which may explain the cerebral signs that appear in some cases without obvious spinal cord involvement. Effects of tetanus toxin have also been ascribed to its affinity for binding at the neuromuscular junction, which may induce direct neuromuscular facilitation prior to the migration of toxin to the CNS. Tetanus toxin may affect sympathetic preganglionic neurons similar to lower motor neurons within the spinal cord and cause signs of autonomic dysfunction. Bradycardia associated with tetanus probably results from vagal hyperactivity. Tetanus toxin is thought to block the presynaptic release of γ-aminobutyric acid, an inhibitory neurotransmitter, in the parasympathetic cardiac inhibitory center of the nucleus ambiguus. Thus, tetanus intoxication may result in increased vagal tone and pronounced bradyarrhythmias. Increased catecholamine release associated with adrenergic stimulation can also cause episodes of tachycardia in tetanus.

CLINICAL FINDINGS

Clinical signs of tetanus usually occur within 5 to 10 days of wounding. Because of the increased resistance of cats and dogs to intoxication, onset may be delayed for up to 3 weeks. This may account for the absence of a detectable wound at the time of examination. However, because of greater innate resistance of cats, the wound required to produce intoxication is so extensive that it is usually obvious. Wounds nearer the head (brain) are associated with more rapid onset and generalized signs of CNS intoxication than injuries to distant extremities.

Localized tetanus is more common in dogs

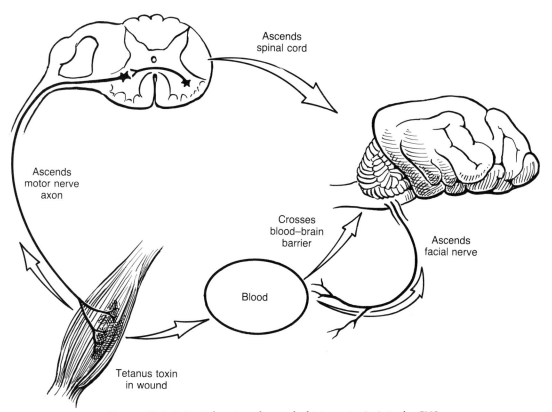

Figure 48–2. Potential routes of spread of tetanus toxin into the CNS.

and cats than in humans, because of the relative resistance of these animals to intoxication. Increased stiffness of a muscle or entire limb is first noted in close proximity to the wound site (Fig. 48–3). The stiffness usually spreads, gradually involving the opposite extremity. This process usually progresses over a variable length of time and eventually involves the entire CNS.[1]

Animals affected with generalized tetanus walk with a stiff gait and generally with an outstretched or dorsally curved tail. They have difficulty in standing or lying down in comfortable positions because of the extreme muscle rigidity (Figs. 48–4 and 48–5). Rectal temperature is usually increased by excessive muscular activity. Postural reaction testing, such as proprioceptive positioning, usually reveals normal initiation but stiff

Figure 48–3. Localized tetanus in the rear right limb of a dog with postpartum metritis. Stiffness progressed to involve all four limbs as well as the facial muscles.

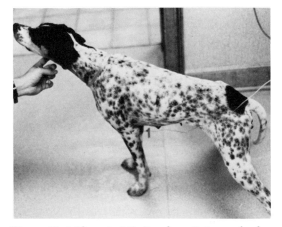

Figure 48–4. Characteristic "sawhorse" stance of a dog with generalized tetanus. (Courtesy of Dr. Wayne Rush, Atlanta, GA.)

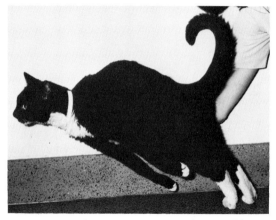

Figure 48–5. Characteristic posture of a cat with generalized tetanus, showing stiff limbs and outstretched tail.

performance of the motor response. Myotactic reflexes are generally accentuated and flexor reflexes depressed, but both may be difficult to elicit because of muscle stiffness.

Intracranial signs develop in the late stages of localized tetanus. They begin earlier in generalized tetanus and usually progress in reverse or descending fashion to produce generalized muscular stiffness. Cranial nerve motor nuclei are affected, causing hypertonicity of respective musculature. Protrusion of the third eyelid and enophthalmos result from involvement of extraocular motor nuclei (Fig. 48–6). The ears are held erect, the lips are drawn back (risus sardonicus), and the forehead is wrinkled as a result of facial muscle spasm. Trismus (lockjaw) is caused by contraction of masticatory muscles. Altered salivation, heart rate, and respiratory rate; laryngeal spasm; and dysphagia can result from involvement of parasympathetic cranial nuclei.

Reflex muscle spasms occur in animals with generalized tetanus or intracranial involvement. Animals become apprehensive and react strongly to tactile or auditory stimulation. Mild stimulation may precipitate periodic generalized tonic contraction of all muscles with opisthotonus or may precipitate grand mal convulsions. If the tonic contractions are first to occur, the interval between spasms decreases until the animal reaches a convulsive state. Dogs and cats usually remain conscious until they develop convulsions. Reflex muscle spasms are painful and animals may vocalize during such episodes. Animals with tetanus usually have a desire to eat, but because of jaw stiffness, they may have trouble in prehending or

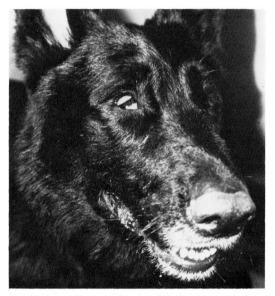

Figure 48–6. German shepherd dog with generalized tetanus, showing protrusion of the third eyelid and contracture of the facial muscles. (From Greene CE, Oliver JE. *In* Ettinger SJ (ed): *Textbook of Veterinary Internal Medicine*, ed 2. WB Saunders Co, 1983, pp 419–460. Reprinted with permission.)

swallowing solid food. Dysuria and urine retention, constipation, and gaseous distention are commonly results of persistent anal and urinary sphincter contractions. The progression of clinical signs culminates in death, which is usually caused by respiratory compromise resulting from rigidity of respiratory musculature, reflex spasms of the larynx, increased airway secretions, and central respiratory arrest from medullary intoxication or anoxia.

DIAGNOSIS

The history of a recent wound and the clinical signs are the primary means of making a diagnosis of tetanus. Hematologic abnormalities, including leukocytosis with neutrophilia and left shift, are the results of wounds that may be present. Serum biochemistry and CSF values are unaffected, except that muscle enzyme activity elevations may be present.

Both tachyarrhythmias and bradyarrhythmias can be seen in tetanus.[3] Rapid heart rates are usually associated with sinus tachycardia. Bradycardia (70 beats/minute) has been characterized by atrioventricular heart block, sinus arrest, and ventricular escape complexes.

Electromyographic findings of tetanus are characteristic. Insertion of the needle or tapping of muscles or tendons is followed by persistent electrical discharges rather than the expected period of electrical silence. Muscle biopsy is usually normal in acute cases of tetanus, and any observed abnormalities have been attributed to muscle trauma as a result of constant hypertonicity or prolonged recumbency.

Measurement of serum antibody titers to tetanus toxin has been used to substantiate the diagnosis of tetanus in a cat.[4] A value of 0.5 U/ml, compared with 0.01 U/ml in a control cat, was considered significant when observed 10 weeks after the initial onset of clinical signs and despite antitoxin administration to both cats. Such measurements might be used in a clinical setting to help confirm the cause of muscle stiffness.

Isolation of C. tetani from wounds can be a difficult procedure and is unrewarding in at least 50% of cases.[5] The organisms are usually present in very low concentrations, and although Gram-stained smears may demonstrate gram-positive rods and dark-staining spherical endospores, the morphology is not unlike that of many other anaerobic bacteria. If culture is attempted, it should be done under strict anaerobic conditions at 37°C for 12 days. Biochemical reactions or bioassays can be evaluated in an attempt to classify the organism. Mouse inoculation with isolates is not readily available.

THERAPY

Therapy for tetanus in severely affected animals is costly and time consuming, and owners must be advised of the possibility of complications and lengthy hospitalization. Fortunately, the disease is often localized or mild in dogs and cats, because of their innate resistance. However, untreated cases can prove fatal. Because of their natural resistance, dogs and cats are not vaccinated with toxoid as a means of prophylaxis or treatment. Recommended dosages for treatment discussed below are summarized in Table 48–2.

Antitoxin

The immediate concern in treating tetanus is administration of antitoxin to neutralize any toxin that is unbound to the CNS or is yet to be formed. The timing and route of antitoxin administration are important in determining the effectiveness of detoxification. Use of antitoxin should be a routine measure. The detoxification of bound toxin in the affected animal is slow, and the administration of antitoxin does little to hasten the process. Thus, recovery in most cases is slow and progressive. The dosage for prophylaxis is much less than that for treatment.

IV administration of antitoxin is superior to IM or SC administration in producing a rapid and marked increase of circulating antitoxin. It takes 48 to 72 hours for antitoxin to reach therapeutic concentrations when given SC.[6] The dose of equine antitoxin is given slowly over 5 to 10 minutes. Larger animals should receive a proportionally lower dosage based on body weight. Total dosages greater than 20,000 units do not appear to be more effective, because they increase the antigenic mass, and they are more costly.

Unfortunately, the use of IV antitoxin is associated with a high prevalence of anaphylaxis; therefore appropriate precautions are warranted during administration. An initial test dose (0.1 to 0.2 ml) of antitoxin should be given SC or intradermally 15 to 30 minutes prior to the administration of the IV dose. A wheal at the site of injection may indicate that an anaphylactic reaction will develop. Glucocorticoids and antihistamines should be readily available in case of an adverse reaction, or they may be given prior to an IV injection of antitoxin if a reaction is anticipated. It is not advisable to repeat the dose at any time during the course of therapy. A therapeutic blood level of antitoxin persists in dogs for 14 days following injection, and repeated administration increases the chance of an anaphylactic reaction.

Local IM injection of a small dose of antitoxin (1000 units) around and proximal to the wound site has been shown to be beneficial in experimental studies of localized tetanus.

Intracisternal (subarachnoid) or intracerebral injection of antitoxin in laboratory animals has been shown to be beneficial in treating tetanus under experimental conditions. Intracisternal or subarachnoid injections of as little as 1% of the recommended IV dose reduced the mortality in dogs with mild or moderate tetanus compared with

Table 48–2. Recommended Drug Dosages for Tetanus[a]

DRUG	SPECIES	DOSE[b] (mg/kg)	Route	INTERVAL (hours)	DURATION (days)
Antimicrobials					
Penicillin G	B	20,000–100,000 U/kg	IV, IM	6–12	10
Metronidazole	D	10	PO	8	10
	C	250 mg total	PO	12–24	10
Tetracycline	B	22	PO, IV	8	10
Clindamycin	B	3–10	PO, IV, IM	8–12	10
Immunotherapy					
Equine antitoxin	B	100–1000 U/kg	IV, IM, SC		Once
		1000 U/site	Intralesional		Once
		1–10 U/kg	Intrathecal		Once
Sedatives					
Acetylpromazine	B	0.02–0.06[c]	IV	2	prn
	B	0.1–0.25[c]	IM	4	prn
	B	1.0	PO	6–8	prn
Chlorpromazine	B	0.5–2.0	IM, IV, PO	8–12	prn
Diazepam	C	2.5–5.0 mg total	PO	2–4	prn
	D	5.0–10.0 mg total	IV, PO, IM	2–4	prn
	B	0.2–1.0	IV	prn	prn
Methocarbamol	B	15–50	PO	6–12	prn
Pentobarbital	B	3–15	IV, IM	2–3	prn
Phenobarbital	B	1–4	PO, IM	6–12	prn
Autonomic Agents					
Atropine		0.05	SC	prn	prn[d]
Glycopyrrolate		0.005	SC, IV	prn	prn[d]
		1 mg total	PO	8	prn

[a]B = dog and cat, D = dog, C = cat, IV = intravenous, IM = intramuscular, PO = oral, SC = subcutaneous, prn = as needed, U = units.

[b]Dose per administration at specified interval, expressed as mg/kg unless otherwise stated. Lowest range value applies to animals with greatest body weight.

[c]Maximum dose IV of 3 mg in any dog.

[d]Use as necessary to control bradyarrhythmias.

similarly affected animals given IV or lumbar intrathecal injections.[7] In severe cases, intracisternal injections prolonged the life of animals but did not reduce the mortality. Antitoxin injected into the CSF has an advantage over a similar systemic dose because it need not penetrate the blood-brain barrier. Toxin that has already bound to nervous tissue has been shown to be partially neutralized if antitoxin is administered intracisternally. Unfortunately, only a portion of bound toxin is neutralized by this method because the signs in experimental animals continue to progress, albeit at a lower rate, following treatment.

Appropriate clinical trials have not been performed to establish the superiority of intracisternal therapy. Furthermore, the antitoxin, being of equine origin, has potential toxicity in the subarachnoid space. For these reasons, intracisternal therapy should be reserved for treatment of severely affected animals. Ammonium chloride and methylamine hydrochloride reduce entry of peripheral nerve-bound toxin into the CNS,[8] but their

utility has not been determined in clinical situations.

Antimicrobial Therapy

Local and parenteral antibiotic therapy should be instituted in an attempt to kill any vegetative *C. tetani* organisms present in the wound. Although antibiotics by themselves may not neutralize circulating toxin, they reduce the amount of antitoxin required to treat experimental tetanus once clinical signs are apparent. Penicillin G, the drug of choice, can be given IV in the form of an aqueous potassium or sodium salt or IM as the procaine salt. A portion of the dosage, in the form of procaine penicillin, can be injected IM in close proximity to an identified wound site. Because the effectiveness of penicillin on the vegetative organisms may vary, tetracycline has been recommended as an alternative. Penicillin derivatives, such as ampicillin, are not as effective against the organism, and their use may cause little or no response to therapy. Metronidazole has been shown to be superior to penicillin and tetracycline in clinical or experimental tetanus.[5,9] Metronidazole may be more active and preferred for treatment of tetanus because it is bactericidal against most anaerobes and achieves effective therapeutic concentrations even in necrotic tissues. Furthermore, because of its inactivity against aerobic and facultative organisms, it is less likely to alter the normal bacterial microflora. It must be remembered that the prognosis for recovery does not always improve, because the degree and site of infection cannot always be determined.

Sedatives

Various drugs alone or in combination have been used to control the reflex spasms and convulsions associated with tetanus. An ideal agent would be one that controls excitability and spasticity without interfering with voluntary motor function or consciousness. Unfortunately, no such drug is available; however, a combination of phenothiazine and barbiturate comes closest to the ideal.

Phenothiazines appear to be highly effective in controlling the hyperexcitable state when used either alone or in combination with barbiturates. Chlorpromazine is the drug of choice, although acetylpromazine and methotrimeprazine can be used as substitutes. Phenothiazines are ineffective against similar-appearing signs caused by strychnine or other causes of convulsions. This is one exception when phenothiazines are used in seizure-prone animals. They are thought to work centrally on the brain stem to depress descending excitatory input on the lower motor neurons within the spinal cord.

Barbiturates can be used successfully to control grand mal convulsions, generalized body stiffness, or opisthotonus that may occur. Pentobarbital may have to be given every 2 to 3 hours, but the actual dose should be adjusted to the clinical signs of the patient as an overdose may unnecessarily suppress respiration and consciousness. Oral or injectable phenobarbital can be given for a longer duration of action. Combination of phenothiazines and pentobarbital can allow a reduction of the amount of barbiturate needed to control tetany.[10] A complication

of the combination of these two drugs is bradycardia. When the heart rate falls below 60 beats/minute, glycopyrrolate can be administered as needed to reverse the bradycardia.

Benzodiazepine derivatives such as diazepam are alternatives to barbiturates in the control of seizures. These drugs work by blocking polysynaptic reflexes within the medulla and spinal cord. Methocarbamol is frequently recommended but is less commonly used as a central-acting muscle relaxant. It has a relatively short duration of action, as does diazepam. Narcotics should never be included in tetanus therapy because they depress the respiratory centers and may stimulate other areas of the CNS. Parasympatholytic drugs such as atropine should also be avoided.

Severely affected animals with respiratory compromise from uncontrollable tetanic spasms may be sedated or anesthetized, intubated, and placed on positive pressure ventilation.

Surgery

Surgery may be required if tissue necrosis or abscess formation is extensive. Antitoxin should be administered prior to surgery because of the release of toxin in the circulation during tissue manipulation. General anesthesia is usually required to debride wounds and remove necrotic tissue. Devitalized tissue and visible foreign material should be removed and the wound irrigated. Hydrogen peroxide may be beneficial in flushing the wound because it increases oxygen tension, which inhibits obligate anaerobes. Foreign bodies should not be overlooked in many wounds associated with tetanus and should be removed at this time.

Autonomic Agents

These are sometimes required to control the cardiac rhythm disturbances that develop. Sympatholytic agents are generally not used in the management of tachyarrhythmias, since other sedatives usually control this complication. Bradyarrhythmias (60 beats/minute) that persist can be controlled by administration of parasympatholytic agents such as atropine or glycopyrrolate as needed on a short-term basis. These arrhythmias often resolve after a few days in animals that begin to show signs of improvement in their muscle stiffness.

Nursing Care

Supportive measures are imperative in the successful management of an animal with tetanus. Constant nursing may be required for severely affected animals. The animal should be placed in a dark, quiet environment with a minimum amount of stimulation. All therapeutic measures should be coordinated for the same time each day so that a minimal amount of handling and stimulation occurs. Soft comfortable bedding should be provided because tetanus causes incapacitation and animals frequently develop decubital ulcers. Animals should be encouraged to eat and drink on their own. They frequently have difficulty in prehending and swallowing solid foods, but they can usually eat blended foods or fluids by sucking through clenched teeth. A stomach tube may be passed if the animal is reluctant to eat, but this is frequently stressful for conscious animals and esophageal spasm may restrict passage of the tube. Only frequent, small amounts of food should be given in this manner because of the high risk of gastroesophageal reflux or vomiting and resultant aspiration pneumonia. A tube gastrotomy may be required for long-term feeding in severely affected animals. The hematocrit, plasma protein, and body weight should be evaluated daily to determine whether adequate fluid balance is being maintained. Balanced polyionic isotonic fluids should be given parenterally to meet any deficits. Parenteral alimentation requires continual IV administration of special fluids and is expensive.

Complications in dogs and cats with tetanus are numerous. Fractures of the long bones, spine, or skull may result from trauma incurred during sudden muscular spasms or convulsions. Other problems include sepsis from IV catheterization and aspiration pneumonia from difficult swallowing. Tracheostomy may be required if obstructive respiration develops from laryngeal spasm. Urinary and fecal retention occurs as a result of hypertonic anal and urethral sphincters. Repeated urinary catheterization may be needed if dysuria or reflex dyssynergia occurs. Simethicone, gastric intubation, and enemas may help relieve gas or obstipation.

Glucocorticoid therapy has never been proved to be beneficial in tetanus and should be avoided. Hyperbaric oxygenation has been used in humans and in dogs with tetanus in an attempt to inactivate *C. tetani*; however, there is little proof of benefit to justify the time and cost of such a procedure. Neuromuscular blocking agents have been used in human tetanus in an attempt to control convulsions or to paralyze the patients, who are then placed on artificial respirators. This therapy, however, is impractical in veterinary medicine because of the intensive monitoring required.

Most dogs and cats have a self-limiting course of tetanus intoxication when rapid and appropriate therapy is instituted. Improvement following institution of treatment is usually noticeable within 1 week, and gradual but complete recovery is noted by 3 to 4 weeks.

PREVENTION

Active immunoprophylaxis with tetanus toxoid is not recommended for dogs and cats as it is for more susceptible species such as humans and horses. Nor are routine tetanus boosters or postexposure prophylaxis required. Appropriate care of infected wounds and rational antibiotic use should minimize the occurrence of tetanus. Epizootics have occurred in veterinary hospitals when sterilization of surgical instruments has not been adequate.

References

1. Gafner F: An atypical progressing case of tetanus in a dog. *Schweiz Arch Tierheilkd* 129:271–276, 1987.
2. Greene CE, Oliver JE: Neurologic examination. *In* Ettinger SJ (ed): *Textbook of Veterinary Internal Medicine*, ed 2. Philadelphia, WB Saunders Co, 1983, pp 419–460.
3. Panciera DL, Baldwin CJ, Keene BW: Electrocardiographic abnormalities associated with tetanus in two dogs. *J Am Vet Med Assoc* 192:225–227, 1988.
4. Baker JL, Waters DJ, deLahunta A: Tetanus in two cats. *J Am Anim Hosp Assoc* 24:159–164, 1988.
5. Ahmadsyah I, Salim A: Treatment of tetanus: an open study to compare the efficacy of procaine penicillin and metronidazole. *Br Med J* 291:648–650, 1985.
6. Mason JH: Tetanus in the dog and cat: a review

with comments. *J S Afr Vet Assoc* 35:209–213, 1964.

7. Firor WM: Intrathecal administration of tetanus antitoxin. *Arch Surg* 41:299–307, 1940.

8. Simpson LL: Ammonium chloride and methylamine hydrochloride antagonize clostridial neurotoxins. *J Pharmacol Exp Ther* 225:546–552, 1983.

9. Freeman WA, McFaszean JA, Whelan JPF: Activity of metronidazole against experimental tetanus and gas gangrene. *J Appl Bacteriol* 31:443–447, 1968.

10. Fleming EJ, Hill B: Nursing the patient through canine tetanus. *Vet Med Small Anim Clin* 79:1357–1361, 1984.

49

ANAEROBIC INFECTIONS

Steven W. Dow

ETIOLOGY

Only recently has the clinical importance of infections caused by anaerobic bacteria been realized. Obligate anaerobes, a frequent component of polymicrobial infection, are often missed in routine aerobic bacteriologic cultures. As laboratory methods for culturing anaerobes have been improved and have become more readily available, an increase in the number of clinically confirmed cases of anaerobic infections in dogs and cats has been found.[1-5] Obligate anaerobes, medically the most important genera of anaerobes, rely on fermentative metabolism and can withstand exposure to atmospheric conditions for only a few minutes. In decreasing order of frequency of isolation are *Bacteroides*, *Fusobacterium*, *Peptostreptococcus*, and some clostridia.[1,3]

Facultative anaerobic bacteria, such as *Escherichia* and *Pasteurella*, are able to survive and grow either aerobically or anaerobically. They are often isolated together with obligate anaerobes from mixed infections and will overgrow the more fastidious anaerobes unless selective culture techniques are used.

PATHOGENESIS

With the exception of some clostridial and cutaneous infections, anaerobic infections are generally endogenous in origin. Under favorable conditions, anaerobic flora are able to invade and destroy tissues and cause infection.

Anaerobes are numerous in the environment as either resistant spores or vegetative bacteria on mucous membranes of the oropharynx, female reproductive tract, and colon. In the colon and the mouth, bacterial numbers may approach 10^{11}/g of feces and 10^8/ml of saliva, respectively. At these sites,

obligate anaerobes greatly outnumber facultative anaerobes and aerobic bacteria. Anaerobes are opportunists and proliferate following damage to the skin or mucosa and underlying tissues. Proper conditions for their survival are met by necrosis in deep tissues, that results from either the initial injury or prior colonization with aerobic or microaerophilic bacteria. Therefore, anaerobic infection, in contrast to aerobic infection, is nearly always polymicrobial and involves complex interactions between different species of bacteria.

Within mixed infections there may be bacteria that function as symbionts, producing necessary bacterial growth factors; others that are simply commensal; and other bacteria that are actually pathogenic to the host. For example, *Bacteroides melaninogenicus* requires vitamin K, produced by nonpathogenic streptococci, in order to grow rapidly and invade tissues.[6] Pathogenic anaerobes elaborate a number of virulence factors, including toxins and enzymes.[7]

CLINICAL FINDINGS

Anaerobic infection is more likely to develop in certain areas of the body, due either to a greater likelihood of contamination by the indigenous flora or to the existence of favorable environmental conditions. Examples of common anaerobic infections in dogs and cats are listed in Table 49–1,[8] and clinical findings that are often associated with anaerobic infection are listed in Table 49–2.

Clostridial Infection

Clostridia are capable of causing various soft tissue infections that range in severity from small, localized, superficial infections to massive wounds with extensive tissue

Table 49–1. Common Sites and Types of Anaerobic Infection in Dogs and Cats

Oropharynx: oropharyngeal and retrobulbar abscesses, ulcerative gingivitis
Skin: bite wounds, infection associated with foreign bodies
Respiratory tract: pyothorax, lung abscess, aspiration pneumonia
Abdomen: intestinal perforation and peritonitis, liver abscess
Reproductive tract: pyometra
Muscles: clostridial fasciitis and myonecrosis
CNS: brain abscess, subdural empyema, chronic otitis media-interna
Bone: chronic osteomyelitis

From Dow SW, Jones RL: *Compend Cont Educ Pract Vet* 9:711–720, 1989. Reprinted with permission.

destruction. Clostridial myonecrosis or gas gangrene, usually caused by *C. perfringens*, is characterized by marked toxin production and muscle necrosis. Fatal clostridial myonecrosis has been reported in dogs.[9,10] Typically, there is a short incubation period followed by rapid onset of illness, including fever; tachycardia; extreme tissue pain; a thin, serosanguineous, foul-smelling wound exudate; and production of tissue gas. Crepitus may be absent or difficult to detect by palpation. Clinical deterioration in dogs often occurs rapidly, progressing to severe septic shock despite treatment.

Clostridial cellulitis or fasciitis without myositis is encountered more frequently, usually as a sequela to penetrating wounds. Often there is extensive subcutaneous crepitus due to liberation of gases, together with a thin, serosanguineous wound exudate and apparent wound pain; systemic toxicity may be present. Gas in tissues is not specific for clostridial infection. Other gas-producing

Table 49–2. Clinical Features of Anaerobic Infection

SUGGESTIVE FINDINGS
  Foul wound odor
  Gas in tissues
  Tissue necrosis
  Blackish exudates
  Sulfur granules in exudate
  Abscess formation
  Infection in closed body spaces
  Lack of response to treatment with aminoglycosides, sulfonamides

DISEASE ASSOCIATIONS
  Bite wounds
  Foreign bodies
  Bone sequestra
  Solid tumor infections
  Aspiration pneumonia
  Postoperative peritonitis

bacteria include anaerobic streptococci, *E. coli*, and *Bacteroides*. A noxious wound odor is strong evidence of anaerobic infection, although it may not be present in all cases.

Infection of the Oropharynx and Skin

Whenever the mucous membrane barriers of the oropharynx are disrupted, there is the potential for anaerobic infection to develop. Necrotizing ulcerative gingivitis occurs in both people and dogs. Affected labial, gingival, and lingual mucous membrane surfaces are covered with painful, ulcerative lesions. Submandibular or retrobulbar abscesses are common sequelae to penetration of the oropharynx by foreign bodies and may result in fever, cervical swelling, and pain on opening the mouth. *Fusobacterium* and *Peptostreptococcus* are frequently cultured from perioral infections of dogs, often together with *Bacteroides* and facultative anaerobes such as *Pasteurella* and *E. coli* (see also Ulcerative Gingivostomatitis, Chapter 9).[11] Bite wound abscesses produced by dogs and cats are commonly infected with these organisms (see Chapter 58).

Pleuropulmonary Infection

Anaerobic bacteria predominate when closed-space infections of the lung and thoracic cavity, particularly lung abscess and pyothorax, are carefully cultured. Those most frequently isolated include *Bacteroides*, *Fusobacterium*, and *Peptostreptococcus*, whereas aerobic pathogens and facultative bacteria are distinctly uncommon.[3,12] Bacterial synergism is undoubtedly important to the development of pyothorax. Pyothorax typically develops weeks to months after penetrating trauma (especially bite wounds) to the chest wall, after migration of foreign bodies from the oropharynx, or after rupture of a lung abscess. Bacteria responsible for pyothorax generally originate from the oropharynx.

Lung abscesses are insidious and often develop after aspiration. Like pyothorax, they often contain anaerobic bacteria originating from the oropharynx, usually as a mixed population of obligate and facultative anaerobes and streptococci.[11]

Intra-abdominal Sepsis

Peritonitis, especially when caused by leakage of large bowel contents, is often a mixed infection. Bacteria are extremely abundant in the colon, where obligate anaerobes, especially *Bacteroides*, *Clostridium*, *Fusobacterium*, and anaerobic streptococci, outnumber facultative bacteria such as *E. coli* by a factor of 10^3 to 10^5 to one. Multiple species of bacteria may be isolated when peritoneal exudates are cultured anaerobically.[1]

Peritonitis tends to proceed through several stages as it develops. In the acute phase, facultative bacteria, especially *E. coli*, proliferate rapidly and release endotoxins, triggering development of septic shock.[13] In patients surviving the initial acute phase of peritonitis, the bacterial flora changes over time, with facultative bacteria eventually being replaced largely by obligate anaerobes such as *Bacteroides* spp. (see Intra-abdominal Infections, Chapter 9).

Anaerobes have been recovered from pyogenic infections of the liver and biliary system in dogs and cats. *Clostridium* may be the most common anaerobic pathogen associated with liver abscesses in dogs, whereas both *Bacteroides* and *Clostridium* have been isolated from biliary specimens of dogs and cats.[11] (Also see Chapter 10.)

Osteomyelitis

Anaerobic bacteria should be suspected in chronic bone infections, particularly when infection develops after traumatic fracture or internal fracture fixation with sequestration or when putrid, dark-colored wound discharges are present. Obligate anaerobes have been found in 74% of cultures obtained from animals with chronic osteomyelitis.[14] Specimens for culture should consist of either surgically harvested sequestra, debrided bone, or adjacent soft tissues.

Anaerobic joint infection occurs infrequently. In persons, most cases are associated with anaerobic bacteremia, whereas in dogs and cats, joint infections are usually monarticular and frequently the result of bite wounds.

Urogenital Infection

Purulent endometritis, vaginal abscess, pyometra, pelvic inflammatory disease, and nonspecific vaginitis are examples of predominately anaerobic genital infections that occur in people. Obligate anaerobes, especially *Bacteroides*, constitute a large portion of the normal vaginal flora of dogs.[15] Uterine infections in dogs and cats have involved obligate anaerobes in up to 38% of cases.[4] Despite the frequency with which pure cultures of *E. coli* are isolated from dogs with pyometra, the presence of obligate anaerobes should not be discounted unless proper anaerobic cultures have been obtained. The characteristic putrid odor associated with pyometra is attributed largely to anaerobic bacterial fermentation. Anaerobic infection of the urinary tract is rare.

Other Infections

As is true of most anaerobic infections, the prevalence of anaerobic bacteremia probably has been underestimated. Anaerobes have been isolated in 9% to 31% of blood cultures from bacteremic dogs and cats.[16,17] Anaerobic endocarditis, though rare, has also been observed in several dogs.[11]

Pyogenic infections of the CNS, especially brain abscess and subdural empyema, often contain anaerobic bacteria. Obligate anaerobes have been recovered from dogs, cats, and other animals with pyogenic infections of the CNS.[18,19] Clinically, animals have been afebrile and displayed signs suggestive of space-occupying lesions, without signs of meningeal involvement.

Anaerobic bacteria may be involved in a number of other infections in animals, including chronic sinusitis, chronic otitis media, periodontal disease, and infections of malignant tumors, especially tumors of the uterus, colon, and lung.

DIAGNOSIS

Whenever possible, cytologic examination of Gram-stained smears of wound exudates should be done as part of the initial evaluation of an animal with suspected anaerobic infection. Multiple morphologic forms of bacteria, together with evidence of neutrophilic inflammation, should be taken as presumptive evidence of anaerobic infection. Bacteria may assume abnormal shapes and have reverse Gram stain affinity when present in long-standing abscesses or after exposure to antibiotics. A brief description of the morphology and Gram-staining characteristics of common anaerobic pathogens is given in Table 49–3.

Anaerobic culture is both expensive and time-consuming for bacteriology laboratories and is not necessary for routine management of most anaerobic infections. Cultures are indicated, though, from animals with suspected anaerobic bacteremia, chronic osteomyelitis, CNS infection, and aggressive soft tissue infections that fail to respond to conventional therapy.

Specimen exposure to oxygen or contaminants must be minimized. Preferred specimens for anaerobic culture are aspirates of tissue fluid or pus, or tissue biopsies of at least 1 ml or 1 g, respectively. These specimens contain sufficient volumes to maintain favorable environmental conditions for anaerobic culture. Specimens for anaerobic culture should be kept at room temperature. Swabbed specimens are discouraged, since very small sample volumes are obtained, oxygen is trapped within swab fibers, and the risk of specimen contamination is high.

Aspirates contained in plastic syringes, from which all the air has been expressed, or tissue biopsy specimens transported in sterile containers are adequate for transport when no delay in processing is anticipated. Large amounts of exudate will usually protect anaerobes if the specimen is kept at room temperature in a plastic syringe for less than 12 hours. If a delay in processing is likely, however, special anaerobic specimen transport devices are necessary. Aspirated specimens can be injected into CO_2-filled vials. Biopsy specimens may be transported following insertion into tubes containing semisolid anaerobic media or into CO_2-filled containers. If used, swabbed specimens must be transported in tubes with semisolid anaerobic media, which should be held upright to prevent escape of oxygen-displacing gases while specimens are being inserted. Some commercial blood culture bottles will support anaerobic growth and are useful for culture of fluids in which bacterial numbers are often low (e.g., CSF, ascitic fluid, joint fluid) (see Collection Devices and Transport, Chapter 42).

THERAPY

With few exceptions, surgical drainage and debridement are essential for optimum treatment of anaerobic infection. Goals of surgical management are to improve tissue circulation, drain collections of pus, eliminate tissue dead space, and thoroughly remove infected and necrotic tissues. Repeated drainage and debridement may be necessary, since anaerobic infections have a tendency to recur and to spread to adjacent healthy tissues.

Antimicrobials

Antimicrobial treatment is given to prevent spread of bacteria to healthy tissues and to eliminate bacteria remaining after surgical treatment. Antibiotics are usually given at higher doses and for longer periods than for aerobic infection, as antibiotic penetration into devitalized tissues is often diminished. Duration of treatment should be based on site and severity of infection, as well as clinical response. Long-term (weeks to months) treatment is generally required for serious anaerobic infections, such as CNS infection, pyothorax, or osteomyelitis.

Selection of antibiotics for treatment of anaerobic infections is usually made empirically because of the slow growth of anaerobic cultures and delay in return of culture results. Suitable specimens for culture can be difficult to obtain, and technical com-

Table 49–3. Characteristics of Common Anaerobic Pathogens

GENUS	GRAM'S STAIN	MORPHOLOGY	COMMENTS
Peptococcus	Positive	Cocci	Singles, pairs, variable groups; resembles *Staphylococcus*
Peptostreptococcus	Positive	Cocci	Pairs, chains, resembles *Streptococcus*
Actinomyces	Positive (variable)	Rods, filaments	Can form tangled mats, branching or radiating
Clostridium	Positive	Large rods	Spores rarely present in clinical specimens
Fusobacterium	Negative	Thin bacilli	Tapered or pointed ends and cigar or needle appearance
Bacteroides	Negative	Coccobacilli	Pleomorphic, beaded or coccoid, difficult to stain

plexities prohibit routine antibiotic susceptibility testing of anaerobic isolates.

In addition, most anaerobic infections are polymicrobial, and it is often unclear whether an isolate is a pathogen, a symbiont, or simply a commensal. Antibiotic treatment directed only against the anaerobic component may lead to responses equal to or better than those obtained with combination antibiotic treatment. This may result from alteration of the delicate ecologic balance that exists between multiple species of bacteria present within a mixed infection. Significant decreases in infection-associated complications may occur in dogs and cats when anaerobic infections are recognized early and treatment with anaerobe-effective antibiotics is instituted promptly.[3]

Furthermore, certain drugs are usually active against anaerobes. Antibiotics considered consistently effective against anaerobes include penicillins, chloramphenicol, clindamycin, metronidazole, some cephalosporins, and imipenem. Predicted susceptibility of pathogenic anaerobes to commonly used antimicrobials is given in Table 49–4. Recommended dosages for treating these infections are listed in Table 49–5.

Penicillins traditionally have been the most widely used and least expensive drugs for treatment of anaerobic infections. Penicillin G is considered the drug of choice for most clostridial infections and for infections involving anaerobic gram-positive cocci.[20] Amoxicillin has a spectrum of activity against anaerobes comparable to that of penicillin G and is preferred over ampicillin or penicillin V for oral administration. Semisynthetic penicillins, such as oxacillin, offer no advantage over penicillin G in treating anaerobic infections. However, expanded-spectrum penicillins, such as piperacillin and ticarcillin, may be somewhat more efficacious than penicillin G against infections caused by B. fragilis.[20]

Penicillin resistance among anaerobes is increasing. Nearly 30% of Bacteroides isolates from veterinary patients have been shown to be penicillin resistant,[2] as have a few strains of Fusobacterium.[22] When penicillin-resistant bacteria are isolated, amoxicillin combined with clavulanic acid may be an effective alternative to penicillin.[22]

Chloramphenicol is effective against most pathogenic anaerobic bacteria, including B. fragilis, penetrates well into most tissues and abscesses, and reaches effective serum concentrations when given orally. Nevertheless, in vivo efficacy of chloramphenicol may not parallel results of in vitro susceptibility testing.

Clindamycin has been used extensively to treat anaerobic infections in persons. Effective concentrations are readily obtained within abscesses.[23] Clindamycin is preferred over penicillin in situations where penicillin resistance is suspected or increased tissue penetrability is desired. Clinical trials in dogs have shown clindamycin effective in treating anaerobic pleuropulmonary infections.[11]

Metronidazole is currently the only readily available antimicrobial with consistent bactericidal activity against B. fragilis and most other medically important anaerobes. Other advantages include excellent oral absorption, effective tissue penetrability, and relative lack of toxicity. Metronidazole is probably the most effective antimicrobial available for treatment of anaerobic infections in relatively inaccessible sites, such as brain and chronically infected bone. At higher doses, serious neurotoxicity has occurred in dogs, manifest by acute onset of

Table 49–4. Susceptibility of Pathogenic Anaerobes to Selected Antimicrobial Drugs[a]

BACTERIA	DRUGS OF CHOICE	ALTERNATIVES
Anaerobic cocci	pen	clin, chlor, cep[b]
Bacteroides fragilis[c]	met, clin, cef	chlor
Bacteroides sp.	pen,[d] clin, met	cef, chlor
Fusobacterium sp.	pen, clin, chlor	met
Actinomyces sp.	clin, chlor, pen	cef
Clostridium perfringens	pen, cep, chlor	clin, met, ery
Clostridium sp.	pen, chlor, met	clin

[a]pen = penicillin, cep = cephalosporins, cef = cefoxitin, chlor = chloramphenicol, clin = clindamycin, met = metronidazole.
[b]First-generation cephalosporins.
[c]Anaerobe most likely to be resistant to penicillin and most cephalosporins.
[d]Penicillins include penicillin G, ampicillin, and amoxicillin.

Table 49–5. Dosages of Drugs for Anaerobic Infections[a]

DRUG	SPECIES	DOSE[b] (mg/kg)	ROUTE	INTERVAL (hours)
Penicillin G	B	20,000 U/kg	IM, IV	6–8
Amoxicillin[c]	B	20	PO, IV	8–12
Cephalexin	B	10–20	PO	8
Cefoxitin	B	10–20	IV, IM	8
Clindamycin	B	5–10	PO, IV	12
Chloramphenicol	D	15–25	PO, SC, IV	8
Metronidazole	B	10	PO, IV	8

[a]B = dog and cat, D = dog, IM = intramuscular, IV = intravenous, PO = orally, SC = subcutaneous, U = units.
[b]Dose per administration at specified interval, expressed as mg/kg unless otherwise stated.
[c]Recommended use with clavulanate for anaerobic infections.

signs suggestive of either cerebellar or central vestibular dysfunction, and has resulted in the death of several animals (see Metronidazole, Chapter 77).[24]

Cefoxitin is one of the most effective cephalosporin antibiotics for treating anaerobic infections. Broad-spectrum coverage, including activity against the Enterobacteriaceae and *B. fragilis*, is achieved with cefoxitin. Cefoxitin has proved effective in dogs as monotherapy for a variety of mixed infections involving anaerobes.[11] Disadvantages include expense and the necessity for parenteral administration.

Imipenem, a derivative of the β-lactam antibiotic thienamycin, has the widest antibacterial spectrum of any antibiotic currently available.[25,26] Nearly all known species of anaerobic bacteria and bacteria of the Enterobacteriaceae family are susceptible.

Trimethoprim-sulfonamides have been shown to be effective in vitro against veterinary anaerobic isolates. Despite this, the two drugs in combination do not appear to be as clinically efficacious in vivo (see Trimethoprim-Sulfonamides, Chapter 43).

MANAGEMENT OF ANAEROBIC INFECTION

Clostridial Infection

Prompt, radical tissue debridement and drainage are indicated for treatment of clostridial infection, particularly if there are signs of systemic toxicity. Removal of infected tissues decreases production and liberation of clostridial toxins.

Oxygen administered under high pressure (hyperbaric oxygen therapy) has been used successfully as adjunctive therapy to treat dogs with gas gangrene.[27] Hypotension often develops rapidly in association with clostridial toxicity. Hemolysis may also occur, and both may precipitate acute renal failure. Maintenance of normal blood pressure by means of volume replacement is essential.

Soft Tissue Infection

Most soft tissue infections are best managed surgically. Antibiotics are indicated as adjunctive therapy when infection is extensive and spreads to surrounding tissues (see also Bite Infections, Chapter 58).

Pleuropulmonary Infection

Successful treatment of pyothorax in dogs and cats requires thorough pleural drainage combined with prolonged antibiotic therapy (see Chapters 8 and 53). Clindamycin may be more effective than penicillin against the usual causative bacteria, possibly owing to greater tissue penetration.[28] Metronidazole may be added to the treatment regimen if penicillin-resistant strains of *Bacteroides* are isolated but should not be used alone if *Actinomyces* or microaerophilic streptococci are present.

Lung abscesses often evolve insidiously and contain a bacterial flora that is predominantly anaerobic. Appropriate antibiotic treatment alone may resolve lung abscess and thereby avoid the need for lobectomy. Accurate specimen collection and cultural methods are very important to ensure optimum antibiotic therapy. Transtracheal aspiration often provides excellent specimens for culture from this site. Several dogs with lung abscess have been observed to respond very well to treatment with clindamycin.[11]

Aspiration pneumonia often involves anaerobic bacteria that have been introduced into pulmonary tissues from the mouth. A transtracheal aspirate is essential for accurate diagnosis and initial antibiotic treatment should include an aminoglycoside or cephalosporin if large, gram-negative rods (likely to be bacteria of the Enterobacteriaceae family) are observed. Follow-up radiographic evaluation is important in monitoring response to treatment and in determining duration of therapy for anaerobic pleuropulmonary infection.

Intra-abdominal Infection

Treatment of peritoneal sepsis generally requires combined medical and surgical management (see Chapter 9). Antibiotic treatment must be broad in spectrum and cover both coliform bacteria and obligate anaerobes.

Bone Infection

Thorough tissue debridement is crucial in the initial management of anaerobic osteomyelitis. Infected bone should be curetted down to the level of healthy, bleeding bone and any infected soft tissues excised (see Chapter 6). Antistaphylococcal penicillins and first-generation cephalosporins, although effective against *Staphylococcus*, are relatively ineffective against β-lactamase-producing anaerobes such as *Bacteroides*. Therefore, these antibiotics should be combined with antibiotics such as metronidazole, which reaches effective concentrations in bone and is bactericidal to all strains of *Bacteroides*. Clindamycin may be effective when given alone, as it penetrates bone well and is active against both *Staphylococcus* and most obligate anaerobes.

Urogenital Infection

Pyometra is the most commonly encountered mixed infection of the reproductive tract in dogs and cats. Although obligate anaerobes can be isolated from nearly one-third of dogs with pyometra, *E. coli* is a much more common isolate. Prostaglandin-induced uterine emptying may be combined with antibiotic administration for treatment of pyometra in valuable breeding animals. Chloramphenicol is a useful antibiotic in these cases, as it provides broad-spectrum coverage and reaches effective tissue concentrations. Ovariohysterectomy is the treatment of choice for nonbreeding animals.

CNS Infection

Although meningitis can be caused by a variety of organisms, intracranial abscesses are usually associated with anaerobic infection. Bacteria isolated from brain abscesses in persons are most often obligate anaerobes and microaerophilic streptococci. In four cases reported in dogs and cats, *Bacteroides*, *Fusobacterium*, and *Peptostreptococcus* have been the most common isolates.[18] Effective antibiotic coverage can usually be attained by combining high doses of a penicillin with chloramphenicol. *Staphylococcus* is much more likely to be present following open head trauma or cranial osteomyelitis, and antibiotics effective against this organism should be selected in those situations. For diagnostic and therapeutic recommendations in managing CNS infections, see Chapter 12.

Bacteremia

Anaerobic bacteria frequently enter the blood stream via infections of the abdomen, following manipulation of mucous membrane surfaces, and occasionally from cutaneous sources. Anaerobic bacteria, especially *C. perfringens*, may sometimes be present in the blood stream of dogs without inducing signs of sepsis (see Time Course of Bacteremia, Chapter 7).[17]

Negative routine blood culture results, despite strong clinical evidence of endocarditis, should prompt consideration of anaerobic endocarditis. Anaerobic endocarditis caused by *Bacteroides* and *Actinomyces* has been documented in dogs.[11] The disease in both cases led to rapid deterioration and death.

References

1. Hirsh DC, Biberstein EL, Jang SS: Obligate anaerobes in clinical veterinary practice. *J Clin Microbiol* 210:188–191, 1979.

2. Hirsh DC, Indiveri MC, Jang SS: Changes in prevalence and susceptibility of obligate anaerobes in clinical veterinary practice. *J Am Vet Med Assoc* 186:1086–1089, 1985.

3. Dow SW, Jones RL, Adney WF: Anaerobic bacterial infections and response to treatment in dogs and cats: 36 cases (1983–1985). *J Am Vet Med Assoc* 189:930–934, 1986.

4. Berg JN, Fales WH, Scanlan CM: Occurrence of anaerobic bacteria in diseases of the dog and cat. *Am J Vet Res* 40:876–881, 1979.

5. MacKintosh ME: Anaerobic bacteria: a cause of infection? *J Small Anim Pract* 28:853–862, 1987.

6. Gorbach SL: The pre-eminent role of anaerobes in mixed infections. *J Antimicrob Chemother* 10(Suppl A):1–6, 1982.

7. Emery DL: Immunity against anaerobic bacterial infections. *Vet Immunol Immunopathol* 15:1–57, 1987.

8. Dow SW, Jones RL: Anaerobic infections. Part 1. Pathogenesis and clinical significance. *Compend Cont Educ Pract Vet* 9:711–720, 1987.

9. Denny HR, Minter H, Osborn AD: Gas gangrene in the dog. *J Small Anim Pract* 15:523–527, 1974.

10. Stead AC, Lawson GHK: A study of the incidence and significance of *Clostridium welchii* in the wounds of dogs undergoing open reduction of fractures. *J Small Anim Pract* 22:1–6, 1981.

11. Dow SW: Unpublished observations. Colorado State University, Fort Collins, CO, 1987.

12. Love DN, Jones RF, Bailey M, et al: Isolation and characteristics of bacteria from pyothorax (empyema) in cats. *Vet Microbiol* 7:455–461, 1982.

13. Bartlett JG: Experimental aspects of intra-abdominal sepsis. *Am J Med* 76(5A):91–98, 1984.

14. Walker RD, Richardson DC, Bryant MJ, et al: Anaerobic bacteria associated with osteomyelitis in domestic animals. *J Am Vet Med Assoc* 182:814–816, 1983.

15. Baba E, Horta F, Fukata T, et al: Vaginal and uterine microflora of adult dogs. *Am J Vet Res* 44:606–608, 1983.

16. Hirsh DC, Jang SS, Biberstein EL: Blood culture of the canine patient. *J Am Vet Med Assoc* 184:175–178, 1984.

17. Dow SW, Curtis CR, Jones RL, et al: Results of blood culture from critically ill dogs and cats: 100 cases (1983–1987). *J Am Vet Med Assoc* 195:113–117, 1989.

18. Dow SW, LeCouteur RA, Henik RA, et al: Central nervous system infection associated with anaerobic bacteria in 2 dogs and 2 cats. *J Am Coll Vet Intern Med* 2:171–176, 1988.

19. Perdrizet JA, Dinsmore P: Pituitary abscess syndrome. *Compend Cont Educ Pract Vet* 8:S311–S318, 1986.

20. Abramowicz M (ed): Drugs for anaerobic infections. *Med Lett* 26:87–89, 1984.

21. Jones RL: Personal communication. Colorado State University, Fort Collins, CO, 1987.

22. Indiveri MC, Hirsh DC: Clavulanic acid-potentiated activity of amoxicillin against *Bacteroides fragilis*. *Am J Vet Res* 46:2207–2209, 1985.

23. Joiner KA, Lowe BR, Dzink JL: Antibiotic levels in infected and sterile subcutaneous abscesses in mice. *J Infect Dis* 143:487–494, 1981.

24. Dow SW, LeCouteur RA, Poss ML, et al: Neurologic dysfunction induced by metronidazole treatment of dogs. *J Am Vet Med Assoc* 195:365–368, 1989.

25. Barza M: Imipenem: first of a new class of beta-lactam antibiotics. *Ann Intern Med* 103:552–560, 1985.

26. Birnbaum K, Kahan FM, Kropp H, et al: Carbapenams, a new class of beta-lactam antibiotics. *Am J Med* 78(Suppl 6A):1–20, 1985.

27. Cooper NA, Unsworth IP, Turner DM, et al: Hyperbaric oxygen used in the treatment of gas gangrene in a dog. *J Small Anim Pract* 17:759–764, 1976.

28. Bartlett JG, Gorbach SL: Penicillin or clindamycin for primary lung abscess? *Ann Intern Med* 98:546–548, 1983.

50

ENTERIC AND OTHER BACTERIAL INFECTIONS

Campylobacteriosis

James G. Fox

ETIOLOGY

Campylobacter is a genus of gram-negative, slender, curved, motile rods (1.5 to 5 μm by 0.2 to 0.5 μm) that occur singularly, in pairs, or in chains with three to five spirals (Fig. 50–1). The cells can also be curve-, S-, or gull-shaped. With the exception of *C. pylori*, *Campylobacter* spp. have a single polar flagellum and microaerophilic growth requirements. *C. jejuni* is the organism routinely associated with diarrheal disease in dogs, cats, and people, as well as other domestic, wild, and laboratory animals. *C. coli*, distinguished from *C. jejuni* on the basis of hippurate hydrolysis, is also isolated from diarrheic animals and people. In addition, a new catalase-negative *Campylobacter* organism has been isolated from asymptomatic and diarrheic dogs, as well as asymptomatic cats.[1,2]

EPIDEMIOLOGY

Privately owned adult dogs and cats generally have a lower isolation rate of the organism than strays or those maintained in kennels or catteries, laboratories, or animal shelters.[3] *C. jejuni* has been isolated from 21% and 29% of diarrheic cats and dogs, respectively, compared with 4% isolation from normal cats and dogs.[4] In other studies, the isolation rate from feces of mature dogs and cats, with and without diarrhea, has varied from 0% to 50%. Puppies and kittens appear more likely to acquire *C. jejuni* and show clinical disease, probably due to lack of previous exposure and development of protective antibody.[4a] Studies of pups show

that shedding of *Campylobacter* sp. ranges from less than 5% to a high of 90%.

As with most enteric microbial pathogens, fecal-oral spread, with foodborne and waterborne transmission, appears to be the principal avenue for infection. Sources of the organism include contaminated meat products, particularly poultry and unpasteurized milk. Nosocomial infection of hospitalized animals is possible, as is exposure from other pets in a household (ferrets, hamsters, birds, rabbits) and rural farm animals that may shed the organism.

PATHOGENESIS

Severity of the disease is dependent on the number of organisms ingested by the host as well as previous exposure and development of protective antibody. Other enteric pathogens, such as parvovirus and coronavirus, *Giardia*, or *Salmonella* may play a synergistic role.[5,6] Environmental, physiologic, or surgical stress may also exacerbate the severity of the disease. A variety of virulence factors, such as enterotoxins, cytotoxins, or adherence or invasion properties, are expressed by different *C. jejuni/coli* isolates. Blood and leukocytes in the feces, congestion, edema, ulcers of mucosa, and occasional sepsis in people suggest that the organism can be invasive. Experimental challenge in laboratory animals also indicates that the organism can be isolated several days postchallenge from blood. Experimental infections of puppies and kittens with strains isolated from people with diarrhea are less severe. Animals appear to be more resistant or better adapted to these

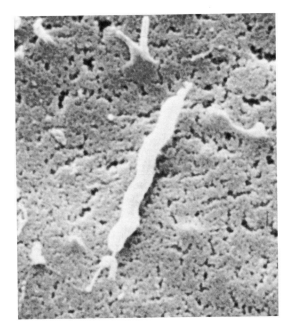

Figure 50–1. Scanning electron microscopic view of C. jejuni adhered to chick embryo cell (× 15,900).

isolates and, at most, develop watery mucoid diarrhea.[7–9]

CLINICAL FINDINGS
Dog

In many cases dogs are asymptomatic carriers of *Campylobacter*. The clinical syndrome, when present, occurs most frequently in dogs less than 6 months of age. Also, animals may be more susceptible to clinical disease when stressed by hospitalization, concurrent disease, pregnancy, shipment, or surgery. *Campylobacter*-associated diarrhea has a wide clinical spectrum in dogs as well as people, ranging from mild, loose feces, to watery diarrhea, to bloody mucoid diarrhea. Acute campylobacteriosis that develops in puppies and some adult dogs is manifest by mucus-laden, watery, or bile-streaked diarrhea (with or without blood and leukocytes) of 5 to 15 days' duration, partial anorexia, and occasional vomiting.[10–12] Elevated temperature and leukocytosis may also be present. In certain cases, diarrhea can be chronic of 2 or more weeks' duration, be intermittent, or in some cases be present for several months.[13]

Cat

In cats, clinical signs of campylobacteriosis are poorly documented in the absence of other pathogens. As with dogs, campylobacteriosis is usually nonsymptomatic, and if clinical signs are evident, the animal generally is less than 6 months of age. In a survey of 159 cats from pounds, 17 shed *C. jejuni* in the feces, but of these only two cats had bloody mucus-laden diarrhea. *Giardia* sp. was present in both, combined with *Isospora* sp. in one cat and *Toxocara* sp. in the other. Another cat concurrently infected with *Salmonella* sp. and *C. jejuni* was depressed and anorectic but not diarrheic. Cultures of the two cats' feces after antibiotic therapy and clinical improvement were negative for *C. jejuni*.[14] Chronic diarrhea in another cat that had serum antibodies to *C. jejuni*, plus positive culture for the organism, abated when treated with chloramphenicol; *C. jejuni* could not be recultured from the stool after therapy.[15]

DIAGNOSIS

Rapid presumptive diagnosis is possible using either darkfield or phase-contrast microscopy. Fresh fecal samples are examined for the characteristic darting motility of *C. jejuni*. This method is especially sensitive in people (and perhaps dogs and cats) during the acute stage of clinical diarrhea. Presence of WBC should be ascertained, since they are a common finding in people who are naturally or experimentally infected with *C.*

jejuni. Rectal swab specimens can be obtained, or fresh feces can be collected. Transport of fecal specimens usually does not present isolation difficulties because *C. jejuni/coli* remains viable in feces at room temperature for at least 3 days and at refrigeration temperatures for at least 1 week. However, higher rates of isolation can be achieved by shorter time delays.[15a] Swabs obtained from fresh feces are streaked onto *Campylobacter* blood agar plates (Campy BAP), which are then placed in an oxygen-reduced atmosphere. The standard method for culture uses commercially available selective medium that inhibits fecal flora; however, it may not be necessary for isolating thermophilic *Campylobacter* strains from acute cases of enteritis. Similarly, broth enrichment procedures have not been more effective than direct plating methods on Campy BAP for isolation of *C. jejuni* from canine feces.[15b] Plates are then incubated at 42°C and examined at 72 to 96 hours. Colonies composed of curved gram-negative rods are round, raised, translucent, and sometimes mucoid. Isolates are identified as *C. jejuni* on the basis of positive oxidase and catalase, susceptibility to nalidixic acid, resistance to cephalothin, and inability to grow at 42°C under aerobic conditions.

Various procedures have been employed, especially in outbreaks, to identify different serotypes of *C. jejuni/coli* by utilizing thermostable and thermolabile surface antigens.[16] Isolates from people and various animal species have shown that extensive serologic heterogeneity exists within *C. jejuni/coli.* Many of the isolates frequently found in diarrheic and normal laboratory beagles and cats have had serotypes frequently encountered in human patients.[17] Six strains obtained from five nondiarrheic cats and one diarrheic cat were also serovars found in people.[18] Plasmid fingerprinting and restriction enzyme mapping can also be used, but these techniques require specialized methodologies.

Serologic Testing

A variety of techniques can be used to detect serum antibodies to various antigens of *Campylobacter.* A specific bactericidal assay has been employed to demonstrate a rising antibody titer in both people and animals. Other serologic assays, such as ELISA, have been developed to survey human populations during outbreaks of campylobacteriosis and to ascertain previous exposure to the organism. Unfortunately, no systematic studies have been performed in dogs and cats to ascertain the importance of antibody titers as an indicator of infection in animals with or without diarrhea.

PATHOLOGIC FINDINGS

Grossly visible findings in naturally and experimentally infected neonates have been abnormally fluid colonic contents and thickening, congestion, and edema of the colonic mucosa.[19] Microscopically, the colon and cecum show decreases in epithelial cell height, brush borders, and numbers of goblet cells; and hyperplasia of epithelial glands results in a thickened mucosa. Subepithelial congestion, hemorrhage, and inflammatory infiltrate have also been seen. Pathologic findings in adult animals inoculated with *C. jejuni* were similar to those in some dogs with natural campylobacteriosis: stunting of intestinal villi, infiltration of the lamina propria with inflammatory cells, and hyperplastic Peyer's patches.[9] Naturally occurring intestinal lesions in adult dogs have consisted of mucosal hyperplasia in the colon, characterized by immature hyperchromatic, hyperplastic epithelial cells with a high mitotic index and deep and irregular crypts.[10] Using Warthin-Starry stain, *Campylobacter*-like organisms have been demonstrated attached to, but not within, colonic epithelium. There has also been a relative increase in the number of lymphocytes infiltrating the lamina propria. Ileal lesions have consisted of focal shallow crypts and blunt and irregular villi, which occasionally have been fused. There has been mild congestion and dilatation of lacteals. Stunting and fusing of intestinal villi and mononuclear cell infiltrate in lamina propria have also been noted in subacute stages of parvovirus infection and in a dog with protracted *Campylobacter*-associated diarrhea.[20]

THERAPY

Efficacy of antibiotic therapy and treatment of *Campylobacter*-associated diarrhea in the dog and cat is not known, nor is it known whether antibiotics indeed effectively alter the course of enteric disease. However, in some cases of severe diarrhea in dogs and cats, antibiotic therapy may be warranted. Antibiotic treatment of infected animals may be instituted to minimize exposure to human household members and other pets. Fortunately, strains of Campylobacter isolated from animals and people are susceptible to several antimicrobial agents (Table 50–1). Erythromycin, the drug of choice for Campylobacter-induced diarrhea in humans, may also be effective in the treatment of the disease in animals. Treatment of clinically affected cats and dogs has resulted in resolution of the illness and elimination of the organism as determined by Campylobacter-negative fecal cultures. It must be cautioned, however, that failure to eliminate C. jejuni with oral erythromycin from ferrets housed in a research environment has also been noted.[23]

Chloramphenicol has been used with mixed results to treat Campylobacter-associated diarrhea in dogs and cats. Treatment in dogs has resulted in abatement of clinical signs. However, the same organism has been reisolated after therapy has been completed. It is possible that these dogs developed an antibiotic-induced carrier state, as recognized in enteric Salmonella infections, or a protracted period of shedding of the Campylobacter sp., or that they became reinfected. A diarrheic cat treated with chloramphenicol showed clinical improvement and fecal cultures after completion of the treatment were negative for C. jejuni.

Several other antibiotics are active against Campylobacter strains isolated from dogs and cats. Campylobacter strains show in vitro susceptibility to furazolidone, as well as gentamicin, neomycin, clindamycin, and tetracycline. However, many strains may carry plasmids that confer resistance to a variety of tetracyclines.

Several antimicrobial agents are usually ineffective in treatment: penicillin, ampicillin, polymyxin B, trimethoprim, and vancomycin. In vitro resistance is also found to metronidazole and sulfadimethoxine.[24] Many Campylobacter strains produce β-lactamase, which accounts for the resistance to penicillin and ampicillin.

PUBLIC HEALTH CONSIDERATIONS

It is now recognized that C. jejuni/coli is a leading cause of enteric disease in people and that puppies and kittens can serve as sources of infection for people. The disease is often severe in people and in addition to diarrhea may be characterized by vomiting, fever, and abdominal discomfort. Usually the incriminated pets have been suffering from diarrhea and have been recently acquired from pet stores or kennels.[3,25,26] However, asymptomatic dogs and cats can also be a source of infection to people.[25,27] Risk factors for acquiring C. jejuni enteritis have included consumption of raw or undercooked chicken or foods contaminated by raw chicken and contact with puppies, cats, or kittens.[28–30] Veterinary practitioners

Table 50–1. Drug Therapy for Nonenteric Salmonellosis and Other Enteric Bacterial Infections in Dogs and Cats[a]

DRUG	SPECIES	DOSE[b] (mg/kg)	ROUTE	INTERVAL (hours)	DURATION (days)	INFECTIONS USED
Erythromycin	D	20	PO	12	5	Campylobacteriosis
	C	10	PO	8	5	
Trimethoprim-sulfonamide	B	12–15	PO, IV	12	7–10	Salmonellosis, shigellosis, yersiniosis
Amox(amp)icillin	B	10–20	PO, IV	8	7–10	Salmonellosis, shigellosis
Chloramphenicol	D	15–25	PO, SC, IV	8	5–7	Salmonellosis, shigellosis,
	C	10–15	PO, SC	12	8	campylobacteriosis[11,15,20]
Metronidazole	B	8–10	PO	8	5–10	Bacterial overgrowth
Tetracycline	B	10–20	PO	8	42	Shigellosis, yersiniosis, bacterial overgrowth
Gentamicin[c]	D	2	IM, SC	12	5	Yersiniosis, salmonellosis
Tylosin	B	11	PO	8	42	Bacterial overgrowth
Cephalosporins	B	10–20	PO	8	7	Yersiniosis

[a]B = both dog and cat, D = dog, PO = oral, IV = intravenous, SC = subcutaneous, IM = intramuscular.
[b]Dose per administration at specified interval, expressed as mg/kg unless otherwise stated.
[c]Monitor for renal failure.

should alert owners of the zoonotic implication of *Campylobacter* infection for other household members and stress the importance of exercising appropriate hygienic measures, especially when pets have diarrhea.

Salmonellosis   Craig E. Greene

ETIOLOGY

Salmonella are primarily motile, non-spore-forming, gram-negative bacilli of the family Enterobacteriaceae. Members of the genus *Salmonella* are pathogens that infect a wide variety of mammals, birds, reptiles, and even insects. Although they occur primarily as intestinal parasites, they can cause systemic disease and can be isolated from other organs and blood. Salmonellae are found worldwide and have important public health implications, as they are capable of causing mild to severe gastroenteritis in humans.

The taxonomy of salmonellae has undergone many changes, with classification schemes being based on both biochemical and serologic differences. The species that are recognized to be of major pathogenic significance in veterinary and human microbiology include *S. choleraesuis*, *S. arizonae* (formerly *Arizona arizonae*), *S. enteritidis*, and *S. typhimurium*. *S. typhi*, which is extremely important as the cause of typhoid fever in people, is not normally pathogenic for animals and is of little, if any, zoonotic importance. *S. enteritidis* has been further divided into more than 1700 bioserotypes, each with a distinguishing name, such as *S. enteritidis dublin*. It is common practice to omit the species name in favor of using the bioserotype alone, that is, *S. dublin*.

Some species or serotypes of salmonellae show a preference for certain animal hosts, and each domesticated farm animal species appears to have an adapted *Salmonella* species (horse—*S. abortus equi*, cow—*S. dublin*, sheep—*S. abortus ovis*, pig—*S. choleraesuis*, fowl—*S. pullorum* and *S. gallinarum*). Rarely, *S. choleraesuis* and *S. dublin* produce disease in humans or other animals.

The remaining serotypes of *Salmonella* show little or no specific host adaptation and are equally pathogenic for people and other animals. Many have been isolated from vertebrates, invertebrates, and the environment. These *Salmonella* serotypes or individual isolates of certain serotypes vary widely in their ability to infect and produce disease within a given animal host, and more virulent serotypes appear to be able to multiply intracellularly. Mucoid and encapsulated strains are more pathogenic than other strains; *S. typhi*, which produces prolonged and systemic infections in its human hosts, is noted for these features. The species most commonly isolated from diseased animals and humans is *S. typhimurium*.

EPIDEMIOLOGY

Source of Infection

Most serotypes of *S. typhimurium* are ubiquitous in nature and are readily transmitted among animals, people, and the environment (Fig. 50–2). The most common source of infection, which occurs through the GI route, is contact with contaminated food, water, or fomites. Airborne transmission, which produces respiratory infection, may occur occasionally, as the organism is able to survive on dried airborne particles in the absence of organic material.

Salmonellae can survive for relatively long periods outside the host. Finding *Salmonella* in the environment usually indicates direct or indirect fecal contamination. A large portion of the aquatic biosphere is now contaminated with *Salmonella* organisms, probably as a result of pollution of streams and lakes with untreated sewage, garbage, or other refuse. Fish and shellfish living in previously infected waters are microbiologic monitors, as they can harbor the organisms in their digestive tracts for extended periods after direct isolation from the water is no longer possible. Dogs and cats may acquire their infections by drinking contaminated water, although this is less of a problem in areas where pets drink from chlorinated municipal water supplies.

Another source of infection for dogs and

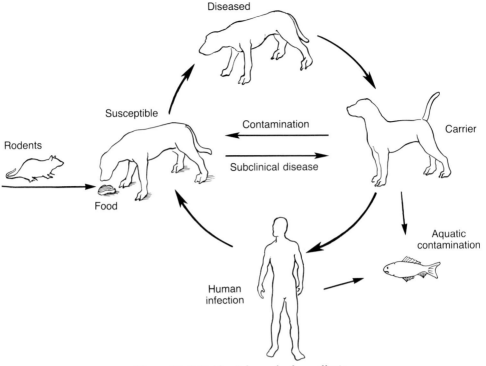

Figure 50–2. Epidemiology of salmonellosis.

cats, as well as for their human owners, is contamination of foodstuffs. This was a major problem in the past because pets were fed uncooked or unprocessed foods.[31] Meat and meat by-products, especially those from contaminated horsemeat, were the foods most commonly incriminated. Isolation of *Salmonella* from infected animals has been most common from swine, cattle, turkeys, and horses, in that order. *S. typhimurium* was by far the most common isolate. Raw or improperly cooked cat food or dog food products prepared from these sources have a higher prevalence of contamination than pelleted and heat-processed foods, which are less likely to be infected because they are adequately sterilized during preparation. *Salmonella* contamination of commercially processed foods poses a problem if these foods are exposed to infected mammals, birds, reptiles, amphibians, or insects or to unsanitary conditions. *Salmonella* can multiply quickly in moistened foodstuffs left at room temperature. Supplementation of processed foods with uncooked food scraps or meat by-products is another common source of infection.

Contaminated fomites such as food dishes, hospital cages, endoscopic equipment, and bathtubs can spread the disease throughout a veterinary hospital. *Salmonella* can occasionally be transmitted by means of contaminated pharmacologic or diagnostic preparations of animal origin, such as pancreatic extracts, liver extracts, bile salts, gelatin, vitamins, and hormonal extracts. Free-roaming dogs and cats have ample opportunity for exposure to *Salmonella* because they are carnivorous and occasionally coprophagous. Cats may have more resistance to infection than dogs, as suggested by the less frequent isolation of *Salmonella* from them.

Infected animal handlers may also be a source of *Salmonella* in a hospital, kennel, or cattery.[31b] Human infections with nontyphoid *Salmonella* are usually self-limiting, and shedding of the organism is usually not a persistent problem. Animal infections are more important in maintaining the organism in animal holding facilities. Human carriers chronically infected with typhoid fever-producing salmonellae pose no health hazard for animals.

Prevalence

Salmonellosis in the dog and the cat is more common than the prevalence of clinical disease would suggest, with numerous serotypes being isolated from each species. The frequency of fecal isolation from clinically healthy or hospitalized dogs is reported to be 1% to 36%[32,33] and from normal cats is 0% to 14%.[34,35] The actual prevalence of infection is probably higher than that estimated on the basis of fecal swab culture results and routine isolation procedures, as culture of intestinal lymph node specimens taken at necropsy yields a much higher prevalence of *Salmonella* organisms.

Host Resistance

The ability to infect animals with *Salmonella* experimentally and to establish clinical illness depends on many factors. Age is an important variable. Puppies and kittens younger than 1 year of age are more susceptible to infection and clinical illness than adult animals. Neonates may acquire infections from contaminated secretions of their dams. In utero transmission may result in death and abortion of the fetuses or birth of weak or ill puppies or kittens.

Nutritional considerations are also important in the establishment of salmonellosis. Obesity and overfeeding decrease the resistance of experimentally infected dogs to salmonellosis. Dietary deficiencies of methionine or choline in pregnant animals increase the susceptibility of their offspring to salmonellosis.

Stress caused by hospitalization, anesthesia, surgical and medical therapy, and overcrowding has been correlated with an increased risk of salmonellosis in dogs and cats.[36] Thiamylal anesthesia enhanced the virulence of *Salmonella* endotoxin for experimentally infected animals.[37]

The impairment of host immune defenses that occurs with malnutrition, malignancy, and glucocorticoid therapy may increase the prevalence of clinically severe salmonellosis. An increased postoperative prevalence of clinical salmonellosis in dogs given high-dosage glucocorticoid therapy for intervertebral disc and intraocular surgery was noted.[38] Salmonellosis has also been reported as a complication of anticancer chemotherapy in dogs with multicentric lymphosarcomas.[39] The severity of salmonellosis is increased in people with chronic or severe hemolytic anemia when the mononuclear phagocyte system is overwhelmed by erythrophagocytosis.

The intestinal tract normally is protected against colonization by enteric pathogens, which explains why the clinical prevalence of gastroenteritis is lower than the frequency of *Salmonella* isolation from the pet population. Normal intestinal motility propels ingested *Salmonella* to the cecum and colon. There, the resident bacterial population produces volatile fatty acids, including acetic and butyric acids, which limit further replication of the pathogens. Thus, any factor that alters the animal's indigenous microbial population increases its susceptibility to infection by *Salmonella*. Intestinal mucus by itself is not bactericidal; however, it contains humoral and cellular immune factors that are important in protection against salmonellosis.

Antibiotic therapy both reduces resistance to salmonellosis and prolongs the course of the illness in experimental animals. A single dose of penicillin or streptomycin greatly increases the susceptibility of mice to salmonellosis by altering the normal intestinal microflora that protects the bowel against colonization by enteric pathogens. Dogs developing salmonellosis in a hospital outbreak were at high risk if they had received antimicrobials, especially ampicillin.[31b]

PATHOGENESIS

Experimentally, a large number of organisms (10^6 to 10^9) must be ingested to produce GI colonization by *Salmonella*, with or without clinical illness.[40] Because a large proportion of ingested organisms are destroyed by the low pH of the stomach, reducing the amount of gastric acidity by administration of buffered compounds or performing vagotomy or partial gastrectomy induces a greater risk of salmonellosis in experimental animals. The organisms that survive passage through the stomach are able to colonize the middle portions of the ileum on the day of ingestion. Here they attach preferentially to the tips of villi, which they invade and in which they multiply. Localization and persistence of the organisms in the intestinal epithelium and lymph nodes account for shedding, which occurs for 3 to 6 weeks in most cases. The shedding is continual for the first week but then becomes intermittent. Intestinal lymph nodes, liver, or spleen may harbor the organism persistently, even in the absence of shedding. Reactivation of shedding or clinical illness may occur following stress, immunosuppression, or concurrent viral infections such as canine distemper and parvoviral infection or feline panleukopenia.[41,42] Reactivation of latent disease or shedding is a common problem in laboratory dogs and cats that are congregated for research purposes.[34]

Cats were also experimentally infected with S. typhimurium by conjunctival inoculation.[43] They developed chronic conjunctivitis and the organism was isolated for up to 1 week. Thereafter, they developed cervical and mesenteric lymphadenopathy and they shed salmonellae intermittently for extended periods. Ocular infection can lead to fecal excretion in the absence of other clinical signs.

Mucosal invasion, host inflammatory response, and resultant GI epithelial injury are more common with salmonellosis than with bacterial diarrhea resulting from other kinds of infections. Salmonella strains differ in their pathogenicity, which correlates with their ability to invade mucosa.[44] However, the extent of injury is not enough to explain the amount of fluid loss associated with diarrhea. There is adequate evidence that some salmonellae cause increases in adenyl cyclase, which stimulates secretion of fluid by the intestinal mucosa, as in diarrheas associated with noninvasive enterotoxigenic bacteria (see Fig. 9–8A).[44]

Endotoxemia or bacteremia may occur during overt enteric infection or in the absence of signs of intestinal illness. Fever, leukopenia, endotoxic shock, and death may result. In surviving animals, focal suppuration with localization of organisms can occur in the biliary tract, kidneys, heart, spleen, meninges, joints, and lungs. A decrease in bacteremia and clearance of organisms from the blood are associated with a rising antibody titer to cell wall (somatic, O) antigen; the flagellar (H) antigen has no role in protection. Prolonged bacteremia or overwhelming sepsis is usually indicative of compromised host defense mechanisms. Prolonged intermittent bacteremia following salmonellosis is not as common a problem in animals as it is with S. typhi in humans. The K or capsular antigen (termed Vi for S. typhi) of this organism allows it to persist intracellularly for long periods despite adequate host defenses.

Endotoxemia from overwhelming salmonellosis is associated with a variety of effects on the host (see Endotoxemia, Chapter 44). Pooling of leukocytes, erythrocytes, and platelets in the peripheral vasculature, hypoglycemia, complement activation, release of vasoactive amines, and the development of DIC may occur.

CLINICAL FINDINGS

Clinical findings in salmonellosis vary according to the number of infecting organisms, the immune status of the host, and complicating factors or concomitant diseases. The syndromes can be artificially divided into gastroenteritis, bacteremia and endotoxemia, organ localization, and persistence of a nonsymptomatic carrier state. The chronic, recurrent enteric fever associated with S. typhi infection of humans is not seen in animals.

Gastroenteritis

The clinical signs associated with Salmonella gastroenteritis are variable. Most acute episodes begin within 3 to 5 days of exposure to the organism or following stress. Very young or old animals show the most severe clinical signs. Fever of 40° to 41.1°C (104° to 106°F), malaise, and anorexia are noted initially, followed by vomiting, abdominal pain, and diarrhea. Cats frequently hypersalivate as a result of persistent vomiting. The diarrhea varies in consistency from watery to mucoid, and fresh blood is present in severe cases. Weight loss and dehydration become evident within several days after the onset of illness. Severely affected animals have pale mucous membranes, weakness, marked dehydration, cardiovascular collapse, shock, and icterus just before death.[31] CNS signs in some animals include hyperexcitability, incoordination, posterior paresis, blindness, and convulsions. Pneumonia can be associated with acute Salmonella gastroenteritis. Coughing, dyspnea, and epistaxis will be seen in affected animals.

Bacteremia and Endotoxemia

Bacteremia and endotoxemia are usually transient subclinical features of Salmonella gastroenteritis in dogs and cats and are generally seen in either very young or immunosuppressed patients. However, dogs and cats have had bacteremia in the absence of GI signs.[45,46] Severe depression, weakness, hypothermia, and cardiovascular collapse may be seen with or without GI signs. Chronic unexplained fever may be the only manifestation in some animals. Because of their incomplete maturation, kittens and puppies affected less than 7 weeks of age may not show a febrile response despite endotoxemia.[46a]

Organ Localization

Metastatic infection may occur following clinical or subclinical bacteremia. Organisms may localize in particular organ systems for many years before producing overt clinical signs. Localization is most likely to occur in tissues previously damaged or devitalized but may spread to involve healthy structures. The clinical signs noted are referable to the organ system of localization.

Subclinical Infections and Clinical Recovery

Only a small proportion (10%) of infected animals die during the acute stages of salmonellosis. Dogs and cats infected with few organisms and those that have otherwise normal defense mechanisms will have transient or no clinical illness. Animals affected by acute diarrhea usually recover after 3 to 4 weeks. Rarely, diarrhea of a chronic or intermittent nature is reported. Recovered and clinically normal animals usually shed the organisms for up to 6 weeks.

Other Syndromes

Abortions, stillbirths, and birth of weak puppies or kittens may result from in utero infection.[47] Vaginal discharges, placentas, and meconia usually contain Salmonella. The bitch or queen generally has prolonged vaginal discharges and delayed postpartum involution. Puppies that survive are weak, unthrifty, and emaciated, and Salmonella can be isolated from various organs. Conjunctivitis has been a major manifestation in some infected cats.[48] For a further discussion of ocular lesions, see Chapter 13.

Songbird Fever

Seasonal bird migrations in the northeastern United States have been associated with an acute febrile illness in cats that usually lasts 2 to 7 days.[49] There is evidence that the birds have been infected with S. typhimurium. Affected cats have primarily been outdoors and have preyed on birds or frequented bird feeders. Acute depression, anorexia, fever (40° to 40.6°C [104° to 105°F]), and diarrhea that was often hemorrhagic developed. Vomiting was variable. Recovery was usually rapid, but in some cases normal feeding behavior did not return for several weeks. Mortality may be as high as 10% and other diseases causing immunosuppression may increase this rate. Therapy and prevention of this syndrome are the same as for other Salmonella infections.

DIAGNOSIS

Salmonellosis should be suspected with any acute or chronic GI illness. It has frequently been overlooked in favor of the more common clinical diagnoses of canine parvovirus or coronavirus infections and feline panleukopenia. The clinical and pathologic features of these diseases may be indistinguishable from those of salmonellosis. Refer to Clinical Findings in Chapters 21 and 23, respectively.

Clinical Laboratory Findings

Hematologic abnormalities are variable, depending on the stage of illness. Nonregenerative hypochromic anemia, lymphopenia, thrombocytopenia, neutropenia with a left shift, and toxic leukocytes are found in animals with severe disease and endotoxemia. Bacterial rods may be found in the leukocytes of dogs or cats with overwhelming sepsis. A mature neutrophilic leukocytosis is more characteristic of localization of infection in a particular organ system.

Biochemical abnormalities are usually present only in animals with severe clinical illness. These abnormalities include hypoproteinemia, especially hypoalbuminemia, hypoglycemia, and moderate prerenal azotemia. Dogs with salmonellosis have had electrolyte abnormalities, hyponatremia, and hyperkalemia typical of primary hypo-adrenocorticism.[50]

Bacterial Isolation

Isolation of *Salmonella* organisms is the most definitive means of confirming infection. However, mere isolation from the oral cavity, vomitus, or feces does not indicate that the organisms are causing clinical disease, because the prevalence of subclinical carriers in dog and cat populations is high. Animals recovering from clinical salmonellosis shed organisms for at least 4 to 6 weeks, and shedding can be reactivated by stress or recurrent illness.

Finding organisms in samples of secretions or body fluids, such as blood, urine, synovial fluid, transtracheal washings, CSF, and bone marrow, may allow a definitive diagnosis of systemic salmonellosis to be made during the acute phases of illness. Samples for culture should be taken from the liver, spleen, lung, mesenteric lymph node, and intestinal tract at necropsy. The gallbladder and bile do not appear to be important sites of localization of infection in animals, although they are in humans infected with S. typhi.

Negative culture results do not necessarily eliminate the possibility of infection, as it is difficult to isolate *Salmonella* in the presence of other organisms. Specimens from normally sterile tissues, such as blood, bone marrow, joint fluid, and CSF, can be cultured on ordinary media. Samples taken from the oral cavity or bowel, both of which have a high concentration of commensal organisms, must be cultured on special media. Enrichment broths (e.g., selenite or tetrathionate) are used to increase the yield and to inhibit growth of competing organisms. After 24 hours, subculturing is performed on an inhibitory medium such as deoxycholate, which favors the growth of *Salmonella*. Following isolation, salmonellae are identified by Gram staining, motility, and biochemical reactions. They ferment certain sugars, including glucose (but not lactose), and react positively with substances such as urea, indole, and methyl red.

Serologic Testing

Serodiagnosis of salmonellosis in human medicine depends on the demonstration of a rise in antibody titer, as measured by the Widal (O and H antigen agglutination) and indirect hemagglutination (HA) tests. Although the HA test has been considered more sensitive for the O antigen, it is relatively nonspecific in detecting clinical illness. Not all subclinically infected dogs and cats have positive serologic titers; thus, serologic testing is not an accurate means of detecting carriers.[36] Cats respond consistently with increased titers only when they are clinically ill. For these reasons, culture of body fluids or secretions is an easier and more definitive means of making a diagnosis.

Cytology

Cytologic examination is helpful in detecting invasive GI pathogens in diarrheal illnesses. The presence of leukocytes in feces can identify diseases that cause disruption of the intestinal mucosa. A wet mount is prepared by mixing small flecks of mucus with a drop of new methylene blue on a microscope slide and covering the mixture with a coverslip. The absence of fecal leukocytes indicates a viral, mild bacterial, or nonspecific diarrhea that does not require extensive therapy. The presence of large numbers of leukocytes is typical of acute salmonellosis and other forms of diarrhea that cause extensive mucosal disruption. These cases usually require intensive parenteral antibiotic therapy.

PATHOLOGIC FINDINGS

Gross lesions are found at necropsy in only a small percentage of infected animals that develop severe clinical illness. Pale mucous membranes and dehydration accompany a diffuse mucoid to hemorrhagic enteritis. Lesions in the intestinal mucosa vary from catarrhal inflammation to mucosal sloughing with extensive denudation of the gut. GI lesions may be extensive but are usually confined to the distal small bowel, cecum, and colon.

Diffusely scattered petechial to ecchymotic hemorrhages present throughout most organ systems are associated with focal thrombosis and necrosis. The lungs are frequently edematous or consolidated, and mesenteric and peripheral lymph nodes are enlarged and hemorrhagic.

Histologically, the lesions are characteristic of a fibrinous to fibropurulent pneumonia, multifocal necrotizing hepatitis, and suppurative meningitis, all of which are associated with hemorrhagic ulcerative gastroenteritis. Histologic or cytologic examination may reveal that bacteria have disseminated to many organs, including the bone marrow, spleen, and lymph nodes.

THERAPY

Appropriate therapy for canine and feline salmonellosis varies according to the type and severity of clinical illness. Acute *Salmonella* gastroenteritis, without systemic signs, is best treated with parenteral polyionic isotonic fluids to replace losses from vomitus and diarrhea. Fluids can be administered orally when vomiting is not a problem. Hypertonic glucose-containing solutions have been effective in reversing fluid loss in infectious diarrhea (see Chapter 9). Transfusion of plasma may be more beneficial than fluid therapy when mucosal disruption and increased GI permeability lower albumin concentration to less than 2.0 g/dl.

Prostaglandin inhibitors such as indomethacin have been effective in reducing fluid losses in animals with experimentally induced *Salmonella* gastroenteritis.[51] Increased net water loss in the lower bowel results from increased intestinal secretion induced by bacterial endotoxin and mediated through prostaglandin synthesis. Prostaglandin inhibitors must be used early in the disease to be effective and must be used cautiously if GI hemorrhage is severe.

Paradoxically, osmotically active laxatives such as lactulose have been recommended for treating acute *Salmonella* gastroenteritis. A nonabsorbable sugar, lactulose produces osmotic diarrhea through the formation of acid metabolites in the distal small bowel and colon. Shortened transit time and an acid environment are deleterious to the survival of *Salmonella* organisms. Such therapy should be used only in cases in which fluid deficits have already been corrected.

Antibiotics reported to be effective against *Salmonella* include chloramphenicol, trimethoprim-sulfonamides, and amoxicillin.[46] Aminoglycosides may be considered when bacterial resistance is anticipated, but the risk of renal toxicity precludes their use. Variable resistance to erythromycin, ampi-cillin, cephapirin, or nitrofurans is reported. The in vivo response of *Salmonella* to antibiotics often correlates poorly with the results of in vitro testing.

Antibiotic therapy has not been advocated for treating uncomplicated *Salmonella* gastroenteritis but, rather, has been recommended for animals with concurrent signs of systemic infection or histories of immunosuppression (see Table 3–3). Because *Salmonella* gastroenteritis is usually self-limiting, such treatment appears to prolong the convalescent excretion period. However, this widely held view has been questioned in studies that demonstrate effective eradication of *Salmonella* from human typhoid carriers by combined antibiotic therapy.

Another inherent problem with routine antibiotic administration for *Salmonella* gastroenteritis is that infecting organisms may acquire transferable (plasmid-mediated) resistance (see Development of Antibacterial Resistance, Chapter 1). An increased prevalence of transferable resistance has been demonstrated among *Salmonella* isolates from dogs, cats, and humans.[34,52] Other disadvantages of routine antibiotic therapy for salmonellosis are that it may enhance susceptibility to infection or activate clinical illness in the latent carrier state.

Animals with more severe signs of endotoxemia or bacteremia should be treated differently from those with simple gastroenteritis. Plasma transfusions of at least 250 ml have reduced mortality in dogs given *Salmonella* endotoxin.[53] Equal volumes of isotonic fluid or smaller volumes of plasma were not helpful. Plasma-treated dogs developed leukopenia, thrombocytopenia, and extensive tissue injury, as did untreated dogs, but had better survival rates.

PREVENTION

Prevention of salmonellosis in dogs and cats is difficult because of their tendency to develop a chronic subclinical carrier state or latent infection. Nontyphoid salmonellae that infect pets are also harbored by many other animals, making eradication difficult. Pets may come in contact with these animals directly in their environments or indirectly through their food. Salmonellae are also well adapted to survive in the environment and resist common forms of disinfection.

Hygiene and strict isolation should be enforced during hospitalization because of the highly infectious and contagious nature of the disease. Infection from food sources can be minimized by using commercially available heat-processed products. Proper sanitation during handling and storing of processed foods is also important, as they frequently become contaminated by contact with utensils, rodents, or insects.

Cages in hospitals, kennels, or catteries should be routinely cleaned and disinfected between uses by different animals (see Chapter 1). Phenolic compounds or household bleach (diluted 1:32 or 4 oz/gal of water) can be used as surface disinfectants. Animals brought into group confinement should be segregated if they have or develop diarrhea or vomiting. Food dishes and utensils should be cold disinfected or, preferably, autoclaved between uses. Using disposable dishes will eliminate this requirement. Endoscopic equipment, shown to be a source of infection in human hospitals, should also be properly disinfected, that is, immersed in ethylene oxide gas, glutaraldehyde (2%), or formalin (20%) for a minimum of 1 hour. The equipment must be thoroughly aerated or rinsed before use (see Chapter 1).

Cats and dogs may shed organisms from their oral cavities or in their feces. Contaminated fur is a ready source of infection for animal handlers or pet owners. Therefore, proper disinfection of hands and clothing after handling animals is important. Human carriers of nontyphoid *Salmonella* may transmit the infection as a reverse zoonosis, and this possibility should not be overlooked if there is a recurrent problem with salmonellosis in an animal holding facility. Long-term boarders or blood donors should not be housed with the transient hospital population because the former may become exposed and then act as sources of salmonellae.

PUBLIC HEALTH CONSIDERATIONS

Salmonellosis is a disease of major zoonotic importance. Considerable emphasis has been placed on foodborne outbreaks in humans by means of contaminated products of animal origin. Sporadic, pet-associated infections have not receive as much attention. Dogs have been recognized as important vectors for nonfoodborne infections because of their habits of coprophagy and ingesting carrion, coupled with their long-term shedding of organisms and their close proximity to people. Dogs and horses have the greatest zoonotic potential for the occupationally exposed.[31] Contact with feces from infected pets has been an inadvertent but important source of exposure for young children. Cats, proved to be important but less frequently infected reservoirs, have been shown to shed organisms orally, conjunctivally, and fecally. Thus, they may contaminate their food, fur, or water source, any of which may serve as a source of infection for humans.

Of increasing concern is the frequency with which antibiotic-resistant *Salmonella* strains have been isolated from dogs and cats.[36] Most of the resistance is plasmid-mediated and is intensified by indiscriminate or frequent use of antibiotics by veterinarians. Antibiotic resistance has made recently acquired salmonellosis more difficult to treat in people. *Salmonella* infections have been more frequent and severe in people infected with human immunodeficiency virus.[54]

Shigellosis   *Craig E. Greene*

ETIOLOGY

Shigella is a genus of nonmotile gram-negative bacteria, morphologically indistinguishable from other enterobacteria, that cause a diarrheal condition known as bacillary dysentery in people and nonhuman primates.[55] On the basis of biochemical and serologic properties, they are divided into four serogroups: *S. dysenteriae*, *S. flexneri*, *S. boydii*, and *S. sonnei*. Each group is further divided into a number of subserotypes that vary in pathogenicity. Shigellae are not as environmentally resistant as salmonellae; they cannot survive a temperature of 55°C for longer than 1 hour, and they are destroyed by dilute (1%) phenol within 30 minutes. They are susceptible to inactivation by sunlight and acid pH but can remain viable for a few days in nonacidic stools maintained in the dark. Shigellae survive best in dried fecal matter on cloth that is kept in a dark, moist place. Because of this short survival, the carrier host is most important in maintaining these organisms in nature.

EPIDEMIOLOGY

Shigellae are principally primate pathogens, causing severe hemorrhagic enteritis (dysentery). The disease, which spreads primarily via fecal-oral contact, is most commonly a problem in nonhuman primate colonies in which substandard sanitation or hygiene is practiced. Waterborne outbreaks in people, although rare, may occur with sewage contamination of domestic water supplies.

Dogs may become infected following contamination of their food or water supplies with infected human feces.[56,57] Because of their coprophagous habits, pets may become exposed in areas where there is improper sewage disposal. Once they contract infection, dogs are probably not carriers but only transient excreters of organisms. Cats have not been reported to be naturally infected.

PATHOGENESIS

Shigella may cause damage in the body because of the gram-negative endotoxin that is produced. Shiga toxin is one of the most toxic biologic agents when given systemically.[58] Certain organisms (e.g., *S. dysenteriae* type 1) produce enterotoxins that increase intestinal fluid secretions and can cause ulceration. Shigellae probably produce diarrhea both by means of intestinal epithelial cell invasion with resultant necrosis and hemorrhage and by effects of the Shiga toxin. Shiga toxin is also synthesized by and may be an important virulence factor of other pathogenic bacterial species. Systemic manifestations of the toxin in infected people include DIC with renal failure, thrombocytopenia, and microangiopathic hemolytic anemia.

CLINICAL FINDINGS

In primates, the organism causes a severe hemorrhagic, mucoid, large bowel diarrhea. Lesions are usually ulcerative, and they spread from the distal to the proximal colon with time.[59] In children and rarely in adults, septicemia may develop with or without diarrhea. Unlike primates, dogs are relatively resistant and cats are highly resistant to infection with *Shigella*. Organisms have been isolated from a small number of clinically normal dogs, but they have not been directly implicated as a cause of diarrhea in this species.

DIAGNOSIS

Demonstration of organisms in cultures is essential to differentiate *Shigella* enterocolitis from diarrhea caused by other bacteria. Owing to the fastidious nature of the organism, samples collected on swabs should be transported to the laboratory immediately and should not be exposed to sunlight. Cytologic examination of the stool will reveal large numbers of inflammatory cellular exudates associated with invasion of the bowel wall by *Shigella*.

THERAPY

Symptomatic treatment with parenteral fluids and antimicrobial therapy are similar to those in salmonellosis and enteropathogenic diarrhea (see Table 50–1). Unlike *Salmonella*, many *Shigella* are still sensitive to ampicillin, sulfonamides, tetracycline, and streptomycin. Antimotility therapy was detrimental to people with experimentally induced shigellosis.[61]

PREVENTION

Control measures are very similar to those outlined for *Salmonella*. Shigellosis is easier to prevent in dogs and cats than salmonellosis because the reservoir of *Shigella* organisms is restricted to the primate host.

Yersiniosis

Craig E. Greene

ETIOLOGY AND EPIDEMIOLOGY

Yersinia enterocolitica is a motile, gram-negative, facultative coccobacillus, measuring 0.5 to 1.0 X 1.0 to 3.0 μm, that causes an enterocolitis in people. An unusual feature of this bacterium is that it replicates in culture at refrigeration temperatures, which allows its selective growth in the laboratory and refrigerated foodstuffs. Heating food at 60°C for a few minutes kills the organism.[62] The bacterium, isolated from the feces of a variety of domestic and wild animal reservoirs and the environment, has a worldwide distribution. The prevalence of isolation of this organism from animals increases in colder months, perhaps because of its affinity for colder temperatures. Differences in virulence exist among various strains of Y. enterocolitica, and serotypes 0:3, 0:8, and 0:9 are the most pathogenic for people.[62a] The organism causes illness by invasion of many body tissues and through the elaboration of a heat-stable enterotoxin. Virulence-related factors of the organism appear primarily at lower temperatures, making human acquisition of infection more likely through contamination of the environment or food rather than directly from the carrier host.[63] People appear to be unnatural hosts for this organism because they develop fever, diarrhea, abdominal pain, septicemia, or skin rashes, all signs that closely mimic those of acute appendicitis. Nonsuppurative arthritis may develop as a sequela following recovery from GI illness. Conditions associated with iron overload appear to predispose to systemic spread of the organism.[64]

CLINICAL FINDINGS

Since Y. enterocolitica has been isolated from feces of clinically normal dogs and cats, it is thought to be a commensal organism.[65] It has also been isolated from people with clinical illness who presumably contracted the organisms from contact with the excreta of infected household pets.[66,67] Experimental infections in adult dogs have produced no clinical illness despite periodic fecal shedding for 52 days and recovery of the organism from mesenteric lymph nodes and other tissues.[62] Y. enterocolitica has also been cultured from the feces of young dogs with symptomatic GI illness.[68,69] The syndrome has been characterized by a several-week history of diarrhea associated with increased frequency of stools, tenesmus, blood, and mucus. In contrast to infected humans, dogs were not systemically ill.

DIAGNOSIS

Diagnosis of yersiniosis has been based on culture of the organism in the feces of affected animals. As with other enteropathogenic bacterial infections, mere isolation from the intestinal tract may not be diagnostic of pathogenicity because the organism can be found in clinically normal animals. Isolation of the organism from deeper tissues such as blood, urine, lymph nodes, wounds, or abscesses would be more meaningful. Yersinia are not usually cultivated on conventional media because they produce small colonies that are later overgrown by normal floral organisms. A selective medium containing cefsulodin, irgasan, and novobiocin greatly improves the ability to isolate Yersinia from enteric specimens.[70] Serotyping of strains of this organism is similar to that for Salmonella. Histologic examination in one clinically affected dog revealed a chronic enteritis with mononuclear and plasma cell infiltrates in the intestinal mucosa and mesenteric lymph nodes.[68]

THERAPY

Therapy of yersiniosis should be attempted in younger dogs or cats, from whose feces the organism has been isolated, that have diarrhea or are in contact with people with confirmed infection. The organism is usually sensitive to routine dosages of chloramphenicol, tetracycline, gentamicin, cephalosporins, and trimethoprim-sulfonamides (see Table 50–1). Penicillin and its derivatives are not usually effective at routinely used dosages.

Tyzzer's Disease

Craig E. Greene
Boyd R. Jones

ETIOLOGY

Tyzzer's disease is caused by *Bacillus piliformis*, a sporeforming, gram-negative obligate intracellular parasite measuring 0.5 X 10 to 40 μm that moves by means of peritrichous flagella. Originally described as a disease of mice, it is now known to affect a wide range of animals. Reports of spontaneous disease have been described for dogs and cats.[71-82]

EPIDEMIOLOGY

B. *piliformis*, which appears to be a commensal organism of the intestinal tracts of laboratory rodents, is found on fecal cultures of normal and diseased animals. Clinical illness in rodents seems to be precipitated by stress, such as crowding, unsanitary conditions, weaning, transportation, irradiation, glucocorticoid therapy, or other forms of immunosuppression.

Dogs and cats may acquire infection by contact with or ingestion of rodent feces containing bacterial spores, although such interspecies transmission has never been documented. Experimental disease has been difficult to produce in normal dogs and cats. Most feline cases have occurred in laboratory-reared cats, some with known contact with domestic or wild rodents. It is possible that dogs and cats harbor the organism

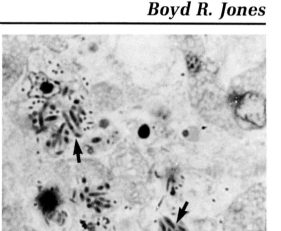

Figure 50–4. Hepatocytes at the margins of a necrotic focus in Tyzzer's disease. Bacteria resembling *Bacillus piliformis* (arrows) are present within viable cells and extracellularly on necrotic tissue (Toluidine blue; × 1500). (From Jones BR, et al: *J Small Anim Pract* 26:411–419, 1985. Reprinted with permission.)

which, under stressful conditions, may produce disease in their intestinal tracts. Immunodeficiency must contribute to the disease, as most cases have been seen in neonates of weaning age. A majority of infected animals have had naturally or experimentally induced familial hyperlipoproteinemia or immunosuppressive diseases, such as canine distemper, feline leukemia, or feline panleukopenia. Severity of experimental disease is enhanced by overcrowding, irradiation, administration of glucocorticoids or cyclophosphamide, splenectomy, partial hepatectomy, or production of mononuclear-phagocyte blockade.[83,84]

PATHOGENESIS

The pathogenic sequence of infection is uncertain. Endogenous or exogenous infection is followed by local proliferation of organisms in the intestinal epithelial cells. Following stress or immunosuppression of the host, organisms spread by the portal circulation to the liver. Colonization in the hepatic parenchyma results in multifocal periportal hepatic necrosis, presumably as the result of an unidentified toxin.

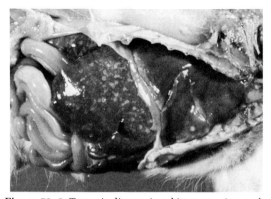

Figure 50–3. Tyzzer's disease in a kitten growing multifocal white spots on the liver from hepatocellular necrosis. Similar-appearing lesions visible through the pericardial sac are caused by focal myocarditis. (From Jones BR, et al: *J Small Anim Pract* 26:411–419, 1985. Reprinted with permission.)

CLINICAL FINDINGS

Clinical signs have been relatively consistent among dogs and cats in which the disease has been reported. A rapid onset of lethargy, depression, anorexia, abdominal discomfort, hepatomegaly, and abdominal distention is followed by hypothermia, a moribund attitude, and death within 24 to 48 hours. Diarrhea has been infrequent; scant amounts of pasty feces are more characteristic. Icterus has been apparent in some animals, especially cats.

DIAGNOSIS

Because of the rapidly fatal course of the disease, diagnosis usually has been made by gross examination of specimens collected at necropsy. Just before death, marked elevations of ALT (formerly SGPT) activity have been found. Characteristically, there are multiple, whitish-gray to hemorrhagic foci, 1 to 2 mm in diameter, on the capsule and cut surface of the liver (Fig. 50–3). Similar lesions may be apparent on other viscera. The intestinal mucosa may be thickened and congested in the region of the terminal ileum and proximal colon. Foamy, dark brown feces are usually present in the lumen, and mesenteric lymph nodes are generally enlarged.

Histologic findings usually include multifocal periportal hepatic necrosis and necrotic ileitis or colitis; other tissues, such as the myocardium, may rarely be affected. Infiltrates of neutrophils and mononuclear cells are usually present at the margins of necrotic lesions. There are numerous intracellular filamentous organisms, only faintly visible by H and E stain, in hepatocytes at the margins of necrotic lesions and in the intestinal epithelial cells. Special stains, such as Giemsa stain or Warthin-Starry or Gomori's silver stain, must be used to confirm the morphology of the organisms, which have a characteristic beaded appearance (Fig. 50–4). The organisms also can be demonstrated in methylene blue-stained impression smears made from lesions in fresh tissues. Both filamentous and spore forms of *B. piliformis* have been found.[82]

B. piliformis cannot be isolated on artificial medium that lacks living cells.[85] Material from hepatic lesions must be inoculated IV or intracerebrally into mice or into embryonating eggs or cell culture.

THERAPY AND PREVENTION

Thus far, treatment has not been successful, as affected animals die before it can have an effect. Antibiotic efficacy is uncertain. Success has been achieved with formalin-inactivated vaccines, which produce immunity to infection in mice. Whenever possible, predisposing factors that have been associated with infection in dogs and cats should be avoided.

Melioidosis   *Craig E. Greene*

Pseudomonas pseudomallei is an aerobic, gram-negative, bipolar-staining, motile bacillus with a single polar flagellum. In Southeast Asia and the South Pacific, it causes a chronic nodular or purulent inflammatory disease, melioidosis, in people, dogs, cats, and other animals. A ubiquitous soil saprophyte in endemic regions, it may be inhaled on dust, or it is introduced into wounds or tissues by bites of arthropod vectors or by direct contact with contaminated soil.[86] Infection results in small, caseous nodules that rupture and spread bacilli to the environment and other animals. Infection may disseminate further as a bacteremia in immunosuppressed animals, resulting in embolic abscess formation in many organs.

Military dogs stationed in Vietnam that became infected developed fever, myalgia, dermal abscesses, and epididymitis.[87] Dogs and cats have also been reported to be infected following insect bites or ingestion of contaminated carcasses.[88,89]

Isolation of the causative agent from blood or lesions is definitive. It grows on routine media used to isolate gram-negative bacteria. Serologic testing for antibodies with a hemagglutination assay is supportive but not as definitive for making a diagnosis as culture of the organism from internal tissues.

The organism is susceptible to tetracyclines, chloramphenicol, or trimethoprim-sulfonamide and novobiocin-tetracycline combinations. Combinations of penicillins and aminoglycosides are ineffective. Therapy may have to be continued for months. For appropriate dosages see Appendix 14.

Public health risk of infected animals is uncertain since no zoonotic transmission has been documented. People in endemic areas become infected from the environment, as do animals.

Glanders

Craig E. Greene

Pseudomonas mallei is a coccoid to filamentous, non–spore forming, unencapsulated, nonmotile, gram-negative organism that is a soil saprophyte of worldwide distribution. It primarily affects solipeds that ingest contaminated food or water or spreads between infected horses via aerosols. Cloven-hoofed animals are relatively resistant. Other animals, such as dogs, cats, or people, have intermediate susceptibility. They are infected by inadvertent contact with diseased horses, by consumption of contaminated horsemeat, or occasionally by wound contamination.

Following intestinal or local wound infection, the organism produces bacteremia and spreads to the lymph nodes, nasal passages, and the lungs, where it produces nodular lesions resembling those of tuberculosis.

The organism grows on laboratory media, a process which can be facilitated by addition of antimicrobials and growth factors. Serologic testing is used to confirm a diagnosis in solipeds, but accuracy in detecting canine and feline infections is uncertain.

P. mallei is sensitive to sulfonamides or tetracyclines. Dosages are listed in Appendix 14.

L-Form Infections

Craig E. Greene

L-forms of bacteria represent cell wall–deficient forms and are morphologically similar to *Mycoplasma*. They are distinguishable from the latter by their variable size (1 to 4 μm diameter), their greater pleomorphism, and their penicillin-binding affinities. Cell wall deficiencies can be induced in vitro or in vivo in many bacteria by exposing them to cell wall-damaging chemicals, antimicrobials, or host immune responses.

Cell wall–deficient bacteria have been isolated from cats with a syndrome of fever and persistently draining, spreading cellulitis and synovitis that often involves the extremities.[90–92] The usual source of infection has been contamination of penetrating bite wounds or surgical incisions. Cats have also presumably been infected from wound exudates from other cats. Infection begins at the point of inoculation, and lesions spread, drain, dehisce, and do not permanently heal. Bacteremic spread of infection can occur, and polyarthritis or distant abscess forma-

tion may develop as a sequela. Progressive polyarthritis, unresponsive to antibiotics and glucocorticoids, occurred in a dog infected with an L-form of *Nocardia asteroides*.[93]

Clinical laboratory abnormalities in cats with polyarthritis may include leukocytosis ($>25,000$ cells/μl) with a mature neutrophilia and nonocytosis, lymphocytosis, and eosinophilia.[92] Hyperfibrinogenemia and hyperglobulinemia may be found. The exudates contain predominantly macrophages and neutrophils with a few lymphocytes. Erythrophagia may be present; organisms *cannot* be detected by numerous cytologic stains. Radiographic abnormalities include periarticular soft tissue swelling and periosteal proliferation.[92] In severe cases, damage occurs to the articular cartilage and subchondral bone.

Diagnosis is difficult since these organisms are hard to demonstrate by light microscopy. The organisms are also difficult to culture on bacterial or mycoplasmal media.

Infection has been transmitted experimentally by SC inoculation with cell-free material from tissues or exudates of affected cats. Electron microscopic evaluation of tissues may show the characteristically pleomorphic, cell wall–deficient organisms in phagocytes.[90]

Cell wall-deficient organisms found in cats have been most responsive to tetracycline at 22 mg/kg given three times daily. Erythromycin and chloramphenicol have been used in canine infections, but these infections do not respond to most antimicrobials. They are characteristically resistant to cell wall–synthesis inhibitors such as the β-lactam antibiotics or many other broad-spectrum antimicrobials often chosen for persistent multifocal infections. Response to therapy should occur within 2 days, and therapy should continue for at least 1 week after discharges have stopped.[90–92]

The public health risk of L-form infections in dogs and cats is uncertain, because all of the cell wall–deficient organisms have not been adequately characterized. Instances of L-form infections in people are rare. In one report, a person developed an L-form infection at the site of a permanent indwelling catheter used for hemodialysis.[94] The L-form isolate was characterized as *Streptococcus sanguis* of animal origin. The same strain of this organism was also isolated from the person's pet dog.

References

1. Sandstedt K, Ursing J, Walder M: Thermotolerent *Campylobacter* with no or weak catalase activity isolated from dogs. *Curr Microbiol* 8:209–213, 1983.
2. Fox JC, Maxwell KO, Taylor NS, et al: "*Campylobacter upsaliensis*" isolated from cats as identified by DNA relatedness and biochemical features. *J Clin Microbiol.* In press.
3. Fox JG, Moore R, Ackerman JI: Canine and feline campylobacteriosis: epizootiology and clinical and public health features. *J Am Vet Med Assoc* 183:1420, 1983.
4. Dillion AR, Boosinger TR, Blevins WT: *Campylobacter* enteritis in dogs and cats. *Compend Cont Educ Pract Vet* 9:1176–1183, 1987.
5. Bruce D, Zochowski W, Fleming GA: *Campylobacter* infections in cats and dogs. *Vet Rec* 107:200–201, 1980.
6. Sandsted K, Wierup M: Concomitant occurrence of Campylobacter and parvovirus in dogs with gastroenteritis. *Vet Res Comm* 4:271–273, 1980/1981.
7. Prescott JF, Karmali MA: Attempts to transmit *Campylobacter* enteritis to dogs and cats. *Can Med Assoc J* 119:1001, 1978.
8. Prescott JF, Barker IK: Campylobacter colitis in gnotobiotic dogs. *Vet Rec* 107:314, 1980.
9. Macartney L, McCandlish IAP, Almasat RR, et al: Natural and experimental infections with *Campylobacter jejuni* in dogs. (Abstr). In Newell DG (ed): Campylobacter; *Epidemiology, Pathogenesis and Biochemistry.* Lancaster, England, MTP Press, 1982, p 172.
10. Fox JG, Krakowka S, Taylor NS: Acute-onset Campylobacter-associated gastroenteritis in adult beagles. *J Am Vet Med Assoc* 187:1268, 1985.
11. Fox JG, Maxwell KO, Ackerman JI: Campylobacter jejuni associated diarrhea in commercially reared beagles. *Lab Anim Sci* 34:151, 1984.
12. Fox JG, Moore R, Ackerman JI: Campylobacter jejuni-associated diarrhea in dogs. *J Am Vet Med Assoc* 183:1430, 1983.
13. Fleming MP: Association of Campylobacter jejuni with enteritis in dogs and cats. *Vet Rec* 113:372–374, 1983.
14. Fox JG, Ackerman JI, Newcomer CE: The prevalence of *Campylobacter jejuni* in random source cats used in biomedical research. *J Infect Dis* 151:743–744, 1985.
15. Fox JG, Claps M, Beaucage CM: Chronic diarrhea associated with *Campylobacter jejuni* infection in a cat. *J Am Vet Med Assoc* 189:455, 1986.
16. Mills SD, Bradbury WC, Penner JL: Basis for serological heterogeneity of thermostable antigens of *Campylobacter jejuni. Infect Immun* 50:284, 1985.
17. Fox JG, Claps MC, Taylor NS, et al: Campylobacter jejuni/coli in commercially reared beagles: prevalence and serotypes. *Lab Anim Sci* 38:262, 1988.
18. Fox JG: Unpublished observation. Massachusetts Institute of Technology, Cambridge, MA, 1987.
19. Collins JE, Libal MC, Brost D: Proliferative enteritis in two pups. *J Am Vet Med Assoc* 183:886, 1984.
20. Davies AP, Gebhart CJ, Meric SA: Campylobacter-associated chronic diarrhea in a dog. *J Am Vet Med Assoc* 184:469, 1984.
21. McOrist S, Browning JW: Carriage of Campylobacter jejuni in healthy and diarrhoeic dogs and cats. *Aust Vet J* 58:33–34, 1982.
22. Holt PE: The role of dogs and cats in the epidemiology of human campylobacter enterocolitis. *J Small Anim Pract* 22:681–685, 1981.
23. Fox JG, Ackerman JI, Newcomer CE: Ferret as a potential reservoir for human campylobacteriosis. *Am J Vet Res* 44:1049–1052, 1983.
24. Fox JG, Dzink JL, Ackerman JI: Antibiotic sensitivity patterns of Campylobacter jejuni/coli isolated from laboratory animals and pets. *Lab Anim Sci* 34:264–267, 1984.
25. Blaser MJ, LaForce FM, Wilson NA, et al: Reservoirs for human campylobacteriosis. *J Infect Dis* 141:665, 1980.
26. Skirrow MB, Turnbull GL, Walker RE, et al: Campylobacter jejuni enteritis transmitted from cat to man. (Letter) *Lancet* 1:1188, 1980.
27. Blaser MJ, Weiss SH, Barret TJ: Campylobacter enteritis associated with a healthy cat. *JAMA* 816:247, 1982.
28. Hopkins RS, Olmsted R, Istre GR: Endemic Campylobacter jejuni infection in Colorado: identified risk factors. *Am J Public Health* 74:249–250, 1984.
29. Deming, MS, Tauxe RV, Blake BA, et al: Campylobacter enteritis at a university: transmission from eating chicken and from cats. *Am J Epidemiol* 126:526–533, 1987.
30. Salfield NJ, Pugh EJ: Campylobacter enteritis in

young children living in households with puppies. Br Med J 294:21–22, 1987.

31. Nation PN: Salmonella dublin septicemia in two puppies. Can Vet J 25:324–326, 1986.

31b. Uhaa IJ, Hird DW, Hirsh DC, et al: Case-control study of risk factors associated with nosocomial Salmonella krefeld infections in dogs. Am J Vet Res 49:1501–1505, 1988.

32. Schaffert RM, Strauch D: Naturally infected dog droppings from public parks and playgrounds as a possible source of infections with salmonellae and helminths. Ann Ist Super Sanita 14:295–300, 1978.

33. Ikeda JS, Hirsch DC, Jang SS, et al: Characteristics of Salmonella isolated from animals at a veterinary medical teaching hospital. Am J Vet Res 47:232–235, 1986.

34. Beaucage CM, Fox JG: Transmissible antibiotic resistance in Salmonella isolated from random-source cats purchased for use in research. Am J Vet Res 40:849–851, 1979.

35. Kaneuchi C, Shyshido K, Shibuya M, et al: Prevalence of Campylobacter, Yersinia, and Salmonella in cats housed at an animal protection center. Jpn J Vet Sci 49:499–506, 1987.

36. Timoney JF: The epidemiology and genetics of antibiotic resistance of Salmonella typhimurium isolated from diseased animals in New York. J Infect Dis 137:67–73, 1978.

37. Walker RI, Parker GA, MacVittie TJ: Evidence for platelet resistance to the synergistic effects of endotoxin and thiamylal in tolerant dogs. Toxicon 17:415–418, 1979.

38. Greene CE: Unpublished observations. University of Georgia, Athens, GA, 1988.

39. Calvert CA, Leifer CE: Salmonellosis in dogs with lymphosarcoma. J Am Vet Med Assoc 180:56–58, 1982.

40. Tanaka Y, Katsube Y, Imaizumi K: Experimental carrier in dogs produced by oral administration of Salmonella typhimurium. Jpn J Vet Sci 38:569–578, 1976.

41. Calvert CA: Salmonella infection in hospitalized dogs: epizootiology, diagnosis, and prognosis. J Am Anim Hosp Assoc 21:499–503, 1985.

42. Hawkins EC, Feldman BF, Blanchard PC: Immunoglobulin A myeloma in a cat with pleural effusion and serum hyperviscosity. J Am Vet Med Assoc 188:876–878, 1986.

43. Fox JG, Beaucage CM, Murphy JC, et al: Experimental Salmonella-associated conjunctivitis in cats. Can J Comp Med 48:87–91, 1984.

44. Murray MJ: Salmonella: virulence factors and enteric salmonellosis. J Am Vet Med Assoc 189:145–147, 1986.

45. Hirsch DC, Jang SS, Biberstein EL: Blood cultures of the canine patient. J Am Vet Med Assoc 184:175–178, 1984.

46. Dow SW, Jones RL, Henik RA, et al: Clinical features of salmonellosis in cats: six cases (1981–1986). J Am Vet Med Assoc 194:1464–1466, 1989.

47. Redwood DW, Bell DA: Salmonella panama: isolation from aborted and newborn fetuses. Vet Rec 112:362, 1983.

48. Fox JG, Galus CB: Salmonella-associated conjunctivitis in a cat. J Am Vet Med Assoc 171:845–847, 1977.

49. Scott FW: Salmonella implicated as a cause of songbird fever. Feline Health Topics. Cornell Feline Health Center, Summer 1988.

50. DiBartola SP, Johnson SE, Davenport DJ, et al: Clinicopathologic findings resembling hyperadrenocorticism in dogs. J Am Vet Med Assoc 187:60–63, 1985.

51. Giannella RA, Rout WR, Formal SB: Effect of indomethacin on intestinal water transport in Salmonella-infected rhesus monkeys. Infect Immun 17:136–139, 1977.

52. MacDonald KL, Cohen ML, Hargrett-Bean NT, et al: Changes in antimicrobial resistance of Salmonella isolated from humans in the United States. JAMA 258:1496–1498, 1987.

53. Walker RI, French JE, Walden DA, et al: Protection of dogs from lethal consequences of endotoxemia with plasma transfusion. Circ Shock 6:190, 1979.

54. Celum CL, Chaisson RE, Rutherford GW, et al: Incidence of salmonellosis in patients with AIDS. J Infect Dis 156:998–1002, 1987.

55. Blaser MJ, Pollard RA, Feldman RA: Shigella infections in the United States 1974–1980. J Infect Dis 147:771–775, 1983.

56. Butler CE, Herd BR: Human enteric pathogens in dogs in central Alaska. J Infect Dis 115:233–236, 1965.

57. Floyd TM: Isolation of Shigella from dogs in Egypt. J Bacteriol 70:621, 1955.

58. Cantley JR: Shigella toxin—an expanding role in the pathogenesis of infectious diseases. J Infect Dis 151:766–771, 1985.

59. Speelman P, Kabir I, Islam M: distribution and spread of colonic lesions in shigellosis: a colonoscopic study. J Infect Dis 150:899–903, 1984.

60. Morduchowicz G, Huminer D, Siegman-Igra Y, et al: Shigella bacteremia in adults: a report of five cases and review of literature. Arch Intern Med 147:2034–2037, 1987.

61. Dupont HL, Hornick RB: Adverse effect of Lomotil therapy in shigellosis. JAMA 226:1525–1528, 1973.

62. Staley LG: Yersiniosis (Yersinia enterocolitica). In Steele JH (ed): CRC Handbook Series in Zoonosis Sect. A. Boca Raton, FL, CRC Press, 1980, pp 257–271.

62a. Cover TL, Aber RC: Yersinia enterocolitica. N Engl J Med 321:16–24, 1989.

63. Buttone EJ: Yersinia enterocolitica. In Ellner PD (ed): Infectious Diarrheal Diseases. Current Concepts and Laboratory Procedures. New York, Marcel Dekker, 1984, pp 13–49.

64. Chiesa C, Pacifico L, Renzulli F, et al: Yersinia hepatic abscesses and iron overload. JAMA 257:3230–3231, 1987.

65. Fukushima H, Nakamura R, Iitsuka S, et al: Presence of zoonotic pathogens simultaneously in dogs and cats. Zentrabl Bakteriol Mikrobiol Hyg [B] 181:430–440, 1985.

66. Gutman LT, Ottesen EA, Quan TJ, et al: An interfamilial outbreak of Yersinia enterocolitica enteritis. N Engl J Med 288:1372–1377, 1973.

67. Wilson HD, McCormick JB, Feeley JC: Yersinia enterocolitica infection in a 4-month old infant associated with infection in household dogs. J Pediatr 89:767–769, 1976.

68. Farstad L, Landsverk T, Lassen J: Isolation of Yersinia enterocolitica from a dog with chronic enteritis. Acta Vet Scand 17:261–263, 1976.

69. Papageorges M, Higgins R, Gosselin Y: Yersinia enterocolitica enteritis in two dogs. J Am Vet Med Assoc 182:618–619, 1983.

70. Lynch JA: Improved Yersinia isolation from enteric specimens. Can Vet J 27:154–155, 1986.

71. Meads EB, Maxie MG, Baker B: Tyzzer's disease in a puppy. Can Vet J 25:134, 1984.

72. Poonacha KB, Smith HL: Naturally occurring Tyzzer's disease as a complication of distemper and mycotic pneumonia in a dog. *J Am Vet Med Assoc* 169:419–420, 1976.

73. Qureshi SR, Carlton WW, Olander HJ: Tyzzer's disease in a dog. *J Am Vet Med Assoc* 168:602–604, 1976.

74. Boschert KR, Allison N, Allen TLC, et al: Tyzzer's disease in an adult dog. *J Am Vet Med Assoc* 192:791–792, 1988.

75. Myerslough N: Tyzzer's disease in puppies. *Vet Rec* 122:238, 1988.

76. Kovatch RM, Zebarth G: Naturally occurring Tyzzer's disease in a cat. *J Am Vet Med Assoc* 162:136–138, 1973.

77. Kubokawa K, Kubo M, Takasaki Y, et al: Two cases of feline Tyzzer's disease. *Jpn J Exp Med* 43:413–421, 1973.

78. Schneck G: Tyzzer's disease in an adult cat. *VM SAC* 70:155–156, 1975.

79. Bennett AM, Huxtable CR, Love DN: Tyzzer's disease in cats experimentally infected with feline leukemia virus. *Vet Microbiol* 2:49–56, 1977.

80. Schmidt RE, Eisenbrandt DL, Hubbard GB: Tyzzer's disease in snow leopards. *J Comp Pathol* 94:165–167, 1984.

81. Jones BR, Johnstone AC, Hancock WS: Tyzzer's disease in kittens with familial primary hyperlipoproteinaemia. *J Small Anim Pract* 26:411–419, 1985.

82. Wilkie JSN, Barker IK: Colitis due to *Bacillus piliformis* in two kittens. *Vet Pathol* 22:649–652, 1985.

83. Nii A, Nakayama H, Fujiwara K: Effect of partial hepatectomy on Tyzzer's disease of mice. *Jpn J Vet Sci* 48:227–235, 1986.

84. Nakayama H, Nii A, Oguihara S, et al: Effect of reticuloendothelial system blocking on Tyzzer's disease of mice. *Jpn J Vet Sci* 48:211–217, 1986.

85. Thunert A: Is it possible to cultivate the agent of Tyzzer's disease (*Bacillus piliformis*) in cellfree media? *Z Versuchstierkd* 26:145–150, 1984.

86. Spotnitz M, Rudnitsky J, Ramboaud JJ: Melioidosis pneumonitis. *JAMA* 202:950–954, 1967.

87. Moe JB, Stedham MA, Jennings PB: Canine melioidosis. *Am J Trop Med Hyg* 21:351–355, 1972.

88. Chooi KF, Omar AR, Lee JS: Melioidosis in a domestic cat with concurrent infestation by nymphs of the cat pentastome, *Armillifer moniliformis*. *Kajian Veterinar* 14:41–43, 1982.

89. Lloyd JM, Suijendorp P, Soutar WR: Melioidosis in a dog. *Aust Vet J* 65:191–192, 1988.

90. Pedersen NC: *Feline Infectious Diseases*. Goleta, CA, American Veterinary Publications, 1988, pp 237–240.

91. Keane DP: Chronic abscesses in cats associated with an organism resembling *Mycoplasma*. *Can Vet J* 24:287–291, 1983.

92. Carro T, Pedersen NC, Beamer BL, et al: Subcutaneous abscesses and arthritis caused by a probable bacterial L-form in cats. *J Am Vet Med Assoc* 194:1583–1587, 1989.

93. Buchanan AM, Beaman BL, Pedersen NC, et al: *Nocardia asteroides* recovery from a dog with steroid- and antibiotic-unresponsive idiopathic polyarthritis. *J Clin Microbiol* 18:702–708, 1983.

94. Chmel H: Graft infection and bacteremia with a tolerant L-form of *Streptococcus sanguis* in a patient receiving hemodialysis. *J Clin Microbiol* 24:294–295, 1986.

51 MYCOBACTERIAL INFECTIONS

Tuberculous Mycobacterial Infections
Craig E. Greene

ETIOLOGY

Mycobacterial infections of dogs and cats are caused by bacteria belonging to the family Actinomycetales. *Mycobacterium* is a genus comprising morphologically similar, aerobic, nonspore-forming, and nonmotile bacteria with wide variations in host affinity and pathogenic potential. They are subdivided into several groups and individual species, according to characteristic biochemical and cultural reactions (Table 51–1).

Mycobacteria have the distinctive property of retaining hot carbolfuchsin stain after subsequent treatment with acid or alcohol. This acid-alcohol fastness is due to the high lipid content of mycolic acid in the cell wall. Cord factor and Wax D, also surface constituents of mycobacterial cells, are partly responsible for the host's granulomatous response to the organism.

Mycobacteria are more resistant to heat, pH changes, and routine disinfection than are other pathogenic non–spore-forming bacteria. Common disinfectants are often added to samples collected for culture of mycobacteria to kill extraneous contaminating organisms. The minimum criteria established for pasteurization and heat disinfection have been developed to kill mycobacteria. Mycobacteria are highly susceptible to dilute (5%) phenol or direct sunlight. Although they are relatively more stable in the presence of organic material, mycobacteria are killed by dilute (5%) household bleach within 15 minutes at room temperature.

Mycobacteria generally produce one of three clinical forms of illness in infected people or animals: internal tubercular granulomas, (tuberculosis), localized cutaneous nodules (leprosy), or spreading, primarily subcutaneous, inflammation (atypical mycobacterial infections). These are discussed under the respective headings that follow.

M. tuberculosis and *M. bovis*, highly pathogenic nodule- or tubercle-producing mycobacteria, are facultative or obligate intracellular parasites. They are closely related species that have been difficult to distinguish using nucleic acid probes. They require infection of reservoir mammalian hosts to be maintained in nature, as environmental survival is limited to a maximum of 1 to 2 weeks on infected fomites.

One of the atypical, saprophytic mycobacteria that occurs as an opportunistic pathogen is *M. avium*. Considerable overlap occurs between the properties of *M. avium* and a closely related pathogen, *M. intracellulare*. Because of this indistinct separation, it has been recommended that *M. avium–M. intracellulare* or *M. avium* complex be used to refer to these organisms. Serotyping by agglutination reactions is used to classify *M. avium*–complex isolates, Groups I through IV being the usual pathogenic subtypes isolated from human and animal infections. This serologic classification should *not* be confused with Runyon's classification system for atypical mycobacteria described in Table 51–1. Since it produces tuberculous lesions indistinguishable from *M. tuberculosis* and *M. bovis*, *M. avium* is discussed with these organisms.

Table 51–1. Characteristics of Selected Species of Mycobacterium of Veterinary Interest

GROUP	REPRESENTATIVE SPECIES	AFFECTED NATURAL HOSTS (EXPERIMENTAL HOSTS)	MEANS OF EXISTENCE[a]	PECULIAR CULTURAL AND BIOCHEMICAL FEATURES
Tuberculous	M. tuberculosis	Human, dog, cat, pig (guinea pig, mouse, hamster)	FI	Niacin-positive, glycerol enhances
	M. bovis	Human, cat, dog, cow, pig (guinea pig, rabbit, mouse)	FI	Niacin-negative, glycerol inhibits
Lepromatous	M. leprae	Human (armadillo, mouse)	OI	Unable to cultivate
	M. lepraemurium	Mouse, cat	OI	Difficult to cultivate, requires complex media
Other	M. paratuberculosis	Cattle	FI	Requires mycobactin
Atypical				**Runyon's Classification[c]**
Slow-growing	M. kansasii	Human, dog (hamster; variable in mouse)	S, FI	I
	M. avium-intracellulare complex[b]	Birds, human, dog, cat (variable in rabbit and mouse)	S, FI	III
Fast-Growing	M. thermoresistible	Cat	S	II
	M. xenopi	Cat	S	III
	M. chelonei	Dog	S	IV
	M. fortuitum	Dog, cat (mouse)	S	IV
	M. phlei	Cat	S	IV
	M. smegmatis	Cat	S	IV

[a]FI = facultative intracellular; OI = obligate intracellular; S = saprophyte.

[b]Included in tuberculous group in this chapter because produces clinically similar disease. Growth enhanced by glycerol and 42° C.

[c]Older (Runyon's) classification system for atypical mycobacteria based on cultural properties:
   I Photochromogens—produce yellow pigment on exposure to light, buff color on growth in dark.
   II Scotochromogens—produce orange pigment, independent of light.
   III Nonchromogens—filamentous forms, buff or yellow regardless of amount of light; slow growth.
   IV Nonchromogens—rapid growth, mature colonies in 4 to 6 days at 37° C, most others require 1–2 weeks.

EPIDEMIOLOGY

Dogs and cats are susceptible to infections by *M. tuberculosis* and *M. bovis* but are relatively resistant to infection by *M. avium*–complex organisms (Table 51–2). Canine and feline infections with *M. tuberculosis* are considered an inverse zoonosis; the direction of transmission is from human to animal (Fig. 51–1). Although pets acquire

Table 51–2. Relative Susceptibility of Dogs, Cats, and Humans to Three Species of Mycobacterium[a]

ORGANISM	DOG	CAT	HUMAN
M. tuberculosis	+ +	+	+ +
M. bovis	+ +	+ +	+ +
M. avium	+	+	+

[a] + + = very susceptible; + = susceptible.

the infection from people, the spread to people from dogs or cats has not been reported. Dogs have had a higher prevalence of infection with *M. tuberculosis* than cats. Dogs with tuberculous pneumonitis discharge organisms in their sputum as do infected people, and aerosolized droplets are the primary means of transmission of this disease. Airborne droplet nuclei from respiratory secretions fall to the ground, where they temporarily remain viable but stationary and thus relatively noninfectious for other people and pets. Only small (3- to 5-μm) diameter particles can successfully bypass upper respiratory clearance mechanisms and deposit in alveoli. Discharges that are not airborne may potentially be infectious to dogs and cats exposed through close contact. In general, tubercle bacilli are not as infectious as other bacterial pathogens

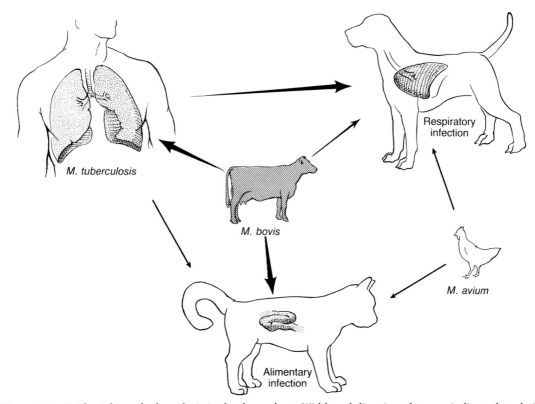

M. tuberculosis

M. bovis

Respiratory
infection

M. avium

Alimentary
infection

Figure 51–1. Epidemiology of tuberculosis in the dog and cat. Width and direction of arrows indicate the relative frequency and usual sources of infection.

since prolonged, frequent exposure or large inocula are usually required. Because of measures imposed to control infection in people, the overall prevalence of human and animal *M. tuberculosis* infections has been decreasing in recent years; relative increases have occurred in densely populated urban areas and in economically depressed areas. The incidence of *M. tuberculosis* infections in the United States is highest in Atlantic coast metropolitan regions and in the southeastern region.

Cats and dogs can be potential disseminators of *M. bovis* when the disease process preferentially localizes in the intestinal or respiratory tracts, respectively. Because of localization of infection, cats usually excrete the organism via feces and dogs via sputum. The GI tract is the most common portal of entry of *M. bovis*. Dogs and cats may be involved in the maintenance of bovine tuberculosis on farms, where it is enzootic, and are probably rarely responsible for transmission of the bovine bacillus to people (see Fig. 51–1). Subclinically infected dogs and cats sometimes remain on farms after reactor cattle have been identified and removed

from the herd, and farms or families with recurrent tuberculosis infections should have their pet animal contacts checked periodically.

Cats are more commonly infected with the bovine bacillus than dogs, and on an experimental basis, cats appear to be more susceptible to bovine than to human tuberculosis.[1,2] Part of this affinity relates to their frequent ingestion of contaminated, unpasteurized milk or uncooked meat or offal from infected cattle. Milk is an ideal medium for the organism because it buffers the gastric acid that normally prevents colonization of the lower GI tract with tuberculous bacilli. Dogs and cats may also acquire tuberculosis from infected organ meat used in cat and dog foods. Owing to eradication measures, the prevalence of bovine tuberculosis is low in the United States.

Infections with avian tubercle bacilli have rarely been reported in dogs[3-5] and cats[6-8] owing to innate resistance to the organism. Poultry are primarily susceptible to *M. avium*–complex infection following contact with infected food or water. Feces of infected birds contain large numbers of bacilli, and infection of dogs and cats occurs from ingestion of infected meat or contact with infected soil or with fomites contaminated by poultry carcasses or feces (see Fig. 51–1). Unlike *M. tuberculosis* and *M. bovis*, *M. avium*–complex organisms remain viable for at least 2 years in the environment, including municipal water supplies, soil, dairy products, and tissues of birds and mammals. The importance of infection with *M. avium*–complex organisms is that they produce granulomas of deeper tissue that are indistinguishable from those caused by mammalian tubercle bacilli.

PATHOGENESIS

Tubercle bacilli enter the body through either the respiratory or alimentary tract, depending on the initial route of exposure. Local multiplication of the bacillus at the initial site of deposition—termed a **primary complex**—as well as in the regional draining lymph node may develop. Granuloma formation occurs at both sites. **Incomplete primary complex** refers to infection and localization in the lymph node without lesion formation at the site of deposition. Cats more commonly form incomplete primary complexes whether tonsils or ileocecal lymph nodes are infected, the latter being the most common site of localization and shedding of *M. bovis* organisms. Dogs, which more commonly acquire *M. tuberculosis*, tend to develop respiratory infections with complete primary complex formation and lesions both in the lungs and hilar lymph nodes. *M. tuberculosis* more readily infects the respiratory tract because of its high oxygen requirements. Infections involving *M. avium*–complex organisms in dogs and cats mainly have been disseminated throughout lymphoid and many other tissues without indications of a primary granuloma at the site of entry.

Not all initial exposure to mycobacteria results in the formation of persistent granulomas, as most immune responses usually limit further multiplication and spread of the agent. The initial inflammatory response may subside and resolve with healing and fibrosis if the remaining tubercle bacilli can be eliminated.

More commonly, with decreased immunologic resistance the mycobacteria merely become confined within phagocytic cells.

They continue to multiply intracellularly because of the body's inefficiency in eliminating these intracellular pathogens. Granuloma formation that results is a reflection of the body's attempt to contain remaining organisms. These viable organisms may remain dormant only to break out later and spread as a result of immunosuppression.

In a certain percentage of animals, the mycobacteria may appear to outpace the host defense mechanism, resulting in progressive disease. This increased virulence may result from alterations in the route of exposure, size of inoculum, organism pathogenicity, and cell-mediated immune defense mechanisms. Having produced primary lesions, the tuberculous mycobacteria may disseminate throughout the body, spreading the infection of the disease into adjacent tissue by direct extension or by mechanical means. Aspiration and gravitation of infectious exudates may spread the disease through other areas of lung tissue. Intracellular multiplication of the bacteria is unimpeded as the infection spreads to other tissues by lymphatic or hematogenous means. A higher prevalence of *M. tuberculosis* infection has been observed in people with AIDS.[9,10] Similarly, certain breeds, such as the basset hound and possibly the Siamese cat, are overrepresented in reports of *M. avium*–complex infection.[5]

It is unclear what factors contribute to mycobacterial resistance by the host. Cell-mediated immunity is typically associated with protection against facultative intracellular pathogens such as mycobacteria. Increased resistance seems to be associated with the enhanced capacity of activated macrophages to kill tubercle bacilli or inhibit their intracellular multiplication.

CLINICAL FINDINGS

Canine and feline tuberculosis is most frequently a subclinical disease. Many pets become inadvertently infected with *M. tuberculosis* while living in the same household with tuberculous owners. Farm pets also may serve as subclinical reservoirs of *M. bovis* for susceptible cattle. The ubiquitous distribution of *M. avium*–complex organisms in the environment compared with the low prevalence of the disease also suggests that subclinical infections are common.

When clinical signs occur in dogs and

cats, they reflect the site of granuloma formation. Bronchopneumonia, pulmonary nodule formation, and hilar lymphadenopathy are most commonly seen in dogs, causing fever, weight loss, anorexia, and harsh, nonproductive coughing. Dogs and cats may develop dysphagia, retching, hypersalivation, and tonsillar enlargement, all the result of ulcerated and chronically draining oropharyngeal lesions. Cats, which develop primary intestinal localization more commonly than dogs, exhibit weight loss, anemia, vomiting, and diarrhea as signs of intestinal malabsorption. Mesenteric lymph nodes are palpably enlarged. Abdominal effusion is present in some cases.

A continuum of clinical signs develop with disseminated disease. Direct extension of lung disease has resulted in pleural or pericardial effusion with signs of dyspnea, cyanosis, and right-sided heart failure. Disseminated disease may be the first sign of illness seen in many dogs and cats, and clinical signs refer to the organ localization in each case. Generalized lymphadenopathy, weight loss, fever, and sudden death may be observed. Masses may be detected in many abdominal organs, including the liver and spleen. Dermal nodules and nonhealing draining ulcers commonly have been seen in cats and sometimes in dogs.[11] Granulomatous uveitis and CNS signs have occurred in some cases. Lameness and spontaneous fractures have been observed with bone localization. Additional clinical signs have included hemoptysis, hematuria, and icterus.

DIAGNOSIS

Clinical laboratory findings in tuberculosis are frequently nonspecific and include a moderate leukocytosis and anemia. Normal-to-reduced serum albumin and hyperglobulinemia are frequently apparent. Radiographically visible masses may be apparent in various organ systems. Abnormalities on thoracic radiography can include tracheobronchial lymphadenopathy and interstitial lung infiltration (Fig. 51–2).[12] Lung consolidation and granuloma formation have been associated with diffuse radiopaque densities in lung lobes. Calcified pulmonary lesions have sometimes been observed in dogs and cats. Metastatic lesions are seen as diffuse miliary densities. Fluid may be present in the pleural or pericardial cavities. Abdominal radiography may reveal enlargement of parenchymatous organs such as the liver and spleen or solitary abdominal masses. Fluid may be present in the abdominal cavity, and calcified mesenteric lymph nodes may be noted. Bony lesions consist of small, circumscribed, radiolucent areas. Thoracic involvement may be associated with hypertrophic pulmonary osteoarthropathy. Discospondylitis or vertebral osteomyelitis may be apparent in the vertebral bodies.

Skin Testing

Intradermal (ID) skin testing has been used as an aid in the detection and diagnosis of

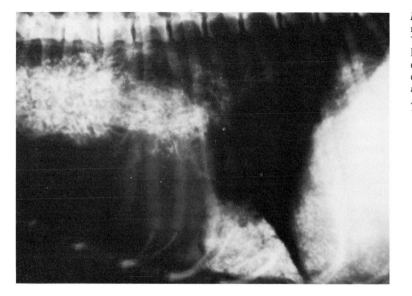

Figure 51–2. Lateral thoracic radiograph of a 3-year-old male Yorkshire terrier with tuberculosis. Note the multiple irregular calcifications of soft tissue in the craniodorsal thorax and cranial abdomen. (From Liu S, et al: *J Am Vet Med Assoc* 177:164–167, 1980, with permission.)

Table 51–3. *Summary of Intradermal Skin Testing for Tuberculosis in Dogs and Cats*[a]

SUBSTANCE	PREFERRED SITE	DOSE
Purified protein derivative (PPD)[13]	Inner surface pinna	250 TU[b] (0.1 ml)
Bacille Calmette-Guérin (BCG)[14–16]	Inner surface pinna	0.1–0.2 ml[c]

[a]See text for information on performance and interpretation of the test.

[b]TU = tuberculin units. PPD for bovine testing from USDA is 30,000 TU/ml (1 mg/ml). To prepare 250 TU/0.1 ml, remove 0.1 ml as supplied; add to 1.1 ml sterile water for injection USP; mix in sterile glass vial.

[c]BCG vaccine USP contains 8–26 million colony-forming units/ml of living bacillus. Reconstitute freeze-dried preparation into 1-ml aliquots according to manufacturer's recommendation.

human tuberculosis and to evaluate delayed-type hypersensitivity in animals. The two types of antigen used for ID testing are summarized in Table 51–3. Depending on a previous history of infection or disease, various strengths (1, 5, or 250 tuberculin units [TU]/0.1 ml) of purified protein derivative (PPD tuberculin) are usually employed in human skin testing. However, the highest concentration is needed to test dogs. ID tuberculin testing in dogs has been reported to be inconsistent and unreliable. However, use of PPD in the pinna was shown to be reliable in detecting dogs previously sensitized with bacille Calmette-Guérin (BCG) vaccine.[13] BCG is an attenuated mutant strain of *M. bovis* that has been used in people as a vaccine to induce resistance to tuberculosis and as a nonspecific immunostimulant. In addition, infected dogs have been shown to respond well to ID skin testing with BCG.[14,15]

Tests are performed by injecting BCG or PPD intradermally on the medial side of the proximal hindlimb or preferably on the inner surface of the pinna. A positive reaction is indicated only if a raised, indurated, and subsequently necrotic swelling appears at the site of injection between 48 and 72 hours later. Necrosis and ulceration may take up to 2 weeks to develop. Mild erythema following ID-BCG injection in dogs is considered to be nonspecific. False-positive results due to cross-reactivity with other bacterial species have been observed.

Unlike many species, cats do not react strongly to ID administered tuberculin.[14,17] Despite their lack of response to PPD, cats still have adequate immunity to tuberculosis. SC or IV challenge with tuberculin is no more reliable, and cats do not respond well to ID-BCG. Cats sensitized to BCG have responded to PPD injected ID in the pinna;[16] unfortunately, the response has usually been inconsistent, infrequent, or transient.

Serologic Testing

Although unreliable compared with skin testing, serologic testing for tuberculosis includes hemagglutination and complement fixation tests. Serologic testing has been used to detect infected dogs and cats when skin testing was inconclusive.

Bacterial Isolation

For culture, tissue samples are usually treated with 4% sodium hydroxide or another disinfectant to eliminate any contaminating microorganisms. Pathogenic mycobacteria are slow-growing, often requiring several weeks to establish visible colonies, and their growth is inhibited unless enrichment media are used. Egg-enrichment media such as Lowenstein-Jensen and Middlebrook (both from Difco Labs, Detroit, MI) are used for isolating tubercle bacilli. Glycerol, which is added to media such as Lowenstein-Jensen to enhance the growth of *M. tuberculosis*, actually inhibits the growth of *M. bovis*, and Stonebrink's media is used when *M. bovis* is suspected. Pathogenic and saprophytic mycobacteria are identified and differentiated by colony growth and biochemical characteristics (see Table 51–1).

Animal inoculation has been used historically to identify mycobacterial species. Laboratory animals such as guinea pigs, rabbits, mice, and hamsters have been inoculated intraperitoneally with suspensions of lymph node, spleen, and granulomas from suspected patients.

Tissue Biopsy

Definitive diagnoses can be made by demonstrating acid-fast organisms within a lesion via biopsy and histologic examination of lesions or with direct smears of exudates or fluids. The acid-fast staining method is ideal for aspirates of tissue and granulomas and for identifying organisms in bacterial cultures (see Appendix 8). Mycobacteria can also be demonstrated using fluorescent dyes on stained preparations. Although often present in low numbers, intracellular tubercle bacilli are recognized by their clubbed shape and beaded appearance.

PATHOLOGIC FINDINGS

In dogs and cats, generalized emaciation is a frequent finding on gross necropsy examination. Multifocal granulomas are grayish-white to yellow circumscribed nodular lesions and appear in many organs (Fig. 51–3). Lung and bronchial lymph nodes are usually the primary lesion sites in dogs, and ileocecal and mesenteric lymph nodes are similarly involved in cats. Generalized spread is more common in dogs than in cats, with pleura, pericardium, liver, kidney, heart, intestine, and CNS lesions being the most frequent (Fig. 51–4). The mesenteric

lymph nodes, spleen, and skin are more commonly involved in cats. Rarely, bone, joint, and genital lesions may be observed in dogs and conjunctival lesions in cats. Unlike larger solitary primary granulomas, metastatic lesions are frequently small (1 to 3 mm) and multifocal or appear as large clusters of coalescing tubercles in many organs.

Histologically, granulomatous lesions consist of areas of focal necrosis surrounded by infiltrations of plasma cells and macrophages. Evidence of encapsulation is apparent by peripheral layers of densely packed fibroblasts in a thin, fibrous, connective tissue capsule. Calcification of the granuloma is sometimes present; however, liquefaction of the necrotic central portion is rarely if ever observed in carnivores (Fig. 51–5). Epithelioid or histiocytic cells usually border the necrotic zone; giant cell formation, which occurs in other species, is uncommon. Short-chained, beaded, slightly pleomorphic, acid-alcohol–fast bacilli may be detected intracellularly in the periphery of necrotic lesions.

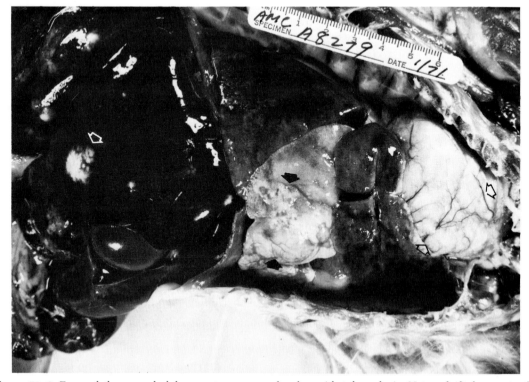

Figure 51–3. Exposed thorax and abdomen at necropsy of a dog with tuberculosis. Note calcified mass in the thorax (*light arrows, right*), calcified granuloma involving the cardiac lung lobe (*dark arrows, center*), and calcified nodules in the liver (*light arrow, left*). (From Liu S, et al: *J Am Vet Med Assoc* 177:164–167, 1980, with permission.)

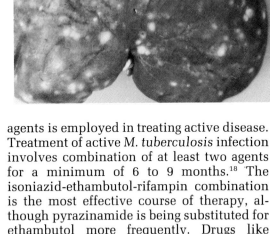

Figure 51–4. Multifocal granulomas in the kidney of a 3.5-year-old male boxer with systemic spread of tuberculous infection. (From Liu S, et al: *J Am Vet Med Assoc* 177:164–167, 1980, with permission.)

THERAPY

Treatment of human tuberculosis involves several drug regimens, depending on whether the patient has been exposed and whether subclinical or active disease has been demonstrated (Table 51–4). Similar guidelines might apply when considering treatment of pets. Long-term (6 months to 1 year) single-drug (isoniazid) regimens are used prophylactically when exposure with concurrent immunosuppression increases the likelihood of producing active disease. Combination chemotherapy using several agents is employed in treating active disease. Treatment of active *M. tuberculosis* infection involves combination of at least two agents for a minimum of 6 to 9 months.[18] The isoniazid-ethambutol-rifampin combination is the most effective course of therapy, although pyrazinamide is being substituted for ethambutol more frequently. Drugs like these have made human tuberculosis a curable disease, and surgical removal of tuberculous granulomas is no longer required. Chemotherapy of spontaneous canine tuberculosis has been successful in certain cases in which it has been used. Rapid regression of experimentally produced lesions in dogs

Figure 51–5. Photomicrograph of a liver from a 2-year-old-female German shepherd showing a caseous tubercle with central necrosis, proliferation of histiocytes and fibroblasts in the middle zone, and encapsulation in the periphery (H and E; × 100). *Inset,* Beaded bacilli (acid-fast stain; × 1000). (From Liu S, et al: *J Am Vet Med Assoc* 177:164–167, 1980, with permission.)

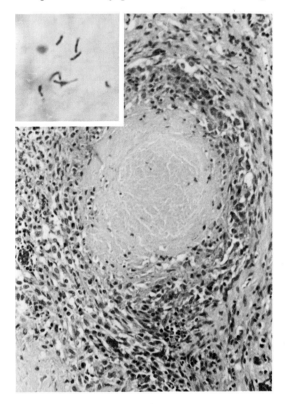

Table 51–4. Dosages of Some Antituberculosis Drugs[a]

DRUG	DOSE[b] (mg/kg)	ROUTE	INTERVAL (HOURS)	TOXICITIES
Chemoprophylaxis[c]				
Isoniazid	10[d]	PO	24	Hepatotoxic
Treatment[e]				
(Minimum of two of the following drugs in combination)				
Isoniazid	10–20[d]	PO	24	Hepatotoxic
Rifampin	10–20[f]	PO	12–24	Hepatotoxic; discolors tears and urine
Ethambutol	15	PO	24	Optic neuritis
Dihydrostreptomycin	15	IM	24	Ototoxic
Pyrazinamide	15–40	PO	24	Hepatotoxic, GL signs, arthralgia

[a]PO = oral, IM = intramuscular. Dosages are extrapolated from human child and adult recommendations.

[b]Dose per administration at specified interval, expressed as mg/kg unless otherwise stated. After daily dosing for weeks to months, switch to twice weekly administration for 6 to 9 months.

[c]For 6 to 12 months.

[d]Maximum 300 mg daily.

[e]*Localized*: isoniazid and rifampin daily for 6 months with pyrazinamide added during the first 2 months or isoniazid and rifampin alone for 9 months.

Disseminated: isoniazid and rifampin, with ethambutol and/or pyrazinamide initially and treat daily beyond 9 months.

[f]Maximum 600 mg daily.

has been achieved by combined IV administration of rifampin and isoniazid and IM administration of streptomycin for 23 months.[19] Increases in coagulation times and liver enzyme activities were side effects of this extended therapy.

The decision to treat infected dogs and cats must be taken seriously because of the obvious human health hazard that exists. Diagnosis by skin or serologic testing is not as reliable in detecting exposed or latently infected animals, and it may be desirable to place dogs or cats exposed to human or bovine tuberculosis on prophylactic chemotherapy.

M. avium may respond to drugs used to treat atypical mycobacterial infections. Increased in vitro activity against this organism has been found with rifapentine, a synthetic analog of rifampin, and liposome-encapsulated amikacin.[20] Unlike atypical and tuberculous mycobacteria, *M. avium* strains are resistant in vitro to the quinolones.

PREVENTION

Tuberculosis is a major human public health problem. Humans are susceptible to *M. bovis*, *M. tuberculosis*, and *M. avium*, which is important with respect to control in animals. Identification of cases of *M. tuberculosis* infection in people should be followed by serologic testing or clinical evaluation of pet contacts as possible reservoirs. Outbreaks of *M. bovis* infection in cattle should also be followed by evaluation of dogs and cats on the farm, and feeding of unpasteurized milk or raw offal to pets should be discontinued. The attempt to control tuberculosis in dogs with modified live vaccines has had moderate success in that some dogs have shown increased resistance to infection,[21] but immunity is partial, and vaccination has not been generally recommended. It also can produce false-positive skin test results as it does in other species.

PUBLIC HEALTH CONSIDERATIONS

Although *M. tuberculosis* and *M. bovis* infections are not maintained in canine and feline reservoirs, infected dogs and cats may serve as temporary sources for dissemination of bacteria in the environment. Since respiratory or intestinal secretions may be contaminated, it is well to recommend that infected animals be either treated or euthanatized. Being a saprophyte, *M. avium* is just as likely to be acquired from environmental sources as it is from infected dogs or cats.

Feline Leprosy

Gail A. Kunkle

ETIOLOGY AND PATHOGENESIS

Feline leprosy is caused by *M. lepraemurium*, the same acid-fast organism responsible for rat leprosy.[22,23] In vitro growth and characterization of these very slow growing, difficult-to-culture organisms have been possible on the surface of 1% Ogawa egg yolk medium.[24] Successful transmission of these nonculturable organisms from spontaneous feline cases into rats and mice has resulted in disease indistinguishable from murine leprosy. Results of experimental transmission of bacillus from spontaneous feline cases into other cats has resulted in equivocal results.[25]

The prevalence of disease is higher in colder wet areas of the world such as New Zealand, parts of Australia, the United Kingdom, and northwestern United States and Canada. Transmission is thought to occur from bites or contact with infected rats.

CLINICAL FINDINGS

Lesions are usually soft, fleshy, focal nodules in the skin and subcutis. They occur most often on the head and extremities and

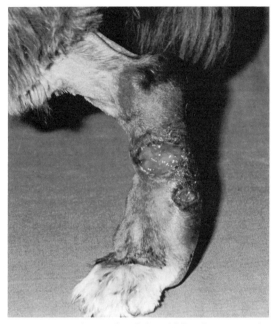

Figure 51–7. Ulcerated nodules of feline leprosy on the limb of a cat. (Courtesy of Dr. Kirk Haupt, Seattle, WA.)

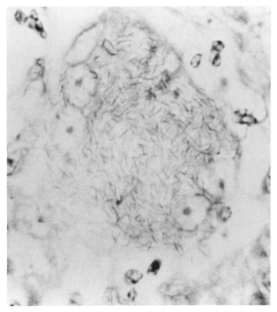

Figure 51–8. Microscopic appearance of nodular lesion from the face of a feline leukemia virus-positive cat. Large numbers of organisms are visible (acid-fast stain; × 100). (Courtesy of Dr. Boyd Jones, Massey University, Palmerston North, New Zealand.)

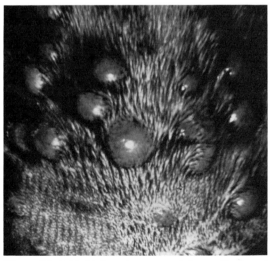

Figure 51–6. Multiple cutaneous nodules on the dorsal neck of a cat with feline leprosy. (Courtesy of Dr. Kirk Haupt, Seattle, WA.)

Table 51–5. Drug Dosages for Lepromatous and Atypical Mycobacterial Infections[a]

DRUG	SPECIES	DOSE[b] (mg/kg)	ROUTE	INTERVAL (hours)	DURATION (weeks)
Lepromatous[c]					
Dapsone	D	1[d]	PO	8	2
	C	50 mg total	PO	12	2
Rifampin	D, H	10–20	PO	12	3–4
Clofazimine[e]	C	8	PO	24	6[f]
Atypical					
Gentamicin	B	2	SC, IM	12	2–4
Amikacin	B	5–7	SC, IM	12	2–4
Kanamycin	B	5–7	SC, IM	12	2–4
Doxycycline	B	5–10	SC, IM	12–24	4–6
Trimethoprim-	D	12–15	PO	12	4–6
sulfonamide	C	10	PO	12	4[g]
Chloramphenicol	D	25	PO	8	4–6
	C	15	PO	8–12	3–4[h]
Enrofloxacin	B	5–15	PO	12	3–4[i]
Clofazimine	B	8	PO	24	3–4[e,f]

[a]D = dog, C = cat, H = human, PO = oral, SC = subcutaneous, IM = intramuscular.
[b]Dose per administration at specified interval, expressed as mg/kg unless otherwise stated.
[c]Surgical removal is the most effective therapy.
[d]For induction therapy; later switch to 0.3 to 0.6 mg/kg per dose.
[e]To achieve proper dose, liquid in commercially available capsules must be aspirated and placed in new capsules. Available from Glaxo, Greenford, Middlesex, UK.
[f]After 6 weeks, begin twice weekly interval of administration.
[g]Monitor BUN weekly for evidence of nephrotoxicity; often combined with other drugs.
[h]Must check hemogram weekly for evidence of myelosuppression.
[i]For the dosage of other quinolones, see Table 43–10.

develop rapidly (Fig. 51–6). They are usually freely movable and nonpainful, and the cat is in good health. They may be haired or superficially ulcerated, and regional lymph nodes may be enlarged (Fig. 51–7). Generalized cutaneous involvement and systemic infection is uncommon.

DIAGNOSIS

The diagnosis is made by the clinical findings in conjunction with the presence of very large numbers of acid-fast bacilli noted on histology or impression smears (Fig. 51–8).[23] Cultures will routinely be negative for tuberculous bacilli and the rapidly growing mycobacteria. When direct impression smears of nodules are stained with an acid-fast stain, most of the bacilli are contained within the cytoplasm of histiocytes. Smears from local lymph nodes also usually contain large numbers of organisms. In some instances, inoculation of infected tissues or laboratory isolates into laboratory animals may be used to further characterize the organism.

Histologic examination shows granulomatous inflammation with large numbers of foamy histiocytes. Neutrophils, lymphocytes, plasma cells, and multinucleated giant cells are usually present. The lesions are not encapsulated and caseation is rare. The cytoplasm of macrophages is densely packed with acid-fast organisms that may push the nucleus against the cell membrane. Although there are exceptions, generally skin tuberculosis and atypical mycobacteriosis in cats result in lesions in which bacilli are infrequent compared with that of feline leprosy.

THERAPY

Surgical removal of lesions is the desired treatment. When surgery is not feasible, cats have been treated with dapsone, a drug used to treat human leprosy (Table 51–5). Toxicity to the drug may occur. The antibiotic rifampin has also been used with mixed clinical results. Clofazimine (Glaxo, Green-ford, Middlesex, UK) may also be useful in the treatment of feline leprosy, but the tox-icity in cats is uncertain.[26]

Atypical Mycobacterial Infections

Gail A. Kunkle

ETIOLOGY

There are numerous saprophytic, nontu-berculous nonlepromatous mycobacterial species called atypical, opportunistic, or anonymous mycobacteria. They are divided into the slow-growing and the rapid-growing species (see Table 51–1). Although the slow-growing atypical mycobacteria are respon-sible for several well-characterized cuta-neous diseases in people, they are less commonly identified as pathogens in the dog and cat, possibly as a result of the lengthy time needed for culture. The exception to this low frequency of isolation is the slow-growing *M. avium* complex, which belongs to the atypical group and has been discussed previously with tuberculosis. The rapidly growing, atypical mycobacteria have been isolated from many cats and several dogs with cutaneous lesions as well as from rare pulmonary infections.[27–32]

EPIDEMIOLOGY

These atypical mycobacteria are ubiqui-tous in nature, especially in water and wet soil, and they are not pathogenic for animals under normal circumstances. Animal-to-animal transmission does not generally oc-cur. Most atypical mycobacteria infecting dogs and cats are acquired from the environ-ment following trauma to the skin or soft tissues. Bite or scratch injuries have also been responsible for human infection (see Chapter 58). The respiratory or alimentary systems rarely are points of entry for these organisms, and the location of bacilli entry in the body is important in determining the type of resulting disease. Most atypical my-cobacterial lesions are localized tissue reac-tions to the presence of acid-fast bacilli in the skin or deeper tissues via puncture or fight wounds. Inoculation of the acid-fast bacilli into an adipose tissue seems to en-hance pathogenicity. The existence of tissue injury, predisposing disease conditions, or impairment of the host's immunologic de-fense mechanism has often been identified in people but not commonly in animals.

M. fortuitum and *M. chelonei* (often known as *M. fortuitum-chelonei* complex) are the commonly isolated species from ca-nine and feline atypical mycobacterial infec-tions in the United States. *M. smegmatis* and *M. phlei* and other similar but as yet uniden-tified species are most common in Australia. Cats seem more susceptible and exhibit a higher infection rate than do dogs, and ab-scesses or granulomas are the typical lesions that develop.

CLINICAL FINDINGS

Atypical mycobacteriosis in cats most commonly occurs with multiple fistulous draining tracts associated with purulent drainage into the caudal abdominal, in-guinal, and lumbar subcutaneous tissues (Fig. 51–9). Cutaneous or subcutaneous nod-ules that periodically drain and recur de-velop with or without punctate ulcers and spreading granulomatous proliferation. By use of careful methodology, *M. fortuitum*[27,28] or *M. smegmatis*[29] can generally be isolated from these lesions. Most cats, even with extensive cutaneous involvement, remain clinically active and somewhat normal ex-cept for serous drainage from the tracts. Fever occasionally occurs, but anorexia, weight loss, and other features of chronic infections are usually absent. Response to antibiotic therapy is usually temporary. These lesions will often wax and wane for years if the owners can tolerate the esthetics of long-term management.

Dogs with atypical mycobacteriosis usu-ally have a history of fight wounds or trauma followed by granulomatous proliferation of cutaneous tissues with serous or seropuru-

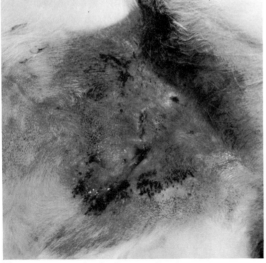

Figure 51–9. Multiple draining fistulas in the inguinal region of a cat caused by chronic infection by M. fortuitum.

lent drainage (Fig. 51–10). The prognosis for remission with surgery and antimicrobial therapy seems to be better for dogs than for cats. Pulmonary infections from M. fortuitum complex have also been reported.[30,31]

DIAGNOSIS

The diagnosis of atypical mycobacteriosis is not always easy, and a diligent search for organisms in impression smears from exudates or tissue biopsy is usually required, especially in infected cats. Tissue biopsies will generally reveal extensive granulomatous to pyogranulomatous inflammation of the dermis and panniculitis. Organisms are not abundant, and they are usually located in the panniculus. Application of acid-fast stains (especially Fite's method), followed by extensive searching, will often reveal a few organisms within extracellular lipid vacuoles surrounded by neutrophils and macrophages. Frozen sectioning of biopsy specimens improves staining capacity and demonstration of organisms.[33] The rapid Ziehl-Neelsen and Kinyoun's carbolfuchsin methods are also useful (see Appendix 8).[27,34] Although finding organisms in tissues is diagnostic, the presence of acid-fast bacteria in exudates alone may be suggestive of infection; however, it is not confirmatory, since other acid-fast saprophytes exist.

Organisms may be difficult to detect because of their scarcity, and repeated biopsies may be necessary to confirm their presence. Pyogranulomatous panniculitis can also be seen with nocardiosis, which should be considered and is more likely than mycobacteriosis if granules are found in the exudate or tissues (see Chapter 53).

Bacterial culture and identification of the organism are essential for definitive diagnosis and future management. Multiple cultures from exudate and tissue samples may be necessary. The rapidly growing mycobacteria will generally begin to grow within 1 week of inoculation into culture. Staphylococcus sp. or other organisms may be secondarily present on the surface and may overgrow the blood agar plate, preventing identification of the pathogen. For these reasons, specific media intended for mycobacterial isolation (see Tuberculous Mycobac-

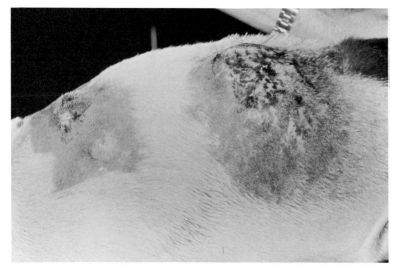

Figure 51–10. Granulomatous draining masses due to M. chelonei infection in a dog.

terial Infections above, Bacterial Isolation) should be used, and the plates should be held for 3 weeks to allow growth to occur. The final identification of acid-fast organisms from culture requires biochemical methods.

THERAPY

Atypical mycobacteria are usually resistant to antituberculous drugs. If a rapidly growing *Mycobacterium* has been isolated, antibacterial susceptibility testing should be performed in vitro or in bioassays. Conventional antibiotic therapy is often beneficial in the management of these patients, and those drugs found most useful both in vitro and in vivo are listed in Table 51–5. Spontaneous improvement is known to occur in people, so reports of successful therapies should always be viewed cautiously. Antibacterial therapy should be used for at least 6 weeks, since these infections are deep. Because the antituberculous drugs (isoniazid, rifampin, and ethambutol) are not usually effective against the atypical mycobacteria and they can be toxic to small animals, their usage is not usually indicated. Quinolones have been shown to be effective against atypical mycobacteria in vitro and can be tried in resistant cases, although higher clinical dosages may be needed. Clofazimine has also been effective in the treatment of some animals (see Table 43–10).

Surgical resection or debulking of large granulomatous masses has been helpful in rare cases, and surgical intervention has appeared to be more beneficial in infected dogs than in cats. Cats may improve with surgery when the lesions are small, but often dehiscence, proliferation of the wound margins, and further progression are sequelae. Glucocorticoid therapy is generally not indicated, especially in the early management of cases when a remission is being attempted. Occasionally, in chronic cases, anti-inflammatory doses on an alternate-day regimen will decrease the granulomatous proliferation in cats. Again, any response to therapy should always be viewed with skepticism.

PROGNOSIS

Even with antimicrobial therapy, the prognosis for atypical mycobacteriosis in cats and dogs is always guarded. Remission has been reported in a few feline cases, but most cases have histories of chronic infections. After years of chronic cutaneous lesions, rare cats have developed visceral masses containing acid-fast rods. Dogs apparently have better prognosis for remission based on current reports. In spite of expensive, long-term therapy, an infected pet who has continual serous drainage must often be euthanatized.

PUBLIC HEALTH CONSIDERATIONS

Since these organisms are free-living saprophytes, there is little or no risk of transmission of these infections.[35] Animal-to-animal or animal-to-people infection has not occurred by direct or indirect transmission. However, wound disinfection and contact precautions are usually advised, especially if immunosuppressed people are present in the same environment. Sodium hypochlorite (100 ppm available chlorine) rapidly kills these organisms on contaminated surfaces or inanimate objects.

Even though zoonotic spread of infection has not been seen, human hospital-acquired infections have occurred. Contamination of multidose-injection syringes, peritoneal and hemodialysis machines, bronchoscopes, and some surgical equipment has led to severe nosocomial infections.[36] Similar problems have not been reported in veterinary hospitals with dogs or cats, but the potential exists.

References

1. Orr CM, Kelly DF, Lucke VM: Tuberculosis in cats, a report of two cases. *J Small Anim Pract* 21:247–253, 1980.
2. Issac J, Whitehead J, Adams JW, et al: An outbreak of *Mycobacterium bovis* infection in cats in an animal house. *Aust Vet J* 60:243–245, 1983.
3. Friend SCE, Russell EG, Hartley WJ, et al: Infection of a dog with *Mycobacterium avium* serotype II. *Vet Pathol* 16:381–384, 1979.
4. Walsh KM, Losco PE: Canine mycobacteriosis: a case report. *J Am Anim Hosp Assoc* 20:295–299, 1984.
5. Carpenter JL, Myers AM, Conner MW, et al: Tuberculosis in basset hounds: four cases (1981–1987). *J Am Vet Med Assoc* 192:1563–1568, 1988.
6. Buergelt CD, Gowler JL, Wright PS: Disseminated avian tuberculosis in a cat. *Calif Vet* 10:13–15, 1982.
7. Suter MM, von Rotz A, Weiss R, et al: Atypical

mycobacterial skin granuloma in a cat in Switzerland. *Zentrabl Veterinarmed* 31:712–718, 1984.

8. Drolet R: Disseminated tuberculosis caused by *Mycobacterium avium* in a cat. *J Am Vet Med Assoc* 189:1336–1337, 1986.

9. Sunderman G, McDonald RJ, Maniatis T, et al: Tuberculosis as a manifestation of the acquired immunodeficiency syndrome (AIDS). *JAMA* 256:362–266, 1986.

10. Saltzman BR, Motyl MR, Friedland GH, et al: *Mycobacterium tuberculosis* in the acquired immunodeficiency syndrome. *JAMA* 256:390–391, 1986.

11. Foster ES, Scavelli TD, Greenelee PG, et al: Cutaneous lesion caused by *Mycobacterium tuberculosis* in a dog. *J Am Vet Med Assoc* 188:1188–1190, 1986.

12. Liu S, Weitzman I, Johnson GG: Canine tuberculosis. *J Am Vet Med Assoc* 177:164–167, 1980.

13. Thilsted JP, Shifrine M: Delayed cutaneous hypersensitivity in the dog: reaction to tuberculin purified protein derivative and coccidioidin. *Am J Vet Res* 39:1702–1705, 1978.

14. Parodi A, Fontaine M, Brion A, et al: Mycobacterioses in the domestic carnivora—present-day epidemiology of tuberculosis in the cat and dog. *J Small Anim Pract* 6:309–326, 1965.

15. Wieselthaler M: Susceptibility of a dog to *Mycobacterium tuberculosis*—a field study. *Wien Tierarztl Monatsschr* 62:357–361, 1975.

16. Pedersen NC: Basic and clinical immunology. *In Proceedings*. 49th Annu Meet, Am Anim Hosp Assoc, 75–84, 1982.

17. Legendre AM, Mallmann VH, Michel RL: Migration-inhibition response of peripheral leukocytes to tuberculin in cats sensitized with viable *Mycobacterium bovis* (BCG). *Am J Vet Res* 38:819–822, 1977.

18. Abramowicz M (ed): Drugs for tuberculosis. *Med Lett* 30:43–44, 1988.

19. Bondanev IM, Ivanov VL, Novoselova VP, et al: Effectiveness of the rapid administration of rifampin and isoniazid and of the intramuscular administration of streptomycin in disseminated destructive pulmonary tuberculosis in dogs. *Antibiotiki* 29:430–434, 1984.

20. Bermudez LEM, Wu M, Young LS: Intracellular killing of *Mycobacterium avium* complex by rifapentine and liposome–encapsulated amikacin. *J Infect Dis* 156:510–513, 1987.

21. Salvioli G, DegliEsposti A, Dino M: Experimental

tuberculosis in puppies vaccinated with live and dead tubercle bacilli. *Acta Tuberc Scand* 28:147–154, 1953.

22. Polema FG, Leiker DL: Cat leprosy in the Netherlands. *Int J Lepr* 42:307–311, 1974.

23. Wilkinson GT: Feline leprosy. *In* Kirk RE (ed): *Current Veterinary Therapy VI*. Philadelphia, WB Saunders Co, 1977, pp 569–571.

24. Pattyn S, Francoise P: In vitro cultivation and characterization of *Mycobacterium lepraemurium*. *Int J Lepr* 48:7–14, 1980.

25. Schiefer HB, Middleton DM: Experimental transmission of a feline mycobacterial skin disease (feline leprosy). *Vet Pathol* 20:460–471, 1983.

26. Mundell AC: The effectiveness of clofazamine in the treatment of feline leprosy. *In Proceedings. Am Acad Vet Dermatol/Am Col Vet Dermatol* 4:44–45, 1988.

27. White SD, Ihrke PJ, Stannard AA, et al: Cutaneous atypical mycobacteriosis in cats. *J Am Vet Med Assoc* 182:1218–1222, 1983.

28. Kunkle GA, Gulbus NK, Fadok V, et al: Rapidly growing mycobacteria as a cause of cutaneous granulomas: report of five cases. *J Am Anim Hosp Assoc* 19:513–521, 1983.

29. Wilkinson GT, Kelly WR, O'Boyle D: Pyogranulomatous panniculitis in cats due to *Mycobacterium smegmatis*. *Aust Vet J* 58:77–78, 1982.

30. Turnwald GH, Pechman RD, Turk JR, et al: Survival of a dog with pneumonia caused by *Mycobacterium fortuitum*. *J Am Vet Med Assoc* 192:64–70, 1988.

31. Jang SS, Eckhaus MA, Saunders G: Pulmonary *Mycobacterium fortuitum* infection in a dog. *J Am Vet Med Assoc* 184:96–97, 1984.

32. Willemse T, Groothuis DG, Koeman JP, et al: *Mycobacterium thermoresistible*: extrapulmonary infection in a cat. *J Clin Microbiol* 21:854–856, 1985.

33. Gross TL, Connelly MR: Nontuberculous mycobacterial skin infection in two dogs. *Vet Pathol* 20:117–119, 1983.

34. Culling CF: Staining organisms, parasites, and fungi in sections. *In* Raphael SS (ed): *Lynch's Medical Laboratory Technology*. Philadelphia, WB Saunders Co, 1976, p 1002.

35. Grange JM, Yates MD: Infections caused by opportunist mycobacteria: a review. *J R Soc Med* 79:226–229, 1986.

36. Brown TH: The rapidly growing mycobacteria—*Mycobacterium fortuitum* and *Mycobacterium chelonei*. *Inf Cont* 6:283–288, 1985.

52 CANINE BRUCELLOSIS

Leland E. Carmichael
Craig E. Greene

ETIOLOGY AND EPIDEMIOLOGY

Brucella canis is a small (1.0 to 1.5 μm), gram-negative coccobacillary organism. However, its rough colonial morphology and differences in biochemical and antigenic reactions make it distinct from other members of the genus *Brucella*. Unlike the smooth *Brucella* organisms that infect several domestic animal species, *B. canis* has a limited host range; only dogs and wild Canidae have been found to be susceptible. Cats can be infected experimentally but are relatively resistant, having a transient bacteremia. Rabbits and nonhuman primates also have been found to be susceptible to experimental infections. No other animal species has developed significant agglutination titers. Human cases have been reported as a result of laboratory accidents and contact with infected dogs, but people appear to be relatively resistant (see Public Health Considerations).

Dogs also are susceptible to infection with *B. abortus*.[1] Natural infection is thought to occur following ingestion of contaminated placentas and aborted fetuses. They usually harbor the organism in the lymph nodes of the GI tract for extended periods. Dogs are not thought to be important in the spread and maintenance of infection.

B. canis infects a susceptible host by penetrating the mucous membranes, especially those of the oral cavity, vagina, and conjunctiva. The minimum oral infectious dose for dogs is about 10^6 bacteria,[2] and the conjunctival dose is 10^4 to 10^5 organisms.[3] Because they contain the highest concentration of organisms, vaginal discharges, semen, or possibly urine are the most likely sources for infection by mucosal contamination.

Natural transmission of canine brucellosis occurs by several routes. Infected female dogs apparently transmit *B. canis* only during estrus, at breeding, or following abortion through oronasal contact with vaginal discharges. Oronasal transmission via aerosols is most common by contact with aborted materials because they contain up to 10^{10} organisms/ml. Shedding of *B. canis* may occur for periods up to 6 weeks following an abortion. Milk of infected bitches contains lower concentrations of organisms and is less important in transmitting infection to surviving pups; most have already been infected in utero.

Seminal fluid and urine have been incriminated as sources of infection from male dogs that harbor the organisms in their prostates and epididymides. The rate of isolation of *B. canis* from the semen of infected dogs is usually high for the first 6 to 8 weeks postinoculation (PI). Intermittent shedding of the organism in low numbers has been noted for up to 60 weeks PI[4] and may continue for a period of at least 2 years. Urinary excretion begins a few weeks after the onset of bacteremia and continues for at least 3 months. Concentrations of 10^3 to 10^6 organisms/ml of urine have been found in male dogs, with lesser numbers of bacteria in the urine of females.[2,3] The urine of infected males was thought earlier to contain too few organisms to be infectious by the oronasal route; however, recent studies have demonstrated that *B. canis* can be transmitted from infected to uninfected mature male dogs after several weeks or months of close contact.[2,3] The propensity of males to shed the organism in the urine probably relates to its localization in the prostate and epididymis, which are in close association with the urinary bladder.

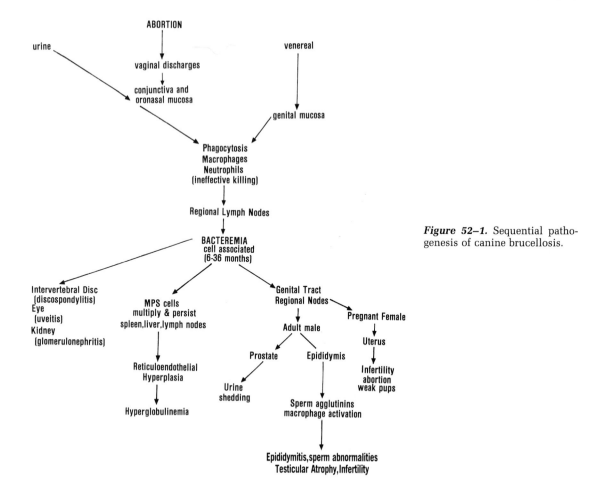

Figure 52–1. Sequential pathogenesis of canine brucellosis.

Alternate means of transmission occur less frequently under natural circumstances. In utero or congenital transmission becomes important as a means of spread of infection to puppies. Transmission via fomites has been reported following vaginoscopy, blood transfusions, artificial insemination, and the use of contaminated syringes.

The prevalence of infection varies according to the animal's age, housing conditions, and geographic location. Pet dogs in suburban environments have a lower prevalence compared with stray dogs in economically depressed areas, which may reflect increased population density and uncontrolled breeding of dogs. A relatively low prevalence has been reported in the United States and Japan (range, 1% to 18%), compared with rates as high as 28% in Mexico and Peru.[5] The southern United States appears to have a relatively higher (≈8%) prevalence of infection. Determination of seroprevalence is strongly influenced by the means of testing and interpretation.

PATHOGENESIS

The general sequence of events following infection by *Brucella* are summarized in Figure 52–1. The bacteria are probably phagocytized at contaminated mucosal sites by tissue macrophages and other phagocytic cells and transported to lymphatic and genital tract tissues, where they multiply. They persist intracellularly within mononuclear phagocytes. A leukocyte-associated bacteremia occurs beginning 1 to 4 weeks PI and can last 6 to 64 months. Generalized lymphoreticular hyperplasia (Fig. 52–2) and development of hyperglobulinemia occur during the course of infection. As with other intracellular parasites, cell-mediated immunity is probably the most important defense

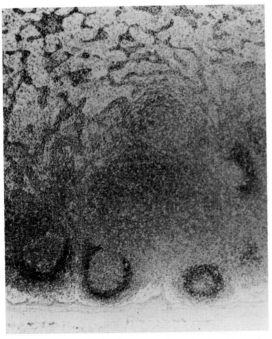

Figure 52–2. Follicular hyperplasia in the lymph node from a dog with chronic *B. canis* infection (H and E; × 40).

involved, including the eye (anterior uveitis), kidney (glomerulopathy), and meninges (meningoencephalitis).

Spontaneous recovery from infection may occur within 1 to more than 5 years PI. Therapy accelerates the recovery process. Bacteremia may be persistent throughout this time in some dogs, whereas others can harbor bacteria in tissues for several months after the bacteremia ceases. Despite tissue persistence, when *B. canis* is no longer detected in the blood, serum agglutination titers decrease.

Dogs that recover have low or negative agglutination titers yet are immune to reinfection, suggesting that protective immunity is cell-mediated. Recovered dogs challenged orally or IV as long as 4 years following spontaneous recovery from experimental infection were completely immune.[7] However, chronically infected dogs that were successfully treated with antibiotics were found to be fully susceptible to oronasal challenge 12 weeks after treatment had been halted.[8] Persistent *B. canis* infection appears to be a requirement to sustain protective immunity. Immunosuppression with glucocorticoids

mechanism against *B. canis*. Persistent nonprotective antibody titers are characteristic of such infections and appear to have little influence on the level of bacteremia or number of organisms in tissues.

Greatest numbers of *B. canis* organisms are found in the lymph nodes, spleen, and tissues of gonadal steroid dependency. In fact, the uterus is not a favored site of growth in the nongravid or diestral female. Although usually confined to mononuclear phagocytes, they may enter other cells such as placental epithelium. Inflammation of the epididymides and testes in males causes sperm leakage, which provokes the immune system to produce a complex of antisperm agglutinating antibodies and delayed-type hypersensitivity reactions against sperm that are unrelated to the antibodies against *B. canis*.[6] The immune responses produced against spermatozoa contribute to the epididymitis, infertility, and eventual spermatogenic arrest seen in most infected male dogs.

B. canis, like other bloodborne bacteria, may localize in nonreproductive tissues such as the endarterial circulation of the intervertebral disc, causing discospondylitis. Other tissues that filter bloodborne organisms or immune complexes may become

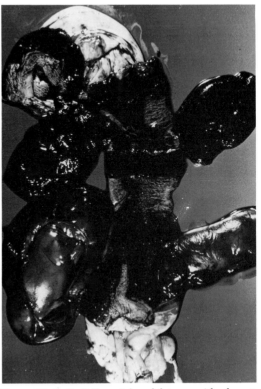

Figure 52–3. Partially autolyzed fetuses with placenta and uterus from a dog infected with *B. canis*. The dog was neutered at 45 days gestation.

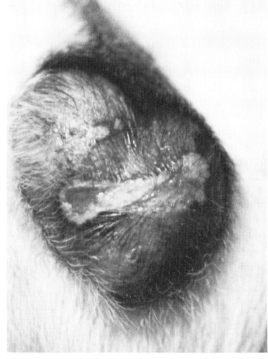

Figure 52–4. Testicular enlargement and scrotal dermatitis in an experimentally infected dog 35 weeks PI.

and antilymphocyte serum appears to increase the susceptibility of dogs to initial infection, but it does not augment the severity of the disease or alter the course of infection in experimentally infected dogs.[9]

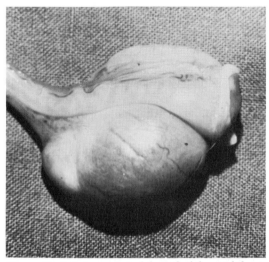

Figure 52–5. Enlargement of the tail of the epididymis on the testicle from an experimentally infected dog 60 weeks PI.

CLINICAL FINDINGS

Despite generalized systemic infection with *B. canis*, adult dogs are rarely seriously ill. Fever is uncommon, and with the exception of males who commonly have epididymitis, most infections will not be diagnosed by routine history or physical examination. Dry, lusterless coats, loss of vigor, and decreased exercise tolerance are occasionally reported by owners of working dogs. Nongravid females show no signs of illness other than lymphadenopathy, which occurs in both sexes.

Overt clinical signs usually involve reproductive disturbances in sexually mature animals. Bitches in late gestation usually abort dead pups between 45 and 59 days of gestation but show no other clinical signs. Pups are usually partially autolyzed, with subcutaneous edema and congestion and hemorrhage of the abdominal subcutaneous region (Fig. 52–3). Moderate quantities of serosanguineous peritoneal effusion are found. Their appearance suggests fetal death in utero some time prior to abortion. Decomposed fetuses are not usually found because they are ingested by the bitch. Abortion is characterized by a brown or greenish-gray vaginal discharge that lasts for periods of 1 to 6 weeks. Brucellosis should be suspected under any circumstance when apparently healthy bitches abort 2 weeks prior to term.

Although abortion of dead puppies is the primary clinical sign reported with brucellosis, conception failures can occur at any time following breeding. In utero death with fetal resorption or abortion and ingestion of fetuses may be suspected if a bitch fails to conceive after an apparently successful mating. Embryonic death may occur as early as 10 to 20 days following mating, although most conception failures are actually undetected abortions. Less commonly, bitches may carry infected puppies to term and whelp both live and dead puppies within a single litter. Most pups that are born alive will die within a few hours or days, but those that survive or that are infected as neonates usually have generalized peripheral lymphadenopathy as the primary clinical manifestation of disease until they reach sexual maturity. Such puppies usually have persistent hyperglobulinemia and some may have transient fever, leukocytosis, or seizures as systemic manifestations of their infections.

As with brucellosis in other species, infections with *B. canis* do not interfere with normal estrous cycles. Up to 85% of bitches that abort may have normal litters subsequently. However, even after having normal litters, some infected bitches experience intermittent reproductive failures.

Because of the prominent testicular abnormalities, male dogs are presented for examination more often than are females, even though impairment of male reproductive performance often is less noticed. Nevertheless, infertility occurs. Males appear to be in good health but may have an enlarged scrotum because of accumulation of serosanguineous fluid in the tunica. Scrotal dermatitis is the result of constant licking and secondary infection with nonhemolytic staphylococci (Fig. 52–4). A major cause of testicular swelling is enlargement of the tail of the epididymis (Fig. 52–5); orchitis and primary testicular enlargement are rarely apparent. In fact, chronically infected males usually develop unilateral or bilateral testicular atrophy. A decreased volume of ejaculate without loss of libido is usually present. Acute pain is not usually evident on scrotal or testicular palpation, but discomfort may be seen at the time of ejaculation.

Nonreproductive abnormalities have been noted less frequently. Splenomegaly may accompany the diffuse lymphadenopathy in some dogs. Dogs with discospondylitis initially experience spinal pain and later paresis and ataxia if spinal cord compression develops.[10] Osteomyelitis of the appendicular skeleton causes lameness of the affected limb.[11] Meningoencephalitis has been reported previously, but only following experimental infection; however, one of the authors[12] has observed a male dog that had confirmed *B. canis* infection with behavioral changes, anisocoria, ataxia, hyperesthesia, head tilt, and circling. Neurologic signs began within 3 weeks following the dog's first breeding. Chronic multifocal pyogranulomatous dermatitis that resembled lick granuloma lesions also has been observed in an infected dog, but a direct causal relationship was not established. Recurrent anterior uveitis with corneal edema has been detected in infected dogs, alone and in combination with other signs. Endophthalmitis has resulted in secondary glaucoma or phthisis bulbi (see Chapter 13).

DIAGNOSIS

Clinical Laboratory Findings

Hematologic and biochemical values are either unaltered or nonspecific in canine brucellosis. Hyperglobulinemia (β and γ) with concomitant hypoalbuminemia has been the most consistent finding in chronically infected dogs. An increased prevalence of positive Coombs' testing in the absence of anemia has been reported.[9] Examination of aspirates or biopsy samples from enlarged lymph nodes usually reveals lymphoid hyperplasia with large numbers of plasma cells. CSF analysis results are pleocytosis, primarily consisting of neutrophils, and increased protein concentration with meningoencephalitis but are unremarkable when discospondylitis alone is present. Urinalysis is usually normal, despite the variable presence of bacteriuria. Radiographic demonstration of intervertebral disc infection (Fig. 52–6) should always be followed by serologic and when possible, bacteriologic confirmation of *B. canis*.

Semen Examination

Semen abnormalities, evident by 5 weeks PI, become pronounced at 8 weeks PI.[13] Abnormalities include immature sperm, deformed acrosomes, swollen midpieces, and retained protoplasmic droplets. By week 15 PI, there are bent tails, detached heads, and head-to-head agglutination. Large aggregates of inflammatory cells, usually consisting of neutrophils, surround adherent macrophages containing phagocytized sperm (Fig. 52–7). More than 90% of the sperm is abnormal by 20 weeks PI. Aspermia without inflammatory cells corresponds with the development of bilateral testicular atrophy. Semen morphology should always be evaluated in dogs with infertility because of the obvious abnormalities that occur with brucellosis.

Serologic Testing

This is the most frequently used diagnostic method for detecting canine brucellosis. These tests are subject to considerable interpretive error because lipopolysaccharide

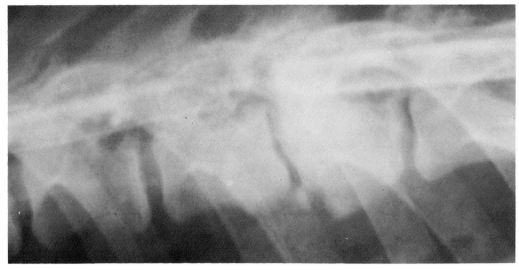

Figure 52–6. Myelogram of a dog with discospondylitis showing thoracic and abdominal hyperesthesia and pelvic limb paralysis. Note obstruction of the flow of radiographic contrast medium over the affected disc space.

(LPS) antigens of several bacterial species cross-react with *B. canis*. Therefore, the problem of false-positive cross-reactions is more common than that of false-negative reactions.[8,14] All sera should be free of hemolysis, as hemoglobin causes false-positive agglutination of the tube test antigen.

Serologic test results often are negative during the first 4 weeks PI, despite the presence of bacteremia by 2 weeks PI. For this reason, newly acquired animals should be sequentially tested at least twice at 30-day intervals before introduction into a breeding kennel. Low or intermediate titers may mean previous disease or very recent infection,

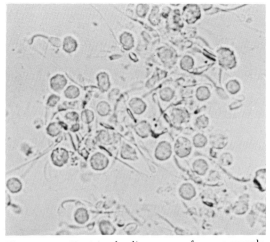

Figure 52–7. Unstained saline smear of semen sample from a dog 35 weeks PI. Large numbers of inflammatory cells are present.

and testing should be repeated or attempts should be made to isolate the organism by hemoculture. Male dogs may harbor the organism in their prostate glands and epididymides for extended periods after bacteremia ceases and agglutination titers have declined. Similarly, female dogs may have diagnostically equivocal antibody titers and negative blood culture results in chronic infections. In females, recrudescence of bacteremia and increased antibody titers develop during estrus, pregnancy, or abortion. These are the most reliable times to screen female dogs for infection.

Antibiotic therapy may contribute to false-negative serology and may result in failure to isolate the organism from infected dogs. Antibacterials should not be given until diagnostic tests have been completed. Tetracycline causes abacteremia and a corresponding decrease in antibody titer that may rebound after treatment is discontinued.

Table 52–1 compares the serologic tests described below. Consult Appendix 8 for information concerning commercially available test kits and submission of laboratory samples. Serologic tests should be evaluated in light of clinical findings in the dog being evaluated. A single high agglutination titer to *B. canis* usually indicates active infection, but this should be substantiated by further tests. Dogs that are asymptomatic but have positive results on agglutination procedures should never be condemned as infected until blood cultures or the more specific agar-gel

Table 52–1. Comparison of Serologic Procedures for Canine Brucellosis

SEROLOGIC TEST	EARLIEST TITER[a] (Weeks PI)	ADVANTAGES	DISADVANTAGES
Mercaptoethanol (ME) rapid slide agglutination test (ME-RSAT)	3 to 4	Quick, high sensitivity, few (1%) false-negative results	False-positive results common; must confirm by other tests
Tube agglutination test (TAT)	3 to 6	Semiquantitative determination	False-positive results similar to RSAT
ME-TAT	5 to 8	Same at TAT, somewhat increased specificity	Longer to get positive titer compared with TAT
Agar-gel immunodiffusion (AGID)			
Cell wall (somatic) antigen	5 to 10	Sensitive. higher specificity possible	Procedure and interpretation complex
Internal (cytoplasmic protein) antigen	8 to 12	Most specific test, detects chronic cases when other tests are negative. Detects infections by other *Brucella* species	Complex procedure, least sensitive

[a]First significant titer to appear. Data based on adult dog.

immunodiffusion (AGID) test confirms the positive findings. All tests, with the exception of the cytoplasmic antigen-AGID method, measure antibodies to LPS antigens and may give nonspecific test results.

Rapid Slide Agglutination Test. The 2-mercaptoethanol rapid slide agglutination test (ME-RSAT) is preferred as an in-office screening procedure because it is inexpensive, rapid, and sensitive and detects antibodies early (D-Tec CB, Pitman-Moore, Washington Crossing, NJ). There is a 99% correlation between a negative test and lack of infection.[5,15] The test kit employs *B. ovis* because it is easier to cultivate. *B. canis* cross-reacts with all rough *Brucella* and with certain other bacterial species, such as mucoid strains of *Pseudomonas*, *Bordetella bronchiseptica*, and *Actinobacillus equuli*, to which serum antibodies may be present. Most causes of cross-reactions, however, have not been identified. The ME-RSAT substantially reduces false-positive reactions by eliminating less specifically reacting IgM antibodies.[16] ME is labile and must be kept in a dark tightly stoppered bottle at 4°C, because use of inactivated ME gives false-positive results. A modification of the RSAT, using a less mucoid (M) variant of *B. canis*, further reduces the rate of false-positive results.[17]

Tube Agglutination Test. The tube agglutination test (TAT) has been the most widely used serodiagnostic procedure for confirmation of infection in ME-RSAT–positive dogs.[8] However, antigen formerly provided by the USDA is no longer available. As with the RSAT, the TAT also is troubled by heterospecific reactions with other infectious agents and by equivocal titers in chronically infected animals. Unfortunately, the ME-TAT also suffers from some lack of specificity, and the increase in ME-TAT antibody titers usually lags 1 to 2 weeks behind those of the TAT and 2 to 4 weeks behind those of the ME-RSAT.

Lack of standardized reagents or methods makes absolute TAT titer comparisons difficult. Nevertheless, a 1:50 titer may indicate either very early (3 weeks) or recovering infections; titer of 1:50 to 1:100 should be considered suspicious for infection; and a titer $\geq$ 1:200 is highly presumptive of active infection since it often correlates with positive hemocultures. However, it must be emphasized that sera from noninfected dogs have been found to have titers from 1:50 to 1:100 and occasionally higher. As semiquantitative tests, the TAT and ME-TAT are most useful in control programs to quantitate serologic responses of dogs over months to determine whether infection has been eliminated with chemotherapy.

Agar-Gel Immunodiffusion Test. An AGID test has been developed as a sensitive procedure for the serodiagnosis of canine brucellosis.[14,18] AGID tests reveal precipitins in the sera of infected dogs 5 to 10 weeks PI, and antibodies persist for several weeks or months after the bacteremia has ceased. Using cell wall (somatic) LPS antigen, the AGID test suffers from the same problems of cross-reactions as do agglutination tests, but those positive sera may be distinguished from false-positive sera by a distinct precipitin band for *B. canis* (Fig. 52–8A).

A second type of AGID test utilizes internal (cytoplasmic protein) antigens liberated by sonication of *B. canis* (Fig. 52–8B). This test has been able to specifically detect precipitins in the sera from dogs after other tests have become equivocal or even negative. A disadvantage of tests utilizing cytoplasmic antigens is the relatively long period between infection and the presence of detectable precipitins (see Table 52–1). Furthermore, one or more precipitin lines may persist up to 12 months after bacteremia has ceased.[14] In contrast to LPS antigens, both rough and smooth *Brucella* share the internal protein antigens. Thus, the possibility of infection with other *Brucella* (e.g., *B. suis* or *B. abortus*) must therefore be considered when cytoplasmic antigen is used. False-positive reactions have not been observed with non-*Brucella* species. False-negative results can occur in some dogs, presumably with early infection, whose sera are RSAT-positive and AGID-negative.[19] Hemoculture is the only definitive way to resolve these differences.

Enzyme-Linked Immunosorbent Assay. An antigen-specific, sandwich ELISA using highly purified *B. canis* cell wall antigen has been developed as a serologic test for *B.*

canis infection.[19a] It is very specific but less sensitive than the TAT in screening for infected dogs.

Bacterial Isolation

Isolation of *B. canis* is time-consuming but not difficult, since the organism grows well aerobically on conventional media used for other *Brucella*.[19] Blood is the most practical tissue or fluid for isolating the organism. Hemoculture should not be used as a sole criterion for infection, because the bacteremia, though generally sustained, is absent in more chronically infected animals. Whole blood must be taken for culture, since the organisms are associated with the leukocyte fraction. Bacteremia is detected 2 to 4 weeks after oronasal infection and if untreated it persists for long (>1 to 2 years) periods of time. Experimentally infected dogs have remained blood culture-positive for as long as 5.5 years. Bacterial numbers in the blood exceed 10^3/ml after 4 to 5 weeks PI and remain high for many (generally > 6) months.[14]

Urine culture is positive in some dogs, especially males, when blood cultures are negative; however, unless cystocentesis is performed, urinary isolation of *B. canis* may be difficult because of overgrowth by contaminants. Collection of semen by ejacula-

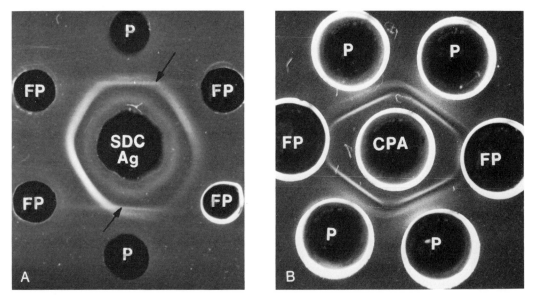

Figure 52–8. AGID patterns using *A*, sodium desoxycholate (SDC)–extracted somatic (LPS) antigens reacted with positive (P) and false-positive (FP) sera. Cross-reactions are evident. Arrows indicate *B. canis*–specific precipitin line. *B*, Cytoplasmic protein antigen (CPA). Precipitin lines occur only with sera from *Brucella*-infected dogs using the CPA.

tion is valuable for culture during the first 3 months of infection, when concentration of organisms is greatest.[13]

B. canis can be isolated at necropsy from several tissues of hemoculture-positive dogs. The lymph nodes, spleen, liver, bone marrow, and male reproductive organs are the most common sources, even though gross lesions are seldom present. In females, the gravid or estral uterus and the placenta and vaginal or uterine fluids are most consistent tissues for isolation.

Laboratory Cultivation

Contamination of specimens for culture of B. canis should be avoided because of overgrowth by faster-growing bacteria. Antibiotics such as bacitracin, polymyxin, and cyclohexamide are usually added to the media prior to cultivation. Whole blood or fluid samples usually are cultured for 4 to 5 days at 37°C in Albimi, Trypticase soy, or Tryptose broth (all from Difco Labs, Detroit, MI), with citrate added as anticoagulant.[20] After 4 to 7 days of growth, cultures are streaked on solid media such as Brucella Broth (BBL, Cockeysville, MD), Tryptose agar (Difco Laboratories, Detroit, MI), horse or cow blood agar, Trypticase soy agar (BBL, Cockeysville, MD), or Thayer-Martin media (Difco, Detroit, MI). Tissue swabs or specimens may be streaked directly onto solid media and incubated aerobically at 37°C. Growth is not usually seen before 48 hours. Initially, colonies appear small and translucent but become mucoid after several days of incubation. Biochemical and immunologic methods and phage typing have been used to type strains of B. canis.[21-23] Strain identity might be used as epidemiologic markers for disease investigations.

PATHOLOGIC FINDINGS

Macroscopic changes in adults or surviving pups are usually confined to lymphadenopathy and splenomegaly.

Histologic changes are relatively uniform, despite the presence or absence of bacteremia.[3] Lymph node enlargement is the result of diffuse lymphoreticular hyperplasia. In dogs with chronic bacteremia, lymph node sinusoids and the spleen are filled with plasma cells and macrophages containing

phagocytized bacteria. Special stains, e.g., Brown-Brenn stain, must be used to detect intracellular organisms.

Diffuse submucosal lymphocytic infiltration occurs in all genitourinary organs. A necrotizing vasculitis occurs in the target tissues of gonadal steroids, including the prostate, scrotum, sheath, or vulva. The prostate, epididymis, renal pelvis, and uterus are the most often affected, whereas milder changes are observed in the testes, ductus deferens, urinary bladder, and ureters. Extensive necrosis of the prostatic parenchyma and seminiferous tubules is caused by inflammatory cell infiltration that eventually results in atrophy or fibrosis (Fig. 52–9). There is a chronic to subacute endometritis in the uterus, with glandular hyperplasia and reticular cell nodules. Focal hepatic necrosis, myocarditis, and meningoencephalitis also have been described.

Renal abnormalities occur in some dogs and consist of hyaline thickening of the basement membrane of glomeruli with minimal cellular infiltration or proliferation. A mild interstitial nephritis has been noted.

Ocular pathology includes granulomatous iridocyclitis and exudative retinitis, consisting of diffuse infiltration of lymphocytes, plasmacytes, and neutrophils.[24] Corneal endothelium has vacuolated cytoplasm with variable plasma cell infiltration; exudates with leukocytes are present in the anterior chamber (see Systemic Bacterial Infections, Chapter 13).

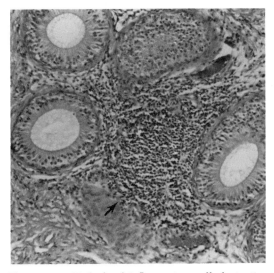

Figure 52–9. Early focal inflammatory cell cluster (*arrow*) in the head of the epididymis from a dog infected with B. canis (H and E; × 40).

THERAPY

Because of the intracellular location of *B. canis*, the outcome of antibiotic therapy of canine brucellosis is uncertain. The organism is susceptible to several antibiotics, but the ineffectiveness of in vivo therapy commonly leads to failures or relapses. Bacteremia often recurs days to months after treatment is discontinued, making follow-up evaluation essential because animals can still harbor infection in some tissues. Aborting females may subsequently produce normal litters, but even in these cases the success of therapy is uncertain. Clinically normal, infected bitches may transmit infection to their surviving offspring. Despite treatment, intact males frequently develop irreversible sterility, making their prognosis as breeding animals poor. Limited studies suggest inability to clear infection in the prostate gland in most instances. For this reason, it is recommended that infected animals, especially males, be eliminated from breeding programs. Infected female dogs have been reinstated in breeding programs, but only after prolonged isolation and therapy and with great risk of failure. The risk of infecting males when breeding to previously infected females has been minimized by judicious use of artificial insemination. Breeding of infected animals should be done only under exceptional circumstances when it is considered essential and after the risk is explained to an owner. Infected pets should be neutered and given a regimen of antibiotic therapy to reduce the chance of infecting family members via genital secretions. Although less likely, the organism can persist in tissues of neutered animals.[25]

Cures of brucellosis must not be assumed, because bacteremia may recur weeks or months after antibiotics are discontinued. Attempted culture of bacteria or serologic testing immediately after treatment is halted is deceiving. Reports of successful cures should be viewed with caution unless cultures and serology have been performed for at least 6 months.

Antibiotic Therapy

Numerous drugs have been used to treat canine brucellosis, but the organism is rarely eliminated if the appropriate antibiotic combination and regimen is not used. By use of mean inhibitory concentration, in vitro susceptibility has been demonstrated for tetracycline, chloramphenicol, aminoglycosides, spectinomycin, rifampin, ampicillin, and sulfonamides. Dogs respond poorly or not at all to these drugs when they are used alone or for a single course of therapy. Relapse occurs within a short period of time after therapy is discontinued. Partial in vitro susceptibility occurs with erythromycin, penicillin, novobiocin, and lincomycin. Decreased susceptibility to cephalosporins, nalidixic acid, and cycloserine exists.[26] None of the antibiotics in these last two groups should be used to treat canine brucellosis. Quinolones such as ciprofloxacin, norfloxacin, and enrofloxacin have been shown to be effective in vitro against *Brucella* spp. but have not been used extensively in treatment of infected dogs.

High-dose oral minocycline therapy combined with IM streptomycin (Table 52–2) gives the highest rate of success in experimentally infected dogs.[8] Lower dosages of this combination or other antibiotics alone or in combination were not as effective. Gentamicin can be substituted for streptomycin and may improve treatment efficacy.[26] Unfortunately, the cost of minocycline treatment may be as high as $500 to $1000 for larger dogs. Treatment regimens that are less expensive but sometimes less effective have been described (Table 52–2).

Localized infections such as in the intervertebral disc should be treated with 2 or more 3-week courses of antimicrobial therapy following neutering. Recurrence of hyperesthetic episodes is common in dogs with canine brucellosis, and owners of infected animals should be cautioned of the potential need for repeated treatment. Decompressive surgery should be avoided in paraparetic dogs when possible by first evaluating the dog's clinical response to antimicrobial therapy. Sequential radiography and titers at 3- to 6-month intervals are used to monitor their progress.

Infected Kennel

Appropriate disinfection procedures should be implemented to arrest spread of infection. Infected animals should be handled with gloves and should be serotested prior to each breeding, even when bred by artificial insemination. If animals are retained as pets

Table 52–2. Recommended Therapy for Canine Brucellosis[a]

DRUG	DOSE[b] (mg/kg)	ROUTE	INTERVAL (hours)	DURATION (weeks)
Minocycline[c,8,26]	25	PO	24	2
	12.5	PO	12	2
and				
Dihydrostreptomycin	5	IM,SC	12	1
or				
Gentamicin	2	IM,SC	12	1
Tetracycline[15]	22	PO	8	4
and				
Dihydrostreptomycin[d]	5	IM,SC	12	Week 1, Week 4
Repositol tetracycline[e,27]	20	IM	1 wk	4
and				
Dihydrostreptomycin	15	IM,SC	12	1

[a]Repeating regimens one to two times after 1- to 4-week lapse may improve therapeutic efficacy. PO = oral, IM = intramuscular, SC = subcutaneous

[b]Dose per administration at specified interval, expressed as mg/kg unless otherwise stated.

[c]Generic doxycycline may be substituted at the same dose and a lower cost.

[d]Ampicillin[28] (20 mg/kg, every 8 hours, for 3 weeks) has been added to this regimen with little apparent improvement in efficacy. Gentamicin may be substituted at 2 mg/kg.

[e]Pain and discomfort are common at the sites of injection. Sometimes easiest treatment program for kennels.

[f]Gentamicin may be substituted at 2 mg/kg.

or working dogs they should be neutered and moved to separate housing, because mere physical separation of infected dogs from the other animals and preventive hygiene has not proved rewarding.[2]

Carrier dogs are important in maintaining *B. canis* in the dog population since its survival outside the host is short-lived. Unfortunately, studies of environmental survival of *B. canis* have not been reported. However, disinfection with quaternary ammonium compounds or iodophors has been effective in killing the bacterium.

PREVENTION

Preventive measures are particularly important in large breeding kennels or wherever large numbers of dogs are kept, but there are no legally mandated control measures, and canine brucellosis is not a reportable disease. There is no vaccine, and results of experimental studies have been unsatisfactory. The desirability of a vaccine is questionable, especially when diagnostic testing is available, since an effective vaccine would be required to provide serviceable immunity but not confound the serodiagnosis.

PUBLIC HEALTH CONSIDERATIONS

Cases of human infection caused by *B. canis* were reported soon after the disease was recognized. More than 35 natural and laboratory-acquired infections have been reported.[5,29,30] Contact with aborting bitches was the source of infection for the majority of infected pet owners, whereas some male dogs and undetermined sources were present in the other cases.

People are relatively resistant to infection with *B. canis*, and the disease is relatively mild compared with infections caused by other *Brucella*. A proportion of cases are asymptomatic, as determined by serotesting, but the overall incidence of infection is low. Fever, chills, fatigue, malaise, lymphadenopathy, and weight loss have been present in symptomatic patients. Rare complications include endocarditis, meningitis, arthritis, hepatitis, and visceral abscesses. Diagnosis of human infections should include bacteriologic examination by blood culture and serologic evaluation. Human antibodies to *B. canis* will react with the antigen used in the ME-RSAT and, as in dogs, they do not cross-react with *B. abortus* antigen used in routine testing for human brucellosis. Titers of 1:200 or more when using the ME-TAT are seen in most active cases. Human infections can be readily and effectively treated with tetracycline therapy. As with infected dogs, people have suffered relapse on ampicillin.

Clients should always be informed of the potential health hazard in keeping *B. canis*–

infected pets. Caution should be used in the laboratory when handling or pipetting samples submitted for diagnostic testing, and veterinarians should use good hygiene when examining suspected dogs, especially aborting bitches.

References

1. Pidgeon GL, Scanlan CM, Miller WR, et al: Experimental infection of dogs with *Brucella abortus*. *Cornell Vet* 77:339–347, 1987.
2. Carmichael LE, Joubert JC: Transmission of *Brucella canis* by contact exposure. *Cornell Vet* 78:63–73, 1988.
3. Serikawa T, Muraguchi T: Significance of urine in transmission of canine brucellosis. *Jpn J Vet Sci* 41:607–616, 1979.
4. George LW: Studies on the immune response in canine brucellosis. PhD diss. Ithaca, NY, Cornell University, 1974.
5. Carmichael LE: Brucellosis (*Brucella canis*): In Steele JH (ed): *CRC Handbook Series in Zoonoses*, vol 1. Boca Raton, FL, CRC Press, 1979, pp 185–194.
6. Serikawa T, Muraguchi T, Yamada J, et al: Spermagglutination and spermagglutinating activity of serum and tissue extracts from reproductive organs in male dogs experimentally infected with *Brucella canis*. *Jpn J Vet Sci* 43:469–490, 1981.
7. Moore JA, Gupta BN: Epizootiology, diagnosis, and control of *Brucella canis*. *J Am Vet Med Assoc* 156:1737–1740, 1970.
8. Flores-Castro R, Carmichael LE: Canine brucellosis: current status of methods for diagnosis and treatment. *In* Proceedings. 27th Gaines Symposium, 17–24, 1977.
9. Ueda K, Magaribuchi T, Saegusa J, et al: Spontaneous *Brucella canis* infection in beagles: bacteriological and serological studies. *Jpn J Vet Sci* 36:381–389, 1974.
10. Kornegay JN: Diskospondylitis. *In* Kirk RW (ed): *Current Veterinary Therapy VIII*. Philadelphia, WB Saunders Co, 1983, pp 718–721.
11. Smeak DD, Olmstead ML, Hohn RB: *Brucella canis* osteomyelitis in two dogs with total hip replacements. *J Am Vet Med Assoc* 191:986–989, 1987.
12. Greene CE: Personal observations. University of Georgia, Athens, GA, 1988.
13. George LW, Duncan JR, Carmichael LE: Semen examination in dogs with canine brucellosis. *Am J Vet Res* 40:1589–1595, 1979.
14. Carmichael LE, Zoha SJ, Flores-Castro R: Problems in the serodiagnosis of canine brucellosis: dog responses to cell wall and internal antigens of *Brucella canis*. *Dev Biol Stand* 56:371–383, 1984.
15. Nicoletti PL, Chase A: The use of antibiotics to control canine brucellosis. *Compend Cont Educ Pract Vet* 9:1063–1066, 1987.
16. Badakhsh FF, Carmichael LE, Douglass JA: Improved rapid slide agglutination test for presumptive diagnosis of canine brucellosis. *J Clin Microbiol* 15:286–289, 1982.
17. Carmichael LE, Joubert JC: A rapid slide agglutination test for the serodiagnosis of *Brucella canis* infection that employs a variant (M-) organism as antigen. *Cornell Vet* 77:3–12, 1987.
18. Zoha SJ, Carmichael LE: Serological responses of dogs to cell wall and internal antigens of *Brucella canis*. *Vet Microbiol* 17:35–50, 1982.
19. Nicoletti PL, Chase A: An evaluation of methods to diagnose *Brucella canis* in dogs. *Compend Cont Educ Pract Vet* 9:1071–1074, 1987.
19a. Serikawa T, Iwaki S, Mori M, et al: Purification of *Brucella canis* cell wall antigen using immunosorbent columns and use of the antigen in enzyme-linked immunosorbent assay for specific diagnosis of canine brucellosis. *J Clin Microbiol* 27:837–842, 1989.
20. Alton GG, Jones LM, Peitz DE: *Laboratory Techniques in Brucellosis*, ed 2. Geneva, WHO, 1975, pp 149–154.
21. Flores-Castro R, Carmichael L: Characterization of different *Brucella canis* strains. *Rev Latinoam Microbiol* 28:145–152, 1986.
22. Forbes LB, Pantekoek JF: *Brucella canis* isolates from Canadian dogs. *Can Vet J* 29:149–152, 1988.
23. Corbel MJ: Use of phage for the identification of *Brucella canis* and *Brucella ovis* cultures. *Res Vet Sci* 38:35–40, 1985.
24. Saegusa J, Ueda K, Goto Y, et al: Ocular lesions in experimental canine brucellosis. *Jpn J Vet Sci* 39:181–185, 1977.
25. Dillon AR, Henderson RA: *Brucella canis* in a uterine stump abscess in a bitch. *J Am Vet Med Assoc* 178:987–988, 1981.
26. Terakado N, Ueda K, Sugawara H, et al: Drug susceptibility of *Brucella canis* isolated from dogs. *Jpn J Vet Sci* 40:291–295, 1973.
27. Zoha SJ, Walsh R: Effect of a two-stage antibiotic treatment regimen on dogs naturally infected with *Brucella canis*. *J Am Vet Med Assoc* 180:1474–1475, 1982.
28. Jennings PB, Crumrine MH, Lewis GE, et al: The effect of a two-stage antibiotic regimen on dogs infected with *Brucella canis*. *J Am Vet Med Assoc* 163:513–514, 1974.
29. Polt SS, Dismukes WE, Flint A, et al: Human brucellosis caused by *Brucella canis*. *Ann Intern Med* 97:717–719, 1982.
30. Swenson RM, Carmichael LE, Cundy KR: Human infection with *Brucella canis*. *Ann Intern Med* 76:435–438, 1972.

53 ACTINOMYCOSIS AND NOCARDIOSIS

Elizabeth M. Hardie

ETIOLOGY

Actinomycetales are branching, filamentous, gram-positive bacteria. Anaerobic or microaerophilic species that produce disease include *Actinomyces viscosus*, *A. hordeovulneris*, *A. odontolyticus*, and *A. meyeri*. The aerobic species are *Nocardia asteroides*, *N. brasiliensis*, *N. otitidiscaviarum* (*N. caviae*), and *Streptomyces griseus*. *Dermatophilus congolensis* is discussed in Chapter 54.

Actinomyces are commensal organisms found in the oral cavities of animals and people. In surveys of anaerobic organisms cultured from lesions in dogs and cats, *Actinomyces* represented 9% of isolates.[1,2] Infection follows puncture wounds or tissue trauma, which create favorable environments for growth. In the western United States, infection with *A. hordeovulneris* commonly occurs secondary to injury by grass awns (foxtails) of the genus *Hordeum*.[3-5,5a] Infection with multiple organisms may also promote growth of *Actinomyces*.[6]

Nocardia are saprophytic organisms that enter the body through soil contamination of wounds or via inhalation. Immunosuppression of the host may enhance the ability of these organisms to cause disease. *Nocardia* have been cultured from canine lesions with one tenth the frequency of *Actinomyces* isolation.[7] *N. asteroides* is the species most often cultured from canine and feline infections.

Streptomyces griseus is a saprophytic organism usually regarded as a cultural contaminant. It has been isolated from cats with actinomycetoma, a localized chronic infection of the extremities associated with multiple draining tracts (Fig. 53–1).[8,9]

CLINICAL FINDINGS

Actinomycosis

Lesions have been found primarily in large breed dogs used for outdoor activities and in cats. *Actinomyces* are usually found in association with other bacteria in localized pyogranulomatous infections. Widely disseminated disease is rare. Lesions include superficial abscesses (particularly around the head and neck), epidural abscesses, chronic draining tracts, thoracic granulomas and empyema, intestinal granulomas and peritonitis, and osteomyelitis of both the vertebrae and long bones (Fig. 53–2).[2,5,6,10-15]

All percutaneous abscesses in dogs and cats can potentially be infected with *Actinomyces*, as many are secondary to bite wounds and almost all wounds will be licked by the animal. Infection with *Actinomyces* should be suspected particularly if the exudate is serosanguineous, if "sulphur granules" are present (Fig. 53–3), if an intense granulomatous reaction surrounds the abscess, or if routine treatment fails to elim-

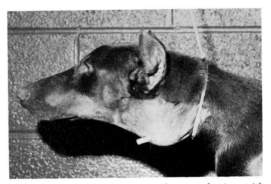

Figure 53–1. A cervical abscess due to infection with *Actinomyces*.

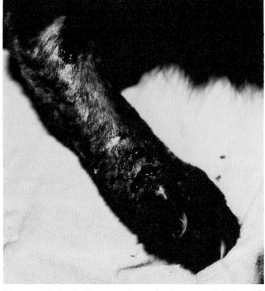

Figure 53–2. Actinomycetoma lesion associated with *Nocardia* infection in a cat.

inate infection. Paraplegia can develop if superficial infection over the lumbosacral region extends into the epidural space.[16,17] Chronic draining tracts infected with *Actinomyces* are often associated with penetrating foreign bodies, particularly plant awns.[3,5]

Lack of exercise tolerance, emaciation, low-grade fever, and dyspnea are common complaints in animals with empyema. Empyema in both dogs and cats may contain *Actinomyces* as part of a mixed bacterial infection. The exudate seen in these cases is

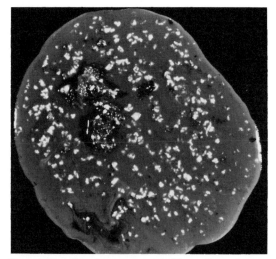

Figure 53–3. Exudates present in *Nocardia* or *Actinomyces* infection are usually serosanguineous and contain clumps of organisms that look like granules on gross examination.

similar to that described for abscesses. Granulomas may be present in association with exudation and will become apparent radiographically once the exudate has been removed.

Lesions ranging from generalized peritonitis to isolated granulomas have been associated with intra-abdominal *Actinomyces* infection.[11] Clinical signs include lethargy, anorexia, abdominal enlargement, vomiting, diarrhea, and anemia. Abdominal masses may be palpable. An abdominal mass in a young (<1 year) dog may be a granuloma rather than a neoplasm.

Osteomyelitis can develop in both the extremities[12,15] and the vertebrae.[6] Fever, lameness, limb swelling, or recurrent draining fistulas will be seen in dogs with extremity lesions. Those with vertebral osteomyelitis show fever, hyperesthesia, weight loss, paresis, or paralysis. Radiographic lesions include osteoporosis, the presence of lytic areas within the bone, reactive osteosclerosis, periosteal proliferation, pathologic fractures, and soft tissue swelling.

Nocardiosis

Nocardia may cause clinical syndromes similar to those listed above, but three major forms have been reported: actinomycetoma, empyema, and a disseminated form.[18–20] Disseminated nocardiosis is a disease of young dogs, whereas empyema and actinomycetoma have been found in both dogs and cats of any age.

Actinomycetoma is a chronic nonhealing wound often involving an extremity (see Fig. 53–1). Often there is a history of a bite or puncture wound at the site of the primary lesion. Numerous draining tracts may be present, with possible extension into lymph nodes, underlying soft tissue, joints, and bone. Occasionally, multiple sites are affected. The exudate produced from the wound is usually serosanguineous, and the presence of granules is variable.

Symptoms of empyema are identical to those of actinomycosis. Only culture or demonstration of an acid-fast organism on cytology will distinguish whether pyothorax is caused by *Nocardia* or *Actinomyces*.

Disseminated nocardiosis usually begins as a respiratory infection that becomes generalized. Clinical signs include anorexia, depression, fever, oculonasal discharges, increased lung sounds, coughing, dyspnea, draining subcutaneous masses, diarrhea, and seizures. In dogs, the disease is easily confused with canine distemper, and in a few cases, distemper has been a concurrent disease. At necropsy abscesses are often noted in a variety of tissues.

DIAGNOSIS

There are no distinct hematologic or serum biochemical findings in either actinomycosis or nocardiosis. Elevated leukocyte counts characterized by neutrophilia and monocytosis are usually present, unless disease is limited to localized abscess formation or osteomyelitis. Animals with empyema or peritonitis may also have severe left shifts and toxic neutrophils. Hypoglycemia and anemia may be present.

If exudate is present (see Fig. 53–2), cytologic examination is the first means of diagnosis. When granules are present in the sample, they should be examined because they consist of colonies of organisms. Several squash preparations of granules should be made between two slides or between a slide and a coverglass and stained with H and E or Gram stain.

Gram-positive, branching, filamentous rods and cocci are typical of actinomycosis or nocardiosis (Fig. 53–4). A specimen should also be stained with Hank's or cold Kinyoun acid-fast stain, using 1% aqueous sulfuric acid as a decolorizing agent.[6,21] If the organism stains acid-fast with this procedure, it may be presumed to be *Nocardia*. A negative stain does not rule out *Nocardia*, as staining may vary. *Actinomyces* and *Streptomyces* do not stain acid-fast. These stains and procedure for their use are described in Appendix 12.

Clostridium villosum, an anaerobic organism common in feline abscesses and pyothorax, is a gram-variable rod with a filamentous pattern of growth. This organism may be mistaken for an actinomycete on cytologic examination.[10]

Definitive diagnosis can be obtained only through culture of the organism. Samples should be obtained anaerobically and should be transported immediately to the laboratory in a stoppered syringe or in anaerobic transport media (see Chapters 42 and 49). A large quantity of exudate containing granules or a

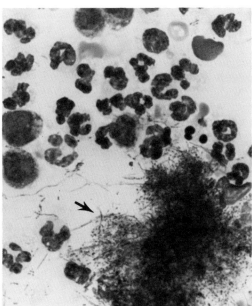

Figure 53–4. Branching, filamentous, gram-positive rods are seen with both *Nocardia* and *Actinomyces* infections. Clump of organisms (*arrow*) looks like a granule on gross examination (see Fig. 53–2) (× 1000). (Courtesy of Dr. Ken Latimer, University of Georgia, Athens, GA.)

large tissue sample gives the best culture results. The laboratory should be informed that an actinomycete is suspected, as special culturing methods are required.[6] Samples cultured for *Actinomyces* should be streaked on blood agar and brain-heart infusion agar and incubated at 37°C under aerobic, anaerobic, and microaerophilic conditions. Samples cultured for *Nocardia* should be placed on blood agar and plain Sabouraud's dextrose agar and incubated at both 25°C and 37°C under aerobic conditions. The plates should be examined daily for 2 weeks. Biochemical features are used to distinguish the isolates. Because of the difficulty in identifying some species, it may be necessary to send specimens to a reference laboratory for final identification.

Lesions compatible with a diagnosis of actinomycosis or nocardiosis should be biopsied if possible, as cultural diagnosis is often difficult. Although one cannot usually distinguish actinomycosis from nocardiosis using microscopic examination of tissues, the presence of the organisms is at least established. Nocardial organisms may not be seen with routine H and E stain and must be demonstrated with Gram, silver, or modified acid-fast stain of tissue.[22]

THERAPY

Treatment principles for the two diseases are similar except in the choice of antibiotics. Lavage and drainage of the affected area, debridement of granulation tissue, and long-term (weeks to months) antibiotic therapy are the major components of treatment.

Localized Lesions

Abscesses should initially be drained and Penrose drains placed. Because drainage may have to be continued for several weeks, drains should not be removed prematurely. The affected area may need to be flushed with povidone-iodine solution while the drain is in place. If extensive granulation tissue is present or if the abscess recurs following drain removal, surgical excision of the affected tissue is recommended. Draining tracts associated with migrating foreign bodies should be followed and the foreign body removed, if possible.

Osteomyelitis requires debridement and removal of infected bone, if possible. In cases of vertebral osteomyelitis, surgical debridement may not be possible, so antibiotic therapy alone must be used. Surgical decompression is usually not needed unless acute fracture or collapse of the vertebral body occurs or the animal fails to respond to medical therapy alone.

Pyothorax

Bilateral large-bore chest tubes should be placed using standard techniques.[23] The thorax is then drained of purulent material, using intermittent aspiration or continuous, closed, underwater suction drainage. Thereafter, twice daily 10 to 20 ml/kg warmed lactated Ringer's solution is placed in the chest, and the animal is rolled to distribute the fluid. The fluid is then removed after 20 to 30 minutes. Lavage and drainage should continue for several days until the aspirated lavage fluid is clear or a faint pink color and no organisms are seen on cytologic examination. Most animals require 5 to 10 days of treatment. If large granulomas are present, or if pleural scarring limits lung expansion, surgical removal of affected tissue and pleural stripping may be indicated.[23]

Abdominal Infection

The abdomen should be explored for a focus of infection. If granulomas or abscesses are found, they should be excised and drained if possible. Often, only copious amounts of exudate are found. The abdomen should then be thoroughly lavaged and drained. Continued lavage and drainage may be accomplished using an indwelling lavage system. Alternatively, an open abdominal drainage technique may be used to remove exudate.[24]

Disseminated Disease

Disseminated disease due to nocardiosis is not treated surgically. Superficial abscesses may be drained, but drainage of multiple abscesses in the body organs and CNS is impossible. Disseminated lesions associated with migrating grass awns may also be difficult to treat surgically because of the extensive involvement of vital body structures in scar tissue and chronic granulation tissue.[25] Chemotherapy alone must be relied upon in these cases.

Antimicrobial Therapy

Antibiotic therapy is usually initiated prior to cultural identification of the organism. The majority of infections containing gram-positive, branching, filamentous bacteria are mixed anaerobic infections with *Actinomyces*, and initial therapy should be directed at a wide variety of anaerobes[26,27] (Table 53–1; see also Chapter 49). In young dogs with disseminated disease or in animals with actinomycetoma lesions, antibiotics active against *Nocardia* should be chosen (Table 53–2).

Actinomycosis. High-dose, long-term penicillin therapy is the preferred treatment. Evidence however indicates that *A. hordeovulneris* forms L-phase (cell-wall deficient) variants in association with the production of calcified sulphur granules (see also L-Form Infections, Chapter 50).[3] Antibiotic penetration into calcified granules is expected to be limited. *A. hordeovulneris* infections responded poorly to ampicillin, indicating that drugs active against cell wall–deficient variants should be combined with

Table 53–1. Drugs Used to Treat Actinomycosis in Dogs and Cats[a]

DRUG	SPECIES	DOSE[b] (mg/kg)	ROUTE	INTERVAL (hours)
Penicillin G[6]	B	100,000 U/kg	IM,SC	12–24
Penicillin G[5a]	D[c]	65,000 U/kg	PO	8
Penicillin V[6,28]	B	50	PO	8
Clindamycin[29]	B	5	SC	12
Erythromycin[28]	B	10	PO	8
Chloramphenicol[28]	D	50	PO,IV,IM,SC	8
	C	50	PO,IV,IM,SC	12
Rifampin[30]	D	10–20	PO	12
Cephaloridine[28]	B	10	IM,SC	8–12
Minocycline[31]	B	5–25	IV,PO	12
Ampicillin[28]	B	20–40	IM,SC,PO	6

[a]B = dog and cat, D = dog, C = cat, IM = intramuscular, SC = subcutaneous, PO = oral, IV = intravenous.
[b]Dose per administration at specified interval, mg/kg unless otherwise stated.
[c]Give medication at least 1 hour before or 2 hours after feeding to facilitate GI absorption.

or substituted for penicillins in this disease.[3] Trimethoprim-sulfadiazine has been recommended to treat L-phase variants,[3] but this drug has a high failure rate in mixed anaerobic infections.[2] Antibiotics active against a wide variety of anaerobes (including *Actinomyces*)[27,36,37] and active against L-phase variants include clindamycin, erythromycin, and chloramphenicol. Other drugs active against a wide variety of *Actinomyces* in vitro are rifampin, cephaloridine, and minocycline.[27,36,37] Drugs to be avoided include aminoglycosides, metronidazole, oral cephalexin, and the semisynthetic penicillins, oxacillin and dicloxacillin.[21,27,36,37]

Nocardiosis. *Nocardia* organisms show marked variation in susceptibility to various antibiotics (even within the same class of antibiotics), and in vitro susceptibility does not necessarily predict in vivo efficacy.[21] The sulfonamides have been used to treat nocardiosis for many years and have proven in vivo efficacy, despite the fact that they are not active in vitro.[21] The efficacy of trimethoprim-sulfonamide is highly controversial.[21] In vitro susceptibility is variable,[38,39] and both clinical successes and failures have been documented. Amikacin and imipenem-cilastatin are highly effective against *Nocardia* organisms in vitro and in experimental infection studies.[38–40] Drugs that are active in vitro but have not been evaluated in experimental animals or clinical studies include cefotaxime, cefmenoxime, ceftriaxone, and cefuroxime.[38,40] Minocycline has marked in vitro activity and has been used successfully on clinical patients but has failed to exhibit efficacy in an experimental infection study.[38,39] Erythromycin combined with ampicillin has been used clinically against *Nocardia*, but in vitro susceptibility to these

Table 53–2. Drugs Used to Treat Nocardiosis in Dogs and Cats[a]

DRUG	DOSE[b]	ROUTE	INTERVAL (hours)
Triple sulfa #4[6]	60[c]	IV	12
Sulfadiazine[6]	80	PO	8
Sulfisoxazole[d,28]	50	PO	8
Amikacin[32,33]	8–12	IV,IM,SC	8
Imipenem-cilastatin[33]	2–5	IV	8
Cefotaxime[34,35]	20–80	IV,IM	6
Minocycline[31,e]	5–25	IV,PO	12
Erythromycin[28]	10	PO	8
Ampicillin[28]	20–40	IV,IM,SC,PO	6

[a]For duration of therapy, see text; usually there is a minimum of 6 weeks with all drugs. IV = intravenous, PO = oral, IM = intramuscular, SC = subcutaneous.
[b]Dose per administration at specified interval, mg/kg unless otherwise stated.
[c]120 mg/kg IV initially.
[d]Also sulfamethizole.
[e]Doxycycline may be substituted.

drugs should be demonstrated first, as resistant strains exist.[11,20] *Nocardia* spp. are generally resistant to many quinolones.

Both actinomycosis and nocardiosis should be treated a minimum of 6 weeks with antibiotic therapy, with the possible exception of localized abscesses that have obviously resolved prior to 6 weeks.[6,11,21] Therapy should be continued until all signs of disease have resolved, and owners should be warned that relapse may occur. Some authors recommend treatment for a minimum of 4 months after all clinical, laboratory, and radiographic evidences of disease have resolved.[5a] Some animals may require lifelong therapy, particularly if migrating foreign bodies that cannot be removed are present.[11,41] Recurrence can be detected by re-evaluating animals 4 to 6 months after discontinuing medication.

Complications associated with treatment of severe disease include hypoalbuminemia leading to dependent edema, persistent hypoglycemia and weakness, cardiac arrhythmias, and self-inflicted damage to drainage tubes.[11] The major long-term complication is relapse following withdrawal of antibiotic therapy.

With actinomycosis and nocardiosis, the prognosis for cure is good in localized infections. Animals with empyema and peritonitis have a fair prognosis, provided they survive the initial diagnostic and therapeutic manipulations. The prognosis for cure in animals with unretrievable foreign bodies is poor, but control may be achieved with long-term antibiotic therapy. The prognosis for cure of disseminated nocardiosis is poor.

References

1. Berg JW, Fales WH, Scanlan CM: Occurrence of anaerobic bacteria in diseases of the dog and cat. *Am J Vet Res* 38:1069–1074, 1977.
2. Dow SW, Jones RL, Adney WS: Anaerobic bacterial infections and response to treatment in dogs and cats: 36 cases (1983–1985). *J Am Vet Med Assoc* 189:930–934, 1986.
3. Buchanan AM, Scott JL: *Actinomyces hordeovulneris*, a canine pathogen that produces L-phase variants spontaneously with coincident calcium deposition. *Am J Vet Res* 45:2552–2560, 1984.
4. Buchanan AM, Scott JL, Gerencser MA, et al: *Actinomyces hordeovulneris* sp. nov. an agent of canine actinomycosis. *Int J Syst Bacteriol* 34:439–443, 1984.
5. Brennan KE, Ihrke PJ: Grass and migration in dogs and cats: a retrospective study of 182 cases. *J Am Vet Med Assoc* 182:1201–1204, 1982.
5a. Edwards DF, Nyland TG, Weigel JP: Thoracic, abdominal, and vertebral actinomycosis: diagnosis and long-term therapy in three dogs. *J Vet Intern Med* 2:184–191, 1988.
6. Attleberger MH: Actinomycosis, nocardiosis, and dermatophilosis. In Kirk RW (ed): *Current Veterinary Therapy VIII*. Philadelphia, WB Saunders Co, 1983, pp 1184–1186.
7. Ackerman N, Grain E, Castleman W: Canine nocardiosis. *J Am Anim Hosp Assoc* 18:147–153, 1982.
8. Reinke SI, Ihrke PJ, Reinke JD, et al: Actinomycotic mycetoma in a cat. *J Am Vet Med Assoc* 189:446–448, 1986.
9. Lewis GE, Fidler WJ, Cromine MH: Mycetoma in a cat. *J Am Vet Med Assoc* 161:500–503, 1972.
10. Love DN, Jones RF, Bailey M, et al: Isolation and characterization of bacteria from pyothorax (empyaemia) in cats. *Vet Microbiol* 7:455–461, 1982.
11. Hardie EM: Actinomycosis and nocardiosis. In Greene CE (ed): *Clinical Microbiology and Infectious Diseases of the Dog and Cat*. Philadelphia, WB Saunders Co, 1984, pp 663–674.
12. McMillan KL, Horne RD, King HA: Osteomyelitis in a dog caused by an anaerobic actinomycete: a case report. *J Am Anim Hosp Assoc* 18:265–268, 1982.
13. Jonas LD: Feline pyothorax: a retrospective study of twenty cases. *J Am Anim Hosp Assoc* 19:865–871, 1983.
14. Robertson SA, Stoddant ME, Evans RJ, et al: Thoracic empyema in the dog; a report of twenty-two cases. *J Small Anim Pract* 24:103–119, 1983.
15. Johnson KA, Lomas GR, Wood AKW: Osteomyelitis in dogs and cats caused by anaerobic bacteria. *Aust Vet J* 61:57–61, 1984.
16. Bestetti G, Buhlmann V, Nicolet J, et al: Paraplegia due to *Actinomyces viscosus* infection in a cat. *Acta Neuropathol (Berl)* 39:231–235, 1977.
17. Stowater JL, Cosner EC, McCoy JC: Actinomycosis in the spinal canal of a cat. *Feline Pract* 8:26–27, 1978.
18. Stead AC: Osteomyelitis in the dog and cat. *J Small Anim Pract* 25:1–13, 1984.
19. Bradney IN: Vertebral osteomyelitis due to Nocardia in a dog. *Aust Vet J* 62:315–316, 1985.
20. Davenport DJ, Johnson GC: Cutaneous nocardiosis in a cat. *J Am Vet Med Assoc* 188:728–729, 1986.
21. Lerner PL: *Nocardia* species, *Actinomyces* and *Arachnia* species. In Mandell GL, Douglas RG Jr, Bennett JE (eds): *Principles and Practice of Infectious Diseases*, ed 2. New York, John Wiley & Sons, 1985, pp 1423–1433.
22. Werczek TW, Trautwein G, Nielsen SW: Canine nocardiosis. *Zentralbl Veterinarmed [B]* 15:171–178, 1968.
23. Orton CE: Pleura and pleural space. In Slatter DA (ed): *Textbook of Small Animal Surgery*. Philadelphia, WB Saunders Co, 1985, pp 547–566.
24. Greenfield CL, Walshaw R: Open peritoneal drainage for treatment of contaminated peritoneal cavity and septic peritonitis in dogs and cats: 24 cases (1980–1986). *J Am Vet Med Assoc* 191:100–106, 1987.
25. Dunbar M, Vulgamott SC: Thoracic and vertebral osteomyelitis caused by actinomycosis in a dog. *VM SAC* 76:1159–1161, 1981.
26. Dow SW, Jones RL: Anaerobic infections. Part I. Pathogenesis and clinical significance. *Compend Cont Educ Pract Vet* 9:711–720, 1987.
27. Dow SW, Jones RL: Anaerobic infections. Part II.

Diagnosis and treatment. *Compend Cont Educ Pract Vet* 9:827–839, 1987.

28. Aronson AL, Kirk RW: Antimicrobial drugs. *In* Ettinger SJ (ed): *Textbook of Veterinary Internal Medicine:* Diseases of the Dog and Cat, ed 2. Philadelphia, WB Saunders Co, 1983, pp 338–366.
29. Weber DJ, Barbier AR, Lollinger AJ, et al: Pharmacokinetics of clindamycin following subcutaneous administration of clindamycin phosphate in the canine. *J Vet Pharmacol Therap* 3:133–143, 1980.
30. American Hospital Formulary Service Drug Information 87. Bethesda, MD, Am Soc Hosp Pharm Inc, 1987, pp 344–348.
31. Pollock RVH: Canine brucellosis: current status. *Compend Cont Educ Pract Vet* 1:255–267, 1979.
32. Baggot JD, Ling GV, Chatfield RC: Clinical pharmacokinetics of amikacin in dogs. *Am J Vet Res* 46:1793–1796, 1985.
33. Aucoin DP: Unpublished observations. North Carolina State University, Raleigh, NC, 1987.
34. McElroy, Ravis WR, Clark CH: Pharmacokinetics of cefotaxime in the domestic cat. *Am J Vet Res* 47:86–88, 1986.
35. Guerrini KH, English PB, Filippich LJ, et al: Pharmacokinetic evaluation of a slow release cefotaxime

suspension in the dog and in sheep. *Am J Vet Res* 47:2057–2061, 1986.
36. Lerner PL: Susceptibility of pathogenic actinomycetes to antimicrobial compounds. *Antimicrob Agents Chemother* 5:304–309, 1974.
37. Sutter VL, Jones MJ, Ghoneim ATM: Antimicrobial susceptibilities of bacteria associated with periodontal disease. *Antimicrob Agents Chemother* 23:483–486, 1983.
38. Gutmann L, Goldstein FW, Kitzis MD, et al: Susceptibility of *Nocardia asteroides* to 46 antibiotics, including 22 β-lactams. *Antimicrob Agents Chemother* 23:248–251, 1983.
39. Gombert ME, Aulicino TM, duBouchet L, et al: Therapy of experimental cerebral nocardiosis with imipenem, amikacin, trimethoprim-sulfamethoxazole, and minocycline. *Antimicrob Agents Chemother* 30:270–273, 1986.
40. Gombert ME: Susceptibility of *Nocardia asteroides* to various antibiotics, including newer β-lactams, trimethoprim-sulfamethoxazole, amikacin, and N-formimidoyl thienamycin. *Antimicrob Agents Chemother* 21:1011–1012, 1982.
41. Walker R: Personal communication, North Carolina State University, Raleigh, NC, 1987.

54

DERMATOPHILOSIS
Craig E. Greene

ETIOLOGY AND EPIDEMIOLOGY

Cutaneous streptothricosis (dermatophilosis) is an exudative skin disease caused by the actinomycete, *Dermatophilus congolensis*. Chronic exposure of the skin to trauma or moisture and immunosuppressive therapy or concurrent debilitating diseases may predispose the skin to overgrowth and colonization by *D. congolensis*. This aerobe or facultative anaerobe is a normal dermal inhabitant of a number of mammalian species, including horses, sheep, goats, and cattle. Although not primary hosts, cats[1–5] and dogs[6,7] can be naturally infected. Contamination of puncture wounds is presumed to occur in infected cats. Acquisition from the soil, contact with another carrier animal, or latent infection with the organism by the affected animal cannot be excluded in reported cases.

Dermatophilosis has been produced experimentally in dogs following inoculation of the organism onto previously damaged skin[8] and in cats by subcutaneous inoculation.[1]

CLINICAL FINDINGS

Dogs

Spontaneous dermatophilosis in dogs has been confined to the skin. As a primary dermatologic disease, dermatophilosis produces minimal signs of systemic illness, although emaciation and debilitation may be associated with an underlying immunosuppressive disease process. Lesions in dogs, which are frequently found on haired portions of the skin, consist of dry, adherent

scabs that become entrapped in surrounding hair (Fig. 54–1). Removal of the crusts reveals underlying erythematous and ulcerated skin.

Cats

In affected cats, deeper abscesses in muscle and lymph nodes and in subcutaneous tissue have been more characteristic. The lesions are submucosal or subcutaneous pyogranulomas that may produce chronic draining fistulas. Fever, anorexia, and regional lymphadenopathy or abscess formation are common. Ulcerative granulomas in cats that involve the tongue or urinary bladder were also described.[5,9]

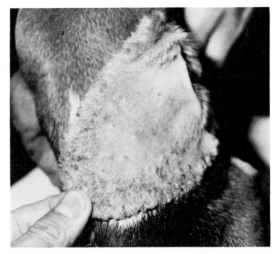

Figure 54–1. Skin lesions of dermatophilosis in a beagle. Note the crusty lesions that surround tufts of hair on the ear margins.

DIAGNOSIS

The simplest and most rapid means of establishing a diagnosis involves removing the dried scabs from epidermal lesions or taking biopsy samples of deeper tissues where abscesses are found. Samples are minced in small amounts of sterile saline or nutrient broth. Some of the material is also used to prepare wet mounts or air-dried smears for microscopic examination, while the remainder is submitted for culture. Wet mounts can be stained with new methylene blue; dried specimens are heat-fixed and are best stained by Giemsa methods, although Wright and Gram stains are suitable. Exudates or minced preparations usually contain large numbers of neutrophils in clusters around gram-positive, branching, filamentous organisms. The filaments are recognized by their characteristic transverse and longitudinal divisions that result in three to eight paired rows of coccoid spores arranged in linear fashion (Fig. 54–2). Monoclonal antibodies to D. congolensis have been used with indirect immunofluorescent staining to specifically identify the organism in clinical samples.[10]

Sterile specimens from scabs or biopsy may be cultured aerobically at 25°C and aerobically or anaerobically at 37°C on solid nutrient agar, such as blood or brain-heart infusion medium. Small grayish, raised colonies surrounded by a zone of hemolysis are typically produced. The organism can be further identified by its biochemical properties or after experimental inoculation in laboratory animals.

PATHOLOGIC FINDINGS

Histologically, the organism produces a suppurative dermatitis characterized by epidermal hyperkeratosis with underlying dermal edema and hemorrhage. There is little involvement of hair follicles. In cats, the lesions consist of pyogranulomas in subcutaneous tissues or lymph nodes. The organism may be identified by H and E stained preparations in the periphery of necrotic lesions. The banded filamentous nature is best demonstrated by Twort's modified Gram stain.

THERAPY

Treatment involves keeping the animal's skin dry and the hair clipped around the periphery of the lesions or, where lesions are extensive, over the entire body. Clipping the hair and subsequent bathing with 2% lime sulfur or organic iodine preparations facilitate the softening and removal of the impervious dry adherent crusts. Bathing and removing crusts should be continued for a minimum of 2 weeks.

The organism also is susceptible to a number of antimicrobial agents in vitro; however, based on cost and efficacy, penicillin derivatives are the most practical choice (Table 54–1). Penicillin may be given alone or in combination with aminoglycoside. Ampicillin has been used successfully to treat cats with abscesses. Attempts must be made to find and eliminate the predisposing causes of dermatophilosis if treatment is to be successful and permanent.

PUBLIC HEALTH CONSIDERATIONS

People are accidental secondary hosts of D. congolensis. People handling infected carcasses or tissues can develop exudative pustular dermatitis.[11] Lesions usually consist of multiple white pustules 2 to 5 mm in diameter at the site of contact. These lesions

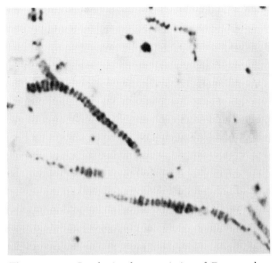

Figure 54–2. Cytologic characteristics of D. congolensis. Note the filaments of paired rows of cocci, which give the appearance of "stacked coins" (Gram stain, × 4300). (Courtesy of Dr. Emmett Shotts, University of Georgia, Athens, GA.)

Table 54–1. Drug Therapy for Dermatophilosis[a]

DRUG	SPECIES	DOSE[b] (mg/kg)	ROUTE	INTERVAL (hours)	DURATION (days)
Penicillin V[c]	B	10	PO	12	7–10
Gentamicin	B	2	IM	12	7
Amp(amox)icillin	B	10–20	PO	12	7–10

[a]B = dog and cat, PO = oral, IM = intramuscular.
[b]Dose per administration at specified interval, expressed as mg/kg unless otherwise stated.
[c]Penicillin may be given alone or in combination with gentamicin.

neither spread nor coalesce but resolve within 2 weeks, more rapidly if the lesions are opened to drain.

References

1. Jones RT: Subcutaneous infection with Dermatophilus congolensis in a cat. *J Comp Pathol* 86:415–421, 1976.
2. Carakostas MC, Miller RI, Woodward MG: Subcutaneous dermatophilosis in a cat. *J Am Vet Med Assoc* 185:675–676, 1984.
3. Miller RI, Ladds PW, Mudie A, et al: Probable dermatophilosis in 2 cats. *Aust Vet J* 60:155–156, 1983.
4. Scott DW: Bacterial disorders. *J Am Anim Hosp Assoc* 16:340–348, 1980.
5. O'Hara JP, Cordes DO: Granulomata caused by dermatophilosis in two cats. *N Z Vet J* 11:151–154, 1963.
6. Blancou J: Infection of a dog with *Dermatophilus congolensis*. *Rev Elev Med Vet Pays Trop* 26:289–291, 1973.
7. Chastain CB, Carithers RW, Hogle RM, et al: Dermatophilosis in two dogs. *J Am Vet Med Assoc* 169:1079–1080, 1976.
8. Richard JL, Pier AC, Gysewski SJ: Experimentally induced canine dermatophilosis. *Am J Vet Res* 34:797–799, 1973.
9. Baker GJ, Breeze RG, Dawson CO: Oral dermatophilosis in a cat: a case report. *J Small Anim Pract* 13:649–653, 1972.
10. How SJ, Lloyd DH: Use of monoclonal antibody in the diagnosis of infection by *Dermatophilus congolensis*. *Res Vet Sci* 45:416–417, 1988.
11. Gordon MA: Characterization of *Dermatophilus congolensis*, its affinities with the Actinomycetales and differentiation from *Geodermatophilus*. In Lloyd DH, Sellers KC (ed): *Dermatophilus Infection in Animals and Man*. London, Academic Press, 1976, pp 187–201.

55

FELINE ABSCESSES
Craig E. Greene

ETIOLOGY AND PATHOGENESIS

Percutaneous abscesses are the most common bacterial infection of feline skin. Abscesses develop more frequently in cats than in dogs owing to the tough, elastic nature of feline skin, which readily seals over contaminated puncture wounds, causing accumulation of subcutaneous exudates. Sharp teeth and fighting behavior, especially of adult males, are important predisposing factors to abscess formation. The size and degree of abscess formation depend upon many factors, including the overlying skin tension, amount of dead space, and gravitation of exudate below the point of penetration. Pus-filled cavities that form above the puncture site drain easily. Cavities that gravitate below the puncture site become overdistended and may repeatedly drain through the puncture site without complete resolution. Abscesses associated with foreign bodies, underlying osteomyelitis, or certain organisms such as *Nocardia* or *Mycobacterium* spp. also tend to recur, persist, or spread in tissues.

Since abscesses usually result from bites and scratches, the most common organisms found within them are resident oral microflora (Table 55–1).[1–8] *Although more difficult to cultivate, anaerobes are more frequently isolated than aerobes.* Cats that sustain bite injuries are more likely to become infected with feline immunodeficiency virus (FIV, see Chapter 26).

CLINICAL FINDINGS

The clinical signs of abscess formation in cats reflect the site and severity of infection. Abscesses are usually located around the cat's legs, face, back, and base of the tail. Some cats have a noticeable swelling with few other signs of illness, whereas more extensive infection is associated with fever (39.7° to 40.6°C [103.6° to 105.2°F]), anorexia, depression, and regional lymphadenopathy. Pain is usually present at the site of infection, and there may or may not be obvious swelling or warmth. Mature abscesses that are ready to discharge are usually tender with a soft fluctuant central area. Feline skin easily stretches over distended abscesses, and redness or discoloration is rarely apparent unless the blood vascular supply has been compromised. Drainage of white, creamy, purulent material occurs spontaneously or following surgical lancing. Foul-smelling, red-brown discharges tend to be associated with anaerobic bacterial infections. Systemic signs often abate once the abscess ruptures, and the only evidence of infection may be matted hair at the site of drainage. Careful examination in the area of swelling usually reveals a small puncture wound covered by a crust.

Additional clinical manifestations reflect various sequelae that can occur. Lameness or paralysis will be apparent with myositis, osteomyelitis, septic arthritis, or discospondylitis. Depression, stiffness, lethargy, nuchal rigidity, or seizures can be seen with meningitis. Osteomyelitis also causes chronic or recurrent draining fistulas that only temporarily respond to antibiotics. Respiratory distress, dyspnea, and stridor are noted with pyothorax, sinusitis, and rhinitis. Vestibular signs can be noted if otitis media or otitis interna develops. Signs of bacteremia and systemic infection include malaise and fever or reflect those of another organ system of hematogenous localization.

DIAGNOSIS

Determining the presence of an abscess is usually based on clinical history and examination. Abscesses should be suspected in cats that develop an acute onset of unexplained fever, anorexia, or lameness, even in the absence of an obvious swelling, as abscess formation may be delayed or hidden. The differential leukocyte count can help in determining the extent of infection and the animal's ability to respond. A low count with an inappropriate shift is associated with diffuse infection or cellulitis. A mature neutrophilia is more characteristic of a walled-off or mature abscess. Severe leukopenia (<4000 cells/μl), with or without an associated anemia, may be present in cats infected with feline leukemia virus (FeLV) or FIV that develop chronic or recurrent abscesses as a result of immunosuppression. Unlike those in FeLV- or FIV-infected cats, the leukogram usually improves in immunocompetent cats after the abscess drains.

Causes of recurrent or nonhealing abscesses in cats include retroviral infections as previously discussed, underlying osteomyelitis, neoplasia or foreign body, or infection with organisms such as *Nocardia, Mycobacterium*, L-forms, fungi, or parasites such as *Cuterebra*. Chronic or recurrent draining abscesses should be evaluated by radiography for underlying osteomyelitis, by cytology and culture for possible fungal infection, or by surgical exploration for the presence of a foreign body or parasite.

THERAPY

Abscesses vary in severity and in the extent of therapeutic intervention required. Small localized abscesses that drain spontaneously by the time animals are presented for examination require that the hair around the wound be clipped and the wound cleaned with hydrogen peroxide or dilute iodophor solutions. More extensive infections that cause signs of systemic illness may require antibiotic administration, surgical drainage, or supportive care.

Antibiotic Therapy

This has a decided but not absolute role in the management of abscesses in cats. Although mortality and complications due to abscesses have been reduced with the use of antibacterials, these agents should not be used indiscriminantly or in the absence of other adjunctive measures. Antibiotics alone

are ineffective in penetrating walled-off abscesses that require drainage. Empiric antibiotic therapy should be discontinued and extensive diagnostic investigation initiated if abscesses or fever persists longer than 1 to 2 weeks or recur following repeated surgical drainage.

Penicillin derivatives are antibiotics of choice for treating abscesses because they are bactericidal and have marked activity against the more frequently encountered organisms (Table 55–2). Penicillin V, amoxicillin, or ampicillin may be dispensed in oral forms to be administered by the client. However, amoxicillin or ampicillin may not always be as effective as penicillin in treating anaerobic infections. Because of similar antibacterial spectrum, chloramphenicol can be substituted for penicillin, but it is bacteriostatic and frequently causes anorexia. If anaerobes are suspected, penicillin, second or third generation cephalosporins, chloramphenicol, clindamycin, and metronidazole have the greatest efficacy. Certain *Fusobacterium* also have been susceptible to erythromycin and doxycycline (see also Therapy, Chapter 49).[9] L-forms are susceptible to tetracycline (see L-Form Infections, Chapter 50). *Rhodococcus* has been primarily susceptible to aminoglycosides, chloramphenicol, and erythromycin (see also Rhodococcal Infections, Chapter 56).[6] Topical application or direct instillation of antibiotics into the abscess cavity is ineffective because, with the exception of nitrofurans, none work in the presence of pus. Hydrogen peroxide or chlorhexidine solutions and nitrofurazone powder or solution are empirically placed in surgically opened abscess cavities without documented efficacy. Systemic antibiotic therapy may be beneficial in minimizing abscess formation when given immediately following bite wound contamination or with diffuse cellulitis (see also Bite Infections, Chapter 58). Within 24 hours of injury, a single injection of procaine penicillin G can thwart the development of an abscess.[10]

Surgery

Surgical intervention is reserved for mature or ruptured abscesses. Diffuse cellulitis or early abscesses should be allowed to mature before surgical drainage is performed. Daily application of warm compresses or

Table 55–1. Bacteria Isolated from Feline Abscesses[a]

GENUS	SPECIES	PERCENT[b]
Anaerobes		
Bacteroides	tectum, heparinolyticus, gingivalis, salivosus, melaninogenicus, corrodens, fragilis, others	27–45
Fusobacterium	nucleatum, necrophorum, russii, others	19–64
Peptostreptococcus	anaerobius	11–45
Clostridium	perfringens, novyi, sordellii, septicum, chauvoei, tetani, villosum	6.5
Propionibacterium	acnes, freudenreichii	4.2
Bifidobacterium	spp.	1.2
Lactobacillus	spp.	1.2
Eubacterium	lentum	0.6
Aerobes/Facultative		
Pasteurella	multocida[c]	13–27
Actinomyces	viscosus, odontolyticus	7–18
Nocardia	spp.	
Rhodococcus	equi	27
Streptococcus	spp.	4.8
Lactobacillus	spp.	1.8
Escherichia	coli	0.6

[a]Summarized from data.[1–8, 8a–8c].

[b]Percentage of those isolates cultured from feline abscesses.[9]

[c]Has been reclassified, see Etiology, Chapter 58.

soaking affected extremities in warm, saturated epsom salt solutions may hasten the maturation process and has been beneficial in keeping already established drainage sites open until proper healing can occur. Surgical therapy usually involves creating drainage openings at the most ventral portion of an abscess cavity. Controversy exists as to the degree and type of surgical closure indicated. Most veterinarians debride the abscess cavity and remove a small portion of overlying skin to prevent premature closure. Placement of soft rubber tubing that exits at the lowest point of incision with partial closure is frequently used to maintain a drainage opening. A few veterinarians, advocating complete primary closure of the abscess cavity following extensive debridement, argue that more rapid healing and less postoperative drainage is achieved with that

method.[11] Systemic antibiotic therapy is probably essential whenever partial or complete surgical closure is performed because the likelihood of organisms remaining in the wound is high, and the risk of systemic spread increases.

Surgical drainage must be established whenever abscess formation occurs within closed cavities. Retrobulbar abscesses must be drained by passing a probe from immediately behind the last upper molar upward into the retrobulbar space. Infraorbital abscesses are usually associated with infection of the upper carnassial tooth, which must be extracted. Sinusal, nasal, and chronic middle ear abscesses also require surgical drainage with debridement of bone because of the loculation of pus within cavities surrounded by bone. Abscesses associated with underlying osteomyelitis must be treated by

Table 55–2. Drug Therapy for Feline Abscesses[a]

DRUG	DOSE[b] (mg/kg)	ROUTE	INTERVAL (hours)	DURATION (days)
Penicillin G	30,000–50,000 U/kg	SC, IM, IV	12	5–7
Penicillin V	20	PO	12	5–7
Amp(amox)icillin	20	PO, SC, IV	8–12	5–7
Chloramphenicol	15	PO, SC, IV	8	5–7
Clindamycin	10	PO, IM	12	5–7
Metronidazole	10	PO, IV	8–12	5–7
Doxycycline	5	PO, IV	12	5–7

[a]See also Drug Therapy for Anaerobic Infections, Table 49–5, and Rhodococcal Infections, Table 56–5. SC = subcutaneous, IM = intramuscular, IV = intravenous, PO = oral.

[b]Dose per administration at specified interval, expressed as mg/kg unless otherwise stated.

surgical debridement of infected bone. Foreign bodies or material must be removed from abscess cavities before they will heal.

Castration is recommended as a preventative measure to abscess formation because it reduces the fighting and roaming behavior of male cats. Progestagens can be used similarly to modify behavior, but the necessity of their continued use induces many undesirable side effects.

References

1. Love DN, Jones RF, Bailey M, et al: Isolation and characterization of bacteria from abscesses in the subcutis of cats. *J Med Microbiol* 12:207–212, 1979.
2. Dobbinson SS, Tannock GW: A bacteriological investigation of subcutaneous abscesses in cats. *N Z Vet J* 33:27–29, 1985.
3. Berg JN, Fales WH, Scanlan CM: Occurrence of anaerobic bacteria in diseases of the dog and cat. *Am J Vet Res* 40:876–881, 1979.
4. Kanoe M, Kido M, Toda M: Obligate anaerobic bacteria found in canine and feline purulent lesions. *Br Vet J* 140:257–262, 1984.
5. Jang SS, Lock A, Biberstein EL: A cat with *Corynebacterium equi* lymphadenitis clinically simulating lymphosarcoma. *Cornell Vet* 65:232–239, 1975.
6. Elliott G, MacKenzie CP, Lawson GHK: *Rhodococcus equi* infection in cats. *Vet Rec* 118:693–694, 1986.
7. Biberstein EL, Knight HD, England K: *Bacteroides melaninogenicus* in diseases of domestic animals. *J Am Vet Med Assoc* 153:1045–1049, 1968.
8. Love DN, Jones FR, Bailey M: Characteristics of *Bacteroides* species isolated from soft tissue infections of cats. *J Appl Bacteriol* 50:567–575, 1981.
8a. Love DN, Jones RF, Bailey M, et al: Bacteria isolated from subcutaneous abscesses in cats. *Aust Vet Pract* 8:87–90, 1978.
8b. Love DN, Bailey M, Johnson RS: Antimicrobial susceptibility patterns of obligatory anaerobic bacteria from subcutaneous abscesses and pyothorax in cats. *Aust Vet Pract* 10:168–170, 1980.
8c. Love DN, Johnson JL, Moore LVH: *Bacteroides* species from the oral cavity and oral-associated diseases of cats. *Vet Microbiol* 19:275–281, 1989.
9. Love DN, Jones RF, Bailey M: Characterization of *Fusobacterium* species isolated from soft tissue infections. *J Appl Bacteriol* 48:325–331, 1980.
10. Joshua JO: Abscesses and their sequelae in cats. Part 1. *Feline Pract* 1:9–12, 1971.
11. Cat abscesses and suturing controversy. *Feline Pract* 2:22–28, 1972.

56

STREPTOCOCCAL AND OTHER GRAM-POSITIVE BACTERIAL INFECTIONS

Streptococci are gram-positive nonmotile, facultatively anaerobic cocci that cause localized to widespread pyogenic infections in animals and people. While certain disease-producing strains exist, many species are commensal microflora of the oral cavity, nasopharynx, skin, and genital and GI tracts. Strain differences of streptococci are responsible for the varying host ranges and degrees of pathogenicity. Several classification systems exist for streptococci, based on cultural characteristics, antigenic composition, and biochemical features. The classification by Lancefield[1] based on antigenic differences in cell wall carbohydrates will be used below to distinguish the groups. The action upon erythrocytes in culture medium has also been used to distinguish the different groups of streptococci. β Hemolysis is characterized by complete lysis of erythrocytes and clearing around the colonies. α Hemolysis is characterized by a greenish-colored zone and intact erythrocytes in the discolored region. γ-(Non)hemolytic organisms produce no hemolytic zone. Lancefield's groups A, B, C, E, G, L, and M are usually β hemolytic. Group D is usually α hemolytic or sometimes nonhemolytic. β-Hemolytic strains tend to be more pathogenic. Organisms in the nonhemolytic group are found on mucous membranes and skin of clinically healthy animals. If present in an infectious process, they are usually regarded as contaminants or secondary invaders.

Rhodococcus equi (previously *Corynebacterium equi*) is a soilborne, pleomorphic, gram-positive bacillus that has been primarily associated with suppurative infections in domestic livestock. Reports of infections in cats are increasing.

Listeriosis and anthrax are less commonly occurring infections of dogs and cats. When they occur, they are typically associated with exposure to domestic farm animals or their by-products.

Group A Streptococcal Infections of Dogs and Cats

Craig E. Greene

People are the principal natural reservoir hosts of group A streptococci, and most human infections are caused by this group. Dermatitis, pharyngitis, scarlet fever, and rheumatic fever are the main syndromes caused by *Streptococcus pyogenes* (Table 56–1). Rarely these organisms produce perianal cellulitis, vaginitis, or localized abscesses. *S. pneumoniae* (formerly *Diplococcus pneumoniae*) can produce pneumonia, bacteremia, otitis media, endocarditis, and meningitis. Of all the streptococcal groups, group A organisms have the greatest virulence for human adults, while organisms of the other groups, such as B, C, D, F, and G, cause the most severe manifestations in neonates. The primary discussion below centers around *S. pyogenes*, although the many fea-

Table 56–1. Summary of Streptococcal Infections of People, Dogs, and Cats[a]

STREPTOCOCCAL SPECIES	HOST SPECIES	MICROFLORAL DISTRIBUTION	DISEASE SYNDROME(S)
Group A			
S. pyogenes	H	Tonsils	Tonsillitis, pharyngitis, otitis, impetigo, bacteremia, toxemia[2,3]
	B	None (human reservoir)	Nonsymptomatic
S. pneumoniae	H	Tonsils	Pneumonia, otitis, bacteremia, polyarthritis, meningitis
	C	None (human reservoir)	Polyarthritis, bacteremia[4]
Group B			
S. agalactiae	H	Anorectum, vagina	Neonate: sepsis[5,6] Immunosuppressed: bacteremia, meningitis, endocarditis[7–9] Postparturient: metritis; septic arthritis; pharyngitis; respiratory, skin, and wound infections
	D	Urogenital	Fatal septicemia in pups, necrotizing pneumonia, bacteremia, pyelonephritis[10,11]
	C	Urogenital	Peritonitis, septicemia, placentitis[12]
Group C			
S. zooepidemicus and S. equisimilis	D	Skin, genitourinary tract	Septicemia, fibrinopurulent bronchopneumonia, acute death,[13,14] urinary tract infections[30a]
	H	None (animal reservoir)	Pharyngitis, glomerulonephritis[15,16]
Group G			
S. canis	H	Tonsils, vagina	Pharyngitis[17–19]
	C		Abscesses, neonatal sepsis, umbilical infections[20–23]
	D	Tonsils, anorectum,[24] genitalia	Otitis media, neonatal sepsis (fading puppy?), umbilical infections, polyarthritis, abscesses, dermatitis, mastitis,[10, 25–28] genital infections:[b] infertility, anestrus, abortion, failure to conceive[30a]
Group L	D	Genitalia	Abortion, fading puppy, sterility in bitch, endometritis[2, 29, 30]
Group M	D	Tonsils[29]	Nonsymptomatic colonization
Group D			
S. faecalis[c] (enterococci)	D,H	Intestine, feces[25]	Nonsymptomatic colonization, urinary tract infections[30a]
Group E	D	Skin, upper respiratory tract[25]	Nonsymptomatic colonization found as mixed flora in mucosal inflammation

[a]H = human, B = dog and cat, C = cat, D = dog.
[b]See Chapter 11.
[c]Also includes S. faecium, S. zymogenes, S. durans; see Group D Streptococcal Overgrowth, Chapter 9.

tures of S. pneumoniae are similar. A report of bacteremia and septic arthritis in a cat attributed the infection to transmission of S. pneumoniae from a human infant in the same household.[4]

The sites of greatest carriage of group A streptococci in people are the caudal aspects of the pharynx and tonsillar region. Group A streptococci can survive extremes in environmental temperature and humidity; however, most infections are associated with direct or close contact between susceptible individuals (Fig. 56–1). Some individuals can harbor the infection for extended periods in the absence of clinical illness. Prevalence rates for group A streptococci are

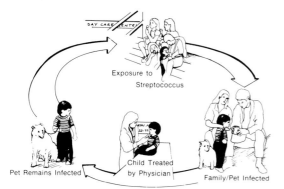

Figure 56–1. Zoonotic aspects of group A streptococcal infection in pets. Children usually acquire infection at school. When the child is treated, reinfection may result if the household pet has acquired infection and is not simultaneously treated. Treatment of additional family contacts is as important in breaking the cycle.

higher in young children, especially those in day-care or classroom situations. The prevalence of positive throat cultures in such circumstances may approach 50% even in the absence of an obvious epidemic. Symptomatic rather than carrier children are most likely to bring infection into the home, and under such circumstances, the isolation rate in other humans in the household approaches 25% to 50%.[31] If the child is nonsymptomatic, the rate is only 9%.[32] Dogs and cats have been suggested as possible sources of reinfection under such circumstances.[32a,32b]

Whenever streptococcal typing has been performed on the oral-pharyngeal region of dogs and cats, groups G, C, L, and M have been present in decreasing frequency.[25,33,34] However, screening for group A streptococcal colonization of the tonsils of dogs and cats from random households in urban environments has shown the prevalence to be 1% to 10%.[35–38] In one study in which recurrent group A streptococcal pharyngitis occurred in people, the prevalence for households was 42% for dogs and 36% for cats.[37] Bacitracin susceptibility was used to distinguish group A from non–group A strains in this study, so the percentages may be inordinately high. With immunologic typing to distinguish between strains, the prevalence of infection would be lower but would still indicate a difference between problem-affected and random unaffected households.

Domestic pets that come into close contact with infected individuals can develop pharyngeal colonization with group A streptococci. Infected pets show no clinical illness or tonsillar enlargement. Since clinical symptomatology is absent in these animals, their presumed danger would be as public health risks. If they were overlooked during treatment, they might serve as a reservoir for reinfection of family members. Pets, however, usually lose their infection within 2 to 3 weeks after they are removed from the household. It is foolish to consider culturing and treating the dog and cat in a household where reinfection occurs without doing so for the human contacts whose infection is undoubtedly more persistent.

The recovery of group A streptococci is affected by the method used in swabbing the throat, since collection of and overgrowth by indigenous microflora can result in the death of group A streptococci. Sedation may be needed, since sterile cotton or Dacron swabs should be rubbed over the surface of the exposed tonsils in their crypts. Swabs that will be unrefrigerated during transport should be kept dry; otherwise overgrowth by contaminating microflora will occur.

Latex agglutination tests are available to pediatricians for rapid detection of group A streptococci in children. Their accuracy in detection of group A infections in dogs and cats is uncertain.

The antimicrobial spectrum for group A streptococcal infection in pets is the same as for human strains. It is judicious to treat pets when they may be a source of recurrent infection of household members. Isolates of

Table 56–2. Drug Therapy for Streptococcal Infections in Dogs and Cats[a]

DRUG	SPECIES	DOSE[b] (mg/kg)	ROUTE	INTERVAL (hours)	DURATION (days)
Penicillin G	B	10,000–20,000 U/kg	IM, SC	12–24	5–7
Penicillin V	B	8–30	PO	8	5–7
Erythromycin	D	3–20	PO	12–24	5–7
Chloramphenicol	D	15–25	PO, IV, SC	8	5–7
	C	10–15	PO, IV, SC	12	5–7
Cephalexin	B	10–40	PO	12	5–7

[a]B = dog and cat, D = dog, C = cat, IM = intramuscular, SC = subcutaneous, PO = oral, IV = intravenous.
[b]Dose per administration at specified interval, expressed as mg/kg unless otherwise stated.

group A streptococci from dogs have shown the greatest susceptibility to penicillin, erythromycin, and chloramphenicol.[35] Recommended total daily dosages are listed in Table 56–2. Resistant strains can be treated with cephalosporins.

Group B Streptococcal Infections of Dogs and Cats   Craig E. Greene

In people, group B streptococci have been associated with neonatal septicemia and postpartum metritis. Skin, pharyngeal, and wound infections can occur. Immunosuppressed individuals can develop disease in many tissues (see Table 56–1). Group B streptococci are more frequently isolated than group G from people with these syndromes. Again, factors at the time of delivery, such as low birthweight or difficult delivery, precipitate the development of clinical illness.

Group B streptococci have been reported to cause septicemia in a dog[11] and endometritis and "fading puppies" that develop bacteremia, pyelonephritis, and necrotizing pneumonia.[10] Group G have been more commonly isolated than group B as causes of neonatal sepsis. Similarly, peritonitis with septicemia and parturient endometritis and placentitis have been described in cats.[12] Whether canine and feline strains are indigenous or of human or other animal origin is uncertain. Therapy is similar to that for group A streptococcal infections (Table 56–2).

Group C Streptococcal Infections of Dogs and Cats   Craig E. Greene

Group C infections have been described only in dogs, although both species have been reported to have these organisms as commensal flora in lower frequency than group G. Acute hemorrhagic and purulent pneumonia has been described to occur primarily in racing greyhounds.[13,14] Weakness, coughing, dyspnea, fever, hematemesis, and red urine have been the predominant clinical signs. Many of the dogs develop septicemia and some die suddenly without signs of clinical illness. Gross lesions at necropsy of fatally affected animals consist of widespread petechial and ecchymotic hemorrhages and pulmonary congestion with mediastinal and free pleural hemorrhage. Microscopically, streptococci are found in clusters intracellularly throughout the lung parenchyma and in the spleen. Injections of the organism into mice have produced abscesses and death, and pure cultures of the organism can be isolated. A commercially available group A and C latex agglutination reagent (PathoDx Kit, Diagnostic Products Corp, Los Angeles, CA) has been accurate in detecting group C streptococci in swabs of clinical specimens from animals.[38a] However, sensitivity and specificity of the test were highest for those streptococci in swabs of equine specimens. Treatment, if given early enough, or prophylaxis in exposed animals may be beneficial. Drugs and dosages recommended are similar to those for group A infections (Table 56–2).

Group G Streptococcal Infections of Cats

Patricia Carey Blanchard
Dennis W. Wilson

ETIOLOGY AND PATHOGENESIS

β-Hemolytic streptococci are commensal microflora of the skin, pharynx, and upper respiratory and genital tracts of cats. The majority of β-hemolytic streptococcal infections in cats are caused by Lancefield group G streptococci (*S. canis*) (see Table 56–1). Whether more virulent disease-producing strains of this organism exist is uncertain. For neonatal kittens, the source of streptococci is the vagina of the queen. Streptococci gain entrance via the umbilical vein and can spread by direct extension into the peritoneal cavity or through the ductus venosus and portal circulation of the liver, resulting in bacteremia.[39] Cervical lymphadenitis caused by this organism in juvenile kittens (3 to 7 months old) follows a subclinical episode of pharyngitis and tonsillitis.[18] Other group G infections that affect cats are often opportunistic and follow wounds, trauma, surgical procedures, viral infections, or immunosuppressive conditions.[40] These suppurative infections can result in septicemia and embolic lesions, most often in the lung and heart.

Infections in juvenile and older cats are sporadic; litters of neonates are most affected. Most kittens affected with the disease are in the first litter of queens less than 2 years of age. More than one kitten in a litter may be affected. Occasional outbreaks of neonatal infections with high mortality can occur in breeding catteries, especially following the introduction of group G streptococci into a naive cattery.

The prevalence of infection is low in kittens born to older or multiparous queens for several reasons. Young queens carry higher numbers of organisms in the vagina and the carrier state persists throughout pregnancy, whereas older, multiparous queens eliminate the carrier state by midgestation.[41] Approximately 50% of female pet cats less than 2 years of age and 70% to 100% of similarly aged queens in breeding catteries may carry group G streptococci in the vagina.[42] Queens in endemically affected catteries can develop protective levels of antibodies by 8 months of age. Kittens receive levels of antibodies equivalent to those of the dam via the colostrum.

Group G streptococci[43] also can be found in the tonsils and pharynx.[43] The tom can carry the organism in the prepuce. Age, exposure, and immune responses are all important in determining whether this commensal organism causes illness.

CLINICAL FINDINGS

The clinical signs vary with the site of infection and host immunocompetence. Sites of streptococcal infections in cats are listed in Table 56–3.[44] Cats are febrile and anorexic with swelling and purulent exudate at the site of infection. Cervical lymphadenitis occurs as a unilateral or bilateral swelling in the ventral cervical lymph nodes (Fig. 56–2).[44a] Although cats of any age may develop streptococcal infections, most cases involve neonatal kittens (<2 weeks of age). Most infected kittens gain less weight than littermates, and occasionally an affected kitten has a swollen, infected umbilicus. Death usually occurs by 7 to 11 days of age, but kittens born to queens with minimal prior exposure may die suddenly at less than 3 days of age with overwhelming sepsis. In kittens with septicemia, the febrile response is transient, occurs within 24 hours prior to death, and frequently goes undetected.

Table 56–3. Anatomic Distribution of β-Hemolytic Streptococcal Isolates[a] from Lesions in Cats[b]

SOURCE	NUMBER OF ISOLATES	NUMBER OF PURE ISOLATES[c]
Integumentary	57	23
Respiratory	38	11
Genital (female)	28	12
Urinary	17	4
Serous cavities	22	9
Neonatal sepsis	12	6
Other[d]	34	13
Total	208	78

[a]34 of 38 isolates tested were Lancefield group G–positive.

[b]Data compiled from cases in a 17-year period presented to the Veterinary Medical Teaching Hospital, University of California, Davis.

[c]Number of times isolated in pure culture (only organism isolated).

[d]Other sites include oral cavity, lymph node, CNS, eye, ear, joint, or mammary gland.

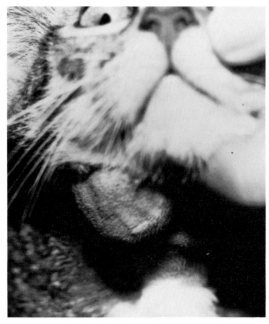

Figure 56–2. Unilateral *Streptococcus canis* cervical lymphadenitis in a 4-month-old kitten. (From Timoney et al [eds]: *Hagan and Bruner's Microbiology and Infectious Diseases of Domestic Animals*, ed 8. Ithaca, NY, Cornell University Press, 1988, with permission.)

DIAGNOSIS AND PATHOLOGIC FINDINGS

The leukogram shows a typical neutrophilic inflammatory response with a left shift. Neonatal kittens (<2 weeks of age) usually have a degenerative left shift in their leukogram due to their limited bone marrow storage pool.[42] With overwhelming sepsis, cocci may be found in the cytoplasm of circulating neutrophils.

Gram staining of exudates from affected tissues reveals single and chains of gram-positive cocci. Confirmation is based on bacteriologic culture of the affected tissues. Aerobic culture of exudates or needle aspirates of enlarged lymph nodes yields β-hemolytic, gram-positive cocci on sheep and bovine blood agar plates. In fatally affected neonates, the organism is found most consistently in the liver, lung, umbilicus, and peritoneal cavity (Fig. 56–3).

Necropsy findings in affected neonatal kittens with septicemia include omphalophlebitis, peritonitis, and, less frequently, embolic hepatitis, pneumonia, and myocarditis.[39] Untreated cases of cervical lymphadenitis in juvenile cats can progress to pleuritis, embolic myocarditis, and embolic pneumonia with secondary pulmonary infarction.[44]

Older cats are less susceptible to systemic spread of streptococci.

THERAPY AND PREVENTION

Group G streptococci are very sensitive to penicillin and its derivatives. Juvenile and older cats with lymphadenitis should be treated immediately with oral or parenteral therapy (see Table 56–4). Draining and flushing the abscesses hasten recovery. These cats should be examined for predisposing conditions such as feline leukemia, infectious peritonitis, immunodeficiency, respiratory viral infections, feline urologic syndrome, or wounds.

For prevention of infection in newborn kittens, dipping the navel and umbilical cord in 2% tincture of iodine and treatment of all kittens at birth with ampicillin, amoxicillin, or with procaine and benzathine penicillin combined have been successful. A much higher dosage of procaine and benzathine penicillin combined should be given immediately to the queen of an infected litter or as a single preventative dose at parturition. Although the population of group G streptococci can be temporarily suppressed by antimicrobial therapy, the carrier state cannot be eliminated.

Treatment of infected juvenile or adult cats with lymphadenitis or arthritis can be accomplished with parenteral or oral therapy (Table 56–4). Dosages are higher than normally recommended because the organ-

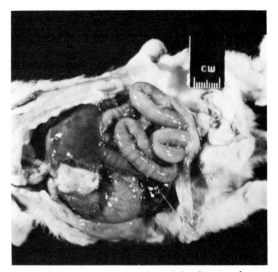

Figure 56–3. Peritonitis and umbilical vein abscess with extension into the liver in a 7-day-old kitten.

Table 56–4. Therapy for Group G Streptococcal Infections in Cats[a]

DRUG	AGE	DOSE[b] (mg/kg)	ROUTE	INTERVAL (hours)	DURATION (days)
Prevention at Parturition					
Amp(amox)icillin	N	25	PO, SC	8	5–7
Procaine and benzathine penicillin	N	6250 IU[c]	SC	48–72	3–5[d]
	Q	150,000 IU[c]	SC	48–72	3–5[d]
Infected (Lymphadenitis or Arthritis)					
Procaine and benzathine penicillin	J,A	75,000–150,000 IU[c]	SC	48–72	3–5[d]
Procaine penicillin	J,A	50,000 IU[c]	SC	24	5
Penicillin V	J,A	20	PO	8	5

[a] N = neonates, Q = queens, J = juveniles, A = adults, IU = international units, PO = oral, SC = subcutaneous.
[b] Dose per administration at specified interval, expressed as mg/kg unless otherwise stated.
[c] Total dose needed for each drug in a fixed combination, based on a 2–3-kg cat.
[d] Only one or two doses usually given during this treatment regimen.

ism can be harbored in the tonsillar crypts and a considerable amount of pus forms in the abscess. Parenteral therapy can be instituted in the veterinarian's office and medication can be dispensed for subsequent oral administration.

PUBLIC HEALTH CONSIDERATIONS

Group G streptococci have received increasing attention as a cause of pharyngitis, tonsillitis, wound infections, cellulitis, neonatal and puerperal septicemia, and endocarditis in people. *Streptococcus canis* is the proposed official name for group G β-hemolytic streptococci of animal origin.[45] The information from biotyping and DNA hybridization studies of animal and human group G streptococci indicates that they are not identical and thus probably do not have a high zoonotic potential.[46]

Group G Streptococcal Infections of Dogs
Craig E. Greene

Group G streptococci are normal inhabitants of the skin, oropharynx, GI tract, and female genital tract of people. Nonsymptomatic pharyngeal carriage of group G streptococci is found in up to 23% of people.[47] The organisms commonly colonize human skin and approximately 5% of nonsymptomatic puerperal women harbor them on the genital mucosa.[47] Group G streptococcal infections in people involve primarily dermatitis and pharyngitis; however, septicemia, endocarditis, peritonitis, and septic arthritis have been reported.

Group G are the major streptococcal type isolated as commensal flora from the skin and mucosa of dogs.[25] Historically, the veterinary literature contains numerous reports of diseases caused by these organisms, including abortion, infertility, and neonatal death. In addition, cellulitis, mastitis, pharyngitis, tonsillitis, and genital infections have been described (Table 56–1). Some of these claims of disease-producing isolates should be evaluated with suspicion because of the frequency with which these organisms are isolated from clinically healthy animals.

Isolation of the organism from the vagina and tonsils of healthy pregnant bitches with production of neonatal death in puppies is thought to result from various factors other than the virulence of the organism. The neonatal puppy becomes contaminated at birth, and stress, lack of warmth, improper navel disinfection, and lack of nursing may increase the susceptibility of puppies to infection. Treatment is similar to that for group A streptococcal infections (Table 56–2).

Other Streptococcal Infections of Dogs

Craig E. Greene

Group L streptococci have been similarly associated with syndromes that parallel those of group G streptococci, although their frequency of isolation from normal and diseased dogs has been low (see Table 56–1). Groups M and E have been found as normal microflora of dogs, although they are isolated with very low frequency from the oral, uro-genital, and respiratory mucosa. Group D streptococci or enterococci are considered normal GI flora of dogs.[25] Group D streptococci have been found responsible for diarrhea in puppies (see Group D Streptococcal Overgrowth, Chapter 9) and are often found in urinary tract infections of dogs.[30a]

Rhodococcus equi *Infection of Cats*

Craig E. Greene

ETIOLOGY

R. equi commonly produces purulent pneumonia in foals, suppurative lymphadenitis in pigs, and granulomatous lymphadenitis in cows. R. equi has also been isolated from lesions in dogs,[48] but abscesses in cats have been most commonly reported.[48–52] R. equi, a saprophyte, can commonly be recovered from soil and from feces of grazing horses and ruminants. The organism may enter the body by a penetrating wound contaminated from the environment and subsequently spread via lymphatics to regional lymph nodes and via the blood to the liver, spleen, and visceral lymph nodes. Underlying immunosuppression may be responsible for this hematogenous dissemination.

CLINICAL FINDINGS

Pyogranulomatous lesions are the characteristic finding and most cats have had primary involvement of an extremity. Localized swelling with ulceration or fistulas and pu-rulent drainage have been found. Pyothorax from mediastinal lymphadenitis is manifest by anorexia, weight loss, and dyspnea. Abdominal distention with a palpable fluid wave, hepatomegaly, and mesenteric lymphadenopathy may be found.

DIAGNOSIS

Hematologic abnormalities may consist of leukocytosis with a left shift. Gram staining of the purulent discharge will show pleomorphic, large, gram-positive bacilli, which may be found intracellularly in macrophages. Thoracic or abdominal effusions are typically exudates with high protein (>3.5 g/dl) and nucleated cell counts (>10,000 cells/μl), with a majority of cells being lymphocytes or nondegenerate neutrophils. Organisms may not be apparent.

PATHOLOGIC FINDINGS

Peripheral abscesses often have many sinus tracts with purulent drainage. Lymph

Table 56–5. Drug Therapy for Rhodococcus equi *Infection in Cats*[a]

DRUG	DOSE[b] (mg/kg)	ROUTE	INTERVAL (hours)	DURATION (days)
Gentamicin	2	SC	12	5[c]
Lincomycin	20	PO	12	7–10[c]
Erythromycin	10	PO	8	14

[a]SC = subcutaneous, PO = oral.
[b]Dose per administration at specified interval, expressed as mg/kg unless otherwise stated.
[c]A second course of therapy may be used with a 1-week interval between courses.

nodes may be enlarged and necrotic with a similar discharge on sectioning. Histologically, the lesions have been pyogranulomatous or granulomatous with necrotic foci. Macrophages contain phagocytized gram-positive bacteria.

THERAPY

Surgical removal of the extremity lesions is only temporarily effective, and they commonly return even after limb amputation. Lincomycin and gentamicin have been most effective,[50] and results with erythromycin have been variable (Table 56–5).[49,52] A poor response has been seen in cats treated with penicillin and streptomycin and in cats whose lesions have become disseminated to many organs.

Listeriosis

Craig E. Greene

Listeria monocytogenes is a pathogenic, β-hemolytic, gram-positive, facultative anaerobe that is morphologically indistinguishable from diphtheroids and may be mistaken for a contaminant in tissues. It is capable of growing over a wide temperature range. Although at least 16 serotypes of the organism exist, most infections are caused by only a few serotypes. As a ubiquitous saprophyte, L. monocytogenes can be isolated from soil, water, sewage, dust, and decaying vegetation. Commonly, it can be found in farm animal feed and silage.[53]

L. monocytogenes differs from nonpathogenic species in that it possesses a hemolytic toxin, a factor that has been implicated in its virulence. It is also able to persist as a facultative intracellular organism indefinitely in macrophages and to escape humoral immune responses. Underlying host immunosuppression, especially of cell-mediated immunity, appears to be an important factor in the intracellular persistence of the organism and in the development of clinical listeriosis.

Natural infection usually results from ingestion of contaminated foodstuffs; damage to the intestinal mucosal integrity is not necessary. Foodborne epidemics are associated with ingestion of contaminated feed or silage by domestic herbivores or of contaminated meat and dairy products by people. Listeria in dogs and cats is uncommon; when it occurs it is usually associated with ingestion of contaminated meat or meat by-products. Pathogenic strains of L. monocytogenes can be recovered from the GI tract of non-symptomatic animals.[54] Exposure in itself does not always produce disease.

Following penetration of the intestinal mucosa, L. monocytogenes produces a blood-borne bacteremia, localization in mononuclear phagocyte tissues, and septic embolization of many organs including the CNS.

Reports of septicemic listeriosis in dogs and cats following oral ingestion of contaminated foodstuffs have been rare.[55,56] Clinical signs depend on the degree of intestinal inflammation and sites of embolic microabscess formation. Fever, diarrhea, and vomiting have been most frequent. Neurologic signs have been apparent in some cases. Abortion was suspected in one bitch.[57] Localized infections have also been infrequently reported. Peritonitis was reported in one cat as a result of a plant awn migrating through the bowel into the peritoneal cavity.[54] Another cat developed an abscess of the front paw 2 weeks after an insect bite at the same location.[58]

In the case of CNS infection, the organism may be recognized premortem with gram-stained sediment of CSF. Organisms appear as short intra- and extracellular gram-positive bacilli to coccobacilli. Diagnosis of infection has usually been made at necropsy, because infected animals often succumb to the septicemia. Microabscess formation may be grossly or microscopically visible. In the absence of contaminating organisms, L. monocytogenes can grow and be identified within 36 hours on routine media at incubation temperatures. Laboratory cultivation of the organism from a nonsterile site is difficult unless special precautions are taken. Selective media and cold cultivation (4°C) have been used to isolate the organism, but weeks of cold enrichment are needed owing to the slow growth at these temperatures. Since the organism can be commonly isolated from the GI tract of nonsymptomatic animals,[59] rectal cultures may not be meaningful.

Antimicrobial agents effective against *Listeria* are penicillin and ampicillin, erythromycin, chloramphenicol, rifampin, tetracyclines, trimethoprim-sulfonamide, and aminoglycosides. Only the latter two are bactericidal, and they are recommended as the first choice for clinical use. Gentamicin and tobramycin have more activity than the other aminoglycosides. Combining gentamicin with ampicillin is considered the most desirable therapy, although high dosages of alternative, widely distributed drugs such as trimethoprim-sulfonamide or rifampin may be needed to reach the CNS or resistant infections.

Listeria in animals has not always been considered a public health risk because animals and people have exposure to the same source of environmental contamination. Nevertheless, human outbreaks have been associated with contact with food-producing animals or their products. Direct transmission from animals has occurred in veterinarians and farm workers through contact of unprotected skin or mucous membranes with infected animal tissues.[60,61] Most infections occur in urban areas, where foodborne contamination is suspected. As a reverse zoonosis, listerial gastroenteritis was suspected in a litter of puppies and a newborn infant that received *Listeria*-infected milk discharged from the child's mother's mammary gland.[62]

Anthrax   *Craig E. Greene*

Bacillus anthracis is a large (1 μm × 3 to 6 μm), gram-positive, spore-forming bacillus that causes anthrax, a soilborne systemic disease of domestic animals. Tropical and subtropical regions of the world have alkaline soils with a high nitrogen content, which allows vegetative growth of spores released into the soil from carcasses of animals that died of anthrax.

Although peracute, fatal infections usually occur in herbivores, carnivores such as the dog and cat are usually infected by ingesting raw meat of contaminated carcasses or animal by-products.

The infection in dogs and cats is usually manifested initially by local inflammation, necrosis, and edema of tissues of the upper GI tract, which are the first to come in contact with the organism. Swelling of the head and neck tissues is usually apparent. Subsequent spread to the local and mesenteric lymph nodes, spleen, and liver usually occurs.

Anthrax is a notifiable disease; however, necropsy of suspected carcasses is not advisable, since resistant aerobic spores are released into the environment. Examination of stained smears of blood from a peripheral vein or of fine-needle aspirates is the most effective and safest means of making a diagnosis.[63] The organisms can be isolated from these samples on routine media, provided materials are fresh.

The organism is very sensitive to penicillin, the treatment of choice if the infection is detected early (see Appendix 14 for dosages). From a public health standpoint, care must be taken in handling infected tissues or carcasses, since the organism can penetrate cuts in the skin, resulting in localized infection with subsequent dissemination.[44a] Infection of people is almost always from infected animals or their by-products.

References

1. Lancefield RC: A serological differentiation of human and other groups of hemolytic streptococci. *J Exp Med* 57:571–595, 1933.
2. Shetty KS: Bacterial flora of the upper respiratory tract of the dog with special reference to streptococci. *Indian Vet J* 29:513–531, 1953.
3. Cone LA, Woodward DR, Schlievert PM, et al: Clinical and bacteriologic observations of a toxic shock-like syndrome due to *Streptococcus pyogenes*. *N Engl J Med* 317:146–149, 1987.
4. Stallings B, Ling GV, Lagenaur LA, et al: Septicemia and septic arthritis caused by *Streptococcus pneumoniae* in a cat: possible transmission from a child. *J Am Vet Med Assoc* 191:703–704, 1987.
5. Dillon HC, Gray G, Pass MA, et al: Anorectal and vaginal carriage of group B streptococci during pregnancy. *J Infect Dis* 145:794–799, 1982.
6. Noya FJ, Rench MA, Metzger TG, et al: Unusual occurrence of an epidemic of type Ib/c group B streptococcal sepsis in a neonatal intensive care unit. *J Infect Dis* 155:1135–1144, 1987.
7. Backes RJ, Wilson WR, Geraci JE: Group B streptococcal infective endocarditis. *Arch Intern Med* 145:693–712, 1985.
8. Lerner PI, Gopalakrishna KV, Wolinsky E, et al:

Group B streptococcus (*S. agalactiae*) bacteremia in adults: analysis of 32 cases and review of the literature. *Medicine* 56:457–473, 1977.

9. Franciosi RA, Kuostman JD, Zimmerman RA: Group B streptococcal neonatal and infant infections. *J Pediatr* 82:707–718, 1973.

10. Davies ME, Skulski G: A study of beta-hemolytic streptococci in the fading puppy in relation to canine virus hepatitis infection in the dam. *Br Vet J* 112:404–410, 1956.

11. Kornblatt AN, Adams RL, Barthold SW, et al: Canine neonatal deaths associated with group B streptococcal septicemia. *J Am Vet Med Assoc* 183:700–701, 1983.

12. Dow SW, Jones RL, Thomas TN, et al: Group B streptococcal infection in cats. *J Am Vet Med Assoc* 190:71–72, 1987.

13. Sundberg JP, Hill D, Wyand DS, et al: *Streptococcus zooepidemicus* as the cause of septicemia in racing greyhounds. *Vet Med Small Anim Clin* 76:839–842, 1981.

14. Wyand DS, Sherman BA: Streptococcal septicemia in racing greyhounds. *J Am Anim Hosp Assoc* 14:399–401, 1978.

15. Skjold SA, Quie PG, Fries LA, et al: DNA fingerprinting of *Streptococcus zooepidemicus* (Lancefield group C) as an aid to epidemiological study. *J Infect Dis* 155:1145–1150, 1987.

16. Barnham M, Thornton TJ, Lange K: Nephritis caused by *Streptococcus zooepidemicus* (Lancefield group C). *Lancet* 1:945–948, 1983.

17. Swindle MM, Narayan O, Luzarrage M, et al: Contagious streptococcal lymphadenitis in cats. *J Am Vet Med Assoc* 177:829–830, 1980.

18. Swindle MM, Narayan O, Luzarraga M, et al: Pathogenesis of contagious streptococcal lymphadenitis in cats. *J Am Vet Med Assoc* 179:1208–1210, 1981.

19. Tillman PC, Dodson ND, Indiveri M: Group G streptococcal epizootic in a closed cat colony. *J Clin Microbiol* 16:1057–1060, 1982.

20. Goldman PM, Moore TD: Spontaneous Lancefield group G streptococcal infection in a random source cat colony. *Lab Anim Sci* 23:565–566, 1973.

21. Wilson D, Blanchard P: Preventing kitten mortality in catteries. *Carnation Res Digest* 22:7–8, 1986.

22. Wilson D, Blanchard P: *Strep canis* bacteria in kittens. *Feline Pract* 16:27, 1986.

23. Reitmeyer JC, Steele JH: The occurrence of β-hemolytic streptococcus in cats. *Southwest Vet* 36:41–42, 1984.

24. DeVriese LA, DePelsmaecker K: The anal region as a main carrier site of *Staphylococcus intermedius* and *Streptococcus canis* in dogs. *Vet Rec* 121:302–303, 1987.

25. Biberstein EL, Brown C, Smith T: Serodiagnosis and biotypes among β-hemolytic streptococci of canine origin. *J Clin Microbiol* 11:558–561, 1980.

26. Minett FA, Ellis AA: Streptococcus infections in dogs. *Vet J* 96:438–449, 1940.

27. Stafseth HJ, Thompson WW, Nev L: Streptococcic infections in dogs. I. "Acid milk," arthritis, and postvaccination abscesses. *J Am Vet Med Assoc* 90:769–781, 1937.

28. Hare T, Fry RM: Preliminary observations of an infection of dogs by beta haemolytic streptococci. *Vet Rec* 50:213–218, 1938.

29. Laughton N: Canine beta hemolytic streptococci. *J Pathol Bacteriol* 60:471–476, 1948.

30. Montovani AR, Restani D, Sciarra D, et al: Streptococcus L infection in the dog. *J Small Anim Pract* 2:185–194, 1961.

30a. Ling GV, Biberstein EL, Hirsh DC: Bacterial pathogens associated with urinary tract infections. *Vet Clin North Am* 9:617–630, 1979.

31. Breese BB, Disney FA: Factors influencing the spread of beta hemolytic streptococci infections within the family group. *Pediatrics* 17:834–838, 1956.

32. James WES, Badger GF, Dingle JH: A study of illness in a group of Cleveland families. XIX. The epidemiology of the acquisition of group A streptococci and of associated illnesses. *N Engl J Med* 262:687–694, 1960.

32a. Greene CE: Zoonotic aspects of group A streptococcal infections in dogs and cats. *J Am Anim Hosp Assoc* 24:218–222, 1988.

32b. Roos K, Lind L, Holm SE: Beta-hemolytic streptococci group A in a cat, as a possible source of repeated tonsillitis in a family. *Lancet* 2:1072, 1988.

33. Thal E, Moberg K: Serological grouping of beta-haemolytic streptococci from animals. *Nord Vet Med* 5:835–846, 1953.

34. Smith JE: The aerobic bacteria of the nose and tonsils of healthy dogs. *J Comp Pathol* 71:428–433, 1961.

35. Kurek C, Rutkowiak B: Dog carriers of *Streptococcus pyogenes* on the mucous membrane of the tonsils. *Epidemiol Rev* 25:234–238, 1971.

36. Crowder HR, Dorn CR, Smith RE: Group A streptococcus in pets and group A streptococcal disease in man. *Int J Zoonoses* 5:45–54, 1978.

37. Cooperman SM: Cherchez le chien—household pets as reservoirs of persistent or recurrent streptococcal sore throats in children. *NY State J Med* 82:1685–1687, 1982.

38. Mayer G, Van Ore S: Recurrent pharyngitis in family of four. *Postgrad Med* 74:277–279, 1982.

38a. Inzana TJ, Iritani B: Rapid detection of group C streptococci from animals by latex agglutination. *J Clin Microbiol* 27:309–312, 1989.

39. Blanchard PC, Wilson DW: Spontaneous *Streptococcus canis* infections of neonatal kittens in a closed cat colony. *Vet Pathol.* In press, 1989.

40. Blanchard PC, Wilson DW: 17 year survey of β-hemolytic streptococcal infections in cats. In preparation.

41. Blanchard PC, Wilson DW: Group G streptococcal infections in kittens. In Kirk RW (ed): *Current Veterinary Therapy X.* Philadelphia, WB Saunders Co, 1989, pp 1091–1093.

42. Blanchard PC: Group G streptococcal infections in kittens: pathogenesis, immunity and maternal carrier state. PhD diss, University of California, Davis, 1987.

43. Blanchard PC: Unpublished observations, University of California, Davis, 1987.

44. Vartian C, Lerner PI, Shlaes DM, et al: Infections due to Lancefield group G streptococci. *Medicine* 64:75–88, 1985.

44a. Timoney JF, Gillespie JH, Scott FW, et al (eds): *Hagan and Bruner's Microbiology and Infectious Diseases of Domestic Animals,* ed 8. Ithaca, NY, Cornell University Press, 1988.

45. Devriese LA, Homme J, Kilpper-Balz R, et al: *Streptococcus canis* sp. nov.: a species of group G streptococci from animals. *Int J Syst Bacteriol* 36:422–425, 1986.

46. Clark RB, Berrafati JF, Janda JM, et al: Biotyping and exoenzyme profiling as an aid in the differentiation of human from bovine group G streptococci. *J Clin Microbiol* 20:706–710, 1984.

47. Rolston KVI: Group G streptococcal infections. *Arch Intern Med* 146:857–858, 1986.
48. Jang SS, Lock A, Biberstein EL: A cat with *Corynebacterium equi* lymphadenitis clinically simulating lymphosarcoma. *Cornell Vet* 65:232–239, 1975.
49. Higgins R, Paradis M: Abscess caused by *Corynebacterium equi* in a cat. *Can Vet J* 21:63–64, 1980.
50. Elliot G, Lawson GH, Mackenzie CP: *Rhodococcus equi* infection in cats. *Vet Rec* 118:693–694, 1986.
51. Barton MD, Hughes KL: Ecology of *Rhodococcus equi*. *Vet Microbiol* 9:65–76, 1984.
52. Oxenford CJ, Ratcliffe RC, Ramsay GC: *Rhodococcus equi* infection in a cat. *Aust Vet J* 64:121, 1987.
53. Fenlon DR: Rapid quantitative assessment of the distribution of *Listeria* in silage implicated in a suspected outbreak of listeriosis in calves. *Vet Rec* 118:240–242, 1986.
54. Turner T: A case of *Listeria monocytogenes* in the cat. *Vet Rec* 74:778, 1962.
55. Decker RA, Rogers JJ, Lesar S: Listeriosis in a young cat. *J Am Vet Med Assoc* 168:1025, 1976.
56. Sholtens RG, Brim A: Isolations of *Listeria monocytogenes* from foxes suspected of having rabies. *J Am Vet Med Assoc* 145:466–469, 1964.
57. Sturgess CP: Listerial abortion in the bitch. *Vet Rec* 124:177, 1989.
58. Jones BR, Cullinane LC, Cary PR: Isolation of *Listeria monocytogenes* from a bite in a cat from the common tree weta (*Hemideina crassidens*). *NZ Vet J* 32:79–80, 1984.
59. Embil JA, Ewan EP, MacDonald SW: Surveillance of *Listeria monocytogenes* in human and environmental specimens in Nova Scotia, 1974 to 1981. *Clin Invest Med* 7:325–327, 1984.
60. Cain DB, McCann VL: An unusual case of listeriosis. *J Clin Microbiol* 23:976–977, 1986.
61. Blenden DC, Kampelmacher EH, Torres-Anjel MJ: Listeriosis. *J Am Vet Med Assoc* 191:1546–1551, 1987.
62. Svabic-Vlahovic M, Pantic D, Pavicic M, et al: Transmission of *Listeria monocytogenes* from mother's milk to her baby and to puppies. *Lancet* 2:1201, 1988.
63. Parry JA, Turnbull PCB, Gibson JR: A colour atlas of *Bacillus* species. London, Wolfe Medical Publications, 1983.

57

STAPHYLOCOCCAL INFECTIONS

Hollis Utah Cox
Johnny D. Hoskins

ETIOLOGY

Staphylococci are spherical, gram-positive, facultatively anaerobic bacteria that are mainly associated with the epidermis and mucous membranes of warm-blooded animals. Most species of staphylococci are potentially pathogenic to people and animals. They display a wide spectrum of virulence, host range, and site specificities, but they are not strictly host or site specific as far as pathogenicity is concerned. Although host-adapted phenotypes occur within some staphylococcal species, transient colonization of a heterologous host may occur when contact between hosts is frequent or infections are present. Transmission is more frequent from people to animals than is the reverse. In addition, staphylococci, which are ubiquitous in nature, are readily acquired from environments (e.g., fomites, soil, air, and water) associated with animals and from a variety of animal products. They survive well in the environment because they are among the more resistant of nonsporulating bacteria to drying and disinfection.

Staphylococci are not inherently invasive and colonize the intact epithelium of healthy animals without causing disease. In this sense, normal animals are subclinical carriers of staphylococci whether they are transient or resident colonizers. Rather, they are opportunistic pathogens, invading epithelium damaged by traumatic insult (e.g., incisions, wounds), other infections (e.g., demodicosis, dermatophytosis), or clinical conditions (e.g., seborrhea, thyroid dysfunction). Therefore, disease results from a disturbance of the natural host-parasite equilibrium. Immuno-compromised hosts are more susceptible to clinical illness as a result of infection.

The pathogenesis of staphylococcal infections, particularly skin disease, is poorly understood. Staphylococcal infections result from the action of virulence factors following tissue invasion. Virulence correlates with a variety of cell envelope components and numerous extracellular toxins and enzymes that produce a wide variety of biological effects on host tissue. With the exception of scalded skin syndrome (epidermolytic toxin), gastroenteritis (enterotoxin), and toxic shock syndrome, no single virulence factor can be consistently implicated in natural clinical infections.

Staphylocoagulase, an enzyme present in most clinically significant staphylococci, polymerizes fibrinogen and clots plasma. Although it is not toxic itself, its presence in a strain correlates with the presence of many other extracellular products or virulence factors. *Staphylococcus aureus*, *S. intermedius*, and some *S. hyicus* produce staphylocoagulase and are generally more pathogenic than *S. epidermidis*, *S. xylosus*, and *S. simulans*, which lack this enzyme. Protein A, an extracellular or cell-bound protein produced by approximately 85% of canine and feline strains of *S. intermedius*, enhances virulence by activating complement and by nonspecifically binding to immunoglobulins. These and other biologic effects provoke various inflammatory and allergic responses, particularly delayed hypersensitivity, that intensify the pyogenic process and heighten the damage produced by staphylococcal infections. Some of these responses may be related to the high concentrations of circulating immune complexes that are found in dogs with recurrent pyoderma and pyo-

611

derma secondary to generalized demodicosis.[1] Complex polysaccharide capsules and slime layers produced by many strains of staphylococci may also enhance virulence by inhibiting or resisting host phagocytosis.

Plasmids, segments of genetic material that are transmissible to other strains of staphylococci and species of bacteria, are found in human strains of S. aureus. They may carry genes for the aforementioned virulence factors and for antimicrobial resistance to penicillin, ampicillin, amoxicillin, lincomycin, erythromycin, tetracycline, chloramphenicol, cephalosporins, kanamycin, and gentamicin. Strains of S. intermedius carry similar plasmids that have not been adequately characterized. Although the antimicrobial susceptibility patterns of clinically important isolates of staphylococci from dogs have not changed considerably in the recent past,[2] the potential exists for transfer of virulent and antimicrobial-resistant strains of S. aureus and S. intermedius between people and animals. Nosocomial transfer is known to modify the staphylococcal flora because nasal carrier rates for coagulase-positive staphylococci increase considerably with prolonged hospitalization of people and dogs.

People are the natural host for S. aureus, which colonizes the nasal passages of up to 40% of healthy adults and rarely other body sites in the absence of dermatosis.[3] Although ecovars adapted to other hosts (e.g., cattle) occur, S. aureus is infrequently isolated from normal dogs and cats and apparently is not indigenous or site-specific in these hosts.[4-6]

The predominant staphylococcal species (40% of isolates) of the resident bacterial microflora of dogs is S. intermedius,[6] which was previously categorized as S. aureus.[7] Specific biotypes can be persistently isolated from the haircoat and mucous membranes of individual dogs for at least 1 year.[6] S. intermedius is not site-specific and, as a percentage of successful isolation, it is most frequently cultured from the prepuce (44%), vagina (34%), mouth (29%), pharynx (28%), haircoat (27%), and anus (24%) and is less frequently isolated from the nares (14%), conjunctiva (12%), and external ear canal (10%).[6] Of 11 coagulase-negative species isolated from normal dogs, S. xylosus is the predominant species (17% of isolates).[6]

The predominant resident staphylococcal species of cats are S. simulans (58%) and S. xylosus (19%).[4,5] S. intermedius and S. au-reus are isolated primarily from the haircoat of household cats and rarely from mucous membranes or from cats confined in a cattery. Apparently, they are transient residents acquired from contact with people or other animals. In general, a less heterogeneous population of staphylococci is associated with cattery cats when compared with household cats or dogs.

CLINICAL FINDINGS

Coagulase-positive staphylococci are the bacteria most frequently isolated from pyogenic infections of dogs and, less commonly, cats.[4,8-10] As significant pathogens, they can affect every organ system independently or concurrently but are most common in abscesses and infections of the skin, eyes, ears, respiratory and genitourinary tracts, skeleton, and joints. In dogs, S. intermedius is the most common staphylococcal species isolated from pyoderma, otitis externa, discospondylitis, bacteremia, and urolithiasis.[8-11] The infection sites are similar for cats; however, S. aureus and S. simulans are isolated more frequently from infections in cats.[4,8,9]

DIAGNOSIS

Staphylococcal infections can be diagnosed presumptively by direct microscopy. Staining of a clinical specimen with Gram stain or rapid cytologic stain will reveal neutrophils and cocci arranged singly or in pairs, short chains, or irregular clusters. For culture, collection methods other than swabbing should be used whenever possible and should be designed to avoid superficial contamination (see Specimen Collection, Chapter 42). Surfaces of intact pustules, furuncles, or abscesses should be gently cleaned with alcohol, and exudate should be directly aspirated or expressed onto a sterile swab without touching the skin (see Diagnosis, Chapter 5). Punch biopsies are suitable procedures for both superficial and deep skin infections. Ear specimens are best obtained with a swab protected by a sterile otoscope cone inserted to the level of the horizontal ear canal. Prior to obtaining blood by venipuncture or urine by cystocentesis for culture, hair should be shaved and the skin scrubbed as for surgery. Respiratory tract specimens should be taken by transtracheal aspiration technique, bronchoscopic wash, or percutaneous transthoracic aspiration to bypass the oral flora. Specimens from deep-seated infections are often taken by direct biopsy or during surgery, such as aspirates or bone fragments curetted in cases of diskospondylitis.

Staphylococci in clinical specimens survive for up to 48 hours when kept cool (4°C [39.2°F]), particularly on commercial swabs containing a holding medium. Clinically significant staphylococci and normal flora contaminants grow best aerobically and may overgrow other pathogens when specimens are cultured on general-purpose nonselective media.

Serologic assays, especially for anti-teichoic acid antibody, are used as a clinical aid in the diagnosis and management of bacteremia, endocarditis, and other deep-seated staphylococcal infections in people; however, their use and interpretation are controversial. None have been adapted for use in animal infections.

THERAPY

Dosages for antimicrobials used to treat staphylococcal infections are listed in Appendix 14 and Table 5–3. Staphylococci are rarely resistant (1% to 4% of isolates) to first-generation cephalosporins (cephalexin, cefadroxil), β-lactamase-resistant synthetic penicillins (oxacillin, dicloxacillin, and clavulanic acid-potentiated amoxicillin), and gentamicin. These should be the drugs of first choice when culture and susceptibility results are unavailable but staphylococcal infection is suspected. Resistance to trimethoprim-potentiated sulfonamides and chloramphenicol is relatively infrequent (6% to 19% of isolates). Resistance to lincomycin, clindamycin, and erythromycin is relatively frequent (20% to 37% of isolates). Clinical isolates of staphylococci from dogs and cats are most frequently resistant (40% to 83%) to penicillin, ampicillin, amoxicillin, and the tetracyclines.[2,9,10,10a] Antimicrobials for which resistance is common should not be used for staphylococcal infections unless an isolate is shown to be susceptible by antimicrobial testing or by lack of β-lactamase production. A history of previous antimicrobial therapy for staphylococcal infection indicates a need to culture regardless of the antimicrobial agent being considered for therapy. Increased resistance of *S. intermedius* to chloramphenicol, clindamycin, and erythromycin has been associated with previous unspecified antimicrobial therapy of canine pyoderma.[11] However, during a 1-year study in which dogs with recurrent folliculitis were treated with repeated courses of cephalexin, antimicrobial susceptibility patterns of *S. intermedius* from lesions and noninfected body sites were unchanged.[12] Clindamycin has been shown to be efficacious in the treatment of experimentally induced *S. aureus* osteomyelitis in dogs.[13]

References

1. DeBoer DJ, Ihrke PJ, Stannard AA: Circulating immune complex concentrations in selected cases of skin disease in dogs. *Am J Vet Res* 49:143–146, 1988.
2. Cox HU, Hoskins JD, Roy AF, et al: Antimicrobial susceptibility of coagulase-positive staphylococci isolated from Louisiana dogs. *Am J Vet Res* 45: 2039–2042, 1984.
3. Kloos WE: Natural populations of the genus *Staphylococcus*. *Annu Rev Microbiol* 34:559–592, 1980.
4. Devriese LA, Nzuambe D, Godard C: Identification and characterization of staphylococci isolated from cats. *Vet Microbiol* 9:279–285, 1984.
5. Cox HU, Hoskins JD, Newman SS, et al: Distribution of staphylococcal species on clinically healthy cats. *Am J Vet Res* 46:1824–1828, 1985.
6. Cox HU, Hoskins JD, Newman SS, et al: Temporal study of staphylococcal species on healthy dogs. *Am J Vet Res* 49:747–751, 1988.
7. Berg JN, Wendell DE, Vogelweid C, et al: Identification of the major coagulase-positive *Staphylococcus* sp. of dogs as *Staphylococcus intermedius*. *Am J Vet Res* 45:1307–1309, 1984.
8. Cox HU, Newman SS, Roy AF, et al: Species of *Staphylococcus* isolated from animal infections. *Cornell Vet* 74:124–135, 1984.
9. Biberstein EL, Jang SS, Hirsh DC: Species distribution of coagulase-positive staphylococci in animals. *J Clin Microbiol* 19:610–615, 1984.
10. Medleau L, Long RE, Brown J, et al: Frequency and antimicrobial susceptibility of *Staphylococcus* species isolated from canine pyodermas. *Am J Vet Res* 47:229–231, 1986.
10a. Medleau L, Blue JL: Frequency and antimicrobial susceptibility of *Staphylococcus* spp. isolated from feline skin lesions. *J Am Vet Med Assoc* 193:1080–1081, 1988.
11. Case LC, Ling GV, Biberstein EL, et al: Staphylococci in canine urolithiasis: species identification using a commercially available tray micromethod. *Am J Vet Res* 46:238–241, 1985.
12. Cox HU: Unpublished observation, Louisiana State University, Baton Rouge, LA, 1988.
13. Bradon TD, Johnson CA, Wakeneil P, et al: Efficacy of clindamycin in the treatment of *Staphylococcus aureus* osteomyelitis in dogs. *J Am Vet Med Assoc* 192:1721–1725, 1988.

58 BITE AND SCRATCH INFECTIONS

Craig E. Greene
Randall Lockwood
Ellie J. C. Goldstein

Dog and Cat Bite Infections

EPIDEMIOLOGY

Although it is estimated that approximately 1 million to 2 million animal bite wounds occur annually, less than half of these are ever reported. Animal bite wounds are fourth among the most commonly reported human illnesses each year in the United States. Bites from family dogs are even more drastically underreported.[1] Nearly 1% of emergency visits of humans to hospitals concern bite injuries.[2] Veterinarians and animal health personnel are at greater risk of being injured by dogs and cats than the general population.[3] Results of a survey of a group of veterinarians in the United States indicated that approximately 65% had sustained a major animal-related injury.[3] Animal bites accounted for 34% and scratches for 3.8% of the trauma. Dogs were involved in 24% and cats in 10% of those injuries. In their careers, 92% of the veterinarians surveyed had sustained dog bites, 81% cat bites, and 72% cat scratches. The following epidemiologic discussion will focus on non–veterinary-related bite injuries for which the veterinarian may be consulted concerning the disposition of the dog or cat responsible for causing the bite, although the information can be applicable to injuries that occur within a veterinary practice setting.

A majority of dog bite injuries occur between April and September, when warm weather is conducive to outdoor activity. Greater than 75% of injuries are in people less than 21 years of age, with peak incidence at 5 to 9 years of age.[4,5,5a] This information may be biased by more frequent attention given to wounds of children as compared with those of adults. Males are more apt to be bitten by dogs than are females, although females are more likely to be bitten by cats.

Dogs account for 80% to 90% of the bites, and cats are responsible for the remaining 10% to 20% of injuries. Other domestic and wild animals account for less than 1% of reported bites. Some dog breeds are more liable to bite than others. Reported bite injuries are highest for large (>50 lb) working and sporting breeds, with young (6 to 11 months of age) male dogs causing most of the injuries.[6] Hound breeds are underrepresented. A disproportionate number of fatal and nonfatal attacks by pit bull terriers, German shepherds, St. Bernards, and dog-wolf hybrids have been reported.[5a,7–10] Intentional or accidental provocation was involved in only 6% of dog bites in one report.[4] Others have noted that approximately 50% of the bites are unprovoked, and the remainder involve threats to the animals' territory or owners. Only 10% or less of attacks are caused by stray dogs; most are caused by neighborhood pets.

The infecting organism in bite or scratch injuries usually corresponds to the normal oral microflora of dogs and cats (compare Table 58–1 with Table 9–1), although organisms from the environment or victim's skin may contaminate the injury. Despite the nu-

Table 58–1. Organisms Isolated from Infected Human Wounds Caused by Dog or Cat Bites or Scratches[a]

ORGANISM	ANIMAL INVOLVED	REPORTED PER CENT OF ISOLATES (DOG [CAT] BITES)
Viruses		
Rabies virus (Chapter 31)	D,C	NA
Motor paralysis agent[11]	C	R
Bacteria		
Gram-negative Aerobes		
Yersinia pestis (Chapter 59)	C	NA
Francisella tularensis (Chapter 60)	C,D	NA
Cat scratch disease agent (Chapter 61)	C	NA
Pasteurella spp.[12–14]	D,C	25–38 [50–75]
Pseudomonas spp.[12]	D	8
Actinobacillus spp.[12]	D	6
Capnocytophaga canimorsus (DF-2)[15, 41–50]	D,C	NA
Capnocytophaga cynodegmi (DF-2-like)[15, 41–50]	D,C	NA
Unclassified rods[c, 16–18] (M-5, EF-4, llj, VE-2)	D	4
Brucella suis[19]	D	NA
Acinetobacter calcoaceticus[20]		
Moraxella spp.[21, 22]	D	NA
Hemophilus spp.[23]	D	4
Streptobacillus moniliformis[21, 24]	D	R
Chromobacterium[21]	D	2
Flavobacterium spp.[22]	D	NA
Neisseria spp.[12]	D,C	2 [25]
Escherichia coli[21]	D	2
Spirillum minor[25]	C	19
Proteus mirabilis[21]	D	2
Klebsiella-Enterobacter[20, 23]	D	2
Mycobacterium fortuitum[26]	D	R
Gram-positive Aerobes		
Streptococcus spp.[d, 12, 13]	D	40 [50]
Staphylococcus (coagulase-positive)[e, 27, 28, 28a]	D	23
Staphylococcus epidermidis[12]	D,C	19 [75]
Corynebacterium spp.[12, 20]	D,C	8–20 [25]
Micrococcus spp.[21]	D	6
Diphtheroids[12]	D,C	4 [25]
Bacillus spp.[20]	D	4
Anaerobes		
Propionibacterium spp.[21]	D	21
Bacteroides spp.[29]	D	11–16
Peptococcus spp.[30]	D	16
Eubacterium spp.[21]	D	11
Fusobacterium spp.[12]	D	5–11
Clostridium spp.[21]	D	5
Clostridium tetani (Chapter 48)	D,C	R
Leptothrix buccalis[12]	D	5
Peptostreptococcus spp.[12]	D	5
Veillonella[12]	D	5
Fungi		
Blastomyces dermatitidis[31, 32] (Chapter 65)	D	R

[a]D = dog, C = cat, NA = not available, R = rare or isolated reports
[b]Percentage based on isolates of those wounds of patients who sought medical attention.
[c]EF-4, VE-2 (Pasteurella- or Actinobacillus-like); llj (Flavobacterium-like); M-5 (Moraxella-like). DF-2 now classified as Capnocytophaga spp.
[d]α-, β-nonhemolytic streptococci included
[e]Includes S. aureus, S. intermedius

merous aerobic and anaerobic organisms that contaminate bite wounds, only a few such as *Pasteurella multocida* and *Capnocytophaga canimorsus* (formerly DF-2) consistently cause systemic manifestations. When present, anaerobic bacteria are usually isolated in mixed cultures. From 4% to 20% of dog bite wounds and 20% to 50% of cat bite wounds for which medical attention is sought become clinically infected.[21] An unusual form of motor neuron disease suspected to be caused by a virus occurred following a cat bite.[11] The public health aspects of rabies, tetanus, and cat scratch disease are covered in Chapters 31, 48, and 62, respectively.

Pasteurella Infections

Pasteurella spp., small, nonmotile, gram-negative, bipolar-staining bacilli, are clinically significant in many dog and cat bite wounds. These organisms normally inhabit the nasal, gingival, and tonsillar regions of approximately 12% to 92% and 52% to 99% of dogs and cats, respectively,[27,28,33,34] as well as many other animals. Pasteurella spp. have been reclassified based on their DNA homology.[35] P. multocida, subsp. multocida and subsp. septica, were the most common isolates from clinically healthy cats, and P. canis was common in both healthy dogs and cats.[34] Strains isolated from cats were more commonly pathogenic (71%) than those from dogs (8%).

Although dog bites account for more than 80% of emergency room visits related to animal bites, cats are responsible for approximately 75% of bites or scratches contaminated with Pasteurella.[36,37,37a] Pasteurella infections also have been reported following bite injuries caused by large exotic Felidae.[38] Scratch injuries produced by dogs are less likely to cause Pasteurella infections than cat scratches, unless the scratch is also associated with a bite injury. The fact that cats frequently lick their paws or that, when they scratch, they also hiss, thereby producing aerosolized secretions that contaminate the wounds, is probably related to the increase in Pasteurella-infected scratches. Pasteurella meningitis developed in a person with extensive dental caries who regularly kissed the family dog.[39] Pasteurella peritonitis developed in a person following a cat scratch or bite that penetrated the tubing of the home dialysis machine.[39a]

Although a majority of human P. multocida infections are related to animal bites, humans also may develop pasteurellosis from nonbite animal exposure, and infections frequently localize in the GI or respiratory tracts or CNS. Patients who are immunosuppressed or who have hepatic dysfunction are more likely to develop bacteremia and die. Most Pasteurella infections occur in people who have frequent contact with farm or pet animals. Presumably, bites in people in urban environments are related to dog or cat or other small animal or rodent exposure.[40]

Capnocytophaga (DF-2 and DF-2-Like) Infections

In 1976, a slow-growing, thin filamentous, nonsporeforming, nonmotile pleomorphic, facultative aerobic, gram-negative bacillus labeled DF-2 (dysgonic fermenter-2) in the Centers for Disease Control (CDC) alphanumeric system was reported to cause fatal septicemia following a dog bite.[41] Until that time, fatal complications following bite injuries were considered uncommon. DF-2 septicemia has also been reported as a result of cat bites.[42] DF-2 has an unusual propensity to cause systemic bacteremia, presumably because of its tropism for endothelial surfaces. Numerous cases of bite-associated DF-2 infection were subsequently reported. Other unclassified bacteria such as M-5, IIj, and EF-4 are also common in the oral cavity of dogs and in bite wounds. The majority of infections with these unnamed species have occurred in immunocompromised individuals. A splenectomized veterinarian died from illness following a dog bite.[43] Most people who developed fatal complications of DF-2 infection had underlying disorders, such as functional or surgical splenectomy, Hodgkin's disease, alcoholism, hemoglobinopathy, granulomatous or other chronic lung disease, chronic arthritis, macroglobulinemia, intestinal malabsorption, or old age.[17,18,44-46] Presumably, these disorders caused defects in their phagocytic immune defenses, and the victims could not eliminate this organism from their blood. As with pasteurellosis, some patients with DF-2 sepsis have had exposure to dogs, cats, or other carnivores or to outdoor environments with no known bites.

Ocular keratitis and blepharitis have developed in people with close association of their pet dogs or cats[47,48] and in people with no known animal exposure.[49] Corneal scratch injuries from cats have also produced keratitis in people.[50] Results from DNA hybridization and biochemical studies have determined that the more virulent species which were isolated from people with septicemia were designated as *Capnocytophaga canimorsus* (DF-2) and those from localized (noninvasive) wound infections or keratitis were distinct species designated as *C. cynodegmi* (DF-2-like).[15]

CLINICAL FINDINGS

The type of injury following dog bite wounds varies, including abrasions, punctures, avulsions, and lacerations. A dog's bite causes severe crushing injuries and laceration with ligamentous tearing and tissue necrosis. A majority of lesions on adults are primarily on the upper extremities and trunk. Young children generally receive facial injuries because of their small stature and lack of experience with dogs and because the dogs tend to bite the face and mouth as part of aggressive behavior.

Cat scratches frequently occur on the handler's extremities and usually are associated with attempts to restrain the animal. Cat bites are deep, and the cats' sharp teeth are more likely to produce wounds that become foci for abscess formation and resultant complications such as osteomyelitis.

Signs indicating wound infection include localized swelling or reddening and pain with or without a purulent drainage. The type of organism and site of bite are most important in determining the clinical course of the injury. Infections caused by the two most clinically significant organisms, DF-2 and *Pasteurella*, are discussed below.

Pasteurella Infections

Pasteurella infections are more progressive than those produced by many other bacteria. Usually within 24 to 48 hours, cellulitis develops at the site of injury. Erythema, tenderness, and swelling occur in association with a serosanguineous to purulent, dark yellow-colored discharge. Lymphadenomegaly and low-grade fever ($>38°C$) develop in some patients. Cellulitis can lead to extensive infection of deeper tissues or potentially fatal septicemia. Septicemia is characterized by persistent chills, fever, and collapse. Chronic osteomyelitis, septic or posttraumatic arthritis, tenosynovitis, and smouldering abscesses also can occur.

Capnocytophaga (DF-2) Infection

Although inconsistent, cellulitis is the most common finding following bite wounds contaminated by DF-2 and DF-2-like strains. In some cases, eschariform lesions, characterized by formation of purplish-black necrotic tissue around the bite site, are seen. Splenectomized or immunosuppressed patients and those infected by DF-2 develop the most severe illness and septicemia, characterized by hypotension, thrombocytopenia with purpura, symmetrical peripheral gangrene, oliguria, DIC, and death. Acute myocardial infarction was reported.[18] Regardless of the clinical spectrum, most patients are continuously bacteremic. Localization of the septic process without death can occur, and some people develop endocarditis, purulent meningitis, and polyarthritis. The organisms may not be demonstrated on microscopic examination of tissues, although they may be seen in blood films of some patients with severe bacteremia and by blood culture.

Capnocytophaga isolates may be detected within 72 hours in culture, but up to 7 to 10 days is typical. Growth is enhanced in the presence of CO_2 and with serum-enriched media. The laboratory should be advised if these organisms are suspected. Since identification of these organisms takes a relatively long time, antimicrobial therapy must be instituted immediately, without microbial identification.

THERAPY

Judging from the discrepancy between the number of reported and the number of estimated bite cases, not all affected people seek medical attention. Bites should be reported to public health officials whose job it is to investigate the incident and to make recommendations concerning the treatment of the bite victim and disposition of the animal. Only a few states have developed formal guidelines for handling these cases.

Although not primarily responsible for the treatment of human victims, veterinarians should be aware of the proper protocols for medical care of bite wounds in people. Thorough washing of all bite wounds and scratches with quaternary ammonium soaps and water is essential. Soaking in an aqueous organic iodine solution may also be beneficial.[14] It is important that wounds be irrigated with physiologic solutions such as lactated Ringer's. Intermittent pulsating high-pressure irrigation which streams isotonic fluids directly into the wound has been most effective in dislodging contaminating bacteria.[2]

The degree of surgical intervention frequently depends on the site and type of bite. Facial injuries bleed profusely and produce highly visible scarring and, therefore, are routinely sutured. Extremity wounds are less visible and often are more contaminated and prone to infection; therefore, they are often treated as open wounds. Puncture wounds that show minimal hemorrhage should be irrigated, although some physicians have excised at the margins of the wound, leaving it open to drain. Any wound that becomes infected should be cultured. The affected extremity should be elevated to prevent swelling.

Antimicrobial therapy with penicillin has been recommended for all penetrating bite injuries, even though studies have questioned routine prophylaxis. This recommendation is based on the fact that most animal bite wound isolates, with the exception of staphylococci, are susceptible to penicillin G.[22] Early initiation of antimicrobial prophylaxis can reduce the severity of infection, but the difference in overall numbers of infections that develop is not statistically significant.[5] Drugs with a gram-positive and anaerobic spectrum, such as penicillins, are usually effective for this purpose. There is generally little need for culture of clinically uninfected bite wounds.[51] Because of their polymicrobic nature, clinically infected bite wounds should be cultured. Resistant bacteria require use of cephalosporins, β-lactamase-resistant antibiotics, or penicillins in combination with β-lactamase inhibitors, such as clavulanate. Use of erythromycin, first-generation cephalosporins, or dicloxacillin is often associated with microbial resistance.

For a discussion of therapy of rabies virus, *Clostridium tetani-*, or anaerobic bacteria-infected wounds, refer to Chapters 31, 48, and 49, respectively.

Pasteurella Infections

Penicillin and its analogs such as ampicillin are the single most effective antibiotics to control this infection in adults. Tetracyclines, chloramphenicol, and some cephalosporins are similarly effective. Bacterial resistance to β-lactamase resistant penicillins and to cephalosporins has been reported in 18% to 50% of animal isolates.[14,22] Erythromycin does not control infection, and relapses can occur following discontinuation of its use.

Capnocytophaga (DF-2) Infections

Many cases of DF-2 sepsis are fatal in immunocompromised hosts; however, some people may completely recover even without antimicrobial therapy. Physicians and veterinarians should realize the risk of dog ownership in potentially immunocompromised people and advise them to seek immediate medical care and antimicrobial treatment following bite injuries. Response to therapy in individuals treated early enough in the course of septicemia has generally been dramatic. The organism shows in vitro susceptibility to many antimicrobials including ampicillin, cephalosporins, tetracycline, carbenicillin, clindamycin, chloramphenicol, erythromycin, and penicillin. Isolates have been resistant to the typical drugs, such as colistin, gentamicin, and kanamycin, selected to treat gram-negative infections. Variable susceptibility has been found to trimethoprim-sulfamethoxazole. Penicillin should be used as a first choice; a third-generation cephalosporin has been recommended to be given concurrently in severely ill people since penicillin-resistant strains of *Capnocytophaga* and *Pasteurella* have been isolated on occasion.[46]

Rat Bite Infections

Two commensal organisms of rodents are responsible for a bacterial disease of dogs, cats, and people who have direct or indirect contact with rodent tissues or their secretions. *Streptobacillus moniliformis* is a small (0.25 to 0.5 μm × 1 to 3 μm), motile, aerobic, pleomorphic gram-negative bacillus with unipolar flagella. *Spirillum minus* is a gram-negative spiral organism (3 to 5 μm) that is motile by means of polar flagellar bundles.

Rodents are the primary reservoir hosts for these organisms. Subclinical infections of rats with *Streptococcus moniliformis* are prevalent worldwide, although in some cases rats develop abscess formation and purulent infections. Other rodents such as mice and guinea pigs more commonly develop clinical illness when infected. With *Spirillum minus*, the prevalence of infection in rats is more variable, depending on the geographic location; however, most are inapparently infected.

Dogs and cats contaminate their oral cavities with these bacteria while catching rodents. They can also harbor these agents subclinically and act as mechanical vectors because they can transmit their recently acquired infection to people by biting. Occasionally, abscesses occur in dogs or cats, presumably as a result of a rat bite.[52]

Infected people have fever, lymphadenitis, and generalized exanthematous eruptions that may develop weeks to months after bites.[53,54] Epidemic infections have rarely been reported after laboratory or foodborne contamination. Endocarditis and polyarthritis are chronic sequelae. With infections caused by *Streptococcus moniliformis*, the site of the original bite usually heals by the time clinical signs are seen. With infections caused by *Spirillum minus*, the healed wound may become reinflamed and later ulcerate during the course of febrile illness. Regional lymphadenitis and lymphangitis are common in the region of the bite.

Streptococcus moniliformis can be isolated in culture on serum-enriched media. Isolation from blood must not be made in blood culture media, since the typical anticoagulant, polyanethol sulfonate, inhibits the organism's growth. *Streptococcus moniliformis* has the propensity to convert to pleomorphic, cell wall-deficient, L-forms in vivo or in vitro, during unfavorable growth conditions or with use of β-lactams in therapy (see also L-Form Infections, Chapter 50). *Spirillum minus* does not grow on laboratory media; therefore, darkfield examination of exudates or inoculation of mice with blood from affected patients is necessary to confirm the infection.

Penicillin is the drug of choice for infection caused by either organism. Tetracyclines are indicated in the event of resistant or L-form infections (see Appendix 14 for dosages). Oral infections of dogs and cats are usually inapparent, so treatment is not necessary. In the case of abscess formation, surgical drainage should accompany antimicrobial therapy.

References

1. Beck AM: The epidemiology of animal bite. *Compend Cont Educ Pract Vet* 3:254–257, 1981.
2. Zook EG, Miller M, van Beek AL, et al: Successful treatment protocol for canine fang injuries. *J Trauma* 20:243–247, 1980.
3. August JR: Dog and cat bites. *J Am Vet Med Assoc* 193:1394–1398, 1988.
4. Beck AM, Loring H, Lockwood R: The ecology of dog bite injury in St. Louis, Missouri. *Public Health Rep* 90:262–267, 1975.
5. Fleisher GR, Boenning DA: The treatment of animal bites in humans. *Compend Cont Educ Pract Vet* 3:366–370, 1981.
5a. Sacks JJ, Sattin RW, Bonzo SE: Dog bite–related fatalities from 1979 through 1988. *JAMA* 262:1489–1492, 1989.
6. Karlson TA: The incidence of facial injuries from dog bites. *JAMA* 251:3265–3267, 1984.
7. Pinckney LE, Kennedy LA: Traumatic deaths from dog attacks in the United States. *Pediatrics* 69:193–196, 1982.
8. Wright JC: Severe attacks by dogs: characteristics of the dogs, the victims and the attack settings. *Public Health Rep* 100:55–61, 1985.
9. Lockwood R, Rindy K: Are "pit bulls" different? An analysis of the pit bull terrier controversy. *Anthrozoos* 1:2–8, 1987.
10. Underman AE: Bite wounds inflicted by dogs and cats. *Vet Clin North Am* 17:195–207, 1987.
11. Hudson AJ, Vinters HV, Povey RC, et al: An unusual form of motor neuron disease following a cat bite. *Can J Neurol Sci* 13:111–116, 1986.
12. Goldstein EJC, Citron DM, Finegold SM: Role of anaerobic bacteria in bite wound infections. *J Infect Dis* 6:S177–S183, 1984.
13. Peeples E, Bostwick JA, Scott FA: Wounds of the hand contaminated by human or animal saliva. *J Trauma* 20:383–389, 1980.
14. Goldstein EJC, Richwald GA: Human and animal bite wounds. *Am Fam Physician* 36:101–109, 1987.
15. Brenne DJ, Hollis DG, Fanning GR, et al: *Capno-*

cytophaga canimorsus sp. nov. (formerly DF-2), a cause of septicemia following dog bite and *C. cynodegmi* sp. nov., a cause of localized wound infection following dog bite. *J Clin Microbiol* 27:231–235, 1989.

16. Dees SB, Powell J, Moss CW, et al: Cellular fatty acid composition of organisms frequently associated with human infections resulting from dog bites: *Pasteurella multocida* and groups EF-4, IIj, M-5, and DF-2. *J Clin Microbiol* 14:612–616, 1981.

17. Kalb R, Kaplan MH, Tenenbaum MJ, et al: Cutaneous infection at dog bite wounds associated with fulminant DF-2 septicemia. *Am J Med* 78:687–690, 1985.

18. Newton NL, Sharma B: Case report: acute myocardial infarction associated with DF-2 bacteremia after a dog bite. *Am J Med Sci* 291:352–354, 1986.

19. Robertson MG: Brucella infection transmitted by dog bite. *JAMA* 225:750–751, 1973.

20. Ordog GJ: The bacteriology of dog bite wounds on initial presentation. *Ann Emerg Med* 15:1324–1329, 1986.

21. Edwards MS: Infections due to human and animal bites. *In* Feign RD, Cherry JD (ed): *Textbook of Pediatric Infectious Diseases*, ed 2. Philadelphia, WB Saunders Co, 1987, pp 2362–2373, 1987.

22. Goldstein EJC, Citron DM, Vagvolgyi AG, et al: Susceptibility of bite wound bacteria to seven oral antimicrobial agents including RU-985, a new erythromycin: considerations in choosing empiric therapy. *Antimicrob Agents Chemother* 29:556–559, 1986.

23. Lavine LS, Isenberg HD, Rubins W, et al: Unusual osteomyelitis following superficial dog bite. *Clin Orthop* 98:251–253, 1974.

24. Gilbert GI, Cassidy SF, Bennett N: Rat-bite fever. *Med J Aust* 2:1131–1134, 1971.

25. Yamato S: Sodoku caused by the bite of a cat. *Jpn J Dermatol Urol* 44:118–119, 1938. (Abstr in *Trop Dis Bull* 36:774, 1939).

26. Ariel I, Hass H, Weinberg H, et al: *Mycobacterium fortuitum* granulomatous synovitis caused by a dog bite. *J Hand Surg* 8:341–345, 1983.

27. Saphir DA, Carter GR: Gingival flora of the dog with special reference to bacteria associated with bites. *J Clin Microbiol* 3:334–349, 1976.

28. Bailie WE, Stowe EC, Schmitt AM: Aerobic bacterial flora of oral and nasal fluids of canines with reference to bacteria associated with bites. *J Clin Microbiol* 7:223–231, 1978.

28a. Talan DA, Staatz D, Staatz A, et al: *Staphylococcus intermedius* in canine gingiva and canine inflicted human wound infections: laboratory characterization of a newly recognized zoonotic pathogen. *J Clin Microbiol* 27:78–81, 1989.

29. Fiala M, Bauer H, Khaleeli M, et al: Dog bite, *Bacteroides* infection, coagulopathy, renal microangiopathy. *Ann Intern Med* 87248–249, 1977.

30. Alpert G, Sutton LN: Brain abscess following a dog bite. *Clin Pediatr* 23:580, 1984.

31. Hiemenz JW, Coccari PJ, Macher AM: Human blastomycosis from dog bites. *Ann Intern Med* 98:1030, 1983.

32. Gnann JW, Bressler GS, Bodet A, et al: Human blastomycosis after a dog bite. *Ann Intern Med* 98:48–49, 1983.

33. Smith JE: Studies on *Pasteurella septica* I. The occurrence in the nose and tonsils of dogs. *J Comp Pathol* 65:239–245, 1955.

34. Baldrias L, Frost AJ, O'Boyle D: The isolation of *Pasteurella*-like organisms from tonsillar region of dogs and cats. *J Small Anim Pract* 29:63–68, 1988.

35. Mutters R, Ihm P, Pohl S, et al: Reclassification of the genus *Pasteurella* Trevisan 1887 on the basis of deoxyribonucleic acid homology. *Int J Sys Bacteriol* 35:309–322, 1985.

36. Arons MS, Fernando L, Polayes IM: *Pasteurella multocida*—the major cause of hand infections following domestic animal bites. *J Hand Surg* 7:47–52, 1982.

37. Tessin I, Brorson JE, Trollfors B: Rapidly fatal *Pasteurella multocida* septicemia in an infant following cat scratch. *Pediatr Infect Dis* 6:425–426, 1987.

37a. Zbenden R, Sommerhalder P, vonWartburg U: Coisolation of *Pasteurella domatis* and *Pasteurella multocida* from cat bite wounds. *Eur J Clin Microbiol Infect Dis* 7:203–204, 1988.

38. Burdge DR, Scheifele D, Speert DP: Serious *Pasteurella multocida* infections from lion and tiger bites. *JAMA* 253:3296–3297, 1985.

39. Rhodes M: *Pasteurella multocida* meningitis in a dog lover (or don't kiss pets). *J Roy Soc Med* 79:747–478, 1986.

39a. Paul RV, Rostad SG: Cat bite peritonitis: *Pasteurella multocida* peritonitis following feline contamination of peritoneal dialysis tubing. *Am J Kidney Dis* 10:318–319, 1987.

40. Carter GR: The epidemiology and pathogenesis of pasteurellosis in man. *Vet Med* 79:629–630, 1984.

41. Bobo RA, Newton EJ: A previously undescribed gram-negative bacillus causing septicemia and meningitis. *Am J Clin Pathol* 65:564–569, 1976.

42. Carpenter PD, Heppner BT, Gnann JW: DF-2 bacteremia following cat bites. Report of two cases. *Am J Med* 82:621–623, 1987.

43. Bacillus isolated by CDC in fatal dog bite case. *J Am Vet Med Assoc* 187:351, 1985.

44. Martone WJ, Zuehl RW, Minson GE, et al: Postsplenectomy sepsis with DF-2: report of a case with isolation of the organism from the patient's dog. *Ann Intern Med* 93:457–458, 1980.

45. Scully RE, Mark EJ, McNeely BU: An asplenic woman with evidence of sepsis and diffuse intravascular coagulation after a dog bite. *N Engl J Med* 315:241–249, 1986.

46. Perez RE: Dysgonic fermenter-2 infections. *West J Med* 148:90–92, 1988.

47. Paton BG, Ormerod LD, Peppe J, et al: Evidence for a feline reservoir for dysgonic fermenter 2 keratitis. *J Clin Microbiol* 26:2439–2440, 1988.

48. Kiel RJ, Crane LR, Anguilar J, et al: Corneal perforation caused by dysgonic fermenter-2. *JAMA* 257:3269–3270, 1987.

49. Glasser DB: Angular blepharitis caused by gram-negative bacillus DF-2. *Am J Ophthalmol* 102:119–120, 1986.

50. Udell IJ, Kelley CG, Wolf TC, et al: Keratitis following corneal cat scratch injury. *Ophthalmology* 94:124, 1987.

51. Jones J, Dougherty J: Routine culture of dog bites. *Ann Emerg Med* 16:730, 1987.

52. Das AM: *Streptobacillus moniliformis* isolated from an abscess of a dog. *Indian J Comp Microbiol Immunol Infect Dis* 7:115, 1986.

53. Brown TM, Nunemaker JC: Rat bite fever: review of the American cases with revaluation of its etiology; report of cases. *Bull Johns Hopkins Hosp* 70:201–227, 1942.

54. Cole JS, Stoll TW, Bulger RJ: Rat bite fever: report of three cases. *Ann Intern Med* 71:979–981, 1969.

59

PLAGUE

Dennis W. Macy
Peter W. Gasper

ETIOLOGY

Plague is caused by *Yersinia pestis*, a nonmotile, non-sporeforming, facultative anaerobic, gram-negative, bipolar-staining coccobacillus of the family Enterobacteriaceae. The organism is nonsaprophytic and is sensitive to desiccation and temperatures above 40°C, which make fomite transmission unlikely.[1,2] It can survive for several weeks to months in organic material, such as infected carcasses, and cold temperatures or freezing may prolong the viability of this organism for years. Three geographic variants of *Y. pestis* (*orientalis*, *antiqua*, and *mediaevalis*) can be distinguished biochemically but are of identical virulence.

EPIDEMIOLOGY

People and domestic animals are alternate hosts for *Y. pestis*, which is maintained in nature by chronic bacteremia in wild rodents and transmitted between these reservoir hosts by fleas. More than 230 species of rodents and 1500 species of fleas infected with the plague organism have been found.[2,3] Despite this wide host range, only 30 to 40 rodent species serve as permanent natural reservoirs for plague, while other species are considered only temporary or amplifying hosts for the organism. Natural reservoir hosts are relatively resistant to plague infections, but susceptibility varies tremendously within a species and is based on geographic location, flea species, and environmental factors. The dog and cat fleas (*Ctenocephalides* spp.) are considered poor vectors for plague.[2] In the United States, prairie dogs (*Cynomys* spp.), rock squirrels (*Spermophilus variegatus*), and ground squirrels such as *Spermophilus richardsonii* are commonly infected wild hosts.[4] Mortality approaches 100% in these species.

Plague exists in various areas on every continent except Australia (Fig. 59–1).[5] These foci of plague are most frequently associated with semiarid, cooler climates usually adjacent to deserts. In the United States, plague foci are located throughout an area bounded on the east by the Rocky Mountains and on the west by the Pacific Ocean, as well as in Hawaii (Fig. 59–2). During epizootics, the geographic area has spread into the High Plains of Colorado, western Kansas, Oklahoma, and Texas.[4] These temporary geographic expansions are due to spread of the disease into highly susceptible ground squirrel populations but are usually not maintained for more than several years because of high mortality in these species. High mountain parks in Colorado and grasslands in California are also susceptible to rapid expansion of plague because of the presence of amplifying rodent species.[4]

Transmission of *Y. pestis* between most hosts occurs by flea bite or less commonly by contact of the organism with mucous membranes or broken skin or by inhalation of droplets from animals with pneumonic plague (Fig. 59–3).[6–8] Following consumption of a blood meal from an infected host, *Y. pestis* multiplies in the stomach of the flea. While consuming blood from a second host, the flea regurgitates its *Y. pestis*-containing contents, thus transmitting the organism into the new host. The flea may remain infected for more than a year, allowing transmission of the disease long after the death of the host.

Rodent burrowing systems maintain plague ecosystems by providing a moist environment for flea reproduction and by housing very large numbers of animals such as prairie dogs. Burrows allow the exchange of

621

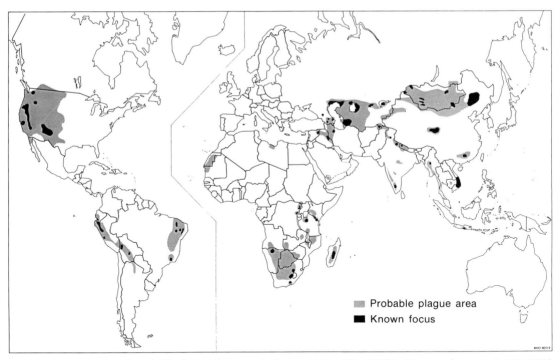

Figure 59-1. Known and probable foci and areas of plague, 1959–1979. (WHO: Human plague in 1979. *WHO Weekly Epidemiological Record* 32:241–244, 1980. Reprinted with permission.)

infected fleas and allow interspecies spread when abandoned burrows are used by another species, such as rabbits, seeking refuge from a predator.

Domestic and wild cats show susceptibil-ity to *Y. pestis* similar to that of people and can be a source of infection for people.[4,4a] Cases in cats have been more common in the summer months, fewer cases being re-ported in the spring and fall. Only rarely

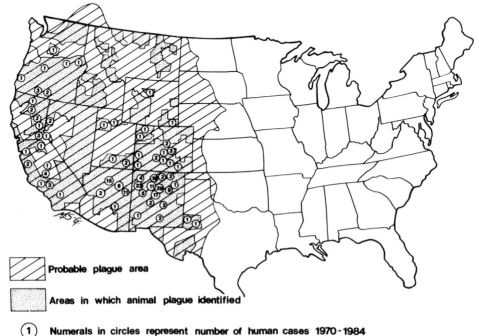

Figure 59-2. Distribution of human plague in the United States from 1970–1984.

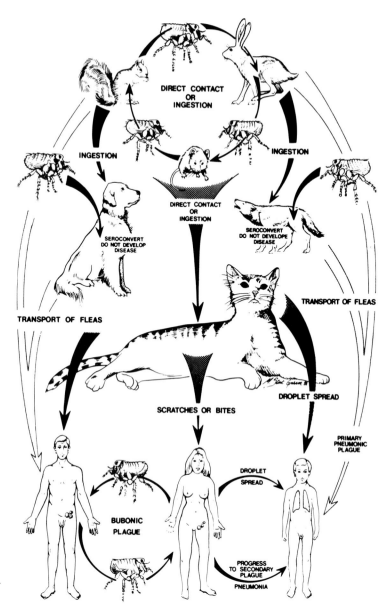

Figure 59–3. Epidemiologic features of plague.

have cases of plague been reported in cats during the winter months.[4a] Raptors and other birds; wild carnivores, including black bears, coyotes, badgers, skunks, and raccoons; and domestic dogs are remarkably resistant to Y. pestis infection but may transport infected fleas or rodent carcasses. Rabbits, although not considered reservoir hosts, may become infected during enzootic outbreaks and serve as a source of infection for hunters.

PATHOGENESIS

Cats and dogs acquire plague by ingestion of infected rodents or lagomorphs or possi-

bly by bites from their prey's plague-infected fleas. Ten days following ingestion of Y. pestis-infected rodents, plague organisms can be isolated from the oropharynx and blood stream in approximately 50% and 20% of dogs, respectively.[9,10] Dogs develop only mild clinical symptomatology, including fever and lymphadenomegaly, and seroconvert. Both wild and domestic cats are more susceptible to plague than dogs or other carnivores.[2,11] In experimental studies, 50% to 80% of cats fed plague-infected meals died within 6 to 20 days.[9,12] Most cats fed infected mice had Y. pestis cultured from their oropharynx and could have transmitted plague.

Depending on whether the organism enters from a flea bite or through mucous membranes or broken skin, two pathogeneses are possible. Following a flea bite, the organism is phagocytized by polymorphonuclear cells and mononuclear cells, multiplies, and is eventually released into the blood stream, which delays bacteremia for 2 to 6 days. Replication in the mononuclear and polymorphonuclear cells renders the organism resistant to further phagocytosis. Therefore, if the organism is ingested or inhaled from contaminated tissues or fluids, which is common in the cat or other carnivores, it has already acquired this resistance to phagocytosis from the rodent's host leukocytes and it spreads more quickly, resulting in a shorter incubation period of 1 to 3 days.

Lesions at the site of inoculation are usually minimal. The most common visible lesions are in the lymph nodes draining the site of inoculation. Marked lymphadenomegaly (bubo formation) develops and nodes may abscess or drain. Both deep and superficial lymph nodes in other parts of the body may become similarly infected following hematogenous or lymphogenous spread of the organism. In the bacteremic state, other tissues, such as eye, liver, kidney, spleen, brain, or lung, may become infected. Y. pestis contains endotoxins that may result in edema, septic shock, and DIC. The clinical course may last between 6 and 20 days. Cats with previous titers to plague by either vaccination or natural infection generally have a more protracted illness but are not protected from bacteremia or death.[9,10]

CLINICAL FINDINGS

In both people and cats, three clinical forms of the disease have been recognized: **bubonic, septicemic,** and **pneumonic** plague.[13] The most common and probably the least fatal form is **bubonic** plague. In cats, bubonic plague is associated with high (40.6° to 41.1°C [105° to 106°F]) fevers, dehydration, and lymphadenomegaly. The submandibular, retropharyngeal, and cervical lymph nodes in the area of inoculation become enlarged, abscess, and may drain. Cats whose abscesses spontaneously drain, survive. If allowed to progress, the bubonic form may spread hematogenously or through the lymphatics to become the septic form. **Septicemic** plague may develop with or

without bubo formation. Hematogenous spread may result in involvement of virtually every organ in the body, although the most frequently involved organs are the spleen in people and lungs in cats.[12] Fever, shock, DIC, and marked leukocytosis are characteristic of the septic form of the disease in the cat. The septic form is usually fatal within 1 to 2 days following the presence of bacteremia. **Pneumonic** plague in cats develops as a result of hematogenous or lymphogenous spread of the organism and may be seen as a sequel to bubonic or septic forms of the disease rather than primary pneumonic plague, which is contracted through droplet transmission. Although cats normally do not contract primary pneumonic plague, they have been responsible for primary pneumonic plague in people caring for them.[14] Pneumonic plague, whether primary or secondary, carries the most severe prognosis. In people, untreated pneumonic plague is considered 100% fatal.[2] In summary, plague should be considered when examining any febrile cat in endemic areas.

DIAGNOSIS

Although a clinician may have a high degree of suspicion for plague based on clinical and epidemiologic information, the diagnosis must be confirmed.

Y. pestis is usually found in large numbers in infected tissues. In the clinical setting it is important to collect samples and start antimicrobial therapy before the disease is confirmed. Needle aspirates from lymph nodes, blood, or infected tissue may be selected, based on the clinical form of the disease in the patient. Aseptically collected samples of fluid, tissues, or blood should be submitted. Cultures of tonsils from experimentally infected cats have given consistently positive results, and the tonsils may serve as a source of infection of the saliva.[12] Four or more slides for bacterial stains should be prepared by making impression smears or cytologic smears, allowing them to air-dry, and then lightly heat fixing them over a flame. Care should be taken to avoid contact with purulent material while taking and preparing these samples.

For immunofluorescent testing, fluid specimens may be applied to clean, thin, glass slides. Place one or two drops of suspected fluid into two circles made with a wax pencil on the slide. Spread with a loop and agitate. With tissue specimens, impression smears are made within each circle. Allow to air-dry. These slides should be frozen if they cannot be examined immediately.

Two serum samples, 10 to 14 days apart, should be collected for antibody titers against Y. pestis. Because dogs and cats in endemic areas frequently have high titers to Y. pestis that persist for a year or longer after exposure, a fourfold rise in titer is needed to distinguish active disease from previous exposure.

Alternatively, specimens may be collected in a sterile syringe by aspiration or placed in blood tubes or inoculated into transport media (Stuarts, Difco, Detroit, MI and Cary-Blair, BBL, Cockeysville, MD are suitable), refrigerated but not frozen, and sent to a reference laboratory for confirmation. Samples should be double-wrapped in plastic and padded to prevent breakage and leakage, to conform with federal requirements for transporting hazardous agents. It is recommended that the State Veterinarian be contacted before shipping samples to the plague branch of the Centers for Disease Control, P.O. Box 2087, Fort Collins, Colorado 80522.[15] A few regional or state laboratories also conduct specialized testing for plague. At the laboratory, Gram stains are performed to determine staining characteristics and Giemsa or Wayson stain is used to detect the bipolarity "safety pin" appearance suggestive of Y. pestis. Y. pestis can be cultured on enriched blood agar but grows slowly, requiring 48 hours of incubation to produce colonies 1 to 2 mm in size at an optimum temperature of 28°C. If growth is observed, suspicious isolates should be shipped to a reference laboratory. See Appendix 8 for a listing of diagnostic laboratories that perform the above tests.

PATHOLOGIC FINDINGS

Cats, of which 50% die acutely, may have focal necrotic lesions of the spleen and liver, with evidence of secondary pneumonic spread of the disease. Those surviving for longer periods of time develop cervical or submandibular abscesses or bubos. Consistent involvement of the medial retropharyngeal lymph nodes has been apparent in experimentally infected cats.[9, 12] In fatal cases,

tonsils and submandibular and cranial thoracic lymph nodes were also affected. The normal nodal architecture was totally replaced by necrosis and hemorrhage. Lymph nodes from cats who were euthanatized after clinical recovery showed only lymphoid hyperplasia. Bacterial infiltration of the lung parenchyma, resulting in pneumonia, is characterized by focal areas of hemorrhage with clusters of bacteria. Since experimentally infected dogs develop only transient fever and lymphadenopathy, no pathologic features have been described.[9]

THERAPY

The decision to treat an animal for plague is seldom based on a definitive diagnosis. When plague is suspected based on clinical or epidemiologic information, specific antimicrobial therapy should be instituted rather than waiting for laboratory confirmation. All plague suspects should be handled with gloves while wearing gowns and high-density surgical masks.[1] Animals with respiratory signs should have thoracic radiographs taken to determine if they have pneumonic plague. Animals should be examined for fleas, and if any are found, patients in surrounding cages, examination rooms, etc., should be treated with carbamates or pyrethrins.[1] Bubos should be lanced and flushed with chlorhexidine diacetate (Nolvasan, Fort Dodge, Fort Dodge, IA). Organic material, including tissues or pus-containing gauzes, should be double-bagged and incinerated.[1] Routine disinfectants are effective in killing the plague organism and should be used as a precautionary measure on cages and examination tables used in the care of infected animals.

Y. pestis is susceptible to a wide variety of antimicrobial agents (Table 59–1). Although Y. pestis appears sensitive in vitro to penicillin and ampicillin, it is resistant to these drugs in vivo.[2, 13] Aminoglycosides such as streptomycin or gentamicin are considered the most effective antibiotic against Y. pestis. Chloramphenicol is used in the treatment of patients with CNS spread of plague organism.[2] Use of tetracyclines has been associated with relapse, presumably owing to the development of bacterial resistance.[22] Tetracyclines are used primarily for the bubonic form of the disease and for prophylaxis. Infected cats should be treated

Table 59–1. Antimicrobial Therapy for Plague[a]

DRUG	DOSE[b] (mg/kg)	ROUTE	INTERVAL (hours)	DURATION (days)
Streptomycin[16]	5	IM	12	21[c]
Kanamycin[17]	5–7.5	IM	12	21[c]
Gentamicin[18]	2–4	IM	12–24	21[c]
Trimethoprim-sulfonamide[19]	15	PO, IV, IM	12	21[c]
Tetracycline[20]	20	PO	8	21
Chloramphenicol[21]	15	PO, SC	12	21

[a]IM = intramuscular, PO = oral, SC = subcutaneous.
[b]Dose per administration at specified interval, expressed as mg/kg unless otherwise stated.
[c]Renal function must be closely monitored because of potential nephrotoxicity.

for a minimum of 21 days, and treatment should continue far beyond the resolution of bubos and pneumonic changes. Prophylactic therapy with tetracycline is indicated in asymptomatic animals exposed to plague and should be continued for a 7-day period.[2] People exposed to plague in the process of caring for plague-infected animals are usually treated in a similar manner, under the direction of a physician. The prognosis depends on the clinical form of the disease and the species infected.

PREVENTION

People and domestic animals have intruded into the natural ecosystem in which plague circulates. Elimination of plague in wild rodent populations is generally impossible. Veterinarians should be especially alert in evaluating sick cats in such outbreaks and take appropriate precautions to protect themselves, their employees, and their clients. Examination of fleas taken from patients may quickly determine if they are of rodent source. Flea control in both dogs and cats should be stressed in enzootic areas, since pets have ample opportunity to share them with their owners. Dogs and cats should not be allowed to come in contact with burrows or have access to carcasses of dead rodents or lagomorphs. Residents in endemic areas should be encouraged to reduce food and habitat, such as rubbish or garbage piles, for peridomestic host species which may become infected during enzootic outbreaks. Local health and state officials may institute rodent control measures but not before flea control has been instituted in an area.[2,4]

Both killed and modified live vaccines for *Y. pestis* have been produced, but only the killed formalin-fixed virulent whole-organism preparation is available in the United States.[21] The vaccine requires multiple inoculations to maintain protective titers, and its use is associated with a high degree of local and systemic reactions. Immunization of cats with this vaccine has not protected them against bacteremia or death but has prolonged the clinical course of the disease. Vaccination is recommended for all laboratory and field personnel who are working with *Y. pestis* and for persons engaged in field operations in areas of enzootic plague.

PUBLIC HEALTH CONSIDERATIONS

The incidence of human plague in the United States is increasing. The 105 cases that occurred in eight Western states during the 1970s represented the largest number in the continental United States in any decade since 1900 to 1909.[23] Ninety percent of human cases of plague have been reported in California, Arizona, and New Mexico. Since 1949, New Mexico annually has reported more than 50% of the cases of plague.[23] In one survey, 82% of human plague cases were transmitted by flea bites, 15% by direct contact with infected wild animals, and 3% by contact with infected domestic cats.[23] In people, the overall death rate in treated patients in the United States is 15% to 22%.

All free-roaming cats in an endemic area must be considered at risk for exposure to plague. Veterinarians and their assistants are at increased risk for exposure to plague as a result of their occupations. People may become infected by inhalation of respiratory droplets from animals infected with secondary pneumonic plague, by handling infected tissues and body fluids via broken skin or mucous membrane contact, or through bites of plague-infected fleas. Plague suspects should be hospitalized and isolated immediately. Attempts should be made to limit the number of individuals caring for infected animals. These individuals should be informed of the mode of transmission of infection and advised to wear protective clothing and gloves in treating and caring for the infected pet. Routine disinfectants should be applied to cages and examination tables, and flea control should be instituted in the area in and around infected animals.[1] After making a diagnosis of plague in cats, veterinarians should advise owners to contact their physicians immediately. Local state health authorities should be notified early in the management of plague-infected animals.

References

1. Kaufmann AF, Mann JM, Gardiner TM, et al: Public health implications of plague in domestic cats. *J Am Vet Med Assoc* 179:875–878, 1981.
2. Poland JD, Barnes AM: Plague. *In* Steele JF (ed): *CRC Handbook Series in Zoonoses*, Section A: *Bacterial, Rickettsial and Mycotic Diseases*. Boca Raton, FL, CRC Press, 1979, pp 515–556.
3. Bahmanyar M, Cavanaugh DC: *Plague Manual*. Geneva, World Health Organization, 1976, p 1.
4. Barnes AM: Surveillance and control of bubonic plague in the United States. *Symp Zool Soc Lond* 50: 237–270, 1982.
4a. Eidson M, Tierney LA, Rollag OJ, et al: Feline plague in New Mexico: risk factors and transmission to humans. *Am J Public Health* 78:1333–1335, 1988.
5. WHO: Human plague in 1979. *WHO Weekly Epidemiological Record* 32:241–244, 1980.
6. Rollag OJ, Skeels MR, Nims LJ, et al: Feline plague in New Mexico: report of five cases. *J Am Vet Med Assoc* 179:1381–1383, 1981.
7. Thornton DJ, Tustin RC, Pienaar BJ, et al: Cat bite transmission of *Yersinia pestis* infection to man. *J South Afr Vet Assoc* 46:165–169, 1975.
8. Infectious Disease Section, California Department of Health Services: death from primary plague pneumonia at South Lake Tahoe. *Calif Morbid Mort Wkly Rep* 48:1–2, 1980.
9. Rust JH Jr, Cavanaugh DC, O'Shita R, et al: The role of domestic animals in the epidemiology of plague. I. Experimental infection of dogs and cats. *J Infect Dis* 24:522–526, 1970.
10. Rust JH, Miller BE, Bahmamyar M, et al: The role of domestic animals in the epidemiology of plague. II. Antibody to *Yersinia pestis* in sera of dogs and cats. *J Infect Dis* 124:527–532, 1971.
11. Poland JD, Barnes AM, Herman JJ: Human bubonic plague from exposure to a naturally infected wild carnivore. *Am J Epidemiol* 97:332–335, 1973.
12. Gasper PW, Benziger J, Barnes AM: Plague in cats: experimental transmission. *J Infect Dis*. Submitted, 1989.
13. Thilsted JP: Plague. *In* Barlough JE (ed): *Manual of Small Animal Infectious Diseases*. New York, Churchill Livingstone, 1988, pp 169–176.
14. Centers for Disease Control: Plague pneumonia. *Calif Morbid Mort Wkly Rep* 33:481–483, 1984.
15. Rosser WW: Zoonosis update: bubonic plague. *J Am Vet Med Assoc* 191:406–409, 1987.
16. Butler T, Bell WR, Linh NN, et al: *Yersinia pestis* infections in Vietnam. I. Clinical and hematological aspects. *J Infect Dis Suppl* 129:78–84, 1974.
17. Quan SF: Effect of kanamycin on *Pasteurella pustis*. *Bacteriol Proc Abstr* M36, 1960.
18. Sites VR, Poland JD: Unpublished data, Centers for Disease Control, Fort Collins, CO, 1988.
19. Meyer RF: Plague. *In* Gellis SS, Kagan BM (eds): *Current Pediatric Therapy, 1966–1967*. Philadelphia, WB Saunders Co, 1966, pp 961–970.
20. Meyer RF, Quan SF, McCrumb FR, et al: Effective treatment of plague. *Ann NY Acad Sci* 55:1228–1230, 1952.
21. Immunization Practices Advisory Committee, Plague Vaccine. *MMWR* 31:301–304, 1982.
22. Culver M: Treatment of bubonic plague in a cat. *J Am Vet Med Assoc* 191:1528, 1987.
23. Kaufman AF, Boyce JM, Martone WJ: Trends in human plague in the United States. *J Infect Dis* 141:522–524, 1980.

60

TULAREMIA*

Arnold F. Kaufmann

ETIOLOGY AND EPIDEMIOLOGY

Tularemia is an acute bacterial infection of many avian and mammalian species, including the dog and cat, and occurs throughout the continental United States.[1] The etiologic agent, *Francisella tularensis*, is a small, pleomorphic, gram-negative, non-spore-forming bacillus. The tularemia bacillus has two biotypes: A and B. Type A strains ferment glycerol and are highly virulent for laboratory rabbits (*Oryctolagus cuniculus*), and type B strains have the opposite characteristics. Type A strains are associated with a tick-rabbit cycle of infection and occur only in North America. Type B strains are more commonly associated with rodents and waterborne infections and occur throughout the Northern Hemisphere. Human illness is generally more severe with type A strain infections.[2]

Because the epidemiology of tularemia is complex,[1] only those aspects important in its transmission to the dog and cat will be discussed here. Various tick species serve as both reservoirs and vectors of tularemia. Infection can pass transovarially in ticks, and infection persists for life. Amplification of the infection rate in a tick population occurs when uninfected ticks feed on bacteremic animals. Although ticks are capable of transmitting tularemia at all three stages of their development, the adult and, less commonly, nymphal stages are most important in transmission to dogs, cats, and people. In the United States, four tick species constitute the primary vectors for dogs and cats: the wood tick (*Dermacentor andersoni*)

found in the Rocky Mountain region; the American dog tick (*D. variabilis*) found in the eastern two thirds of the country as well as in the Pacific coastal states; the Pacific coast tick (*D. occidentalis*) found in California and Oregon; and the Lone Star tick (*Amblyomma americanum*) found in the south central and southeastern states. Cats and dogs may also be infected when they hunt or eat infected rabbits or rodents.

PATHOGENESIS

Dogs

The severity of illness following experimental infections varies with age, puppies being more susceptible than young adult dogs. Ingestion of infected tissues or intradermal challenge produced milder disease than intranasal challenge.[3,4] When dogs were fed on infected tissues, an acute 5-day illness began after a 48-hour incubation period.[4] Fever to 40.2°C (104.4°F) and a mucopurulent discharge from the nose and eyes was present. Transient ulceroglandular tularemia follows intradermal challenge with concomitant development of fever, pustules at the inoculation site, and regional lymphadenomegaly.

More serious illness characterized by septicemia and high mortality follows SC or IM inoculation. Draining abscesses develop at the inoculation sites and are associated with regional lymphadenomegaly and high fever, with systemic dissemination of the disease after 1 week. At this time, the dogs appear obviously ill, have a mucopurulent ocular and nasal discharge, and develop a vesiculopapular skin rash.

---

*All material in this chapter is in the public domain, with the exception of any borrowed figures or tables.

Cats

Cats have become ill after eating infected guinea pigs.[5] Although some cats appear unaffected, younger cats primarily succumb to systemic infection characterized by generalized lymphadenomegaly and miliary abscess formation involving the liver and spleen.

Following SC inoculation, similar findings have been apparent, and young kittens appear most susceptible.[5] In addition, some SC and intranasally inoculated cats have had areas of bronchopneumonia, from which *F. tularensis*, as well as splenomegaly and multifocal hepatic necrosis, was isolated.[4]

CLINICAL FINDINGS

Dogs

Despite the ability to produce experimental infections and high seroprevalence indicating exposure in endemic areas, naturally acquired cases have been rare,[1,3,6–8] and dogs are considered resistant to tularemia.[2,9,10] Typically, a dog develops a brief episode of anorexia, listlessness, and low-grade fever. Sudden death of uncertain cause has occurred in a dog a few days after sniffing a dead, infected rabbit. Another dog developed multifocal draining abscesses in the subcutaneous tissue and superficial lymph nodes in addition to fever, anorexia, myalgia, and shivering. Uveitis and conjunctivitis developed in the left eye, with subsequent transient conjunctivitis and corneal clouding in the right eye.

Cats

Based on the number of reports, cats appear to be more susceptible to tularemia than dogs but are still considered relatively resistant to infection. Clinical information on spontaneous feline tularemia has generally been limited to brief mention in epidemiologic reports of human cases, and not all the cats were ill.[1,5,11–16] Infected cats have frequently eaten or mouthed wild rabbits prior to the onset of clinical signs. Variable signs of fever, anorexia, listlessness, lymphadenomegaly, draining abscesses, and occasionally, icterus and death have been noted.

DIAGNOSIS

Testing for serologic evidence of agglutinating antibody is the most commonly used diagnostic procedure. Both dogs and cats develop antibodies, but titers tend to be lower than would be observed in people. Titers from 1:40 to 1:160 are typical of recent infections in dogs.[2,4,10] Enzyme immunoassays have been developed to detect antibodies to specific *F. tularensis* antigens in infected people,[16a] but their usefulness for testing canine and feline sera is uncertain. Fluorescent antibody methods can be used to detect the coccobacillary organisms in exudates and tissues, even with paraffin-embedded tissues.

The isolation of *F. tularensis* from exudates or tissue specimens is the definitive method of diagnosis. This may be performed by culture on special media, such as supplemented chocolate agar, or through initial inoculation of a susceptible laboratory animal with subsequent culture of the test animal's liver and spleen. The infectious dose for humans is less than 100 organisms, inhaled as an aerosol, accidentally inoculated, or splashed in the conjunctival sac. Therefore, cultures of *F. tularensis* and necropsies of animals with suspected tularemia should be performed only in laboratories with adequate biosafety equipment.

See Appendix 8 for a listing of the laboratory that performs these diagnostic tests.

PATHOLOGIC FINDINGS

Gross necropsy findings in affected dogs and cats are similar. Most of this information has been obtained in experimentally infected animals. Generalized lymphadenomegaly, hepatomegaly, and splenomegaly may be present, and draining sinuses may be apparent from severely affected lymph nodes. Multiple white spots may be found in the liver and spleen, and bronchopneumonia may be apparent. The foci are areas of acute inflammation or microabscesses containing numerous coccobacillary organisms.

THERAPY

No reports have been made on antimicrobial therapy of canine or feline tularemia. In people, streptomycin and gentamicin are currently considered the drugs of first choice.[17] Tetracycline and chloramphenicol are alternative drugs, but relapses occur frequently with these drugs. Both streptomycin and tetracycline have been used successfully in controlled trials of antibiotic prophylaxis in experimental human tularemia.[18] Antimicrobial susceptibility tests suggest that erythromycin, rifampin, and some cephalosporins, such as ceftazidime, ceftriaxone, and moxalactam, may also be effective.[19]

PUBLIC HEALTH CONSIDERATIONS

In the United States, human tularemia occurs at a low incidence, fewer than 200 cases annually in the past decade. Most cases have resulted from tick-borne infection and to a lesser extent contact with tissues of wild animals such as rabbits. Only 26 cat-associated cases and eight dog-associated cases have been reported in North America, and some of these cases have not been well substantiated.

Cat-associated cases usually have involved bites or scratches, with the initial lesion typically developing at the trauma site. Although the cats often have no obvious illness, a common feature has been a history of hunting or eating wild animals, particularly rabbits.

None of the eight dog-associated cases have involved bites or scratches. In one case, a young girl developed typhoidal tularemia 3 days after the onset of a vague illness in her pet puppy, which presumably had contact with rabbits.[1] The dog frequently licked the young girl, and its saliva was considered her probable source of infection. In another instance, a family of seven persons staying at a cottage with their dogs during a 1-week period developed pulmonary tularemia.[20] The weather was rainy, and after returning from hunting rabbits, the dogs would shake the water from their hair when they entered the cottage. The dogs never appeared ill but subsequently were found to have antibodies to F. tularensis. The aerosol generated when the dogs shook off the rainwater after catching infected rabbits was considered the most likely source of infection for the human cases.

In people, tularemia occurs in two main syndromes: ulceroglandular and typhoidal.[21,22] Both syndromes have an incubation period of 2 to 10 days, followed by acute onset of high fever, chills, and other nonspecific constitutional symptoms. Ulceroglandular tularemia is characterized by a skin ulcer developing at the portal of infection with associated regional lymphadenopathy. In typhoidal tularemia, few localizing signs occur, pneumonia is more common, and the case-fatality ratio can exceed 30% if the illness is untreated.

Although no cases have been associated with removing ticks from pets, finding of infected ticks on dogs does indicate a potential hazard.[2,10] Proper removal of ticks from pets is discussed in Chapter 38, Rocky Mountain Spotted Fever, under Public Health Considerations.

References

1. Jellison WL: Tularemia in North America. Missoula, University of Montana Printing Department, 1974.
2. Schmid GP, Kornblatt AN, Connors CA, et al: Clinically mild tularemia associated with tick-borne Francisella tularensis. J Infect Dis 148:63–67, 1983.
3. Ey LF, Daniels RE: Tularemia in dogs. JAMA 117:2071–2072, 1941.
4. Johnson HN: Natural occurrence of tularemia in dogs used as a source of canine distemper virus. J Lab Clin Med 29:906–915, 1944.
5. Simpson WM: Tularemia. New York, Paul B Hoeber, 1929.
6. Calhoun EL, Mohr CO, Alford HI Jr: Dogs and other mammals as hosts of tularemia and of vector ticks in Arkansas. Am J Hyg 63:127–135, 1956.
7. Coffee WM, Miller J: Acute canine tularemia: a case report. J Am Vet Med Assoc 102:210–212. 1943.
8. Martone WJ, Marshall LW, Kaufmann AF, et al: Tularemia pneumonia in Washington, D.C.: a report of three cases with possible common-source exposures. JAMA 242:2315–2317, 1979.
9. Calhoun EL: Natural occurrence of tularemia in the Lone Star tick, Amblyomma americanum (Linn.), and in dogs in Arkansas. Am J Trop Med Hyg 3:360–366, 1954.
10. Markowitz LE, Hynes NA, de la Cruz P, et al: Tickborne tularemia: an outbreak of lymphadenopathy in children. JAMA 254:2922–2925, 1985.
11. Evans ME, McGee ZA, Hunter PT, et al: Tularemia and the tomcat. JAMA 246:1343, 1981.
12. Gallivan MVE, Davis WA, Garagusi VF, et al: Fatal cat-transmitted tularemia: demonstration of the organism in tissue. South Med J 73:240–242, 1980.
13. Miller LD, Montgomery EL: Human tularemia transmitted by bite of cat. J Am Vet Med Assoc 130:314, 1957.

14. Packer RM, Harrison LR, Matthews CF, et al: Tu-
    laremia associated with domestic cats—Georgia,
    New Mexico. *MMWR* 31:39–41, 1982.
15. Quenzer RW, Mostow SR, Emerson JK: Cat-bite
    tularemia. *JAMA* 238:1845, 1977.
16. Shaffer JH: Tularemia: a report of four cases with
    unusual contacts. *Ann Int Med* 18:72–80, 1943.
16a. Bevanger L, Maeland JA, Naess AI: Competitive
    enzyme immunoassay for antibodies to a 43,000-
    molecular weight *Francisella tularensis* outer
    membrane protein for the diagnosis of tularemia. *J
    Clin Microbiol* 27:922–926, 1989.
17. Murphy TM: Tularemia. *In* Rakel RE (ed): *Conn's
    Current Therapy 1986*. Philadelphia, WB Saunders
    Co, pp 99–100.
18. Sawyer WD, Dangerfield HG, Hogge AL, et al:
    Antibiotic prophylaxis and therapy of airborne tu-
    laremia. *Bacteriol Rev* 30:542–548, 1966.
19. Baker CN, Hollis DG, Thornsberry C: Antimicrobial
    susceptibility testing of *Francisella tularensis* with
    a modified Mueller-Hinton broth. *J Clin Microbiol*
    22:212–215, 1985.
20. Teutsch SM, Martone WJ, Brink EW, et al: Pneu-
    monic tularemia on Martha's Vineyard. *N Engl J
    Med* 301:826–828, 1979.
21. Evans ME: Tularemia. A 30-year experience with
    88 cases. *Medicine* 64:251–269, 1985.
22. Boyce JM: *Francisella tularensis* (tularemia). *In*
    Mandell GL, Douglas RG Jr, Bennett JE (eds): *Prin-
    ciples and Practice of Infectious Diseases*, ed 2.
    New York, John Wiley & Sons, 1985, pp 1290–
    1294.

61 CAT SCRATCH DISEASE*

Douglas J. Wear
Charles K. English
Andrew M. Margileth

ETIOLOGY

Cat scratch disease (CSD) also known as cat scratch fever, benign nonbacterial lymphadenitis, or Parinaud's oculoglandular syndrome (POGS) is a disease affecting people who have previously been in contact with cats. A gram-negative bacterium has been identified in lymph node,[1] skin,[2] and conjunctiva of CSD patients.[3] A similar bacterium has been found in feline lymph nodes.[4] The CSD bacillus is 0.2 μm wide, 0.5 to 2.5 μm long, forms long chains or filaments, branches (Y forms) (Fig. 61–1), stains gram-negative, and forms wall-defective variants both in human tissue and in culture.[5] The bacteria are more abundant in early lesions at cool sites such as the skin and conjunctiva. In culture it grows best in brain-heart infusion biphasic bottles at 32°C.[5] Colonies on blood agar are gray-white, glistening, convex, opaque, 1.5 mm wide with entire edges. Bacilli are nonhemolytic, motile, oxidase-positive, reduce nitrate to nitrite, produce urease, and are assacharolytic.

EPIDEMIOLOGY

Although CSD probably occurs worldwide, the authors have only confirmed ba-

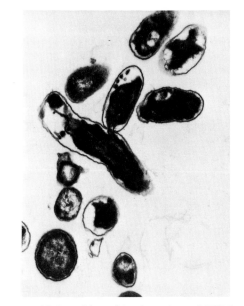

Figure 61–1. Y-shaped branching bacterium of CSD in culture (uranyl acetate and lead acetate; × 21,000).

cillus-infected cases in the United States, Canada, Japan, Europe, and Turkey. Men are more frequently infected, and the patients are usually less than 21 years old.[6] Approximately 5% of families are found to have CSD in several members; the onset of illness in each additional member usually begins within 3 weeks of the onset of that of the first member. CSD occurs more frequently in the cooler months in temperate climates. Although human contact with cats as with scratches, licking of wounds, bites, and kissing occurs, many other sources of human infection have been identified. Dog, goat, or squirrel scratches; scratches while handling crab claws and fish; horse contact; and splinter, barbed wire, thorn, and cactus wounds have been reported by the authors' patients.

*All material in this chapter is in the public domain, with the exception of any borrowed figures or tables.

The opinions or assertions contained herein are the private views of the authors and are not to be construed as official or as reflecting the views of the United States Navy, the United States Army, the United States Department of Defense, the Uniformed Services University of the Health Sciences, or the Armed Forces Institute of Pathology.

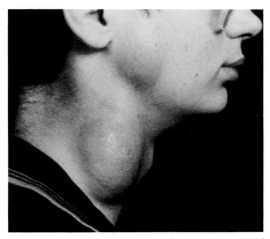

Figure 61–2. Enlarged lymph nodes in a person with CSD.

Animal handlers, including veterinarians and owners of kittens, are at higher risk.[6]

CLINICAL FINDINGS

CSD is characterized by dermal or conjunctival lesions, regional (usually single) or chronic (3 weeks to years) peripheral lymphadenopathy (Fig. 61–2). Other signs include fever, malaise, fatigue, myalgia, arthralgia, skin eruptions, weight loss, and occasionally hepatomegaly, splenomegaly, encephalitis, neuroretinitis, pleurisy, arthritis, and mediastinal and abdominal lymphadenopathy (Tables 61–1 and 61–2).[7] A case with unusual history follows.

Case History

A 20-year-old white woman had fever, chills, nausea, dizziness, and right cervical

Table 61–1. Cat Scratch Disease: Clinical Presentation of 1352 Patients, January 1957 to December 1987

CLINICAL FEATURES	ABNORMALITY (%)
Typical presentation	88.6
Inoculation lesion (skin, eye, mucous membrane)	59.7
Unusual manifestation	11.3
Parinaud's oculoglandular syndrome	6.0
Encephalopathy	2.2
Systemic disease, severe, chronic	1.7
Erythema nodosum	0.8
Atypical pneumonia	0.2
Breast tumor	0.1
Thrombocytopenic purpura	0.2

Table 61–2. Clinical Features in 1008 Patients with Cat Scratch Disease and a Positive Skin Test, April 1975 to December 1987

SYMPTOMS AND SIGNS	PERCENTAGE	DURATION (days)
Adenopathy	100.0	14–365
Adenopathy only	48.9	14–365
Fever (38.3° to 41.1° C)	31.9	1–60
Malaise/fatigue	30.0	1–21
Headache	13.1	1–7
Anorexia, emesis	14.2	3–30
Splenomegaly	11.5	7–30
Sore throat	8.4	1–5
Exanthem	4.6	5–17
Conjunctivitis	3.4	1–11
Parotid swelling	1.5	7–28

lymphadenopathy following a thorn scratch on her wrist while walking through the woods in France. Skin test for CSD was positive. Over the next 4 months she developed a persistent rash on her extremities; nodules over her tibia; an intermittent arthralgia of her hands and feet; and partial reduction in the size of her enlarged cervical lymph nodes. Seven months after initial scratch she began to have a recurrence of signs which consisted of severe headache that persisted for 11 days, myalgia, malaise, arthralgia, continued periodic rash, and recurrent right cervical lymphadenopathy. The patient was treated with trimethoprim-sulfamethoxazole and the headache resolved. Indirect fluorescent antibody staining determined an eightfold rise in antibody titers between sera collected before and after the onset of recurrent signs. Cultures of blood revealed wall-defective variants of CSD bacillus.

DIAGNOSIS

A clinical diagnosis of CSD in humans is made when three of four criteria have been met: (1) cat contact, with the presence of a scratch or a primary dermal or eye lesion, (2) a positive skin test using heated pus removed from a patient known to have CSD,[6] (3) regional lymphadenopathy with negative laboratory studies for other causes of lymphadenopathy, and (4) characteristic histologic changes in a biopsied lymph node. Presence of the bacilli in Warthin-Starry silver impregnation-stained sections histologically proves CSD. In the research laboratory, the diagnosis can also be made by a fourfold rise in antibody titer to the CSD bacillus.

Most of the patients in a recent study of CSD had antibody titers of 1:32 or greater.[5] Three had fourfold or greater rises in antibody titers. Antibody titers in ten healthy volunteers ranged from 1:2 to 1:16.

PATHOLOGIC FINDINGS

The histologic reactions in CSD-affected people extends from anergy to hyperergy. In the anergic patient, bacilli are massed in vessel walls (Fig. 61–3). The walls are widened and eosinophilic. The endothelial cells are swollen, and the lumen may be obliterated. On electron microscopy, the bacilli are in the collagen bundles, separating and in parallel with the collagen fibers. As the lesion develops, there is karyorrhexis, necrosis, and neutrophil and macrophage invasion to form abscesses. Bacilli may completely fill these macrophages. Other macrophages ring the abscess. In the hyperergic patient, macrophages mass around a few bacilli (probably in dendritic cells). Central karyorrhexis and occasional neutrophils appear. At this stage, both types of lesions appear similar and progress to stellate granulomas with central suppuration and, finally, central caseation necrosis. Bacilli are centered in necrosis. Lesions with bacilli are found in peripheral lymph nodes, skin, con-

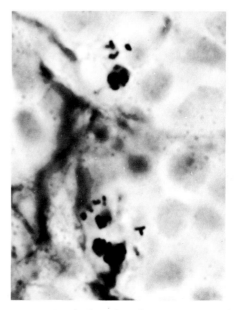

Figure 61–4. Similar branching bacteria in macrophage found in a lymph node of cat (Modified Dieterli's method; × 1400.) (From Kirkpatrick CE, Whiteley HE: *J Infect Dis* 156:690–691, 1987. Reprinted with permission.)

junctiva, liver, abdominal lymph nodes, and spleen.

In the cat, bacilli indistinguishable from CSD bacilli have filled macrophages, and were also found in vascular endothelial cells and free along collagen fibers in mandibular lymph nodes, the architecture of which was obliterated by an extensive proliferation of lymphocytes. In one cat, the process was mistakenly diagnosed as lymphoma (Fig. 61–4).[4] Similar bacilli have been seen in dilated ducts of the parotid gland of a cat that transmitted CSD to the owner. Experimental infection in the armadillo reproduces the early lesions seen in human skin. Bacilli not only fill macrophages at the inoculation site but occur in the dermal collagen and can be cultured from the lesions.

THERAPY

The majority of infections resolve spontaneously in 2 to 4 months. Surgical excision removes the offending bacilli and may lead to a definite diagnosis but is NOT necessary in patients with typical case histories. In culture CSD-bacilli are susceptible to cefoxitin, cefotaxime, gentamicin, and amikacin; are partially sensitive to trimethoprim-sulfamethoxazole; and are resistant to penicillin, ampicillin, erythromycin, tetracycline,

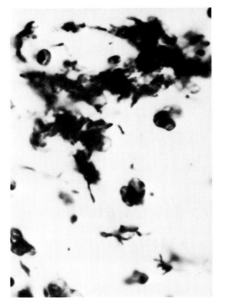

Figure 61–3. Branching, filamentous, and clumped bacilli of CSD around vessel and along sinuses in lymph node of a veterinarian (Warthin-Starry method; × 1200.)

chloramphenicol, clindamycin, and cephalothin.[5] See Appendix 14 for dosages.

References

1. Wear DJ, Margileth AM, Hadfield TL, et al: Cat scratch disease: a bacterial infection. *Science* 221:1403–1405, 1983.
2. Margileth AM, Wear DJ, Hadfield TL, et al: Cat scratch disease. Bacteria in skin at the primary inoculation site. *JAMA* 252:928–931, 1984.
3. Wear DJ, Malaty RH, Zimmerman LE, et al: Cat scratch disease bacilli in the conjunctiva of patients with Parinaud's oculoglandular syndrome. *Ophthalmology* 92:1282–1287, 1985.
4. Kirkpatrick CE, Whiteley HE: Argyrophilic, intracellular bacteria in the lymph node of a cat: cat-scratch disease bacilli? *J Infect Dis* 156:690–691, l987.
5. English CK, Wear DJ, Margileth AM, et al: Cat scratch disease: isolation and culture of the bacterial agent. *JAMA* 259:1347–1352, 1988.
6. Margileth AM: Cat scratch disease: a therapeutic dilemma. *Vet Clin North Am* 17:91–103, 1987.
7. Margileth AM, Wear DJ, English CK: Systemic cat scratch disease: report of 23 patients with prolonged or recurrent severe bacterial infection. *J Infect Dis* 155:390–402, 1987.

FUNGAL AND ALGAL INFECTIONS

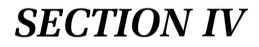

SECTION IV

62 LABORATORY DIAGNOSIS OF FUNGAL AND ALGAL INFECTIONS

Spencer S. Jang
Ernst L. Biberstein

Specific diagnosis of fungal and algal infections in animals requires laboratory procedures that include direct microscopic examination and culture, frequently supported by serologic tests. Many such direct examinations and primary cultures and some serologic tests are now well within the scope of in-office diagnostic procedures for a veterinary practice. Currently, the development of improved methods for mycologic diagnosis is directed at rapid procedures utilizing prepackaged identification sets and reagents as well as serologic kits. In a high proportion of such cases, confirmation by a specialty laboratory will still be necessary to establish a definitive diagnosis.

SPECIMENS FOR LABORATORY DIAGNOSIS

A satisfactory sample should be representative of the focus of infection and of an adequate size to permit direct examination and culture. Except in systemic infections suggesting fungemia and requiring blood culture, samples should be obtained from the site of infection as indicated by lesions, signs, or symptoms. Because systemic mycoses are usually acquired via the respiratory tract, lung tissue or airway exudates are preferred samples.[1] In certain disseminated mycotic infections, urine may also be an appropriate specimen to culture.

Sample Collection

Surface antisepsis, when feasible, aids in the collection of uncontaminated samples and thereby ensures a significant result.

Swabs are of limited value in fungal isolation. If no alternative collection method is available, any swabs used for direct smears preferably should not consist of cotton as recovery rates are poor and cotton fibers may be mistaken for hyphae by inexperienced observers.[2] Transport media should not be used routinely for shipment of swabs or other specimens intended for mycological study.[2]

Blood for cultures can be collected in conventional blood culture bottles (Becton Dickinson Microbiology Systems, Cockeysville, MD) or special culture systems (see Isolation). Blood for culture, about 8 ml, may also be collected in yellow-stoppered vacuum tubes (Vacutainer, Sherwood Medical, St. Louis, MO) containing 0.05% Liquoid.[3] Before venipuncture, the skin must be sterilized by swabbing with 70% alcohol followed by 2% iodine. A fresh needle is used for transfer of blood, 1 ml per 10 ml of culture medium, from syringe to the culture bottle.

Urine is best taken by percutaneous cystocentesis, which ensures a sample uncontaminated by bacterial or fungal flora in the lower genitourinary tract (see Chapter 11).

When collecting skin scrapings for dermatophyte culture, briefly clean the lesion, particularly the periphery with 70% alcohol; iodine is harmful to dermatophytes. Scrapings are obtained with a scalpel or the edge of a microscope slide from the marginal, most active portion of the ringworm lesion. Use of a Wood's lamp may identify hairs infected with certain dermatophyte species. Such hairs are then plucked with forceps for culture. Nails are collected by clipping. The surface of heavily keratinized structures is scraped away for access to deeper portions. Sterile water or saline may be used to prepare a site if yeast infection is suspected.[3]

The surface of skin pustules, nodules, vesicles, etc. is disinfected and aspiration is done with sterile needle and syringe. A biopsy may be required if fungi fail to grow from an aspirate or scraping and should include normal tissue along with portions from all zones of the lesion.[3] Opened skin lesions are not disinfected or cleaned, as such procedures may remove or kill the organisms.

Fluids and contents of abscesses are collected through aspiration by needle and syringe. Large volumes, adequate for centrifugation, are best. Any granules should be included and characterized. Bone marrow is likewise sampled by needle and syringe or core needle biopsy. At least 3 ml of CSF is obtained via lumbar or cisternal puncture. For lung sampling, a transtracheal or bronchial wash or bronchial brushing is done.

Necrotic material or curettings and other surgically collected material should be handled aseptically pending examination and culture. Corneal lesions are sampled by scraping with a sterile spatula (see Fig. 13–1). Slide preparation and culturing are done at the site and time of collection.

Transportation and Preservation

For referral to a diagnostic laboratory, tissue and fluid samples are shipped by the most expeditious route in secure, sturdy, leakproof containers. Accompanying information on the type of sample submitted and any clinical and other circumstances will assist the laboratory in selecting appropriate methods of processing the submittal, including media, conditions of incubation, and safety precautions.

Specimens that cannot be promptly processed are generally refrigerated but not frozen for periods up to 12 to 15 hours.[1] Refrigeration may delay proliferation of slow-growing fungi for 1 to 2 days. Aspergillus spp. and zygomycetes are sensitive to refrigeration.[2] If a specimen suspected of harboring a zygomycete cannot be promptly cultured, overnight storage at room temperature in a bacteriologic transport medium is permissible.[2] Some fungi have been re-

covered from specimens up to 2 weeks in transit, but this type of delay is not recommended.[4]

Urine specimens may be kept under refrigeration for no longer than 18 to 24 hours prior to culture. Most bacteria and yeasts will multiply in urine kept at room temperature. A Urine C & S Transport Kit (Becton Dickinson, Rutherford, NJ) delays growth of bacteria and Candida albicans for up to 48 hours at room temperature.

CSF and blood cultures, if subject to delay in processing, are held at room temperature or in an incubator at 30°C. The presence of protein and carbohydrates in CSF contributes to its qualities as a maintenance medium.[1] Fluids from serous cavities and joints, bone marrow samples, and vaginal swabs may be refrigerated 18 to 24 hours if necessary.

Nasal curettings and excised polyps may be divided between sterile containers for culturing and jars of 10% buffered formalin for histologic preparation aimed at detection of rhinosporidiosis (Fig. 62–1). Impression smears of nasal tissue should be made prior to fixation of specimens (see Fig. 70–1).

Skin scrapings, nails, and hairs can be collected in a clean envelope for mailing. Skin scrapings also can be held in place between glass slides taped at both ends. Such samples should not be kept in tightly

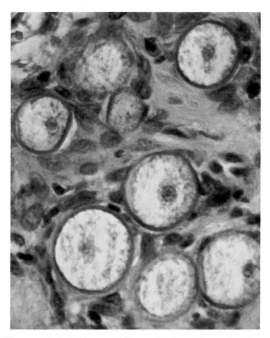

Figure 62–1. Rhinosporidium. Section of nasal polyp, dog. Thick-walled proliferating spherules (sporangia) (H and E; × 500).

sealed containers, since resulting accumulation of moisture can lead to overgrowth by saprophytes.

PROCESSING OF SPECIMENS

The complete processing of specimens involves three steps. In the following sections some of the procedures will be considered with particular reference to their feasibility as in-office tests. No special equipment, beyond that required for basic clinical bacteriology, is needed for fungal diagnosis. For incubation purposes, an undisturbed area where room temperature (about 25°C) remains fairly constant is adequate. A hand lens (8 to 10×) or a dissecting microscope is helpful in the early recognition of fungal colonies.

Direct Microscopic Examination

The search for diagnostically significant fungal structures may involve preparation of stained or unstained wet mounts, fixed stained smears, and histologic sections. Some of these techniques are simple and rapid and may provide the clinician with a presumptive or even definitive diagnosis and a timesaving guide to therapy.

Wet Mounts. Specimen material may be suspended on a slide in saline, water, or, preferably, 10% KOH, which clears the preparation of tissue admixtures, leaving fungal elements intact. Examination should begin under low power (100×) and with subdued light, with the condenser racked down to achieve maximum contrast. When structures suggestive of fungal elements are seen, higher magnification (400×) is used for confirmation.

The KOH digestion method is used universally in preparation of cutaneous samples suspected of harboring dermatophytes (see Chapter 64). The hair or skin scraping to be examined is placed into a drop of 10% KOH on a clean slide (Fig. 62–2A). The crusty material is teased with forceps or a dissecting needle and covered with a coverslip. This preparation is passed over an open flame several times, but care must be taken not to boil the mixture. This slide is examined immediately for the presence of arthrospores or fungal chains embedded in the

material (Fig. 62–2B and C). If no organisms are initially observed, the slide is reexamined in 30 minutes.

India ink (Pelikan) or nigrosin (1% aqueous), when mixed on a slide with fluids containing *Cryptococcus neoformans*, provides a dark background outlining the large capsules surrounding the yeast cells (see Fig. 67–6A). Less than 50% of culture-positive human CSF samples are proved to be infected by this method.[5]

Less generally available useful methods of unstained wet-mount study include phase microscopy, which improves the visibility of fungal structures against a background of tissue debris, and fluorescent microscopy, where a specimen is prepared by mixing with 1 to 2 drops of 10% KOH-0.5% calcofluor white (Difco, Detroit, MI) on a slide. The specimen is examined on a fluorescent microscope equipped with a 365-nm exciter filter and a barrier filter that will transmit light at 410 nm. The fungal wall will fluoresce brilliantly.

Fixed Smears. Gram stain (Difco, Detroit, MI) is of limited use in differentiating fungi because most fungi stain gram positive or unpredictably, and it produces distortion in cell morphology. Yeasts often can be detected because they retain the primary crystal violet stain (Fig. 62–3). Fungal cell walls often appear as unstained halos. The usefulness of the Gram stain is generally limited to smears in which *Candida*, *Malassezia* (Fig. 62–4), *Geotrichum*, *Trichosporum*, or the yeast form of *Sporothrix* spp. (Fig. 62–5) is suspected.

Romanowsky-type stains such as Wright, Giemsa, Leishman, and Diff-Quick (American Scientific Products, McGraw Park, IL), will stain many fungi, especially yeasts, and are the stains of choice for the tissue phase of *Histoplasma capsulatum* (see Fig. 66–7). As with the Gram stain, fungal cell walls remain unstained by these procedures.

A special fungal stain applicable to direct smears is a modified periodic acid-Schiff (PAS) stain, which colors mycotic structures and some other extraneous and tissue components selectively red.[6] It is beyond the scope of most routine office laboratory work but should be obtainable as a service through any histology laboratory.

Fluorescent antibody (FA) microscopy has had some limited application in mycologic diagnosis. At present, no FA diagnostic re-

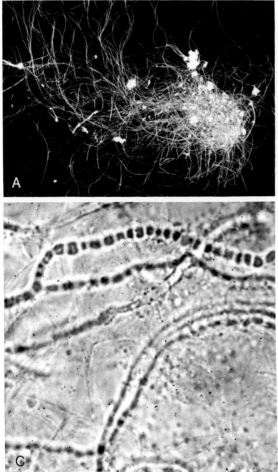

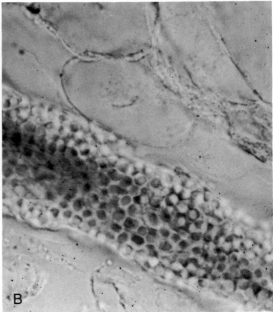

Figure 62–2. Unstained KOH preparation (A) of hairs from a crusty skin lesion under 40× magnification with (B) arthrospores along or on the hair shaft or (C) chains of arthrospores embedded in crusty material.

agents are available commercially and no diagnostic services utilize this approach.[6]

Histology. Stained sections from biopsy and necropsy specimens often provide critical diagnostic information on mycotic infections. Routine H and E stain permits detection of the tissue phase of dimorphic fungi causing systemic mycoses (coccidioidomycosis, histoplasmosis, blastomycosis, cryptococcosis) and with filamentous fungi may demonstrate hyphae in tissue, often providing an indication as to their septate or nonseptate nature and thereby helping with their classification. More specific for fungi are the Grocott-Gomori methenamine silver method, which stains fungal structures brownish black against a pale green background, and a number of PAS stains, which make mycotic elements appear dark red against a contrasting background, depending on the counterstain.[7] Many laboratories use H and E as a counterstain, which permits better pathologic characterization of the lesion than do other procedures.

Isolation

Inoculation of a suitably prepared specimen on an appropriate medium is required. Preparation may include centrifugation of fluid samples, grinding of biopsied and other tissues, surface sterilization of necropsy specimens by searing, repeated washing of granules from mycetomas with saline, or filtration of CSF and blood. Scrapings, swabs, and blood may be inoculated directly without further preparation.

Since many pathogenic fungi, when propagated on agar media, constitute airborne health hazards, laboratories often prefer tubes and bottles over petri plates for isolation purposes.[3] If plates are used, they should be securely taped. All examinations of cultures producing aerial mycelium

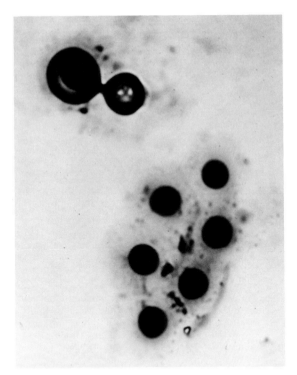

Figure 62–3. *C. neoformans.* Nasal granuloma of a cat. Budding forms, *top center,* hazy zone around the six cells below represent capsules (Gram stain; × 2000).

should be carried out in biologic safety cabinets. Most fungi grow on media used routinely in microbiologic diagnosis. These media should be used when the sample is obtained from an uncontaminated site, that is, one that has no resident flora and is not exposed to the external environment such as CNS, internal organ, or joints. Samples originating from cutaneous sources or mucous membranes that harbor such flora are cultured on selective media that may contain broad-spectrum antibacterial and antimycotic agents (Table 62–1) for the suppression of bacteria and nonpathogenic fungi, respec-

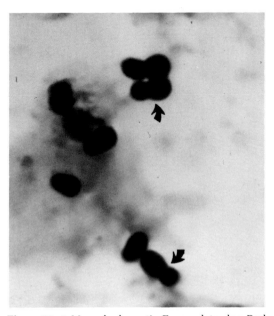

Figure 62–4. *M. pachydermatis.* Ear exudate, dog. Budding yeast cells (*arrows*) have "shoe print" appearance (Gram stain; × 2000).

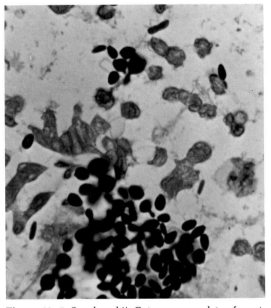

Figure 62–5. *S. schenckii.* Cutaneous exudate of a cat. Note budding yeasts, oval, rod, and cigar-shaped forms (Gram stain; × 1000).

Table 62–1. Isolation Media for Fungi

MEDIUM (COMMERCIAL SOURCE)	SELECTIVE FEATURES	PRINCIPAL USE/LIMITATIONS IN MYCOLOGIC DIAGNOSIS
Blood agar (Remel, Lenexa, KS)	Highly nutritious for most fungi	General purpose, converts some dimorphic fungi to yeast form./ Noninhibitory, nonselective, easily overgrown.
Blood/MacConkey agar (Remel, Lenexa, KS)	MacConkey inhibits gram-positive and some gram-negative bacteria	General purpose, blood agar portion for fungal isolation./ Reduced surface area, insufficient to obtain isolated colonies.
Inhibitory mold agar (Remel, Lenexa, KS)	Gentamicin and chloramphenicol for bacterial suppression	General purpose./ Not for dermatophytes.
Sabouraud dextrose agar with inhibitors (Mycosel, BBL, Cockeysville, MD, or Mycobiotic, Difco Lab, Detroit, MI)	Low pH, modest nutritional quality, chloramphenicol and cycloheximide inhibit bacteria and some fungi	Isolation from contaminated environments./ Cycloheximide inhibits *Cryptococcus, Aspergillus, Scedosporium apiospermum (Pseudallescheria boydii)*, some *Candida* spp. Chloramphenicol inhibits some yeasts.
Dematophyte test medium DTM (Fungassay, Pitman-Moore, Washington Crossing, NJ)	Gentamicin, tetracycline, and cycloheximide are inhibitors. Glucose and phenol red are indicators.	Isolation of dermatophytes, which turn the yellow medium to red in 48 hours./ Not for sporulation, may produce atypical colonical growth; natural pigmentation obscured. Nondermatophytes turn yellow medium to red eventually.
Rapid sporulation medium RSM (marketed as DERM DUET with DTM in a two-compartment plate by Bactilab, Mountain View, CA)	Cycloheximide and chloramphenicol are inhibitors. Glucose and bromothymol blue are indicators.	For dermatophytes, which turn medium blue-green early. Prompt conidial and pigment development permit identification./ Color change of RSM not as intense as with DTM with some dermatophytes.

tively. A low pH (≤ 6.0) of the medium may further limit bacterial overgrowth. Yeasts can be selectively recovered from specimens heavily contaminated with bacteria by propagation on a medium of pH 3.5 to 4.0.[3] Fungal cultures are optimally incubated at 25° to 30°C.

Blood can be collected either directly by IV catheter or via syringe into a suitable medium. Blood cultures are preferably done in Bi-Phasic medium (Becton Dickinson Microbiology Systems, Cockeysville, MD) or Isolator system (E. I. Dupont Inc., Wilmington, DE).[8] Bi-Phasic bottle contains 50 ml of brain heart infusion broth and brain heart infusion agar. Bi-Phasic bottle is inoculated with 10 ml of blood, vented, and incubated in an upright position. After daily examination, it is tilted so that the broth floods the agar surface. The Isolator system has improved the number and rate of fungal isolations from blood.[9] It involves lysis and centrifugation of 10 ml of blood. The supernatant is removed from the upper stopper,

and the concentrate is removed from the bottom stopper and plated.

Identification

Microscopic morphology of fungal reproductive structures is the most helpful criterion for identification. Other criteria are macroscopic colonial features under different conditions of incubation, nutritional and metabolic properties, antigenic characteristics, and pathogenicity for experimental animals.

Agar cultures are examined daily during the first 2 weeks of incubation and twice weekly thereafter. Some common zygomycetes (*Mucor, Rhizopus* spp.) grow rapidly and abundantly, filling a tube or petri dish within 2 or 3 days. Fruiting bodies may be visible as black specks in the colorless mycelium (Fig. 62–6). Aerial mycelium is grossly less prominent but more intensely pigmented by the presence of fruiting struc-

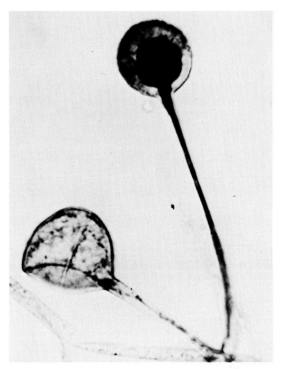

Figure 62–6. Mucor in culture. Sporangia form on sporangiophores, nonseptate, broad hyphae (LPCB; × 500).

tures with *Aspergillus* and *Penicillium* spp. (Fig. 62–7). Some fungi produce soluble pigment that diffuses through the medium (e.g., *Microsporum canis*). In others, pigment is

confined to parts of the organism and may be best observed either on the surface or on the reverse side of the colony. The colony surface varies according to mycelial growth patterns from smooth ("glabrous") to powdery, velvety, and cottony. Yeasts, which form no or little (pseudo)mycelium, produce mucoid, creamy, pasty, or waxy colonies.

Low-power (25 to 50 ×) microscopy helps in early detection of mycelial growth and such diagnostic features as macroconidia and microconidia of dermatophytes (Figs. 62–8, 62–9, 62–10). Once colonial growth is established, identification is based largely on microscopic examination for hyphal characteristics—septate vs. nonseptate, pigmented (Fig. 62–11) vs. nonpigmented—and conidia and their supporting structures. This obviously involves opening of a culture vessel and should be done only by trained, experienced personnel and under conditions where exposure of people and animals and contamination of the environment can be avoided.

At the office laboratory level, it is feasible to make "teased preparations" or scotch tape lactophenol cotton blue mounts (LPCB)[1] from mold cultures by using appropriate precautions (see Appendix 12). Diagnostic features are usually better preserved in their natural interrelationships in scotch tape mounts (Figs. 62–12 and 62–13). In the absence of a laminar-flow hood, such attempts

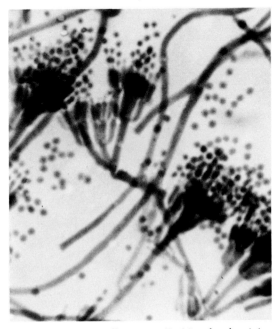

Figure 62–7. *Penicillium* sp. Fruiting heads giving brushlike appearance (LPCB; × 500).

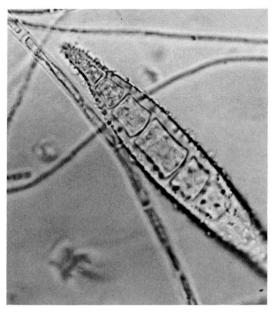

Figure 62–8. *Microsporum canis.* Rough and thick-walled multicellular spindle-shaped macroconidia. Note curved, pointed ends (LPCB; × 500).

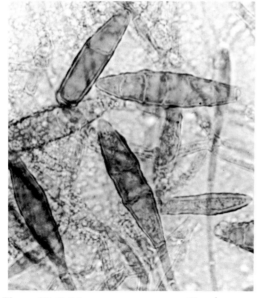

Figure 62–9. *Microsporum gypseum.* Numerous multicellular, fairly thin-walled macroconidia with rounded ends (LPCB; × 500).

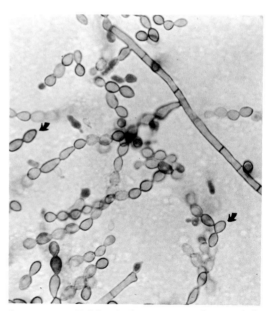

Figure 62–11. *Xylohypha bantiana* in culture. (*Cladosporium trichoides*). Oval-shaped conidia occurring in chains. Note dematiacous (dark-pigmented) appearance of some conidia and mycelium (*arrows*) (LPCB; × 500).

should be restricted to macroscopically positive dermatophyte cultures.

The slide culture procedure[1] probably exceeds the capabilities of most veterinary practices and should be left to clinical lab-

oratories. This procedure permits study of undisturbed fungal structures by utilizing LPCB (Figs. 62–14 and 62–15).

The germ-tube test allows rapid differentiation of *Candida albicans* (see Chapter 72) from most of the other, usually nonpathogenic, *Candida* spp. Serum, 0.5 to 1 ml, is inoculated lightly with suspect growth and incubated at 35°C for 2 to 3 hours. A drop of the suspension is then examined micro-

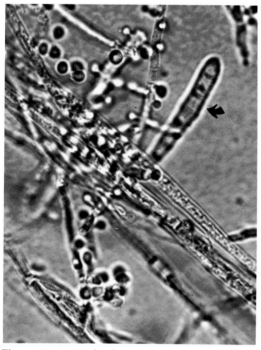

Figure 62–10. *Trichophyton mentagrophytes.* Spherical microconidia and one thin-walled, multicellular, cigar-shaped macroconidium (*arrow*) (LPCB; × 500).

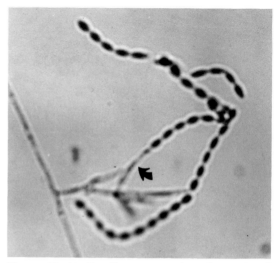

Figure 62–12. *Paecilomyces* sp. in culture. Ovoid chains of conidia attached to a phialide (*arrow*) that is usually tapered (not visible) (LPCB; × 500).

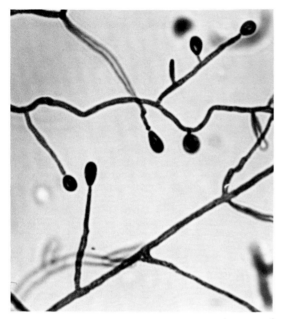

Figure 62–13. *Scedosporium apiospermum* (= asexual stage of *Pseudallescheria boydii*) in culture. Single elliptical conidia attached to tips of conidiophores arising along the hyphae (LPCB; × 500).

scopically (100× and 400×) for the presence of germ tubes sprouting from yeast cells of *C. albicans* (Fig. 62–16).

Commonly used differential media include Czapek agar (Difco Laboratories,

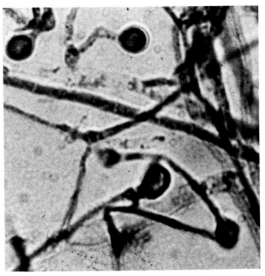

Figure 62–15. *Blastomyces dermatitidis* in culture. One-celled conidia on short conidiophores, "lollipop" appearance (LPCB; × 500).

Detroit, MI) for the differentiation of *Aspergillus* spp.; cornmeal agar for the demonstration of chlamydospores in *C. albicans* and their absence in most other *Candida* spp.; and *Trichophyton* agars (Remel, Lenexa, KS) for the identification of *Trichophyton* spp. by their growth factor needs.

For definitive identification of the dimorphic fungi *Coccidioides immitis*, *Histoplasma capsulatum*, and *Blastomyces dermatitidis* antisera are commercially available (ImmunoMycologics, Norman, OK) for use in agar immunodiffusion exoantigen

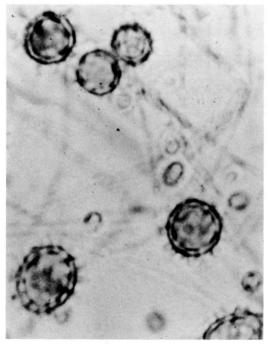

Figure 62–14. *Histoplasma capsulatum* in culture. Tuberculate macroconidia (LPCB; × 1000).

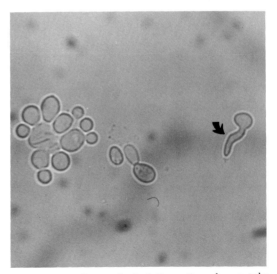

Figure 62–16. Germ tube test. Formation of germ tube (*arrow*) characteristic of *Candida albicans*. Blastoconidia on left. (Wet mount; × 1000).

tests. The antigen is prepared from an extract of mycelial growth.

Among miniaturized prepackaged identification sets for yeast and *Prototheca* isolates are API Yeast-Ident and API 20C (API, Plainview, NY) and Uni-Yeast-Tek plate (Flow, McLean, VA).[10] All rely on tests that are scored to yield a single number, which is listed in a code book and translates into a yeast species. Identification can be completed within 4 hours to several days and more conveniently and generally more rapidly than by conventional methods.

SEROLOGY

Reagents designed to detect antigens and antibodies in body fluids are becoming commercially available in increasing numbers. An antigen detection kit, the *Cryptococcus neoformans* latex agglutination test (Meridian Diagnostics, Cincinnati, OH), has been adapted for use in office laboratories (see Chapter 67 and Appendix 8). For a discussion of serologic testing of particular fungal infections, see the respective chapters.

References

1. Koneman EW, Roberts GD: *Practical Laboratory Mycology.* Baltimore, Williams & Wilkins, 1985.
2. Lennette EH, Balows A, Hausler WJ Jr, et al: *Manual of Clinical Microbiology.* Washington, DC, American Society for Microbiology, 1985.
3. McGinnis MR: *Laboratory Handbook of Medical Mycology.* New York, Academic Press, 1980.
4. Sarosi GA, Armstrong D, George RB, et al: Laboratory diagnosis of mycotic and specific fungal infections. *Am Rev Respir Dis* 132:1373–1379, 1985.
5. McGowan KL: Practical approaches to diagnosing fungal infections in immunocompromised patients. *Clin Microbiol Newslett* 9(5):33–36, 1987.
6. Haley LD, Trandel J, Coyle MB: Practical methods for culture and identification of fungi in the clinical microbiology laboratory. *CUMITECH 11.* Washington, DC, American Society for Microbiology, 1980.
7. Sheehan DC, Hrapchak BB: *Theory and Practice of Histotechnology.* Detroit, Lipshaw, 1980.
8. Billie J, Edson RS, Roberts GD: Clinical evaluation of the lysis-centrifugation blood culture system for the detection of fungemia and comparison with a conventional biphasic broth blood culture system. *J Clin Microbiol* 19:126–128, 1984.
9. Henry NK, McLimans CA, Wright AJ, et al: Microbiological and clinical evaluation of the isolator lysis centrifugation blood culture tube. *J Clin Microbiol* 17:864–869, 1983.
10. Salkin IF, Land GA, Hurd NJ, et al: Evaluation of YEASTIdent and UNI-YEAST-TEK yeast identification systems. *J Clin Microbiol* 25:624–627, 1987.

63

ANTIFUNGAL CHEMOTHERAPY
Craig E. Greene

SYSTEMIC ANTIFUNGALS

Table 63–1 summarizes the properties of the systemic antifungal drugs and the circumstances of their use. Table 63–2 lists the drug dosages. See Chapters 64 to 75 for further discussions of their clinical applications.

Griseofulvin

This orally administered antifungal drug is produced by *Penicillium griseofulvum*. It inhibits protein and nucleic acid synthesis of fungi, and eventually causes destruction of intracellular organelles. The absorption of griseofulvin from the GI tract is facilitated by the addition of fat to the diet and has also been improved by the production of microsized and ultramicrosized drug formulations. It is effective against infections caused by dermatophytes but not yeast infections.

Griseofulvin is deposited in the epidermal layers of the skin and dermal appendages as they are formed. Several weeks of therapy are required for complete drug distribution throughout cell layers and for inhibition of fungal growth. Griseofulvin is effective against all dermatophytes, and resistance rarely develops during the course of therapy. The dose recommended by manufacturers of microsized products (11 to 22 mg/kg/day) is much less than that currently recommended for use in dogs or cats (see Tables 63–2, 64–6, and Appendix 14). The manufacturer's dosage rate did not account for the more rapid hepatic clearance of the drug in animals.[1] Therapy in skin infections should be continued until fungal cultures are negative or for at least 2 weeks following resolution of signs and for at least 5 months for onychomycosis. Refer to Chapter 64 for more information concerning its clinical applications.

With the exception of nausea, vomiting, and diarrhea, signs of toxicity of griseofulvin are relatively minimal. Anemia and panleukopenia with bone marrow suppression, anorexia, dehydration, edema of the skin and mucosae, pruritus, and ataxia have been noted in griseofulvin-treated cats.[1] Occasionally these side effects have been fatal, and they may be responses to high-dose, long-term therapy or may be idiosyncratic reactions since they have not been consistently reproduced in experimental cats.[2] Griseofulvin may interfere with spermatogenesis and produce teratogenic and mutagenic effects in a number of species. Its use is contraindicated in pregnant animals.

Iodides

A solution of 20% sodium or potassium iodide has been given orally to treat cutaneous sporotrichosis (also see Chapter 69). The mechanism of action is uncertain; this drug is not directly toxic to *Sporothrix* in vitro. Either drug is less toxic than amphotericin B, which should be reserved for second choice. Iodism, manifested clinically as dermal eruption with hair loss, may occur as a result of therapy.

Amphotericin B

Amphotericin B (AMB) is a lipophilic polyene, isolated from *Streptomyces nodosus*, that binds to sterols present in the cell

Table 63–1. Systemic Antifungal Drugs[a]

GENERIC NAME (TRADE NAME)	ROUTE OF ADMINISTRATION	CLINICAL FORMULATION	SUSCEPTIBLE ORGANISMS (MOST TO LEAST)
Griseofulvin (Fulvicin, Grisactin)	PO	Capsules (125, 250 mg) Tablets (500 mg) Suspension (125 mg/ml)	Dermatophytes, *Sporothrix*
Sodium or potassium iodide	PO	Solution (20%)	*Sporothrix*
Amphotericin B (Fungizone)	IV	Vial (50 mg lyophilized)	*Blastomyces, Histoplasma, Cryptococcus, Coccidioides,* Mucoraceae, *Candida, Aspergillus*
Flucytosine (Ancobon)	PO	Capsules (250, 500 mg)	*Cryptococcus, Candidia, Cladosporium,* phaeohyphomycosis organisms[b]
Miconazole (Monistat I.V.)	IV	Ampules (10 mg/ml in 20 ml)	*Coccidioides, Candida, Histoplasma, Cryptococcus, Aspergillus, Blastomyces*
Ketoconazole (Nizoral)	PO	Oral suspension (100 mg/5 ml) Tablets (200 mg)	*Candida, Coccidioides, Histoplasma, Blastomyces, Cryptococcus, Sporothrix, Aspergillus,* dermatophytes
Itraconazole (R51,211)	PO, IV	NA	*Aspergillus, Sporothrix, Candida, Cryptococcus, Blastomyces, Coccidioides*
Fluconazole (UK 49,858)	PO	NA	*Histoplasma, Cryptococcus, Candida*
Vinbunazole (BAY-n-7133)	PO	NA	*Aspergillus, Sporothrix*
ICI 195,739	PO	NA	*Blastomyces, Candida, Cryptococcus,* dermatophytes

[a]PO = oral, IV = intravenous, NA = not available for clinical use.
[b]See Table 74–1 for a listing of the genera causing phaeohyphomycosis.

membranes of eukaryotic organisms and causes increased permeability and leakage of nutrients and electrolytes. AMB has a greater binding affinity for ergosterol, the major sterol of fungal cell membranes, than for cholesterol, which is present in mammalian host cells. Because it is poorly absorbed across the GI mucosa or skin, AMB must be given IV for the treatment of systemic mycoses. IV preparations contain lyophilized AMB combined with deoxycholate and buffer in a colloidal state. Occasionally, the drug is used for topical therapy of mycotic disease.

Pharmacology. In vivo, AMB appears to be strongly bound to lipoprotein sites on cell membranes, as serum concentration is relatively low compared with the amount of drug administered. Most of the drug is metabolized locally at tissue sites, and lesser amounts are excreted in the urine. Following a single dose, small amounts of the drug are found in the urine daily for up to 3 weeks and in tissues for longer periods. Because of this unusual metabolic processing of the drug, there is little increase in serum con-

centration even in the presence of renal insufficiency. AMB penetrates relatively well into most inflammatory exudates and tissues, with the exception of normal or inflamed meninges, vitreous humor, and amniotic fluid.

Indications. The fungal organisms affected by AMB are listed in Table 63–1. Zygomycetes (Mucoraceae) are variably susceptible, and *Aspergillus* is usually resistant. In vitro studies have suggested that drugs such as minocycline and flucytosine, when given concomitantly, reduce the concentration of AMB needed to inhibit growth of *Candida* and *Cryptococcus neoformans*. Similarly, rifampin potentiates the effect of AMB on *Aspergillus, Candida,* and *Histoplasma capsulatum.* AMB may alter the permeability of the cell membrane, enabling these other drugs to enter the cell and disrupt fungal metabolism.

Until recently, AMB has been the first line of therapy in the treatment of rapidly progressive or disseminated deep mycotic infections. Resistance rarely, if ever, develops during treatment; however, relapses may oc-

Table 63–2. Dosages of Systemically Administered Antifungal Drugs[a]

GENERIC NAME	SPECIES	ROUTE	DOSE[b] (mg/kg)	INTERVAL (hours)	DURATION (weeks)
Griseofulvin (microsized)	B	PO	50–150[c]	24	6
	B	PO	25–75[c]	12	6
Sodium iodide	D	PO	20–40	8–12	4–6
	C	PO	20	24	4–6
Amphotericin B	D	IV	0.5	48[d]	6–8[e]
	C	IV	0.25	48[d]	4–6[f]
Flucytosine[g]	B	PO	25–50	6	6
	B	PO	50–65	8	6
Ketoconazole	B	PO	5–15	12	8–12
	D	PO	10–30	24	8–12
	C	PO	10–15	24–48	8–12
Ketoconazole and amphotericin B	D	PO	10–30	24[h]	8–12
		IV	0.25	48	6–8[e]
Itraconazole	B	PO	5–10	12–24	8–12
Fluconazole	D	PO	2.5–5	24	8–12

[a]B = dog and cat, D = dog, C = cat, PO = oral, IV = intravenous.
[b]Dose per administration at specified interval, expressed as mg/kg unless otherwise stated. See text for an explanation of which dose to use when more than one dose level is indicated.
[c]Ultramicrosized formulations require 50% or less of this dose. Also see Table 64–6 and Appendix 14.
[d]Often given on a Monday-Wednesday-Friday schedule.
[e]Given until a cumulative dose of 8 to 12 mg/kg is reached for dogs.
[f]Given until a cumulative dose of approximately 4 mg/kg is reached for cats.
[g]Only given in combination with AMB, except for treatment of phaeohyphomycosis.
[h]Given until a cumulative dose of 4 to 6 mg/kg is reached.

cur when drug therapy is discontinued. Newer drugs such as ketoconazole (KTZ), added to the treatment regimen to control relapses and to facilitate antifungal activity, are not routinely recommended as substitutes for AMB. However, KTZ has become an adjunctive mode of therapy in the treatment of systemic mycoses.

Administration and Dosage. AMB, which is insoluble in water, is prepared as an IV solution by forming a colloidal dispersion with sodium deoxycholate. Even the undiluted powder should be stored in the dark because of inactivation by sunlight. The drug will precipitate from saline solutions and those containing preservatives, and if this develops the drug should be discarded.

Commercially available vials containing 50 mg of AMB powder should be reconstituted with 10 ml of sterile water for injection. The drug is recommended to be diluted with relatively large volumes of 5% glucose to produce a final concentration of not more than 10 mg of AMB/100 ml, at which local irritating effects will be reduced. The manufacturer recommends that the calculated dose of solution should be given over a range of 2 to 6 hours. In cases in which the large-

volume infusion is desired, an indwelling catheter should be placed and the dose, depending on the amount, diluted in 300 ml to 1 L of 5% dextrose. However, clinical experience in treating dogs and cats and experimental research have shown that the dose may be diluted in small volumes (10 to 60 ml) of 5% dextrose, which can be conveniently placed in a syringe and infused through a butterfly catheter over a 2- to 5-minute period. A 5% dextrose flush of approximately 10 ml should be infused immediately before and after the AMB is given. In dogs, rapid bolus infusion of 1 mg/kg in 25 ml of 5% dextrose was compared with the same dose given in 1 L of 5% dextrose over 5 hours; the bolus infusion was associated with greater nephrotoxicity.[2a] The difference noted in toxicity may reflect the supplemental fluids given to the dogs medicated by slow infusion rather than the more rapid rate of injection in the dogs given bolus infusion. For this reason, supplemental fluid diuresis should *always* be given to dogs receiving treatment by the bolus method. In cats, indwelling catheters are preferable because of the difficulty in repeated venipuncture.

A wide range of dosages of AMB used in

IV therapy has been described in veterinary literature. No particular dosage regimen has proved superior; all attempt to reduce the side effects associated with treatment. A frequently used initial regimen in dogs or cats divides a total dosage of 4 to 12 mg/kg into alternate-day or Monday-Wednesday-Friday treatments (Table 63–2). The drug has been given on these days at a daily dose ranging from 0.15 to 0.5 mg/kg, which is continued until the final calculated total dosage is reached or toxicity occurs. The 0.5 mg/kg daily dose for dogs probably should be used cautiously, as it has been associated with an increased risk of nephrotoxicity. Daily doses as high as 1 mg/kg, given 2 to 3 times weekly, have been used in particularly resistant infections. A lower total dosage of 4 mg/kg is commonly used in dogs if adjunctive therapy with KTZ or flucytosine is desired. Renal toxic effects are monitored at *least* weekly by examination of the urine for specific gravity, protein, casts, and hematuria. Urine sediment examination detects toxicity earlier than serum biochemical alterations. BUN and electrolyte concentrations should be checked as well. Therapy should be temporarily discontinued if toxic signs (anorexia or vomiting) occur or if the BUN becomes abnormal (>30 mg/dl). Therapy with AMB or alternative drugs is reinstituted after the clinical signs and laboratory findings of nephrotoxicity disappear. Maintenance therapy with weekly or monthly injections of AMB or daily oral KTZ is recommended to avoid relapses. Animals are monitored periodically to ensure that non-regenerative anemia and weight loss, which develop as complications of long-term therapy with AMB, do not occur. The normochromic, normocytic anemia that occurs on long-term therapy is thought to be caused by the drug's inhibition of erythropoietin either directly or as a result of renal failure.[3]

Several adjunctive measures can be taken during IV therapy to minimize side effects of the drug. Hypokalemia, a complication in humans receiving AMB, has not been a problem in dogs and cats. Even if potassium or other electrolytes are needed, solutions containing them should never be added to AMB because the colloid will precipitate. The fever, nausea, and vomiting that occur during or immediately following drug administration are less severe if a *physiologic* dose of hydrocortisone sodium succinate, 0.5 mg/kg IV, or diphenhydramine, 0.5 mg/kg IV, or

aspirin, 10 mg/kg orally, is given prior to administering the AMB. Anti-inflammatory or immunosuppressive dosages of glucocorticoids should not be given because they predispose to fungal dissemination. Starting at the low daily dose of AMB (0.15 to 0.25 mg/kg) and gradually increasing the dose administered over several treatments until a slightly higher level is reached has been recommended. Alternatively, a small (1 mg total) test dose is given for the first few treatments with gradually increasing doses per administration.[4] Muscular fasciculations and rigors that develop in people during IV infusions have been controlled with dantrolene sodium (10 to 50 mg total IV) or meperidine (0.5 mg/kg IV).[5]

Toxicity. Causes of nephrotoxicity have included vasoconstriction, impaired acid excretion, and direct tubular injury. Mannitol (0.5 to 1 g/kg), sodium bicarbonate (1 to 2 mEq/kg), and dopamine (3 to 10 μg/kg/min) were given experimentally and empirically to dogs at the time of therapy to help overcome these toxic effects, but controlled clinical studies of their efficacy have not been conclusive.[6] Beneficial effects were obtained when sodium-containing fluids or furosemide (5 mg/kg) or aminophylline was given to dogs just prior to administration of AMB.[7] Adding heparin to AMB to control phlebitis that develops following repeated infusions has been advocated, but there is no conclusive evidence that its use decreases the reaction. In-line micropore filters, used to remove particulate matter and bacteria from solutions of AMB, should not be less than 0.45 μm in diameter or they will remove the drug from solution. Because of this size limitation, the smallest bacteria cannot be eliminated from the contaminated colloidal suspension.

The methyl ester of AMB has been developed in an attempt to make the drug less toxic. It is more water-soluble and less nephrotoxic, but unfortunately it also has less therapeutic activity and has produced side effects of leukoencephalopathy.[8] AMB has been administered experimentally in the form of liposomes, lipid complexes, or biopolymers, which are taken up selectively by the mononuclear phagocyte system. Larger dosages with less toxicity and longer survival were noted in people and experimental animals.[9,9a,9b,9c]

Alternative Routes of Administration. AMB

may be given topically, intra-articularly, or intrathecally in the bladder or renal pelvis if the locus of infection requires additional chemotherapy. Topical administration of the drug has been successful in treating refractory candidiasis. Total dosages at these sites are low.

For bladder infusions, AMB is mixed in sterile water at a concentration of 200 mg/L. This is infused once daily for 5 to 15 days. The bladder is distended, and the animal is permitted to void spontaneously. Alternatively, a constant drip infusion of 50 mg/L has been used. For intrathecal administration while the animal is under anesthesia, 0.2 to 0.5 mg of drug is diluted in 10% dextrose or in 5 ml of CSF that has just been removed from the animal. It is injected into the lumbar or cisternal space and the head is kept in a lowered position for a few minutes if signs of intracranial involvement are apparent. This procedure must be repeated 2 to 3 times weekly.

Flucytosine

Flucytosine or 5-fluorocytosine (5FC) is a fluorinated pyrimidine that was originally synthesized as an antineoplastic agent. It interferes with pyrimidine metabolism and resultant DNA synthesis in yeasts. 5FC is well absorbed from the GI tract, but its distribution within body tissues is uncertain. It enters the CSF in high concentration, approximately 75% of that found in serum. Most of the drug is excreted unchanged in the urine. Dosage adjustments must be made when concurrent AMB administration causes renal insufficiency.

The selective toxicity of 5FC results from the ability of host and fungal cells to convert the drug to fluorouracil. Although less than 4% of the administered drug is converted, it probably accounts for the bone marrow toxicity that is noted with its use.

5FC is effective against C. neoformans, Candida, and other yeasts, but has little or no effect on other deep mycotic agents or on Aspergillus. Localized candidiasis or cryptococcal infections respond best, but resistance to 5FC frequently develops during the course of therapy. For this reason, the drug is always given in combination with AMB. As a single agent, 5FC has minimal side effects, but with AMB and decreased renal function, more complications such as leukopenia with or without thrombocytopenia, diarrhea, nausea, and abdominal pain are seen.[4] Combination therapy with 5FC and KTZ has proved especially toxic to cats.[10]

Azole Derivatives

Synthetic imidazole derivatives were originally produced as broad-spectrum anthelmintics with activity against some gram-positive bacteria and protozoa. Like AMB, they inhibit sterol synthesis as one of their main effects, but, in general, they are less toxic. It was noticed that they possessed broad-spectrum antifungal activity, apparently causing inhibition of nucleic acid, triglyceride, and fatty acid synthesis and altered oxidative enzyme biochemistry. At low concentrations they are fungistatic and at higher concentrations, which cannot be achieved systemically, they are fungicidal. Thiabendazole was initially recognized as being effective in treating human dermatophytoses. It now has a limited role in the treatment of nasal aspergillosis. Miconazole, clotrimazole, and econazole are available in creams and lotions for the topical treatment of fungal infections of the skin, such as dermatophytosis and candidiasis. Oral therapy with griseofulvin or KTZ is needed for nail infections. KTZ, an orally administered azole, is becoming widely used in human and veterinary medicine to treat systemic and opportunistic fungal infections. In vitro susceptibility testing of the drugs shows variable efficacy against different fungi; however, fungal susceptibility testing in vitro does not always parallel in vivo efficacy.[11,12] Itraconazole and fluconazole are triazoles, derivatives with better absorption, longer duration of activity, less toxicity, and more potency than ketoconazole. The azole derivatives are covered under systemic or topical antifungal therapy below, based on their respective usages.

Miconazole. Miconazole is partially absorbed following oral administration but is more effective when given parenterally; thus, it is more valuable than clotrimazole in treatment of systemic fungal infections. The drug penetrates joint and ocular fluids and CSF at variable rates. It is primarily metabolized by the liver and is excreted in the urine in a metabolized form. Miconazole has been used topically to treat dermatophyte and yeast infections and is a second choice in therapy for aspergillosis. Thrombophlebitis, pruritus, nausea, leukopenia, thrombocytopenia, and increased hepatic enzyme activities have made miconazole a second choice to AMB alone or in combination with 5FC in treating human aspergillosis.

Ketoconazole. This has been the most widely used imidazole. It is less active than miconazole, but absorption from the GI tract is better, making it convenient for the treatment of systemic mycoses and chronic mucocutaneous candidiasis. Absorption is improved in acid media, so antacids and H_2-receptor antihistamine antagonists should not be given concurrently. Dividing the daily dose and giving it with meals helps produce an acidic gastric environment that favors absorption. The drug is predominantly bound to plasma albumin and thus it enters all tissues and body fluids in therapeutic concentrations with the exception of the seminal, CNS, and ocular tissues. The drug has been found to be distributed throughout the skin and subcutaneous tissues, consistent with the observed beneficial effect it has in treating superficial fungal infections of the skin and hair. The liver metabolizes the drug into metabolites that lack antifungal activity. Potential side effects of KTZ include reduced production of adrenal and sex hormones and the effects resulting from their deficiency. An increase in serum progesterone and deoxycorticosterone concentrations and a reduction in serum testosterone and cortisol concentrations have been seen in male dogs,[13] and only a transient decrease in testosterone has been seen in male cats[14] given KTZ at 30 mg/kg daily. The hormonal side effects of KTZ have made it somewhat useful in people and dogs for the management of endocrine diseases such as hyperadrenocorticism and prostatic disorders.[15]

Occasional nausea, partial anorexia, and vomiting in dogs can be overcome if the drug is given with meals and by dividing the daily dose into three or four administrations. Pruritus and alopecia have been seen when the drug is given at increased dosages for extended periods. Lightening of the coat, a more consistent side effect, frequently develops in dogs receiving higher dosages because of loss of guard hairs and a more visible undercoat.[16] Cats develop dry hair-

coats and weight loss as the most consistent findings.[14] Other side effects of KTZ are similar to those of other azoles. Frequently, reversible subclinical increases in serum activities of hepatic transaminases and serum ALP occur as manifestations of hepatotoxicity. Less commonly, clinical hepatitis develops, and if the drug is not discontinued or dosages are high enough, it may be fatal.[17-19] At clinical dosages (10 to 30 mg/kg/day), cats are more sensitive to the hepatotoxic effects of the drug than are dogs, although one cat with cryptococcosis was treated with 72 mg/kg/day for over 10 months without obvious signs of toxicity.[20] Histologic findings in the liver of animals developing hepatotoxicity include enlarged portal tracts, bile duct proliferation, and infiltration with mononuclear cells.

Mummified fetuses and stillbirths have been found in bitches being treated with KTZ. It should not be given to pregnant or lactating animals for this reason.

KTZ is most effective in vitro against yeast and dimorphic fungi such as *Candida*, *Malassezia (Pityrosporon) pachydermatis*, *C. immitis*, *H. capsulatum*, and *Blastomyces dermatitidis* and is less effective against *C. neoformans*, *Sporothrix schenckii*, and *Aspergillus fumigatus*.[21] Evidence suggests that in rapidly progressing systemic mycoses, such as many cases of blastomycosis, patients should first be treated with AMB, followed by maintenance therapy with KTZ (see Amphotericin B). The action of KTZ alone often occurs so slowly (5 to 10 days) that the disease progresses before the drug has a chance to take effect. In contrast, KTZ has been used alone in dogs and cats to treat coccidioidomycosis and some cases of histoplasmosis and cryptococcosis successfully, although relapses are common when host defenses are inadequate. Where underlying immunosuppression is thought to be responsible for the fungal disease, concurrent treatment with AMB is recommended, although the expense of therapy is greater. There is no evidence that KTZ provides synergistic effects with other antifungals except AMB, and even then such evidence is inconclusive.[22]

The total daily dose of KTZ in dogs and cats ranges from 10 to 30 mg/kg, depending on the species being treated and the type of fungal infection (see Table 63–2 and therapy tables in Chapters 64 to 75). Total daily doses of 40 mg/kg/day are required for measurable amounts of the drug to be found in CSF, although even then therapeutic concentrations may not be reached.[23,24] Once the disease process is under control, the dosage can be reduced and therapy continued for months or even years with minimal toxicity. Hepatomegaly and increased ALT (formerly SGPT) and serum ALP activities can develop during therapy but are reversible after treatment is discontinued. Only occasional nonregenerative anemia has been noted. Alternate-day therapy with 20 mg/kg given twice daily or with a lower single daily dose (50 mg) has been used in cats to reduce signs of toxicity. Signs of toxicity in cats on daily therapy usually include anorexia and, less commonly, fever, depression, and diarrhea. The development of resistant fungi has been a problem with many of the imidazole drugs. KTZ has not been used extensively, so the degree of resistance to it is uncertain at present. Unfortunately, as noted with many of the other antifungal drugs, eradication of the systemic fungi with azole drugs often is not complete, and relapses can occur when maintenance therapy with KTZ is discontinued. Infections in areas where the drug cannot reach, such as the bone and CNS, are especially difficult to treat. Therapy should always be continued for at least 4 weeks after disease can no longer be detected clinically.

Itraconazole. This broad-spectrum azole has more potent activity than KTZ against *Candida, Aspergillus,* and dermatophytes.[25] It can be given orally or parenterally; it is widely distributed with the exception of the CNS. Absorption is substantially improved from the GI tract by giving it with meals. The drug is highly protein bound and concentrations in CSF and urine are minimal in the absence of inflammation. The best success in treating human patients has been with (in decreasing order) paracoccidioidomycosis, blastomycosis, sporotrichosis, noninvasive aspergillosis, meningeal cryptococcosis, and aspergilloma.[26,27] In veterinary practice it has been most effective in treatment of cryptococcosis (Chapter 67), blastomycosis (Chapter 65), and nasal aspergillosis (Chapter 71). Toxicity of this drug appears less than that of KTZ, probably because it more selectively inhibits fungal as compared with mammalian enzymes. Nausea and edema have been commonly observed side effects. Unlike KTZ, itraconazole has been

effective as the first and sole agent in the management of systemic mycotic infections of dogs and cats. Higher dosages should be expected to cause side effects similar to those of KTZ. Dosage adjustments do not appear to be necessary in the presence of renal dysfunction.

Fluconazole. This orally active agent has use in the treatment of systemic mycoses including cryptococcal meningitis, blastomycosis, and histoplasmosis and of superficial infections such as candidiasis and dermatomycoses.[28–31] Because of low protein binding, fluconazole crosses the blood-brain and blood-CSF barriers better than any of the other azole derivatives. It also is water soluble, is well absorbed orally, and has a long half-life, making it a potentially more desirable drug for treating susceptible fungal infections. Toxicity appears to be less than that of KTZ in experimental animals, and inhibition of hormone synthesis appears minimal.[32]

Other Azoles. Vibunazole is a derivative with oral and topical activity. Its activity is most impressive in treating aspergillosis following oral administration.[27] ICI 195,739 is an investigational compound with more potent activity than any of the presently available drugs. It readily penetrates fungal cell walls and in animal experiments has been effective in treating superficial and systemic mycotic and some protozoal infections.[31]

Other Drugs

Terbinafine. An antifungal allylamine derivative has been extremely effective in the treatment of people with chronic dermatophytosis of the nails.[32a] A dosage of 250 mg daily was used for 6 to 12 months for the treatment of finger or toe nail infections, respectively. Improvement or resolution of infection usually occurs by 3 to 6 months of therapy. Side effects have been minimal. This drug would have a potential benefit for treatment of canine and feline onchomycosis.

Combination Therapy. Simultaneous use of antifungal agents is indicated under selected circumstances. Combined use of AMB and 5FC is beneficial in treating cryptococcal infections; presumably AMB facilitates penetration of 5FC into the fungal cell. Synergism has also been subjectively assessed in treatment of blastomycosis, coccidioidomycosis, and histoplasmosis by combining AMB and KTZ.

TOPICAL ANTIFUNGALS

Many formulations are used in the treatment of dermatophytosis and superficial yeast infections (Table 63–3). Undecylenic acid is an unsaturated fatty acid that has been used in combination with zinc to treat dermatomycoses. Its mechanism of action is unknown. Mercaptans, which are organic mercurial compounds, have been used as plant fungicides. They can be applied in dilute concentrations as a dip for affected animals at relatively low cost. Tolnaftate, a highly effective synthetic lipid-soluble compound, has also been used. Hyperkeratotic plaques must be removed prior to application of the drug if it is to be effective. Topical cuprimyxin, a copper-containing compound, is highly effective against *Malassezia (Pityrosporon)*. Iodochlorhydroxyquin is a

halogenated oxyquinoline that has been given orally as an antifungal, antiprotozoal, and antibacterial agent in dogs. Overdosages have caused CNS toxicity. Chlorhexidine solution (0.5%) can be used as a daily dip or shampoo for persistent dermatophyte infections.[33] Haloprogin is a broad-spectrum topical antifungal drug that may be more useful in treating dermatophyte and *Candida* infections.

Nystatin is a polyene antibiotic, closely related to AMB, that is produced by *Streptomyces noursei*. It is poorly absorbed following oral administration or topical application to skin or mucous membranes. Because it is very toxic to internal tissues, parenteral use must be avoided. Although nystatin is somewhat effective against dermatophytes and *Aspergillus*, its primary use has been to treat candidiasis.

The azole derivatives were discussed with the systemic antifungal drugs. **Thiabendazole** (13%) has been used as a three-times-weekly dip solution for 3 weeks in treating cats with dermatophytosis.[34] **Clotrimazole** is one of the most effective of these drugs against dermatophytes, but because of its

Table 63–3. Commonly Used Topical Antifungal Drugs[a]

GENERIC NAME (TRADE NAME)	CLINICAL FORMULATION (% activity)	SUSCEPTIBLE ORGANISMS (MOST TO LEAST)
Undecylenic acid (Desenex, Crux)	Powder, ointment, cream (2–10%)	Dermatophytes
Amphotericin B (Fungizone)	Cream, lotion, ointment (3%)	*Candida*[b]
Mercaptans (Captan)	45% technical grade powder[c]	Dermatophytes
Ciclopirox olamine (Loprox)	Cream (1%)	*Malassezia*,[d] dermatophytes, *Candida*
Haloprogin (Halotex)	Cream, solution (1%)	Dermatophytes, *Malassezia*
Tolnaftate (Tinactin)	Cream, powder, solution, aerosol (1%)	Dermatophytes
Iodochlorhydroxyquin (Vioform)	Cream, ointment (3%)	Dermatophytes, bacteria
Chlorhexidine (Nolvasan)	Solution (1%)	Dermatophytes
Nystatin (Mycostatin, Candex)	Powder (100,000 U/g); Suspension (100,000 U/ml); Tablets (500,000 U); Cream or ointment (100,000 U/g)	*Candida*, dermatophytes, *Aspergillus* (variable)
Thiabendazole (many)	Solution (13%)	Dermatophytes, *Candida*, *Aspergillus*
Clotrimazole (Lotrimin, Veltrim, Mycelex)	Cream, solution, lotion (1%); vs (100, 200, 500 mg)	Dermatophytes, *Candida*
Miconazole (Micatin, Conofite)	Powder, cream, lotion (2%); vs (200 mg)	Dermatophytes, *Candida*, *Malassezia*
Ketoconazole (Nizoral, Fungarol)	Cream, solution (2%)	Dermatophytes, *Malassezia*
Enilconazole (Imaverol)	Solution (10%)	*Aspergillus*[e]
Econazole (Spectazole, Pevaryl)[f]	Cream, spray, powder (1%)	Dermatophytes, *Candida*
Butoconazole (Femstat)[g]	Cream (2%); vs (100 mg)	*Candida*

[a]vs = vaginal suppositories.
[b]Sensitivity of *Candida* often includes other yeasts.
[c]Dilute powder 1:200 w/v with water and apply as rinse twice weekly.
[d]Previously called *Pityrosporon*.
[e]See Topical Therapy, Nasal *Aspergillus*, Chapter 71.
[f]Similar formulations and susceptibilities seen with bifonazole (Mycospor), croconazole (Pilzcin), fenticonazole (Lomexin), tioconazole (Trosyd), isoconazole (Travogen), oxiconazole (Oceral, Myfungar), sulconazole (Exelderm).
[g]Similar formulations and susceptibilities seen with terazol (Fungistat).

limited absorption and systemic toxicity, it has been confined to topical use. It is ineffective when given parenterally and is poorly absorbed when administered orally, producing severe GI irritation. Its use is restricted to topical therapy of dermatophyte and yeast infections. It was more effective than miconazole in treating experimental dermatomycosis in dogs[35] and in naturally infected dogs and cats when a 1% solution was applied twice daily for 2 weeks.[36] **Enilconazole** is a topically applied derivative that has been effective in the treatment of nasal aspergillosis (see Chapter 71). A number of commercially available topical azoles used in human medicine are listed in Table 63–3.

References

1. Helton KA, Nesbitt GH, Caciolo PL: Griseofulvin toxicity in cats: literature review and report of seven cases. *J Am Anim Hosp Assoc* 22:453–458, 1986.
2. Kunkle GA, Meyer DJ: Toxicity of high doses of griseofulvin in cats. *J Am Vet Med Assoc* 191:322–323, 1987.
2a. Rubin SI, Krawiec DR, Gilberg H, et al: Nephrotoxicity of amphotericin B in dogs: a comparison of two methods of administration. *Can J Vet Res* 53:23–28, 1989.
3. MacGregor RR, Bennett JE, Erslev AJ: Erythropoietin concentration in amphotericin B-induced anemia. *Antimicrob Agents Chemother* 14:270–273, 1978.
4. Drugs for treatment of deep fungal infections. *Med Lett* 30:30–32, 1988.
5. Prevention of amphotericin B induced rigors by dantrolene. *Arch Intern Med* 146:1587–1588, 1986.
6. Reiner NE, Thompson WL: Dopamine and saralasin antagonism of renal vasoconstriction and oliguria caused by amphotericin B in dogs. *J Infect Dis* 140:564–575, 1979.
7. Gerkens JF, Heidemann TH, Jackson EK, et al: Effect of aminophylline on amphotericin B nephrotoxicity in the dog. *J Pharmacol Exp Ther* 224:609–613, 1983.
8. Ellis WG, Sobel RA, Nielsen SL: Leukoencephalopathy in patients treated with amphotericin B methyl ester. *J Infect Dis* 146:125–137, 1982.
9. Graybill JR, Craven PC, Taylor RL, et al: Treatment of murine cryptococcosis with liposome-associated amphotericin B. *J Infect Dis* 145:748–752, 1982.
9a. Clark JM, Whitney RR, George RJ, et al: Amphotericin B lipid complex: efficacy in systemic *Candida* infections in mice. Abstr 28th Intersci Conf Antimicrob Agents Chemother, Los Angeles, Oct 1988, p 165.
9b. Whitney RR, Kunselman L, Clark JM, et al: Efficacy of amphotericin B lipid complex in cryptococcal meningitis in normal or immunocompromised mice. 29th Intersci Conf Antimicrob Agents Chemother, Houston, Sept 1989, p 128. (Abstr.)
9c. Meunier F, Sculier JP, van der Auwera P, et al:

10. Pukay BP, Dion WM: Feline phaeohyphomycosis: treatment with ketoconazole and 5-fluorocytosine. *Can Vet J* 25:130–134, 1984.
11. Shadomy S, White SC, Hung PYL, et al: Treatment of systemic mycoses with ketoconazole: in vivo susceptibilities of clinical isolates of systemic and pathogenic fungi to ketoconazole. *J Infect Dis* 152:1249–1256, 1985.
12. Galgiani JN: Antifungal susceptibility tests. *Antimicrob Agents Chemother* 31:1867–1870, 1987.
13. Willard MD, Nachreiner R, McDonald R, et al: Ketoconazole-induced changes in selected canine hormone concentrations. *Am J Vet Res* 47:2504–2509, 1986.
14. Willard MD, Nachreiner RF, Howard VC, et al: Effect of long-term administration of ketoconazole in cats. *Am J Vet Res* 47:2510–2513, 1986.
15. Stevens DA: Ketoconazole metamorphosis, an antimicrobial becomes an endocrine drug. *Arch Intern Med* 145:813–815, 1985.
16. Jeffery KL: Personal communication, Mesa Veterinary Hospital, Mesa, AZ, 1983.
17. Duarte PA, Coow CC, Simmons F, et al: Fatal hepatitis associated with ketoconazole therapy. *Arch Intern Med* 144:1069–1070, 1984
18. Heel RC: Toxicology and safety studies. In Levine HB (ed): *Ketoconazole in the Management of Fungal Diseases.* New York, ADIS Press, 1982, pp 74–76.
19. Tabor E: Hepatotoxicity of ketoconazole in men and in patients under 50. *N Engl J Med* 316:1606, 1987.
20. Hansen BL: Successful treatment of severe feline cryptococcosis with long term high doses of ketoconazole. *J Am Anim Hosp Assoc* 23:193–196, 1987.
21. Gabal MA: Antifungal activity of ketoconazole with emphasis on zoophilic fungal pathogens. *Am J Vet Res* 47:1229–1234, 1986
22. Schaffner A, Frick PG: The effect of ketoconazole on amphotericin B in a model of disseminated aspergillosis. *J Infect Dis* 151:902–910, 1985.
23. Craven PC, Graybill JR, Jorgensen JH: High-dose ketoconazole for treatment of fungal infections of the central nervous system. *Ann Intern Med* 98:160–167, 1983.
24. Goodpasture HC, Hershberger LRE, Barnett AM: Treatment of central nervous system fungal infection with ketoconazole. *Arch Intern Med* 145:879–880, 1985.
25. Graybill JR, Ahrens J: Itraconazole treatment of murine aspergillosis. *Sabouraudia: J Med Vet Mycol* 23:219–223, 1985.
26. Cauwenbergh G, De Doncker P: The clinical use of itraconazole in superficial and deep mycoses. In Fromtling RA (ed): *Recent Trends in the Discovery, Development and Evaluation of Antifungal Agents.* Barcelona, JR Prous Publishers, 1987, pp 273–284.
27. Plempel M: Antimycotic activity of BAY N 7133 in animal experiments. *J Antimicrob Chemother* 13:447–463, 1984.
28. Graybill JR: Fluconazole efficacy in animal models of mycotic diseases. In Fromtling RA (ed): *Recent Trends in the Discovery, Development and Evaluation of Antifungal Agents.* Barcelona, JR Prous Publishers, 1987, pp 113–124.

29. Troke PF, Andrews RJ, Marriott MS, et al: Efficacy of fluconazole against experimental aspergillosis and cryptococcosis in mice. *J Antimicrob Chemother* 19:663–670, 1987.
30. Kobayashi GS, Travis SJ, Medoff G: Comparison of fluconazole and amphotericin B in treating histoplasmosis in immunosuppressed mice. *Antimicrob Agents Chemother* 31:2005–2006, 1987.
31. Fromtling RA: Overview of medically important antifungal azole derivatives. *Clin Microbiol Rev* 1:187–217, 1988.
32. Tachibana M, Noguchi Y, Monro AM: Toxicology of fluconazole in experimental animals. *In* Fromtling RA (ed): *Recent Trends in the Discovery, Development and Evaluation of Antifungal Agents.* Barcelona, JR Prous Publishers, 1987, pp 93–102.
32a. Evanx EGV, Roberts ST: Oral treatment of dermatophytosis of nails with terbinafine, a new allylamine antifungal agent. Abstr 28th Intersci Conf Antimicrob Agents Chemother, Los Angeles, Oct 1988, p 211.
33. Van Winkle GD: Chlorhexidine treatment of ringworm in a cat. *Mod Vet Pract* 68:310, 1987.
34. Heymann LD: Thiabendazole treatment of ringworm in a cat. *Mod Vet Pract* 67:545, 1986.
35. McCurdy HD, Hepler DI, Larson KA: Effectiveness of a topical antifungal agent (clotrimazole) in dogs. *J Am Vet Med Assoc* 179:163–165, 1981.
36. Refai M, Abdel-Halim M, Itman RH: Successful treatment of ringworm in dogs and cats with clotrimazole 1% solution. *Vet Med Rev* 2/86:123–129, 1986.

64 DERMATOPHYTOSIS
Carol S. Foil

ETIOLOGY

Normal Microflora

Dogs and cats harbor many saprophytic molds and yeasts on their haircoats and probably on dermatitic skin as well.[1] The most common of these fungi isolated from the haircoats of clinically healthy dogs are *Alternaria* (14% to 60%), *Cladosporium* (25% to 97%), and *Aspergillus* spp. (0% to 12%).[1a] In cats, the same genera are isolated with somewhat lower frequencies. Other isolates have included *Mucor, Rhizopus, Penicillium, Cephalosporium, Stemphylium, Aureobasidium, Botrytis, Curvularia,* and *Phialophora* sp. and a high prevalence of unidentifiable molds. Only *Alternaria, Cladosporium,* and the yeasts have been suggested as a cause of dermatitis. Dermatophyte species have also been isolated from the haircoats of normal dogs and cats. To what extent dermatophytes represent resident flora or transient flora is uncertain. Most of the saprophytic isolates probably represent transient contamination of the pelage by airborne or soil-acquired spores. *Microsporum canis* causes a persistent nonsymptomatic infection of long-haired cats.[2] In one report 88.5% of culture results from nonsymptomatic cats were positive for dermatophytes[3] and carriage rates as high as 35% have been found in show cats.[4] In the author's experience, *M. gypseum* is likely to be cultured from pododermatitis in dogs, which probably is a result of incidental contamination of existing lesions. Therefore, positive dermatophyte identification in a skin lesion should always also be considered as possible nonsymptomatic colonization.

Pathogenic Dermatophytes

Dermatophytosis is a cutaneous infection with one of a number of keratinophilic species of fungi. The list of unusual dermatophytes that have been reported to infect domestic dogs and cats is extensive (Table 64–1). However, the great majority of canine and feline dermatophytosis is caused by *M. canis, Trichophyton mentagrophytes,* or the geophilic species *M. gypseum.* In cats, 98% of cases are reportedly caused by *M. canis.*[16] However, in a more recent survey 9% of feline cases were caused by *M. gypseum.*[17] In dogs, the prevalence of infections caused by each of the three common etiologic agents may also vary geographically (see Table 64–2).

Simultaneous infection of dogs with more than one dermatophyte species may occur.[19] Of combined infections, those caused by *M. gypseum* and *T. mentagrophytes* have been the most common.

EPIDEMIOLOGY

Prevalence

Fungal skin disease is overdiagnosed in veterinary medicine, especially in the dog. In all studies of skin diseases of dogs and cats where fungal cultures have been performed, the prevalence of dermatophyte infection may be as low as 2% of all dermatologic cases.[8] The percentage of positive culture results among specimens submitted from suspected ringworm cases has ranged from 11%[17] to 22%.[11] In Norway, a survey showed that culture results were positive from only 5% of 780 canine specimens and

659

Table 64–1. Unusual Dermatophyte Species Reportedly Isolated from Dogs and Cats

SPECIES	HOST[a]	SOURCE[a]	SELECTED REFERENCES
Epidermophyton floccosum	B	A	5–7
Microsporum audouini	B	A	8–10
M. cookei	B	G	11
M. distortum[b]	B	Z	9
M. nanum	B	Z	13
M. persicolor[b]	D	Z	7
M. vanbreuseghemii	B	?	8, 14
Trichophyton ajelloi	B	G	8, 9, 11
T. erinacei[b, c]	B	Z	11, 12
T. equinum	B	Z	7, 12
T. megnini[b]	B	A	7, 12
T. quinckeanum[b, d]	B	Z	12
T. rubrum	B	A	9, 15
T. schoenleini	B	A	10, 12
T. simii[d]	D	Z,G	7
T. terrestre	B	G	11, 15
T. tonsurans	B	A	10
T. verrucosum	B	Z	7, 12
T. violaceum	B	A	7, 12

[a]B = dog and cat, D = dog, A = anthropophilic, Z = zoophilic, G = geophilic, ? = uncertain.
[b]Rare and geographically limited distribution.
[c]T. erinacei = T. mentagrophytes var. erinacei.
[d]T. quinckeanum = T. mentagrophytes var. quinckeanum.

31% of 279 feline specimens from animals suspected of having dermatophytosis.[20]

Transmission

Dermatophytes spread between animals by direct contact or by contact with infected hair and scale in the environment or on fomites. The source of M. canis infections is usually an infected cat. Trichophyton sp. infections are generally acquired directly or indirectly by exposure to the typical reservoir host, which might be determined by specific identification of the fungal species or subspecies. In most Trichophyton infections, dogs and cats are suspected of being exposed by contact with rodents. M. gypseum is a geophilic organism that inhabits rich soil. Dogs and cats are exposed by digging and rooting in contaminated areas. Infections with anthropophilic species are

acquired as reverse zoonoses by direct contact with infected persons.

Dermatophyte infections of dogs and cats involve the hair shaft and follicle. Infected hair shafts are fragile and dislodged hair fragments containing infectious arthrospores are the most efficient means of transmission to other hosts. Such material may remain infectious in the environment for many months.

Host Factors

Susceptibility to infection is poorly understood, but the ability to mount an inflammatory response plays a crucial role in terminating an infection. Dermatophyte infections in healthy dogs are usually self-limiting. Glucocorticoid therapy is particulary likely to increase suceptibility to dermatophytosis by means of inhibiting local inflammation. Other more subtle aberrations

Table 64–2. Relative Frequency (%) of Dermatophyte Species Isolated from Clinically Affected Dogs in the United States and New Zealand

LOCATION	M. canis	M. gypseum	T. mentagrophytes
United States[16]	70	20	10
Indiana[8]	63	5	32
Louisiania[17]	32	45	23
Florida[18]	2	28	69
New Zealand[11]	75	8	11

in the immune response may influence the likelihood of acquiring and retaining a dermatophyte infection. For example, atopic people are at increased risk for dermatophytosis due to local inhibition of T lymphocyte function and inflammation.[21]

As with many infectious diseases, young animals are predisposed to acquiring symptomatic dermatophyte infections. This is partly due to a delay in development of adequate host immunity. Immunodeficient hosts will be at greater risk for acquiring infections and their infections may be more serious, more widespread, or more prolonged. The minimal inflammatory response of most feline ringworm lesions is probably related to the relative adaptation of this natural host species to *M. canis*.

CLINICAL FINDINGS

It is dangerous to diagnose dermatophytosis on the basis of clinical signs alone, not only because of the protean nature of the dermatologic findings but also because there are several other skin diseases, such as demodicosis and staphylococcal folliculitis, which mimic the classical ringworm lesion. Since the infection is follicular in dogs and cats, the most consistent clinical sign is one or more circular patches of alopecia with variable scaling. Some patients may develop a classic ring lesion with central healing and fine follicular papules on the periphery. Generally, though, signs and symptoms are highly variable and depend on the host-fungus interaction and thus the degree of inflammation. Some of the clinical presentations of dermatophytosis are characterized in Table 64–3.

Cat

The nonsymptomatic carrier plays an important role in the epidemiology of feline dermatophytosis. Culturing for fungi should be considered a part of the minimum data base in the work up of virtually every feline skin disease because the lesions caused by dermatophytes are so variable.

Feline dermatophytosis often appears as irregular patchy alopecia (Fig. 64–1); this is the most common presentation in long-haired cats. Other syndromes include classic circular patches of alopecia with scaling, miliary dermatitis, focal or multifocal pruritic dermatitis, onychomycosis, and granulomatous dermatitis.

Granulomatous dermatitis, which takes the form of a well circumscribed, ulcerated dermal nodule, frequently has been recognized in the cat (Fig. 64–2).[23,24] The lesions usually occur on cats afflicted with more generalized typical *M. canis* infection. These lesions have been called mycetomas, pseudomycetomas, and Majocchi's granulomas.

Dog

Dogs often develop classical foci of alopecia with follicular papules, scales, and crusts. However, dermatomycosis should be considered in any papular or pustular eruption. Facial folliculitis and furunculosis, superficially mimicking an autoimmune skin disease, can develop (Fig. 64–3). Nodular skin lesions (kerion) may also be caused by dermatophytosis (Fig. 64–4). Kerion is a common presenting sign of *M. gypseum* infection. Onychomycosis may be manifested by chronic ungual fold inflammation, with or without footpad involvement, or the claw

Table 64–3. Clinical Features of Canine and Feline Dermatophytosis[a]

SYNDROME	HOST[b]	FUNGAL SPECIES[c]	COMMENTS
Classical	B	Mc	Circular patch of alopecia, scale, central healing
Alopecia	C	Mc, Tm	Irregular to widespread; long-haired cats
Miliary dermatitis	C	Mc	Always consider dermatophytosis
Folliculitis	D	Mc, Mg, Tm	May be localized, regional (facial), or generalized; often with furunculosis
Onychomycosis	B	Mg, Tm	Rare; often with paronychia
Kerion	D	Mg, Tm	Highly inflamed, single or multiple
Granulomas	B	Mc, Mg, Tm	Rare (also called pseudomycetoma, Majocchi's granuloma)
Asymptomatic	C	Mc	Especially long-haired cats

[a]Modified from Foil CS: In Nesbitt GH (ed): *Dermatology*. Churchill Livingstone, 1987, Table 6–1.
[b]B = dog and cat, C = cat, D = dog.
[c]Mc = *Microsporum canis*, Tm = *Trichophyton mentagrophytes*, Mg = *Microsporum gypseum*.

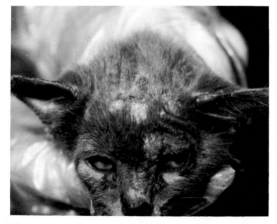

Figure 64–1. Dermatophytosis in this kitten with *Microsporum canis* is characterized by patchy alopecia with marked scaling and hyperkeratosis.

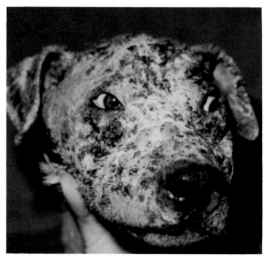

Figure 64–3. Facial folliculitis and furunculosis in this dog was caused by *Trichophyton mentagrophytes*. This dog was referred as a suspected pemphigus foliaceus case.

alone may be infected, which causes claw deformity and fragility.

Demodicosis and dermatophytosis can be clinically indistinguishable but can be reliably differentiated by a skin scraping. Superficial folliculitis, especially when it is accompanied by the spreading rings of erythema and exfoliation that have been characterized as "staphylococcal hypersensitivity," is more often mistaken for dermatophytosis. Also, staphylococcal skin lesions of seborrheic spaniels are often misdiagnosed as ringworm.

DIAGNOSIS

Direct Microscopic Examination

Hair and scales may be mounted in 10% KOH overnight for clearing (see Appendix 12). Even in experienced hands, this technique is time consuming and may be diagnostic in only a few cases. It may lead to misinterpretation if saprophytic fungal spores are present in the specimen. Dermatophytes never form macroconidia in tissue (Fig. 64–5), but rather form hyphae and arthroconidia on hair and scale (see Fig. 62–2).

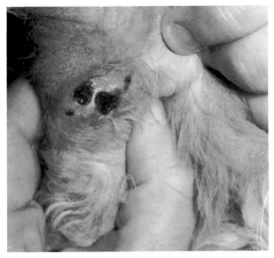

Figure 64–2. Granulomatous dermatitis has developed in this cat with generalized dermatophyte infection caused by *Microsporum canis*. Microscopically, this lesion resembled a mycetoma. (Courtesy of Dr. Gail Kunkle, University of Florida, Gainesville, FL.)

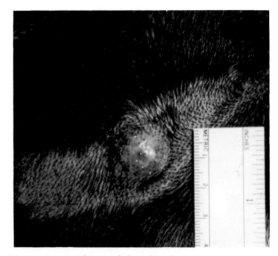

Figure 64–4. This nodular skin lesion on a dog is a kerion caused by *Microsporum gypseum*.

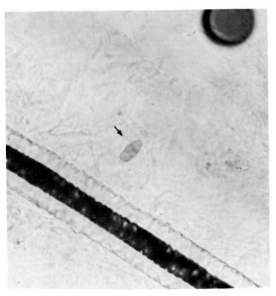

Figure 64–5. This KOH-digested microscopic preparation of hair and scale from a dog contains a multiloculated fungal spore that may be mistaken for a dermatophyte macroconidium. It is an *Alternaria* spore. Dermatophytes never produce macroconidia in tissue.

Wood's Light Examination

This technique can be very valuable in the hands of an experienced diagnostician. *M. canis* infections may be positive on a Wood's light examination. However, a negative result should never be used to rule out dermatophytosis, as not all infections exhibit fluorescence. It is easy for the less experienced clinician to mistake scale and medication for a positive result. True fluorescence is quite bright, apple green, and should only be within the shafts of infected hairs.

Fungal Culture

Definitive diagnosis of dermatophytosis is made by culture. Several important principles should be followed to ensure accurate specimen collection.

Specimen Collection. If done properly, clipping and cleaning the lesions to be cultured will reduce contaminant growth. The hair should be clipped to 0.5-cm length and the area patted clean with an alcohol-moistened gauze and then allowed to dry.

The hair stubble should be collected from several sites with hemostats by grasping the hair shafts close to the skin and rolling the hairs from the follicles. Hairs that fluoresce in UV light or that are broken and that are near active inflammation should be selected when possible. Scales should be included in the sample to be cultured. Exudates or antiseptics should not be transferred to the medium. If surgical biopsy is performed on nodular lesions, aseptically collected and transported tissue should be submitted for cultural as well as histologic examination.

Media and Incubation. Culture can readily be performed as an in-office procedure using dermatophyte test medium (DTM) (see also Table 62–1). DTM consists of Sabouraud's dextrose agar, phenol red as pH indicator, and antimicrobials to inhibit bacterial and saprophytic mold growth. For incubation, DTM containers should be loosely capped at room temperature and protected from UV light and desiccation. They should be inspected daily for a color change of the medium to red and simultaneous growth of a cottony mycelium. If the color change occurs later, which may be a result of saprophyte growth exhausting the carbohydrate in the medium, the result will be a false-positive reading.

After 7 to 10 days of growth, most colonies will begin to produce spores, which will allow specific identification (see Figs. 62–8 to 62–10). A suspect colony that fails to produce spores or is difficult to identify, as is often the case in *Trichophyton* spp., should be sent to a qualified diagnostic laboratory.

Zoophilic dermatophyte colonies are white to buff-colored. Anthropophilic species may be pinkish to yellow. If blue, green, dark brown, or black fungal contaminants have overgrown a colony suspected of being a dermatophyte, subculturing will be necessary.

Culturing Nonsymptomatic Animals. Brush culturing is the preferred method of obtaining such specimens. A sterilized toothbrush or a surgical scrub brush is satisfactory for this technique. The animal's haircoat is brushed thoroughly and extensively. The bristles are then impressed directly onto the culture medium in several sites.

Onychomycosis. When dermatophytosis is suspected as a cause of chronic paronychia, special culture techniques may be needed. In many cases the hair surrounding the un-

Table 64–4. Treatment Recommendations for Various Forms of Small Animal Dermatophytosis[a]

DERMATOPHYTE SPECIES	LESION TYPE	PATIENT CHARACTERISTICS	TREATMENT
Microsporum gypseum	Localized	Dog or cat	Topical, anti-inflammatory
M. gypseum	Multifocal	Dog or cat	Topical, griseofulvin
Microsporum canis	Localized	Dog	Topical
M. canis	Localized	Young, short-haired cat	Topical
M. canis	Any form	Long-haired cat	Topical, griseofulvin
M. canis	Generalized	Dog or cat	Topical, griseofulvin
Trichophyton mentagrophytes	Any form	Dog or cat	Topical, griseofulvin
Any species	Onychomycosis	Dog or cat	Long-term griseofulvin; remove nails; ketoconazole
Any species	Any lesion	Immunocompromised host	Topical griseofulvin

[a]From Foil CS: In Kirk RW (ed): Current Veterinary Therapy IX. WB Saunders, 1986, pp 560–565.

gual fold may be infected and may be cultured as for elsewhere on the body, taking special care to clip and clean to reduce contaminant growth. However, in dogs, geophilic fungi may contaminate preexisting foot lesions, so it may be necessary to correlate cultural findings with histologic demonstration of fungi in hair or claw. Otherwise, repeated isolation of fungus from the lesions may be regarded as evidence of causation. If the claws alone are affected, a scalpel blade may be used to shave fine pieces from the proximal end of clipped or surgically excised specimens for culture. In this case, untreated Sabouraud's dextrose agar as well as DTM should be used.

PATHOLOGIC FINDINGS

Biopsy examination is not as sensitive as culture in diagnosis of dermatophytosis. However, in cases where the true significance of culture results is questioned, demonstration of the organism in biopsy specimens is more definitive. Histologic examination is most useful in detecting the nodular forms of dermatophytosis, i.e., the kerion and granulomatous ringworm. With nodular lesions, it may be impossible to culture from hair and scale the organisms causing the inflammation. Shaved, clipped, or surgically excised specimens of claws may be submitted for histologic examination in cases of paronychia, onychorrhexis, or onychomadesis. If fungal organisms are present, they will be readily visible within the substance of the claw.

THERAPY

All animals with dermatomycosis should receive topical therapy; however, not every animal needs systemic treatment. For specific recommendations, see Table 64–4. In particular, long-haired cats should always be treated by whole-body clip followed with systemic therapy until culture results are negative. Trichophyton infections should always be treated systemically as well, since spreading and generalized infections are common.

Topical Therapy

See Table 64–5 for a summary of the appropriate topical therapy for each condition. Dermatomycotic lesions should always be clipped widely. Baths and rinses will remove the scale, crusts, exudate, and infected hairs, reducing the potential for spread of infection both on the patient and to other animals and people. When sparsely haired sites are infected and when the infection is localized, topical therapy alone may be sufficient. In highly inflamed lesions, topical treatment with low-potency glucocorticoids in combination with antifungal agents may hasten resolution of clinical disease. For localized treatment, creams or lotions are available.

Kerions and granulomatous lesions do not require specific antifungal therapy unless more widespread disease is also present. The kerion should be cleansed gently to remove exudate and avoid potentiation of scarring. Systemic antibiotics may be required if extensive purulent exudation has developed.

Systemic Therapy

Drugs and dosage regimens are summarized in Table 64–6.

Table 64–5. Products Recommended for Topical Therapy in Dermatophytosis in Dogs and Cats[a]

PRODUCT	ADMINISTRATION	COMMENTS
Povidone-iodine[b]	1:4 in water daily	Irritating, sensitizing
Chlorhexidine		
Solution[c]	0.5–2% rinse daily	
Shampoo[d]	Bathe every 5 days	Author's preference
Lime-sulfur[e]	2% rinse every 5–7 days	Odorous, not for white animals
Sodium hypochlorite (bleach)	1:20 (0.5%) rinse every 5–7 days	Not for black animals
Captan[f]	2% (2 tbs/gal) rinse or spray	Inexpensive
Miconazole[g] (cream, lotion)	Apply twice daily	For localized lesions, can be irritating
Clotrimazole[h] (cream)	Apply twice daily	For localized lesions, can be irritating
Ketoconazole[i] (cream)	Apply twice daily	Nonirritating, minimal systemic absorption

[a]Modified from Foil CS: In Kirk RW (ed): *Current Veterinary Therapy IX.* WB Saunders, 1986, pp 560–565.
[b]Betadine solution (Purdue-Fredrick, Norwalk, CT).
[c]Nolvasan solution (Fort Dodge, Fort Dodge, IA).
[d]Nolvasan shampoo (Fort Dodge, Fort Dodge, IA).
[e]Lym Dyp (Dermatologic for Veterinary Medicine, Miami, FL).
[f]Orthocide spray (Chevron [Ortho] Chemical, San Francisco, CA).
[g]Conofite cream, lotion (Pitman-Moore, Washington Crossing, NJ).
[h]Veltrim (Haver, Shawnee, KS), Lotrimin (Schering, Kenilworth, NJ).
[i]Nizoral cream (Janssen, Piscataway, NJ).

Griseofulvin. Treatment with griseofulvin is expensive and long-term and side effects are common. It should be used only when diagnosis is certain. Fortunately, dermatophytosis is rare in adult dogs, which would require the largest dosages. Like many antifungal agents, griseofulvin is poorly water soluble and thus GI absorption after oral dosing is variable and incomplete. Absorption is enhanced by administration with a fat-containing meal or by formulations containing polyethylene glycol. Particle size (micronization) also greatly affects oral absorption and bioavailability.

Dosages recommended for use in dogs and cats are not based on modern pharmacologic studies. Dosages that have proved to be effective in the largest numbers of cases are higher than manufacturer's recommendations and significant toxicities may be encountered.[26] The most common side effects are vomiting, diarrhea, and anorexia. These can be partially avoided by dividing the daily dosage into two administrations. Bone marrow suppression and neurologic signs have occured, probably as idiosyncratic reactions.[26,27] The author recommends performance of CBC every 2 weeks throughout griseofulvin therapy. Griseofulvin is teratogenic and must never be given during the first two-thirds of pregnancy. For a further discussion of toxicity, see Griseofulvin, Chapter 63.

Ketoconazole (KTZ). KTZ has been shown to be a moderately effective fungistatic drug against *M. canis* and *T. mentagrophytes.*[28] There have been several uncontrolled studies of the successful use of KTZ in canine and feline dermatophytosis.[29–31] In one, 85 cats and 124 dogs were treated with

Table 64–6. Drugs for Systemic Therapy of Dermatophytosis in Dogs and Cats[a]

DRUG	DOSE[b] (mg/kg)	ROUTE	INTERVAL (hours)	DURATION (weeks)
Griseofulvin				
Microsized[c]	25–60	PO	12	4–6[d]
Ultramicrosized[e]	2.5–5	PO	12–24	4–6[d]
Ketoconazole[f]	10	PO	24	3–4[d]

[a]PO = oral.
[b]Dose per administration at specified interval, expressed in mg/kg unless otherwise stated.
[c]Trade names: Grifulvin V, Fulvin U/F, Grisactin.
[d]Follow-up brush culture should be negative before discontinuing therapy.
[e]Dose is approximately two-thirds that of microsized preparation. Some preparations contain polyethylene glycol to facilitate absorption. Trade names: Fulvicin P/G, Grisactin Ultra, Gris-PEG.
[f]Effectiveness is not well established. Trade name: Nizoral.

10 mg/kg for either 10 or 20 days.[32] The 20-day treatment protocol was much more successful, having been associated with a 97% cure rate in cats and a 90% cure rate in dogs as tested 6 weeks after the initiation of treatment. However, by 3 weeks only 22% of cats and 22% of dogs were mycologically cured, so some of the favorable results seen at 6 weeks may have represented spontaneous remission. In the same study, less favorable results were reported in long-haired animals.

There is concern about less than favorable fungicidal activity of KTZ and the fact that the drug is not licensed for use in dogs and cats in the United States. Since griseofulvin is a fairly safe and effective approved drug for the treatment of dermatophytosis in these species, KTZ should be reserved for cases in which resistance to griseofulvin is strongly suspected or in which the patient cannot tolerate griseofulvin. In vitro susceptibility testing of the isolate with KTZ would be ideal, but such studies do not always correlate with in vivo efficacy.

Side effects of KTZ are GI and hepatotoxic and inhibition of steroidal hormone synthesis (see Ketoconazole, Chapter 63).

Environmental Control

In each confirmed case of dermatophytosis in dogs and cats, there is an environmental cleanup problem to be handled. The veterinarian must be prepared to advise the client about environmental contamination and recommend appropriate measures to prevent spread of infection. Dermatophyte arthrospores, liberated from broken and shedding hairs of infected pets, are quite long-lived. Household bleach (1:20) or chlorhexidine (2%) may be used to disinfect surfaces and utensils. Carpets and furnishings must be vacuumed thoroughly or steam-cleaned. Contaminated air-conditioning filters in households where there are many infected cats must be changed regularly. Clothing and bedding should be laundered with bleach.

Control in the Cattery

The prevalence of dermatophytosis in breeding establishments for the long-haired breeds is probably quite high. The following principles may be helpful when the veterinarian undertakes to help the breeder eliminate the problem from the cattery.[33] All animals in the cattery should be presumed to be infected unless culture results are negative. Infected animals must be segregated from all others throughout the course of treatment and until culture results prove negative. In addition, all utensils and grooming equipment should be separated, and airflow patterns must be controlled to avoid cross-contamination. Handlers must change clothing and move only from uninfected to infected quarters. Alternatively, the colony can be closed and all members assumed to be infected.

Treatment of infected individuals should include clipping, topical rinses, and systemic treatment with griseofulvin or KTZ, at recommended doses until culture results for each animal are negative. As KTZ and griseofulvin both adversely affect fertility and griseofulvin is teratogenic, breeding activities must be halted throughout the treatment period. An alternative is to treat queens with griseofulvin during the last week of pregnancy and during lactation. After weaning, the kittens should be segregated and treatment continued until they are proved culture negative.

Brush culturing should be used to test cats who are receiving therapy and any new cat entering the household. All cats suspected of being infected should be kept segregated until their culture status is known. Also, any culture-negative queen who has been known to produce infected kittens should be recultured.

PUBLIC HEALTH CONSIDERATIONS

Pet Owners

Nonsymptomatic carriage by cats of a zoonotic pathogen such as M. canis represents an unsuspected threat to exposed people. A 35% prevalence of nonsymptomatic carriage of M. canis has been found in long-haired show cats.[2,33a] Approximately 50% of people exposed to symptomatic or nonsymptomatic infected cats have acquired the infection.[34] In 69.6% of all households with infected cats, at least one person in the household became infected.[34]

The importance of zoophilic dermatophytosis has been slowly recognized in human medicine because the numbers of infections with anthropophilic species overwhelm the numbers of zoophilic infections. However, in one survey, 15% of all cases of ringworm in children were caused by zoophilic dermatophytes.[35] In reported cases of pet-associated zoonoses among people in United States Air Force communities, dermatophytes have been the most frequently reported zoonotic agents, with cats being responsible for the majority of infections.[36] Worldwide, the reported cases of human infection with M. canis is increasing.[37]

Animal Health Workers

The occupational risk of acquiring dermatophytosis is great. In a study of government veterinarians and animal health workers conducted in Great Britain, animal ringworm was the most commonly reported zoonosis; the overall prevalence was 24%.[38] Veterinary practitioners must be vigilant in protecting themselves and their employees from this troublesome and potentially serious zoonosis (see Environmental Control).

Person-to-Animal Transmission

This is possible, as illustrated in the isolation of the anthropophilic dermatophyte species in Table 64–1. M. canis may be transmitted from children to household pets as well.[36]

References

1. van Cutsem J, DeKeyser H, Rochett F, et al: Survey of fungal isolates from alopecic and asymptomatic dogs. Vet Rec 116:568–569, 1985.
1a. Philpot CM, Berry AP: The normal fungal flora of dogs. A preliminary report. Mycopathologia 87:155–157, 1984.
2. Woodgyer AJ: Asymptomatic carriage of dermatophytes by cats. NZ Vet J 25:67–69, 1977.
3. Zaror L, Fischmann O, Borges M, et al: The role of cats and dogs in the epidemiological cycle of Microsporum canis. Mykosen 29:185–188, 1986.
4. Quaife RA, Womar WM: Microsporum canis isolates from show cats. Vet Rec 110:333–334, 1982.
5. Stenwig H, Taksdal T: Isolation of Epidermophyton floccosum from a dog in Norway. Sabouraudia 22:171–172, 1984.
6. Terreni AA, Gregg WB Jr, Morris PR, et al: Epidermophyton floccosum infection in a dog from the United States. Sabouraudia 23:141–142, 1985.
7. Rebell G, Taplin D: Dermatophytes, Their Recognition and Identification, revised. Coral Gables, FL, University of Miami Press, 1970.

8. Blakemore JC: Dermatomycosis. In Kirk RW (ed): Current Veterinary Therapy V. Philadelphia, WB Saunders Co, 1974, pp 422–437.
9. Kaplan W, Georg LK, Ajello L: Recent developments in animal ringworm and their public health implications. Ann NY Acad Sci 70:636–649, 1958.
10. Scott DW, Horn RT Jr: Zoonotic dermatoses of dogs and cats. Vet Clin North Am 17:117–144, 1987.
11. Carman MG, Rush-Munro FM, Carter ME: Dermatophytes isolated from domestic and feral animals. NZ Vet J 27:136, 143–144, 1979.
12. Muller GH, Kirk RW, Scott DW: Small Animal Dermatology, ed 3. Philadelphia, WB Saunders Co, 1983, cited in Table 7–2.
13. Muhammed SI, Mbogwa S: The isolation of M. nanum from a dog with skin lesion. Vet Rec 21:573, 1974.
14. Rippon JW: Medical Mycology. The Pathogenic Fungi and the Pathogenic Actinomycetes, ed 2. Philadelphia, WB Saunders Co, 1982, cited in Table 8–9.
15. Connole MD: Keratinophilic fungi on cats and dogs. Sabouraudia 4:45–48, 1965.
16. Kaplan W: Dermatophytosis (ringworm, dermatomycosis). In Kirk RW (ed): Current Veterinary Therapy III. Philadelphia, WB Saunders Co, 1968, pp 279–283.
17. Case material, Louisiana State University School of Veterinary Medicine, 1980–1986.
18. Bone WJ, Jackson WF: Pathogenic fungi in dermatitis. Incidence in two small animal practices in Florida. Vet Med/Small Anim Clin Feb;140–142, 1971.
19. Wilkinson GT: Multiple dermatophyte infections in a dog. J Small Anim Pract 20:111–115, 1979.
20. Stenwig H: Isolation of dermatophytes from domestic animals in Norway. Nord Vet Med 37:161–169, 1985.
21. Jones HE: The atopic-chronic dermatophytosis syndrome. Acta Dermatovener (Stockholm) Suppl 92:81–85, 1980.
22. Foil CS: Cutaneous fungal diseases. In Nesbitt GH (ed): Dermatology. New York, Churchill Livingstone, 1987, Table 6–1.
23. Yager JA, Wilcock BP, Lynch JA, et al: Mycetoma-like granuloma in a cat caused by Microsporum canis. J Comp Pathol 96:171–175, 1986.
24. Miller WH Jr, Goldschmidt MH: Mycetomas in the cat caused by a dermatophyte: a case report. J Am Anim Hosp Assoc 22:255–260, 1986.
25. Foil CS: Antifungal agents in dermatology. In Kirk RW (ed): Current Veterinary Therapy IX. Philadelphia, WB Saunders Co, 1986, pp 560–565.
26. Helton KA, Nesbitt GH, Caciola PL: Griseofulvin toxicity in cats: literature review and report of seven cases. J Am Anim Hosp Assoc 22:453–458, 1986.
27. Kunkle GA, Meyer DJ: Toxicity of high doses of griseofulvin in cats. J Am Vet Med Assoc 191:322–323, 1987.
28. Gabal MA: Antifungal activity of ketoconazole with emphasis on zoophilic fungal pathogens. Am J Vet Res 47:1229–1234, 1986.
29. Woodward DC: Ketoconazole therapy for Microsporum spp. dermatophytes in cats. Feline Pract 13:28–29, 1983.
30. Hall EJ, Miller WH, Medleau L: Ketoconazole treatment of generalized dermatophytosis in a dog with hyperadrenocorticism. J Am Anim Hosp Assoc 20:597, 1984.

31. Angarano DW, Scott DW: Use of ketoconazole in treatment of dermatophytosis in a dog. *J Am Vet Med Assoc* 190:1433–1434, 1987.

32. DeKeyser H, Vanden Brande M: Ketoconazole in the treatment of dermatomycosis in cats and dogs. *Vet Quart* 5:142–144, 1983.

33. Foil CS: Diagnosis and management of dermatophytosis in dogs and cats. *In* Proceedings. 53rd Annu Mtg Am Anim Hosp Assoc, pp 174–177, 1986.

33a. Thomas ML, Scheidt VJ, Walker RL: Inapparent carriage of *Microsporum canis* in cats. *Compend Cont Educ Pract Vet* 11:563–580, 1989.

34. Pepin GA, Oxenham M: Zoonotic dermatophytosis (ringworm). *Vet Rec* 118:110–111, 1986.

35. Srejgaard E: Epidemiology and clinical features of dermatophytomycoses and dermatophytoses. *Acta Dermatovener (Stockholm) Suppl* 121:19–26, 1986.

36. Warner RD: Occurrence and impact of zoonoses in pet dogs and cats at US Air Force bases. *Am J Public Health* 74:1239–1243, 1984.

37. Alteras I, Fuerman EJ, David M, et al: The increasing role of *Microsporum canis* in the variety of dermatophyte manifestations reported from Israel. *Mycopathologia* 94:105–107, 1986.

38. Constable PJ, Harrington JM: Risks of zoonosis in a veterinary service. *Br Med J* 284:246–248, 1982.

65

BLASTOMYCOSIS
Alfred M. Legendre

ETIOLOGY

Blastomycosis is a systemic mycotic infection caused by the dimorphic fungus *Blastomyces dermatitidis*. In nature, *Blastomyces* grows as a saprophytic mycelial form that produces infective spores (see Fig. 62–15). At body temperatures, the organism transforms into the yeast form in tissues. Budding yeasts are 5 to 20 μm in diameter and have a thick, refractile, double-contoured cell wall. Dogs and people most commonly are infected with *Blastomyces*, but cats, horses, sea lions, lions, ferrets, and polar bears can also develop systemic blastomycosis.

EPIDEMIOLOGY

Natural Reservoir

The reservoir for *Blastomyces* is thought to be the soil. Recovery of the organism from sites of suspected exposure is uncommon. Growth of *Blastomyces* in the environment appears to require sandy, acid soil and proximity to water. Environmental survival of *Blastomyces* is further restricted because normal soil organisms in most areas will destroy *Blastomyces* inoculated into the soil. A special set of environmental conditions, an "ecologic niche," is required for proliferation of the organism. *Blastomyces* organisms have been recovered from a beaver dam where a number of schoolchildren became exposed to the organism.[1] Results of a Wisconsin study indicated that 69% of dogs with blastomycosis lived near water.[2]

Even within endemic regions, *Blastomyces* does not seem to be widely distributed. Most people and dogs living in such areas show no serologic or skin test evidence of exposure. A "point source" where exposure occurs within an enzootic area is more likely.[3] For example, it is not unusual to find neighborhoods in which a number of canine cases of blastomycosis have occurred over a short period of time. Some owners have had a number of dogs develop blastomycosis, suggesting a focus in their immediate environment.[4] Suspected common-source exposure of dogs and people while duck and raccoon hunting has been reported.[5,6]

Blastomycosis differs from other fungal infections such as histoplasmosis, aspergillosis, and coccidioidomycosis, to which many are exposed but few develop significant disease. Subclinical infection in dogs is uncommon or rarely recognized. When tissues from pound-source dogs in endemic areas have been cultured for fungal organisms, *Blastomyces* has been recovered from 2% and *Histoplasma* from 50% of dogs cultured.[7]

Geographic Distribution

Blastomycosis is principally a disease of North America, but it has been identified in Africa and Central America. South American blastomycosis is caused by a different organism, *Paracoccidioides brasiliensis*. Blastomycosis has a well-defined endemic distribution that includes the Mississippi, Missouri, and Ohio River valleys and the mid-Atlantic states (Fig. 65–1)[8]; however, these areas may be enlarging.[2] Blastomycosis also occurs sporadically outside this region. Pets visiting or hunting in enzootic areas may become infected. A history of travel to an endemic area should increase the clinician's index of suspicion for blastomycosis.

Mode of Infection

Most cases of blastomycosis are acquired by inhalation of the spores from mycelial

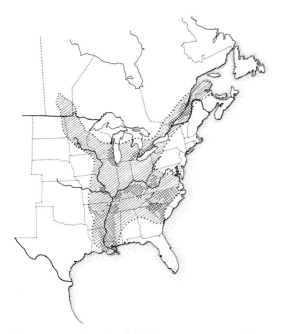

Figure 65–1. Area in which blastomycosis is endemic is within the dotted lines. Areas of highest incidence are stippled. (From Rippon JW: Medical Mycology, ed 3. WB Saunders, 1988, pp 474–505. Reprinted with permission.)

growth in the environment. The spores enter the terminal airway and establish a primary infection in the lungs. The size of the yeast when it grows at body temperature precludes its entering the terminal airway in an aerosol. Inoculation of *Blastomyces* from soil into a wound appears to be uncommon in the dog, but in solitary skin infections without systemic disease the possibility of direct inoculation cannot be excluded. Because of the rarity of focal skin disease, cutaneous blastomycosis in the dog should be considered a manifestation of disseminated disease.

Dissemination of Organisms

After *Blastomyces* becomes established in the lungs, it disseminates throughout the body. The preferred sites in the dog are the skin, eyes, bones, lymph nodes, subcutaneous tissues, external nares, brain, and testes. Less commonly affected sites are mouth, nasal passages, prostate, liver, mammary gland, vulva, and heart. Dissemination is thought to occur via blood and lymphatic routes. Although lung entry occurs in almost all cases, lung lesions may resolve by the

time the sites of disseminated infection become apparent.

Host Response

There appear to be distinct species differences in susceptibility to *Blastomyces*. The dog appears to be most susceptible to infection. In enzootic areas, the canine disease incidence is at least 10 times the incidence in people. Dogs appear to have a shorter prepatent period and tend to develop disease before people when exposed at the same time.[5] Dogs may inhale a larger inoculum of organisms than people because they are closer to the ground. The larger the dose of inoculum, the earlier the progression of the disease and death of the host.[9] Considerable variation in pathogenicity of isolated strains has also been demonstrated.[10] Cats have uncommonly been infected with *Blastomyces*. A 5-year survey of the Veterinary Medical Data Program identified 3 cats compared with 324 dogs with blastomycosis.[11]

Sex and breed differences in susceptibility also have been noted in dogs. Male dogs are more frequently infected than female dogs, and in dogs with equally severe blastomycosis, a greater percentage of females survive treatment.[12] In people, there is a 9:1 male-to-female ratio, which has, in part, been attributed to the increased exposure of males while hunting. There appears to be difference in breed susceptibility, with Doberman pinschers and Labrador retrievers over-represented.[11] Large breeds of dogs, in general, are more commonly infected than small breeds. This may reflect increased exposure from outdoor activities and roaming in larger dogs.

The highest prevalence is in 2-year-old dogs, with most cases occurring in dogs 1 to 5 years of age. There does not appear to be a seasonal occurrence in the southeastern United States, but a greater number of cases have been found from late spring through late fall in Wisconsin.[2]

Many factors in innate resistance of the host to blastomycosis are still unclear. Recovery from symptomatic blastomycosis without treatment rarely occurs in dogs, but it has been noted to occur in people.[13] A majority of dogs experimentally infected by exposure to contaminated soil recover from blastomycosis without treatment.[14] It is likely that under natural circumstances many infected dogs become mildly symptomatic and that the respiratory disease resolves spontaneously. However, nearly all dogs with clinical signs that have warranted veterinary attention have disseminated disease and should be aggressively treated.

Recovery from mycotic diseases is attributed to cell-mediated immunity. Although antibody production occurs in most cases, it is not protective. Dogs with severe disseminated disease appear to have the greatest concentration of antibodies.

Dogs with disseminated disease are probably immunosuppressed, which hinders their immune response. Forty percent of dogs with blastomycosis are lymphopenic. There is also a significant reduction in lymphocyte reactivity to mitogens when the lymphocytes are cultured in autologous sera, suggesting a circulating factor that suppresses immune response.[15] Whether this reduced lymphocyte response is a cause or effect is uncertain.

CLINICAL FINDINGS

Dogs

Dogs with blastomycosis usually have clinical signs that include anorexia, weight loss, coughing, dyspnea, ocular disease, lameness, or skin lesions. Signs of disease usually have been present for a few days to a week but may have been apparent for up to a year. In some dogs, the disease process seems to stabilize; animals may show minimal signs for weeks to months, and then the disease suddenly progresses with worsening of signs. In many cases, there has been a history of antibiotic therapy with minimal or temporary improvement.

The physical findings in blastomycosis vary greatly. Mental depression is frequent but inconsistently noted. About 40% of dogs have a fever of 39.4°C (103.0°F) or greater. Dogs with chronic lung disease are often severely emaciated. Lymphadenomegaly of one or more nodes is a frequent finding.

A majority (85%) of dogs with blastomycosis have lung lesions with characteristic dry, harsh lung sounds. Dogs with mild lung disease show exercise intolerance, while severely affected dogs have dyspnea at rest. Coughing is a variable finding. Thoracic radiographs are indicated for dogs suspected of having blastomycosis because some dogs

have lung changes without respiratory signs. Diffuse, nodular interstitial and bronchointerstitial lung changes are most commonly seen (Fig. 65–2). Other less common manifestations include well-marginated solitary to multiple cystic or solid nodules to masses. Tracheobronchial lymphadenomegaly occurs in some dogs.[16] Pleural effusion, pneumomediastinum, and cavitary lung lesions are also seen. Chylothorax and solid fibrous masses are uncommon manifestations of thoracic blastomycosis.[4,17] Solid fibrous masses may partially occlude the great vessels.

Up to 40% of dogs with blastomycosis have ocular lesions, the most common of which is uveitis. Early signs of uveitis are aqueous flare, miosis, blepharospasm, and photophobia (Fig. 65–3). Retinal separation with detachment, retinal granulomas, and vitreal hemorrhage are also seen (Fig. 65–4). Severe corneal edema may prevent good visualization of the internal ocular structures. Glaucoma secondary to angle closure occurs in blastomycosis. Periorbital cellulitis and involvement of the nictitating membrane also occur. Uveitis in conjunction with signs of respiratory or skin disease should alert the clinician to consider blastomycosis. Early diagnosis and appropriate treatment are essential to preservation of vision in blastomycosis (see also Blastomycosis, Chapter 13).

Skin lesions, found in 20% to 40% of dogs with blastomycosis, may be ulcerated with drainage of a serosanguineous or purulent fluid (Fig. 65–5). Other lesions may be gran-

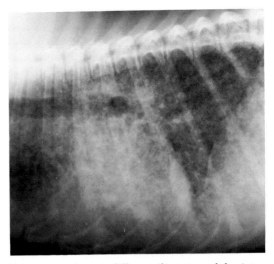

Figure 65–2. Severe, diffuse miliary to nodular interstitial pulmonary infiltrate. (Courtesy of Dr. Bill Adams, University of Tennessee, Knoxville, TN.)

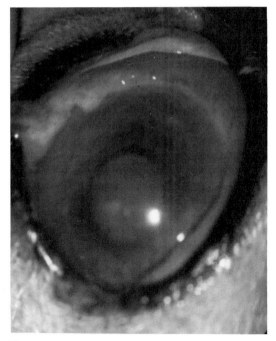

Figure 65–3. Conjunctival hyperemia and anterior uveitis associated with blastomycosis. (Courtesy of Dr. Dennis Brooks, University of Tennessee, Knoxville, TN.)

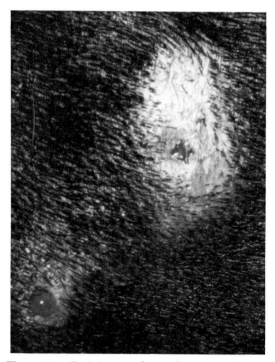

Figure 65–5. Draining tract from subcutaneous abscess producing a serosanguineous discharge. (Courtesy of Dr. Lynn Schmeitzel, University of Tennessee, Knoxville, TN.)

ulomatous, proliferative, and meaty. There may be well-defined subcutaneous abscesses. Although the skin lesions may be found anywhere, the planum nasale (Fig. 65–6), the face, and the nail beds (Fig. 65–7) appear to be preferred sites.

Bone involvement occurs in up to 30% of dogs with blastomycosis. Lameness is the primary sign in affected animals and may be

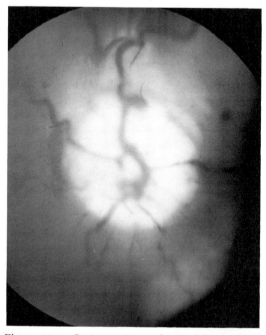

Figure 65–4. Optic neuritis and retinal hemorrhages associated with blastomycosis of the eye and central nervous system. (Courtesy of Dr. Dennis Brooks, University of Tennessee, Knoxville, TN.)

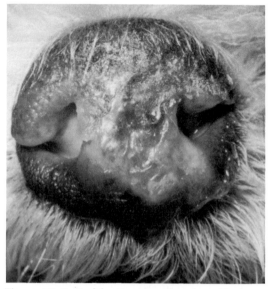

Figure 65–6. Proliferative granulomatous blastomycosis lesion of the nose causing distortion. (Courtesy of Dr. Lynn Schmeitzel, University of Tennessee, Knoxville, TN.)

the only sign of disease. Special procedures, such as bone scans, may identify a greater percentage of dogs with bone involvement. Lesions usually involve the appendicular skeleton or vertebrae; they are usually osteolytic with periosteal proliferation and soft tissue swelling (Fig. 65–8). A majority of the bone lesions are solitary and occur distal to the stifle and elbow. Fungal osteomyelitis must be differentiated from primary and metastatic bone tumors and bacterial osteomyelitis.

A variety of other tissues may be less commonly infected, including testes, prostate, kidney, bladder, brain, and nasal passages. The testes and epididymis may be greatly enlarged and painful. Involvement of the prostate gland produces swelling and pain. Dogs with involvement of the kidneys, bladder, and prostate may have organisms in the urine. Brain involvement usually occurs with widely disseminated disease but may develop without multisystemic manifestations.[4] Depression, seizures, and neurologic deficits are noted with CNS infection. Nasal discharge and obstruction of airflow through the nose occur when blastomycosis involves the nasal passages. Lesions have been found in most organs of infected dogs except the stomach and intestinal tract.

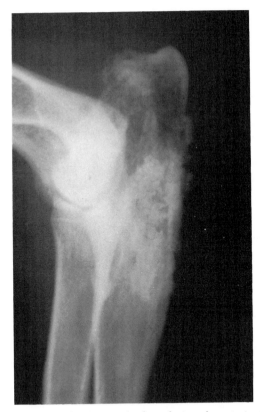

Figure 65–8. Semiaggressive bone lesion characterized by osteolysis and amorphous bone production of the proximal ulna. (Courtesy of Dr. Bill Adams, University of Tennessee, Knoxville, TN.)

Cats

There does not seem to be a breed, age, or sex predisposition in the cat.[18] Cats have lesions similar to those of dogs, but too few cats have been evaluated to derive a good characterization of the predominant signs. Dyspnea, draining skin lesions, and weight loss are the most prominent findings, and posterior paralysis also is reported.[19–23]

DIAGNOSIS

Clinical Laboratory Testing

Preliminary laboratory evaluation shows a mild normocytic, normochromic anemia attributed to chronic inflammation. Most dogs have a moderate leukocytosis (WBC 17,000 to 30,000 cells/μl) with a mild left shift, and lymphopenia is common. Serum biochemical profiles show hyperglobulinemia and hypoalbuminemia. The increased

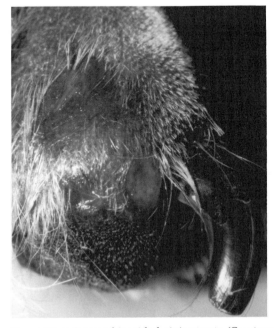

Figure 65–7. Paronychia with draining tracts. (Courtesy of Dr. Lynn Schmeitzel, University of Tennessee, Knoxville, TN.)

globulin levels are due to increases in α_2-globulin and a polyclonal increase in immunoglobulins.[15] The only other biochemical change that may be seen is hypercalcemia (12.5 to 17.5 mg/dl), which may occur without bone lesions.[24] Elevated serum calcium concentrations return to normal after treatment of the blastomycosis. Hypercalcemia may be associated with renal failure.

Diagnosis should be made by identification of the organism by cytologic or histologic evaluation. Any of the commonly used cytologic stains can be used. Because of the potential for severe treatment complications and the cost of therapy, a definitive cytologic rather than a serologic diagnosis is preferred. The combination of aspirates of enlarged lymph nodes and impression smears of skin lesions or cytology of draining exudate will yield organisms in over half of the cases. Organisms are usually plentiful in fulminating disease. When the disease is primarily ocular and less invasive diagnostic procedures have failed, vitreous aspirates or histologic examination of enucleated blind eyes will identify the disease as blastomycosis. In dogs with productive coughs, a tracheal wash may identify the organism but is less reliable than other procedures, probably because of the primarily interstitial site of infection. Lung aspirates can be used when the lung is the only affected site and results of tracheal wash are negative. Pneumothorax is a potential complication of lung aspiration, although severe complications are uncommon. Premedication with atropine is recommended prior to lung aspiration to prevent excessive vagal stimulation. In dogs with urinary tract or prostatic blastomycosis, the organism may be found on urinalysis. In dogs with brain involvement, organisms rarely may be found on examination of the CSF. Culture of cytologic specimens is not recommended for in-hospital laboratories because of the danger of infection from the mycelial form of the organism.

Atypical pulmonary fibrous masses containing organisms in small inflammatory foci may develop in lieu of the usual granulomatous reaction. These fibrous masses have few organisms and cytology of aspirates is usually unrewarding. Surgical biopsies are required, and multiple histologic sections with fungal staining are needed to find the organism.

Serologic Testing

Only after an extensive search for the organisms has been made should serologic testing be used to help establish a diagnosis. Although serologic testing alone is not definitive, a combination of compatible history, clinical signs, and suggestive radiographs in conjunction with positive serology may be substituted for identification of the organism.

The agar-gel immunodiffusion test (AGID), which has replaced the complement fixation test, is currently the most used serologic test available for diagnosis of blastomycosis (see Appendix 8). It has a sensitivity and specificity in the dog of over 90%.[25,26] AGID test results may be negative early in the development of infections. Although the intensity and the number of bands seen on the AGID tend to decrease after successful treatment, the persistence of antibodies in cured animals precludes the use of the AGID for evaluating response to therapy or relapse following treatment. The counterimmunoelectrophoresis test has a similar sensitivity and specificity to the AGID, and it is a more rapid test.[27]

An enzyme-linked immunosorbent assay (ELISA) has been developed which appears very promising in the serologic diagnosis of blastomycosis. In people, the ELISA test has a sensitivity of 77% to 100%.[28-31] Titers of 1:8 or greater are considered positive, but titers of 1:8 to 1:32 may show cross-reactivity with other fungal infections.[31] Titers of 1:32 or greater are strongly supportive of a diagnosis of blastomycosis but can be seen in exposed animals that have recovered from infection. The specificity of the ELISA in people is lower (78% to 92%) than that of the AGID (100%).[28-30] ELISA results with sera from 6 dogs with active blastomycosis and 31 asymptomatic dogs showed a sensitivity of 100% and a specificity of 97% when a 1:8 or greater titer was considered positive.[31] When the ELISA test becomes commercially available, the ideal serologic testing would be a combination of the AGID and the ELISA to maximize sensitivity and specificity. In vitro lymphocyte stimulation testing utilizing soluble *Blastomyces* antigen has been used on a limited basis to detect human infection,[29] but there is no data for its validity in diagnosing canine infection. Intradermal skin testing has no place in clinical evaluation of canine blastomycosis.

See Appendix 8 for a listing of diagnostic laboratories that perform the above tests.

PATHOLOGIC FINDINGS

Blastomycosis produces purulent to pyogranulomatous lesions in infected tissues of dogs and cats. The yeasts are admixed with neutrophils, macrophages, and multinucleated giant cells. Lymph nodes are hyperplastic with increased numbers of plasma cells and macrophages. In tissue, the broad-based, budding yeasts are best demonstrated by special stains (PAS, Gridley's fungal, or Gomori methenamine silver stain).[32] Filamentous forms in lieu of the yeast form have been found in the tissue of people and dogs.[33]

THERAPY

Amphotericin B (AMB)

This is an effective, rapidly acting, fungicidal drug for the treatment of blastomycosis. In the past, AMB was given alone at a relatively high dose of 1 mg/kg IV three times a week to a cumulative dose of 8 to 9 mg/kg.[12] At this dosage, it was diluted in large quantities (200 to 500 ml) of 5% dextrose and given over a 3- to 6-hour period. In response to AMB alone, clinical signs improved in 4 or 5 days. This high-dose treatment, though effective, is not currently preferred because of nephrotoxicity (Table 65–1).

With AMB, hydration prior to therapy is important to reduce the likelihood of renal toxicity. Monitoring of renal function is recommended before each treatment, and therapy should be discontinued if the BUN concentration exceeds 50 mg/dl to prevent severe persistent renal dysfunction.[12] Giving AMB by slow IV drip over a long period of time reduces renal toxicity. The addition of 0.5 g/kg of mannitol to the AMB drip has also been shown to decrease the renal toxicity.[12] These kidney-sparing measures should be considered especially in animals with preexisting renal impairment (also see Amphotericin B, Chapter 63).

AMB is irritating and will result in phlebitis, making venipuncture difficult after prolonged therapy. Fever occurs after administration of the first dose of AMB in about 30% of dogs, and seizures have occurred in one dog.[12] AMB does not cross an intact blood-brain barrier. In spite of these shortcomings, AMB used alone remains a reference for comparison in the evaluation of efficacy of other drugs. A relapse rate of 17% of treated dogs is expected with AMB treatment.[12]

Ketoconazole (KTZ)

This oral imidazole, which alters the ergosterols of the fungal cell membrane, is fungistatic at tolerated doses (see Ketoconazole, Chapter 63). It is generally well tolerated in the dog but may produce anorexia, liver toxicity, and increases in ALT (formerly SGPT) activity.[34] Cats appear more sensitive to KTZ than dogs and rarely tolerate doses of 20 mg/kg/day. A total dose of 10 mg/kg/day is a good starting dose in cats to establish a tolerance level to the drug. KTZ at high doses will penetrate the blood-brain barrier and has been effective in treatment of fungal infections of the CNS in people.[35] KTZ does not appear to be completely effective as a sole agent in the treatment of canine blastomycosis. In nine dogs treated with KTZ at 10 mg/kg/day for 60 days, 62% responded to therapy, but 33% of those treated had a relapse after discontinuation of treatment.[12] This relatively poor cure rate may reflect the low dose of KTZ given. A dog with bony blastomycosis was cured with KTZ at 30 mg/kg/day for 61 days.[36] Studies in people have shown that higher dosages produced significantly greater cure rates than lower dosages; however, toxicity was increased.[37]

Although KTZ has been shown to be an effective treatment for blastomycosis in people, AMB is the recommended treatment for life-threatening disease.[38] Response to therapy with KTZ is much slower than that to AMB, and relapse is more likely in dogs treated with KTZ. KTZ has been shown to depress hormone concentrations significantly and cause lightening of the haircoat, and it should be used cautiously in dogs used for breeding.[39] Because of its relatively low toxicity and the convenience of oral administration, KTZ plays a significant role in the treatment of blastomycosis.

Sequential Therapy

The sequential use of AMB and KTZ is a regimen of choice for treating canine blas-

Table 65–1. Drug Therapy for Blastomycosis[a]

DRUG	SPECIES	DOSE[b] (mg/kg)	ROUTE	INTERVAL (hours)	DURATION (days)
Systemic Disease					
Initially					
Amphotericin B	D	0.5[c]	IV	3 times weekly	[d]
	C	0.25	IV	3 times weekly	[d,e]
Followed by					
Ketoconazole	D	10–15	PO	12	60[f]
	C	10	PO	12–24	60[f]
Or Alone					
Itraconazole	B	5	PO	12	60[f]
or					
Amphotericin B	D	0.5[c]	IV	3 times weekly	[g]
Neurologic Disease					
Amphotericin B	D	0.5[c]	IV	3 times weekly	[h]
and					
Ketoconazole		15–20	PO	12	60[f]

[a]D = dog, C = cat, B = both dog and cat, IV = intravenous, PO = oral.

[b]Dose per administration at specified interval, expressed as mg/kg unless otherwise stated.

[c]Reconstituted and calculated dose diluted in 60 to 120 ml of 5% dextrose as a slow infusion over 5 to 10 minutes.

[d]Until cumulative dose reaches 4 mg/kg, then start ketoconazole therapy. Stop amphotericin B if BUN exceeds 50 mg/dl.

[e]In non-life-threatening blastomycosis in the cat, therapy with ketoconazole alone may be advantageous.

[f]Side effects of anorexia, vomiting, or diarrhea may require dosage reduction.

[g]Alternative regimen requiring prolonged IV dosing, may have to be discontinued if nephrotoxicity develops. Otherwise continue until 8 to 9 mg/kg cumulative dose is reached.

[h]Until cumulative dose reaches 6 mg/kg.

tomycosis (Table 65–1). Initiation of therapy with AMB, a rapidly acting drug, is especially important to save vision in dogs with ocular blastomycosis and to save dogs with severe, life-threatening pulmonary or disseminated disease. This initial therapy should be followed by KTZ. This combination therapy reduces the likelihood of severe renal dysfunction from AMB because a lower total dose is used, but it can produce cure rates similar to those with AMB alone.[12] The cost of combining AMB and KTZ simultaneously may be prohibitive.

Dogs with severe lung disease should receive a longer course of AMB (cumulative dose of 6 mg/kg), and dogs with neurologic disease should be started simultaneously on AMB and KTZ at 30 to 40 mg/kg/day. This high dose of KTZ must be reduced if signs of toxicity occur. Blind eyes should be enucleated as soon as the dog is capable of tolerating anesthesia. Clearance of ocular tissues is difficult with drug therapy, and these serve as a nidus for reinfection after therapy is discontinued.

Itraconazole

Itraconazole (ITZ), a newer azole derivative (see Itraconazole, Chapter 63), is more effective than KTZ against blastomycosis. ITZ can be used *alone* in treatment and appears to produce cure rates comparable to those of AMB therapy (Table 65–1). The onset of improvement appears to be comparable to that with AMB. As with KTZ, anorexia and increases in ALT activity reflect the degree of hepatic damage produced by ITZ and should be used to monitor liver damage. Lower dosages of ITZ are effective compared with those of KTZ, so that the risk of toxicity may be reduced with its use. Therapy should be discontinued if significant elevations in liver enzyme activities are noted, especially if they are accompanied by anorexia. Occasionally, dogs have also developed vasculitis while on therapy. Vasculitis produces ulcerative skin lesions and limb edema. ITZ promises to be an excellent drug for the treatment of blastomycosis, but further studies will be needed to evaluate the overall efficacy and potential toxicity of ITZ.

Prognosis

Approximately 80% of dogs with blastomycosis can be effectively treated. The severity of lung disease evaluated by thoracic radiography is the major factor that determines the likelihood of death or relapse in dogs with blastomycosis.[12] With severe pulmonary involvement, most deaths occur during the first week of therapy. With the same degree of lung disease, female dogs are more likely to survive than male dogs. Even in dogs with moderate lung involvement, a guarded prognosis is warranted. Some dogs will have a worsening of lung disease after the initiation of therapy, which may be attributable to an inflammatory response from dying fungal organisms. Brain involvement warrants a more guarded prognosis.

Treatment of Relapse

Approximately 20% of the animals will relapse after AMB alone or AMB plus KTZ therapy.[12] Relapse following apparently successful treatment usually occurs in the first 6 months after completion of therapy.[12] Dogs that are well at a year are considered cured, although rarely a dog will relapse after more than a year. Likelihood of relapse is related to severity of the initial lung disease. Reinfection after cure does not appear to occur.

Reinstitution of the full course of therapy is probably necessary to achieve a cure following relapse. Greater care must be given to proper hydration and monitoring of renal function, because there is usually residual renal damage from the initial AMB therapy. An increased incidence of prostatic involvement in dogs that have relapsed suggests that this is another site of inadequate drug penetration.[12]

PREVENTION

The ecologic niche for growth of *Blastomyces* has not been identified; therefore, preventive measures are not possible. Even if the site were identified, sterilization of the soil is impossible. Restriction of the animals from lakes and creeks in areas where other dogs have become infected may be helpful. There is no vaccine available for prevention of blastomycosis.

PUBLIC HEALTH CONSIDERATIONS

There is no danger from aerosol transmission of the organism from animals to people or from people to people. Penetrating wounds contaminated by the organism have produced infections in people. Care should be taken to avoid getting bitten when handling a dog with blastomycosis.[40] Accidental inoculation of organisms by contaminated knives or needles should be avoided at necropsy or during fine-needle aspiration.[41] Culturing of the organism should be reserved to laboratories with proper facilities. Primary pulmonary blastomycosis has occurred in a laboratory worker exposed to a culture of the mycelial form of *Blastomyces dermatitidis*.[42]

References

1. Klein BS, Vergeront JM, Weeks RJ, et al: Isolation of *Blastomyces dermatitidis* in soil associated with a large outbreak of blastomycosis in Wisconsin. N Engl J Med 314:529–534, 1986
2. Archer JR, Trainer DO, Schell RF: Epidemiologic study of canine blastomycosis in Wisconsin. J Am Vet Med Assoc 190:1292–1295, 1987.
3. Furcolow ML, Smith CD: A new hypothesis on the epidemiology of blastomycosis and the ecology of *Blastomyces dermatitidis*. Trans NY Acad Sci 35:421–430, 1973.
4. Legendre AM: Unpublished observation. University of Tennessee, Knoxville, TN, 1988.
5. Sarosi GA, Eckman MR, Davies SF, et al: Canine blastomycosis as a harbinger of human disease. Ann Intern Med 91:733–735, 1979.
6. Armstrong CW, Jenkins SR, Kaufman L, et al: Common-source outbreak of blastomycosis in hunters and their dogs. J Infect Dis 155:568–570, 1987.
7. Turner C, Smith CD, Furcolow ML: Frequency of isolation of *Histoplasma capsulatum* and *Blastomyces dermatitidis* from dogs in Kentucky. Am J Vet Res 33:137–141, 1972.
8. Rippon JW: *Medical Mycology*, ed 3. Philadelphia, WB Saunders Co, 1988, pp 474–505.
9. Williams JE, Moser SA: Chronic murine pulmonary blastomycosis induced by intratracheally inoculated *Blastomyces dermatitidis* conidia. Am Rev Respir Dis 135:17–25, 1987.
10. Moser SA, Koker PJ, Williams JE: Fungal-strain dependent alterations in the time course and mortality of chronic murine pulmonary blastomycosis. Infect Immun 56:34–39, 1988.
11. Legendre AM: Systemic mycotic infections of dogs

and cats. *In* Scott FW (ed): *Infectious Diseases.* New York, Churchill Livingstone, 1986, pp 29–53.

12. Legendre AM, Selcer BA, Edwards DF, et al: Treatment of canine blastomycosis with amphotericin B and ketoconazole. *J Am Vet Med Assoc* 184:1249–1254, 1984.

13. Sarosi GA, Davies SF, Phillips JR: Self-limiting blastomycosis: a report of 39 cases. *Semin Respir Infect* 1:40–44, 1986.

14. Smith CD, Furcolow ML, Hulker P: Effects of immunosuppressants on dogs exposed two and one-half years previously to *Blastomyces dermatitidis. Am J Epidemiol* 104:299–305, 1976.

15. Legendre AM, Becker PU: Immunologic changes in acute canine blastomycosis. *Am J Vet Res* 43:2050–2053, 1982.

16. Walker MA: Thoracic blastomycosis: a review of its radiographic manifestations in 40 dogs. *Vet Radiol* 22:22–26, 1981.

17. Willard MD, Conroy JD: Chylothorax associated with blastomycosis in a dog. *J Am Vet Med Assoc* 186:72–73, 1985.

18. Legendre AM: Systemic mycotic infections. *In* Sherding R (ed): *Diseases of the Cat.* New York, Churchill Livingstone, 1989, pp 427–437.

19. Alden CL, Mohan R: Ocular blastomycosis in a cat. *J Am Vet Med Assoc* 164:527–528, 1974.

20. Breider MA, Walker TL, Legendre AM, et al: Five cases of feline blastomycosis. *J Am Vet Med Assoc* 193:570–572, 1988.

21. Hatkin JM, Phillips WE, Utroska WR: Two cases of feline blastomycosis. *J Am Anim Hosp Assoc* 15:217–220, 1978.

22. Jasmin AM, Carroll JM, Baucom JN: Systemic blastomycosis in Siamese cats. *Vet Med/Small Anim Clin* 64:33–37, 1969.

23. Nasisse MP, vanEE RT, Wright B: Ocular changes in a cat with disseminated blastomycosis. *J Am Vet Med Assoc* 187:629–631, 1985.

24. Dow SW, Legendre AM, Stiff M, et al: Hypercalcemia associated with blastomycosis in dogs. *J Am Vet Med Assoc* 188:706–709, 1986.

25. Legendre Am, Becker RU: Evaluation of the agar-gel immunodiffusion test in the diagnosis of canine blastomycosis. *Am J Vet Res* 41:2109–2111, 1980.

26. Phillips WE, Kaufman L: Cultural and histopathologic confirmation of canine blastomycosis diagnosed by an agar-gel immunodiffusion test. *Am J Vet Res* 41:1263–1265, 1980.

27. Barta O, Hubbert NL, Pier AC, et al: Counterimmunoelectrophoresis (immunoelectroosmosis) and serum electrophoretic pattern in serologic diagnosis of canine blastomycosis. *Am J Vet Res* 44:218–222, 1983.

28. Klein BS, Kuritsky JN, Chappell WA, et al: Comparison of the enzyme immunoassay, immunodiffusion, and complement fixation tests in detecting antibody in human serum to the A antigen of *Blastomyces dermatitidis. Am Rev Respir Dis* 133:144–148, 1986.

29. Klein BS, Vergeront JM, Kaufman L, et al: Serological tests for blastomycosis: assessments during a large point-source outbreak in Wisconsin. *J Infect Dis* 155:262–268, 1987.

30. Lambert RS, George RB: Evaluation of enzyme immunoassay as a rapid screening test for histoplasmosis and blastomycosis. *Am Rev Respir Dis* 136:316–319, 1987.

31. Turner S, Kaufman L, Jalbert M: Diagnostic assessment of an enzyme-linked immunosorbent assay for human and canine blastomycosis. *J Clin Microbiol* 23:294–297, 1986.

32. Buyukmichi NC, Moore PF: Microscopic lesions of spontaneous ocular blastomycosis in dogs. *Comp Pathol* 97:321–328, 1987.

33. Kaufman AF, Kaplan W, Kraft DE: Filamentous forms of *Ajellomyces* (*Blastomyces*) *dermatitidis* in a dog. *Vet Pathol* 16:271–273, 1979.

34. Moriello KA: Ketoconazole: clinical pharmacology and therapeutic recommendations. *J Am Vet Med Assoc* 188:303–306, 1986.

35. Craven PC, Graybill JR, Jorgensen JH, et al: High-dose ketoconazole for treatment of fungal infections of the central nervous system. *Ann Intern Med* 98:160–167, 1983.

36. Dunbar M, Pyle RL: Ketoconazole treatment of osseous blastomycosis in a dog. *Vet Med/Small Anim Clin* 76:1593–1595, 1981.

37. National Institute of Allergy and Infectious Diseases Mycoses Study Group: Treatment of blastomycosis and histoplasmosis with ketoconazole. *Ann Intern Med* 103:861–872, 1985.

38. McManus EJ, Jones JM: The use of ketoconazole in the treatment of blastomycosis. *Am Rev Respir Dis* 133:141–143, 1986.

39. Willard MD, Nachreiner R, McDonald R, et al: Ketoconazole-induced changes in selected canine hormone concentrations. *Am J Vet Res* 47:2504–2509, 1986.

40. Gnann JW, Bressler GS, Bodet CA: Human blastomycosis after a dog bite. *Ann Intern Med* 98:48–49, 1983.

41. Graham WR, Callaway JL: Primary inoculation blastomycosis in a veterinarian. *J Am Acad Dermatol* 7:785–786, 1982.

42. Baum GL, Lerner PI: Primary pulmonary blastomycosis: a laboratory-acquired infection. *Ann Intern Med* 73:263–265, 1970.

66

HISTOPLASMOSIS
Alice M. Wolf

ETIOLOGY AND PATHOGENESIS

The etiologic agent of American histoplasmosis is the soil-borne, dimorphic fungus *Histoplasma capsulatum*. This organism can survive wide fluctuations in environmental temperature and prefers areas with moist, humid conditions. It grows best in soil containing nitrogen-rich organic matter such as bird and bat excrement.[1,2]

H. capsulatum is endemic throughout large areas of the temperate and subtropical regions of the world (Fig. 66–1).[3] The fungus has been isolated from soil in 31 of the continental United States, with most clinical cases occurring in the central United States in the region of the Ohio, Missouri, and Mississippi rivers. Histoplasmosis can appear in traditionally nonendemic regions if local environmental conditions are altered to favor fungal growth.[4] In addition, obtaining a detailed travel history is important in order to identify patients that may have acquired infection while traveling through endemic regions.

The life cycle of *H. capsulatum* is similar to that of other dimorphic fungi: the free-living, mycelial stage in soil produces macroconidia (5 to 18 μm) (see Fig. 62–14) and microconidia (2 to 5 μm) that are the source of infection for mammals. Histoplasmosis is probably acquired by inhalation of microconidia that are small enough to reach the lower respiratory tract. The conidia convert to the yeast phase in the lung and reproduce by budding. The yeast organisms are phagocytized by cells of the host's mononuclear phagocyte system and undergo further intracellular replication. Infection may be grossly limited to the pulmonary tree; however, lymphatic and hematogenous dissemination of

H. capsulatum can occur early in the course of the disease because of the intracellular location of the fungus.[5] Severe clinical disease can result if the dose of infective spores is large or if the immune system of the host is compromised. The cellular immune system in most patients will rapidly bring the infection under control.

The occurrence of GI histoplasmosis without respiratory tract involvement suggests

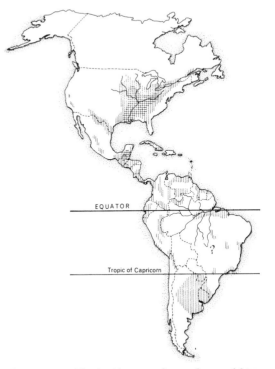

Figure 66–1. The incidence and prevalence of histoplasmosis in North and South America based on skin testing surveys. The darker shaded areas indicate zones of very high endemicity. (From Rippon JW: *Medical Mycology*, ed 3. WB Saunders Co, 1988. Reprinted with permission.)

679

that the GI tract may also be a primary site of infection. However, experimental studies have failed to produce GI disease following oral administration of H. capsulatum spores.[6] It is difficult to determine true infection rates for histoplasmosis in companion animals because most infections are subclinical. The prevalence of infection probably parallels that in the human population in endemic regions.

CLINICAL FINDINGS

Cat

Evidence suggests that cats are a very susceptible host and are at least as likely as dogs to develop clinical histoplasmosis.[4,7–13] The age range of cats affected with histoplasmosis has been 4 months to 13.5 years, with the majority of cases in young cats (<4 years of age). There is no apparent breed or sex predilection.

Most infected cats have disseminated disease and exhibit a wide range of nonspecific clinical signs including depression, weight loss, fever, anorexia, and pale mucous membranes. Coughing is uncommon but dyspnea, tachypnea, and abnormal lung sounds are found in over half of affected cats. Other frequent findings include peripheral or visceral lymphadenomegaly and hepatomegaly. Occasionally, Histoplasma affects the eye, causing conjunctivitis, granulomatous chorioretinitis, retinal detachment, and optic neuritis. Some cats have had osseous lesions causing soft tissue swelling and lameness. The skin is infrequently affected with nodular or ulcerated lesions. Rare clinical findings include splenomegaly, oral ulcers, nasal polyps, vomiting, and diarrhea.

Dog

Histoplasmosis has been reported in dogs ranging in age from 2 months to 14 years.[2,6,14–21] Like the disease in cats, it usually affects young dogs (<4 years) with no apparent sex predilection. With respect to breed, pointers, weimaraners, and Brittany spaniels are over-represented in some published reports.[2,6]

Inappetence, weight loss, and fever unresponsive to antibiotic therapy occur in most cases of canine histoplasmosis. In some

dogs, the clinical signs may be limited to the respiratory tree and include dyspnea, coughing, and abnormal lung sounds. However, in most dogs, clinical signs result from disseminated histoplasmosis with GI involvement. Signs of large bowel diarrhea with tenesmus, mucus, and fresh blood in the stool are the most common clinical findings (Fig. 66–2). Pale mucous membranes often are found with extensive blood loss. Extensive Histoplasma infiltration of the small bowel can cause a voluminous, watery stool with an accompanying protein-losing enteropathy (Fig. 66–3A and B). Hepatomegaly, visceral lymphadenomegaly, splenomegaly, icterus, and ascites are frequent associated findings (Fig. 66–4). Unusual signs include vomiting, peripheral lymphadenomegaly, and lameness due to osseous infection. Ocular lesions and skin lesions described above for cats have also been reported in the dog. Neurologic involvement has been recognized with dissemination of infection in dogs; however, it is rare.

DIAGNOSIS

Clinical Laboratory Testing

The most common hematologic abnormality in both dogs and cats with dissemi-

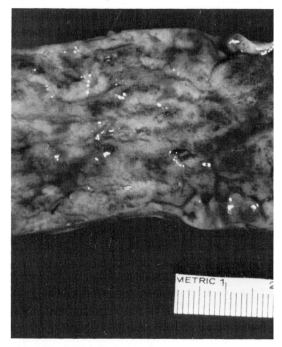

Figure 66–2. Thickening and ulceration of the colonic mucosa due to histoplasmosis results in large bowel diarrhea containing mucus and fresh blood.

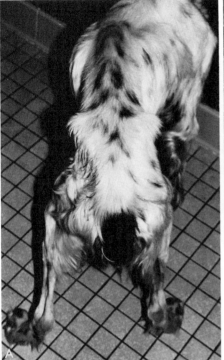

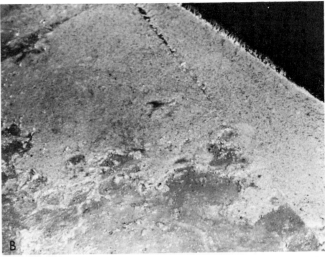

Figure 66–3. A, Emaciation in a dog with chronic small bowel diarrhea and malabsorption due to *Histoplasma* infiltration of the bowel. B, Small bowel–type diarrhea fills the dog's kennel run.

nated histoplasmosis is normocytic, normochromic, nonregenerative anemia. The anemia probably results from chronic inflammatory disease, *Histoplasma* infection of the bone marrow, and intestinal blood loss. Leukocyte counts are variable. Neutrophilic leukocytosis with monocytosis and eosinopenia is found most frequently; leukopenia and

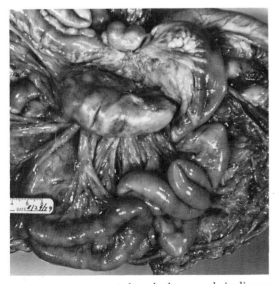

Figure 66–4. Mesenteric lymphadenomegaly in disseminated histoplasmosis.

thrombocytopenia have also been reported.[6] Severe pancytopenia has been observed in some cats.[3,6,8] *Histoplasma* organisms may be found during routine blood film examination in circulating monocytes, neutrophils, and, rarely, eosinophils.[15] Performing 1000 cell differential counts and examining buffy-coat smears will enhance detection of infected cells.

Abnormal coagulation function tests have been found in some thrombocytopenic dogs with disseminated histoplasmosis, suggesting the presence of microangiopathic hemolysis.[6,14,16] DIC in these dogs may occur as a result of extensive *Histoplasma* infiltration of the liver. Hemolysis and an increased bleeding tendency associated with DIC may enhance the severity of the anemia seen in these patients.

Biochemical profiles are usually unremarkable in dogs with pulmonary histoplasmosis. Hypoalbuminemia is a fairly consistent finding in cats with disseminated histoplasmosis.[8] Some cats have had hyperproteinemia, hyperglobulinemia, and mild elevations of serum glucose and ALT (SGPT) activities.[8,22] Dogs with disseminated disease may have hypoproteinemia and severe hypoalbuminemia due to intestinal blood loss or a protein-losing enteropathy. Liver dysfunction in affected dogs may cause hypoalbuminemia, hyperbilirubinemia, elevated SAP and ALT values, and abnormal results on liver function tests.[6]

Urinalyses are usually normal in dogs and cats with histoplasmosis. Most cats tested have been negative for feline leukemia virus infection.[8]

Radiography

Thoracic radiographs of dogs and cats with active pulmonary histoplasmosis usually exhibit a linear or diffuse pulmonary interstitial pattern.[23] These infiltrates often are coalescing and may appear miliary or grossly nodular (Fig. 66–5). True alveolar involvement in pulmonary histoplasmosis is rare. Hilar lymphadenomegaly is a common finding in dogs but is rare in the cat.[11] Pleural effusion occurs infrequently in the dog. Pulmonary calcification, indicative of inactive pulmonary histoplasmosis, is occasionally seen in dogs.

The interpretation of abdominal radiographs in dogs with GI histoplasmosis may be difficult because of the emaciated condition and presence of abdominal fluid. Noncontrast studies may demonstrate hepatomegaly, splenomegaly, or ascites. Barium-contrast examination may reveal irregulari-ties of the intestinal mucosa and thickening of the intestinal walls.

Osseous involvement with histoplasmosis is rare in the cat and even less common in the dog. The typical radiographic appearance of bony lesions is a mixed pattern of osteolysis, subperiosteal bone proliferation, and periosteal new bone formation (Fig. 66–6). In the cat, *Histoplasma* most frequently affects the metaphyses of long bones with a predilection for the bones of and adjacent to the carpal and tarsal joints.[12]

Cytologic and Histologic Findings

Histoplasma organisms are usually numerous in affected tissues and a definitive diagnosis can often be made by fine-needle aspiration and exfoliative cytology. The organisms are usually contained within cells of the mononuclear phagocyte system; single or multiple yeast cells may be present within each phagocytic cell. Routine hematologic stains demonstrate the organism as a small (2 to 4 μm) round body with a basophilic center and lighter halo caused by shrinkage of the yeast during staining (Fig. 66–7A and B). In the cat, *Histoplasma* organisms are most easily recovered from bone marrow, lung, and lymph node aspirates. Rectal scrapings, imprints of colonic biopsy specimens, and aspirates of liver, lung, spleen,

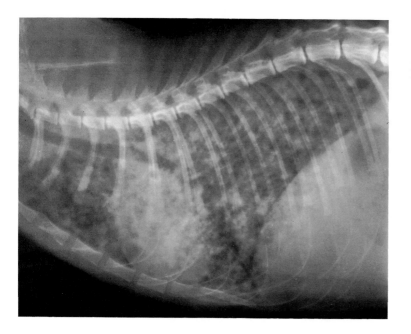

Figure 66–5. Thoracic radiograph of a 2-year-old cat with disseminated histoplasmosis showing coalescing interstitial pulmonary infiltrates.

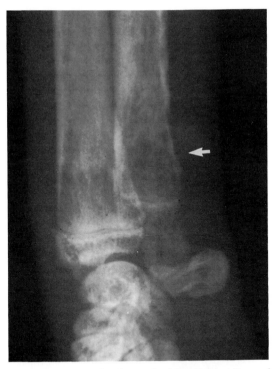

Figure 66–6. Lateral radiograph of the distal radius and ulna of a 5-year-old cat showing diffuse osteolysis and reactive new bone formation (*arrow*) characteristic of osseous histoplasmosis.

and bone marrow are most productive in the dog. Other tissues or body fluids should be examined as warranted by the clinical signs in each case.

Tissue biopsy may be required if exfoliative cytology is not diagnostic. Affected tissues demonstrate granulomatous inflammation but *Histoplasma* organisms are difficult to detect with routine H and E stain.[1,6] Special fungal stains (PAS, Gomori methenamine silver, Gridley's fungal stain) should be used if histoplasmosis is suspected.

Fungal Isolation

H. capsulatum can be cultured from tissue specimens, fine-needle aspirates, and body fluids. The yeast phase produces white, moist colonies when inoculated on blood agar and incubated at 30°C or 37°C (see Chapter 62). The mycelial phase will develop within 7 to 10 days on routine fungal culture media incubated at room temperature. Microconidia produced by the mycelial phase are infectious, and cultures exhibiting fluffy white or buff-brown mycelial growth should be handled with caution. Attempts

to culture *H. capsulatum* in a routine practice setting are not recommended because of the pathogenic potential of this organism.

Immunodiagnosis

Intradermal skin tests for reactivity to histoplasmin are unreliable in companion animals and cannot be used to confirm the diagnosis of histoplasmosis. Serologic tests for antibodies directed against *Histoplasma* antigens are usually falsely negative in animals with naturally occurring disease. They also may be falsely positive in animals with prior exposure that have recovered from infection. At present, no reliable immunodiagnostic test is available for the diagnosis of histoplasmosis in companion animals.

THERAPY

Pulmonary histoplasmosis in the dog may be self-limiting and can resolve without treatment. However, antifungal chemotherapy is recommended because dissemination can occur early in the course of infection. Ketoconazole (KTZ) is currently the drug of choice for dogs with early or mild pulmonary infections (Table 66–1).[2,24] Acute side effects of KTZ treatment include vomiting, diarrhea, and inappetence. These effects usually subside if drug administration is stopped for a few days. Ketoconazole therapy can then be reinstituted at a lower dose and, if the drug is well tolerated, the dose can be increased to required therapeutic levels after 7 to 10 days. Long-term effects of KTZ include elevation of liver enzyme concentrations, alopecia, lightening of haircoat color, and suppression of adrenal cortical function (see Ketoconazole, Chapter 63). These effects are reversible when drug therapy is discontinued.

In dogs or cats with severe or fulminating pulmonary histoplasmosis, combination therapy with amphotericin B and KTZ may provide more rapid control of the fungal infection (see Table 66–1). Slow drip administration of amphotericin B and concurrent use of mannitol, furosemide, or salt loading may decrease the nephrotoxicity of this drug. KTZ treatment is initiated at the same time as amphotericin B administration and is continued after termination of the amphotericin B regimen.

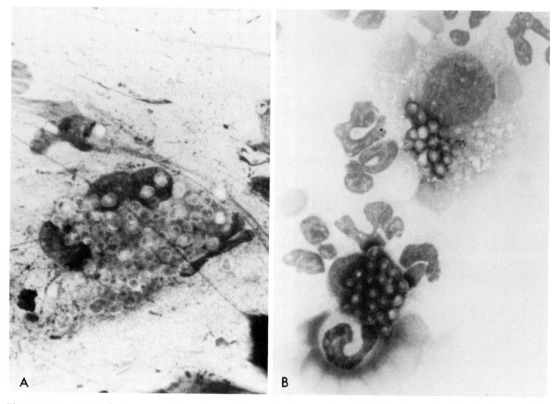

Figure 66–7. *A,* Cytologic preparation of a rectal scraping from a dog with histoplasmosis showing intracellular organisms in a macrophage (Wright's stain; × 800). This is one of the best and most common ways to confirm a diagnosis of histoplasmosis. *B, H. capsulatum* in circulating blood monocytes. This organism can also be found in neutrophils and, rarely, in eosinophils. (Wright's stain; × 1000) (Courtesy of Dr. Ken Latimer, University of Georgia, Athens, GA.)

Dogs with GI histoplasmosis and most cats have extensive, disseminated fungal involvement at the time their disease is recognized. Aggressive antifungal chemotherapy with KTZ alone or in combination with amphotericin B is recommended for these animals, although treatment is frequently unrewarding in these patients due to their debilitated condition and widespread fungal involvement.

The duration of antifungal treatment required for each patient is variable and is determined by the severity of infection and the clinical response of the patient. The response to therapy should be evaluated by monitoring the resolution of clinical signs,

Table 66–1. Therapy for Histoplasmosis[a]

DRUG	SPECIES	DOSE[b] (mg/kg)	ROUTE	INTERVAL (hours)	DURATION (months)
Ketoconazole[2, 23]	B	10–15	PO	12	4–6[c]
	C	50 (total)	PO	24	4–6[c]
Amphotericin B[d]	B	0.25–0.5	IV	48[e]	f
Itraconazole[26]	B	5–10	PO	24	4–6[c]
Fluconazole	B	2.5–5	PO	12–24	4–6[c]

[a]C = cat, B = both dog and cat, PO = oral, IV = intravenous.
[b]Dose per administration at specified interval, expressed as mg/kg unless otherwise stated.
[c]Minimum time; each case must be evaluated independently; see text. Treat for at least 2 months after resolution of clinical signs.
[d]Given in conjunction with ketoconazole in severe cases; see text.
[e]Monday-Wednesday-Friday schedule usually employed.
[f]Continue until cumulative dose of 5 to 10 mg/kg is reached in dogs, 4 to 8 mg/kg in cats.

hematologic and biochemical abnormalities, and radiographic lesions.

A new triazole, itraconazole (ITZ), has shown good efficacy in the treatment of people with naturally occurring histoplasmosis and in mice and guinea pigs with experimentally induced histoplasmosis.[25–30] Itraconazole is given orally and, although poorly absorbed from the GI tract, it is 5 to 100 times more active than KTZ (see Table 66–1).[31,32] The ratio of tissue and plasma drug levels shows that ITZ has a high affinity for the majority of tissues usually involved in fungal infections.[32] Pharmacologic studies in dogs have demonstrated no significant toxicity in doses up to 40 mg/kg/day given for 3 months.[32] The usual dose recommended is listed in Table 66–1. This dose is also suitable for cats and appears to be less toxic than KTZ.[33] Itraconazole is teratogenic and embryotoxic and should not be used in pregnant animals.[32]

Another orally administered triazole, fluconazole, has been as effective as KTZ and amphotericin B in the treatment of experimental histoplasmosis in mice.[28,34] Both ITZ and fluconazole exhibit fewer GI and hepatotoxic side effects than KTZ.[26,32] In addition, they do not significantly inhibit testicular and adrenal steroidogenesis.[26,32] Newer azoles, such as Bay R3783 under investigation,[25, 25a] appear to have promise in the treatment of systemic mycoses, although additional studies are needed to determine the efficacy and safety of these newer azole antimycotic agents in naturally occurring histoplasmosis in companion animals.

Dogs with pulmonary histoplasmosis have a fair to good prognosis, depending on the severity of the fungal involvement. The prognosis for all cats and for dogs with disseminated histoplasmosis is guarded to grave.

PREVENTION

Effective immunoprophylaxis is not available for histoplasmosis. Prevention consists of avoiding exposure to Histoplasma-infected soil in endemic areas. Soil containing bird or bat excrement enhances the growth of Histoplasma and is particularly dangerous. Formalin (3%) or formaldehyde solution may be used for soil decontamination if small, focal sources of infection can be identified.[5,6]

PUBLIC HEALTH CONSIDERATIONS

Both companion animals and people residing in or traveling through endemic regions of the country are at risk of exposure to H. capsulatum. Direct transmission of histoplasmosis from animal to animal or animal to people has not been reported.[6,35] Fungal cultures containing mycelial growth of H. capsulatum are highly infectious and should be handled with extreme caution.

References

1. Larsh HW, Hall NK: Histoplasma capsulatum. In Braude AI, Davis CE, Fierer J (eds): Infectious Diseases and Medical Microbiology, ed 2. Philadelphia, WB Saunders Co, 1986, pp 580–583.
2. Wolf AM, Troy GC: Deep mycotic diseases. In Ettinger SJ (ed): Textbook of Veterinary Internal Medicine, ed 3. Philadelphia, WB Saunders Co, 1989, pp 351–354.
3. Rippon JW: Medical Mycology, ed 3. Philadelphia, WB Saunders Co, 1988.
4. Kabli S, Koschmann JR, Robertstad GW, et al: Endemic canine and feline histoplasmosis in El Paso, Texas. J Med Vet Mycol 24:41–50, 1986.
5. Sarosi GA, Davies SF: Histoplasmosis. In Braude AI, Davis CE, Fierer J (eds): Infectious Diseases and Medical Microbiology, ed 2. Philadelphia, WB Saunders Co, 1986, pp 863–867.
6. Barsanti JA: Histoplasmosis. In Greene CE (ed): Clinical Microbiology and Infectious Diseases of the Dog and Cat, ed 1. Philadelphia, WB Saunders Co, 1984, pp 687–699.
7. Aronson E, Bendickson JC, Miles KG, et al: Disseminated histoplasmosis with osseous lesions in a cat with feline lymphosarcoma. Vet Radiol 27:50–53, 1986.
8. Clinkenbeard KD, Tyler RD, Cowell RL: Disseminated histoplasmosis in cats: 12 cases (1981–1986). J Am Vet Med Assoc 190:1445–1448, 1987.
9. Gabbert NH, Campbell TW, Beiermann RL: Pancytopenia associated with disseminated histoplasmosis in a cat. J Am Anim Hosp Assoc 20:119–122, 1984.
10. Wolf AM, Belden MN: Feline histoplasmosis: a literature review and retrospective study of 20 new cases. J Am Anim Hosp Assoc 20:995–998, 1984.
11. Wolf AM, Green RW: The radiographic appearance of pulmonary histoplasmosis in the cat. Vet Radiol 28:34–37, 1987.
12. Wolf AM: Histoplasma capsulatum osteomyelitis in the cat. J Vet Intern Med 1:158–162, 1987.
13. Wolf AM: Successful treatment of osseous histoplasmosis in two cats. J Am Anim Hosp Assoc 24:511–516, 1988.
14. Carakostas MC, Miller RI, Gossett KA: Clinical laboratory evaluation of deep mycotic diseases in dogs. J Small Anim Pract 25:687–693, 1984.
15. Clinkenbeard KD, Cowell RL, Tyler RD: Identification of intracellular Histoplasma organisms in cir-

culating eosinophils of a dog. *J Am Vet Med Assoc* 192:217–218, 1988.

16. Clinkenbeard KD, Cowell RL, Tyler RD: Thrombocytopenia associated with disseminated histoplasmosis in dogs. *Compend Cont Educ Pract Vet* 11:301–306, 1989.

17. Echols JT: Histoplasmosis in a dog. *Mod Vet Pract* 61:1009–1011, 1980.

18. Forjaz MH, Fischman O: Animal histoplasmosis in Brazil. *Mykosen* 28:191–194, 1985.

19. Hoffman D, Norton J, Mudie A, et al: Suspected *Histoplasma capsulatum* of the intestine in a dog. *Aust Vet J* 62:390–391, 1985.

20. VanSteenhouse JL, DeNovo RC Jr: Atypical *Histoplasma capsulatum* infection in a dog. *J Am Vet Med Assoc* 188:527–528, 1986.

21. Clinkenbeard KD, Cowell RL, Tyler RD: Disseminated histoplasmosis in dogs: 12 cases (1981–1986). *J Am Vet Med Assoc* 193:1443–1447, 1988.

22. Lenarduzzi RF, Jones L: Diagnosing pulmonary histoplasmosis despite nonspecific signs. *Vet Med* 81:412–418, 1986.

23. Ackerman N, Spencer CP: Radiologic aspects of mycotic diseases. *Vet Clin North Am* 12:175–191, 1982.

24. Moriello KA: Ketoconazole: clinical pharmacology and therapeutic recommendations. *J Am Vet Med Assoc* 188:303–306, 1986.

25. Wolf AM: Unpublished observations, Texas A & M University, College Station, TX, 1988.

25a. Pappagianis D, Zimmer BL, Hector RF: Comparative efficacy of the triazole Bay R3783 in murine models of deep mycoses. 29th Intersci Conf Antimicrob Agents Chemother, Houston, Sept 1989, p 223 (Abstr).

26. Dupont B, Drouhet E: Early experience with itraconazole in vitro and in patients: pharmacokinetic studies and clinical results. *Rev Infect Dis* 9 (Suppl 1):s71–s76, 1987.

27. Ganer A, Arathoon E, Stevens DA: Initial experience in therapy for progressive mycoses with itraconazole, the first clinically studied triazole. *Rev Infect Dis* 9 (Suppl 1):s77–s85, 1987.

28. Graybill JR, Palou E, Ahrens J: Treatment of murine histoplasmosis with UK 49,858 (fluconazole). *Am Rev Respir Dis* 134:768–770, 1986.

29. Negroni R, Palmieri O, Koren F, et al: Oral treatment of paracoccidioidomycosis and histoplasmosis with itraconazole in humans. *Rev Infect Dis* 9 (Suppl 1):s47–s50, 1987.

30. Van Cutsem J, Van Gerven F, Janssen PA: Activity of orally, topically, and parenterally administered itraconazole in the treatment of superficial and deep mycoses: animal models. *Rev Infect Dis* 9 (Suppl 1):s15–s31, 1987.

31. Phillips P, Fetchick R, Weisman I, et al: Tolerance to and efficacy of itraconazole in treatment of systemic mycoses: preliminary results. *Rev Infect Dis* 9 (Suppl 1):s87–s93, 1987.

32. Van Cauteren H, Heykants J, De Coster R, et al: Itraconazole: pharmacologic studies in animals and humans. *Rev Infect Dis* 9 (Suppl 1):s43–s46, 1987.

33. Medleau L: Personal communication, University of Georgia, Athens, GA, 1988.

34. Kobayashi GS, Travis S, Medoff G: Comparison of in vitro and in vivo activity of the bis-triazole derivative UK 49,858 with that of amphotericin B against *Histoplasma capsulatum*. *Antimicrob Agents Chemother* 29:660–662, 1986.

35. Larsh HW: The epidemiology of histoplasmosis. In Al-Doory Y (ed): *The Epidemiology of Human Mycotic Diseases*. Springfield, Charles C Thomas, 1975, pp 52–73.

67 CRYPTOCOCCOSIS

Linda Medleau
Jeanne A. Barsanti

ETIOLOGY

Although there are several different species of the genus *Cryptococcus* in the environment, only one, *C. neoformans*, causes disease. The ability of *C. neoformans* to grow at 37°C may explain its pathogenicity in mammals, since other cryptococcal species grow poorly at this temperature. The growth of the organism is inhibited as temperature increases above 39°C. *C. neoformans* is a saprophytic, round, yeast-like fungus (3.5 to 7 μm in diameter) with the ability to form a large (1 to 30 μm thick) heteropolysaccharide capsule (Fig. 67–1). The organism may or may not produce the capsule when grown on artificial media or when growing naturally in the environment, but it always produces the capsule in tissues.[1] Not a true yeast, *C. neoformans* is related to the rust and smut fungal pathogens of higher plants. It reproduces by forming one or two buds

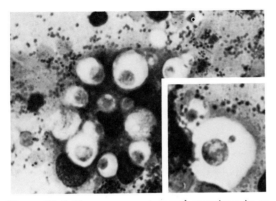

Figure 67–1. Numerous cryptococcal organisms in an impression smear of the nasal exudate from a cat. The thick nonstaining capsule is visible (Wright's stain; × 1000). *Inset*, which has been enlarged: typical budding appearance of *Cryptococcus*.

(blastoconidia) that are connected to the parent cell by a narrow isthmus (Fig. 67–1). The buds may break off when small; as a result, the yeast population varies in size. Unlike other dimorphic fungi, the yeast phase of *C. neoformans* is always found under normal laboratory conditions and in infected tissues. The sexual reproductive phase can be demonstrated only under controlled laboratory conditions.

Although *C. neoformans* has been isolated from several sources, it is most frequently found associated with droppings and accumulated filth and debris of pigeon roosts. The organism passes through the gut of pigeons, but spontaneous avian cryptococcosis is extremely rare. Presumably the pigeon's high body temperature (42°C [107.6°F]) protects it from infection. In pigeon droppings, cryptococci may remain viable for at least 2 years unless exposed to drying or sunlight.[2] It has been suggested that the high concentration of creatinine in pigeon droppings favor cryptococcal growth. However, pigeon feces provide an alkaline, hyperosmolar environment that is rich in many nitrogen-containing compounds besides creatinine.

C. neoformans is worldwide in distribution and in addition to people, infects a variety of domestic and wild mammals, including the cat and the dog. In contrast to the other systemic mycoses, the prevalence of cryptococcosis in cats is equal to or greater than that in dogs.

Four serotypes of *C. neoformans* have been identified. Serotypes A and D are found in pigeon feces.[3] The ecologic sites of types B and C are unknown. Type A is most frequently associated with disease in people, except in southern California, where types B and C are the cause of half of human

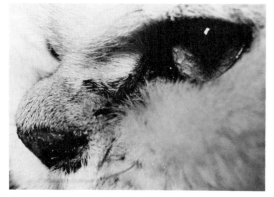

Figure 67–2. Cat with nasal swelling due to cryptococcosis.

illness. The serotypes involved in animal cryptococcosis have not been determined.

PATHOGENESIS

The exact mode of infection is unknown. Based on circumstantial evidence, the most likely route is through inhalation of airborne organisms in geographic areas where infected pigeon droppings are abundant. Following inhalation, the organism may deposit in the upper respiratory tract, inducing nasal granulomas (Fig. 67–2), or reach the alveoli, causing pulmonary granulomas (Fig. 67–3). Encapsulated organisms (5 to 20 μm) are too large to enter terminal airways, but shrunken, unencapsulated cryptococci that are small enough for alveolar deposition have been isolated from pigeon feces and soil.[4] It is theoretically possible to inhale the basid-

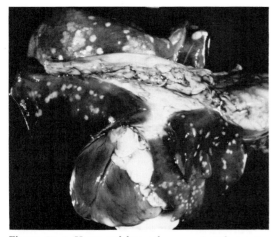

Figure 67–3. Heart and lungs from a cat with cryptococcosis, showing multiple white pulmonary nodules.

iospores of the sexual (mold) stage, but whether this mode of infection occurs naturally has not been proved.[1]

Cryptococcosis has been experimentally induced in cats by intranasal and intrathecal administration of organisms, but not by oral or SC administration.[5] Under natural circumstances, primary GI infection is unlikely. Drinking unpasteurized milk from cattle with cryptococcal mastitis did not induce disease. However, under certain circumstances, direct inoculation of the organisms could result in disease in animals.[6] The organism is not transmitted between people or animals, a feature common to the other systemic mycoses.

Cryptococcosis can disseminate from the respiratory system, usually to the CNS by local extension through cribriform plates or by hematogenous spread. When CNS signs appear, there may be no evidence of respiratory infection.

The establishment and spread of infection are highly dependent on host immunity. As with most fungal infections, cell-mediated immunity is most important in preventing or eliminating cryptococcal infection. Acquired antibody provides no protection. The natural resistance of people to cryptococcosis is so strong that the presence of the disease is a signal to look for another predisposing cause. About 50% of humans with cryptococcal meningitis have another disease, primarily lymphoreticular malignancy.[7] Immunosuppression, as seen with glucocorticoid therapy, sarcoidosis, and AIDS, also predisposes patients to cryptococcal meningitis. As in people, both experimental and natural cases of cryptococcal infection in dogs and cats have been accelerated or worsened by glucocorticoid therapy.[5,8] In cats, infection with feline leukemia virus (FeLV) or feline immunodeficiency virus (FIV) may be a predisposing factor for feline cryptococcosis. However, underlying diseases are often not detected in cats with cryptococcosis. In dogs, immunosuppressive diseases such as ehrlichiosis have been associated with fatal disseminated cryptococcosis.[8a]

The organism also has features that contribute to its virulence. The capsule is essential to its pathogenicity, inhibiting plasma cell function, phagocytosis, and leukocyte migration. It also decomplements serum and absorbs opsonins.[1]

CLINICAL FINDINGS

Cats

Cryptococcosis is the most common of the systemic mycoses in the cat. There is no sex predisposition, and the age range of affected cats is broad (1 to 13 years, average 5.0 years). Cats with cryptococcosis usually have one or more of the following organ systems affected: respiratory, cutaneous, CNS, and ocular (Table 67–1). Upper respiratory signs are most common and include sneezing, snuffling, and a mucopurulent, serous or hemorrhagic, unilateral or bilateral chronic nasal discharge. In about 70% of these cases, a flesh-colored, polyp-like mass is visible in the nostril, or a firm, hard, subcutaneous swelling over the bridge of the nose is evident (Fig. 67–2), and often there is submandibular lymphadenomegaly. Ulcerated or proliferative lesions in the oral cavity are occasionally seen in conjunction with upper respiratory tract infections.[9,18] Lower respiratory signs are rare. Radiographs of the nasal passages may show homogeneous infiltrates and possible destruction of the nasal turbinates. Thoracic radiographs are usually normal, although small lesions may be present. Rarely, a secondary bronchopneumonia or pulmonary nodules may be found.

Cutaneous lesions are also commonly seen in cats with cryptococcosis. The skin or subcutaneous tissues have been affected in approximately 40% of reported cases. In most cats, either multiple lesions have been present or other organ systems were affected, suggesting that the skin lesions are the result of dissemination from another site rather than a direct infection of the skin caused by trauma. The firm swelling over the bridge of the nose previously described usually involves the subcutaneous tissue. Cutaneous lesions elsewhere on the body are usually characterized by papules and nodules that palpate fluctuant to firm and range from 1

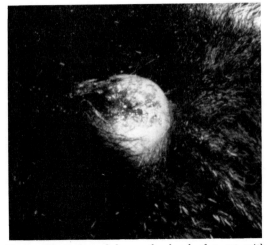

Figure 67–4. A nodule on the head of a cat with cutaneous cryptococcosis.

to 10 mm in diameter (Fig. 67–4). Larger lesions tend to ulcerate, leaving a raw surface with a serous exudate. Pruritus is usually nonexistent to mild, and peripheral lymphadenomegaly is common.

Neurologic signs associated with CNS cryptococcosis in cats are variable, depending on lesion location, and include depression, changes in temperament, seizures, circling, head pressing, ataxia, paresis, apparent loss of smell, and blindness. These signs may occur alone or in association with other clinical signs and may result from the presence of a mass (granuloma) or from meningoencephalitis. Cranial nerve involvement is common. Upper motor neuron limb deficits are usually present owing to brain involvement, although lower motor neuron spinal cord or nerve root lesions also have been described.

Ocular abnormalities occur in some affected cats, especially those with CNS signs. The most common ocular signs are dilated, unresponsive pupils and blindness due to exudative retinal detachment, granulomatous chorioretinitis, panophthalmitis, or optic neuritis (see Systemic Fungal Infections, Chapter 13). The fundus also can be affected without apparent visual loss. Chorioretinitis is probably a consequence of hematogenous spread and suggests that there is systemic involvement, whereas optic neuritis usually is associated with CNS involvement.[18] An anterior uveitis is also present in some cats (Fig. 67–5).

Fever is uncommon in affected cats and when present, is mild, usually 39.5°C (103°F). Cryptococcosis is often chronic, causing list-

Table 67–1. Frequency of Clinical Signs Reported in 63 Cats with Cryptococcosis[6, 9–17]

CLINICAL SIGNS	NUMBER AFFECTED
Sneezing, snuffling, nasal discharge	35
Nasal mass	26
Skin lesions	25
Abnormal ocular signs	15
Abnormal CNS signs	11

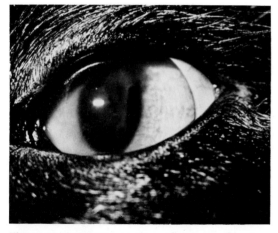

Figure 67–5. Anterior uveitis with aqueous flare in a cat with disseminated cryptococcosis.

lessness and anorexia with resultant weight loss. Other reported signs are peripheral lymphadenomegaly unassociated with skin lesions, bone lysis associated with subcutaneous infection, chronic cough, and rarely, uremia due to renal involvement.

Dogs

No sex predisposition has been reported in dogs with cryptococcosis. The average age of affected dogs was 3 years (range, 2 weeks to 8 years). Most cases have been reported in larger breeds.

The major organ systems affected by canine cryptococcosis are the CNS and the eyes (Table 67–2). CNS signs include head tilt, nystagmus, facial paralysis, paresis to paraplegia or tetraplegia (usually upper motor neuron), ataxia, circling, seizures, and neck pain. These signs are usually related to

Table 67–2. Frequency of Clinical Signs Reported in 28 Dogs with Cryptococcosis[11, 16, 19–22]

CLINICAL SIGNS	NUMBER AFFECTED
Abnormal CNS signs	21
Abnormal ocular signs	18
Anorexia/emaciation	12
Skin lesions	6
Fever	5
Peripheral lymphadenomegaly	5
Nasal discharge	4
Dry cough	3
Vomiting	3
Lytic bone lesions	3
Vaginal discharge	1

a meningoencephalomyelitis. The most common ocular abnormalities are exudative granulomatous chorioretinitis and optic neuritis, associated with dilated pupils, and blindness (see Chapter 13). An anterior uveitis is occasionally present. A retrobulbar abscess with lysis of the bone of the orbit has been reported in one dog.

Cutaneous involvement may also be seen in association with systemic disease. Skin lesions are usually characterized by ulcers that may involve the nose, tongue, gums, hard palate, lips, or nail beds. Other rarely reported lesions have included a pharyngeal abscess formation or skin wounds with multiple draining sinuses.

Fever (39.4° to 40.5°C [103° to 105°F]) is noted in about 25% of natural infections. Less common clinical signs include a dry cough, vomiting, lameness due to lytic bone lesions, a serous to hemorrhagic nasal discharge, weight loss due to anorexia, and peripheral lymphadenomegaly.

DIAGNOSIS

Cytologic Examination

The most rapid method of diagnosis is cytologic evaluation of nasal exudate, skin exudate, CSF, tissue aspirates, and samples obtained by paracentesis of the aqueous or vitreous chambers of the eye. Although Wright's stain has been used most often in diagnosing cryptococcosis, this stain can cause the organism to shrink and the capsule to become distorted. New methylene blue (Fig. 67–6) and Gram stains (see Fig. 62–3) are considered to be better than Wright's stain for this reason. With Gram stain the organism retains crystal violet whereas capsule stains lightly red with safranin.[1] The organism can be seen with low (× 100) power. India ink may also be used to visualize the organism, which appears unstained and silhouetted against a black background (Fig. 67–6). It is not as definitive as the other stains unless budding is seen, as lymphocytes, fat droplets, and aggregated India ink particles may be confused with the organism. Cytologic examination can also be performed on tissue biopsy samples. Impression smears may be made directly, or part of the biopsy can be macerated with a scalpel, mixed with 1 ml of 15% potassium hydroxide (KOH), incubated at 37°C for 30 minutes,

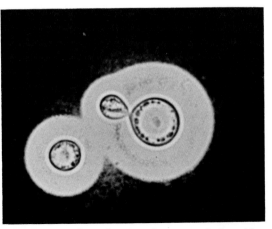
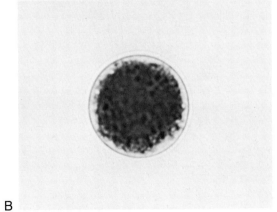

A   B

Figure 67–6. India ink (A) and new methylene blue (B) preparations of CSF from a dog with cryptococcal meningoencephalitis. Budding is evident in the India ink preparation. Capsule is not well visualized and only internal structure stains.

and examined microscopically for budding organisms (see Appendix 12). The KOH will digest all other cells and debris. Cytologic examination of nasal or cutaneous exudates, masses, or ocular fluid has revealed organisms in a majority of cases. Organisms have been missed in approximately 25% of cases, so negative cytology does not rule out cryptococcosis.

Serologic Testing

The detection of cryptococcal capsular antigen using a latex agglutination procedure is the *only* clinically useful serologic test. This commercially available test detects cryptococcal capsular antigen in serum, urine, or CSF and is a rapid diagnostic method in suspected cases in which the organism has not been visualized or cultured (see Appendix 8). In people, false-negative titers can be seen if the disease is localized, and false-positive titers may be seen in *Klebsiella* infections or if rheumatoid factor is present.[2] The specificity of this test has been improved by modification in which the serum to be tested is pretreated with a protease.[22a] The test can be used in cats to support a diagnosis made by cytologic or histologic methods.[10,11] Its use, which has not been documented in canine infections, should be similarly valuable. Titers can be quite high (>1:2048) in affected cats, although even a titer of 1:1 is considered to be a positive result. A cryptococcal antigen titer has been useful in evaluating the progress of cats during therapy.[10–12] A good prog-

nosis is indicated by a decrease in antigen titer during the course of therapy, whereas a persistent titer following treatment suggests continued infection.

Tissue Biopsy

Because of the rapidity of cytologic evaluation, impression smears or KOH preparations should always be made from biopsy samples. If no organisms are seen, part of the sample can be used for culture, and the rest can be processed for routine histologic examination. On H and E staining, the organism stains as a faint, eosinophilic, round to oval body surrounded by a clear halo, because the capsule does not stain (Fig. 67–7). The organism is more easily visualized with PAS, methenamine silver, or Masson-Fontana stain, but the capsule still does not stain. Mayer's mucicarmine is the definitive stain of choice, because the cryptococcal capsule appears a rose-red color and the organism appears pink against a blue background. Other fungi that have similar morphologic characteristics do not stain with this method.[1] The large capsule and the thin cell wall of *Cryptococcus* differentiate it from *Blastomyces*. Its budding and lack of endospores distinguish it from *Coccidioides immitis*.

Fungal Isolation

The organism can be cultured from exudate, CSF, urine, joint fluid, and tissue sam-

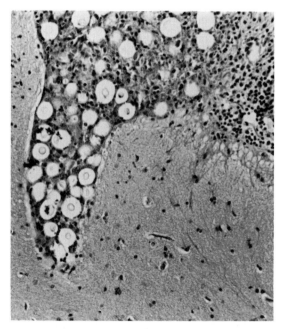

Figure 67–7. Histologic section of brain and meninges from a dog with cryptococcal meningoencephalitis showing numerous organisms and an inflammatory response (H and E; × 400).

ples fairly easily if a large enough sample volume is obtained. Sabouraud's agar with antibiotics is used when bacterial contamination is likely. *Cryptococcus* is sensitive to media containing cycloheximide.[1] The organism should be cultured at both 25° and 37°C; growth will occur in 48 hours to 6 weeks, depending on the amount of inoculum. The organism forms white, creamy colonies that yellow with age, are mucoid when the organism forms its capsule, and are dry when it is unencapsulated. Characteristics used to identify the organism are its morphology (i.e., presence of the capsule), growth at 37°C, hydrolysis of urea, response to various assimilation tests, and virulence for mice. Culture of CSF reveals cryptococcosis more frequently than does cytologic examination, so fungal culture of abnormal CSF is always recommended in cases of possible cryptococcosis when the organism cannot be demonstrated cytologically or serologically.

PATHOLOGIC FINDINGS

The lesion associated with cryptococcosis varies from a gelatinous mass, consisting of numerous organisms with minimal inflammation to granuloma formation. In people,

the degree of granuloma formation has been directly related to the duration of the lesion. The lesion usually is composed of aggregates of encapsulated organisms within a connective tissue reticulum (Fig. 67–7). The primary cellular response is composed of macrophages and giant cells with a few plasma cells and lymphocytes. Epithelioid and giant cells and areas of caseation are less common than with the other systemic mycoses.

Cats

In cats that die or are euthanatized, the respiratory system is most often affected. The nasal cavity most frequently has contained a granulomatous lesion, but in many, the lungs also have granulomas (see Fig. 67–3). Pulmonary granulomas rarely will be suspected prior to death and only then because of respiratory signs or by visualization on thoracic radiographs.

The ocular system and CNS are next most commonly affected. Lesions are usually meningitis, peripheral neuritis, most frequently involving the optic nerve, and granulomatous chorioretinitis. Occasionally, a granulomatous mass rather than a diffuse meningoencephalitis is found. Other affected organs are skin and subcutaneous tissues, kidneys, and lymph nodes draining infected areas. Renal granulomas have been found in approximately 30% of cases. Granulomas have also been found occasionally in the spleen, adrenal glands, thyroid glands, and liver.

Dogs

In contrast with cats, dogs that die or are euthanatized because of cryptococcosis usually have severe disseminated disease, and most have CNS or ocular involvement. The lesions are usually meningoencephalitis; peripheral neuritis of the optic, facial, or vestibular nerves; and granulomatous chorioretinitis. Approximately 50% of dogs in reported cases had lesions in the respiratory tract, usually in the lungs. A small proportion have had lesions in the nasal cavity, and rarely is there sinus involvement. Other affected organs, in decreasing order of frequency, have been kidneys, lymph nodes, spleen, liver, thyroid gland, adrenal glands, pancreas, bone, GI tract, muscle, myocardium, prostate gland, heart valves, and tonsils. In one instance, a dog had an acute eosinophilic periportal hepatitis associated with cryptococcal organisms.

THERAPY

Amphotericin B and Flucytosine

Amphotericin B (AMB) has been used alone to successfully treat cats with cryptococcosis (Table 67–3). Lower dose rates should be given initially and then gradually increased when it is determined that the cat has not become azotemic (see also Chapter 63).

Because cats require such a small amount per dose, a bottle of AMB can be reconstituted in sterile water, divided into small aliquots, and frozen. Each week an aliquot can be thawed, with a portion diluted for treatment, and the remainder refrigerated for use later that week. For each treatment, the AMB is diluted in a small volume of 5% dextrose solution and then administered by bolus IV infusion rather than by IV drip.

There are several disadvantages of using AMB in treating cryptococcosis. It must be given IV and is potentially nephrotoxic. Long-term hospitalization and constant monitoring are often necessary during treatment. Even cats successfully treated with AMB have developed transient renal failure that necessitated parenteral fluid administration and delayed further treatment.

Flucytosine can be used alone or in combination with AMB (Table 67–3).[23] When flucytosine is used alone, however, the development of drug resistance may occur, so combination therapy with AMB and flucytosine is recommended.

There are few reports of treatment of infected dogs with AMB, with or without flucytosine. The meningoencephalitis frequently observed in dogs is more like the disease in humans and carries a more guarded prognosis than does the disease in cats. Neurologic signs in dogs have progressed during treatment or after it has been discontinued.[19] The inability of AMB or flucytosine to cross the blood-brain and blood-CNS barriers explains the limited efficacy of these drugs in cases of cryptococcal meningoencephalitis. Intrathecal AMB has been used in severe cases of cryptococcal meningitis in humans.

Ketoconazole

Ketoconazole (KTZ), an imidazole derivative, has been used to successfully treat cats with cryptococcosis.[9–14,24] In general, the dosage is given once or twice daily but may have to be given less frequently in cats that

Table 67–3. Therapy for Cryptococcosis[a]

DRUG	SPECIES	DOSE[b] (mg/kg)	ROUTE	INTERVAL[c] (hours)	DURATION (months)
Amphotericin B	C	0.1–0.5	IV	3 times/week	[d]
	D	0.25–0.5	IV	3 times/week	[d]
and/or					
Flucytosine	C	30	PO	6	1–9
		50	PO	8	1–9
		75	PO	12	1–9
	D	50–75	PO	8	1–12
Ketoconazole	C	5–10[e]	PO	12	4–5[f]
		10–20[e, g]	PO	24	4–5[f]
	D	5–15	PO	12	3–5
		30	PO	24	3–5
Itraconazole[h]	C	5–10	PO	12	4–5[f]
		20	PO	24	4–5[f]
Fluconazole[h]	B	5–10	PO	12–24	4–5

[a]C = cat; D = dog; B = both dog and cat; PO = by mouth; IV = intravenous.
[b]Dose per administration at specified interval, expressed as mg/kg unless otherwise stated.
[c]Expressed in hours unless otherwise stated.
[d]Until a cumulative dosage of 4 to 10 mg/kg is reached.
[e]If toxicity develops, the dose should be changed to 50 mg/cat every other day.
[f]Range may vary from 3 to 10 months.
[g]Rarely, can require up to 60 to 70 mg/kg/day for cure if the dose can be tolerated.
[h]Investigational drug.

develop toxicity (Table 67–3). Because KTZ is fungistatic and, therefore, slow-acting, treatment may need to continue for several months until serum cryptococcal antigen titers are negative or for 1 month past resolution of all clinical signs.

KTZ's absorption from the GI tract is greatly enhanced by giving it with food. Side effects of KTZ in cats include anorexia, vomiting, diarrhea, elevated serum liver enzyme activities, and icterus.[14,25] Giving KTZ with food and dividing the daily dosage may help alleviate signs of anorexia or vomiting. If anorexia persists, KTZ therapy should be stopped until the cat is eating normally, and then reinstituted at a lower dosage or on an alternate day basis.

KTZ has also been used less commonly to treat infected dogs, but the response has not been as consistent as in cats.[11,15,22] Presumably, this relates to the tendency for dogs to have disseminated or neurologic manifestations that are difficult to treat. Dogs with disseminated cryptococcosis have not improved or have relapsed, whereas those with primarily cutaneous manifestations recovered after 3 months of treatment.

Itraconazole

Itraconazole (ITZ) is a triazole antifungal agent that is currently investigational (see Table 67–3). It shares its basic principles of activity with KTZ and is also administered orally but appears to have fewer side effects in cats. ITZ has been used to successfully treat experimental cryptococcosis in mice, rabbits, and cats.[26–28] Response in spontaneously infected cats is promising.[26] Although it has been used in dogs with other systemic mycoses, its efficacy for canine infections is uncertain. Newer triazoles such as fluconazole may have better efficacy of penetrating the blood-CSF barrier and have been more effective than the other azoles but similar to AMB in treating cryptococcal meningitis (see Chapter 63)[29].

PREVENTION

The major means of prevention is restricting animal contact with areas of high concentrations of pigeon droppings, especially those inside shaded, damp buildings.[1] The number of organisms can be greatly reduced by repeated cleaning of pigeon habitats with hydrated lime diluted in water 40 g/L (1 lb/ 3 gal) plus 1.5 g/L NaOH. This solution should be applied at a rate of 1.36 L/m² (1 gal/30 ft²).[30]

PUBLIC HEALTH CONSIDERATIONS

Unlike culture of other systemic fungi, culture of Cryptococcus is not a public health hazard, because only the yeast form is routinely grown and this form does not aerosolize from media. Contact with infected pets is also not a risk, as the organism does not aerosolize from sites of tissue infection. The major public health significance of infected pets is that their source of exposure is also a potential source of exposure for associated humans.

References

1. Davis CE: Cryptococcus. In Braude AI, Davis CE, Fierer J (eds): Medical Microbiology and Infectious Diseases. Philadelphia, WB Saunders Co, 1986, pp 564–571.
2. Rippon JW: Medical Mycology. The Pathogenic Fungi and the Pathogenic Actinomycetes, ed 3. Philadelphia, WB Saunders Co, 1988, pp 582–609.
3. Diamond RD: Cryptococcus neoformans. In Mandell GL, Douglas RG, Bennett JE (eds): Principles and Practice of Infectious Diseases. New York, John Wiley & Sons, 1985, pp 1460–1468.
4. Powell KE, Dahl BA, Weeks RJ, et al: Airborne Cryptococcus neoformans: particles from pigeon excreta compatible with alveolar disposition. J Infect Dis 125:412–415, 1972.
5. Turnquest RU: Experimental feline cryptococcosis. MS thesis. Ithaca, Cornell University, 1968.
6. Pal M, Mehrotra BS: Occurrence and etiologic significance of Cryptococcus neoformans in a cutaneous lesion of a cat. Mykosen 26:608–610, 1983.
7. Schimpff SC, Bennett JE: Abnormalities in cell-mediated immunity in patients with Cryptococcus neoformans infection. J Allergy Clin Immunol 55:430–441, 1975.
8. MacDonald DW, Stretch HC: Canine cryptococcosis associated with prolonged corticosteroid therapy. Can Vet J 23:200–202, 1982.
8a. Collett MG, Doyle AS, Reyers F, et al: Fatal disseminated cryptococcosis and concurrent ehrlichiosis in a dog. J S Afr Vet Med Assoc 58:197–202, 1987.
9. Emms SG: Ketoconazole in the treatment of cryptococcosis in cats. Aust Vet J 64: 276–277, 1987.
10. Pentlarge VW, Martin RA: Treatment of cryptococcosis in three cats, using ketoconazole. J Am Vet Med Assoc 188:536–538, 1986.
11. Noxon JO, Monroe WE, Chinn DR: Ketoconazole

therapy in canine and feline cryptococcosis. *J Am Anim Hosp Assoc* 22:179–183, 1986.

12. Hansen BL: Successful treatment of severe feline cryptococcosis with long-term high doses of ketoconazole. *J Am Anim Hosp Assoc* 23:193–196, 1987.

13. Medleau L, Hall EJ, Goldschmidt MH, et al: Cutaneous cryptococcosis in three cats. *J Am Vet Med Assoc* 187:169–170, 1985.

14. Schulman J: Ketoconazole for successful treatment of cryptococcosis in a cat. *J Am Vet Med Assoc* 187:508–509, 1985.

15. Willard MD: Cryptococcosis. *Calif Vet* 12:13–16, 1982.

16. Barsanti JA: Cryptococcosis. In Greene CE (ed): *Clinical Microbiology and Infectious Diseases of the Dog and Cat*. Philadelphia, WB Saunders Co, 1984, pp 702–703.

17. Dye JA, Campbell KL: Cutaneous and ocular cryptococcosis in a cat: case report and literature review. *Companion Anim Pract* 2:34–44, 1988.

18. Blouin P, Conner MW: Cryptococcosis. In Holzworth J (ed): *Diseases of the Cat: Medicine and Surgery*. Philadelphia, WB Saunders Co, 1987, pp 332–342.

19. Stampley AR, Barsanti JA: Disseminated cryptococcosis in a dog. *J Am Anim Hosp Assoc* 24:17–21, 1988.

20. Jergens AE, Wheeler CA, Collier LL: Cryptococcosis involving the eye and central nervous system of a dog. *J Am Vet Med Assoc* 189:302–304, 1986.

21. Hodgin EC, Corstvet RE, Blakewood BW: Cryptococcosis in a pup. *J Am Vet Med Assoc* 191:697–698, 1987.

22. Panciera DL, Bevier D: Management of cryptococcosis and toxic epidermal necrolysis in a dog. *J Am Vet Med Assoc* 191:1125–1127, 1987.

22a. Gray LD, Roberts GD: Experience with the use of pronase to eliminate interference factors in the latex agglutination test for cryptococcal antigen. *J Clin Microbiol* 26:2450–2451, 1988.

23. Wilkinson GT, Bate MJ, Robbins GM, et al: Successful treatment of four cases of feline cryptococcosis. *J Small Anim Pract* 24:507–514, 1983.

24. Legendre AM, Gompf R, Bone D: Treatment of feline cryptococcosis with ketoconazole. *J Am Vet Med Assoc* 181:1541–1542, 1982.

25. Greene CE, Miller DM, Blue J: Trichosporon infection in a cat. *J Am Vet Med Assoc* 187:946–948, 1985.

26. Itraconazole: Basic Medical Information Brochure. Janssen Pharmaceutica, 1984.

27. Prefect JR, Savani DV, Durack DT: Comparisons of itraconazole and fluconazole in the treatment of cryptococcal meningitis and *Candida* pyelonephritis in rabbits. *Antimicrob Agents Chemother* 29:579–583, 1986.

28. Medleau L, Greene CE: Unpublished data. University of Georgia, Athens, GA, 1988.

29. Dismukes W, Cloud G, Thompson S, et al: Fluconazole versus amphotericin B therapy of acute cryptococcal meningitis. 29th Intersci Conf Antimicrob Agents Chemother. Houston, Sept 1989, p 282 (Abstr).

30. Walter JE, Coffee EG: Distribution and epidemiologic significance of the serotypes of *Cryptococcus neoformans*. *Am J Epidemiol* 87:167–172, 1968.

68 COCCIDIOIDOMYCOSIS

Jeanne A. Barsanti
Kenneth L. Jeffery

ETIOLOGY

Coccidioides immitis is a soil organism restricted to certain geographic regions. It grows in the soil as a mycelium that forms square to rectangular multinucleate arthrospores, 2 to 4 μm wide and 3 to 10 μm long (Fig. 68–1).[1] These arthrospores are easily detached and dispersed into the air by wind. Following inhalation or, rarely, by contamination of a skin wound, the arthrospores transform into spherules that gradually enlarge to 20 to 200 μm in diameter. The wall of the spherule seems to act as a germinal center, resulting in endospore production through cleavage.[2] Intact spherules are poorly chemotactic for neutrophils.[3] Those neutrophils that do attach cannot penetrate the wall of the spherule (Fig. 68–2).[3] When released from the spherule, each endospore forms a new mature spherule at 37°C or a mycelium at room temperature. The endospore, the vulnerable stage of *C. immitis* in the body, attracts large numbers of neutrophils and is of sufficiently small size to be phagocytized.[3] In the body, endospores preferably mature in the lungs, although dissemination to other tissues via lymphatics or blood is possible.

EPIDEMIOLOGY

The mycelial phase of *C. immitis* has been found in nature only in a specific ecologic area, the Lower Sonoran life zone. This zone is characterized by sandy, alkaline soils, high environmental temperature (summer mean > 26.6°C; winter mean 4° to 12°C), low rainfall (3″ to 20″), and low elevation (sea level to a few hundred feet).[4] During pro-

longed periods of high temperature and low soil moisture, *C. immitis* survives below the soil surface at depths as great as 20 cm, where competitive organisms are few. After a period of rainfall, *C. immitis* returns to the soil surface, sporulates, and releases large numbers of arthrospores to be disseminated by the wind. Epidemics in people have occurred after dust storms following the rainy season. Geographically, this area is within the southwestern United States (Fig. 68–3), Mexico, and Central and South America (Guatemala, Honduras, Colombia, Vene-

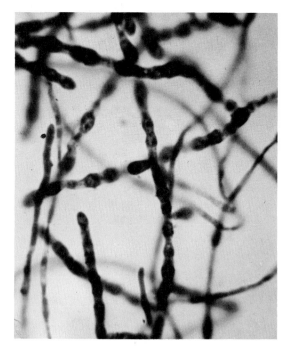

Figure 68–1. Arthrospores arising from a mycelial culture of *C. immitis* (H and E; × 970). (From Maddy KT: *J Am Vet Med Assoc* 132:483–489, 1958. Reprinted with permission.)

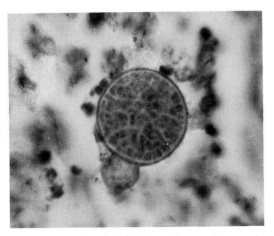

Figure 68–2. Spherule of *C. immitis* containing endospores (H and E; × 970). (From Maddy KT: *J Am Vet Med Assoc* 132:483–489, 1958. Reprinted with permission.)

zuela, Paraguay, Argentina). In the United States, the disease was named San Joaquin Valley fever after an endemic area in California, but it is also prevalent in Arizona and southwestern Texas. The disease is less common in New Mexico, Nevada, and Utah.

Although the vast majority of cases in animals and people are from the southwestern United States, an occasional case may be identified outside the endemic area. Usually, the animals have a history of previous residence in or contact with fomites from the endemic area. Serologic surveys indicate that most human and canine inhabitants of the endemic area become infected. Most human infections are subclinical or cause only mild, transient respiratory signs. However, in dogs that develop clinical respiratory disease, disseminated disease and death are more common.[5]

Cases have been described in all species of domestic animals and a variety of wild animals, but of the spontaneous cases, the disease in dogs resembles most closely that occurring in people. Case descriptions of affected cats have been rare.

PATHOGENESIS

The major route of infection is by inhalation, and in dogs, very few (<10) arthrospores must be inhaled to produce disease.[6] Primary localized infection via skin lesions following penetrating wounds has rarely been reported. Experimentally, intradermal inoculation or skin scarification produces only localized infection in a small percentage of animals.[2] The incubation period from inhalation to onset of abnormal respiratory signs is 1 to 3 weeks in people and dogs.

Following inhalation, the spores first enter the bronchioles and alveoli, then extend into the peribronchiolar tissue. Subsequently, the

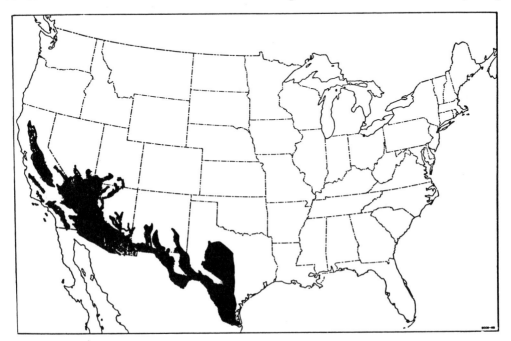

Figure 68–3. Areas in the United States in which coccidioidomycosis is endemic. (From Maddy KT: *J Am Vet Med Assoc* 132:483–489, 1958. Reprinted with permission.)

organisms move toward the lung surface, eventually causing subpleural lesions. The first cellular response is neutrophilic, followed by monocytes, lymphocytes, and plasma cells. Although humoral antibody production is stimulated, cell-mediated immunity is more important in elimination of the infection.[7] Recovery from infection in people results in life-long immunity, but resistance to reinfection in dogs is uncertain. With massive exposure or depressed cellular immunity, pulmonary infection can become more extensive, and the organisms can disseminate to other tissues. This process involves the cycle from spherule to endospores to new spherules.

The mediastinal and tracheobronchial lymph nodes are the first extrapulmonary tissues in dogs to be affected, as soon as 10 days after exposure. If the infection spreads beyond these lymph nodes, the disease is considered disseminated. Signs referable to other organs usually occur about 4 months after pulmonary signs, but this period is variable, and the respiratory infection may never have been noticed.[8]

Once they develop respiratory infection, boxer and Doberman pinscher dogs have been noted to have a greater prevalence of disseminated disease.[1] Male dogs may be at greater risk than female dogs.[9] If the disease disseminates from the pulmonary system, the organs that are usually affected are, listed in decreasing order, bones and joints, visceral organs (primarily spleen, liver, kidney), heart and pericardium, testicles, eyes, brain and spinal cord. Ocular lesions begin as a chorioretinitis and extend into the anterior chamber.[10] Disseminated cases usually have a chronic course of months to years.

CLINICAL FINDINGS

Dogs

The high prevalence of positive skin test reactions in epidemiologic surveys of healthy dogs indicates that the most common form of coccidioidomycosis is an asymptomatic or mild, undiagnosed respiratory infection. When clinical respiratory disease develops, it is usually characterized by a dry harsh cough, similar to that associated with tracheobronchitis; however, like pneumonia, fever, partial anorexia, and weight loss are more typical of coccidioido-

mycosis. The pulmonary disease can then resolve or progress, the latter course leading to severe generalized lung disease with a worsening of respiratory signs.

Clinical signs frequently associated with progressive pulmonary or disseminated disease include, in order of decreasing frequency, cough or dyspnea, persistent or fluctuating fever, anorexia and weight loss, depression and weakness, localized peripheral lymphadenomegaly, lameness, draining skin lesions, keratitis, uveitis or acute blindness, and diarrhea. Generalized peripheral lymphadenomegaly is uncommon. The type of cough is variable, from dry and harsh to soft and moist, depending on the type of pulmonary lesion. Dyspnea with wheezing is associated with compression of bronchi by markedly enlarged tracheobronchial lymph nodes. Signs of right-sided or left-sided congestive heart failure can also occur. Cardiac dysfunction arises from disturbances in blood flow, conduction, and myocardial contractility, resulting from lesions in the myocardium and conduction system, heart valves, epicardium, and pericardium. The latter lesion often results in constrictive pericarditis. Involvement of the liver can result in icterus; GI and neurologic signs can result from uremia due to renal involvement. Renal involvement is characterized by renomegaly due to pyogranulomas.[11] Seizures, ataxia, behavioral changes, and coma have been associated with lesions in the CNS.

Lameness usually is accompanied by painful bone swelling or joint enlargement (Fig. 68–4). Bone lesions usually are initially localized to one bone but progress to involve multiple sites. The lesions generally occur in the long bones in the distal diaphysis, metaphysis, and epiphysis and are more productive than lytic. Lesions occur in the axial skeleton but only at a 10% prevalence compared with the appendicular skeleton.

Skin lesions that begin as small bumps and progress to abscesses, ulcers, or draining tracts are almost always found over sites of infected bone (Fig. 68–5). Naturally occurring primary cutaneous infection is extremely rare in dogs.[12] Most cutaneous involvement results from systemic spread of the organism.

Cats

Only five cases have been reported in cats,[10–13] and only a few have been seen by

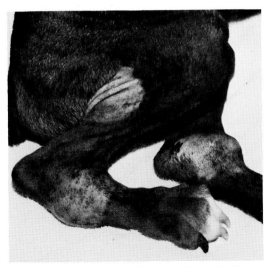

Figure 68–4. Rear limb swelling in a dog with disseminated coccidioidomycosis. The popliteal lymph nodes, over which the hair was clipped prior to aspiration, were also enlarged.

the authors. Signs include chronic draining skin lesions without fever, progressive anorexia and weight loss, cough, dyspnea, lameness with productive osteomyelitis of the appendicular skeleton, and uveitis.

DIAGNOSIS

Clinical Laboratory Findings

Hematologic changes may include increased erythrocyte sedimentation rate, mild

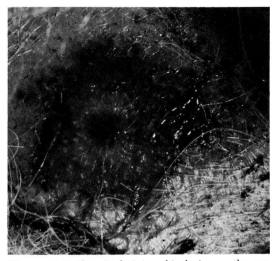

Figure 68–5. Chronic draining skin lesion on the ventral thorax of a dog with disseminated coccidioidomycosis. The underlying sternebrae were affected by osteomyelitis. The exudate contained large numbers of spherules of *C. immitis*.

nonregenerative anemia, and a moderate neutrophilic leukocytosis, often with a left shift. Eosinophilia of blood and CSF has been reported in people.[16]

Azotemia, isosthenuria, and proteinuria have been described with renal involvement.[8] Hypoalbuminemia has been common, and hyperglobulinemia can occur. Hypercalcemia unassociated with bone lesions has been found in some human patients, and an osteotropic factor similar to humoral hypercalcemia of malignancy has been postulated.[17]

Radiography

Thoracic radiographic findings vary with the severity of the disease. A diffuse interstitial pattern is most common but is often mixed with a bronchovascular pattern (Fig. 68–6). Miliary to nodular interstitial densities may be found, and alveolar disease is less frequent. Pulmonary abscess formation, fibrosis, bronchiectasis, (and rarely calcification) may be sequelae to severe pulmonary infection. Hilar lymphadenopathy is quite common, affecting most dogs with chronic illness, but calcification of the hilar lymph nodes or sternal lymphadenopathy is rare. Pericardial and pleural effusion may occur secondary to right-sided myocardial failure or to pericarditis. Radiographs of affected bones show osteomyelitis that is more productive than lytic (Fig. 68–7).

Cytology

Coccidioidomycosis is conclusively diagnosed by visualization of the organism by cytology or biopsy. However, cytologic demonstration of the organism is often not possible. In such cases, a diagnosis is based on history, clinical findings, and results of serologic testing.

As with other nodular interstitial diseases, falsely negative results are common with transtracheal or bronchial washings. The organism may be sometimes found in lymph node aspirates or by cytology of exudate from draining skin lesions (Fig. 68–8).

The organism can be seen in unstained preparations under reduced light as a large (10 to 80 μm), round, double-walled structure with endospores. Ten percent potassium hydroxide (KOH) can be used to clear

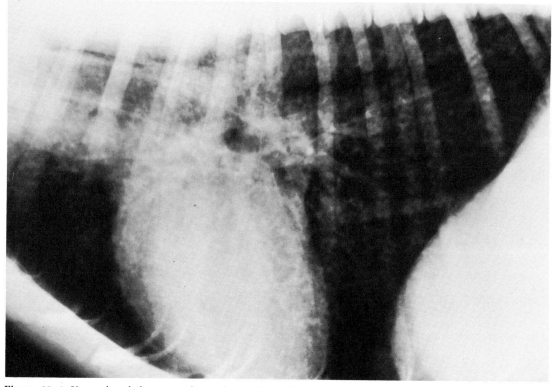

Figure 68–6. Ventrodorsal thoracic radiograph of a dog with pulmonary coccidioidomycosis, showing a diffuse interstitial pattern.

an unstained specimen; stained preparations can also be used (see Appendix 12). The best stains are Papanicolaou's (PAP) and PAS. With PAP stain, the capsular wall is refractile and purple-black, the cytoplasm yellow, and the endospores red-brown. Not all spherules will contain recognizable endospores.[18] Smaller spherules may have a crumpled, transparent wall. With PAS stain, the wall is deep red to purple and the endospores are bright red. Large numbers of neutrophils may surround the spherules, making them difficult to visualize.

Biopsy

In biopsy samples, the organism usually can best be found in microabscesses. Routine H and E stain can be used, but the organism is better visualized with special stains such as PAS or Grocott-Gomori methenamine silver. Identification of the organism from bone biopsies is difficult; repeated biopsies may be necessary to find a positive sample.[8] Fluorescent antibody techniques can also be used to identify *C. immitis* spherules in

tissues or cytologic preparations, but false-negative results can occur.

Fungal Isolation

C. immitis will grow on a wide range of commonly used fungal culture media or blood agar. The mycelial phase grows best at 25° to 30°C. It usually grows within 3 days but may require longer if the number of organisms in the sample is low. There are both in vitro and in vivo methods to identify the organism.[4] *It must be remembered that arthrospores from mycelial growth are highly infectious.* Attempts should *not* be made to culture this organism in veterinary practices but only in laboratories familiar with it (see Appendix 8). As a general rule, diagnosis is *not* confirmed by culture because of the public health risk.

Serology in Dogs

For suspected cases in which the organism cannot be demonstrated by cytology or bi-

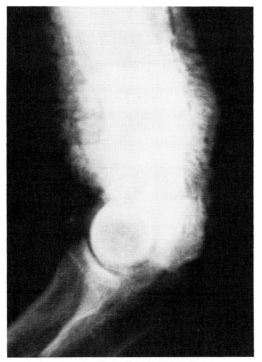

Figure 68–7. Radiograph of the distal humerus of a dog with disseminated coccidioidomycosis. The lesion is mainly osteoproductive.

opsy, precipitin and CF tests are useful as presumptive tests for coccidioidomycosis, although anticomplementary factors in dog serum make the CF test difficult to perform and interpret.[19–21] For interpretation of precipitin and CF titers in naturally infected dogs refer to Table 68–1. In enzootic areas, diagnosis often depends on recognition of suspect clinical signs and on serologic re-

sults. Precipitin and CF tests in commercial laboratories are screened by agar-gel immunodiffusion (see Appendix 8). Serologic titers normally increase during the course of active clinical disease. The precipitin test becomes positive about 2 weeks after exposure and then negative after 4 to 5 weeks. The precipitin test may become positive again with dissemination of a chronic (≥ 5 weeks) infection. An increase in the CF titer usually parallels the increase in the precipitin test titer early in infection. However, the CF titer usually remains elevated for months after the disease is either successfully treated or arrested. With successful resolution of the disease, the CF titer gradually falls. Titers may be falsely negative in immunosuppressed or anergic animals.

An electroimmunodiffusion test that is similar to but more rapid than the CF test has been evaluated for use in dogs.[21] Since the result is qualitative rather than quantitative, its usefulness is limited to a crude screening test. Latex agglutination and fluorescent immunoassays are also available but have not been as thoroughly investigated.[22] Tests to detect antigenemia (rather than antibody titers) have been developed and used on an investigational basis in people.[23,24] Interference by various components in serum is a major problem with antigen tests.[24] Appendix 8 should be consulted for information concerning the submission of samples for serologic testing of coccidioidomycosis.

Serology in Cats

CF tests performed on three of four reported feline cases have been negative.[12–14] One cat with cutaneous infection had positive precipitin test results,[12] but a cat with ocular infection had negative results for precipitin as well as CF tests.[13]

Skin Testing

The accuracy of intradermal testing with coccidioidin is subject to antigen variability.[4] Skin testing is used for epidemiologic surveys and evaluation of immunocompetence to *C. immitis* rather than as a diagnostic test. A positive reaction is an induration of 5 mm or greater in diameter 24 to 36 hours after injection. A positive test indi-

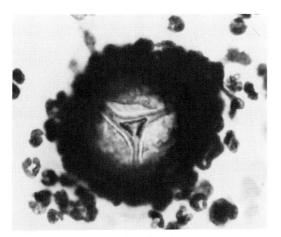

Figure 68–8. Cytology of exudate from chronic draining skin lesions in Figure 68–6, showing a large *C. immitis* spherule surrounded by neutrophils (Wright's stain; × 1000).

Table 68–1. Interpretation of Results of Serologic Testing for Canine Coccidioidomycosis

	PRECIPITIN TEST RESULTS: NEGATIVE[b]	PRECIPITIN TEST RESULTS: POSITIVE[b]
CF TEST RESULTS: NEGATIVE[a]	1. No infection 2. Rapidly fatal, fulminating infection in severely immunocompromised animal 3. Early infection; if disease suspected, repeat test in 2 to 5 weeks to detect positive precipitin or CF test results	1. Early infection: probably pulmonary, although variable; precipitin test results may become positive 2 weeks postexposure and may become negative after 4 to 5 weeks
CF TEST RESULTS: POSITIVE[a]	1. Past exposure or disease, healing or localized lesions, long-standing residual titer (weak CF titer, 1:4 or 1:8) 2. Later infection: precipitin titer frequently decreases after 5 to 6 weeks; CF titers $\geq 1:4 \leq 1:32$ with primary pulmonary lesion 3. Higher CF titers $\geq 1:64$, frequently with disseminated lesions	1. Early active infection: the greater the CF titer, the more likelihood of dissemination 2. Chronic infection: occasionally, positive precipitin tests occur later, at the time of dissemination

Data from Bartsch RC, 1988.[19]
[a]CF = complement fixation, primarily detects IgG.
[b]Precipitin test primarily detects IgM.

cates past or present infection. In people, the test result becomes positive within 1 week, following development of respiratory signs, whereas in dogs a positive test result has been found within 3 to 8 weeks of natural exposure. In healthy people, a positive skin test indicates past exposure and resistance to infection and remains positive for years. About 5% of people and 10% of dogs with disseminated disease have a negative skin test owing to severe immunosuppression. Skin testing is not specific since cross reactions with histoplasmin and blastomycin can occur. Development of an antigen from the spherule phase, spherulin, has not proved diagnostically superior to coccidioidin in people.

PATHOLOGIC FINDINGS

The lesion induced by *C. immitis* can be granulomatous, suppurative, or pyogranulomatous. On gross inspection, the lesion may vary from miliary to massive, from red to gray to white, from nodular to diffuse, and from firm to caseous or liquefactive (Fig. 68–9). Lesions are most often seen in the lungs. Tracheobronchial lymph nodes are often increased in size and firmness. Bone enlargement is found in dogs with coccidioidal osteomyelitis. At the time bone lesions are observed, lung lesions may have resolved. With CNS involvement, granulomas

have been found in the cerebrum and midbrain. A granulomatous uveitis, retinitis, and keratitis may be present. In dogs with granulomatous pericarditis, the organism can be found in pericardial fluid. Coccidioidal pericardial disease is a more common cause of right-sided heart failure than primary coccidioidal myocarditis.

On histologic examination, the organism is usually easier to see with PAS or methenamine silver staining than with H and E. The organism is most often in the center of the lesion. In addition to the organs listed above, microscopic granulomas occasionally

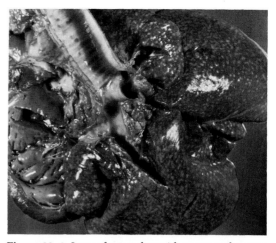

Figure 68–9. Lungs from a dog with severe pulmonary coccidioidomycosis showing multiple light-colored densities throughout the lung lobes.

occur in the kidneys, adrenal glands, liver, and spleen.

THERAPY

Treatment is recommended for acute respiratory coccidioidomycosis in dogs since the disease often disseminates to other tissues. This contrasts with acute respiratory infections in people, which are usually self-limiting. Dogs in enzootic areas should be treated when clinical respiratory signs and a CF titer of > 1:8 are present. A titer of 1:8 is suspicious but not confirmatory, and the test should be repeated in 3 to 4 weeks to determine whether the titer is rising.

Proper therapy of coccidioidomycosis involves long-term antifungal chemotherapy. Immunotherapy has been tried with little or variable success in people using transfer factor or dinitrochlorobenzene. Similarly, levamisole has been given to infected dogs with little success. All immunosuppressive drugs, including glucocorticoids, should be avoided or withdrawn prior to and during therapy.

If the eye is the only site of active infection and is nonresponsive to antifungal therapy, enucleation should be performed in conjunction with antifungal therapy.[10] In one cat, enucleation alone was apparently successful as treatment.[13]

Ketoconazole (KTZ)

The current drug of choice to initially treat coccidioidomycosis is KTZ, a member of the azole group (see Chapter 63). KTZ has been used to treat coccidioidomycosis in a large number of dogs in the southwestern United States. Treatment of infected cats has not been reported, but one of the authors has treated two cats successfully.[5] Except where noted, most of the discussion below refers to therapy of infected dogs.

Minimal side effects, including temporary anorexia or depressed appetite, have been noted for the first 30 days that the drug is administered. Lightening or graying of the hair coat is a temporary side effect developing after 3 to 4 months of therapy. Hair-coat color generally returns to normal once treatment is discontinued or the dosage is reduced. Reproductive disorders, including abortions and mummified fetuses, have been

seen with the use of the drug in pregnant bitches. Significant hepatotoxicity is uncommon unless underlying hepatic disease exists. A biochemical profile is recommended prior to initiation of therapy to evaluate this possibility.

The overall cost of KTZ for treating dogs has been similar to amphotericin B (AMB); however, it is easier to administer, since it is given orally and requires less monitoring. Owners are more willing to comply with this therapy protocol than with that of AMB. The cost of therapy is sufficient so that confirmation of the diagnosis by serology, cytology, or histology is essential.

The recommended dosages for KTZ are listed in Table 68–2. The duration of therapy has been variable, depending on the site and extent of disease. Relapses are common if the drug is not administered for an adequate period of time on a daily basis. Treatment of animals with disseminated infection should continue for a minimum of 1 year, even if observable lesions such as those in the skin clear up after 2 to 3 months of therapy.

Poor response and relapses are possible with ketoconazole. Serologic tests should be repeated after 3 to 4 weeks of therapy. If the titer using the CF test has continued to rise or clinical signs are deteriorating, AMB should be used in addition to KTZ (Table 68–2). Relapses can be controlled by placing the animal on a lower maintenance oral dosage after the animal has been on the higher dosage for 12 months. Deciding whether to terminate therapy is based upon resolution of the clinical disease and radiographic appearance of bone and lung lesions. Serologic titers cannot be used to determine whether the disease is in remission because CF titers may stabilize or decrease only slightly within short time periods. However, long-term monitoring of serologic response may be beneficial to determine whether the titer is rising. Rising titers suggest poor therapeutic response or relapse, and therapy should be reinstituted or continued at higher dosages, or AMB should be added.

In people with nonmeningeal coccidioidomycosis, KTZ appears to be fungistatic; most patients improve, but relapses are common even at higher than recommended dosages, and cures occur in only approximately 30%.[25]

For meningeal disease, KTZ has been considered a poor choice for treatment because

Table 68–2. Antifungal Therapy of Coccidioidomycosis[a]

DRUG	SPECIES	DOSE[b] (mg/kg)	ROUTE	INTERVAL (hours)	DURATION (months)
Induction (achieve remission)					
Ketoconazole	D	5–10	PO	8–12	6–12[c]
(KTZ)	C	50 mg (total)	PO	12–24	6–12[c]
Amphotericin B (AMB)					
Alone[d]	D	0.4–0.5	IV	48–72[e]	f
Combined with KTZ[g]	D	0.4–0.5	IV	48–72[e]	h
Maintenance (prevent relapses)					
KTZ	D	2–5	PO	24	prn
AMB	D	0.4–0.5	IV	30 days	prn

[a]D = dog, C = cat, PO = oral, IV = intravenous, prn = as needed.
[b]Dose per administration at specified interval, expressed in mg/kg unless otherwise stated.
[c]Minimum duration with dissemination: treat for at least 12 months, then use maintenance to control relapses if necessary.
[d]Use alone if unable to tolerate KTZ.
[e]Given Monday and Thursday or Monday, Wednesday, and Friday.
[f]Until cumulative dose is 8 to 11 mg/kg.
[g]Repeat CF tests after 3 to 4 weeks of therapy with KTZ; if titer rises or disease not responding, AMB should be added.
[h]Until cumulative dose is 4 to 6 mg/kg.

of its decreased penetration into the CSF. Success with high-dose KTZ (1200 mg/day) in human cases of meningeal coccidioidomycosis has been variable.[26] A new oral triazole, fluconazole, does achieve relatively high CSF concentrations and has been shown to be effective in treating coccidioidal meningitis in people (see Fluconazole, Chapter 63).[27,27a]

Amphotericin B

AMB, previously the drug of choice for treating canine coccidioidomycosis, is still indicated in animals that are unable to tolerate KTZ or that do not improve on KTZ alone. The toxicities and difficulties of administering AMB make it less desirable than KTZ for dogs (see Chapter 63). In people, AMB remains the drug of choice.[28]

The dose of AMB to induce remission when used alone or in combination is listed in Table 68–2. Periodic, once-monthly maintenance injections of AMB, given at the same daily dosage, may be required over extended periods to prevent relapses.

Coccidioidal meningitis in people requires intrathecal AMB (see Chapter 63). Dosage recommendations have been increased.[29] Intrathecal injections must be given at least 3 times a week for months. Studies have not been done in dogs or cats.

PROGNOSIS

Although the prognosis for localized respiratory coccidioidomycosis in people is good without treatment, all affected dogs should be treated to decrease the chance of dissemination, since the prognosis for disseminated coccidioidomycosis in dogs is guarded. Many dogs will die or have to be euthanatized without treatment, but more than 90% of these cases *improve* with KTZ therapy.[5] However, complete recovery rates in animals that require no further maintenance therapy are much lower and vary with the severity of the disease, from 90% with only pulmonary involvement to 0% with multiple bone involvement. An overall recovery rate of approximately 60% has been noted.[5]

Of five reported feline cases, one recovered without treatment,[12] and one after enucleation of the affected eye,[13] whereas the other three died or had to be euthanatized.[14,15] Two cats treated by one of the authors with KTZ recovered.[5]

PREVENTION

Vaccines have been developed experimentally to prevent *C. immitis* in people and nonhuman primates, but the organism has been difficult to attenuate, as avirulent strains reverted unpredictably to virulence, and killed preparations have not prevented infection. Vaccines are still under study.[30]

The only means of prevention, although impractical, is to avoid the endemic area, especially during dust storms following the rainy season. Laboratory workers should always be extremely cautious with a suspect mycelial growth of *C. immitis*.

PUBLIC HEALTH CONSIDERATIONS

There is no known direct spread from animal-to-animal; thus, infected dogs are not considered public health hazards. *Handling of mycelial cultures of the organism in the laboratory, on the other hand, is dangerous,* and precautions must be taken to prevent arthrospore release into the air. Laboratory technicians have developed primary cutaneous lesions while working with the mycelial phase or while injecting suspected cultures into laboratory rodents.

References

1. Maddy KT: Disseminated coccidioidomycosis of the dog. *J Am Vet Med Assoc* 132:483–489, 1958.
2. Gabal MA: Pathogenesis and electron microscopic changes of spherulogenesis of *Coccidioides immitis* (valley fever). *Am J Vet Res* 46:671–675, 1985.
3. Huppert M: *Coccidioides immitis*: structure and function or know thy adversary. In Einstein HE (ed): *Coccidioidomycosis.* Washington, DC, National Foundation of Infectious Disease, 1985, pp 77–87.
4. Walch HA: *Coccidioides immitis.* In Braude AI (ed): *Medical Microbiology and Infectious Diseases.* Philadelphia, WB Saunders Co, 1981, pp 658–664.
5. Jeffery KL: Unpublished observations, Mesa Veterinary Hospital, Phoenix, AZ, 1988.
6. Converse JL, Reed RE, Kuller HW, et al: Experimental epidemiology of coccidioidomycosis. I. Epizootiology of naturally exposed monkeys and dogs. In Ajello L (ed): *Coccidioidomycosis.* Tucson, University of Arizona Press, 1965, pp 397–402.
7. Burch WM, Synderman R: Induction of cellular immunity to *Coccidioides immitis* after sensitization to dinitrochlorobenzene. *Ann Intern Med* 96:329–331, 1982.
8. Armstrong PJ, DiBartola SP: Canine coccidioidomycosis: a literature review and report of 8 cases. *J Am Anim Hosp Assoc* 19:937–945, 1983.
9. Selby LA, Becker SV, Hayes HW: Epidemiologic risk factors associated with canine systemic mycoses. *Am J Epidem* 113:133–139, 1981.
10. Angell JA, Merideth RE, Shively JN, et al: Ocular lesions associated with coccidioidomycosis in dogs: 35 cases (1980–1985). *J Am Vet Med Assoc* 190:1319–1322, 1987.
11. Ingram KA, Hatch RL, Ingram IA: Atypical presenting signs in three cases of coccidioidomycosis in dogs. In Einstein HE (ed): *Coccidioidomycosis.* Washington, DC, National Foundation of Infectious Disease, 1985, pp 282–287.
12. Wolf AM: Primary cutaneous coccidioidomycosis in a dog and a cat. *J Am Vet Med Assoc* 174:504–506, 1979.
13. Angell JA, Shively JN, Merideth RE, et al: Ocular coccidioidomycosis in a cat. *J Am Vet Med Assoc* 187:167–169, 1985.
14. Reed RE, Hoge RS, Trautman RJ: Coccidioidomycosis in two cats. *J Am Vet Med Assoc* 143:953–956, 1963.
15. Schwartz W: *Coccidioides immitis* infection in a cat. *Southwest Vet* 34:94, 1981.
16. Schermoly MJ, Hinthorm DR: Eosinophilia in coccidioidomycosis. *Arch Intern Med* 148:895–896, 1988.
17. Parker MS, Dokoh S, Woolfenden JM, et al: Hypercalcemia in coccidioidomycosis. *Am J Med* 76:341–344, 1984.
18. Layton DR, Volh TL: Criteria for the identification of *Coccidioides immitis* for cytology specimens. In Einstein HE (ed): *Coccidioidomycosis.* Washington, DC, National Foundation of Infectious Disease, 1985, pp 250–263.
19. Bartsch RC: Personal Communication, Southwest Veterinary Diagnostic Lab, Phoenix, AZ, 1988.
20. Yturraspe DJ: Clinical evaluation of a latex particle agglutination test and a gel diffusion precipitin test in the diagnosis of canine coccidioidomycosis. *J Am Vet Med Assoc* 158:1249–1256, 1971.
21. Shifrine M, Pappagianis D, Neves J: Double electroimmunodiffusion: a rapid diagnostic test for canine coccidioidomycosis. *Am J Vet Res* 36:819–820, 1975.
22. Jackson JA, Mauldin RA, Bauman DS, et al: Treatment of canine coccidioidomycosis with ketoconazole: serologic aspects of a case study. *J Am Anim Hosp Assoc* 21:572-578, 1985.
23. Salgiani JN, Dugger DO, Ito JI, et al: Antigenemia in primary coccidioidomycosis. *Am J Trop Med Hyg* 33:645–649, 1984.
24. Galgiani JN, Ito JI, Dugger KO: Enzyme-linked immunosorbent assay detection of coccidioidal antigens in human serum. In Einstein HE (ed): *Coccidioidomycosis.* Washington, DC, National Foundation of Infectious Disease, 1985, pp 239–249.
25. Galgiani JN, Stevens DA, Graybill JR, et al: Ketoconazole therapy of progressive coccidioidomycosis. *Am J Med* 84:603–610, 1988.
26. Craven PC, Graybill JR, Jorgensen JH, et al: High-dose ketoconazole for treatment of fungal infections of the central nervous system. *Ann Intern Med* 98:160–167, 1983.
27. Tucker RM, Williams PL, Arathoon EG, et al: Pharmacokinetics of fluconazole in cerebrospinal fluid and serum in human coccidioidal meningitis. *Antimicrob Agents Chemother* 32:369–373, 1988.
27a. Classen DC, Burke JP, Smith CB: Treatment of coccidioidal meningitis with fluconazole. *J Infect Dis* 158:903–904, 1988.

28. Einstein HE: Therapy of nonmeningeal disseminated coccidioidomycosis. *In* Einstein HE (ed): *Coccidioidomycosis*. Washington, DC, National Foundation of Infectious Disease, 1985, pp 458–465.

29. Labadie EL, Hamilton RH: Survival improvement in coccidioidal meningitis by high-dose intrathecal amphotericin B. *Arch Intern Med* 146:2013–2018, 1986.

69

SPOROTRICHOSIS

Edmund J. Rosser
Robert W. Dunstan

ETIOLOGY AND EPIDEMIOLOGY

Sporotrichosis is caused by the dimorphic fungus *Sporothrix schenckii*. *S. schenckii* exists in a mycelial form at environmental temperatures (25° to 30°C) and as a yeast form in body tissues (37°C [98.6°F]). The organism is distributed worldwide and can be found preferentially in soils that are rich in decaying organic matter. It has also been isolated from sphagnum moss and tree bark.[1]

The traditionally accepted method of acquiring sporotrichosis is via the inoculation of the infectious organism into tissues.[2–4] Frequently, clinical disease is associated with a puncture wound from a thorn or wood splinter. Sporotrichosis is most commonly identified in hunting dogs. In cats, sporotrichosis is most commonly identified in intact males that roam outdoors, presumably because of their exposure to puncture wounds received in cat fights and subsequent inoculation of the organism from contaminated claws.[2] Although contamination of a puncture wound by organisms in the environment is considered an important mechanism in acquiring the disease in people, contact exposure of people to cats infected with *S. schenckii* is now considered a significant means by which a zoonotic infection can be established.[5] (see Public Health Considerations.)

CLINICAL FINDINGS

Sporotrichosis can occur in three clinical forms: cutaneolymphatic, cutaneous, and disseminated. In many instances, more than one of these forms may be present concurrently. Sporotrichosis in the dog is usually in the cutaneous or cutaneolymphatic form; the disseminated form of the disease is ex-

tremely rare.[4a,4b] The **cutaneous** form is a multinodular condition, typically occurring on the trunk or head (Fig. 69–1), with the nodules in the dermal and subcutaneous layers. The nodules may or may not be ulcerated. Ulcerated nodules are associated with purulent exudate and crust formation. Animals with the **cutaneolymphatic** form usually develop nodules on the distal aspect of one limb. The infection then ascends proximally following lymphatic vessels, and secondary nodules develop that may also ulcerate and drain a purulent exudate. The cutaneolymphatic form is usually associated with a regional lymphadenomegaly.

In the cat, lesions usually occur on the distal aspects of the limbs, head, or tail base region.[2,5] Draining puncture wounds that first appear are similar to fight wound ab-

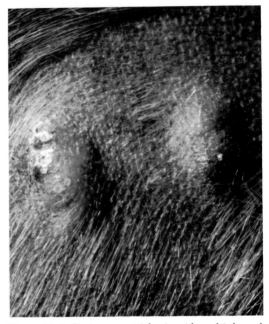

Figure 69–1. Canine sporotrichosis with multiple nodules in the abdominal region.

scesses or cellulitis. Subsequently, ulcerated, crusted nodules that drain a purulent exudate develop (Fig. 69–2).[5] The lesions in cats may have extensive zones of necrosis, exposing muscle and bone. The disease process may be further complicated by autoinoculation, occurring when the animal licks and scratches the lesions and then continues with normal grooming behavior, which result in multiple lesions on the extremities, face, and ears. The involvement of the lymphatic system may or may not be apparent during the physical examination of affected cats. However, with necropsy or biopsy of internal organs, most have evidence of **disseminated** disease with lymph node and lymphatic vessel involvement, and organisms are commonly present.

In addition to the cutaneous manifestations, dogs and cats may have a history of lethargy and anorexia, and upon physical examination may be depressed and febrile. These signs, if referable to disseminated sporotrichosis, can develop in previously immunocompromised hosts.[3,4]

DIAGNOSIS

The initial presentation of dogs or cats with sporotrichosis is similar to that of animals with deep cutaneous bacterial infec-

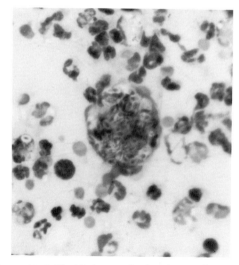

Figure 69–3. Photomicrograph of an impression smear from an ulcerated nodule in a cat with sporotrichosis. Notice the numerous fungal organisms within a macrophage (Wright-Giemsa stain; × 27). (Courtesy of Dr. Patricia White, Charlotte, MI).

tions. Sporotrichosis should be one of the diagnoses to be ruled out if the appropriate use of systemic antibiotics for a deep pyoderma results in minimal or partial improvement. It is also important to note that when bacterial cultures have been performed, the ulcerative and exudative lesions of sporotrichosis are often secondarily infected with bacterial organisms, especially *Staphylococcus intermedius*.

Cytology

Exudates from draining lesions should first be examined cytologically and stained for the presence of fungal organisms using either periodic acid-Schiff (PAS) or Gomori's methenamine silver (GMS) stain. The organism is often difficult to find in exudates from dogs but as a rule is easily identified in exudates from cats. When present, *S. schenckii* appears as a pleomorphic yeast that is round, oval, or cigar-shaped and either may be present within macrophages and inflammatory cells or may be found extracellularly (Figs. 62–5 and 69–3).

Fungal Isolation

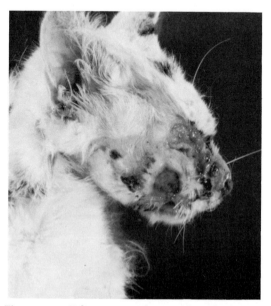

Figure 69–2. Feline sporotrichosis with multiple nodules, ulceration, and draining tracts. (From Dunstan RW, et al: *J Am Acad Dermatol* 15:37–45, 1986. Reprinted with permission.)

When culturing for the presence of *S. schenckii*, samples of the exudate deep within a draining tract and a piece of tissue surgically removed for a macerated tissue culture should be submitted. This is especially important in the dog, in which there usually are very few organisms present in the infectious process. It is also advisable that the laboratory to which samples have been submitted be alerted to the fact that a diagnosis of sporotrichosis is being considered (see Appendix 8).

Histologic Findings

Sporotrichosis of the dog and cat is a nodular to diffuse pyogranulomatous inflammatory reaction. It is primarily located in the dermal and subcutaneous tissues and may extend to involve the underlying skeletal muscle. As with cytologic examination, it is easier to find the organism in lesions of cats as compared to those of dogs. In the feline lesions, organisms are so numerous that they are readily demonstrated within the pyogranulomatous reaction, even on H and E–stained sections. Because there are usually only a few organisms in canine tissues, slides should be counterstained with a fungal stain such as PAS or GMS, and even then, each section of tissue should be carefully examined.

Immunofluorescent Testing

Specific fluorescent antibody detection of the organism in samples is most useful in establishing the diagnosis in dogs when the results of the above procedures have been negative or when attempts at culturing the organism have failed.[6] This diagnostic procedure can be performed by the Centers for Disease Control, Atlanta, GA, on a sample of exudate or preferably on affected tissue from a patient suspected of having the disease (see Appendix 8).

THERAPY

In treating sporotrichosis in dogs and cats, the use of glucocorticoids or any immunosuppressive drug is contraindicated, both during and after the treatment of the disease. Immunosuppressive doses of glucocorticoids have been shown to cause a recurrence of the clinical disease after it has apparently resolved.[7]

Dog

The treatment of choice for dogs is administration of a supersaturated solution of potassium iodide (SSKI, Upsher-Smith Labs, Minneapolis, MN) with food for 30 days beyond the apparent clinical cure (Table 69–1). When sporotrichosis is not treated for an adequate period of time it can often recur. Care should be taken to observe the dog for any signs of iodism (ocular and nasal discharge, a dry haircoat with excessive scaling, vomiting, depression, and collapse). If iodism is observed, the medication should be discontinued for 1 week. If the side effects were mild, they may not recur, and therapy should be reinstituted. Should the side effects recur or if the initial reactions were severe, an alternative treatment should be considered. Ketoconazole can be used in dogs that do not tolerate SSKI, as well as those that are refractory to iodide therapy. The authors have successfully treated a dog with sporotrichosis using ketoconazole at 15 mg/kg, given every 12 hours for 1 month beyond the apparent clinical cure (which required 3.5 months of treatment). Itraconazole has also been shown to be effective in treatment of experimental sporotrichosis.[7a]

Cat

The treatment of sporotrichosis in the cat is more difficult than in the dog because of the cat's greater sensitivity for the development of toxic side effects from iodides and ketoconazole. The treatment of choice, as for dogs, is oral administration of SSKI with food and should be continued for 30 days beyond the apparent clinical cure (Table 69–1). Cats should be carefully observed for any signs of iodism such as vomiting, anorexia, depression, twitching, hypothermia, and cardiovascular failure.[8] Should these signs be observed, the medication should be discontinued, and an alternative mode of therapy should be considered. The next treatment of choice is ketoconazole and as with SSKI, its administration should be continued for 30 days beyond the apparent clinical cure. The cat should be closely observed for the development of any toxic side effects of ketoconazole, including anorexia, fever, depression, diarrhea, and jaundice.[9,10] If any of these signs are observed, the medication should be discontinued. As problems of tox-

Table 69–1. Drug Therapy for Sporotrichosis[a]

DRUG	SPECIES	DOSE[b] mg/kg	ROUTE	INTERVAL (hours)
SSKI[c]	D	40	PO	8
	C	20	PO	12
Ketoconazole	D	5–30	PO	12–24
	C	5–10	PO	12–24

[a]Continue treatment at least 30 days beyond resolution of all clinical signs, usually involving 2 or more months of treatment.
[b]Dose per administration at the specified interval, expressed as mg/kg unless otherwise stated.
[c]SSKI (potassium iodide, oral solution, USP), Upsher-Smith Labs, Inc, supplied in 30-ml bottles with 1 g KI/ml.
D = dog, C = Cat, PO = oral.

icity are observed in the cat, it may be necessary to alternate between the above-mentioned drug regimens.

PUBLIC HEALTH CONSIDERATIONS

Traditionally, sporotrichosis has been considered to have minimal zoonotic potential. However, there have been several reports documenting the transmission of sporotrichosis to people by contact with an ulcerated wound or the exudate from an infected cat.[2,5] The ready transmission of sporotrichosis from animals to people appears to be a feature limited to feline sporotrichosis, presumably due to the copious numbers of organisms found in examined tissues, exudates, and feces of infected cats. Theoretically, transmission from infected dogs or people seems less likely since it is often difficult to demonstrate the presence of the organism.

The population that is potentially at greatest risk for acquiring sporotrichosis from an infected cat includes veterinarians, their assistants, and anyone exposed during treatment. In some instances, infection has occurred after exposure to an infected cat, although there had been no known preexisting injury or penetrating wound on the person prior to contracting the disease. With these considerations in mind, it is advisable that people handling cats **suspected** of having sporotrichosis should wear gloves. Afterward, they should remove the gloves carefully and wash their forearms, wrists, and hands with either a chlorhexidine or povidone-iodine scrub.

References

1. Barsanti JA: Sporotrichosis. In Greene CE (ed): Clinical Microbiology and Infectious Diseases of the Dog and Cat. Philadelphia, WB Saunders Co, 1984, pp 722–727.
2. Dunstan RW, Reimann KA, Langham RF: Feline sporotrichosis. J Am Vet Med Assoc 189:880–883,1986.
3. Chandler FW, Watts JC: Pathologic Diagnosis of Fungal Infections. Chicago, ASCP Press, 1987.
4. Rippon JW: Subcutaneous and systemic fungal infections. In Moschella SL, Hurley HJ (eds): Dermatology, vol 1. Philadelphia, WB Saunders Co, 1985, pp 774–779.
4a. Moriello KA, Franks P, Delany-Lewis D, et al: Cutaneous lymphatic and nasal sporotrichosis in a dog. J Am Anim Hosp Assoc 24:621–626, 1988.
4b. Iwasaki M, Hagiwara MK, Gandra CR, et al: Skeletal sporotrichosis in a dog. Companion Anim Pract 2:27–31, 1988.
5. Dunstan RW, Langham RF, Reimann KA, et al: Feline sporotrichosis: a report of five cases with transmission to humans. J Am Acad Dermatol 15:37–45, 1986.
6. Kaplan W, Ochoa AG: Application of the fluorescent antibody technique to the rapid diagnosis of sporotrichosis. J Lab Clin Med 62:835, 1963.
7. Raimer SS, Ewert A, MacDonald EM, et al: Ketoconazole therapy of experimentally induced sporotrichosis infections in cats: a preliminary study. Curr Ther Res 33:670–680, 1983.
7a. Kan VL, Bennett JE: Efficacy for four antifungal agents in experimental murine sporotrichosis. Antimicrob Agents Chemother 32:1619–1623, 1988.
8. Macy DW, Small E: Deep mycotic diseases. In Ettinger SJ (ed): Textbook of Veterinary Internal Medicine, vol 1. Philadelphia, WB Saunders Co, 1983, pp 257–258.
9. Moriello KA: Ketoconazole: clinical pharmacology and therapeutic recommendations. J Am Vet Med Assoc 188:303–306, 1986.
10. Noxon JO, Digilio K, Schmidt DA: Disseminated histoplasmosis in a cat. J Am Vet Med Assoc 181:817–820, 1982.

70 RHINOSPORIDIOSIS

Edward Breitschwerdt

ETIOLOGY AND EPIDEMIOLOGY

Rhinosporidiosis, a mycotic disease caused by *Rhinosporidium seeberi*, induces tumor-like growths of epithelial tissues in domestic animals, birds, and people.[1,2] It is endemic in India, Sri Lanka, and Argentina and is reported sporadically from other parts of the world. Infection most frequently involves mucous membranes of the nasal cavity, but infrequently, infection can involve the ear, pharynx, larynx, trachea, esophagus, genital and urinary mucosa, and skin. Reported cases of canine rhinosporidiosis have involved only the nasal cavity.[3-8] Rhinosporidiosis has not been reported in cats.

R. seeberi is a fungal organism of uncertain classification.[1] Previous attempts to culture it utilizing conventional fungal culture media have not been successful. The organism was grown in tissue culture, utilizing an epithelioid rectal tumor cell line.[9] Complete development of *R. seeberi* appears to require interaction with epithelial cells; this may explain previous failures to propagate the organism. It is of interest that the organism appears to induce in vitro cellular proliferation.

A small, round, 8-μm sporangiospore (endospore) is the infective unit, and it proliferates in epithelial tissue to produce sporangia (spherules; 300 to 400 μm) that are grossly visible on the superficial surface of the polyp. Sporangia undergo a maturation process resulting in the production of 16,000 to 20,000 spores that are expelled, leaving an empty sporangial case.

PATHOGENESIS

The pathogenesis of canine rhinosporidiosis has not been characterized in detail owing to difficulties associated with propagation of the organism. In contrast with the human disease, in which dissemination develops, although rarely, reported canine cases have been limited to nasal involvement.

Reports from endemic areas suggest that infection is acquired by mucosal contact with stagnant water. Mucous membrane trauma is a predisposing factor. In arid countries, most human infections are ocular, and dust is postulated to be a fomite.[1] In the United States, canine rhinosporidiosis has been reported only in southern states; however, occurrence of the disease in a dog native to Ontario[5] suggests the possibility of more widespread distribution in North America. The disease occurs in large-breed dogs, many being exposed to flowing or impounded fresh water. In the dog, there appears to be a sex predilection for males, as is true of infections in people and horses.[1] Behavioral as well as biologic factors may be responsible for this apparent predilection.

CLINICAL FINDINGS

Clinical findings include wheezing, sneezing, unilateral seropurulent nasal discharge, and epistaxis. Polyps may be visible in the nares or may be visualized by rhinoscopy in the rostral nasal cavity. Single or multiple polyps ranging in size from a few millimeters up to 3 cm are pink, red, or pale gray and are covered with numerous pinpoint, white sporangia. Polyps may be sessile or pedunculated, and the superficial surface is irregular and glistening and may be ulcerated.

DIAGNOSIS

Cytologic examination of nasal exudate or histologic examination of the polyp should allow diagnosis by visualization of *R. seeberi*

711

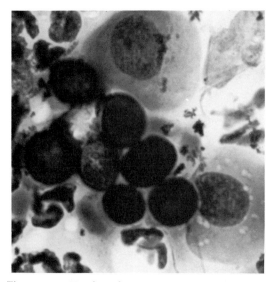

Figure 70–1. Nasal exudate containing sporangiospores of *R. seeberi* (× 1000). (Courtesy of Drs. Roger Easley and Donald Meuten, North Carolina State University, Raleigh, NC.)

spores (Fig. 70–1). The organism can be grown in tissue culture.[9]

PATHOLOGIC FINDINGS

Microscopically, polyps are composed of fibrovascular tissue lined by squamous or

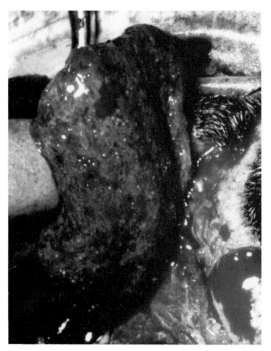

Figure 70–2. Surgically excised nasal polyp. Miliary white foci on the surface are sporangia of *R. seeberi*.

columnar epithelium that is frequently ulcerated.[2,8] Sporangia (spherules) are visualized and may be releasing sporangiospores (endospores) through the epithelium to the superficial surface (see Fig. 62–1). A superficial exudate, most prominent in areas of spore extrusion, is composed of spores, neutrophils, epithelium, and erythrocytes. A mixed inflammatory response, consisting predominantly of plasma cells and lymphocytes and to a lesser extent, macrophages, is scattered throughout the tissue.[8]

THERAPY

Surgical excision is the treatment of choice and may be curative in those instances in which a single polyp is excised. Owing to the frequent rostral location of the polyps, surgical excision through the nares or by an anterior lateral approach to the nares generally is possible, negating the necessity for the more invasive dorsal nasal flap procedure. Recurrence has been reported following surgery in dogs with single or multiple polyps. Dapsone (1 mg/kg every 8 hours for 2 weeks, followed by 1 mg/kg every 12 hours for 4 months) was likely curative in a dog that had recurrence of polyps following surgical extirpation.[7] Dapsone has been utilized to treat human rhinosporidiosis with variable success.[1,10] Ketoconazole (8.7 mg/kg every 8 hours for 21 days) eliminated nasal discharge in a dog after 4 days, and visual and cytologic resolution of the polyps occurred after 21 days of therapy.[11] The dog was treated with ketoconazole (8.7 mg/kg every 8 hours) for an additional 21 days; however, recurrence 6 months later necessitated surgical excision of a polyp (Fig. 70–2). The utility of medical therapy in canine rhinosporidiosis requires additional evaluation.

PUBLIC HEALTH CONSIDERATIONS

There is no evidence to support the possibility of direct transmission of *R. seeberi* from animals to people. Dogs and people are infected from common environmental sources.

References

1. Rippon JW: *Medical Mycology: The Pathogenic Fungi and the Pathogenic Actinomycetes*, ed 3. Philadelphia, WB Saunders Co, 1982, pp 362–372.
2. Chandler FW, Kaplan W, Ajello L: *Histopathology of Mycotic Diseases*. Chicago, Year Book Medical Publishers, 1980, pp 109–111.
3. Castellan MC, Idiart Jr, Martin AA: Rhinosporidiosis in a dog. *VM SAC* 79:45–46, 1984.
4. Mosier DA, Creed J: Rhinosporidiosis in a dog. *J Am Vet Med Assoc* 185:1009–1010, 1984.
5. Hoff B, Hall DA: Rhinosporidiosis in a dog. *Can Vet J* 27:231–232, 1986.
6. Fox SM: Surgical extirpation for rhinosporidiosis in a dog. *Compend Cont Educ Pract Vet* 8:152–156, 1986.
7. Allison N, Willard MD, Bentinck-Smith J, et al: Nasal rhinosporidiosis in two dogs. *J Am Vet Med Assoc* 188:869–871, 1986.
7a. Wilson RB, Pope RW, Sumrall R: Canine rhinosporidiosis. *Compend Cont Educ Pract Vet* 11:730–734, 1989.
8. Easley JR, Meuten DJ, Levy MG, et al: Nasal rhinosporidiosis in the dog. *Vet Pathol* 23:50–56, 1986.
9. Levy MG, Meuten DJ, Breitschwerdt EB: Cultivation of *Rhinosporidium seeberi* in vitro: interaction with epithelial cells. *Science* 234:474–476, 1986.
10. Mahakrisnan A, Rajasekaram V, Pandian PI: Disseminated cutaneous rhinosporidiosis treated with dapsone. *Trop Geogr Med* 33:189–192, 1981.
11. Breitschwerdt EB: Unpublished observations. North Carolina State University, Raleigh, NC, 1986.

71 ASPERGILLOSIS AND PENICILLIOSIS

Canine Nasal Aspergillosis/Penicilliosis

N. J. H. Sharp

ETIOLOGY

Canine nasal aspergillosis is encountered much more frequently than is nasal penicilliosis. The two conditions are indistinguishable other than by culture and subsequent differentiation by the appearance of the conidial heads (Fig. 71–1; also see Fig. 62–7). *Aspergillus fumigatus* is the most common species encountered, although *A. niger, A. nidulans,* and *A. flavus* are occasionally involved. The species of *Penicillium* causing penicilliosis have not been defined. Both groups of fungi are ubiquitous saprophytes and are regarded as opportunistic pathogens.

PATHOGENESIS

In people and probably in dogs and cats as well, two broad categories of aspergillosis exist, excluding the Arthus type of allergic responses.[1] The **disseminated** (systemic) form is seen in severely immunocompromised patients in whom the primary focus is the lung or, less commonly, the paranasal sinuses or GI tract. The **localized** form, or colonization aspergillosis, involves cavities such as the nose, ears, paranasal sinuses, or even old cavitating tuberculous lesions. Although the term *localized disease* is used, infection of the paranasal sinuses in people can be invasive or noninvasive, and the invasive form can simulate malignant disease by causing obstruction of the nasal passages and erosion of bone. The noninvasive form of disease has been described in one dog, in which at surgery a "fungal ball" was found within the nasal chamber without radiographic or gross evidence of tissue destruction.[2]

Invasion with destruction and necrosis of

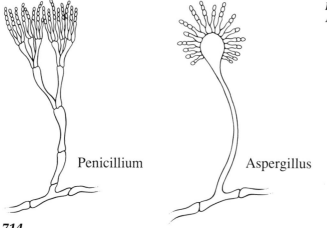

Figure 71–1. Conidial heads of *Penicillium* and *Aspergillus* organisms.

Penicillium

Aspergillus

nasal mucosa and underlying turbinate bones usually occur with canine nasal aspergillosis and penicilliosis, probably as a result of vasculitis and vascular necrosis of submucosal vessels.[3] A. fumigatus has been shown to produce an endotoxin that is both hemolytic and dermonecrotic. Bony invasion is usually restricted to destruction of the turbinate bones but may occasionally extend through the cribriform plate, palatine bones, or into the orbit.

In most instances, no predisposing factor for infection can be identified in affected dogs. Severe lymphopenia is a common feature but may be secondary to the infection itself. Lymphocyte transformation and immune testing has shown both T and B cell dysfunction in nasally infected dogs.[4] It is also not clear, however, if this is a cause or a result of the infection. Indeed, products of A. fumigatus have been shown to inhibit lymphocyte transformation of both B and T cells in vitro.[5]

CLINICAL FINDINGS

Dolichocephalic and mesocephalic breeds are more susceptible to infection. Dogs of any age may be affected, but 40% are 3 years old or less, and 80% are 7 years old or less.[4] The clinical features of nasal aspergillosis are listed in Table 71–1. The three hallmarks are a profuse sanguinopurulent nasal discharge that may alternate with periods of frank epistaxis; ulceration of the external nares (Fig. 71–2); and pain or discomfort in the facial region.[4]

DIAGNOSIS

Many techniques have been employed for the diagnosis of nasal aspergillosis. Blind

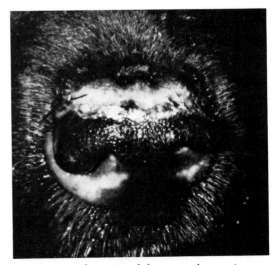

Figure 71–2. Ulceration of the external nares in association with A. fumigatus infection.

culture or cytologic examination of discharge is often unrewarding and can erroneously suggest the disease to be a bacterial rhinitis. Heavy growth of Pseudomonas spp. or other Enterobacteriaceae are common; however, these are considered to be opportunistic microflora that proliferate in the necrotic tissue within the nasal chamber. Caution should also be employed in interpreting a positive fungal culture result. Following culture of nasal swabs taken without direct visualization from 15 clinically normal dogs, 40% had positive culture results for either Aspergillus or Penicillium spp.[3] Histologic examination performed on tissue obtained by blind biopsy through the nares may also result in a diagnosis of nonspecific rhinitis if fungal colonies are missed.[6] The three most informative tests are radiographic, rhinoscopic, and serologic examinations.

The radiographic features of aspergillosis have been reviewed (Fig. 71–3).[7] Of 71 dogs with nasal aspergillosis, all showed destruction of turbinate bones, and 80% also showed associated areas of increased radiolucency; 30% showed mixed density, and only one dog showed an overall increase in radioopacity.[7,8] Frontal sinus osteomyelitis, demonstrated in the rostrocaudal or "skyline" frontal sinus projection, occurred in 80% of 29 dogs evaluated.[7]

Rhinoscopy has proven invaluable in the diagnosis of aspergillosis, particularly when a 3- to 5-mm (diameter) flexible pediatric bronchoscope is available.[9] A working channel considerably facilitates biopsy for my-

Table 71–1. Clinical Features of 35 Dogs with Nasal Aspergillosis/Penicilliosis

CLINICAL FINDING	AFFECTED (%)
Profuse nasal discharge	91
Nasal pain	85
Rhinarial ulceration	77
Sanguinopurulent discharge	76
Frontal sinus osteomyelitis	65
Epistaxis	63
Mucopurulent discharge	24
Sparse nasal discharge	9
Mild radiographic changes	8
Chemosis	7

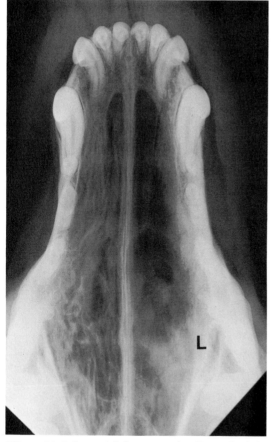

Figure 71–3. Intra-oral dorsoventral radiograph of the nasal cavity of a dog with aspergillosis, showing typical turbinate destruction and increase in radiolucency in the left (L) nasal chamber.

cologic confirmation. An arthroscope also can be employed but is less versatile and because of its rigid nature is more likely to cause friable tissues to bleed. An otoscope with a bright light source is useful,[9] even as the sole means of guiding biopsy of fungal plaques (colonies). Fungal plaques appear as a white, yellow, or light green mold lying on the turbinates. The turbinate destruction characteristic of nasal aspergillosis facilitates rhinoscopic evaluation owing to the large, air-filled cavities that result.

Serologic diagnosis is possible using agar gel immunodiffusion (AGID), counter immunoelectrophoresis (CIE),[10] and ELISA techniques (see Appendix 8). The AGID test has been reliably used for many years but has given 6% false-positive results from 250 clinically normal dogs, 100 of which were subjected to necropsy examination.[11] Fifteen percent of false-positive results were found from the same group of dogs when using

CIE, although others have reported no false-positive or false-negative results with this technique.[10] Corresponding data are unavailable for ELISA, but this test has given reliable results over the previous 2 years of clinical use in the United States.[4] It is still advisable to use a mixture of *Aspergillus* and *Penicillium* spp. antigenic extracts to detect dogs with penicilliosis by use of either AGID or ELISA tests.[3, 4]

For clinical diagnosis in a patient prior to the institution of therapy, the previously defined criteria serve as sensible guidelines.[12] These are fungal invasion of the host and serologic and mycologic or serologic and radiologic confirmation. Fungal invasion can best be documented by rhinoscopic examination. Surgical visualization or histologic evidence is also suitable, but both are more invasive techniques.

Mycologic confirmation is possible by either cytologic examination or culture on a fungal medium such as Sabouraud's dextrose agar. Specimens should ideally be obtained by direct rhinoscopic biopsy of fungal colonies. This will help prevent both false-positive results due to contaminating environmental spores[3] and false-negative results from examination of the nasal discharge alone.

The most important differential diagnosis for nasal aspergillosis is nasal neoplasia. Rhinoscopic examination is often very frustrating in nasal neoplasia[9] and up to 15% of dogs with this condition may have positive results on serologic testing for aspergillosis.[6] Differentiation is best made by radiographic examination followed by tissue biopsy through the nostril. Although both nasal neoplasia and aspergillosis cause consistent turbinate destruction, the soft tissue mass of nasal neoplasia causes a marked increase in radio-opacity but rarely if ever an increase in radiolucency.[8] Furthermore, initial turbinate destruction in nasal neoplasia predominates in the caudal nasal chamber, whereas the rostral chamber is primarily affected in aspergillosis.[7] Endoscopy may be more difficult in animals with nasal neoplasias than in those with aspergillosis owing to the space-occupying nature of the tumors. Although limited to use at referral institutions, computed tomography can also help to differentiate these two conditions. Other causes of nasal disease such as foreign bodies, dental disease, or chronic rhinitis do not cause the turbinate destruction seen in aspergillosis or neoplasia. Idiopathic destructive rhinitis has been encountered when the clinical features are identical to aspergillosis/penicilliosis but no fungal organisms can be found on rhinoscopic, mycologic, or serologic examination.[9]

THERAPY

Systemic

Effective treatment regimes are presented in Table 71–2. All orally administered drugs should be used for a minimum period of 6 weeks. Nausea and vomiting can be a side effect with thiabendazole,[12] but withdrawal and then gradual reintroduction back to the full dose usually overcomes this problem. Ketoconazole may also cause nausea and anorexia.[13] Both drugs should be given with food to enhance absorption. Two new azole derivatives, fluconazole[4] and itraconazole,[14] have shown encouraging results in experimental studies in treating aspergillosis but are not yet commercially available. Topical treatment appears to provide the most encouraging results at this time.

Topical

Both natamycin and amphotericin B have been instilled locally, but the results were no better than either oral ketoconazole or thiabendazole.[15] The most successful regimen appears to be enilconazole (Imaverol, Janssen Pharmaceuticals, Oxfordshire, UK) administered topically for 7 to 10 days through tubes implanted into each nasal chamber via the frontal sinus.[16] Two indwelling tubes are surgically implanted through trephine holes in the frontal sinuses so that they lie in the midnasal chamber. In cases with active infection of the frontal sinus, an additional tube is passed through the trephine hole to end in the frontal sinus (Fig. 71–4).

The calculated dose of stock solution of 10% (100 mg/ml) enilconazole is drawn into a syringe and mixed into an emulsion with an equal volume of water or isotonic saline. The drug is more active when diluted equally with water, and the dose to be given must be used within 2 to 3 minutes or the emulsion solidifies. The total daily dose is 20 mg/kg. Ten mg/kg of enilconazole emulsion is administered twice daily, divided between the two tubes, at each treatment. Any liquid remaining in the tubes is flushed with air. The animal's nose is lowered during the flush to assist the liquid to flow or be sneezed into the nasal passages rather than the nasopharynx. Profuse salivation may accompany each dosage administration owing to the bad taste of the drug. An Elizabethan collar is used throughout the course of therapy. Enilconazole is active against both *Aspergillus* and *Penicillium* spp. and is ideal as a topical agent because it is also active in the vapor phase, possibly enhancing its distribution throughout the nasal chamber.

Topical therapy fails when the disease involves soft tissue structures outside the nasal cavity such as those of the orbit. These cases require a combination of topical with systemic treatment.

Surgery

Rhinotomy and turbinectomy have traditionally been combined with medical management of this disease. Evidence suggests, however, that surgery is of no benefit in controlling the nasal discharges and may even be detrimental.[12] It is the author's opin-

Table 71–2. Therapy for Nasal Aspergillosis[a]

GENERIC DRUG (TRADE NAME)	SPECIES	DOSE[b] (mg/kg)	ROUTE	INTERVAL (hours)	DURATION (weeks)	EFFICACY (%)
Thiabendazole (Mintezole)	D	10–20	PO	12	6–8	43
Ketoconazole	D	5–10	PO	12	6–8	43
(Nizoral)	C	10–15	PO	12	6–8	NA
Fluconazole	D	2.5–5	PO	12	6–8	60
Itraconazole	D	5	PO	12	6–8	60–70
Enilconazole	D	10	Topical	12	1	80–90

[a]D = dog, C = cat, PO = oral, NA = data not available.
[b]Dose per administration at the specified interval, expressed as mg/kg unless otherwise stated.

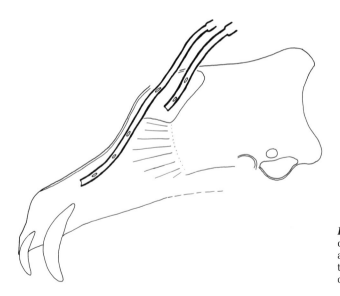

Figure 71–4. Diagram showing tube placement on one side for topical treatment of canine nasal aspergillosis with enilconazole. The end of one tube is in the midnasal cavity and that of the other is in the frontal sinus.

ion that surgery other than the tube placement described above should not be employed.

Prognosis

Serology is of limited value in assessing the response to treatment. Although both AGID and ELISA titers tend to decline over 1 to 2 years, this is not a reliable indicator. Positive titers may persist for more than 2 years (ELISA) or 5 years (AGID), in dogs that remain nonsymptomatic.[4]

Thirty dogs successfully treated by various regimens were then reexamined under anesthesia and showed no evidence of fungal infection. These dogs have remained nonsymptomatic for an additional 3 to 6 years

at the time of writing.[4] Therefore, reinfection would not appear to be a problem once the fungus has been eliminated.

PUBLIC HEALTH CONSIDERATIONS

There are no documented instances of infection in people arising from dogs or cats. Infection is obtained from common environmental sources. It would seem prudent, however, for the veterinarian to inform an owner that immunosuppressed individuals should not be exposed to affected animals discharging large quantities of nasal exudate containing fungal spores. Precautions should also be taken when trephining an infected frontal sinus.

Feline Nasal Aspergillosis/ Penicilliosis

N. J. H. Sharp

Although rare in the cat, both organisms have been incriminated in frontal sinusal infections on two occasions and have extended into the soft tissues of the orbit.[17,18] In these two cats, ophthalmic signs such as

proptosis predominated, and one cat also demonstrated *Penicillium* pneumonitis. The immune status of these animals was not evaluated. A third cat with aspergillosis of the nasal cavity and frontal sinus was FeLV-positive.[19] This cat had a positive result on AGID testing and was successfully treated by rhinotomy and turbinectomy. Daily doses of ketoconazole up to 30 mg/kg have been safely used in some cats,[20] and the drug may, therefore, prove valuable in the therapy for this condition. There is no information on the topical use of enilconazole in the cat.

Canine Disseminated Aspergillosis

Michael J. Day

ETIOLOGY AND PATHOGENESIS

Most cases of canine disseminated aspergillosis have occurred in German shepherd dogs (age range, 2 to 8 years) and have been reported from Western Australia or California, although unreported cases have occurred elsewhere. In those cases where the species has been identified, infection has involved, in decreasing frequency, *Aspergillus terreus, A. deflectus, A. flavipes,* or *A. fumigatus.* The portal of entry of *Aspergillus* is thought to be via the respiratory tract with subsequent hematogenous spread.[21] Disseminated aspergillosis in people is usually secondary to immunodeficiency or immune suppression. Predisposing factors for canine aspergillosis may include a combination of optimum climatic conditions, access to particular strains of *Aspergillus,* and a subtle defect in mucosal immunity that may have a genetic basis.[21–23]

CLINICAL FINDINGS

Disease involves multiple organ systems and develops over several months, but most dogs are terminally ill when presented. The most consistent clinical features are vertebral pain progressing to paraparesis or paraplegia or limb lameness with pronounced swelling and discharging sinus tracts.[21,22]

Other nonspecific clinical signs include anorexia, weight loss, muscle wasting, pyrexia, weakness, lethargy, and vomiting. Occasionally, dogs have clinical evidence of CNS involvement,[24,25] lymphadenomegaly with cutaneous edema, or pyometra.[21] Uveitis or endophthalmitis may be clinically apparent some months before generalized illness develops and thus may be important in early diagnosis.[21]

DIAGNOSIS

The most consistent hematologic abnormality is the presence of mature neutrophilia. Biochemical analysis may reveal elevations in total protein concentration, BUN, and serum ALP, ALT (formerly SGPT), and amylase activities.[21,22] Radiography of affected long bones reveals areas of lysis and cortical destruction, with similar changes in vertebral bodies associated with discospondylitis (Fig. 71–5).[21]

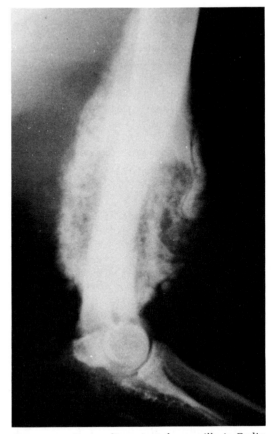

Figure 71–5. Canine disseminated aspergillosis. Radiograph of humeral lesion. Note extensive cortical destruction and new bone formation.

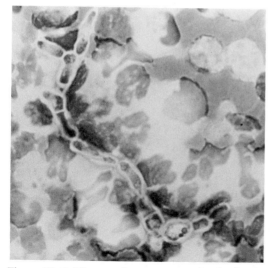

Figure 71–6. Microscopic appearance of stained urine sediment from a dog with disseminated aspergillosis. Branching hyphal elements amid leukocytes and erythrocytes (Wright's stain; × 1000). (Courtesy of Drs. E. Mahaffey and A. Kaufman, University of Georgia, Athens, GA.)

An effective and simple diagnostic test involves examination of a catheterized urine sample for the presence of hyphal elements (Fig. 71–6).[21] Fungal elements may also be observed on cytologic examination of blood, synovial fluid, lymph node, bone, or intervertebral disc material. Confirmation of fungal involvement by culture on Sabouraud's dextrose agar requires 5 to 7 days. Several serologic tests, including AGID, CIE, ELISA, and IFA, may provide rapid serologic confirmation, but not all dogs with disseminated infection have detectable *Aspergillus* antibodies (see Appendix 8).[22]

PATHOLOGIC FINDINGS

Gross changes include focal osteomyelitis and multiple, pale granulomata in kidneys and spleen that also may be seen in lymph nodes, myocardium, pancreas, and liver. Occasionally, pulmonary congestion or GI mucosal reddening or erosions may be found.[24–26] Microscopic granulomata may be associated with areas of slow vascular flow in liver, lungs, eyes, and pancreas and occasionally in prostate, thyroid, uterine submucosa, and brain.[27] Infarcted areas secondary to thrombi containing fungal elements have been found in spleen, kidneys, and liver (Fig. 71–7).[27] Lesions contain varying

numbers of septate, branching hyphae that may have characteristic lateral branching aleuriospores (Fig. 71–8A). Intralesional hyphae are best visualized by PAS or Gomori's methenamine silver stain[27] and have been identified by immunostaining with specific antisera (Fig. 71–8B).[28] The cellular infiltrates may be predominantly neutrophilic or may also include macrophages, giant cells, lymphocytes, and plasma cells.[27,28]

THERAPY AND PROGNOSIS

Terminally ill dogs have a poor prognosis. Treatments, including supportive therapy of fluids and antibiotics, together with thiabendazole or ketoconazole with and without concurrent 5-fluorocytosine, have been unsuccessful.[21,24] The use of amphotericin B generally is contraindicated by pre-existing renal damage. One dog was reported to be alive 4 months after amputation of an affected foreleg.[24]

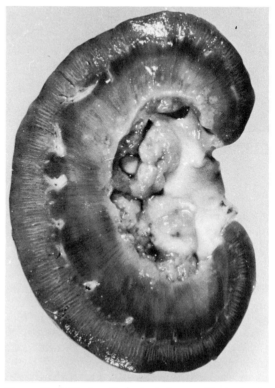

Figure 71–7. Canine disseminated aspergillosis. Sagittal section of kidney with fungal mass in renal pelvis and scattered fungal granulomata (*A. terreus*).

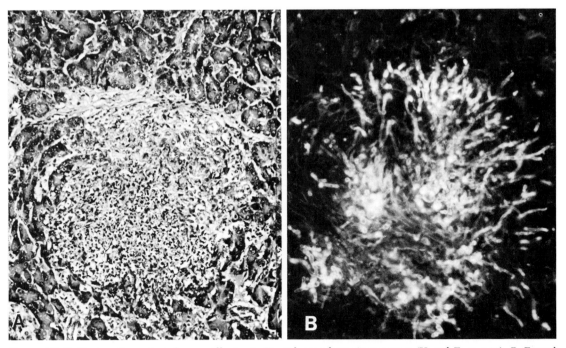

Figure 71–8. Canine disseminated aspergillosis. *A,* Fungal granuloma in pancreas (H and E; × 140). *B,* Fungal hyphae within a granuloma marked with antiserum to *A. terreus* (IFA; × 320).

Feline Disseminated Aspergillosis

Michael J. Day

Feline aspergillosis largely occurs in cats up to 2 years of age that often are in terminal illness. Unlike dogs with aspergillosis, most affected cats have concurrent immunosuppressive disease such as panleukopenia, feline infectious peritonitis, feline leukemia virus infection, or multiple diseases, or they have had dystocia or have been receiving glucocorticoid or antibiotic therapy.[29] Clinical signs are referrable to GI or pulmonary involvement, with nonspecific findings similar to those seen in dogs. Hematologic findings are variable and may reflect other underlying diseases.

Necropsy findings may include pulmonary granulomata, GI ulcers or pseudomembranes, and involvement of urinary system or CNS. These lesions are characterized by hemorrhage and necrosis, with variable numbers of inflammatory cells and fungal hyphae that may invade blood vessels, leading to thrombosis.[30]

References

1. Myrvik QN, Weiser RS: *Fundamentals of Medical Bacteriology and Mycology.* Philadelphia, Lea & Febiger, 1988, pp 551–552.
2. Hargis AM, Denny Liggitt H, Lincoln JD, et al: Noninvasive aspergillosis (fungus ball) in a six-year-old standard poodle. *J Am Anim Hosp Assoc* 22:504–508, 1986.
3. Harvey CE, O'Brien JA, Felsburg PJ, et al: Nasal penicilliosis in six dogs. *J Am Vet Med Assoc* 178:1084–1087, 1981.
4. Sharp NJH, Harvey CE, Sullivan M: Unpublished observations. North Carolina State University, Raleigh, NC, 1987.
5. Chaparas SD, Morgan PA, Holobaugh P, et al: Inhibition of cellular immunity by products of *Aspergillus fumigatus. J Med Vet Mycol* 24:67–76, 1986.
6. Harvey CE, O'Brien JA: Nasal aspergillosis/penicilliosis. *In* Kirk RW (ed): *Current Veterinary Therapy VIII.* Philadelphia, WB Saunders Co, 1983, pp 236–241.
7. Sullivan M, Lee R, Jakovljevic S, et al: The radio-

logical features of aspergillosis of the nasal cavity and frontal sinuses in the dog. *J Small Anim Pract* 27:167–180, 1986.

8. Gibbs C, Lane JG, Denny HR: The radiological features of intra-nasal lesions in the dog: a review of 100 cases. *J Small Anim Pract* 20:515–535, 1979.

9. Sullivan M: Rhinoscopy, a diagnostic aid? *J Small Anim Pract* 28:839–844, 1987.

10. Richardson MD, Warnock DW, Bovey SE: Rapid serological diagnosis of *Aspergillus fumigatus* infection of the frontal sinuses and nasal chambers of the dog. *Res Vet Sci* 33:167–169, 1982.

11. Cervantes-Olivares RA: Studies on antigens of *Aspergillus*; their use in veterinary mycology. PhD diss., Glasgow University, UK, 1983.

12. Harvey CE: Nasal aspergillosis and penicilliosis in dogs: results of treatment with thiabendazole. *J Am Vet Med Assoc* 184:48–50, 1984.

13. Sharp NJH, Sullivan M: Use of ketoconazole in treatment of canine nasal aspergillosis. *J Am Vet Med Assoc* 194:782–786, 1989.

14. Legendre A: Personal communication. University of Tennessee, Knoxville, TN, 1988.

15. Venker van Haagan AJ: Personal communication. University of Utrecht, Utrecht, The Netherlands, 1988.

16. Sharp NJH: Nasal aspergillosis. In Kirk RW (ed): *Current Veterinary Therapy X*. Philadelphia, WB Saunders Co, 1989, pp 1106–1109.

17. Peiffer RL, Belkin PV, Janke BH: Orbital cellulitis, sinusitis and pneumonitis caused by *Penicillium* spp in a cat. *J Am Vet Med Assoc* 176:449–451, 1980.

18. Wilkinson GT, Sutton RH, Grono LR: *Aspergillus* spp infection associated with orbital cellulitis in a cat. *J Small Anim Pract* 23:127–131, 1982.

19. Goodall SA, Lane JG, Warnock DW: The diagnosis and treatment of a case of nasal aspergillosis in a cat. *J Small Anim Pract* 25:627–633, 1984.

20. Pentlarge VW, Martin RA: Treatment of cryptococcosis in three cats, using ketoconazole. *J Am Vet Med Assoc* 188:536–538, 1986.

21. Day MJ, Penhale WJ, Eger CE, et al: Disseminated aspergillosis in dogs. *Aust Vet J* 63:55–59, 1986.

22. Day MJ, Eger CE, Shaw SE, et al: Immunologic study of systemic aspergillosis in German shepherd dogs. *Vet Immunol Immunopathol* 9:335–347, 1985.

23. Day MJ, Penhale WJ: Humoral immunity in disseminated *Aspergillus terreus* infection in the dog. *Vet Microbiol* 16:283–284, 1988.

24. Jang SS, Dorr TE, Biberstein EL, et al: *Aspergillus deflectus* infection in four dogs. *J Med Vet Mycol* 24:95–104, 1986.

25. Mullaney TP, Levin S, Indrieri RJ: Disseminated aspergillosis in a dog. *J Am Vet Med Assoc* 182:516–518, 1983.

26. Marks DL: Systemic aspergillosis in a dog. *Canine Pract* 10:49–52, 1983.

27. Kabay MJ, Robinson WF, Huxtable CRR, et al: The pathology of disseminated *Aspergillus terreus* infection in dogs. *Vet Pathol* 22:540–547, 1985.

28. Day MJ: A study of the immune response in canine disseminated aspergillosis, PhD diss. Murdock University, Murdoch, Western Australia, 1987.

29. Ossent P: Systemic aspergillosis and mucormycosis in 23 cats. *Vet Rec* 120:330–333, 1987.

30. Bolton GR, Brown TT: Mycotic colitis in a cat. *Vet Med Small Anim Clin* 67:978–981, 1972.

72

CANDIDIASIS

Craig E. Greene
Francis W. Chandler

ETIOLOGY

Candida is a genus of dimorphic fungi in the family Cryptococcaceae. In the yeast phase, *Candida* normally inhabits the alimentary, upper respiratory, and genital mucosa of mammals. A sexual stage has not been identified, and the small (2 to 6 μm), thin-walled, ovoid, yeastlike cells reproduce by budding. Candidas, especially *C. albicans* and *C. parapsilosis*, have been the most commonly isolated fungal organisms cultured from the ears, nose, oral cavity, and anus of clinically normal dogs.[1] Occasionally, *C. tropicalis*, *C. pseudotropicalis*, *C. guilliermondii*, and *C. krusei* have been found on human and animal body surfaces. Only rarely are the *Candida* spp. isolated from soil or as laboratory contaminants. *Torulopsis glabrata*, which had been tentatively merged with the genus *Candida* as *Candida glabrata*, is now considered to be taxonomically distinct.[2]

EPIDEMIOLOGY

The *Candida* spp., first acquired by the neonate as it passes through the birth canal, colonize the oral, GI, upper respiratory, and genital mucosa for the life of the animal, but their presence normally evokes no reaction. The skin is an abnormal site for *C. albicans* except at mucocutaneous junctions of body orifices. Opportunistic infections may result if the skin becomes chronically traumatized or moistened.[3] Under certain circumstances, the *Candida* spp. can also invade deeper host tissues and proliferate as blastoconidia, pseudohyphae, and branched, septate hyphae (Fig. 72–1). In other instances, they may disseminate via the blood stream to many tissues (Fig. 72–2).

PATHOGENESIS

Local proliferation of *Candida* in wounds or on mucosal surfaces is the first step in spread of infection. Overgrowth of *Candida* is probably inhibited under most circumstances by a variety of factors, including intestinal, genital, and skin microflora. Factors that upset the normal endogenous microflora, such as prolonged broad-spectrum antibiotic therapy, may allow *Candida* to proliferate, especially in the oropharynx and GI tract. Similarly, disruption of cutaneous or mucosal barriers by burns, surgery, trauma, or indwelling vascular or urinary catheters allows a pathway for *Candida* to enter the body from the body surfaces or the environment.[4,5] Once in the body, further spread of infection correlates with cell-mediated immunocompetence. Cell-mediated immunity appears to be an important determinant of further spread of infection. Prolonged immunosuppression, cytotoxic chemotherapy causing persistent neutropenia, diabetes mellitus, long-term glucocorticoid therapy, and prolonged antibiotic therapy have resulted in an increased prevalence of both localized and disseminated candidiasis.[6] Circulating neutrophils appear to be a major defense against candidiasis; candidiasis has occurred in neutropenic persons,[7] in dogs with experimentally induced neutropenia,[8,9] and in a dog with neutropenia from parvoviral infection.[10] A similar correlation has not been made for the occurrence of disseminated candidiasis in cats.[10a]

In disseminated infection, the microcirculation of tissues, such as lung, skin, kidneys, liver, brain, myocardium, eyes, and skeletal muscle, acts to filter and clear the blood. This results in embolic colonization and microabscess formation at these sites.[11,12]

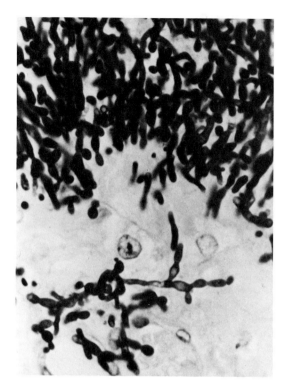

Figure 72–1. Invasive candidiasis. Budding yeastlike cells (blastoconidia) and segmentally constricted pseudohyphae of *C. albicans* invade the esophageal mucosa (PAS; × 700).

CLINICAL FINDINGS

Localized candidiasis is found in chronically immunosuppressed dogs and cats or those with nonhealing ulcers of the oral, GI, or genitourinary mucosa.[10,13,14] Lesions are characterized by nonhealing ulcers covered by whitish-gray plaques with hyperemic margins (Fig. 72–3). A white vaginal or preputial discharge may be seen in candidiasis of the genital mucosa. Chronic lesions of the skin or nail beds may appear as nonhealing,

erythematous, moist, exuding, and crusting lesions.[15]

Systemic candidiasis has been recognized in dogs and cats. Although clinical signs frequently reflect involvement of particular organ systems, lesions in dogs and cats with disseminated infection are often widespread. Fever and the sudden appearance of multiple raised erythematous to hemorrhagic skin lesions have been described in canine systemic candidiasis.[15] The lesions begin as small wheals or macules that eventually ul-

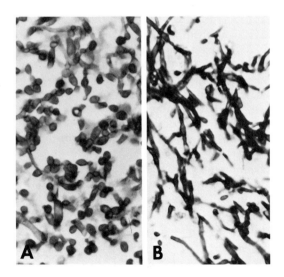

Figure 72–2. Hematogenous renal candidiasis caused by *C. albicans. A*, A cortical abscess contains sperical to oval blastoconidia and few pseudohyphae. (Gomori's methenamine-silver nitrate stain; × 700). *B*, Branched, septate hyphae with parallel contours proliferate within a necrotic renal papilla (PAS; × 560).

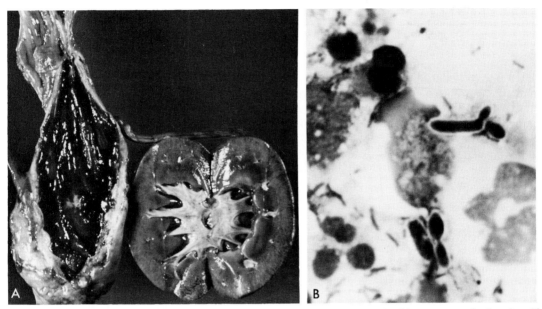

Figure 72–3. A, Bladder from a dog with secondary *Candida* cystitis as a result of long-term cyclophosphamide therapy. B, Stained urinary sediment contains blastoconidia with leukocytes (Wright's stain; × 1000).

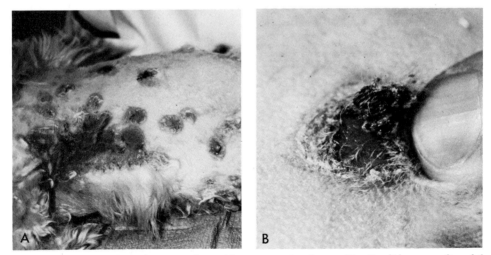

Figure 72–4. A, Ulcerative dermatitis in a dog with concurrent polymyositis. *Candida* was cultured from the lesions, and the disease responded to therapy with ketoconazole. B, Closer view of a skin lesion.

Table 72–1. Recommended Drugs for Topical Treatment of Candidiasis and Trichosporosis[a]

GENERIC (BRAND) DRUG	FORMULATION	INTERVAL (hours)	DURATION (weeks)
Nystatin (Nilstat)	100,000 U/g	8–12	1–2
Miconazole (Conofite)	2%	241	2–4
Clotrimazole	1%	6–8	1
Amphotericin B (Fungizone)	3%	6–8	1

[a]U = units.

cerate (Fig. 72–4A and B). Pain and reluctance to move are common manifestations of myositis. Systemic candidiasis also has been reported in a dog that developed peripheral lymphadenomegaly and fistulous drainage resulting from osteomyelitis of the humerus.[16] Cats with systemic infection have developed uveitis, neurologic deficits, and pleural effusions.[10a,16a,16b]

DIAGNOSIS

Hematologic findings usually are normal in localized infections; however, leukopenia and thrombocytopenia may occur with disseminated disease. Muscle and liver enzyme activities may be increased, depending on the tissues affected. Antemortem blood samples for culture should be obtained from peripheral arteries since most of the organisms, effectively filtered out by tissues, never reach the systemic venous circulation.[17] Because consistent renal embolization occurs with disseminated infection, *Candida* spp. are more easily isolated from the urine than from the blood. Organisms may sometimes be cultured from many tissues at surgery or necropsy (see Fig. 62–16). Culture of *Candida* from cutaneous or mucosal surfaces or exudates alone should not be considered an absolute indicator of infection. Histologic confirmation of deeper tissue invasion is essential. Cutaneous or mucosal tissue biopsy samples should be submitted for histologic and cultural examinations simultaneously. A definitive histologic diagnosis

can sometimes be made in the face of negative cultures.

PATHOLOGIC FINDINGS

Animals that die of disseminated candidiasis have gross lesions consisting of multiple white foci in the heart, liver, spleen, lymph nodes, CNS, kidneys, or other organs. Microscopic evaluation reveals multifocal abscesses or areas of necrosis that contain abundant blastoconidia, pseudohyphae, and true hyphae surrounded by mixed cellular infiltrates (Fig. 72–2). Infiltrates are usually minimal in profoundly immunosuppressed or leukopenic animals. Occasionally, hyphal angioinvasion or occlusion of small and medium-size arteries by systemic candidal emboli results in nodular, hemorrhagic infarcts. Caution must be exercised in diagnosing localized, superficial candidal infections based on cytologic or histologic study of mucocutaneous lesions unless hyphal elements and numerous inflammatory cells are present (see Fig. 72–3). Individual *Candida* organisms are morphologically and tinctorially indistinguishable in clinical specimens. Culture is needed for definitive identification.

THERAPY

Treatment of superficial candidiasis involves drying of nonmucosal lesions. Antifungal susceptibility testing is unreliable. Mucosal lesions can be treated with topical nystatin, gentian violet (1:10,000), micona-

Table 72–2. Recommended Drugs for Systemic Treatment of Candidiasis and Trichosporosis[a]

SYSTEMIC DRUG	SPECIES	DOSE[b] (mg/kg)	ROUTE	INTERVAL (hours)	DURATION (weeks)
Ketoconazole (Nizoral)	D	5–11	PO	12	4
	C	50–100 mg (total)	PO	12–24	4
Itraconazole	B	5–7	PO	12	4

[a]D = dog, C = cat, B = dog and cat.
[b]Dose per administration at specified interval, expressed as mg/kg unless otherwise stated.

zole creams, or topical amphotericin B lotions (Table 72–1). Systemic candidiasis can be treated with IV amphotericin B, but the drug's nephrotoxicity in otherwise compromised hosts can be fatal. Ketoconazole and other related benzimidazoles are presently the drugs of choice for treating infected dogs (see Table 72–2).[18] Liposome-encapsulated amphotericin B has been relatively effective and nontoxic in preliminary studies.[19] Supplemental administration of oral vitamin A might be recommended since it has been shown to increase resistance to infection by *Candida*.

References

1. Ishihara H: Studies on canine mycosis. *Bull Nippon Vet Zootech Col* 24:109–127, 1975.
2. Bodey GP, Fainstein V (eds): *Candidiasis.* New York, Raven Press, 1985.
3. Maksymiuk AW, Thongprasert S, Hopfer R, et al: Systemic candidiasis in cancer patients. *Am J Med* 77(4D):20–27, 1984.
4. Rotrosen D, Gibson TR, Edwards JE: Adherence of *Candida* species to intravenous catheters. *J Infect Dis* 147:594, 1983.
5. McCaw D, Franklin R, Fales W, et al: Pyothorax caused by *Candida albicans* in a cat. *J Am Vet Med Assoc* 185:311–312, 1984.
6. Hughes WT: Systemic candidiasis: a study of 109 fatal cases. *Pediatr Infect Dis* 1:11–18, 1982.
7. Haron E, Feld R, Tuffnell P, et al: Hepatic candidiasis: an increasing problem in immunocompromised patients. *Am J Med* 83:17–26, 1987.
8. Ehrensaft DV, Epstein RB, Sarpel S, et al: Disseminated candidiasis in leukopenic dogs. *Proc Soc Exp Biol Med* 160:6–10, 1979.
9. Chow HS, Sarpel SC, Epstein RB: Experimental candidiasis in neutropenic dogs: tissue burden of infection and granulocyte transfusion effects. *Blood* 59:328–333, 1982.
10. Andersonn PG, Pidgeon G: Candidiasis in a dog with parvoviral enteritis. *J Am Anim Hosp Assoc* 23:27–30, 1987.
10a. Miller WW, Albert RA: Ocular and systemic candidiasis in a cat. *J Am Anim Hosp Assoc* 24:521–524, 1988.
11. Barnes JL, Osgood RW, Lee JC, et al: Host-parasite interactions in the pathogenesis of experimental renal candidiasis. *Lab Invest* 49:460–467, 1983.
12. Montes LF, Wilborn WH: Fungus-host relationship in candidiasis. *Arch Dermatol* 121:119–124, 1985.
13. Lorenzini R, DeBernardis F: Antemortem diagnosis of an apparent case of feline candidiasis. *Mycopathologica* 93:13–14, 1986.
14. McKeever PJ, Klausner JS: Plant awn, candidal, nocardial and necrotizing ulcerative stomatitis in the dog. *J Am Anim Hosp Assoc* 22:17–22, 1986.
15. Pilcher ME, Gross TL, Kroll WR: Cutaneous and mucocutaneous candidiasis in a dog. *Compend Cont Educ Pract Vet* 7:225–230, 1985.
16. Holoymoen JI, Bjerkas I, Olberg IH, et al: Disseminated candidiasis (moniliasis) in a dog. A case report. *Nord Vet Med* 34:362–367, 1982.
16a. McCousland IP: Systemic mycosis of two cats. *NZ Vet J* 20:10–12, 1972.
16b. McCaw D, Franklin R, Fales W, et al: Pyothorax caused by *Candida albicans* in a cat. *J Am Vet Med Assoc* 185:311–312, 1984.
17. Stone HH, Kolb LD, Currie CA, et al: Candida sepsis: pathogenesis and principles of treatment. *Ann Surg* 179:697–711, 1974.
18. Weber MJ, Keppen M, Gawith KE, et al: Treatment of systemic candidiasis in neutropenic dogs with ketoconazole. *Exp Hematol* 13:791–795, 1985.
19. Lopez-Berestein G, Bodey GP: Treatment of hepatosplenic candidiasis in cancer patients with liposomal amphotericin B. (Abstr). *Proc Am Soc Clin Oncol* 5:259, 1986.

73 TRICHOSPOROSIS

Craig E. Greene
Francis W. Chandler

ETIOLOGY

Trichosporon spp., yeast-like fungi that exist in nature as soil saprophytes, are members of the family Cryptococcaceae. In culture they form hyaline yeast-like cells, mycelia, and characteristic arthroconidia. Trichosporon spp. are not considered to be primary pathogens since they are widely distributed in the environment and form a minor component of normal skin and mucosal flora of people and animals.

T. beigelii (T. cutaneum), a transient skin commensal, is recognized as the agent of white piedra, a nodular mycosis of hair shafts affecting people, monkeys, and horses in temperate to tropical climates. T. capitatum has been incriminated as causing abortion in a cow and horse. Both T. beigelii and T. capitatum have caused systemic infection in people, especially in patients being treated for acute leukemia or lymphoma[1] and in recipients of renal and bone marrow transplants.[2] T. pullulans and T. beigelii have caused infections in three cats.[4,5]

PATHOGENESIS

Most cases of trichosporosis in people have been disseminated and fatal and have occurred in patients with severe immunosuppression who were also neutropenic; many had received multiple or broad-spectrum antibiotics for documented or presumed bacterial infections. Presumably, the organism invades the mucosal surfaces of the respiratory, GI, or urogenital tracts of immunosuppressed hosts, with subsequent dissemination.

Feline infections have been characterized by mixed suppurative and granulomatous inflammation of the mucosal and submucosal or subcutaneous tissues. Evidence for immunosuppression has not been apparent in all affected cats, but one had multicentric lymphosarcoma.

CLINICAL FINDINGS

One cat was reported to have fever, inspiratory stertor, and a protruding unilateral nasal mass similar to that caused by Cryptococcus neoformans (Fig. 73–1).[3] Later spread to regional lymph nodes and pulmonary tissue was suspected. Another was affected by a chronic ulcerative subcutaneous lesion at the site of a bite wound.[4] A cat suffered from chronic hematuria and dysuria as a result of chronic cystitis complicated by the yeast infection.[4] In people, clinical findings are usually of fungal sepsis, with fever that is unresponsive to antibiotic therapy.[5,6]

DIAGNOSIS

Mere culture of Trichosporon spp. from cutaneous or mucosal surfaces can be mis-

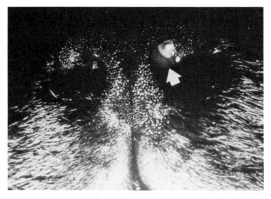

Figure 73–1. Mass (arrow) protruding from the nostril of the cat with nasal trichosporosis. (From Greene CE, et al: *J Am Vet Med Assoc* 187:946–948, 1985, with permission.)

728

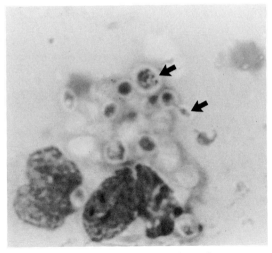

Figure 73–2. Macrophage with multiple intracytoplasmic yeasts (*arrows*) in an impression smear of the biopsied mass shown in Figure 73–1 (Wright's stain; × 800). (From Greene CE, et al: *J Am Vet Med Assoc* 187:946–948, 1985, with permission.)

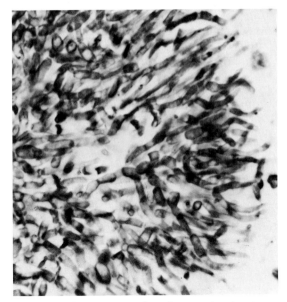

Figure 73–4. Disseminated trichosporosis. A microcolony of *Trichosporon beigelii* consists of true hyphae and arthroconidia formed by septal disarticulation of hyphae (Gomori's methenamine-silver stain; × 850).

leading because the organism is a normal constituent of the microflora in these areas. Impression smears of lesions may reveal intracellular yeasts (Fig. 73–2) that suggest their role in the disease process. Biopsy with histologic confirmation of invasion of the deeper tissues by fungal elements is more specific for documentation of fungal pathogenicity.

Trichosporon spp. can be grown on Sabouraud's or Mycosel agar (Becton Dickinson Microbiology Systems, Cockeysville, MD) at 25°C, and after several days, spreading cream-colored yeast-like colonies are formed. Wet-mount lactophenol blue-stained preparations show hyaline, septate hyphae, arthroconidia (10.4 × 2.5 μm), and pleomorphic blastoconidia (2.5 to 8 μm in diameter). The characteristic arthroconidia are produced by segmentation and fragmentation of hyphae. Unlike those of *C. neoformans*, blastoconidia of the *Trichosporon* spp. do not show a thick capsule when stained with mucin stains or India ink. The species is determined by specific biochemical reactions.

T. beigelii produces a heat-stable, cell-wall antigen that is antigenically similar to the capsular polysaccharide of *C. neoformans*.[7] The latex agglutination test, used to detect cryptococcal capsular polysaccharide antigen (see Chapter 67), has been used to diagnose disseminated *T. beigelii* infection in people.[8] In a case of nasal infection caused by *T. pullulans* in a cat, cryptococcal antigen testing of serum was negative prior to clinical evidence of dissemination.[3]

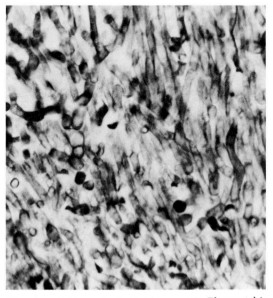

Figure 73–3. Disseminated trichosporosis. Pleomorphic blastoconidia and branched, septate hyphae of *Trichosporon beigelii* occupy a nodular splenic infarct (Gomori's methenamine-silver stain; × 850).

PATHOLOGIC FINDINGS

Histologic findings in trichosporosis consist of abscesses and hemorrhagic infarcts, with mycotic vascular invasion and infiltration of neutrophils and macrophages. Spherical to oval yeast-like organisms (blastoconidia), arthroconidia, and septate hyphae can be seen in tissue sections or in impression smears (Figs. 73–3 and 73–4). All fungal elements stain positively with PAS and Gomori's methenamine-silver stains due to polysaccharides in the fungal cell walls.

THERAPY

Trichosporon spp. are more susceptible in vitro to benzimidazole compounds than to amphotericin B or flucytosine. Cats should be treated orally with ketoconazole (see Table 72–2). Cats that develop anorexia, vomiting, or diarrhea may need to have this dosage reduced to 50 mg on alternate days. However, reduction of the dosage has been associated with relapse of disease. In contrast, itraconazole should be effective and has seemingly not been as hepatotoxic as ketoconazole in cats. Surgical removal of a nasal granuloma in one cat was incomplete, and the infection later disseminated.[3]

References

1. Gold JWM, Poston W, Mertelsmann R, et al: Systemic infection with *Trichosporon cutaneum* in a patient with acute leukemia. *Cancer* 48:2163–2167, 1981.
2. Gardella S, Nomdedeu B, Bombi JA, et al: Fatal fungemia with arthritic involvement caused by *Trichosporon beigelii* in a bone marrow transplant recipient. *J Infect Dis* 151:566, 1985.
3. Greene CE, Miller DM, Blue JL: Trichosporon infection in a cat. *J Am Vet Med Assoc* 187:946–948, 1985.
4. Doster AR, Erickson ED, Chandler FW: Feline trichosporonosis. *J Am Vet Med Assoc* 190:1184–1186, 1987.
5. Yung CW, Hanauer SB, Fretzin D, et al: Disseminated *Trichosporon beigelii* (*cutaneum*). *Cancer* 48:2107–2111, 1981.
6. Haupt HM, Merz WG, Beschorner WE, et al: Colonization and infection with *Trichosporon* species in the immunosuppressed host. *J Infect Dis* 147:199–203, 1983.
7. Melcher GP, Rinaldi MG, Frey CL, et al: Demonstration by immunoelectronmicroscopy of a cell wall antigen of *Trichosporon beigelii* that cross-reacts with *Cryptococcus neoformans* capsular polysaccharide. *J Infect Dis* 158:901–902, 1988.
8. McManus EJ, Bozdech MJ, Jones JM: Role of the latex agglutination test for cryptococcal antigen in diagnosing disseminated infections with *Trichosporon beigelii*. *J Infect Dis* 151:1167–1169, 1985.

74 MISCELLANEOUS FUNGAL INFECTIONS

Carol S. Foil

This chapter discusses pythiosis, which is common but not easily classified with other mycoses, and several fungal infections that only sporadically infect dogs and cats as opportunistic infections. The infections are covered in a roughly taxonomic order and are summarized similarly in Table 74–1. The confirmation of infections with rare and primarily saprophytic fungi must be made on the basis of concomitant isolation of the organism *from tissue* (not exudate) and demonstration of *tissue invasion* of a morphologically compatible organism. Eumycotic mycetoma is treated separately as a unique clinical syndrome caused by a variety of organisms.

Oömycosis (Pythiosis)

ETIOLOGY

More careful mycologic evaluation of previously reported cases of "phycomycosis" in animals and people has revealed that several agents, belonging to diverse taxonomic groups, produce fungal granulomas containing superficially similar, wide, nonseptate hyphae. Phycomycosis is now more properly classified as either oömycosis (pythiosis) or zygomycosis. It is not acceptable to classify uncultured lesions as zygomycosis (phycomycosis) on the basis of pathologic morphology, as the epidemiology and treatment of pythiosis and zygomycosis are dissimilar.

The organism causing pythiosis in dogs initially was assumed to be a zygomycete based on the morphology in tissue and on study of sterile in vitro cultures. However, further studies of the life cycle of the agent placed it in the genus *Pythium* of the order Peronosporales, class Oömycetes, kingdom Protista. *Pythium* isolates from dogs, as well as from horses, cattle, and people, have been described as a new species, *P. insidiosum*.[1,2] Oömycetes do not share the cell wall characteristics of the true fungi,[3] which many antifungal chemotherapeutic agents are directed against.

There have been many published cases of "phycomycosis," mostly of the GI tract, in dogs. Unfortunately, most have not been accompanied by cultural evaluations. Because of this and morphologic similarities with the agents of zygomycosis in tissue, much of the older literature on canine "phycomycosis" must be viewed cautiously. The organisms that cause pythiosis must be specifically differentiated from those that cause zygomycosis by cultural studies or IFA or ELISA tests. Some cases described prior to the recognition of these facts are likely to represent canine pythiosis, but only the most recent reports have included culturally confirmed cases.[4–8]

EPIDEMIOLOGY

Large-breed, male dogs are affected most frequently. Affected dogs have been from subtropical regions of the United States and Australia, many becoming infected during the warm and wet months of the year. These

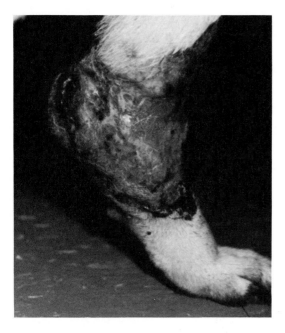

Figure 74–1. Canine subcutaneous pythiosis is the cause of this lesion on the hock of a German shepherd. The swelling and ulceration surround the limb. The lesion is infarcted in several sites.

patterns generally imply a sylvatically acquired infection.

Pythium spp. have aquatic motile zoospores and are infective to plants, the primary hosts of other parasitic members of this genus. The zoospores demonstrate chemotaxis toward damaged plant or animal tissues, which is undoubtedly the natural mode of infection in most cases. It is not known, however, whether infection can occur from direct inoculation of mycelial elements present in infected tissue. Animals are probably exposed by standing in or drinking stagnant fresh water containing newly emerged zoospores. It is not known whether the zoospore can penetrate intact oropharyngeal or GI mucosa. One observer has suggested that ingestion of large foreign

bodies might be associated with location of the lesions in the GI tract.[8]

CLINICAL FINDINGS

Cutaneous Form

Large boggy and proliferative lesions with ulceration and draining tracts may develop from dermal ulcerated nodules. Lesions may enlarge rapidly and become quite destructive; some cases develop necrosis. The most common sites are on the extremities and the tail-head or perineum. Occasionally the nodules are pruritic; early lesions on the limbs may resemble lick granulomas. Some limb lesions will progress to involve the entire

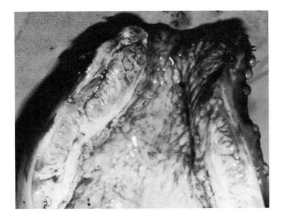

Figure 74–2. A surgically resected gastric pylorus demonstrating marked infiltration of the wall caused by gastric pythiosis. This dog was cured with this surgical procedure.

circumference of the limb (Fig. 74–1). The face may become involved as an extension of oropharyngeal disease.

GI Form

Affected dogs have a recent history of vomiting that is suggestive of an upper GI obstruction. Most often there is a palpable abdominal mass. Diarrhea is uncommon. Any part of the GI tract may be affected with a markedly infiltrative granulomatous enteritis (Fig. 74–2); the stomach and duodenum are the most common sites. Occasionally, the infiltration is diffuse, but often it is localized to one region of the tract. Oropharyngeal infection is less common. In that site, infarction and necrosis are prominent features.

Systemic Form

Rarely, dogs with either the cutaneous or GI or oropharyngeal form may develop disseminated disease with granulomatous foci developing in any organ. Rapid death is accompanied by signs suggestive of particular organ involvement. The use of glucocorticoids may be associated with rapid dissemination, either locally or systemically. Other host factors associated with dissemination are not known.

DIAGNOSIS

Cytology

Diagnosis can occasionally be established cytologically if lesions are accessible. Macerated tissue fixed in 10% KOH may be examined by direct microscopic inspection for the presence of typical wide, poorly septate, and branching hyphal elements (see Appendix 12).

Histology

Pathologic diagnosis will often require silver stains as the organism is difficult to see in routine H and E stains in canine specimens. As the organism in tissue is quite similar to the zygomycetes, it is necessary to have cultural as well as histologic infor-

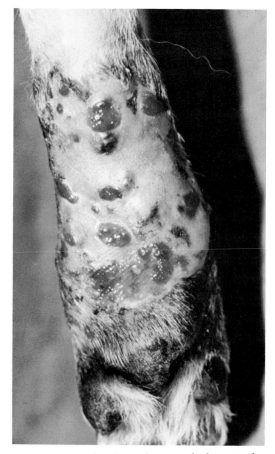

Figure 74–3. The split-thickness graft that was done following a resection of a subcutaneous pythiosis lesion has become infiltrated with new granulomatous nodules. The leg was amputated, resolving the disease.

mation to establish the diagnosis. Fluorescent antibody techniques have been used for specific detection of the organism in tissues, but they are not widely available.

Cultural Identification

The organism is not fastidious and will grow rapidly on both Sabouraud's dextrose and blood agar media when bits of aseptically obtained tissue are inoculated. The tissue should not be ground with mortar and pestle prior to being placed on the agar. It is advisable to submit specimens to veterinary diagnostic laboratories, where the microbiologist is more likely to be familiar with *Pythium* and its characteristic growth patterns. Unless specialized culture techniques are employed, the organisms will not produce diagnostic spores, and familiarity with the organism will be necessary for identification.

Serologic Findings

An immunodiffusion test has been developed for the serologic identification of anti-*Pythium* antibody production.[9] To date, this test has been used only in infected horses and is not commercially available.

THERAPY

The prognosis in pythiosis is poor unless the affected tissue can be completely excised. In the GI tract, this often requires radical resection. When lesions are on an extremity, amputation can be curative. Wide and deep excision of skin lesions followed by skin grafting may be successful, but if excision is not complete the graft may become reinfected (Fig. 74–3).

As *Pythium* spp. do not share cell wall characteristics with true fungi, it is not surprising that antifungal chemotherapeutic agents have been disappointing in the treatment of this disease. Limited in vitro testing with some agents has also indicated that the organism is not susceptible. Preliminary studies with the agricultural chemical metalaxyl show that this drug may be useful. Fungal "vaccines" have been tried with little success in infected dogs.

Zygomycosis

ETIOLOGY

Diseases caused by fungi in the class Zygomycetes are classified herein. There are two orders that cause diverse types of diseases in people and animals. The order Mucorales includes the genera *Rhizopus*, *Mucor*, *Mortierella*, and *Absidia* among others. The term "mucormycosis" has been applied to this group of infections. The order Entomophthorales contains the genera *Conidiobolus* (*Entomophthora*) and *Basidiobolus*. Entomophthoromycosis is the term applied to their infections of animals and people.

There has been only one confirmed report of disseminated *Basidiobolus haptosporus* infection in a dog,[10] but more reports of entomophthoraceous infections may be expected as the cultural identification of this and similar organisms becomes better understood. GI and pharyngeal entomophthoromycosis caused by undetermined species has been defined on the basis of fungal morphology in tissue by a skilled investigator in two additional dogs.[7]

A chronically infected cervical bite wound in a dog was culturally confirmed as infected by *Absidia corymbifera*.[11] In another report of canine zygomycosis of the pancreas, however, the diagnosis was based on morphologic description of the pathology and organism, without confirmation by fungal culture.[12]

As reviewed previously,[13] the systemic phycomycosis in dogs from western Europe and the northeastern United States in some older reports was likely to have been caused by zygomycetes. Lesions in these affected animals involved the kidney, GI tract, heart muscle, or disseminated tissues.

Some reports have been made of mucormycosis in cats with diabetes or with immunosuppressive diseases such as feline leukemia virus infection or panleukopenia.[14] *Mortierella parasitica* was isolated from a tracheal lesion in a cat.[15] *Mucor pusillus* was associated with cerebral zygomycosis in another cat.[16]

EPIDEMIOLOGY

Zygomycetes are ubiquitous in nature and are common contaminants in cultures. Infectious material probably consists of either vegetative or reproductive spores. The portal of entry may be GI or respiratory tracts or via wound inoculation. In people and animals, a compromised immune system is necessary for invasion to occur in most cases. In most confirmed and suspected cases in dogs, such factors have not been documented, whereas in some the disease has been associated with long-term antibiotic use, distemper infection, and prior bite wounds.

CLINICAL FINDINGS

The disease is poorly defined in dogs and cats, and most diagnoses have been obtained by the necropsy examination. It is difficult to draw conclusions about typical clinical findings; most reported cases have involved the GI tract and have had acute to subacute courses. Many patients have vomited and have had palpable abdominal masses, and some have been moribund on presentation. In disseminated disease, local granulomatous lesions have associated local and generalized lymphadenomegaly. The rhinocerebral form of zygomycosis seen in immunocompromised people does not appear to occur commonly in dogs and cats.

DIAGNOSIS

There must be the demonstration of tissue invasion and the concomitant cultural identification of a morphologically compatible organism (see Fig. 62–6). The gross morphologic appearance of granulomatous lesions mimics that of a neoplasm. For this reason, tissue from masses must be saved for cultural studies pending cytologic and histologic evaluation.

Rapid analysis of impression smears or tissue macerated in 10% KOH may provide a tentative diagnosis of a mycotic disease (see Appendix 12). In most reported cases of zygomycosis, fungal elements are abundant within necrotic centers of tissue masses and, thus, would be expected to be readily accessible for cytologic preparations. The broad, poorly septate hyphae characteristic of zygomycosis are confused only with those seen in pythiosis.

THERAPY

The prognosis is grave in the case of disseminated and abdominal disease. When GI lesions can be completely excised, there is some hope of a cure. The susceptibility of most of the Mucorales to antimycotic agents is quite variable; for the Entomophthorales it is largely unknown. Since the latter infections may be confined to the skin, surgical resection may be attempted with or without follow-up chemotherapy. In people, these infections may be successfully treated with KI. If antifungal chemotherapy is to be attempted, it should be based on results of in vitro susceptibility tests.

Hyalohyphomycosis

ETIOLOGY

The term "hyalohyphomycosis" has been proposed to encompass all opportunistic infections caused by nondematiacious fungi whose basic tissue form is hyaline hyphal elements (Table 74–1).[17] These forms may be septate, branched or unbranched, or toruloid. Some infections have been covered elsewhere in this volume (see Aspergillosis and Penicilliosis, Chapter 64).

Paecilomyces fumosoroseus, P. varioti, and other *Paecilomyces* species have been associated with cutaneous and disseminated lesions in dogs and cats.[18,19] *Pseudallescheria (Allescheria) boydii* has been isolated from a dog with mycotic pneumonia[20] and with disseminated diseases.[21] *Geotrichum candidum* infection has been reported in a dog[22] and a cat.[23]

Paecilomyces is a ubiquitous saprophytic mold and a common contaminant of laboratory cultures (see Fig. 62–12). *Geotrichum* and *Pseudallescheria* are likewise common soil saprophytes (see Fig. 62–13). *Geotrichum* may also be considered a normal part of the oral and GI flora.

CLINICAL FINDINGS

In dogs and cats, paecilomycosis seems to begin in the skin or ear and later to disseminate. Signs, which vary with the organ system affected, have involved the nasal passages, CNS, respiratory system, and bone marrow. No predisposing feature has been identified in any reported case.

In the case of pseudallescheriosis, fungal pneumonia has been diagnosed.[20] The agent has been cultured from transtracheal exudate rather than tissue, and no tissue biopsy

Table 74–1. Miscellaneous Fungi Reported to Cause Disease in Dogs and Cats

GROUP CLASSIFICATION	GROUP CHARACTERISTICS	DISEASE	FUNGAL GENERA INVOLVED	PRIMARY ORGAN SYSTEM OR TISSUES INVOLVED
Oömycetes	Broad, poorly septate hyphae	Pythiosis	*Pythium*	GI tract, subcutaneous, disseminated
Zygomycetes	Broad, sparse, or nonseptate hyphae	Zygomycosis Mucormycosis	*Mucor, Rhizopus, Mortierella, Absidia*	GI tract, CNS, skin, disseminated
		Entomophthoromycosis	*Basidiobolus*	Skin, disseminated
Hyaline Hyphomycetes (nondematiacious)	Septate mycelia with no brown pigment in cell walls	Hyalohyphomycosis Aspergillosis	*Aspergillus*	Nasal cavity, disseminated
		Penicilliosis	*Penicillium*	Nasal cavity
		Paecilomycosis	*Paecilomyces*	CNS, disseminated
		Adiaspiromycosis	*Chrysosporium*	Lung
		Pseudallescheriosis (no grains)	*Pseudallescheria*	Respiratory
		Geotrichosis	*Geotrichum*	Disseminated
		Eumycotic mycetoma (white grains)	*Acremonium Pseudallescheria*	Abdominal cavity
Dematiacious Hyphomycetes	Septate mycelia with brown pigment in cell walls	Phaeohyphomycosis	*Xylohypha (Cladosporium) Bipolaris (Drechslera) Exophiala Moniliella Phialemonium Phialophora Pseudomicrodochium Stemphylium Alternaria Scolecobasidium*	Subcutaneous, occasional CNS, disseminated
		Eumycotic mycetoma (black grains)	*Curvularia Madurella*	Subcutaneous

has been obtained. However, the response to antifungal therapy has been supportive of the diagnosis. Disseminated disease in another dog was manifest by lethargy, intermittent fever, and forelimb swelling and lameness.[21] At necropsy, the dog had a large mediastinal mass, lymphadenopathy, and granulomas in many tissues.

Disseminated disease has been reported in a dog with geotrichosis; the dog had fever, respiratory distress, icterus, and uremia.[22] The disease progressed rapidly to a fatal outcome.

THERAPY

None of the reported animals with paecilomycosis have survived. A cat and a dog have been treated with ketoconazole unsuccessfully. However, one of the isolates was susceptible in vitro to amphotericin B, 5-fluorocytosine, nystatin, and natamycin; showed intermediate susceptibility to ketoconazole; and showed resistance to miconazole and griseofulvin.[10] A dog with pseudallescheriosis has been treated successfully with amphotericin B.[20]

Animals with disseminated or CNS disease would be expected to have a grave prognosis. If treatment of more localized forms of infections with these and similar agents is to be attempted, the isolate should be subjected to in vitro susceptibility testing in order to formulate a rational therapeutic plan. Where possible, surgical removal is the treatment of choice, although dissemination might be expected.

Phaeohyphomycosis

ETIOLOGY AND EPIDEMIOLOGY

Phaeohyphomycosis is caused by a number of saprophytic and ubiquitous molds that have the characteristic of forming pigmented (dematiacious) hyphal elements in tissue. These are uncommon to rare opportunistic infections. The organisms that have been isolated from canine and feline infections include *Xylohypha bantiana (Cladosporium trichoides, C. bantianum), Bipolaris (Drechslera) spicifera, X. emmonsii, Exophiala jeanselmei, Moniliella suaveolens, Phialemonium obovatum, Phialophora verrucosa, Alternaria alternata, Pseudomicrodochium suttonii, Scolecobasidium humicola,* and *Stemphylium sp.* Several cases have been reported on the basis of histologic descriptions without cultural identification of the causative agent. *Xylohypha, Bipolaris, Exophiala, Phialemonium, Phialophora,* and *Stemphylium* are ubiquitous wood and soil saprophytes. *Moniliella* has been recovered from cheese, butter, and margarine. *Scolecobasidium* is usually a cause of phaeohyphomycosis in cold-blooded vertebrates. *Alternaria* has been cultured from the skin of clinically healthy people and dogs. Animals and people presumably are exposed to infection with dematiacious fungi by wound contamination, although initial respiratory tract colonization cannot be ruled out in systemic cases.

CLINICAL FINDINGS

The superficial forms (piedra and tinea nigra) and cutaneous forms of phaeohyphomycosis have not been documented in dogs and cats. Most cases have been subcutaneous.[24-26] In systemic cases, *Xylohypha* has been implicated and most have involved the CNS, possibly by extension from nasal cavity or pulmonary infection (Fig. 74–4).[27-30] In several of these systemic and cerebral cases, previous systemic problems, such as chronic renal disease, have been associated with the infection.[31] Keratomycosis in a cat has been associated with *Xylohypha* sp.[32] Dissemination was seen in a dog infected with *Pseudomicrodochium*.[33]

Subcutaneous phaeohyphomycosis consists of solitary ulcerated nodules to widespread ulcerative and nodular disease with crusting and fistulous tract formation.[24] In advanced cases, lesions may coalesce to form large ragged ulcers (Fig. 74–5). In cats, the lesions may resemble chronic bacterial abscesses.[26] The disease may evolve over a period of weeks to months. Lesions often recur after surgical excision. A skin lesion in a dog has been associated with underlying mycotic osteomyelitis of the limb.[34]

Systemic disease usually has an acute to subacute course with symptoms referable to the organ system involved. As noted above, CNS disease is prominent and is invariably fatal.

DIAGNOSIS

Direct examination of exudate or macerated tissue mounted in KOH may reveal the pigmented fungal elements (see Appendix 12). As with other opportunistic mycoses, confirmation of the diagnosis is based on the concomitant demonstration of hyphae in tissue and culture of a morphologically compatible organism from tissue. These organisms grow readily on Sabouraud's dextrose

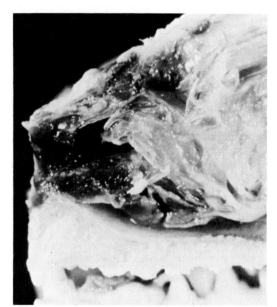

Figure 74–4. This necropsy specimen of a cat with nasal phaeohyphomycosis illustrates the darkly pigmented nature of the infiltrate. The pigment is imparted by the dark fungal growth. (Courtesy of Dr. Richard I. Miller, Australia.)

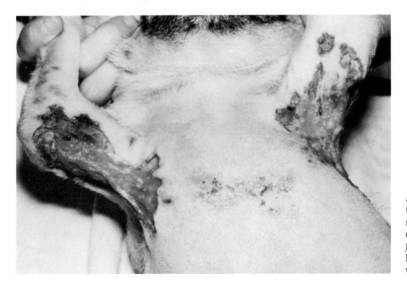

Figure 74–5. This extensive cutaneous ulceration is caused by subcutaneous phaeohyphomycosis due to *Drechslera spicifera*. (Courtesy of Dr. Kenneth Kwochka, The Ohio State University, Columbus, OH.)

agar, although specialized agar may be required to encourage production of the identifying fruiting bodies (see Fig. 62–11).

THERAPY

Prognosis in systemic or widespread cutaneous disease is grave, although in localized cutaneous forms, successful therapy has been described. When the lesions are excisable, surgery may be curative, but recurrence at the same or at new sites is common. In unexcisable or in recurrent cases, antifungal chemotherapy may be helpful but, depending on the agent, the response may be unpredictable. Drugs should be chosen on the basis of in vitro susceptibility testing if at all possible. The azoles show variable in vitro activity against saprophytic organisms. A cat apparently has been cured after multiple excisions and treatment with ketoconazole,[35] while another has been treated successfully with amphotericin B.[36] In other feline cases, treatment with both ketoconazole and 5-fluorocytosine was unsuccessful.[37] A cat with two lesion caused by infection with *Scolecobasidium humicola* was treated unsuccessfully with oral ketoconazole therapy alone.[24a] For appropriate dosages of antifungal drugs, see Table 63–2.

Eumycotic Mycetoma

Mycetomas are granulomatous nodules of the subcutaneous tissues that contain tissue grains or granules. Within the grains are dense colonies of the organism along with host-derived matter, usually necrotic debris. When such lesions are caused by fungi, they are known as eumycotic mycetomas to distinguish them from actinomycotic lesions (see Chapter 53) and botryomycosis. Eumycotic mycetomas may be caused by pigmented fungi that impart their pigmented appearance to the grains in tissue. These are called black- or dark-grain mycetomas.

Black-grain mycetomas have been associated with infections by *Curvularia* and *Madurella*. When the agents are unpigmented they cause white-grain mycetoma. White-grain mycetomas have been found with infections caused by *Acremonium* and *Pseudallescheria*.

Most eumycotic mycetomas are confined to the subcutaneous tissue, but white-grain mycetomas may be extensions of abdominal cavity disease. Granulomas with grains within the abdominal cavity have also been referred to as mycetomas.

ETIOLOGY

Fungal isolation from affected dogs and cats has not been done in all cases. Several species of saprophytic fungi have been associated with mycetomas in dogs. Of the black-grain mycetomas, *Curvularia geniculata* is the most common isolate.[38–40] In abdominal and body-wall white-grain mycetoma of the dog, *Pseudallescheria* (*Allescheria*) *boydii*[41,42,42a] and *Acremonium hyalinum*[43] have been isolated. *Madurella grisea* has been isolated from a cat with mycetoma.[14] The color of the tissue grains has not been described, but this agent is pigmented.

CLINICAL FINDINGS

In white-grain mycetoma, most infections have involved abdominal cavity organs. Dogs have developed peritonitis or abdominal masses after surgical wound dehiscence.[41,42,42b] Contamination of viscera following dehiscence is a likely source of infection. Lesions within the abdomen have had tissue grains and were associated with *Pseudallescheria boydii*. It will be necessary to analyze more cases to confirm whether these infections are associated with nonabsorbable suture materials left in the abdomen.

Cutaneous mycetoma has been the typical finding of black-grain infection. Infections probably develop at the site of a superficial wound, possibly contaminated by a plant foreign body. In one cat, a black mycetoma developed following a bite wound.[44] Lesions are cutaneous nodules, relatively poorly circumscribed, usually on the extremities or the face. They do not often ulcerate widely, but fistulas may form within the nodule. Most become surmounted by alopecic and hyperkeratotic epidermis. Cycles of healing and ulceration may lead to firm swelling and scarring. Black tissue grains may be visible within the exudate, or the exudate or the tissue itself may appear black. Some nodules are so heavily pigmented that they are mistaken for cutaneous melanomas. On the limbs and feet, the infectious process may involve underlying bone.[40,45]

DIAGNOSIS

A presumptive diagnosis of mycetoma may be made if there are grains within exudate from any draining tract. Cytologic investigation must be directed at the tissue grains, for the organism is often scant or absent elsewhere within exudate or tissue. Grains may be crushed and smeared on a slide for staining in some cases. Black grains are often gritty and may require digestion in 10% KOH before they can be mounted for microscopic study (see Appendix 12). The fungal elements are usually quite evident in thinly smeared or flattened grains. Serum may be tested for specific antibodies by agar-gel immunodiffusion.[42b] Formalin-fixed, paraffin-embedded tissue may be stained with fluorescein-conjugated immunoglobulins specific for *P. boydii*.[42a]

Cultural investigation is necessary to confirm the cytologic findings and to identify the causative organism. Tissue grains may be collected from exudate and washed in sterile saline for culturing. Alternatively, surgically excised tissue, if it contains grains, may be cultured. Fungal isolates should be retained for possible in vitro susceptibility testing. The agents associated with mycetomas in dogs and cats are readily cultured on standard media.

THERAPY

The prognosis in abdominal mycetoma is guarded, as cases described to date have had extensive involvement of abdominal organs. Cutaneous mycetoma is not a life-threatening disease but is difficult to resolve. Radical surgical excision has been the treatment most often employed in human cases. Amputation of affected limbs may be necessary; spontaneous resolution does not occur. Any attempt at antifungal chemotherapy should be based on in vitro susceptibility testing of the isolate. Even if an antifungal chemotherapeutic agent that may be helpful is identified, it is apparently difficult to attain effective levels within the tissue grains where the organism resides. Successful outcomes have been reported in human cases with local hyperthermia treatments.

References

1. DeCock AWAM, Mendoza L, Padhye AA, et al: *Pythium insidiosum* sp. nov., the etiologic agent of pythiosis. *J Clin Microbiol* 25:344–349, 1987.
2. Shipton WA: *Pythium destruens* sp. nov. an agent

of equine phythiosis. *J Med Vet Mycol* 25:137–151, 1987.

3. Shipton WA, Miller RI, Lea IR: Cell wall, zoospore and morphological characteristics of Australian isolates of a *Pythium* causing equine phycomycosis. *Trans Br Mycol Soc* 79:15–23, 1982.

4. Miller RI, Qualls CW Jr, Turnwald GH: Gastrointestinal phycomycosis in a dog. *J Am Vet Med Assoc* 182:1245–1246, 1983.

5. Foil CS, Short BG, Fadok VA, et al: A report of subcutaneous pythiosis in five dogs and a review of the etiologic agent *Pythium* spp. *J Am Anim Hosp Assoc* 20:959–966, 1984.

6. English PB, Frost AJ: Phycomycosis in a dog. *Aust Vet J* 61:291–292, 1984.

7. Miller RI: Gastrointestinal phycomycosis in 63 dogs. *J Am Vet Med Assoc* 186:473–478, 1985.

8. Troy GC: Canine phycomycosis: a review of twenty-four cases. *Calif Vet* 39:12–17, 1985.

9. Mendoza L, Kaufman L, Standard PG: Immunodiffusion test for diagnosing and monitoring pythiosis in horses. *J Clin Microbiol* 23:813–816, 1986.

10. Miller RI, Turnwald GH: Disseminated basidiobolomycosis in a dog. *Vet Pathol* 21:117–119, 1984.

11. English MP, Lucke VM: Phycomycosis in a dog caused by unusual strains of *Absidia corymbifera*. *Sabouraudia* 8:126–132, 1970.

12. Mezza LE, DuFort RM, King JM: A new manifestation of canine zygomycosis: zygomycotic pancreatitis. *Vet Med* May:34–41, 1985.

13. Barsanti JA: Miscellaneous fungal infections. *In* Greene CE (ed): *Clinical Microbiology and Infectious Diseases of the Dog and Cat*. Philadelphia, WB Saunders Co, 1984, pp 738–746.

14. Holzworth J, Blouin P, Conner MW: Mycotic diseases. *In* Holzworth J (ed): *Diseases of the Cat. Medicine and Surgery*, vol 1. Philadelphia, WB Saunders Co, 1987, pp 320–358.

15. Constantin: Note sur un cas do pneumomycose observé sur un chat par M. Neumann. *Bull Soc Mycol Fr* 8 (1892):57–59, as cited in Holzworth J (ed): *Diseases of the Cat. Medicine and Surgery*, vol 1. Philadelphia, WB Saunders Co, 1987, p 348.

16. Ravisse P, Fromentin H, Destmobes, et al: Mucormycose cérébrale du chat due a *Mucor pusillus*. *Sabouraudia* 16:291–298, 1978.

17. Ajello L, McGinnis MR, 1984, as cited in Matsuda T, Matsumoto T: Disseminated hyalohyphomycosis in a leukemic patient. *Arch Dermatol* 122:1171–1175, 1986.

18. Elliot GS, Whitney MS, Reed WM, et al: Antemortem diagnosis of paecilomycosis in a cat. *J Am Vet Med Assoc* 184:93–94, 1984.

19. Littman MP, Goldschmidt MH: Systemic paecilomycosis in a dog. *J Am Vet Med Assoc* 191:445–450, 1987.

20. Tuntivanich P: First report on fungal pneumonia caused by *Monosporium apiospermum* (*Allescheria boydii*) in a dog and the effective treatment. *J Am Anim Hosp Assoc* 16:269–272, 1980.

21. Baszler T, Chandler FW, Bertoy RW, et al: Disseminated pseudallescheriasis in a dog. *Vet Pathol* 25:95–97, 1988.

22. Lincoln SD, Adcock JL: Disseminated geotrichosis in a dog. *Pathol Vet* 5:282–289, 1968.

23. Gray J: Personal comunication, 1958, as cited in Holzworth J (ed): *Diseases of the Cat. Medicine and Surgery*, vol 1. Philadelphia, WB Saunders Co, 1987, p 342.

24. Kwochka KW, Calderwood Mays MB, Ajello L, et al: Canine phaeohyphomycosis caused by *Drechslera spicifera*: a case report and literature review. *J Am Anim Hosp Assoc* 20:625–633, 1984.

24a. VanSteenhouse JL, Padhye AA, Ajello L: Subcutaneous phaeohyphomycosis caused by *Scolecobasidium humicola* in a cat. *Mycopathologia* 102:123–127, 1988.

25. McKenzie RA, Connole MD, McGinnis MR, et al: Subcutaneous phaeohyphomycosis caused by *Moniliella suareulens* in two cats. *Vet Pathol* 21:582–586, 1984.

25a. Padhye AA, McGinnis MR, Ajello L, et al: *Xylohypha emmonsii* sp. nov., a new agent of phaeohyphomycosis. *J Clin Microbiol* 26:702–708, 1988.

26. Bostock DE, Coloe PJ, Castellani A: Phaeohyphomycosis caused by *Exphiala jeanselmei* in a domestic cat. *J Comp Pathol* 92:479–482, 1982.

26a. Dhein CR, Leathers CW, Padhye AA, et al: Phaeohyphomycosis caused by *Alterneria alternata* in a cat. *J Am Vet Med Assoc* 193:1101–1103, 1988.

27. Shinwari MW, Thomas AD, Orr JS: Feline cerebral phaeohyphomycosis associated with *Cladosporium bantianum*. *Aust Vet J* 62:383–384, 1987.

28. Fiske RA, Choyce PD, Whitford HW, et al: Phaeomycotic encephalitis in two dogs. *J Am Anim Hosp Assoc* 22:327–330, 1986.

29. Dillehay DL, Ribas JL, Newton JC, et al: Cerebral phaeohyphomycosis in two dogs and a cat. *Vet Pathol* 24:192–194, 1987.

30. Newsholme SJ, Tyrer MJ: Cerebral mycosis in a dog caused by *Cladosporium trichoides* Emmons 1952. *Onderstepoort J Vet Res* 47:47–49, 1980.

31. Migaki G, Casey HW, Bayles NB: Cerebral phaeohyphomycosis in a dog. *J Am Vet Med Assoc* 191:997–998, 1987.

32. Miller DM, Blue JL, Winston SM: Keratomycosis caused by *Cladosporium* sp. in a cat. *J Am Vet Med Assoc* 182:1121–1122, 1983.

33. Ajello L, Padhye AA: Phaeohyphomycosis in a dog caused by *Pseudomicrodochium suttonii* sp. nov. *Mucotaxon* 12:131–136, 1980.

34. Lomax LG, Cole JR, Padhye AA, et al: Osteolytic phaeohyphomycosis in a German shepherd dog caused by *Phialemonium obovatum*. *J Clin Microbiol* 23:987–991, 1986.

35. Sousa CA, Ihrke PJ: Subcutaneous phaeohyphomycosis caused by *Phialophora gougerotti*. *Cornell Vet* 67:467–471, 1977.

36. McKeever PJ, Caywood DD, Perman V: Chromomycosis in a cat: successful medical therapy. *J Am Anim Hosp Assoc* 19:533–536, 1983.

37. Pukay BP, Dion WM: Feline phaeohyphomycosis: treatment with ketoconazole and 5-fluorocytosine. *Can Vet J* 25:130–134, 1984.

38. Bridges CH: Maduromycotic mycetomas in animals. *Curvularia geniculata* as an etiologic agent. *Am J Pathol* 33:411–427, 1957.

39. Brodey RS, Schryver HF, Deubler MJ, et al: Mycetoma in a dog. *J Am Vet Med Assoc* 151:442–451, 1967.

40. Coyle V, Isaacs JP, O'Boyle DA: Canine mycetoma: a case report and review of the literature. *J Small Anim Pract* 25:261–268, 1984.

41. Jang SS, Popp JA: Eumycotic mycetoma in a dog caused by *Allescheria boydii*. *J Am Vet Med Assoc* 157:1071–1076, 1970.

42. Kurtz HJ, Finco DR, Perman V: Maduromycosis (*Allescheria boydii*) in a dog. *J Am Vet Med Assoc* 157:917–921, 1970.

42a. Allison N, McDonald RK, Guist SR, et al: Eumycotic mycetoma caused by *Pseudallescheria boydii* in a dog. *J Am Vet Med Assoc* 194:794–799, 1989.

42b. Walker RL, Monticello TM, Ford RB, et al: Eumycotic mycetoma caused by *Pseudallescheria boydii* in the abdominal cavity of a dog. *J Am Vet Med Assoc* 192:67–70, 1988.

43. Hay CEM, Loveday RK, Spencer BMT, et al: Bilateral mycotic myositis, osteomyelitis and nephritis in a dog caused by *Cephalosporium*-like hyphomycete. *J S Afr Vet Assoc* 49:359–361, 1978.

44. Van den Broek AHM, Thoday KL: Eumycotoma in a British cat. *J Small Anim Pract* 28:827–831, 1987.

45. Mezza LE, Harvey HJ: Osteomyelitis associated with maduromycotic mycetoma in the foot of a dog. *J Am Anim Hosp Assoc* 21:215–218, 1985.

75

PROTOTHECOSIS

David E. Tyler

ETIOLOGY

Protothecosis is caused by *Prototheca*, microorganisms that are morphologically similar to the green algae of the genus *Chlorella*. Unlike *Chlorella*, which possess chlorophyll, *Prototheca* are thought to be achlorophyllous mutants. In culture or in tissue, the cells are spherical to oval and range from 1.3 to 13.4 μm in diameter and from 1.3 to 16.1 μm in length. Size varies with the stage of development, the species, and the medium used for culture. Organisms have a hyaline cell wall approximately 0.5 μm thick; a granular, basophilic cytoplasm; and a small, centrally located nucleus. In smaller immature forms, a nucleus may not be evident. Reproduction is by endosporulation, with irregular nuclear and cytoplasmic cleavage resulting in 2 to 20 or more endospores. The mother cell ruptures, discharging tiny replicas that enlarge, mature, and repeat the life cycle. Empty cell casings scattered among intact algal cells may be seen in lesions. Typical *Prototheca* in tissue are seen in Figure 75–1.

Of the three species of *Prototheca* now recognized, *P. stagnora*, *P. zopfii*, and *P. wickerhamii*, the last two have been incriminated as pathogens. The species can be differentiated either by sugar and alcohol assimilation tests or by IFA.

EPIDEMIOLOGY AND PATHOGENESIS

Ecologically, *Prototheca* are primary inhabitants of raw and treated sewage, slime flux of trees, and animal wastes.[1] From these sources *Prototheca* secondarily contaminate water systems, soil, and food, from which they may be ingested by people and animals. Although *Prototheca* occasionally can be isolated from freshly voided human and animal feces, they are regarded as transient contaminants and only rarely cause disease. Protothecosis is considered to be acquired exogenously and is not transmissible between hosts. Its low incidence indicates an infection with minimal pathogenicity that occurs when the host's immune resistance is suppressed or altered, often by preexisting or concurrent disease. Lack of cell-mediated immunity (CMI) seems to be more important than decreased humoral responses in allowing entrance of *Prototheca* into tissues and establishment of infection. Extremely high serum concentrations of *Prototheca*-specific IgG may, in fact, cause a blockade of CMI, allowing dissemination of *Prototheca* throughout the body. Additional evidence for the proposed inhibitory effect of antibody on CMI is substantiated in canine protothecosis, where the cellular response is minimal but usually contains an abnormally large component of plasma cells.

Another possible pathogenetic mechanism noted in some infected people is a deficiency in the ability of the host's neutrophils to specifically destroy *Prototheca* after phagocytosis. There has been no evidence of failure of either humoral immunity or CMI in such patients. Evaluation of immune function in a dog with disseminated protothecosis revealed depressed T lymphocyte function and neutrophil inhibition.[2] A single serum inhibitory factor may have been responsible for both findings.

In nearly all canine cases, evidence of colitis and a history of intermittent bloody diarrhea over a prolonged period are reported. This suggests that the colon may be the common site of entry for *Prototheca* in this species and may explain why the disease is usually disseminated throughout the viscera rather than a localized infection, the form most frequently seen in people and cats.

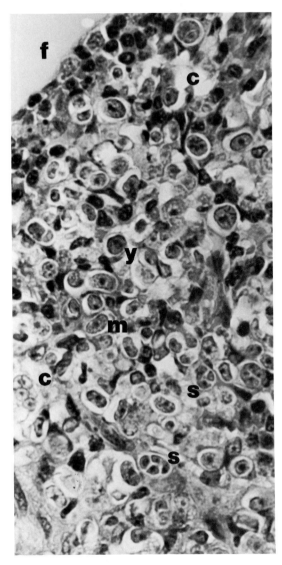

Figure 75–1. *Prototheca* in various stages of development. The lesion is in the thyroid gland. y = young spherical cell; m = more mature oval cell; s = sporulating cells; c = empty casings of cells that have discharged their spores; f = follicle (H and E; × 400).

Virulence of the organism may differ between species of *Prototheca*. In cutaneous cases in both dogs and cats, only *P. wickerhamii* has been isolated. In contrast, *P. zopfii* is nearly always isolated from disseminated cases in dogs. Breed susceptibility may be a factor in dogs. A disproportionate number of cases have occurred in collies. There is no age predilection, but a majority of the cases have been in female dogs.

CLINICAL FINDINGS

Dog

Protothecosis in the dog is generally a widely disseminated disease with clinical signs varying in kind and severity depending on the tissues involved. The most frequently reported clinical observation is bloody diarrhea, which is usually intermittent and protracted. Weight loss and debility become progressively more pronounced over the course of the disease. Clinical signs attributed directly to involvement of the CNS have been reported in about 40% of the cases and have included marked depression, ataxia, circling, incoordination, and paresis. Deafness has been observed in three cases, as have signs of renal failure. Only a few cases of the cutaneous manifestation of the disease have been reported in dogs. Skin lesions are chronic and characterized by draining ulcers and crusty exudates of the skin of the trunk and extremities and mucosal surfaces of many months' duration (Fig. 75–2). Even in cutaneous cases, lesions may be disseminated, involving other organs such as the lymph nodes and lungs.

The eyes are involved in two-thirds of the cases and in some animals blindness may be the only sign noted. Leukocoria due to vitreous clouding is seen frequently when dogs are first presented for examination.[3] Generally, ophthalmoscopic examination reveals exudative clouding of the fluid in one or both chambers and multiple white, raised foci or streaks in the retina (Fig. 75–3), often accompanied by small hemorrhages. Retinal detachment is usually evident.

Cat

Only the cutaneous form of protothecosis has been reported in the cat.[4–7] Lesions usually occur as large, firm cutaneous nodules on the limbs or feet but have also been reported on the nose, forehead, pinna, and base of the tail. All cats were reported to be in good health otherwise.

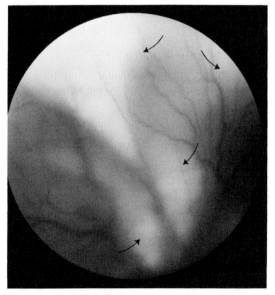

Figure 75–3. Ophthalmoscopic appearance of the ocular fundus from a dog with protothecosis. The retina contains multiple white foci (*arrows*). (Courtesy of Dr. Susan M. Winston, Marietta, GA.)

DIAGNOSIS

Whenever a dog is presented with a history of protracted bloody diarrhea coupled with ocular lesions, protothecosis should be considered as a highly probable cause.

Clinical Laboratory Findings

Laboratory data have not been well documented in the cases of canine and feline protothecosis. Generally, the results of CBC are within reference ranges, and serum enzymes are rarely slightly elevated. If present, abnormalities in the CSF may include marked pleocytosis (>100 cells/μl) with granulocytes or lymphocytes being the predominant nucleated cell types and increased protein (>100 mg/dl).[2,8]

Algal Identification and Isolation

Clinically, organisms have been found by culture of fluid obtained by vitreous centesis or of CSF, examination of Wright's-stained rectal scraping (Fig. 75–4), and histologic evaluation of biopsied lesions. Since *Prototheca* commonly invade Bowman's space and renal tubules, evaluation of urinary sediment has revealed the organism in some

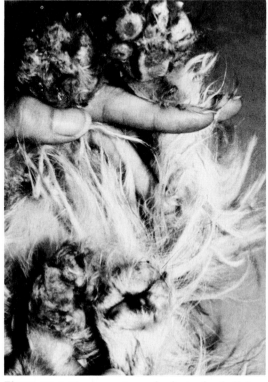

Figure 75–2. Heavy crusts on the footpads of all four feet of a dog with a rare cutaneous form of protothecosis.

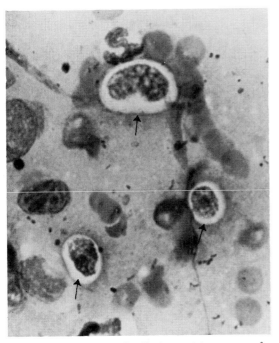

Figure 75–4. Protothecal cells (*arrows*) in a smear of a rectal scraping from a dog with disseminated protothecosis (Wright's stain; × 1008). (Courtesy of Dr. Ken Latimer, University of Georgia, Athens, GA.)

infected dogs.[2] Finding the organism in the urinary sediment would be an accurate way to determine that dissemination of infection has occurred.

Because organisms in tissues stained with H and E show variability in staining, Gomori's methenamine-silver (GMS) or PAS stains are preferred. Since *Prototheca* and *Chlorella* species are morphologically indistinguishable when stained with H and E, the GMS or PAS stains should be used. With these stains, large starch granules are readily seen in *Chlorella* sp. but not in *Prototheca* sp. Infections with *Chlorella* have not been reported in the dog or cat; however, they have been observed in several other species and frequently have been improperly identified as *Prototheca*.

Prototheca grow readily on a variety of laboratory media, such as Sabouraud's cyclohexamide-free dextrose agar at 25° to 37°C, forming white to light tan colonies within 2 to 7 days. Characteristic organisms in all stages of development can be recognized easily by staining a smear from the colony with Gram's iodine stain (Fig. 75–5).

Ribostamycin-impregnated discs have been used to differentiate *Candida* and *Prototheca* colonies on Sabouraud's glucose agar[9]; *Prototheca* show a halo of inhibition around the discs, while *Candida* are not inhibited. *Prototheca* species have been differentiated by the use of clotrimazole-impregnated discs, since *P. wickerhamii* are susceptible to clotrimazole while *P. zopfii* are resistant.[10]

There may be sufficient morphologic differences between *P. zopfii* and *P. wickerhamii* to establish histologic identification of species[11]; however, these are too subtle for pathologists seeing these organisms infrequently to appreciate. It is recommended, therefore, that preserved biopsy and necropsy tissues and unstained histologic sections be sent to the Histopathology Laboratory, Center for Infectious Diseases, Centers for Disease Control, Atlanta, GA, for specific identification by the IFA technique (see Appendix 8). Formalin-fixed tissues may be examined by this method. The slower but acceptable method of culturing followed by sugar and alcohol assimilation testing can be done in most diagnostic laboratories.

PATHOLOGIC FINDINGS

Dog

Protothecosis occurs predominantly as a disseminated disease producing lesions in a

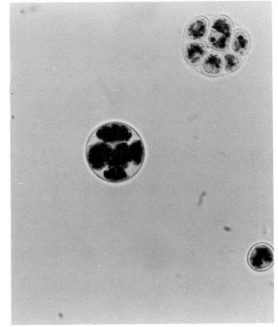

Figure 75–5. Sporulating and nonsporulating forms of *P. zopfii* isolated from canine CSF (Gram's iodine stain; × 1000). (From Tyler DE, et al: *J Am Vet Med Assoc* 176:987–993, 1980. Reprinted with permission.)

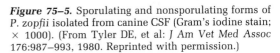

wide variety of tissues. Lesions in parenchymatous organs and on serosal surfaces are diffusely scattered throughout the tissue and are seen as white to tan granular foci measuring 0.5 to 2 mm in diameter or streaks measuring 0.5 × 2 to 3 mm in length. This pattern is especially seen in the myocardium, skeletal muscle, intestinal muscularis, lymph nodes, thyroid, liver, and loose connective tissues.[12] In the kidney, lesions tend to be larger, often measuring up to several centimeters in size, and are surrounded by a peripheral ring of hemorrhage. They also have a radiating linear pattern and may appear in either the cortex or medulla. Gross lesions have been reported throughout the intestinal tract, but the colon is most commonly affected. The lesions in the mucosa may vary from diffuse reddening to marked nodular thickening with scattered ulcerations, which are often hemorrhagic. Tiny white foci, as just described, are frequently seen in the muscularis and serosa. Gross sectioning of the eye reveals a gray-white cloudy exudate, often with red streaks in one or both chambers and beneath the retina, which is detached.

Microscopically, a variety of host reactions may be seen. Usually, there is little evidence of necrosis and only a minimal mixed inflammatory cell infiltration at the periphery of *Prototheca* cell clusters. The infiltrate consists mostly of macrophages, lymphocytes, neutrophils, and plasma cells, which may be present in inordinately large numbers. Infrequently, the inflammatory reaction is more pronounced and may be granulomatous or pyogranulomatous. In such lesions many *Prototheca* cells are contained within macrophages and multinucleate giant cells. Hemorrhage and necrosis more commonly are seen in the kidneys, heart, and intestines.

In the colon, lesions consist of masses of organisms often arranged in cords or nodules, replacing most of the mucosa and extending into and filling the submucosa (Fig. 75–6). Small focal colonies of organisms are seen throughout the muscularis and serosa. Inflammatory cell response is mixed but usually is minimal. Focal ulcerations of the mucosal surface and hemorrhage are frequently encountered. When there has been a history of prolonged diarrhea, granulation tissue may be seen intermingled with organisms in the mucosa and submucosa (Fig. 75–6). Fibrous connective tissue proliferation in

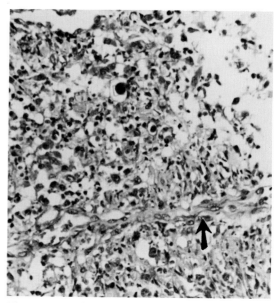

Figure 75–6. The mucosa of the colon from a dog has been replaced by masses of *Prototheca* cells. Only a few mixed mononuclear inflammatory cells are scattered throughout the lesion. A wisp of granulation tissue is seen at the arrow (H and E; × 100).

colonic lesions is probably an indication of a longer-standing infection and suggests that the colon was the likely site of entry for the *Prototheca*.

In the kidney, multiple focal aggregates of *Prototheca* cells are seen in the interstitium of the cortex, medulla, and occasionally the papillae. Minimal to marked necrosis and inflammatory cell infiltrate occur at the periphery of the organism cluster. The cellular infiltrate consists of plasma cells (which often predominate), lymphocytes, macrophages, and occasionally granulocytes.

Lesions in the brain and spinal cord usually occur as widely scattered, small foci of necrosis with an infiltration of mixed inflammatory cells. Numbers of *Prototheca* cells in these foci vary from none to large aggregates. Similar findings may be present in the inner ear.

Focal to diffuse granulomatous chorioretinitis with retinal detachment and severe retinal degeneration are the most common ocular lesions seen microscopically. Masses of organisms are seen within the vitreous and between the retina and choroid; lesser numbers occur focally in the choroid. The inflammatory infiltrate is mixed and may be pyogranulomatous.

In cutaneous lesions, masses of *Prototheca* occur in the dermis, subcutis, and subjacent skeletal muscles. The epidermis has zones

Table 75–1. Proposed Drug Therapy for Prototothecosis[a]

DRUG	SPECIES	DOSE[b] (mg/kg)	ROUTE	INTERVAL (hours)	DURATION (days)
Amphotericin B	D	0.25–0.5	IV	3 times weekly	[c]
and	C	0.25	IV	3 times weekly	[d]
Tetracycline	B	22	PO	8	[e]
Ketoconazole[f]	B	10–15	PO	12	28–42
Itraconazole[f]	B	10	PO	12	28–42
Clotrimazole	B		Topical		

[a]Although these regimens have been used to treat people and experimental animals, none has yet been extensively used in treating affected dogs and cats; see text. D = dog, C = cat, B = dog and cat, IV = intravenous, PO = oral.
[b]Dose per administration at specified interval, expressed as mg/kg unless otherwise stated.
[c]Until cumulative dose = 8 mg/kg.
[d]Until cumulative dose = 4 mg/kg.
[e]Continued while receiving amphotericin B.
[f]Effective against *P. wickerhamii* but not against *P. zopfii*.

of hyperkeratosis, ulceration, atrophy, and the typical inflammatory cell response. Ulcerated surfaces are necrotic and secondarily infected with bacteria. Where cutaneous lesions extend into the nasal mucosa, necrosis, ulceration, hemorrhage, and infiltration of neutrophils and plasma cells mixed with large masses of proliferating *Prototheca* are seen.[13] Regional lymph nodes commonly are invaded secondarily.

Cat

Localized cutaneous lesions in cats are gray-white subcutaneous or dermal masses of variable consistency that extend deeply into the underlying tissue and intermesh with tendons, nerves, and blood vessels. Histologically, they are granulomas characterized by densely packed epithelioid cells and sparse multinucleated giant cells. Neutrophils and plasma cells may be prominent in some lesions. Masses of *Prototheca* in all stages of reproduction constitute the bulk of the lesion.

THERAPY

Since protothecosis usually occurs as a single focal cutaneous lesion in people and cats, excision has been successful and the preferred therapeutic approach. A variety of antimicrobials has been tried therapeutically in infected people and animals; however, in most instances, treatment has failed. These have included systemic administration of various antibacterial drugs, amphotericin B, griseofulvin, potassium iodide, and pentam-idine isothionate and topical applications of antibiotics, copper sulfate, amphotericin B lotion, gentian violet, brilliant green, and chlorinated lime. However, in the treatment of the only reported human case of disseminated protothecosis, amphotericin B and transfer factor were used successfully.[14] Treatment of human cutaneous protothecosis with amphotericin B alone has been successful. In vitro studies have shown a synergistic effect between amphotericin B and tetracycline in growth inhibition of *P. wickerhamii*. There has been a report of successful treatment of human cutaneous protothecosis with amphotericin B and tetracycline.[15] See Table 75–1 for appropriate dosages.

Successful treatment of a wrist wound infected with *P. wickerhamii* in a human by use of orally administered ketoconazole has been reported.[16] Hepatoxicity, which developed in response to the treatment, spontaneously resolved after cessation of the therapy. Ketoconazole was effective in causing regression of multifocal cutaneous abscesses caused by infection with *Prototheca* sp. in a dog.[16a] Treatment was continued for 4 months. Although long-term follow-up is not available, the organism showed marked in vitro susceptibility to ketoconazole.

Amphotericin B was not effective in the treatment of ocular protothecosis (*P. zopfii*) in a dog.[17] Initial treatment reduced the lesion in the eye and blood culture results became negative, but due to development of renal toxicity the therapy was discontinued. Subsequently, lower doses failed to stop the progression of the lesions. In the same dog simazine, an algicidal drug used to clean fish tanks, gentamicin, and ketoconazole also were tried without success. In vitro, clotrimazole has no activity against *P. zopfii* but is highly efficacious against *P. wickerhamii*.[10] Since *P. zopfii* is the most common species infecting dogs, clotrimazole probably might not be of value in treating canine protothecosis. On the other hand, since cutaneous protothecosis in both dogs and cats is caused by *P. wickerhamii*, topically applied clotrimazole might be the drug of choice for this form of protothecosis.

Ribostamycin, an aminoglycoside antibiotic, closely related to kanamycin, is an effective in vitro agent against all species of *Prototheca*, especially *P. zopfii*.[18] Although not commercially available, ribostamycin was used on an experimental basis to treat a dog with chorioretinitis as the primary manifestation of the disease caused by *P. zopfii*.[19] The drug was administered at a dose of 12.5 mg/kg given IM twice daily. Ocular manifestations improved but later the dog died with disseminated lesions.

References

1. Pore RS, Barnett EA, Barnes WC, et al: *Prototheca* ecology. Mycopathologia 81:49–69, 1983.
2. Rakich PM, Latimer KS: Altered immune function in a dog with disseminated protothecosis. *J Am Vet Med Assoc* 185:681–683, 1984.
3. Merideth RE, Givin RM, Samuelson DA, et al: Systemic protothecosis with ocular manifestations in a dog. *J Am Anim Hosp Assoc* 20:153–156, 1984.
4. Coloe PJ, Allison JF: Protothecosis in a cat. *J Am Vet Med Assoc* 180:78–79, 1982.
5. Finnie JW, Coloe PJ: Cutaneous protothecosis in a cat. *Aust Vet J* 57:307–308, 1981.
6. Kaplan W, Chandler FW, Holzinger EA, et al: Protothecosis in a cat: first recorded case. *Sabouraudia* 14:281–286, 1979.
7. Dillberger JE, Homer B, Daubert D, et al: Protothecosis in two cats. *J Am Vet Med Assoc* 192:1557–1559, 1988.
8. Tyler DE, Lorenz MD, Blue JL, et al: Disseminated protothecosis with central nervous involvement in a dog. *J Am Vet Med Assoc* 176:987–993, 1980.
9. Casal M, Gutierrez J: Simple new test for presumptive differentiation between genus *Candida* and genus *Prototheca*. Mycopathologia 94:3–5, 1986.
10. Casal M, Guteirrez J: Simple new test for rapid differentiation of *Prototheca zopfii*. *J Clin Microbiol* 18:992–1003, 1983.
11. Chandler FW, Kaplan W, Libero A: *Histopathology of Mycotic Diseases: A Color Atlas and Text.* Chicago, Year Book Medical Publishers, 1980, pp 96–100.
12. Cook JR, Tyler DE, Coulter DB, et al: Disseminated protothecosis causing acute blindness and deafness in a dog. *J Am Vet Med Assoc* 184:1266–1272, 1984.
13. Sudman MS, Majika JA, Kaplan W: Primary mucocutaneous protothecosis in a dog. *J Am Vet Med Assoc* 163:1372–1374, 1973.
14. Cox EG, Wilson JD, Brown P: Protothecosis: a case of disseminated algal infection. *Lancet* 2:379–382, 1974.
15. Venezio FR, Lavoo E, Williams JE, et al: Progressive protothecosis. *Am J Clin Pathol* 77:485–493, 1982.
16. Pegram SP, Kerns FT, Wasilauskas BL, et al: Successful ketoconazole treatment of protothecosis with ketoconazole hepatotoxicity. *Arch Intern Med* 143:1802–1805, 1983.
16a. Macartney L, Rycroft AN, Hammil J: Cutaneous protothecosis in the dog: first confirmed case in Britain. *Vet Rec* 123:494–496, 1988.
17. Moore FM, Schmidt GM, Desai D, et al: Unsuccessful treatment of disseminated protothecosis in a dog. *J Am Vet Med Assoc* 186:705–708, 1985.
18. Casal M, Gutierrez J: In vitro activity of ribostamycin against *Prototheca* sp. *Mycopathologia* 83:21–23, 1983.
19. Scagliotti RH: Personal communication. Sacramento, CA, 1989.

PROTOZOAL AND OTHER INFECTIONS

SECTION V

76 LABORATORY DIAGNOSIS OF PROTOZOAL INFECTIONS

Michael R. Lappin
Janet P. Calpin
Annie K. Prestwood

Successful diagnosis of a protozoal infection is dependent on the careful choice of diagnostic procedures. For example, saturated sodium nitrate fecal flotation is not useful for many enteric protozoal infections because the specific gravity of most protozoal cysts is greater than that of the flotation solution. Trophozoites, on the other hand, are killed by the sodium nitrate solution. Furthermore, accurate diagnosis of a protozoal infection, whether it is caused by an enteric, a systemic, or a blood-borne organism, also depends on the proper collection and preservation of the clinical sample. Radiographic techniques involving barium sulfate many hinder detection of intestinal protozoa for a week or more.[1] Antibiotics and other medications also may affect the recovery of protozoa from stool and blood samples. Also, many enteric organisms are shed intermittently, requiring examination of multiple samples.

The reader is referred to Appendix 12 for formulas and detailed procedures for the diagnostic tests described in this chapter that can easily be performed in the veterinary office. More sophisticated diagnostic laboratory techniques are discussed briefly; however, only the collection and preservation of the clinical sample to be sent to specialized testing laboratories are emphasized.

FECES

Sample Collection and Storage

About 50 g of fresh feces should be collected and placed in a clean, dry container that is sealed with a tight-fitting lid. The sample should be free of contaminants such as urine and litter. If blood or mucus is present in the stool, it should be included in the sample.

Microscopic examination of the sample should be done as soon as possible, especially if the feces is diarrheic. Diarrheic stool samples should be maintained at room temperature and examined within 30 minutes of collection because they may contain fragile trophozoite stages of the infectious agent, which cannot survive refrigeration. If immediate examination is impossible, the sample should be mixed with a preservative (see Preservation of Feces). Formed stools, which do not usually contain trophozoites, should be refrigerated if there is any delay in examination. If the container is tightly sealed to prevent desiccation, the sample may be usable for up to 1 week.

Examination of Feces

Table 76–1 lists the recommended microscopic procedures for the diagnosis of GI protozoal infections.

Direct Smear. The direct smear technique is usually reserved for diarrheic samples or for examination of mucus in the sample. The substage condenser of the microscope must be adjusted to maximum contrast, as the unstained organisms appear transparent. When available, the use of phase-contrast or darkfield microscopy may aid in the demonstration of motile trophozoites.

Table 76–1. Recommended Procedures for the Diagnosis of Gastrointestinal Protozoans of the Dog and Cat

ORGANISM	STAGE	PROCEDURE
Entamoeba histolytica	Trophozoites	Direct smear
	Cysts	Direct smear
Giardia	Trophozoites	Direct smear
	Cysts	Zinc sulfate centrigutation flotation technique or formalin-ether sedimentation
Pentatrichomonas	Trophozoites	Direct smear
Balantidium coli	Trophozoites	Direct smear
	Cysts	Zinc sulfate centrifugation flotation technique
Coccidia (Toxoplasma, Isospora, Sarcocystis, Hammondia, Besnoitia, and Cryptosporidium)	Oocysts	Sheather's sugar centrifugation flotation technique

Fresh Saline Smear. The saline smear is made by placing a drop of physiologic saline on a clean microscope slide. The amount of feces that adheres to the end of an applicator stick is mixed evenly with the saline so that the smear is thin. A coverslip is applied, and the slide is systematically scanned using low power (10× objective). It may be necessary to warm the smear to enhance the motility of *Entamoeba histolytica*. Motility and structural features of protozoa are best examined using the high-dry objective (40 or 43×). Generally, use of the oil immersion objective is not recommended for examining fresh wet mounts. After motility has been observed, stain may be added to the saline smear to aid in the specific identification of the organism.

Stained Smear. Adding stain to the wet mount through the edge of the coverslip will aid in visualizing internal structures of protozoa. Because staining the preparation kills the organism, the examination for motility must be done first. Table 76–2 describes the appearance of trophozoites found on direct smears from dogs and cats.

Iodine stains have traditionally been used to reveal the internal structural detail of protozoans. Lugol's solution is the most popular (Appendix 12). When used correctly, iodine stains the cytoplasm of cysts yellow-gold, whereas the nuclei are paler and refractile. Methylene blue in acetate buffer (pH 3.6) has been used to stain trophozoite stages, especially those of *E. histolytica*.[1] An aqueous solution of eosin will stain fecal debris bright red, but trophozoites and cysts will remain colorless. Acid methyl green is recommended for staining the macronucleus of *Balantidium coli* (see Appendix 12).[2]

Fecal Flotation. Fecal concentration methods are employed to confirm the presence of protozoal cysts or oocysts. Protozoal cysts are more frequently found in formed stools, whereas coccidian oocysts, especially *Cryptosporidium*, are more frequently found in diarrheic feces. The following techniques are described in Appendix 12.

Sheather's sugar centrifugation technique is recommended as a routine diagnostic procedure for intestinal parasites that can be performed in the veterinary clinic. The solution is inexpensive, and the technique is effective in revealing *Toxoplasma*, *Cryptosporidium*, and other coccidia. The hypertonicity of the solution will distort the cysts of *Giardia*; however, the distortion itself may be diagnostic. Most *Giardia* cysts are oval, and the cytoplasm is pulled to one side so that a half- or quarter-moon is presented.

The **zinc sulfate centrifugation technique** reveals protozoal and helminthic parasites in feces. Although it causes some distortion of protozoans, it distorts *Giardia* cysts less than the sugar solution. For this reason, zinc sulfate should be used to verify the identity of *Giardia*-like cysts revealed by sugar flotation. *Giardia* cysts also take up iodine, which helps distinguish them from coccidian oocysts which do not stain.

Fecal sedimentation will recover protozoal and helminthic parasites present in the feces; however, the resultant sample will also contain debris. The formalin-ether and formalin-ethyl acetate sedimentation techniques are recommended for concentrating *Giardia* cysts. The sedimentation procedure is similar for the two techniques; the only difference is whether ethyl acetate or ether is used. Although ether is extremely flammable and explosive, it is especially effec-

Table 76–2. Protozoal Trophozoite Identification by Direct Fecal Smear

ORGANISM	SIZE (μm)	DISTINGUISHING MORPHOLOGY	
		Fresh Smear	Stained Smear
Entamoeba histolytica	12–50	Constantly changes shape when active; moves by means of finger-like projections of cytoplasm; one nucleus that is difficult to see; may contain erythrocytes	Nucleus usually has evenly distributed peripheral chromatin and centrally located, compact karyosome
Giardia	9–21 × 5–15 × 2–4	Bilaterally symmetric; pear-shaped on dorsoventral view; crescentic on lateral view; rolling movement by means of flagella; contains two nuclei	Two large nuclei, each with prominent karyosomes and axonemes and median bodies, give monkey-faced appearance
Pentatrichomonas	5–20 × 3–14	Oval to pear-shaped; wobbly, jerky, rapid movement by means of flagella; undulating membrane visible	Oval nucleus in anterior half of body; axostyle protruding from posterior end
Balantidium coli	50–150	Oval shape; revolving movement by means of cilia; macronucleus may be visible	Large kidney bean-shaped macronucleus is prominent; occasionally micronucleus may be seen

tive in concentrating cysts from stools that have a high fat content.[3]

Preservation of Feces

If there is a delay in examining a fecal sample for protozoa or if the sample is to be sent to a diagnostic laboratory for further analysis, a preservative must be added to it. It is important that the fecal sample be broken up and thoroughly mixed with the preservative prior to shipment to the laboratory. Procedures discussed below are described in detail in Appendix 12.

Polyvinyl Alcohol Preservation. The greatest advantage of the polyvinyl alcohol (PVA) technique is that permanent-stained slides may be made at a later date from a stool sample that has been fixed in PVA. Another advantage is that the formalin-ether sedimentation technique can be performed on PVA-fixed specimens. The fixative remains stable for years; however, it contains mercury, and care must be exercised in handling and storing the solution. PVA can be used to fix large volumes of feces or individual smears on microscope slides.

Merthiolate-Iodine-Formalin Preservation. The merthiolate-iodine-formalin (MIF) preservation procedure has the advantage of both preserving the sample and staining any protozoans that may be present. This technique involves mixing two stock solutions immediately before use. The Lugol's solution (iodine) used can also be used to stain direct smears (see Direct Smears). The disadvantages of this method are that the iodine solution does not have a long shelf life and that permanent-stained slides cannot be made from MIF-preserved material.

10% Formalin Preservation. This technique is effective in preserving protozoal cysts; however, it is not recommended for trophozoites. Several grams of feces are mixed with 10% formalin that has been warmed to 60°C. As with the MIF procedure, the major disadvantage is that permanent-stained smears cannot be prepared from formalin-fixed specimens.

Permanent Staining of Fecal Smears. Frequently, positive identification of intestinal protozoa can be made only by specialized laboratories using a permanent-staining method. Samples that have been fixed in PVA can be submitted to a diagnostic laboratory, where trichrome or iron-hematoxylin stains can be used. See Appendix 8 for a listing of diagnostic laboratories that perform these tests.

BLOOD

Collection

Films to be used for the diagnosis of blood-borne protozoal infections may be made from either fresh blood or blood that has been collected into EDTA. Care should be taken in handling the sample since hemolysis of the erythrocytes and destruction of the parasites will hinder positive identification. If fresh blood is used, the film must be made before the blood clots. Some blood-borne protozoans, especially *Babesia*, are more readily demonstrated if blood from microcapillary beds (i.e., ear margin, toenail) is used to make films. Table 76–3 lists the protozoans that may be seen on blood films or tissue smears.

Preparation of Blood Films

When diagnostic blood films are made, the microscope slide must be completely clean. If slides are to be sent to a diagnostic laboratory for protozoal identification, both thick and thin films (*at least* two of each) should be prepared.

Thick Films. A larger amount of blood is examined with a thick film, thereby increasing the chances of detecting parasites, especially when the parasitemia is mild. However, organisms may be distorted in thick films, so thin films should be made for proper identification.

Two to three small drops of blood are placed on a clean microscope slide and spread in a circular motion over a 2-cm area with the corner of another slide. When fresh blood is used, it should be stirred on the slide for 30 seconds to prevent formation of fibrin strands. If EDTA-anticoagulated blood is used, additional stirring is unnecessary. The film should be air dried at room temperature with the slide kept on a flat surface. The choice of stain will determine whether the film will have to be laked, i.e., immersed in distilled water to rupture and remove the erythrocytes (see Staining Blood Films). Thick films to be stored for later examination or shipped to a diagnostic laboratory should be laked. Films should be stored in a cool (27°C), dry, clean place.

Thin Films. A small drop of blood is placed at one end of a clean microscope slide. The short edge of another clean slide (the spreader slide) is placed in the middle of the slide at a 30 degree angle and pulled back toward the blood. The blood is allowed to spread along the width of the spreader slide; then, in a fairly rapid, even motion, the spreader slide is *pushed* across the length of the slide, dragging the blood along. The blood should not be pushed across the slide, as this will rupture many cells and parasites. The blood film should be air dried at room temperature. As with thick films, the staining method will determine the need for prior fixation (see Staining Blood Films). If the films are not stained within 48 hours, they should be fixed in 100% methyl alcohol (methanol). Slides should be stored as for thick films.

Table 76–3. Practical Techniques for the Diagnosis of Blood-Borne and Systemic Protozoal Infections[a]

ORGANISM	BLOOD FILMS	ASPIRATE IMPRESSIONS	TISSUE IMPRESSIONS
Toxoplasma	+[b]	+	+
Neospora	?	+	+
Trypanosoma	+	+	+
Leishmania	−	+	+
Hepatozoon	+	−	+
Encephalitozoon	−	+[c]	−
Cytauxzoon	+	−	+
Babesia	+	−	−
Entamoeba histolytica	−	+	−
Pneumocystis	−	+	+

[a]+ = useful or indicated; − = not used; ? = uncertain.
[b]Rare.
[c]May give negative results in seropositive animals.

Staining Blood Films

Both Giemsa stain and Wright's stain are available commercially in ready-to-use form. The choice of stain is a matter of personal preference. Generally, however, Giemsa stain is used for differentiation of blood protozoans and Wright's stain is used for differential leukocyte counts.

When treated properly with Giemsa stain, erythrocytes should be pale gray-blue; leukocyte cytoplasm should stain blue, and the nucleus should be purple; eosinophilic granules should be a bright pink, and neutrophilic granules should stain a deep blue, whereas the nucleus should be red. Giemsa stain is a permanent stain, and slides can be kept for years when properly stored.

With Wright's stain, erythrocytes are light tan; the nuclei of leukocytes are bright blue, and the cytoplasm is lighter; eosinophilic granules are red, and neutrophilic granules are pink. Protozoal cytoplasm stains a light blue, whereas the nucleus is a deeper blue. Wright's stain has a tendency to fade with time.

Examination of Blood Films

Thin blood films can be examined with or without coverslips. If a coverslip is used, only the number 1 size is thin enough to allow proper focusing with a microscope. A neutral mounting medium should be used to prevent the stain from bleaching. Use of mounting medium will also aid in viewing the cells with low and high-dry objectives and will prevent the coverslip from moving when the oil immersion objective is used. If the thin film is not coverslipped, a small drop of oil may be placed on the slide and thinly spread over the blood film. This procedure eliminates the diffraction of light around blood cells during scanning with the low and high-dry objectives. After scanning, another drop of oil should be added, and with the oil immersion objective the film should be systematically examined for blood parasites, which usually are located and best visualized at the feathered end and edges of the film.

Thick films may be examined with or without coverslips. After the microscope is focused and the slide scanned with low power, oil may be applied and the film examined for parasites.

ASPIRATES, TISSUE IMPRESSIONS, AND BIOPSY SPECIMENS

Aspirates

Fine-needle aspirates from lymph nodes, spleen, liver, bone marrow, and CSF are used to detect systemic protozoa and should be examined immediately using the direct smear technique to reveal motile protozoa that may be present (Table 76–3). If aspirated material is compressed between two slides, the impression that results when the slides are pulled apart can be stained and examined for the internal morphology of protozoa. Alternatively, a small amount of aspirated material is placed on a microscope slide and then spread by repeatedly passing the tip of a 22-gauge needle through the material, drawing it along the slide. This technique may lessen the destruction of cells. If bronchial washings are obtained by transtracheal aspiration biopsy (transtracheal wash) or bronchoscopy to aid in the diagnosis of *Toxoplasma* or *Pneumocystis* pneumonia, the aspirate should be concentrated by centrifugation at 2000 × g for 5 minutes before making impressions or smears. The procedure for staining aspirate impressions is identical to that for staining thin blood films (see Staining Blood Films).

Tissue Impressions

A tissue impression should be made from any biopsy material. The cut edge of the tissue should be blotted on a paper towel to remove the excess blood, and then the specimen should be touched to a clean microscope slide. The resulting impression is one cell layer thick and, when stained, should reveal parasitized cells (see Table 76–3). The staining procedure is the same as for thin blood films (see Staining Blood Films).

Biopsy Specimens

If possible, a biopsy specimen should be examined as a fresh preparation (using frozen sectioning and staining) so that a rapid diagnosis can be made. However, the accessibility of the diagnostic laboratory will influence the usefulness of this technique. If there will be a delay in the examination of biopsy material, it should be preserved in 10% buffered formalin; then, on arrival at the diagnostic laboratory, the tissue can be handled as for routine histologic processing.

CULTURE, ANIMAL INOCULATION, XENODIAGNOSIS, AND OOCYST SPORULATION

Because these tests require fresh (unpreserved) specimens, the diagnostic laboratory should be contacted before the sample is shipped. The sample should be sent by the most rapid means available.

Culture

Often, protozoa are suspected as the disease agent but are not detectable on routine laboratory tests because they are so few in number. If blood, aspirate, or tissue is inoculated into a medium that will enhance the growth of protozoa, the chances of isolating the organism are improved. It may require 5 days or longer to obtain results. Specific media have been developed that will support the growth of *E. histolytica*, *B. coli*, *Pentatrichomonas*, *Trypanosoma*, and *Leishmania*.

Animal Inoculation

Material that has been collected under sterile conditions may be inoculated orally, intraperitoneally, or IV into a susceptible recipient animal. It may be necessary to sporulate coccidial oocysts to the infectious stage prior to animal inoculation (see Oocyst Sporulation). If tissue is being used, cysts may be concentrated by density centrifugation after tissue digestion. Months may be required for infection to develop. Because of the space and expense required to maintain inoculated animals, this diagnostic tool has limited use.

Xenodiagnosis

Xenodiagnosis utilizes a laboratory-reared, parasite-free arthropod vector of the

disease in question. The vector is allowed to feed on a suspected infected host. Following feeding, the vector must be maintained until the parasite has had sufficient time to develop (which may be 6 weeks). Then it is examined for the parasitic stage of the organism. Historically, xenodiagnosis has been used in the detection of trypanosomiasis.

Oocyst Sporulation

If it should be necessary to submit feces to a laboratory for coccidial identification, a simple procedure will enhance oocyst sporulation. The stool is mixed with 2.5% potassium dichromate and strained through cheesecloth to remove large debris. The suspension is sporulated at room temperature in an open container, but the dichromate solution should not be allowed to decrease in volume. Sporulation takes 3 to 5 days or longer, after which the specimen should be refrigerated until identification is completed. Sporulated oocysts of *Toxoplasma* are highly infectious; therefore, great caution should be used during sporulation and subsequent handling of this material. If *Toxoplasma* is suspected, the diagnostic laboratory should be contacted *before* sporulation for instructions regarding shipment of material, as it is *not* recommended that infectious material be sent via parcel post.

IMMUNODIAGNOSTIC PROCEDURES

A number of different immunologic procedures have been developed to aid in the diagnosis of protozoal infections. Techniques using serum, feces, and tissue have been assessed. Some tests have limited commercial availability or are performed only at research institutions. The reader is referred to the chapters on specific protozoal diseases and Appendix 8 for discussion of specific tests and listing of the commercial, state, and federal laboratories that run them.

Serologic Testing

Serodiagnosis of protozoal diseases involves the testing of serum for the presence of either antibodies against the parasite or antigens of the parasite. Parasite-specific serum antibody testing has been used as a diagnostic aid in most blood-borne and systemic protozoal diseases. The major advantages of antibody testing include ease of sample collection, inexpense of most procedures, and wide availability of most assays. IgG-class antibody responses have been studied most extensively. Unfortunately, IgG develops to detectable levels well after clinical disease has begun and then remains elevated for months to years with most protozoal infections. Diagnosis of recent or active infection using IgG measurement necessitates demonstration of a fourfold rising titer.

Preliminary work with parasite-specific IgM-class antibody response to *Toxoplasma gondii* infection indicates that the presence of this antibody in a single serum sample may correlate with active infection (see Chapter 86). The major problem associated with measurement of either antibody class is correlation of results with clinical illness. Also, sensitivity and specificity vary with different assays. If immunosuppression is present concurrently with protozoal infection, parasite-specific antibody responses may be diminished.

The detection of parasite-specific circulating serum antigens has been used in the diagnosis of pneumocystosis and toxoplasmosis. Antigen detection can be beneficial for the diagnosis of protozoal infection, especially in cases with concurrent immunosuppression and poor specific antibody production. Problems include the presence of antigen in clinically normal individuals and the potential presence of cross-reactive antigens.

Blood should be collected for serum antibody or antigen tests as described earlier in this chapter except that blood is dispensed into a clean tube that does not contain an anticoagulant. It should be processed to prevent hemolysis. Separated serum samples may be frozen prior to testing. Thawing during shipment to a diagnostic laboratory should not affect the outcome of antibody or antigen testing as long as bacterial growth is minimized. Sodium azide should be added to the tube if transport will take more than a few days.

Feces

The use of immunodiagnostic procedures such as ELISA to detect parasite antigens in feces has been studied in some enteric protozoal infections. Primary problems have been associated with sensitivity and specificity of individual assays, leading to both false-positive and false-negative reactions.

Tissue

Special immunofluorescent or immunoperoxidase staining techniques can be performed at some diagnostic and research laboratories. These procedures can aid in the specific identification of tissue forms of protozoans.

References

1. Garcia LS, Ash LR: *Diagnostic Parasitology Clinical Laboratory Manual*, ed 2. St. Louis, CV Mosby, 1979.
2. Adam KMG, Paul J, Zaman V: *Medical and Veterinary Protozoology*. London, Churchill Livingstone, 1971.
3. Traunt AL, Elliot SH, Kelly MT, et al: Comparison of formalin-ethyl ether sedimentation, formalin-ethyl acetate sedimentation, and zinc sulfate flotation techniques for detection of intestinal parasites. *J Clin Microbiol* 13:882–884, 1981.

77

ANTIPROTOZOAL CHEMOTHERAPY

Craig E. Greene

Table 77–1 summarizes the properties of antiprotozoal drugs. Respective Chapters 78 to 89 should be consulted for the chemotherapy of specific diseases. Dosages are summarized in Table 77–2 and Appendix 14.

AZO-NAPHTHALENE DRUGS

Trypan blue was one of the first compounds used to treat babesiosis. Because local irritation and abscesses develop following SC injection, it is administered IV. Trypan blue does not completely eliminate *Babesia*, but rather infected animals recover from illness and remain in a state of premunition. They must be treated with aromatic diamidines within 1 month to effect a cure. A disadvantage of trypan blue is that it stains all body tissues and secretions for several weeks.

ACRIDINE DYES

Quinacrine, developed as a human antimalarial drug, is now commonly used in dogs as a alternative treatment for giardiasis. It becomes incorporated into the DNA of the organism and inhibits nucleic acid synthesis. Evidence of toxicity includes vomiting, fever, pruritus, neurologic signs, yellow discoloration of urine or tissues, and hepatic dysfunction.

QUINOLINE DERIVATIVES

Quinuronium sulfate is a relatively effective babesiacide that has been used to treat infections in a number of species. This drug has marked parasympathomimetic effects, inhibits cholinesterase, and stimulates histamine release. Any of these actions may produce toxic side effects. Salivation, nausea, vomiting, dyspnea, cyanosis, and death have been noted. Quinuronium sulfate has had limited use in recent years.

Primaquine and moxipraquine are antimalarial 8-aminoquinolines that have efficacy against *Trypanosoma* and *Leishmania*.

Diiodohydroxyquin and iodochlorhydroxyquin are halogenated oxyquinolines that are discussed more thoroughly with the topical antifungal drugs (see Chapter 63). They are also amebicidal when administered orally. They are not absorbed and have a relatively low toxicity. Signs of toxicity are abdominal pain, diarrhea, and neurologic signs, all of which have been reported in dogs.

AROMATIC DIAMIDINES

Phenamidine, pentamidine, diminazene, amicarbalide, and imidocarb, which are diamidine derivatives, are the drugs of choice for treatment of *Babesia* infections of dogs and cats, and they are effective against other organisms (Table 77–1). Usually administered IM or SC, they act by interfering with nucleic acid metabolism. The free drug is combined as a salt to reduce irritating effects that occur following parenteral administration. The diamidines are rapidly effective and usually reverse clinical signs and parasitemia within 24 hours of administration. They do not completely eradicate the organisms but have a residual effect following a single injection. Drugs such as pentamidine are excreted unchanged and are avidly concentrated in organs such as the liver and brain.[1] Use of subtherapeutic dosages is not

Table 77–1. Properties of Antiprotozoal Drugs

GENERIC NAME (TRADE NAME)	SUSCEPTIBLE ORGANISMS FIRST (SECOND) CHOICE
Azo-Naphthalene Dyes	
Trypan blue	None *(Babesia)*
Acridine Dyes	
Quinacrine hydrochloride (Atabrine, Keybrin)	None *(Giardia)*
Quinoline Derivatives	
Quinuronium sulfate (Acaprin, Ludobal)	None *(Babesia)*
Diiodohydroxyquin [iodoquinol] (Diodoquin, Yodoxin)	*Balantidium (Entamoeba)*
Iodochlorhydroxyquin [clioquinol] (Cliquinol, Vioform)	*Balantidium (Entamoeba)*
Aromatic Diamidines	
Pentamidine isethionate (Lomidine, Pentam, NebuPent)	*Babesia (Leishmania, Pneumocystis)*
Diminazene aceturate (Berenil, Ganaseg)	*Babesia* (none)
Imidocarb dipropionate (Imizol)	*Babesia (Ehrlichia)*
Amicarbalide (Diampiron)	*Ehrlichia* (none)
Nitroimidazoles	
Metronidazole (Flagyl, Stomorgyl[a])	*Giardia, Pentatrichomonas,*
Dimetridazole (Emtryl)	*Entamoeba, Balantidium*
Tinidazole (Fasigyn)	*(Babesia)*
Ionophores	
Monensin (Rumensin, Coban)	*Coccidia (Toxoplasma)*
Lasalocid (Bovatec)	*Coccidia* (none)
Salinomycin (Bio-cox)	*Coccidia* (none)
Antimonials	
Sodium stibogluconate (Pentostam)	*Leishmania* (none)
Meglumine antimonate (Glucantime)	*Leishmania* (none)
Antibacterials	
Paromomycin (Humatin)	None *(Entamoeba)*
Furazolidone (Furoxone)	*Coccidia (Giardia)*
Nifurtimox (Lampit)	None *(Trypanosoma)*
Tetracycline (many)	*Balantidium* (none)
Trimethoprim-sulfonamide (Tribrissen, Ditrim, Bactrim, Septra)	*Pneumocystis,* coccidia (none)
Pyrimethamine (Daraprim)	*Toxoplasma* (none)
Spiramycin (Rovamycin, Stomorgyl[a])	*Cryptosporidium (Toxoplasma)*
Clindamycin (Antirobe, Cleocin)	*Toxoplasma (Babesia)*
Miscellaneous	
Thiacetarsamide sodium (Caparsolate)	*Haemobartonella* (none)
Bismuth-N-glycollylarsanilate (Milibis-V)	None *(Entamoeba, Giardia)*
Amprolium (Amprol, Corid)	None (coccidia)
Amphotericin B (Fungizone)	*Acanthamoeba (Leishmania)*
Toltrazuril	*Coccidia (Toxoplasma)*

[a]Combination of 125 mg metronidazole and 174 mg spiramycin per tablet.

advised because organisms will develop resistance to these drugs. The slow metabolism and elimination of the diamidines contribute to their prophylactic effects.

Toxic effects of phenamidine and pentamidine include impairment of the circulatory system characterized by vasodilation and reduced blood pressure. Hypotension has been associated with IV and IM administration; however, its occurrence was reduced by infusing the drug IV over at least 60 minutes.[2] The drugs may cause local pain and swelling at the site of injection and systemic anaphylaxis, nausea, salivation, vomiting, and diarrhea. Pretreatment with antihistamines is advisable. Hypoglycemia, hypocalcemia, and hypokalemia are frequent biochemical alterations.[3] Because renal clearance of pentamidine accounts for such a small proportion of total body clearance, its elimination is unaffected by renal failure in dogs.[1] The drug, however, may produce azotemia as a side effect. To reduce systemic toxicity of the drug, pentamidine is available as a solution for aerosol administration (NebuPent, LyphoMed, Rosemont, IL) to treat people with pulmonary pneumocystosis.

To ensure its stability, diminazene should be kept refrigerated in sealed glass contain-

Table 77–2. Selected Drug Dosages for Antiprotozoal Chemotherapy[a]

GENERIC NAME	SPECIES	ROUTE	DOSE[b] (mg/kg)	INTERVAL (hours)	DURATION (days)
Trypan blue	D	IV	4	Once	NA
Quinacrine	D	PO	6–11	12	3[c]
Primaquine	B	PO, IM	0.5	Once	NA
Phenamidine	B	SC	15	24	2
Diminazene	B	IM	3.5	Once	NA
Imidocarb	D	IM	2–6	Once	NA
Metronidazole	B	PO	15	12	5[d]
Paromomycin	H	PO	10	8	3–5
Spiramycin	D	PO	8	12	6–10
	C	PO	10	12	6–10
Clindamycin	D	PO	5–20	12	7–10
	C	PO	25	12–24	7–10
Furazolidone	B	PO	8–10	12–24	7
Nifurtimox	H	PO	8–10	24	4 months
Tetracycline	B	PO	22	8	7
Trimethoprim-sulfonamide	D	PO	30–60	24	5
	C	PO	15–30	24	5
Pyrimethamine and sulfonamide	B	PO	0.5–1	24	7–14
	B	PO	60	24	7–14
Meglumine antimonate	D	IV, SC	100	24	21–28
Sodium stibogluconate	D	IV, SC	30–50	24	21–28
Toltrazuril	C	PO	10	24	4

[a]D = dog, B = dog and cat, H = human, C = cat, IV = intravenous, PO = oral, IM = intramuscular, SC = subcutaneous, NA = nonapplicable.

[b]Dose per administration at specified interval, expressed as mg/kg unless otherwise stated.

[c]Maximum dose is 50–100 mg per administration, not to exceed a total of 200 mg daily.

[d]Prolonged or higher dosages may result in CNS toxicity; see text.

ers and protected from light. Following a single injection, the drug accumulates in the liver, brain, and kidneys. It is not detoxified in the body but is gradually excreted in the urine. Acute anaphylaxis is less likely to occur with diminazene than has been observed when other drugs of this class are used. Like the other diamidines, diminazene may produce CNS signs, including behavioral changes, nystagmus, ataxia, extensor rigidity, and opisthotonus and death. Acute hemorrhagic gastroenteritis and cardiac muscle failure have been reported.

Imidocarb is a diamidine of the carbanilide series that has been shown to be safe for treatment and prophylaxis of babesiosis and ehrlichiosis in dogs. Some variation in species and strain susceptibility to the drug has been noted. The drug is slowly metabolized and excreted following a single IM injection and protects dogs from infection for up to 5 weeks. The less toxic dipropionate salt produces hypotension and signs similar to those of organophosphate intoxication when administered IV and occasionally IM, but this effect can be counteracted by prior administration of atropine. Hypersalivation and diarrhea have been the main side effects noted in dogs.[4]

Amicarbalide is a derivative that was developed for treatment of anaplasmosis. Its mechanism of action and side effects are similar to those of imidocarb, although its availability is limited.

NITROIMIDAZOLES

These drugs are effective in treating the anaerobic enteric protozoa that cause trichomoniasis, amebiasis, giardiasis, and balantidiasis. They affect both the intraintestinal and the invasive parasites. Anaerobic protozoa and bacteria contain highly efficient enzymes that reduce the nitrogroup after penetration of the antimicrobial drug into the cell. These drugs are less effective against microaerophilic or aerobic microorganisms. Metronidazole, tinidazole, nimorazole, dimetridazole, and ornidazole are close structural analogs marketed in various regions of the world. Metronidazole is the most widely used of these compounds. In addition to protozoa, it is active against obligate spore-forming anaerobes such as clostridia, some non-spore-forming anaerobes such as *Campylobacter fetus*, and microaerophilic organisms such as the Enterobacteriaceae.

Metronidazole is almost completely absorbed following oral administration. Food does not interfere with complete absorption but may delay the onset to peak serum concentration. To facilitate the medication of small cats, the standard 250-mg tablet can be ground and the appropriate dosage given.[5] The drug distributes widely and penetrates into body tissues, extracellular fluids, and even pus-filled cavities. It achieves good concentrations in the CNS even in the absence of inflammation. It is primarily eliminated by hepatic metabolism. IV administration of metronidazole is recommended in severely ill patients.

The drug diffuses into anaerobic microorganisms and converts to toxic free radicals, which damage the microbial cell through inhibition of DNA synthesis, leading to cell necrosis. Metronidazole has been used alone to treat stomatitis and in combination with aminoglycosides to treat mixed infections associated with bowel perforation and intraabdominal sepsis (see Chapter 9). In people, the drug is effective in the treatment of intraabdominal, pelvic, pleuropulmonary, CNS, and bone and joint infections. In a number of countries, metronidazole (125 mg) is marketed combined with spiramycin (174 mg) (Stomorgyl, Rhone Merieux, Lyon, France) for treatment of gram-positive and anaerobic infections such as stomatitis, abscesses, and genital and cutaneous infections.

Side effects of metronidazole include GI irritation with signs of vomiting and anorexia, glossitis, and stomatitis. Neurologic signs may be seen after 7 to 10 days of treatment with high (≥ 66 mg/kg/day) dosages and may be reversed when therapy is discontinued, but dogs have developed fatal encephalopathy, persistent seizures, or cerebellar and central vestibular ataxia. CSF abnormalities have included mild increases in protein concentration. Necropsy findings have shown degenerative changes in Purkinje's cells and associated cerebellar and vestibular axons in the brain.[6,7] Some dogs have improved gradually over several months. Long-term use of metronidazole may cause Candida overgrowth in the GI tract. The urine may be discolored a deep red-brown. Evidence of mutagenicity and carcinogenicity in laboratory rodents has generally restricted the use of this drug to adult humans.

IONOPHORES

These compounds form lipid-soluble complexes with cations, which facilitates the transport of these ions across biological membranes. They are antibiotics isolated from Streptomyces spp. and are used primarily as coccidiostats. Monensin, lasalocid, and salinomycin, the compounds of veterinary interest, cause accumulation of intracellular ions within the parasite, interfering with its metabolism. Their use has primarily been as growth promoters in food animal practice, although monensin has been used experimentally to reduce shedding of Toxoplasma oocysts by cats. The ionophores also have antibacterial spectra and have been used experimentally to treat endotoxic shock in dogs. Because of their stimulatory effects on cardiac contractility and myocardial perfusion, their toxicity may be increased by concurrent use of cardiac glycosides.

ANTIMONIALS

Sodium stibogluconate and meglumine antimonate are the primary therapeutic agents for the treatment of leishmaniasis. They are both pentavalent antimony compounds. The dosage used is based on the amount of antimony compound administered. Meglumine antimonate solutions usually contain 85 mg/ml, whereas sodium stibogluconate solutions usually contain pentavalent antimony at 100 mg/ml. Treatment with these drugs is not curative and two or three courses of therapy may be necessary. Side effects with either drug include anorexia, vomiting, nausea, myalgia, and lethargy. Electrocardiographic abnormalities and nephrotoxicity can develop at higher dosages.

ANTIBACTERIALS

Paromomycin and furazolidone are nonabsorbable antibacterials, previously discussed under antibacterial therapy (Chapter 43), that are effective in treatment of infections caused by pathogenic intestinal protozoa. Because of potential intestinal absorption and nephrotoxicity, paromomycin, an aminoglycoside, must be used with caution in treating amebiasis when bowel lesions are extensive. Furazolidone and sulfonamides are effective in treating intestinal coccidial infections. Nifurtimox, a nitrofuran derivative, is suppressive but not curative for *Trypanosoma cruzi* infections. Nausea, vomiting, and convulsions may be side effects. Several newer antifolate drugs (see Chapter 86) are under development for toxoplasmosis.[8]

Trimethoprim, a previously discussed antibacterial diaminopyrimidine compound that inhibits folic acid synthesis, has broad-spectrum antimicrobial activity (see Trimethoprim-Sulfonamide, Chapter 43). Combined with sulfonamides, it has been used to treat *Pneumocystis* and coccidial infections. Pyrimethamine is closely related but is more effective against protozoa than trimethoprim. It has been used in combination with sulfonamides to treat toxoplasmosis.

SPIRAMYCIN

Spiramycin, a macrolide antibiotic, has an antibacterial spectrum similar to that of erythromycin but is less effective. Absorption following oral administration is adequate for therapeutic purposes, and it achieves wide tissue distribution. It differs from other macrolides in that it is eliminated principally in the urine. Although it has limited use for bacterial infections, spiramycin has been found to be the most effective drug for treating intestinal cryptosporidiosis[9] and in utero toxoplasmosis.[9a] Spiramycin is irritating following IM injection. It has produced cutaneous irritation in some veterinarians who have been exposed to it in drug preparations.

Clindamycin, a macrolide previously described in Chapter 43, has been shown to be effective against *Toxoplasma* when used in much higher dosages than those recommended to treat anaerobic bacterial infections.

MISCELLANEOUS DRUGS

Thiacetarsamide sodium, an organic arsenical, has been used to treat *Haemobartonella*, which is actually considered to be a rickettsia. Bismuth-N-glycollylarsanilate is an anthelmintic drug that is a second choice in treating giardiasis. Amprolium is a thiamine inhibitor that is commonly used to treat coccidiosis in dogs, although not approved by the Food and Drug Administration for this purpose (see Chapter 87). Overdoses may produce neurologic signs. Toltrazuril is a new anticoccidial agent that is unrelated to the others.[10] It appears to be very effective in eliminating coccidia in most species without interfering with a persistent host immune response. It has been used to control oocyst shedding by cats acutely infected with *Toxoplasma gondii*.[11] The drug can be given orally in the water or feed or systemically by SC injection or by topical application.

References

1. Navin TR, Dickinson CM, Adams SR, et al: Effect of azotemia in dogs on the pharmacokinetics of pentamidine. *J Infect Dis* 155:1020–1026, 1987.
2. Navin TR, Fontaine RE: Intravenous versus intramuscular administration of pentamidine. *N Engl J Med* 311:1701–1702, 1984.
3. Ganda OP: Pentamidine and hypoglycemia. *Ann Intern Med* 100:464, 1984.
4. Abdullah AS, Baggot JD: Pharmacokinetics of imidocarb in normal dogs and goats. *J Vet Pharmacol Ther* 6:195–199, 1983.
5. Zimmer JF: Treatment of feline giardiasis with metronidazole. *Cornell Vet* 77:383–388, 1987.
6. Shaarer K: Selektive Purkinje-zellschädigungen nach oraler vebrechung grosser Dosen von Nitroimidazolderivaten am Hund. *Folia Dtsch Ges Pathol* 56:407–410, 1972.
7. Dow SW, LeCouteur RA, Poss ML, et al: Central nervous system toxicity associated with metronidazole treatment in dogs: five cases (1984–1987). *J Am Vet Med Assoc* 195:365–368, 1989.
8. Araujo FG, Guptill DR, Remington JS: In vivo activity of piritrexin against *Toxoplasma gondii*. *J Infect Dis* 156:828–830, 1987.
9. Sez-Llorens X, Odio CM, Umaña MA, et al: Spiramycin vs. placebo for treatment of acute diarrhea caused by *Cryptosporidium*. *Pediatr Infect Dis J* 8:136–140, 1989.
9a. Daffos F, Forestier F, Capella-Pavlovsky M, et al: Prenatal management of 746 pregnancies at risk for congenital toxoplasmosis. *N Engl J Med* 318:271–275, 1988.
10. Haberkorn A, Stoltefuss J: Studies on the activity of toltrazuril, a new anti-coccidial agent. *Vet Med Rev* 1/87:22–32, 1987.
11. Rommel M, Schnieder T, Krause HD, et al: Trials to suppress the formation of oocysts and cysts of *Toxoplasma gondii* in cats by medication of the feed with toltrazuril. *Vet Med Rev* 2/87:141–153, 1987.

78

AMERICAN TRYPANOSOMIASIS

Stephen C. Barr

ETIOLOGY AND LIFE CYCLE

Trypanosoma cruzi, the etiologic agent of American trypanosomiasis, is a hemoflagellate protozoan of the class Zoomastigophorea and family Trypanosomatidae. The organism exists in three morphologic forms. The trypomastigote, or blood form, is 15 to 20 μm long, with a flattened spindle-shaped body and a centrally placed vesicular nucleus. A single free flagellum originates from a basal body near the large subterminal kinetoplast (situated posterior to the nucleus) and passes along the body to project anteriorly (Fig. 78–1). The intracellular or amastigote form is approximately 1.5 to 4.0 μm in diameter, ovoid, and contains a large round nucleus and rod-like kinetoplast. The flagellum is too small to be obvious under light microscopy. Epimastigotes, the third morphologic form, are found in the reduviid vector (subfamily Triatominae) commonly known as the kissing bug. This flagellate and spindle-shaped form has a kinetoplast situated anterior to the nucleus.

Infection usually occurs when trypomastigotes are deposited in the insect vector's feces at the bite site (Fig. 78–2). Oral ingestion of infected insects will cause infection in opossums and might be a possible route of infection for dogs. Other less common routes include blood transfusions, congenital, or ingestion of meat or milk from infected lactating animals. Trypomastigotes usually enter macrophages and myocytes, either locally or systemically after hematogenous spread. Once intracellular, trypomastigotes transform into amastigotes, which multiply by binary fission. These transform into trypomastigotes prior to rupture of and release from the cell. Rapid intracellular multiplication cycles ensure a rapid rise in parasitemia before effective immunity develops. The vector becomes infected by ingesting circulating trypomastigotes, which transform to epimastigotes and multiply by binary fission. Transformation of the epimastigotes back into trypomastigotes occurs in the vector's hindgut before the trypomastigotes are passed in the feces (Fig. 78–2).

EPIDEMIOLOGY

T. cruzi infects humans and a wide range of domestic and wild animal species in the Americas. It is a major human health problem in South America, especially Brazil, Venezuela, and Argentina, although the disease rarely has been reported in people or dogs in the United States (Fig. 78–3).

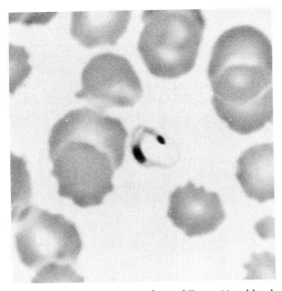

Figure 78–1. Trypomastigote form of *T. cruzi* in a blood film (Wright's stain; × 1000).(From Barr et al: *J Am Vet Med Assoc* 188:1307–1309, 1986, with permission.)

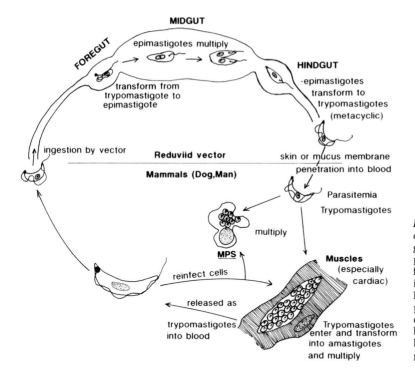

Figure 78–2. Life cycle of T. cruzi. Replication by epimastigotes occurs in the vector. Trypomastigotes in the vector's feces infect the host and divide intracellularly as amastigotes. Host cells rupture, releasing trypomastigotes, which enter other cells or the blood stream. Vectors become infected by ingesting blood containing trypomastigotes.

Transmission of T. cruzi depends on the confluence of reservoirs, vectors, parasites, and the host (people or animal) in a single habitat. There are two extremes of vector behavior: those that are habitually domiciliated and those that are habitually sylvatic, with many species being intermediate in behavior. Because of this variation, vectors tend to have either domestic or sylvatic cycles with crossover between the two occurring occasionally. Of the many Triatominae species that can feed on people in South America, only three, *Triatoma infestans*, *T. dimidiata*, and *Rhodnius prolixus*, are related to the epidemiology of human infections. They are efficient human vectors because they feed on both people and domestic reservoir mammals (dog, cat, guinea pig), cohabit prolifically close to people, and defecate soon after taking a blood meal.[2] Infection rates in these vectors can be as high as 100% south of the equator. In comparison, infection rates of the two principal vectors in the United States, *T. protracta* and *T. sanguisuga*, are 20%. These latter vectors are peridomestic and their inability to adapt to living in human dwellings, their different feeding and defecation habits, and their association with a higher standard of housing are some reasons for low infection rates in the United States.

Infection rates in wild animals in the United States are highest in raccoons (16%),[3] opossums (38%),[4] and armadillos,[5] although a wide range of mammals are reported to be infected. The few T. cruzi isolates from infected vectors, animal reservoirs, and people show in vivo and in vitro characteristics similar to those of isolates from South America.[4,6] South American and a few North American T. cruzi isolates have been characterized by their isoenzyme pattern. Three

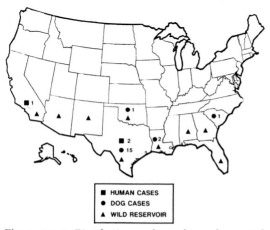

Figure 78–3. Distribution and numbers of reported human and canine trypanosomiasis cases in the United States. Infected wild reservoir hosts occupy most southern states.

main groups or zymodemes have been described,[7,8] although heterogeneity and exceptions exist. Two zymodemes have been isolated from people, mammals, and vectors in areas where sylvatic *T. cruzi* transmission occurs, and another group has been found in areas of domestic transmission.

PATHOGENESIS

T. cruzi trypomastigotes enter host cells soon after infection, multiply unhindered, escaping the immune response, and are transported throughout the body primarily within macrophages. Parasitemia develops within a few days and peaks 2 to 3 weeks postinfection (PI), coinciding with acute clinical disease.[9] The time period from infection to development of acute disease is variable but, experimentally, is 2 to 5 weeks. Young pups 8 to 10 weeks of age receiving a high SC inoculation of a zymodeme isolated from North American opossums developed parasitemia by 3 to 6 days PI and acute myocarditis 14 to 26 days PI. Parasitemia peaks at the time of acute disease and drops to zero over the next 14 days in surviving dogs.[9,10] Dogs infected at an older age may show no signs of acute disease other than slight depression and a rising parasitemia.

Cardiomyopathy may be caused by muscle fiber damage by toxic parasite products, cardiac adrenergic destruction, or autoimmune-mediated mechanisms.[11] Mechanical destruction of myofibrils by parasites occurs during the acute phase of illness, and other indirect mechanisms, such as autoimmunity, may play important roles in chronic disease.[12]

Finally, although some *T. cruzi* isolates from the United States have been shown to be less pathogenic in mice than South American isolates, others produce as severe disease in dogs as South American isolates.[13]

CLINICAL FINDINGS

Dogs

The acute form of illness is more commonly seen. Generalized lymphadenomegaly develops in most cases prior to the development of clinical signs. Signs referable to acute myocarditis, such as sudden collapse and death of a previously normal young dog, have been reported most frequently. Pale mucous membranes, a slowed capillary refill time, weak pulse with deficits, tachyarrhythmia, and terminal hypothermia and respiratory distress are common. Most infected dogs that do not die suddenly develop ascites and hepatomegaly due to right-sided heart failure. Anorexia and diarrhea are also common during acute disease. Neurologic signs including profound weakness and ataxia suggestive of distemper have been found in naturally and experimentally infected dogs. An older dog with laryngeal paralysis was found incidentally to have trypanosomiasis, which may have been caused by a less pathogenic strain.[1]

Electrocardiographic (ECG) changes during acute disease are highly variable and include alteration in ST-T segments, T wave inversion, low-amplitude QRS complexes, positive polyphasic ventricular premature contractions, and first- and second-degree heart block. Survivors of acute myocarditis will become aparasitemic, asymptomatic, and develop chronic myocarditis with cardiac dilation over the following 8 to 36 months.[9, 14] During the long asymptomatic period between acute and chronic disease in the dog, the ECG may be normal except for the intermittent occurrence of ventricular arrhythmias, which can be exacerbated by exercise or excitement. Sudden death during this stage can occur and is thought to be due to fatal cardiac arrhythmias. As cardiac dilation occurs, ECG abnormalities become more prevalent and clinical signs referable to right-sided and eventually left-sided chamber failure occur. These cases are indistinguishable from chronic dilational cardiomyopathy seen in large breeds of dogs and often are diagnosed as such until histology is done.[13] Trypanosomiasis should be considered in any dog while signs of myocarditis or cardiomyopathy are present.

Cats

Cats are reported to be susceptible to South American isolates of *T. cruzi*, but little information is available regarding clinical disease. There are no reports of domestic feline trypanosomiasis from North America.

DIAGNOSIS

Thoracic radiography is of value in the diagnosis of pleural effusion, pulmonary edema, and chamber dilation in both acute and chronic myocarditis. Echocardiography can provide valuable information on the state of the myocardium including contractility, cardiac output, and septal and left ventricular free wall thickness.

Hematology is of little specific diagnostic value. A lymphocytosis may occur in the acute phase in a small number of cases. ALT (SGPT) activity may be elevated as a result of hepatic hypoxia. Creatine kinase (CK) and lactate dehydrogenase (LDH) activities are rarely elevated during acute disease. Elevations of serum CK (isoenzyme MB) do occur but are too variable and transient to be of any diagnostic value in the dog.[13] The abdominal effusion is typically a modified transudate from cardiac causes.

Cytology

Trypomastigotes can be identified in the blood just prior to and during acute disease (Fig. 78–1). Although organisms are identified in most cases of acute trypanosomiasis, rarely are they found in chronic cases. Parasitemias are often so low, however, that organisms can be missed during routine examination of Wright's stained blood films. High-power (400×) examination of the buffy coat-plasma interface of a centrifuged microhematocrit tube may reveal characteristically motile parasites. A thick-film buffy coat smear, stained with Wright's or Giemsa stain or examined as a wet preparation for trypomastigote movement, is also an effective means of concentrating trypomastigotes. Lymph node aspirates or impression smears of enlarged lymph nodes may be positive even when parasitemias are very low. Abdominal effusions may contain organisms that can be identified cytologically.

Isolation

Isolation of organisms into germ-free hosts or cell culture systems is a sensitive but time-consuming practice. Blood agar slants overlaid with liver infusion tryptose (LIT) medium or LIT alone are effective for isolating trypomastigotes from blood of an infected animal[15] but can take from 2 to 20 weeks to become positive for epimastigotes. Direct inoculation of blood into a Vero cell monolayer will usually result in the development of intracellular amastigote forms and trypomastigotes in media after 2 to 4 weeks.

Weanling laboratory mice inoculated intraperitoneally or SC with the patient's blood will usually develop detectable parasitemias 10 to 30 days later. The sensitivity depends on the strain of the mouse and parasite present and can be increased by treating mice with glucocorticoids prior to and after inoculation.

Serologic Testing

The IFA, direct hemagglutination, and complement fixation tests are most commonly used.[16] These tests confirm the presence of antibodies to T. cruzi and, although most cross-react with antibodies to Leishmania and T. rangeli in South America, they are sensitive and specific for North American use. A central laboratory is available in North America for T. cruzi serologic assays (Appendix 8). Serial changes in IgM and IgG levels have not been reported in the dog, but all clinically affected dogs that have been serologically tested to date have had positive test results.

PATHOLOGIC FINDINGS

In acute disease, lesions usually are confined to the heart, especially the right side. Subendocardial and subepicardial hemorrhages as well as multiple yellow to white myocardial spots and streaks mainly involve the coronary groove.[17] Hepatic, splenic, and renal congestion as well as pulmonary edema may be present secondary to cardiac failure. Microscopically, a diffuse granulomatous inflammation, hydropic degeneration and necrosis of myofibrils, and a mononuclear cellular infiltrate typify acute cases. Numerous pseudocysts containing amastigotes are often associated with the inflammatory response. Mild granulomatous myositis and organisms can be found in other organs including the smooth muscle of the stomach, small intestine, bladder, and skeletal muscle. A nonsuppurative encephalitis has also been found.

Chronic disease is characterized by a bilaterally enlarged flaccid heart with areas of thinning of the ventricular walls due to fibrous plaques.[10] Histologically, there are multifocal coalescing areas of lymphoplas-

Table 78–1. Therapy for Trypanosomiasis[a]

DRUG	DOSE[b] (mg/kg)	ROUTE	INTERVAL (hours)	DURATION (months)
Nifurtimox[c]	2–7	PO	6	3–5
Benznidazole	5	PO	24	2

[a]PO = oral.

[b]Dose per administration at specified interval, expressed as mg/kg unless otherwise stated.

[c]Lampit (Bayer) is an investigational drug in the United States. Available only from the Centers for Disease Control, Atlanta, GA, for treatment of human infections.

mocytic inflammation and mild necrosis with extensive loss of myocardial fibers and replacement by fibrous tissue. Organisms are seldom found in tissues. The apex of the heart is one of the more likely areas to find them.

THERAPY

The investigational drug nifurtimox (Bayer 2502 or Lampit, Bayer AG, Leverkusen-Bayerwerk, West Germany) has been reported to be successful in treating experimental and natural cases of canine trypanosomiasis (Table 78–1).[18] Improved survival has been shown to occur in dogs treated concurrently with anti-inflammatory doses of glucocorticoids.[19] Benznidazole has been shown to produce cures in acute Chagas' disease in people.[20]

Supportive therapy including furosemide and theophylline is indicated in cases of dilational myocarditis. Cardiac arrhythmias may require specific therapy depending on the source and severity of the disturbance. If the disease is diagnosed and treated early enough, the mortality rate of acute disease can be decreased. However, dogs surviving acute disease invariably progress to chronic cardiac disease, the prognosis of which must be guarded, as the outcome is usually fatal. Without therapy, progression to chronic disease occurs 8 to 20 months after the acute illness.

PREVENTION

Preventing contact between dogs and infected vectors by upgrading dog housing will do much to limit infection. Residual insecticides should be sprayed monthly in peridomiciliary structures (woodpiles, chicken houses) and dog kennels. Limiting contact between dogs and infected reservoir hosts (opossums, raccoons, skunks) in the wild

and their vectors is virtually impossible. Most cases in the United States have been reported in hunting dogs, which do have an increased risk of exposure. Dogs should not be fed raw meat of reservoir hosts. Blood donors in endemic areas should be screened serologically to determine previous exposure to *T. cruzi*.

PUBLIC HEALTH CONSIDERATIONS

An estimated 10 million to 12 million Latin Americans are infected with Chagas' disease, but only three human cases have been reported in the United States (Fig. 79–3).[6] Several factors are probably responsible for this low prevalence of Chagas' disease. First, the North American species of *Triatoma* have usually left the host when they defecate, unlike the South American insect, which defecates while still on the host.[6] Since contact with infected feces is the usual mode of transmission, this limits the chance of contact. Second, the density of infected *Triatoma* in human dwellings is much less in the United States than it is in endemic areas of South America. Third, more cases of human Chagas' disease may have occurred in the United States but have gone unrecognized because of a low index of suspicion.

Chagas' disease in dogs and wild hosts is of considerable public health significance because of the severity of and difficulty in treating the disease in people. Veterinarians should take particular care in treating such cases and make owners aware of the potential zoonotic risk. Blood samples taken from infected dogs are potentially infective and laboratory staff should be appropriately instructed in their handling.

References

1. Barr SC, Baker D, Markovits J: Trypanosomiasis and laryngeal paralysis in a dog. *J Am Vet Med Assoc* 188:1307–1309, 1986.

2. Carcavallo RU: The subfamily Triatominae (Hemiptera, Reduviidae): systematics and some ecological factors. *In* Brenner RR, Stoke A (ed): *Chagas' Disease Vectors*, Vol 1. Boca Raton, FL, CRC Press, 1987, pp 13–18.

3. McKeveer S, Gorman GW, Norman L: Occurrence of a *Trypanosoma cruzi*-like organisms in some mammals from southwestern Georgia and northwestern Florida. *J Parasitol* 44:583–587, 1958.

4. Barr SC, Dennis VA, Klei TR: Biological characterization of *Trypanosoma cruzi* isolated from Louisiana mammals. *Proceedings*. Am Soc Trop Med Hyg, No 66, 1986.

5. Yaeger RG: The prevalence of *Trypanosoma cruzi* infection in armadillos collected at a site near New Orleans, Louisiana. *Am J Trop Med Hyg* 38:323–326, 1988.

6. Navin TR, Roberto RR, Juranek DD, et al: Human and sylvatic *Trypanosoma cruzi* infections in California. *Am J Public Health* 75:366–369, 1985.

7. Miles MA: The epidemiology of South American trypanosomiasis—biochemical and immunological approaches and their relevance to control. *Trans R Soc Trop Med Hyg* 77:5–23, 1983.

8. Apt W, Aguilera X, Arribaba A: Epidemiology of Chagas' disease in northern Chile: isozyme profile of *Trypanosoma cruzi* from domestic and sylvatic transmission cycles and their association with cardiopathy. *Am J Trop Med Hyg* 37:302–307, 1987.

9. Barr SC, Holmes BA, Dennis VA, Klei TR: Experimental *Trypanosoma cruzi* infections in dogs. *Proceedings*. Anim Dis Res Work South States, No 59, 1987.

10. Anselmi A, Pifano CF, Suarex JA, et al: Myocardiopathy in Chagas' disease. 1. Comparative study of pathologic findings in chronic human and experimental Chagas' myocarditis. *Am Heart J* 72:469–481, 1966.

11. Kierszenbaum F: Autoimmunity in Chagas' disease. *J Parasitol* 72:201–211, 1986.

12. Andrade ZA: Mechanisms of myocardial damage in *Trypanosoma cruzi* infections. *In* Ciba Foundation Symposium No 99: *Cytopathology of Parasitic Diseases*. London, Pitman Books, 1983, pp 214–233.

13. Barr SC: Unpublished observations, Louisiana State University, Baton Rouge, LA, 1988.

14. Andrade ZA, Andrade SG, Sadigursky M, et al: Experimental Chagas' disease in dogs. *Arch Pathol Lab Med* 105:460–464, 1981.

15. Logan LL, Hanson WL: *Trypanosoma cruzi*: morphogenesis in diffusion chambers in the mouse peritoneal cavity and attempted stimulation of host immunity. *Exp Parasitol* 36:439–454, 1974.

16. Voller A: Serological methods in the diagnosis of Chagas' disease. *Trans R Soc Trop Med Hyg* 71:10–11, 1977.

17. Williams GD, Adams LG, Yaeger RG, et al: Naturally occurring trypanosomiasis (Chagas' disease) in dogs. *J Am Vet Med Assoc* 171:171–177, 1977.

18. Haberkorn A, Gonnert R: Animal experimental investigations into the activity of nifurtimox against *Trypanosoma cruzi*. *Arzneimittelforsch* 22:1570–1582, 1972.

19. Andrade SG, Andrade ZA, Sadigursky M: Combined treatment with a nitrofuranic and a corticoid in experimental Chagas' disease in the dog. *Am J Trop Med Hyg* 29:766–773, 1980.

20. Krettli AU, Cancado JR, Brener Z: Effects of specific chemotherapy in the levels of lytic antibodies in Chagas' disease. *Trans R Soc Trop Med Hyg* 76:334–340, 1982.

79

LEISHMANIASIS

Robbert J. Slappendel
Craig E. Greene

Leishmaniasis is an infectious disease of people and wild and domestic animals with worldwide distribution in the temperate, subtropical, and tropical areas.[1,2] It is caused by a diphasic protozoan microorganism of the genus *Leishmania*. Different leishmanial species occur in various parts of the Old World and the New World and are responsible for a spectrum of diseases in people, with 400,000 to 1,200,000 new cases being diagnosed annually (Fig. 79–1).[3–5]

Knowledge of leishmaniasis is important for the small animal clinician because the infection may cause clinical disease in dogs and cats and because these animals are reservoirs of the disease for people in some countries where the disease is endemic. In other endemic areas, rodents and other wild animals are the reservoir hosts. Because of the chronic insidious nature of the disease, isolated cases in dogs and cats have occurred in nonendemic regions where infected pets have been imported.

ETIOLOGY

Classification of *Leishmania* species traditionally has been based on geographic distribution, clinical symptoms, and serology in people and on the clinical symptoms and pathologic findings of the disease in experimentally infected hamsters. According to a simplified but utilitarian classification, Old World leishmaniases can be divided into the cutaneous form, the mucocutaneous form, and the visceral form, each caused by a different leishmanial complex (Table 79–1). New World leishmaniasis is also broadly separable into the same forms caused by distinct leishmanial complexes. The word "complex" implies a group of various subspecies and the taxonomic relationships are

probably oversimplified. New biochemical methods, including isoenzyme patterns, DNA peptide mapping, and immunologic reactivity to monoclonal antibodies and membrane-shed antigens, have revealed that the taxonomy is much more complicated.[6]

EPIDEMIOLOGY

The natural cycle of infection is usually a zoonosis with bloodsucking sandflies as vectors transmitting the parasite among wild or domestic animals, especially rodents and dogs. Sandflies of the genus *Phlebotomus* in the Old World and *Lutzomyia* in the New World are the primary vectors. Wild and domestic dogs are reservoirs for the disease because they develop cutaneous lesions that allow the vector access to parasitized macrophages during feeding. Domestic dogs and wild Canidae are considered reservoir hosts in Central Asia, Erithrea, parts of China, northeast Brazil, Portugal, and the Mediterranean area. People and cats are generally incidental hosts, though humans appear to be their own reservoir in some regions, such as northeast India and some parts of China and East Africa.[5]

In the vertebrate host, *Leishmania* is found in macrophages only as a nonflagellate form, the amastigote, which is ovoid or round, 2.5 to 5.0 μm long by 1.5 to 2.0 μm wide. Apart from a reddish nucleus, a characteristic purple rod-shaped kinetoplast is generally visible when the amastigote is stained with Wright's or Giemsa stain (Fig. 79–2).[7]

Amastigotes multiply by binary fission, rupture out of the macrophage, and infect new cells. Sandflies can ingest the amastigotes when they suck blood from an infected host. In the sandfly, the organism multiplies and undergoes a series of morphologic alter-

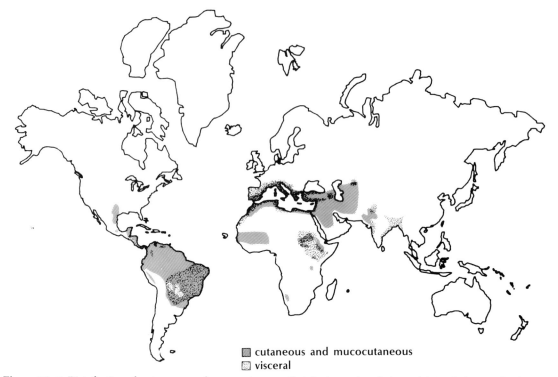

Figure 79–1. Distribution of cutaneous and mucocutaneous (hatched areas) and visceral (stippled areas) leishman-iasis. (Adapted by permission from *The Leishmaniases*. The WHO Expert Committee. WHO Technical Report Series No. 701. Geneva, WHO, 1984.)

ations including transformation into a flag-ellate form, the promastigote. These may be injected into the skin of a vertebrate host when the fly feeds again. After inoculation into the host, the promastigotes lose their flagella and again change into amastigotes (Fig. 79–3).

Sandflies are active mainly at sunset, more rarely at night, from early spring to late autumn. Since they have a limited flight range, people must come into their habitat to become infected, or the vector and reser-voir host must both live in close proximity to people.

Old World

The geographic distribution of visceral leishmaniasis in people (Fig. 79–1), which

Table 79–1. Leishmanial Species and the Diseases They Cause in Humans Worldwide

CLINICAL DISEASE	OLD WORLD	NEW WORLD
Cutaneous	L. tropica complex L. tropica (L. t. minor) L. t. major L. aethiopica aethiopica	L. mexicana complex L. m. mexicana L. m. amazonensis L. m. pifanoi L. m. garnhami L. braziliensis complex L. b. braziliensis L. b. panamensis L. b. guyanensis L. peruviana
Mucocutaneous	Rare[3]	L. braziliensis complex L. b. braziliensis L. b. panamensis
Visceral	L. donovani complex L. d. donovani L. d. archibaldi L. d. infantum	L. donovani complex L. d. chagasi

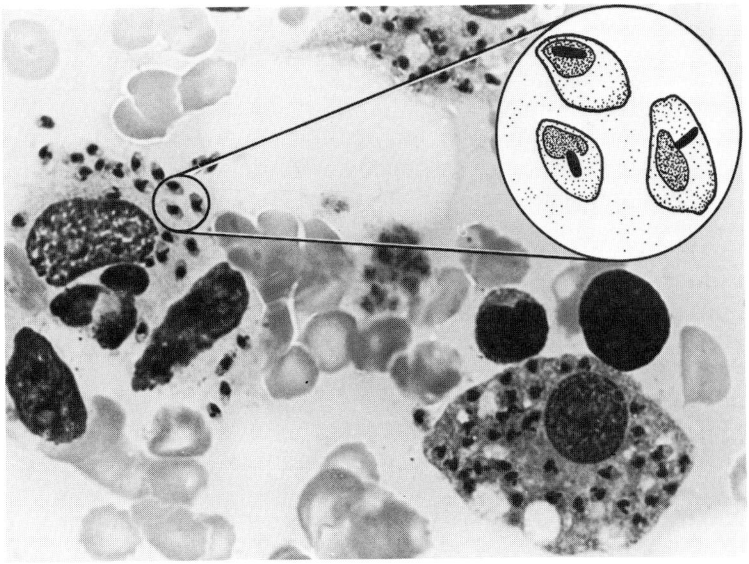

Figure 79–2. Amastigotes in macrophages in stained smear of bone marrow aspirate (May-Gruenwald-Giemsa stain). Insert: schematic drawing of amastigotes. (From Slappendel RJ: *Vet Q* 10:1–16, 1988, with permission.)

is caused mainly by parasites of the *L. donovani* complex (Table 79–1), coincides in broad outline with the distribution of leishmaniasis in dogs. In the past, human visceral leishmaniasis was widespread in China and cases were also reported from Mongolia. Following the mass destruction of dogs in the 1950s, visceral leishmaniasis was largely eliminated in these areas.[5] In India visceral leishmaniasis is an anthropozoonosis caused by *L. d. donovani*, which does not occur in dogs. In West Africa (Sénégal, Nigeria) canine leishmaniasis is well known but human infection seems to be extremely rare.[5]

Infection of dogs with parasites of the *L. tropica* complex seems to occur more inci-

dentally. Yet dogs are probably involved in the epidemiology of the urban type of dermal leishmaniasis, caused by *L. t. tropica*.[8]

L. t. major, hitherto thought to occur exclusively in rodents and people, was detected in dogs in Egypt[9] and Saudi Arabia.[10]

Clinical reports on leishmaniasis in small animals have been mainly of dogs infected in countries around the Mediterranean basin and Portugal. Sporadic autochthonous cases have also been reported in the northern parts of France, Switzerland, and The Netherlands.

The inciting organism primarily has been *L. d. infantum*, but *L. t. tropica* may have been involved occasionally. Both species oc-

Figure 79–3. The infectious cycle of *Leishmania infantum*. (The relative incidence of contamination is indicated by the boldness of the arrows.)

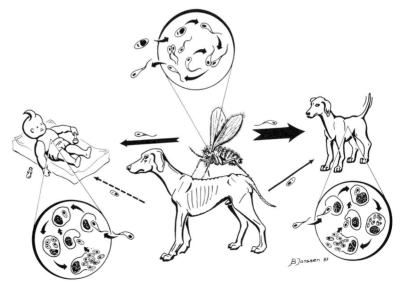

cur in the Mediterranean area and are morphologically indistinguishable. In dogs, the two species cannot be discriminated by clinical signs. In humans, *L. d. infantum* causes visceral leishmaniasis (kala-azar), whereas *L. t. tropica* is usually associated with dermal leishmaniasis (oriental sore).

The prevalence of leishmanial infections in dogs in endemic areas varies, ranging from 20% to 40% in some countries. Not all dogs are clinically ill, but approximately 90% of the infected dogs ultimately will develop clinical signs. In the Mediterranean, dogs are more commonly infected than people. In areas with a high infection rate among dogs, the prevalence of infection of human native inhabitants does not exceed 1% to 2% and includes mainly young children and babies.

It is difficult to estimate the prevalence of imported leishmaniasis in dogs in nonendemic countries. Imported leishmaniasis has been diagnosed in the United States, Canada, and many countries in Europe. In the United Kingdom at least 7 cases have been recognized among 4000 dogs that had been imported from all over the world.[4] Cats have been found to be infected on a limited basis, and their role as a reservoir for infection is uncertain.[11]

New World

The distribution of leishmaniasis in the New World is indicated in Figure 79–1. As in the Old World, domestic and wild dogs are considered reservoir hosts for a majority of the leishmanial species.[12] *Leishmania* of people, dogs, and cats in the New World is an endemic, sporadic infection in South and Central America. The endemic region is extending northward into Mexico. Isolated foci of infection have been found in Texas, Oklahoma, and Ohio.

Although parasites of the *L. donovani* complex are considered the primary viscerotropic subspecies of the Americas,[13] they can also produce primarily cutaneous lesions in people and dogs.[14] Parasites of the *L. braziliensis* complex produce a cutaneous form of the disease, usually manifested by single ulcerated lesions on the ears.[14a] The reports of cases in dogs,[15,16,16a,16b] cats,[17] or people[16,18] in Texas, Oklahoma, and Ohio may represent newly established endemic foci where diseased hosts from other areas

may have infected native sandfly populations. The strain of *Leishmania* involved in the canine infection in Oklahoma was thought to be *L. d. infantum*. The isolate from the cat infected in Texas was classified by isoenzyme determinations as *L. m. mexicana* and was thought to be the same strain associated with the human infections in Texas.

PATHOGENESIS

In susceptible dogs, local infection of the skin is usually followed by spread of the parasites throughout the body before symptoms develop. Depending on host immunocompetence, clinical signs become evident within a period of 1 month to several years[19,19a]; incubation times of up to 7 years have been reported.[7] Since *Leishmania* is an obligatory intracellular parasite, host defenses are strongly dependent on T lymphocyte activity. T lymphocyte regions in the lymphoid organs become depleted and B cell regions proliferate in response to the infection.[20] Without support of T cells, macrophages are not able to kill amastigotes; hence parasites disseminate intracellularly all over the body. Proliferation of B lymphocytes, histiocytes, and macrophages results in generalized lymphadenopathy and hepatosplenomegaly.

The resultant immunoglobulin response is usually enormous; however, it is detrimental and nonprotective. Specific antibodies may opsonize amastigotes, thus enhancing their phagocytosis by macrophages, within which the parasite continues to survive. Also, numerous coincidental antibodies are produced, including autoantibodies that may be associated with the development of pathologic phenomena such as immune-mediated thrombocytopenia and anemia.

A potential hazard of impaired T lymphocyte regulation and exuberant B lymphocyte activity is the generation of large amounts of circulating immune complexes (CIC). CIC deposition in the walls of blood vessels may cause vasculitis, polyarthritis, and glomerulonephritis. CIC may also bind complement to blood cells and hence shorten their life span. In dogs, CIC deposition in the kidneys eventually results in renal failure, which is the main cause of death of dogs with leishmaniasis.[7] The serum of patients with CIC often contains so-called cryoglobulins. These proteins may precipitate in the blood vessels of the extremities when exposed to cold, thus causing ischemic necrosis.[7]

Dogs with leishmaniasis may have epistaxis or other signs of a hemorrhagic diathesis for various reasons: hyperglobulinemia and paraglobulinemia may interfere with fibrin polymerization; uremia inhibits thrombocyte function; and CIC, autoantibodies, splenic pooling, and bone marrow failure may induce thrombocytopenia. Anemia may develop as a sequel of blood loss or erythrolysis and decreased erythropoiesis.

CLINICAL FINDINGS

Cats

Cats are rarely clinically affected.[2] In some studies, cats have been seropositive without clinical disease.[11] In a case of cutaneous leishmaniasis, nodules on the pinna were the only clinical finding, and they were locally recurrent following surgical removal (Fig. 79–4).[20]

Dogs

Leishmania infection usually causes chronic systemic disease. The clinical findings in canine leishmaniasis are presented in Table 79–2.

Almost 90% of dogs with leishmaniasis

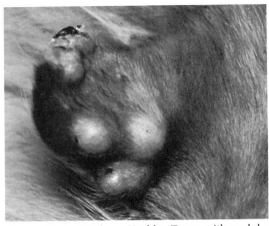

Figure 79–4. Cat from Uvalde, Texas with nodular lesions of *Leishmania* on the ear pinna. (Courtesy of Drs. TM Craig and CL Barton, Texas A & M University, College Station, TX.)

have cutaneous involvement; however, dermatologic abnormalities in the absence of other signs of disease are rare (Fig. 79–5). Therefore, any animal with dermal manifestations of the disease should be presumed to have visceral involvement. The skin problems are variable in character and extent. The most prominent feature is hyperkeratosis, presenting as excessive scaling of the epidermis and thickening, depigmentation, and chapping of the muzzle and the footpads. Scaling may be most prominent on the nose, around the eyes, and on the pinna but also may be diffuse over the body. The haircoat is mostly dry and brittle with diffuse hair loss. Some dogs develop dermatitis, mucocutaneous ulcers, and small intradermal nodules. Abnormally long or brittle nails, a rather specific finding, is present in a minority of the patients.

Weight loss and muscle atrophy are the most common signs of visceral involvement. Some dogs lose weight despite having ravenous appetites, but serious loss of condition is usually associated with anorexia and other signs of renal failure, including mental depression, polyuria, polydipsia, and vomiting.

Decreased physical activity is obvious and related to somnolence, decreased endurance, and locomotion disturbances. The latter may be due to neuralgia, polyarthritis, polymyositis, clefts in the footpads, interdigital ulcers, or even osteolytic lesions or proliferative periostitis.[7,21,22] Body temperature may fluctuate but is usually normal or subfebrile.

DIAGNOSIS

Clinical and Laboratory Testing

The abnormalities (and percentages) observed are shown in Table 79–3. A primary feature of canine leishmaniasis in some endemic foci in the New World has been radiographic and clinical evidence of interstitial pneumonia.[23]

Organism Identification

Leishmanial amastigotes are found free or in macrophages, in Wright's- or Giemsa-stained smears from lymph nodes or bone marrow. Detection of parasites in other tis-

Table 79–2. Clinical Findings in 80 Dogs with Leishmaniasis[a]

HISTORICAL SIGNS	%	PHYSICAL EXAMINATION ABNORMALITIES	%
Decreased endurance	67.5	Lymphadenomegaly	90
Weight loss	64	Skin involvement	89
Somnolence	60	Cachexia	47.5
Increased fluid intake	40	Abnormal locomotion	37.5
Anorexia	32.5	Hyperthermia	36
Diarrhea	30	Conjunctivitis	32.5
Vomiting	26	Palpable spleen	32.5
Polyphagia	15	Abnormal nails	20
Epistaxis	15	Rhinitis	10
Melena	12.5	Keratitis	7.5
Sneezing	10	Pneumonia	2.5
Coughing	6	Icterus	2.5
Fainting	6	Uveitis	1.3
		Panophthalmitis	1.3

[a]Modified from: Slappendel RJ: Vet Q 10:1–16, 1988.

sues such as liver or skin biopsies is possible but more difficult and less practical. An immunoperoxidase staining method has been described[24] that may facilitate the identification of amastigotes in tissues. *Leishmania* has been found in synovial fluid of infected dogs.[25] Sometimes the diagnosis has to be established by the culture of parasites from lymph node or bone marrow aspirates or other tissues in Novy-MacNeal-Nicolle (NNN) media or Schneider's *Drosophila* medium, or by the inoculation of hamsters.

Serologic Testing

A wide range of immunodiagnostic tests has been developed using complement fixation, IFA, direct hemagglutination, and ELISA methods.[25a] Serologic tests verify the presence of antibodies but do not prove or disprove active disease. As stated before, however, infected dogs rarely eliminate the parasite spontaneously without showing signs of disease, so a positive titer should indicate current infection. Depending on the

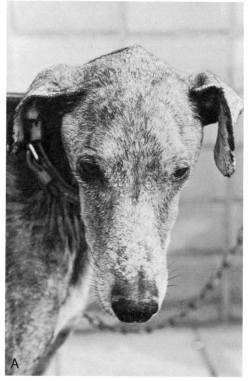

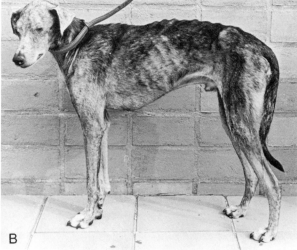

Figure 79–5 A and B. Dog with characteristic features of leishmaniasis. Notice the thin haircoat, excessive scaling, cachexia and muscle atrophy. (From Slappendel RJ: Vet Q 10:1–16, 1988, with permission.)

Table 79–3. Clinical Laboratory Abnormalities in Dogs with Leishmaniasis[a]

ABNORMALITY	% OF DOGS
Hyperglobulinemia	100
Hypoalbuminemia	94
High total serum protein	91
Proteinuria	85
Positive Coombs' test result (mostly weak)	84
High alanine aminotransferase activity	61
High serum alkaline phosphatase activity	51
Thrombocytopenia	50
Azotemia	45
Hypercreatininemia	38
Positive results for antinuclear antibody	31
Leukopenia, associated with low normal or decreased lymphocyte count	22
Positive results for lupus erythematosus cells	13
Leukocytosis with left shift	8

[a]Modified from Slappendel RJ: *Vet Q* 10:1–16, 1988.

sensitivity and specificity of the test methods used, false-positive or false-negative results may be obtained. Improved serodiagnosis in people has been achieved by using purified parasite proteins in the assay procedure.[25b] Experimentally infected dogs have had IgG antibody titers detected by 14 to 28 days postinfection (PI) with maximum titers by 45 to 80 days.[26] IgG titers detected by IFA have decreased 60 to 90 days after treatment had been instituted, which allows monitoring for the reactivation of infection.[26] Serum samples should be submitted to laboratories that have considerable experience with these serologic tests to ensure accuracy in the results and interpretation. See Appendix 8 for a listing of diagnostic laboratories that perform these tests.

PATHOLOGIC FINDINGS

Severely affected patients are cachectic. The organs mainly affected are the skin and elements of the mononuclear-phagocyte system in diverse sites. Generalized enlargement of lymph nodes is usually present. Hepatosplenomegaly may be present but is less common, as in human patients with visceral leishmaniasis. These organs and tissues enlarge from increased numbers of cells made up of histiocytes, macrophages, which may be parasitized, eosinophils, lymphocytes, and plasma cells. Small, light-colored nodular foci, which are granulomas, may occur in various organs, including the skin and the kidneys. Mucosal ulcerations in the

stomach, intestine, and colon occasionally have been seen. Petechiae and ecchymotic bleeding in mucosal and serosal membranes are rare. Kidney lesions include CIC-induced glomerulonephritis, interstitial nephritis, and occasionally amyloidosis. Amyloid deposits may also be present in other organs. The bone marrow is usually red and abundant, but erythropoiesis is ineffective. Osteolytic or proliferative periosteal processes may be found in various parts of the skeleton in some patients.

THERAPY

Leishmaniasis in dogs is more resistant to therapy than the disease in people, and drugs used in human medicine are often ineffective in treating dogs. It should be assumed that the organism will never be eliminated and that retreatment will be necessary. At present, pentavalent antimonials, that is, meglumine antimonate (Glucantime, Specia, Paris, France; Rhodia, New York, NY) and sodium stibogluconate (Pentostam, Wellcome, Beckenham, U.K.), are considered the most effective drugs for the treatment of canine leishmaniasis. Meglumine should produce less side effects than stibogluconate. Dosage regimens vary. In the author's experience,[7] good results have been obtained if meglumine is given at the dosage schedule in Table 79–4. Antimonials should be injected SC or IV but not IM in the thigh, as the latter may result in abscess formation and severe lameness due to muscle fibrosis. Treatment of experimentally infected dogs with liposome-encapsulated antimonate has been shown to be more effective at lower dosages with reduced toxicity as compared with the commercially available drugs,[27] but the results of such treatment were disappointing in spontaneous cases, at least in the hands of the senior author. The drugs also have been used experimentally for topical application to cutaneous nodules with some success. Other drugs that are coupled to carrier substances specifically taken up by macrophages have been effective in treatment of experimental leishmaniasis.[27a,27b]

Relapses, which usually occur a few months to a year after therapy, should be treated with another course of daily injections. In some cases, antimicrobial treatment seems to shift the immunopathologic state

Table 79–4. Antimicrobial Therapy for Canine Leishmaniasis[a]

DRUG	DOSE[b] (mg/kg)	ROUTE	INTERVAL (hours)	DURATION[c] (weeks)
Meglumine antimonate	100	IV, SC	24	3–4
Sodium stibogluconate[d]	30–50	IV, SC	24	3–4

[a]IV = intravenous, SC = subcutaneous.

[b]Dose per administration at specified interval, expressed as mg/kg unless otherwise stated. Therapy should be given on the basis of active antimony and should not fluctuate because of generic or trade name.

[c]All long-term survivors will have to be treated on multiple occasions because of relapses.

[d]Available in the United States for treatment of human infections by special request from the Centers for Disease Control, Atlanta, GA.

of the patient from anergic toward allergic without accomplishing a definite cure, a situation comparable to that of people with so-called post–kala-azar dermal lesions. In dogs, this results in the development of granulomatous dermal nodules and iridocyclitis.[7]

If dogs are seriously ill at the start of treatment, especially in case of severe renal failure, antimicrobial treatment should be started in reduced doses, and prednisolone (1 mg/kg) should be given in addition during the first days. It is also necessary to restore fluid and acid-base balances before treatment with antimonial drugs is started.

Surgical removal of cutaneous nodules offers only temporary resolution in cutaneous infections and instead, they should be expected to resolve with chemotherapy. In an affected cat where surgical management was used alone,[14] the lesions recurred at the incision site 2 years following radical pinnectomy.[28]

Prognosis is dependent on kidney function at the start of treatment. In dogs with renal insufficiency, the prognosis is very poor.[7]

PREVENTION

At present there are no prophylactic drugs or commercially available vaccines effective against canine leishmaniasis. Use of a crude vaccine to protect people against cutaneous leishmaniasis has had limited evaluation.[29] A partially purified extract of L. d. infantum has produced neutralizing antibodies and suppressed development of infection with L. t. major.[30] Prevention of the disease in areas where it is endemic is difficult and depends on control of the insect vectors, detection and extermination of animal reservoirs, and early detection and treatment of infected pets.

Measures to protect the individual dog include keeping the animal indoors from 1 hour before sunset to 1 hour after dawn during the vector season and the use of repellants, insecticides, and fine wire gauze to keep dogs, kennels, and houses free of sandflies. In addition, eradication of the breeding places of the sandflies has resulted in limited control of the disease. Owners who live in Leishmania-free countries should leave their pets at home when visiting endemic areas.

PUBLIC HEALTH CONSIDERATIONS

In people, visceral leishmaniasis is a serious disease that may be fatal when untreated. Children under 5 years of age and adults on cytostatic or immunosuppressive drugs are most severely affected.[31]

In endemic areas, sandflies may pass the disease from dog to people. Considering the low prevalence of leishmaniasis among tourists who have visited endemic regions, the risk of such an infection is low. In areas where sandflies are absent, the risk of infection of people is remote, even when they live in close contact with infected dogs. However, very incidental infections by direct contact from animals to people have been reported.[4,7] Therefore, direct contact with contaminated injection needles or with open wounds with organic material from dogs with leishmaniasis should be strictly avoided. The risk of direct transmission seems to be greater between dogs than from dogs to people.

References

1. Chapman WL, Hanson WL: Leishmaniasis. In Greene CE (ed): Clinical Microbiology and Infec-

tious *Diseases of the Dog and Cat*. Philadelphia, WB Saunders Co, 1984, pp 764–770.

2. Holzworth J: Leishmaniasis. *In* Holzworth J (ed): *Diseases of the Cat. Medicine and Surgery*. Philadelphia, WB Saunders Co, 1987, p 397.

3. World Health Organization: *The Leishmaniases*. Geneva, WHO, 1984.

4. Longstaffe JA, Guy MW: Canine leishmaniasis—United Kingdom update. *J Small Anim Pract* 27:663–671, 1986.

5. Molyneux DH: *The Biology of Trypanosoma and Leishmania*. London, Taylor & Francis, 1983.

6. Neva FA: Leishmaniasis. *In* Wijngaarden JB (ed): *Cecil Textbook of Medicine*, ed 17. Philadelphia, WB Saunders Co, 1985, pp 1786–1792.

7. Slappendel RJ: Canine leishmaniasis. A review based on 95 cases in The Netherlands. *Vet Q* 10:1–16, 1988.

8. Soulsby EJL: *Helminths, Arthropods and Protozoa of Domesticated Animals*, ed 7. London, Balliere Tindall, 1982, pp 544–552.

9. Morsy TA, Schnur LF, Feinsod FM, et al: Natural infections of *Leishmaina major* in domestic dogs from Alexandria, Egypt. *Am J Trop Med Hyg* 37:49–52, 1987.

10. Elbihar S, Cheema AH, El-Hassan AM: *Leishmania* infecting man and wild animals in Saudi Arabia. 4. Canine cutaneous leishmaniasis in the eastern province. *Trans R Soc Trop Med Hyg* 81:925–927, 1987.

11. Michael SA, Morsey TA, Abou El Seoud SF, et al: Leishmaniasis antibodies in stray cats in Ismailiya Governate, Egypt. *J Egypt Soc Parasitol* 12:283–286, 1982.

12. Falqueto A, Coura JR, Barros GC, et al: Participation of the dog in the cycle of transmission of cutaneous leishmaniasis in the municipality of Viana, Estado do Espirito Santo, Brazil. *Mem Inst Oswaldo Cruz* 81:155–163, 1986.

13. Grimaldi JG, Momen H, Pacheco RS, et al: Canine visceral leishmaniasis in Rio de Janeiro, Brazil. Clinical, parasitological, therapeutic, and epidemiological findings (1977–1983). *Mem Inst Oswaldo Cruz* 80:349–357, 1985.

14. Oliveira NMP, Grimaldi G, Momen LI, et al: Active cutaneous leishmaniasis in Brazil, induced by *Leishmania donovani chagasi*. *Mem Inst Oswaldo Cruz* 81: 303–309, 1986.

14a. Permez C, Coutinho SG, Marzochi MC, et al: Canine American cutaneous leishmaniasis: a clinical and immunological study in dogs naturally infected with *Leishmania brazilensis* in an endemic area of Rio de Janeiro Brazil. *Am J Trop Med Hyg* 38:52–58, 1988.

15. Anderson DC, Buckner RG, Glenn BL, et al: Endemic canine leishmaniasis. *Vet Pathol* 17:94–96, 1980.

16. Kocan KM, MacVean DW, Fox JC: Ultrastructure of a *Leishmania* sp. isolated from dogs in an endemic focus in Oklahoma. *J Parasitol* 69:624–626, 1983.

16a. Swenson CL, Silverman J, Stromberg PC, et al: Visceral leishmaniasis in an English foxhound from an Ohio research colony. *J Am Vet Med Assoc* 193:1089–1092, 1988.

16b. Johnson JB: More on leishmaniasis in Ohio. *J Am Vet Med Assoc* 194:375, 1989.

17. Craig TM, Barton CL, Mercer SH, et al: Dermal leishmaniasis in a Texas cat. *Am J Trop Med Hyg* 35:1100–1102, 1986.

18. Gustafson TI, Reed CM, McGreevy PB, et al: Human cutaneous leishmaniasis acquired in Texas. *Am J Trop Med Hyg* 34:58–63, 1985.

19. Keenan CM, Hendricks LD, Lightner L, et al: Visceral leishmaniasis in the German shepherd dog. I. Infection, clinical disease and clinical pathology. *Vet Pathol* 21:74–79, 1984.

19a. Pospischel A, Fiebiger I, Krampitz HE, et al: Experimental infection with *Leishmania* in a dog: clinical, pathologic, parasitologic and serologic findings. *Zentralbl Veterinarmed B* 34:288–304, 1987.

20. Keenan CM, Hendricks LD, Lightner L, et al: Visceral leishmaniasis in the German shepherd dog. II. Pathology. *Vet Pathol* 21:80–86, 1984.

21. Turrell JM, Pool RR: Bone lesions in four dogs with visceral leishmaniasis. *Am Coll Vet Radiol* 23:243–249, 1982.

22. Macri B, Guarda F: A case of dermatomyositis due to leishmaniasis in a dog. *Schweiz Arch Tierheilkd* 129:265–266, 1987.

23. Duarte MI, Laurenti MD, Brandao-Nunes VL, et al: Interstitial pneumonitis in canine visceral leishmaniasis. *Rev Inst Med Trop Sao Paulo* 28:431–436, 1986.

24. Ferrer L, Rabanal R, Domingo M, et al: Identification of leishmania amastigotes in canine tissues by immunoperoxidase staining. *Res Vet Sci* 44:194–196, 1988.

25. Yamaguchi RA, French RQ, Aimpaon CF: *Leishmania donovani* in the synovial fluid of a dog with visceral leishmaniasis. *J Am Anim Hosp Assoc* 19:723–726, 1983.

25a. Harith AE, Slappendel RJ, Reiter I, et al: Application of a direct agglutination test for detection of specific anti-*Leishmania* antibodies to the canine reservoir. *J Clin Microbiol* 27:2252–2257, 1989.

25b. Jaffe CL, Zalis M: Use of purified parasite proteins from *Leishmania donovani* for the rapid serodiagnosis of visceral leishmaniasis. *J Infect Dis* 157:1212–1220, 1988.

26. Reiter I, Kretzschmar A, Boch J, et al: Leishmaniasis in dogs. Clinical course of infection, diagnosis and therapy following experimental infection of beagles with *Leishmania donovani*. *Berl Munch Tierarztl Wochensch* 98:40–44, 1985.

27. Chapman WL, Hanson WL, Alving CR, et al: Antileishmanial activity of liposome-encapsulated meglumine antimonate in the dog. *Am J Vet Res* 45:1028–1030, 1984.

27a. Mukhopadhyay A, Chaudhuri G, Arora SK, et al: Receptor-mediated drug delivery to macrophages in chemotherapy of leishmaniasis. *Science* 244:705–707, 1989.

27b. Murray WH, Nathan CF: In vitro killing of intracellular visceral *Leishmania donovani* by a macrophage-targeted hydrogen-generating system. *J Infect Dis* 158:1372–1375, 1988.

28. Craig TM: Personal communication. Texas A & M University, College Station, TX, 1988.

29. Monjour L, Monjour E, Vovldoukis I, et al: Protective immunity against cutaneous leishmaniasis achieved by partly purified vaccine in a volunteer. *Lancet* 1:1490, 1986.

30. Ogunkolade BW, Vouldoukis I, Frommel D, et al: Immunization of dogs with a *Leishmania infantum* derived vaccine. *Vet Parasitol* 28:33–41, 1988.

31. Kirmse P, Mahin L, Lahrech TM: Canine leishmaniasis in Morocco with special reference to infantile kala-azar. *Trans R Soc Trop Med Hyp* 81:212–213, 1987.

80 HEPATOZOONOSIS

Thomas M. Craig

ETIOLOGY AND EPIDEMIOLOGY

Hepatozoon canis infects dogs throughout Africa, southern Europe, and Asia, including the Middle East and islands of the Pacific and Indian oceans where the tick vector, *Rhipicephalus sanguineus*, is found. In the United States, hepatozoonosis was initially described in the Texas Gulf Coast; however, its apparent range appears to be wider since infected dogs have been reported from Louisiana[1] and Oklahoma.[2]

The geographic distribution of *H. canis* in the Eastern Hemisphere is essentially that of *R. sanguineus*. In the Western Hemisphere, *R. sanguineus* has adapted to urban environments, but many reported cases are from rural or suburban areas and other vectors may be implicated.[3]

H. canis is classified in the family Haemogregarinidae, order Eucoccidiida, class Sporozoasida in the phylum Apicomplexa. Although some authors consider each host to have separate species of *Hepatozoon*, others describe infections in nondomestic Felidae and other carnivores as caused by *H. canis*. Rodents are the most commonly infected group of mammals, although infection has also been reported in marsupials, insectivores, and ungulates.

The life cycle of *H. canis*, as it is currently understood, is similar to that of other *Hepatozoon* species (Fig. 80–1).[4] The primary vector tick for *H. canis*, *R. sanguineus*, ingests isogamonts, which have also been described as macrogamonts and microgamonts, in monocytes or neutrophils as part of its blood meal. Syngamy occurs in the gut of the tick. The ookinete (zygote) penetrates the gut wall and sporogony occurs in the hemocoelom of the tick. The oocyst that is formed consists of numerous sporocysts each containing 12 to 24 sporozoites. There is no evidence that the sporozoites migrate to the salivary gland or mouth parts of the

tick, so, to become infected, the dog must ingest the tick. After the tick is ingested the sporozoites are released, penetrate the dog's intestinal wall, and are carried by blood or lymph to mononuclear phagocyte or endothelial cells of the spleen, bone marrow, lungs, liver, or muscle, where merogony occurs.

Meronts have been found in a number of tissues, predominantly the lung, myocardium, and skeletal muscle, and have also been detected in the liver, spleen, and lymph nodes. A cyst is a thick-walled structure containing a meront (macromeronts or micromeronts), which develops into merozoites. Macromeronts and micromeronts have been described, although the relationships of the various stages of meront development are uncertain. Macromeronts may produce a few large merozoites, which become meronts. Micromeronts may, in turn, produce a large number of micromerozoites, giving rise to gamonts in leukocytes. Meront and cystic stages described in the Texas strain of *Hepatozoon* varied from those previously described; however, forms resembling both macromeronts and micromeronts have been found.[5]

Two types of vertebrate hosts are recognized. In one type (predator host), all stages of the organism (meronts, gamonts, and endogenous cysts) are formed. In the other type (prey host), only cysts are formed.[6] When sporozoites enter the predacious host, meronts are formed. These meronts give rise to either gamonts, which in turn infect arthropods, or long-lived cysts, which can be freed from the host only if it is eaten. The host with only the cyst forms cannot infect arthropods but may serve as a source of infection for an animal that preys on it.

Although transmission of *H. canis* to the dog usually occurs via ingestion of the vector tick, there may be other means. Disease has not resulted from SC or IP inoculation of

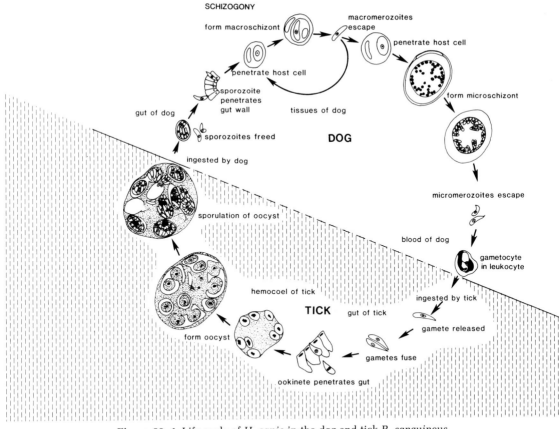

Figure 80–1. Life cycle of *H. canis* in the dog and tick *R. sanguineus*.

tissues or blood from infected dogs,[4] but inoculation of emulsified ticks will transmit the organism.

Various vectors have been incriminated in the transmission of *Hepatozoon* in other hosts. If vectors that fed on one host are eaten by another host, the second host may become infected by an unusual species of *Hepatozoon*. Vector or cyst ingestion with predation seems a likely method of transmission in the case of carnivorous hosts.

The host range of *H. canis* in mammalian carnivores includes the domestic dog, jackals, coyote, fox, hyena, lion, leopard, genet, palm civet, and cheetah.[7–10] *Hepatozoon* species isolated from other feline hosts include those from ocelots and bobcats.[3,11] The relationships among carnivorous hosts of *Hepatozoon* and their common arthropod vectors are uncertain.

PATHOGENESIS

Observations of naturally and experimentally infected dogs indicate that the hepato-

zoonosis syndrome is complex and factors other than the presence of the organism are necessary to induce the clinical syndrome. Concurrent infection or immunosuppression appears to be important inasmuch as experimentally infected dogs have been given glucocorticoids or have been from a litter of puppies having congenital defects in their neutrophil function. The age of the dog at the time of infection apparently influences clinical manifestations, especially that of periosteal bone proliferation. Susceptibility may also be related to age since dogs older than 4 to 6 months are resistant to experimental infection.

The progression of the infection in dogs from ingestion of sporozoites in the tick until the onset of clinical signs has not been well studied. A bloody diarrhea beginning 2 or 3 days postinoculation (PI) lasted for 2 days to 2 weeks in 50% of experimentally infected dogs.[12] An elevated rectal temperature initially occurred on day 7 PI and remained elevated for 24 weeks. The lymph nodes became visibly swollen 3 weeks PI. Leukocytosis occurred 4 weeks PI, as did ocular discharge and cachexia.

The progression of the various tissue stages of the organism is not known. The first recognizable meronts, seen approximately 2 months PI, were well developed. Amyloid deposits have occurred in multiple organs, and vasculitis and glomerulonephritis have developed in fatal cases, which suggests that immune complexes may be important in the pathogenesis of disease.[13] Humoral immunity is stimulated by *H. canis*,[14] but there is no evidence that antibodies are protective, and instead they may predispose to immune-complex formation.

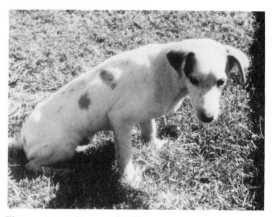

Figure 80–2. Six-month-old terrier mix with hepatozoonosis. Notice the extreme emaciation and "master's voice" posture.

CLINICAL FINDINGS

Some authors consider *H. canis* infections in Africa to be nonsymptomatic and any observed signs should be attributed to other infectious agents.[1,15] In these multiple infections it is questionable which agent gives rise to clinical signs. Intermittent fever and emaciation are two clinical signs reported most frequently.[13,15a,16] Other signs such as anemia, diarrhea, anorexia, and paraparesis or paraparalysis have been noted in some reports.[16a] The syndrome associated with the Texas strain of *H. canis* seems to be clinically distinct, even if other infections are concurrently seen in the affected dogs.

Fever (unresponsive to antibiotics), cachexia, depression, muscular hyperesthesia (especially noticeable over the paraspinal regions), purulent ocular and nasal discharges, mild anemia, and occasionally bloody diarrhea were seen in most of the cases.[13]

Hyperesthesia has been manifest by a reluctance to move, and cervical and trunk rigidity and probably resulted from periosteal reaction and muscle inflammation. The dogs often assumed a "master's voice" stance (Fig. 80–2). Pain, particularly in the lumbar region, may resemble that in traumatic or degenerative disease of the spine. Because of fever, lumbar pain, and leukocytosis, a few cases initially were suspected of having pyelonephritis.

The course of the disease often has been prolonged, with periods of apparent remission interspersed with episodes of fever and pain. In responding cases, the periods of remission become longer and the painful episodes occur less often. In fatal cases, the reverse seemed to be true. Perhaps the most unusual observation of this chronic febrile disease has been the normal appetite exhibited by many dogs until near the time of death.

In dogs that appear to be in a state of remission, using glucocorticoids or allowing noninfected *R. sanguineus* to feed on the dog usually results in recurrence of a febrile episode within a few days. A few days following the cessation of glucocorticoids or removal of ticks, the dogs again may go into remission. Dogs apparently may overcome the clinical disease spontaneously, even though organisms may still be found in their tissues years later.

DIAGNOSIS

Clinical Laboratory Findings

An elevated leukocyte count is typical of the naturally occurring disease, with the count ranging from 20,000 to 200,000 cells/μl.[2,13,17,18] Infection with the Texas strain is usually associated with a neutrophilia with an occasional left shift.[13,18] In other cases, a normal leukocyte count with an increase in eosinophils of up to 20% of the total leukocyte count has been found. A mild regenerative anemia has been a consistent finding with reported cases of hepatozoonosis.

Abnormalities of serum chemistry include lowered glucose and albumin concentrations and increased serum alkaline phosphatase (ALP) activity and inorganic phosphorus concentration.[13,18] Slight alterations in other serum constituents, such as elevated BUN concentration, have been encountered. The most consistent abnormalities have been the low serum glucose concentration and increased ALP activity. The extremely low (10 to 15 mg/dl) glucose concentration is considered to be an artifact of the extreme neutrophilia and its effect on increasing glucose catabolism from the time of collection until the time of serum separation; this may be overcome by collection of blood in sodium fluoride.[14]

Radiography

Radiographic findings may be spectacular or nonexistent. Periosteal bone proliferation was associated with the attachment of muscle on most bones of the body except the skull[17] (Figs. 80–3 and 80–4). Bony changes have been noted in the vertebrae, pelvis, radius, ulna, humerus, femur, fibula, and tibia. Not all infected dogs develop this unique lesion. Radiographic lesions are more common in younger dogs (<1 year) than in older dogs. It is not known at this time whether the radiographic changes are associated with rapid skeletal growth or indicative of a more severe infection in the young.

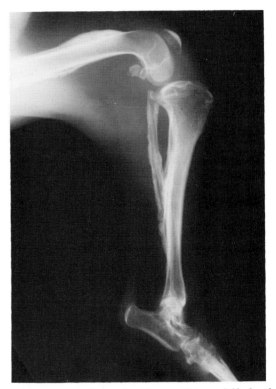

Figure 80–4. Radiograph of femur, tibia, and fibula of dog infected with *H. canis.*

Cytology and Biopsy

A definitive diagnosis of *H. canis* infection can be made if the organism is found in Romanovsky's-stained blood films. The gamonts, found in both neutrophils and monocytes, stain an ice-blue color with Giemsa or Leishman's stain (Fig. 80–5). Parasites, especially in low concentrations, can be better identified with special staining, which is

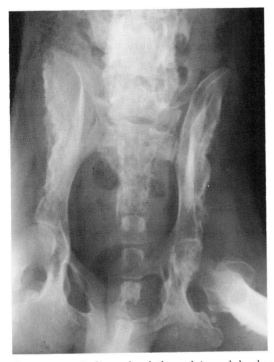

Figure 80–3. Radiograph of the pelvis and lumbar vertebrae of a dog with periosteal new bone proliferation associated with *H. canis.*

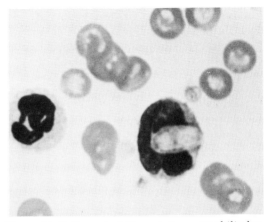

Figure 80–5. Gamont of *H. canis* in neutrophilic leukocyte on a peripheral blood smear (Giemsa stain; × 1200).

unfortunately time consuming.[19] If films are not made shortly after blood collection, many gamonts appear to leave host cells and a nonstaining capsule is all that remains. Unless the capsules are present in great numbers, they can easily be overlooked. Although other reports indicate higher parasitemias,[16,20] usually the gamonts of the Texas strain are very difficult to find in peripheral blood films.[17] When a dog does have a detectable parasitemia, only 1 or 2 cells per 1000 leukocytes are infected.

Muscle biopsy is a convenient means of establishing a diagnosis of hepatozoonosis. Both macromeronts and micromeronts are located in the muscles of dogs infected with the Texas strain.

PATHOLOGIC FINDINGS

The consistent gross lesion of dogs infected with *H. canis* is cachexia. Muscle atrophy is especially evident in the temporal region. Dogs are often anemic and may have an enlarged liver and spleen. There may be pulmonary congestion, lymphadenopathy, congestion of the gastric mucosa, and pale kidneys.

Microscopically, meronts have been found in the skeletal and cardiac muscles, lymph nodes, spleen, liver, kidneys, or skin of various hosts. Meronts are named for the size of the merozoites that they contain: the micromeront, which contains micromerozoites, is actually larger than a macromeront. The vast majority of organisms that have been identified in the tissues of infected dogs are micromeronts. Micromeronts with a characteristic wheel-spoke pattern have not been seen in the canine cases from the Texas Gulf Coast. Instead, large cysts similar to those described in Felidae[7] have been found. A cyst-like micromeront averaging 250 μm in diameter is a unique stage that is seen with the Texas infections (Fig. 80–6). This structure contains a nucleus (15 to 60 × 30 to 90 μm) surrounded by bluish, mucinous, or often granular material and fine laminar membranes (Fig. 80–6).

Occasionally, accumulations of small structures are seen which may represent developing macromeronts (Fig. 80–7). The individual structures are approximately 10 μm in diameter with the total grouping about the size of a cyst (250 μm). Whether a cyst

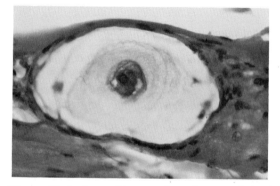

Figure 80–6. Cyst with central nucleus in skeletal muscle. The nucleus is surrounded by fine laminar membranes (H and E; × 1200).

always gives rise to multiple macromeronts is unknown.

Pyogranulomas composed of macrophages and neutrophils are seen in the muscle, but there is no evidence of encapsulation, and inflammatory cells are often seen in fascial planes away from the organism. The granulomas are similar to those seen in Chagas' disease (see American Trypanosomiasis, Chapter 78), from which hepatozoonosis must be differentiated. During the growth and maturation of the meront there is no inflammatory response. However, on release of merozoites, an intense granulomatous response, composed of equal numbers of macrophages and neutrophils with varying numbers of eosinophils, is seen. Few lymphocytes or plasma cells are associated with the lesions, and giant cells have not been found. In tissues, especially the muscles, there are large accumulations of neutrophils, which may account for the pain, fever, and stimulation of periosteal bone proliferation (Fig. 80–8).

The Texas strain has a predilection for

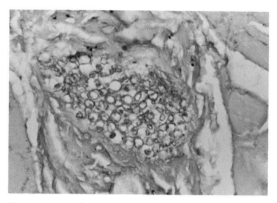

Figure 80–7. Skeletal muscle with developing macromeronts (H and E; × 400).

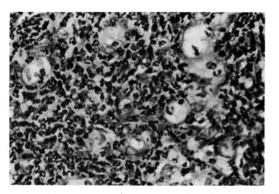

Figure 80–8. Pyogranuloma, thought to be associated with the invasion of a group of macromeronts of *H. canis*. Several meronts, each containing one to three macromerozoites, are incorporated within the granuloma (H and E; × 1200).

cardiac muscles; however, organisms are numerous in skeletal muscle and, occasionally, the smooth muscle of the intestine. The organism has not been observed in the liver or kidneys and only rarely in spleen, lymph nodes, or skin of dogs infected with the Texas strain. The granulomatous response to the Texas strain of *H. canis* appears to be more striking than that ascribed to others.

The cause of death has not always been established in fatal cases of hepatozoonosis. As noted previously, amyloidosis and immune-complex disorders may develop. Concomitant diseases or, in other cases, the chronic progressive debilitation leads to a point of cachexia and death.

THERAPY

Several antiprotozoal agents have been used in an effort to control hepatozoonosis, although none are known to cause an improvement in the clinical outcome of the infection even though parasitemias may be reduced (Table 80–1). Clearance of blood forms has been found with imidocarb dipropionate.[21] The response to imidocarb therapy has been inconsistent, both with and without other chemotherapeutic agents.[13b] Treatment with diminazene aceturate was followed by a remission of clinical signs, although drug therapy may have been coincidental to recovery.[17] Treatment of hepatozoonosis with a combination of oxytetracycline and primaquine resulted in recovery of a cat.[23] A combination of tetracycline and imidocarb was reported to cause a clinical remission and clearance of a parasitemia;

however, at least some of the dogs so treated were concurrently infected with *Ehrlichia canis*.[16] Whether the response was a direct effect of the drug on *Hepatozoon* or an indirect effect on *Ehrlichia* is unknown. Primaquine phosphate has also been used with apparent success in dogs when given PO or IM.[22] This drug is being evaluated for its effect on clinical hepatozoonosis.

Toltrazuril, a coccidiostat (see Miscellaneous Drugs, Chapter 77), has been administered to voles, and it protected them from experimental hepatozoonosis but did not clear them of infection.[23a] The drug is safe for use in dogs, but there is no data on its effect on *H. canis*.

The criteria for effectiveness of a drug in a disease like hepatozoonosis are difficult to ascertain because of the chronicity of the bone and muscle lesions.

Symptomatic palliative treatment with nonsteroidal anti-inflammatory agents seems to be the most important aspect of therapy at this time. Drugs such as aspirin, phenylbutazone, or flunixin seem to be of value in relieving discomfort in clinical cases. In many instances, administration of these drugs will provide clinical relief, and the owner can adjust the dosage and frequency of administration to the reappearance of clinical signs.[13] Each individual dog seems to respond to palliative treatment uniquely, and the ideal treatment must be adjusted depending on the degree of pain and extent of side effects caused by treatment. Glucocorticoids give temporary clinical relief[17] but should probably be avoided for long-term therapy as they apparently exacerbate the disease.[4]

PREVENTION

Control of ticks by routine dipping of dogs from infected premises is important to limit the spread of disease. The transmission of *H. canis* occurs transstadially or by male ticks; transovarial transmission is unknown. Therefore, environmental control of the vector and keeping it from feeding on infected dogs will help to break the chain of spread. Home or kennel environments should be sprayed on a routine basis. Regular dipping of dogs in infected premises will kill any of the three stages of the tick feeding at that time.

If vectors other than *R. sanguineus* are

Table 80–1. Antiprotozoal Therapy for Hepatozoonosis[a]

DRUG	SPECIES	DOSE[b] (mg/kg)	ROUTE	INTERVAL (hours)	DURATION (days)
Diminazene aceturate[17]	D[c]	3.5	IM	24	1
Imidocarb dipropionate[21]	D	5	SC	24	1
Imidocarb dipropionate[16]	D	6	SC	14 days	
and					
tetracycline		22	PO	8	14
Primaquine phosphate[22]	D	0.5	SC	Once	
Primaquine phosphate[23]	C	2	PO	Once	
and					
oxytetracycline		50	PO	12	7
Toltrazuril	B[d]	5–10	SC, PO	24	3–5

[a]Drugs may clear parasitemia but do not always reverse clinical signs of infection. Supportive anti-inflammatory therapy may be needed. See text. D = dog, C = cat; B = dog and cat; IM = intramuscular, SC = subcutaneous, PO = oral.

[b]Dose per administration at specified interval, expressed as mg/kg unless otherwise stated.

[c]Clinical response, no change in parasitemia.

[d]Dose extrapolated from studies in rodents and with use of the drug in treating other protozoal infections. See also Tables 86–1 and 87–2.

involved, they will have to be identified for control programs to be instituted. In a few instances where the disease was recognized, careful scrutiny of the dog's home environment failed to reveal *R. sanguineus*.[14] Kissing bugs (family Reduviidae) were found, but no oocysts of *H. canis* have been recovered from these insects. Large numbers of *Dermacentor variabilis*, American dog ticks, were associated with bobcats and ocelots infected with *Hepatozoon* sp.[3] Further research into the potential vectors of this disease is required.

Until the development of an effective antiprotozoal agent and a serologic test that is sensitive enough to identify inapparent carriers, the prevention of hepatozoonosis will be largely a matter of controlling known vectors. Direct transmission via predation seems less likely in infected house pets; however, it may have a role in the spread of infection in wildlife hosts. Control of wildlife reservoir hosts is unlikely to be successful.

PUBLIC HEALTH CONSIDERATIONS

Infection with *Hepatozoon* sp. was described in a patient with occasional chills, anemia, and jaundice in the Philippines.[24] Hypersegmentation of the nucleus of unparasitized neutrophils, as is seen in many canine infections, was noted in this case. Morphologically the gamonts resemble *H. canis*, but the identification is far from certain. Whether the scarcity of reports of in-

fection in people is due to the rarity of instances in which they ingest suitable vectors or is due to natural resistance is unknown. Attempts to infect primates experimentally are not known.

References

1. Gossett KA, Gaunt SD, Aja DS: Hepatozoonosis and ehrlichiosis in a dog. *J Am Anim Hosp Assoc* 21:265–267, 1985.
2. Baker JL, Craig TM, Barton CL, et al: *Hepatozoon canis* in a dog with oral pyogranulomas and neurologic disease. *Cornell Vet* 78:179–183, 1988.
3. Mercer SH, Jones LP, Rappole JH, et al: *Hepatozoon* sp in wild carnivores in Texas. *J Wildl Dis* 24:574–576, 1988.
4. Nordgren RM, Craig TM: Experimental transmission of the Texas strain of *Hepatozoon canis*. *Vet Parasitol* 16:207–214, 1984.
5. Craig TM, Jones LP, Nordgren RM: Diagnosis of *Hepatozoon canis* by muscle biopsy. *J Am Anim Hosp Assoc* 20:301–303, 1984.
6. Landau I: A comparison of the life cycles of *Toxoplasma* and *Hepatozoon*, with reference to the general phenomenon and the role of cyst formation in the coccidia. *Ann Trop Med Parasitol* 67:403–407, 1973.
7. McCulley RM, Basson PA, Bigalke RD, et al: Observations on naturally acquired hepatozoonosis of wild carnivores and dogs in the Republic of South Africa. *Onderstepoort J Vet Res* 42:117–134, 1975.
8. Klopfer U, Nobel TA, Neumann F: *Hepatozoon*-like parasite (schizonts) in the myocardium of the domestic cat. *Vet Pathol* 10:185–190, 1973.
9. Ewing GO: Granulomatous cholangiohepatitis in a cat due to protozoan parasite resembling *Hepatozoon canis*. *Feline Pract* 7:37–40, 1977.
10. Maede Y, Ohsugi T: Hepatozoon infection in a wild fox (*Vulpes vulpes schrenchi*, Kishida) in Japan. *Jpn J Vet Sci* 44:137–142, 1982.
11. Lane JR, Kocan AA: *Hepatozoon* sp infection in bobcats. *J Am Vet Med Assoc* 183:1323–1324, 1983.

12. Nordgren RM: Experimental infection of *Hepatozoon canis* in the dog. MS Thesis, Texas A&M University, College Station, TX, 1981.

13. Barton CL, Russo EA, Craig TM, et al: Canine hepatozoonosis: a retrospective study of 15 naturally occurring cases. *J Am Anim Hosp Assoc* 21:125–134, 1985.

14. Nordgren RM: Personal communication. Texas A&M University, College Station, Texas, 1982.

15. Ogunkoya AB, Adeyanju JB, Aliu YO: Experiences with the use of imizol in treating canine blood parasites in Nigeria. *J Small Anim Pract* 22:775–777, 1981.

15a. Ezekoli CD, Ogunkoya Ab, Abdullahi R, et al: Clinical and epidemiological studies on canine hepatozoonosis in Zaria, Nigeria. *J Small Anim Pract* 24:455–460, 1983.

16. Elias E, Homans PA: *Hepatozoon canis* infection in dogs: clinical and haematological findings; treatment. *J Small Anim Pract* 29:55–62, 1988.

16a. Beaufils JP, Martin-Gravel J, Bertrand F: Hepatozoonose canine 2ᵉ porte. A propos de 28 cas. *Pratiq Med Chirug L'anim Cie* 23:281–293, 1988.

17. Craig TM, Smallwood JE, Knauer KW, et al: *Hepatozoon canis* infection in dogs: clinical, radiographic and hematologic findings. *J Am Vet Med Assoc* 173:967–972, 1978.

18. Gaunt PS, Gaunt SD, Craig TM: Extreme neutrophilic leukocytosis in a dog with hepatozoonosis. *J Am Vet Med Assoc* 182:409–410, 1983.

19. Mercer SH, Craig TM: Comparison of various staining procedures in the identification of *Hepatozoon canis* gamonts. *Vet Clin Pathol* 17:63–65, 1988.

20. Rajamanickam C, Wiesenhutter E, Zin FMD, et al: The incidence of canine haematozoa in peninsular Malaysia. *Vet Parasitol* 17:151–157, 1984/85.

21. Ogunkoya AB, Adeyanju JB, Aliu YO: Experiences with the use of imizol in treating canine blood parasites in Nigeria. *J Small Anim Pract* 22:775–777, 1981.

22. Potgeiter FT: Personal communication. Veterinary Research Institute, Onderstepoort, South Africa, 1982.

23. van Amstel S: Hepatozo'o'nose in n' Kat. *J S Afr Vet Assoc* 50:215–216, 1979.

23a. Krampitz HE, Haberkorn A: Experimental treatment of *Hepatozoon* infections with anticoccidial agent toltrazuril. *J Vet Med* 35:131–137, 1988.

24. Carlos ET, Cruz FB, Cabiles CC, et al: *Hepatozoon* sp in the WBC of a human patient. *Univ Philipp Vet* 15:5–7, 1971.

81 ENCEPHALITOZOONOSIS

J. R. Szabo
V. Pang
J. A. Shadduck

ETIOLOGY

Encephalitozoon cuniculi is a small (1.5 by 2.5 μm) intracellular parasite in cytoplasmic vacuoles of renal tubular epithelial cells, endothelial cells, tissue macrophages and less frequently, glial cells, myocytes, and hepatocytes. *E. cuniculi* undergoes asexual division within the host cell, and five major forms of the microsporidian are recognized (Fig. 81–1). The spore is a resistant, extracellular structure, the contents of which are extruded through the polar filament. The sporoplasm, which is released, is round (700 to 800 μm in diameter) with a large nucleus. It is confined within a single, limiting membrane and is considered the infective particle for a new cell. Once intracellular, the parasite develops into a schizont, one of two proliferative stages. Schizonts have two distinct nuclei, the characteristic that distinguishes *E. cuniculi* from other microsporidia such as *Nosema*. Schizonts either divide by binary fission to form more schizonts or mature into the next proliferative stage, the sporont, a thick-walled structure detached from the wall of the parasitophorous vacuole. Sporonts divide only once and then mature into sporoblasts, which have a thicker outer membrane than sporonts, a single nucleus, and a developing polar filament. Sporoblasts develop into ovoid spores, which possess one nucleus, a polaroplast, a polar cap, and a polar filament (Fig. 81–2). In the case of the kidney, these are released into the renal tubular lumen and are passed in the urine.

EPIDEMIOLOGY

Natural infection with *E. cuniculi* has been reported sporadically in dogs, foxes,

domestic cats, and wild carnivores. Widespread and marked economic loss attributable to *E. cuniculi* infection in farm-reared blue-fox cubs in Nordic countries suggests that the blue fox may be extremely sensitive to encephalitozoonosis.

The method by which microsporidia naturally infect animals is presently unknown, but the most likely route is oronasal from contaminated urine. Neonatal dogs may ingest spores by suckling urine-contaminated mammae of a bitch harboring *E. cuniculi*, or they may be infected in utero. Infection also may occur through ingestion of tissues from rabbits or mice with latent encephalitozoonosis. Experimentally, animals can be infected orally and by intracranial, intravenous, or intraperitoneal injection. Host factors must be important in determining the course of the disease since infection is not consistently produced following ingestion of spores. Canine encephalitozoonosis occurs primarily as a kennel problem when large numbers of animals are confined and less intensive sanitation procedures are used compared with those for the household pet.

CLINICAL FINDINGS

Dogs

A plethora of signs is present in dogs infected with *E. cuniculi*, depending upon the time course and location of tissue damage. Clinical signs in the neonate appear within a few weeks postpartum, and several pups in a litter may be affected with stunted growth and general unthriftiness. As the course of the infection progresses, animals show signs of renal failure and neurologic abnormalities such as depression, ataxia,

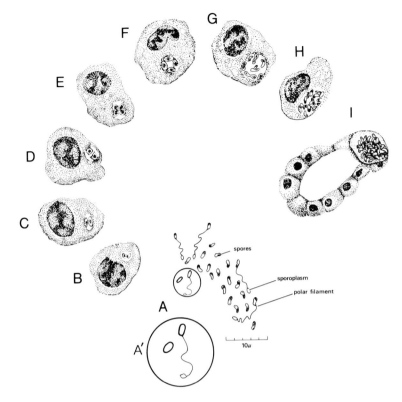

Figure 81–1. Diagram of the intracellular life cycle of *E. cuniculi* in a renal tubular epithelial cell. The diagram is based on light and electron microscopic examination of parasites. *A*, Mature spores, some with sporoplasm extruded by means of the polar filament. *B* to *G*, Proliferative forms of the parasite (schizonts) in parasitophorous vacuole. Binary fission occurs in contact with the membrane of the vacuole. As maturation progresses, spores collect in the center of the vacuole. *H* to *I*, Parasitophorous vacuole containing spores and proliferative forms. These stages are visible under the light microscope. The vacuole (*I*) ruptures and releases its spores (*A*) into the renal tubule lumen. *A′*, Enlargement showing how sporoplasm is attached to the spore by means of the polar filament.

convulsions, and blindness. Animals may develop signs of aggressive behavior, consisting of viciousness, biting, and abnormal vocalization. Sera from dogs with azotemia have a higher frequency of anti–*E. cuniculi* antibodies than a control group, suggesting that *E. cuniculi* may contribute to chronic renal disease in the dog.[2]

Cats

Clinical signs in feline encephalitozoonosis are variable. Severe muscle spasms, depression, paralysis, and death have been found in natural infections;[3,4] however, kittens experimentally infected by the authors of this chapter showed no clinical signs.[5] Superficial corneal infection with blepharospasm represents an unusual site of infection and course of the disease.[6]

DIAGNOSIS

Clinical laboratory findings are not available for feline encephalitozoonosis, and those abnormalities seen in infected dogs

are nonspecific. A normochromic, normocytic anemia is a consistent finding and may result from severe renal lesions with depression of erythropoietin production. In contrast, leukocytes, especially lymphocytes and monocytes, are increased. Bone marrows in experimentally infected animals are hypercellular, with a preponderance of large mononuclear cells. Serum biochemical findings reflect tissue damage caused by parasite replication. Increases in ALT (formerly SGPT) and serum ALP activities are expected; however, increases may be only high normal or slightly above reference range. BUN and creatinine values are variable but are usually increased in animals with severe renal lesions.[7] Increases in total serum proteins have been seen in infected Canidae. No individual serum fraction dominates the general increase in serum proteins in dogs. In blue foxes, however, the immunoglobulin fraction is selectively increased, which may reflect polyclonal activation of lymphocytes.

Analysis of CSF may be abnormal in those animals displaying behavioral and neurologic signs with increased protein and nucleated cell concentrations. Immunoglobulin-specific *E. cuniculi* is present in the CSF,

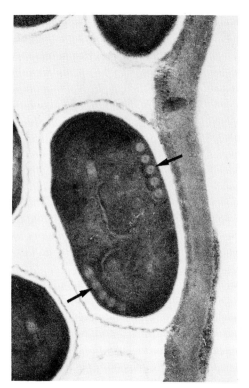

Figure 81–2. Cross-section of a mature spore of *E. cuniculi.* Polar filaments (*arrows*) and electron-lucent spore wall are demonstrated. The sporoplasm is contained within the electron-dense material, although it does not appear in the micrograph (lead citrate/uranyl acetate; × 35,000). (From Shadduck JA et al: *Vet Pathol* 15:449–460, 1978. Reprinted with permission.)

although usually at titers lower than in the serum.

On urinalysis, hematuria and pyuria may be present. Spores shed into the urine from parasitized renal tubular epithelial cells are readily identifiable in the sediment with either Gram or Ziehl-Neelsen staining.[8] Stained spores are gram-positive, whereas the proliferative stages are gram-negative. When viewed with cross-polarizing filters, *Encephalitozoon* and other microsporidia are birefringent in appearance, unlike the coccidians, *Toxoplasma* and *Isospora*.[8a] Positive identification requires use of a direct or an indirect immunochemical procedure (Fig. 81–3).

Serologic Testing

Intradermal testing, an in vivo assay for cell-mediated immunity, works reasonably well in determining infection in rabbits and mice but not in dogs, so that serologic testing

is required. Antibody directed by IFA against *E. cuniculi* is seen as early as 3 days postinoculation (PI) in experimentally infected dogs (Fig. 81–3). Inoculated dogs produce an IgM response to *E. cuniculi* for the first 1.5 months PI.[8b] Thereafter, titers decline and are indistinguishable from the background fluorescence associated with lower dilutions of canine sera. IgG titers are increased within a few days PI, corresponding to the IgM increase, but the IgG titers remain elevated for at least 1 year. In contrast, infected cats develop low titers 2 weeks PI with increased titers only 4 to 5 weeks PI.[5] The immunofluorescence and dot-ELISA tests are fairly sensitive and specific tests for canine encephalitozoonosis.[9,10,10a] Titers vary with each testing laboratory; however, the authors consider a reciprocal IgG-IFA titer of ≥ 20 to indicate past or present infection and titers of > 40 are considered to be diagnostic of active canine encephalitozoonosis.[9] Serologic observations must be critically examined and correlated with clinical observations owing to the fact that *E. cuniculi* has been shown to cross-react with antibodies to other microsporidia.[11] See Appendix 8 for a listing of diagnostic laboratories that perform these tests.

PATHOLOGIC FINDINGS

Gross lesions of canine encephalitozoonosis vary from animal to animal, reflecting the degree of individual organ involvement. Hepatomegaly and petechiae throughout the surface of multiple organs are commonly found. Other frequently detected lesions are

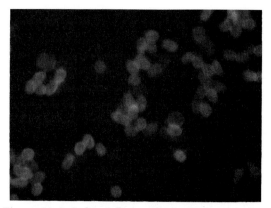

Figure 81–3. Indirect fluorescent antibody test of *E. cuniculi* spores in urine sediment (fluorescein isothiocyanate; × 2400).

patchy consolidation of lung parenchyma, pulmonary edema, fibrinous pericarditis, regional enteritis, focal myocardial degeneration, swollen kidneys, hemorrhagic cystitis, and splenomegaly. In the kidney, lesions may be as mild as cortical petechiae or as severe as renal cortical cysts or infarcts (Fig. 81–4). Similarly, gross brain lesions may be absent or as severe as thrombosis of meningeal blood vessels and focal encephalomalacia. Resolution of a focus of encephalomalacia may result in cystic spaces within the brain parenchyma. Certain gross lesions reported with greater frequency in naturally infected blue foxes include nodular thickening of the extramural coronary arteries, fibrinous hemopericarditis, renal infarcts, splenomegaly, lymphadenopathy, and microhemorrhages in the meninges and choroid plexus.

Histologically, dogs and blue foxes with encephalitozoonosis consistently have nonsuppurative meningoencephalitis. Lesions may range from parasitophorous vacuoles without an inflammatory reaction to glial nodules of microglia and astrocytes to mononuclear perivascular cuffs and multifocal granulomas (Fig. 81–5). Organisms may reside in neurons or more commonly in endothelial cells, where at times they appear to occlude the lumina of blood vessels. Fibrinoid necrosis of small- and medium-sized arteries of the brain can result in thrombosis and encephalomalacia.[12] Nonsuppurative meningitis is found in conjunction with parenchymal lesions. Venous thrombosis occurs in the larger veins of the leptomeninges

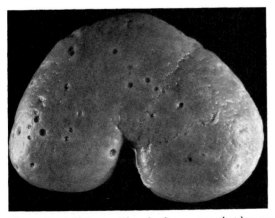

Figure 81–4. Kidney with pale, firm cortex that has an irregular subcapsular surface and numerous projecting cysts filled with clear fluid. (From Shadduck JA et al: *Vet Pathol* 15:449–460 1978. Reprinted with permission.)

and extends to the vessels of the more superficial sulci and gyri.

Nonsuppurative interstitial nephritis is a consistent histologic feature of encephalitozoonosis in dogs, cats, and foxes. The canine renal lesions consist of plasma cells, lymphocytes, macrophages, and epithelioid cells in the interstitium adjacent to the cortex and extending to the renal pelvis. Foxes have an acute to chronic nonsuppurative interstitial nephritis that with time progresses to interstitial fibrosis. Experimentally infected cats have mild to moderate interstitial nephritis, consisting of lymphoplasmacytic infiltrates in the interstitium.[5]

Focal myocardial necrosis, vasculitis, and fibrinoid necrosis of small and medium-sized arteries occur. Within arteries undergoing fibrinoid necrosis, E. cuniculi organisms are evident in endothelial cells and smooth muscle cells. Polymorphonuclear leukocyte infiltrates are seen early in the course of infection; however, older lesions consist of mononuclear cell aggregations, predominantly plasma cells, and a fibrocellular replacement of the muscle wall.

The authors have produced hepatic lesions in both dogs and cats experimentally infected with E. cuniculi. The parasites reside in hepatocytes and Kupffer and endothelial cells. The predominant parenchymal lesion consists of a mild to moderate lymphoplasmacytic infiltrate in periportal connective tissue. Focal hepatic necrosis is present. Nodular lesions, oriented along hepatic vessels, consist of fibrinoid necrosis with mononuclear cell infiltration in the media and adventitia and macroscopically and microscopically resemble periarteritis nodosa.

Ocular lesions in blue foxes include lens, choroidal, iridociliary, and retinal lesions and are attributable to arterial lesions of the short and long ciliary arteries and retinal vessels.[13] E. cuniculi organisms are within arterial lesions. Organisms can be demonstrated in situ by immunochemical techniques.[14]

Other organ systems of the dog, cat, and blue foxes are affected; however, these lesions are mild or nonspecific. Pulmonary edema, nonsuppurative interstitial pneumonia, lymphadenopathy, reticulo-endothelial hyperplasia in the spleen, infiltration of lymphocytes and macrophages into the intestinal lamina propria, and hyperplasia of the bone marrow have been found.

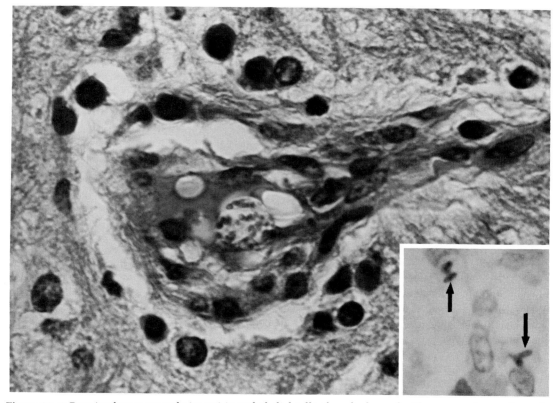

Figure 81–5. Parasitophorous vacuole (*arrow*) in endothelial cells of cerebral vessel with mononuclear perivascular cuff from a dog (H and E; × 1300). *Inset, E. cuniculi* spores (*arrows*) free in brain parenchyma of an experimentally infected kitten. Note the lack of an inflammatory response (Gram stain; × 2000). (From Shadduck JA et al: *Vet Pathol* 15:449–460, 1978. Reprinted with permission.)

THERAPY

Currently, no treatment exists for either canine or feline encephalitozoonosis. In vitro experiments demonstrate that the antibiotic fumagillin inhibits the replicative ability of the organism without damaging the host cell,[15] but the drug in its present formulation is toxic to animals.

PREVENTION AND PUBLIC HEALTH CONSIDERATION

Human microsporidiosis has been reported.[16,17] Antibodies to *E. cuniculi* (measured by IFA) have been reported in human sera,[18] but the importance of encephalitozoonosis as a zoonotic disease has been questioned.[19] Human infections with other genera of microsporidia have been reported with increasing frequency, especially in patients with AIDS.[20]

Sanitation is of the utmost importance in suspected encephalitozoonosis. Spores can readily be rendered uninfective by a variety of disinfectants; the most commonly available are 2% phenol, 10% formalin, and 70% ethyl alcohol.[21] Infectivity is unaffected by sonication, freezing and thawing, or by pH ranging from 4 to 9.[22] Infectivity of spores stored in neutral buffer at 4°C and 20°C is retained after 24 days, indicating spore survival is possible in a humid environment at ambient temperatures. In the event of encephalitozoon infection, serologic monitoring of contact animals is beneficial.

References

1. Shadduck JA, Bendele R, Robinson GT: Isolation of the causative organism of canine encephalitozoonosis. *Vet Pathol* 15:449–460, 1978.
2. Stewart CG, Reyers F, Synman H: The relationship between primary renal disease in dogs and antibodies to *Encephalitozoon cuniculi. J S Afr Vet Assoc* 59:19–21, 1989.
3. VanRensburg IBJ, DePlessis JL: Nosematosis in a cat: a case report. *J S Afr Vet Med Assoc* 42:327–331, 1971.

4. Varva J, Blazek K, Lavicka N, et al: Nosematosis in carnivores. J Parasitol 57:923–924, 1971.

5. Pang V, Shadduck JA: Susceptibility of cats, sheep, and swine to a rabbit isolate of Encephalitozoon cuniculi. Am J Vet Res 46:1071–1077, 1985.

6. Buyukmihci N, Bellhorn RW, Hunziker J, et al: Encephalitozoon (Nosema) infection in the cornea in a cat. J Am Vet Med Assoc 171:355–357, 1977.

7. Botha WS, Dormehl IC, Goosen DJ: Evaluation of kidney function in dogs suffering from canine encephalitozoonosis by standard clinical pathological and radiopharmaceutical techniques. J S Afr Vet Assoc 57:79–86, 1986.

8. Goodman DG, Garner FM: A comparison of methods for detecting Nosema cuniculi in rabbit urine. Lab Anim Sci 22:568–572, 1972.

8a. Tiner JD: Birefringent spores differentiate Encephalitozoon and other microsporidia from coccidia. Vet Pathol 25:227–230, 1988.

8b. Szabo JR, Shadduck JA: Immunologic and clinicopathologic evaluation of adult dogs with Encephalitozoon cuniculi. J Clin Microbiol 26:557–563, 1988.

9. Beckwith C, Peterson N, Liu JJ, et al: Dot enzyme-linked immunosorbent assay (dot-ELISA) for antibodies to Encephalitozoon cuniculi. Lab Anim Sci 38:573–576, 1988.

10. Hollister WS, Canning EU: An enzyme-linked immunosorbent assay (ELISA) for detection of antibodies to Encephalitozoon cuniculi and its use in determination of infections in man. Parasitology 94:209–219, 1987.

10a. Hollister WS, Canning EU, Viney M: Prevalence of antibodies to Encephalitozoon cunicula in stray dogs as determined by an ELISA. Vet Rec 124:332–336, 1989.

11. Niederkorn JY, Shadduck JA, Weidner E: Antigenic cross reactivity among different microsporidian spores as determined by immunofluorescence. J Parasitol 66:675–677, 1980.

12. Botha WS, Stewart CS, Van Dellen AF: Observations on the pathology of experimental encephalitozoonosis in dogs. J S Afr Vet Assoc 57:17–24, 1986.

13. Arnesen K, Nordstoga K: Ocular encephalitozoonosis (nosematosis) in blue foxes. Polyarteritis nodosa and cataract. Acta Ophthalmol (Copenh) 55:641–651, 1977.

14. Gannon J: The immunoperoxidase test diagnosis of Encephalitozoon cuniculi in rabbits. Lab Anim 12:125–127, 1978.

15. Shadduck JA: Effects of fumagillin on in vitro replication of Encephalitozoon cuniculi. J Protozool 27:202–208, 1980.

16. Connor DH, Strano AJ, Neafie RC: Nosema—a recently recognized pathogen of man. Lab Invest 30:371, 1974.

17. Sprague V: Nosema connori n. sp., a microsporidian parasite of man. Trans Am Microsc Soc 93:400–403, 1974.

18. Berqquist R, Morfeldt-Manssar L, Pehrson PO, et al: Antibody against Encephalitozoon cuniculi in Swedish homosexual men. Scand J Infect Dis 16:389–391, 1984.

19. Bywater JEC: Is encephalitozoonosis a zoonosis? Lab Anim 13:149–151, 1979.

20. Shadduck AJ: Human microsporidiosis and AIDS. Rev Infect Dis 11:203–207, 1989.

21. Waller T: Sensitivity of Encephalitozoon cuniculi to various temperatures, disinfectants, and drugs. Lab Anim 13:227–230, 1979.

22. Shadduck JA, Polley MB: Some factors influencing the in vitro infectivity and replication of Encephalitozoon cuniculi. J Protozool 25:491–496, 1978.

82

CYTAUXZOONOSIS
Ann B. Kier

ETIOLOGY AND EPIDEMIOLOGY

Cytauxzoonosis is a fatal blood protozoal disease of domestic cats in the United States that has been reported from several south central and southeastern states (Fig. 82–1). Cytauxzoonosis was first reported in a number of African ungulates, but the reservoir host for *Cytauxzoon felis*, the organism found in cats in the United States, is uncertain.

Cytauxzoon is classified in the order Piroplasmida and family Theileriidae. This family has both an erythrocytic and a leukocytic, or tissue, phase. In the case of *C. felis*, the leukocytic, or tissue, phase consists of large schizonts that develop within macrophages or monocytes,[1] while *Theileria*, a more familiar genus of this family, has its exoerythrocytic phase primarily within lymphocytes. No serologic cross-reactivity exists between *C. felis* and the South African parasites *Theileria taurotragi* and *Babesia felis*.[2]

Information concerning the life cycle of *Cytauxzoon* is limited. In infected cats, schizonts develop primarily within mononuclear phagocytes, first as indistinct vesicular structures within the cytoplasm of infected cells and later as mature, distinct, nucleated macroschizonts that actively undergo division by schizogony and binary fission. The phagocytes line the lumens of veins within almost every organ and become huge and numerous, often occluding the vessel like a thrombus. Multiplication of macroschizonts within host cells is observed ultrastructurally to be true schizogony, without host cell division. Later in the course of the disease, macroschizonts develop buds (merozoites) that separate off and eventually fill the entire host cell. The host cell probably ruptures, releasing the merozoites into the blood or tissue fluid. Merozoites appear in macrophages 1 to 3 days before they are observed in erythrocytes. These organisms,

which then invade uninfected erythrocytes, produce late-stage parasitemias, usually 1 to 3 days prior to death, that are detected on examination of blood films.[1]

The apparently sporadic occurrence, short course of illness, and consistently fatal nature of the disease in cats indicate that the domestic cat is likely an incidental dead-end host. Since the bobcat (*Lynx rufus*) is known to inhabit all of the geographic areas where the disease in the domestic cat has been reported, it could be implicated as being the natural host for *C. felis*. A survey of 20 wild-trapped bobcats in Oklahoma revealed a 60% prevalence of infection of erythrocytes by a piroplasm indistinguishable by light microscopy from the intraerythrocytic forms of the feline *Cytauxzoon* organisms.[3] Blood from these naturally infected bobcats when subinoculated into domestic cats did not however cause fatal cytauxzoonosis; rather, a persistent erythroparasitemia developed. The cats remained asymptomatic. In contrast, infections of bobcats induced by inoculation of tissues or blood collected from domestic cats in the final stages of the fatal disease have shown that bobcats will develop either a fatal or nonfatal form of the disease.[4] Attempts to infect numerous other domestic, laboratory, and wildlife species have been unsuccessful.[5]

Ticks likely are the natural vector for *Cytauxzoon* since most cases have been associated with the presence of ticks on the hosts, and most recently tick (*Dermacentor variabilis*) transmission between wild-caught, splenectomized bobcats with parasitemia and two splenectomized domestic cats was accomplished.[6] Both domestic cats died of the fatal form of the disease. In contrast, when blood from this same bobcat was inoculated directly into a domestic cat, a persistent but nonfatal erythroparasitemia developed. Thus, subinoculation of blood

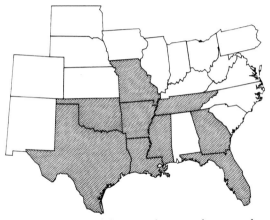

Figure 82–1. Distribution of reported cases of cytauxzoonosis in domestic cats. Cases have been reported in the states that are shaded.

from bobcats to cats appears to transmit only the erythrocytic piroplasm stage. The fatal form of the disease with extraerythrocytic stages develops only after tick transmission of the organism or inoculation of tissues from fatally infected cats.

PATHOGENESIS

Rapid multiplication of the tissue phase of the parasite may cause mechanical obstruction of blood flow, especially through the lungs. By-products of tissue parasites may be toxic, pyrogenic, and vasoactive, whereas the blood phase may induce destruction and phagocytosis of erythrocytes.[1] Infected cats appear to die from a shock-like state.

CLINICAL FINDINGS

In the naturally occurring disease, after an unknown incubation period, affected cats develop nonspecific clinical signs that lead to a rapid course of illness and death. Anorexia, dyspnea, lethargy, dehydration, depression, icterus and pallor, and high fever (39.4° to 41.6°C [103° to 107°F]) have been observed.[7] The percentage of parasitized erythrocytes during illness ranges from 1% to 4%. Mild to moderate regenerative anemias and variable leukocyte counts, occasionally with a left shift and thrombocytopenia, have been found.[8] The number of nucleated erythrocytes may increase slightly. Although BUN and ammonia concentrations

and hepatic enzyme activities may be elevated in febrile or comatose animals, they are not elevated earlier in the course of disease. Hemoglobinuria and bilirubinuria are only rarely observed.

Clinical signs in experimentally induced cytauxzoonosis have been similar to those of naturally occurring cases. Incubation periods have varied from 5 to 20 days.[1,9] The variation was apparently attributable to type and dose of inoculum, method of cryopreservation, and individual cat response. After a febrile period (39.9° to 40.1°C [103.8° to 104.2°F]), the temperature may become subnormal, and the cat may have difficulty breathing. Parasitized erythrocytes are observed late (6 days postinoculation) in the disease, during the febrile episode. Cats usually die 2 or 3 days after the temperature peak, and the entire course of clinical illness usually takes less than a week.

DIAGNOSIS

Cytauxzoonosis should be considered in the differential diagnosis when a cat that is allowed access to rural wooded areas becomes depressed, develops high fever and possibly anemia and jaundice. Diagnosis is made by demonstrating the erythrocyte phase (piroplasms) in Wright's- or Giemsa-stained thin blood films and the tissue phase

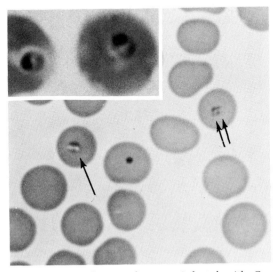

Figure 82–2. Feline erythrocytes infected with *Cytauxzoon* piroplasms: ring (*single arrow*) and dividing forms (*double arrows*). The Howell-Jolly body is included for comparison of size and structure (Giemsa-Triton stain; × 1000). *Inset*, Enlarged view of ring forms in parasitized erythrocytes.

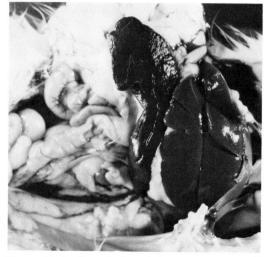

Figure 82–3. Gross lesions in a cat experimentally infected with *C. felis* include a greatly enlarged spleen and a slightly enlarged liver with rounded edges and distended veins.

in Wright's- or Giemsa-stained bone marrow aspirates or impression smears of spleen and lymph node (see Appendix 12).[8] Histologic confirmation should be made from standard formalin-fixed tissues (lung, any lymph node, spleen, liver) that are sent to a veterinary pathology laboratory for parasite evaluation since the major differential diagnoses, haemobartonellosis and babesiosis, do not have a tissue stage (see Appendix 8). The ring form of *Haemobartonella* may appear

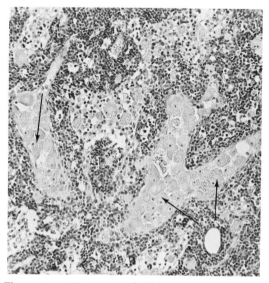

Figure 82–4. Numerous infected mononuclear phagocytes filling the lumina and lining the walls of veins (*arrows*) within a lymph node from a cat experimentally infected with *C. felis* (H and E; × 400).

similar to the erythrocytic stage of *Cytauxzoon*.

The piroplasms within erythrocytes appear as round "signet ring"–shaped bodies 1 to 1.5 μm in diameter, bipolar oval "safety pin" forms 1 by 2 μm, or anaplasmoid round "dots" less than 1 μm in diameter (Fig. 82–2). All forms may occur in a single blood film. The cytoplasm of the piroplasm stains light blue and the nucleus dark red or purple. The number of parasitized cells varies from cat to cat and with the stage of the disease. In experimental inoculations, piroplasms first appear with the onset of fever, and infected cells may range from only a few per film to 25% before death.[1] A single cell usually contains only one parasite, but pairs and tetrads (Maltese crosses) are observed occasionally.

An IFA test has been developed for the detection of the tissue phase of feline cytauxzoonosis; however, it is not commercially available.[10]

PATHOLOGIC FINDINGS

Gross findings in domestic cats include dehydration; pallor; icterus; hydropericardium; enlarged, edematous, and hemorrhagic lymph nodes; intra-abdominal venous distention; splenomegaly; and hemorrhages on the serosal surfaces of abdominal organs and lungs.[1,9] The lungs are frequently congested and edematous, often with petechiae throughout (Fig. 82–3).

The characteristic lesion on histologic examination of feline cytauxzoonosis is the accumulation of large numbers of parasitized mononuclear phagocytes containing schizonts in various stages of development. These cells are particularly prevalent within the lumens of veins of the lungs, liver, lymph nodes, and spleen, making these vessels appear partially or completely occluded (Fig. 82–4). Spleen and lymph node should be used for tissue impression films, which should be stained with Wright's or Giemsa stain.

THERAPY

Preliminary attempts to treat cats that have either natural and experimentally induced disease have had very limited success. In approximately 500 naturally and experimen-

Table 82–1. Therapy for Cytauxzoonosis[a]

DRUG	DOSE[b] (mg/kg)	ROUTE	INTERVAL (hours)	DURATION (days)
Parvaquone	10–30	IM, SC	24	2–3
Buparvaquone	10	IM, SC	24	2–3
Thiacetarsamide	0.1	IV	12	2

[a]IM = intramuscular, SC = subcutaneous, IV = intravenous.
[b]Dose per administration at specified interval, expressed as mg/kg unless otherwise stated.

tally induced cases known to the author, six cats have recovered, and of these, four experimentally infected cats appeared to be immune to reinfection. Of the six recovered cats, two were untreated, whereas four were treated with either supportive fluids (1) or drugs (3). A total of approximately 30 cats with documented cytauxzoonosis have been treated. Four drugs have been used to treat infected cats, but only two appear to be effective (Table 82–1). Parvaquone (Clexon, Cooper's Animal Health, Hertz, England or Wellcome Research Labs, Beckenham, Kent, England) has been used, beginning 2 to 12 days postinfection.[2,11] Two of 18 treated cats survived. One of two cats treated by a practitioner with sodium thiacetarsamide (Caparsolate, Ceva Laboratories, Overland Park, KS) has survived.[11]

Buparvaquone (Butalex, Cooper's Animal Health), a drug related to parvaquone, does not appear to be as effective as parvaquone.[11] Four of four treated cats died. Six cats were given tetracycline orally from the onset of fever; all died.[12]

Intensive supportive care with fluids and broad-spectrum antibiotics by a practitioner resulted in survival of one cat. Thus, success with drug therapy to date is about the same as with aggressive supportive care, and in either case, chance of survival is low.

PREVENTION

A conscientiously applied ectoparasite control program and confinement of cats indoors during tick season could be beneficial in preventing cytauxzoonosis, since all naturally occurring cases known to the author have involved cats that were free to roam in rural, wooded, tick-infested areas.

References

1. Kier AB, Wagner JE, Kinden DA: The pathology of experimental cytauzxoonosis. *J Comp Pathol* 97: 415–432, 1987.
2. Uilenberg G, Franssen FFJ, Perie NM: Relationships between *Cytauxzoon felis* and African piroplasmids. *Vet Parasitol* 26:21–28, 1982.
3. Glenn BL, Rolley RE, Kocan AA: *Cytauxzoon*-like piroplasms in erythrocytes of wild-trapped bobcats in Oklahoma. *J Am Vet Med Assoc* 181:1251–1253, 1982.
4. Kier AB, Wagner JE, Morehouse LG: Experimental transmission of *Cytauxzoon felis* from bobcats (*Lynx rufus*) to domestic cats (*Felis domesticus*). *Am J Vet Res* 43:97–101, 1982.
5. Kier AB, Wightman SF, Wagner JE: Interspecies transmission of *Cytauxzoon felis*. *Am J Vet Res* 43:102–105, 1982.
6. Blouin EF, Kocan AA, Glenn BL, et al: Transmission of *Cytauxzoon felis* (Kier, 1979) from bobcats, *Felis rufus* (Schreber), to domestic cats by *Dermacentor variabilis* (Say). *J Wildl Dis* 20: 241–242, 1984.
7. Kier AB: Cytauxzoonosis. In Greene CE (ed): *Clinical Microbiology and Infectious Diseases of the Dog and Cat.* Philadelphia, WB Saunders Co, 1984, pp 791–795.
8. Franks PT, Harvey JW, Shields RP, et al: Hematological findings in experimental feline cytauxzoonosis. *J Am Anim Hosp Assoc* 24:395–401, 1988.
9. Wagner JE: A fatal cytauxzoonosis-like disease in cats. *J Am Vet Med Assoc* 168:585–588, 1976.
10. Shindel N, Dardiri AH, Ferris DH: An indirect fluorescent antibody test for the detection of Cytauxzoon-like organisms in experimentally infected cats. *Can J Comp Med* 42:460–465, 1978.
11. Motzel S: Personal communication. University of Missouri, Columbia, MO, 1988.
12. Kier AB: Unpublished observations. University of Missouri, Columbia, MO, 1978.

83

BABESIOSIS
Edward B. Breitschwerdt

Babesiosis is a tick-borne hematozoan disease of domestic and wild animals and humans. Several *Babesia* species can infect the dog or cat and result in progressive anemia as the primary clinical finding. Canine babesiosis has been reported in domestic dogs, wolves, and striped and black-backed jackals and is known to occur throughout the world, particularly in tropical, subtropical, and temperate zones.[1]

Feline babesiosis occurs within a wide host range in the cat family. Feline babesiosis is enzootic along the coastal regions of South Africa, and a large portion of the information regarding this disease has been reported from that region.[2]

ETIOLOGY

Dog

Of the 71 species of *Babesia*, three are known to infect members of the canine family. They are *B. canis*, *B. gibsoni*, and *B. vogeli*. The geographic distribution and morphologic characteristics of these organisms are summarized in Table 83–1. *B. canis* organisms are frequently encountered as paired piriform trophozoites in an erythrocyte as depicted in Figure 83–1. Organisms also can be found in endothelial cells of the lungs and liver, in macrophages of the mononuclear phagocyte system, and in neutrophils of peripheral blood. *B. gibsoni* is also pleomorphic.

Following ingestion by ticks, *Babesia* organisms undergo a complex developmental cycle involving a series of binary fissions that give rise to numerous infective parasites. Vector ticks that transmit the various species of canine *Babesia* are listed in Table 83–1. Both transstadial and transovarial transmissions of *B. canis* and *B. gibsoni* occur in vector ticks.

Cat

Four species of *Babesia*, *B. cati*, *B. felis*, *B. herpailuri*, and *B. pantherae*, are known to infect domestic and wild cats. The geographic distribution and morphologic characteristics of the organisms are summarized in Table 83–1.

PATHOGENESIS

Dog

The pathogenesis and disease entity caused by the three species of canine *Babesia* are very similar (Fig. 83–2). Differences in pathogenicity among different strains within a species of *Babesia*, the degree of parasitemia, and the immunologic response and age of the host are important factors that contribute to the variation in severity of the clinical syndrome.[3] The incubation period following tick exposure is thought to range from 10 days to 3 weeks. Babesiosis may be acquired by transplacental transmission or inadvertently by blood transfusion.

Following experimental infection of susceptible dogs with *B. canis*-infected blood, a transient parasitemia began on day 1 postinoculation (PI) and lasted approximately 4 days. Organisms then disappeared from peripheral blood for about 10 days, and a second, more intensive parasitemia developed about 2 weeks PI. The number of organisms within erythrocytes increases by binary fission and appears to peak in experimental infections around day 20 PI. Rapid clinical deterioration has been observed in most dogs with circulating parasitemia, although the severity of the disease is not always proportional to the degree of parasitemia. Dogs that recovered from the initial infection have shown variable and unpre-

Table 83–1. Characteristics of Babesial Parasites Infecting Canidae and Felidae

SPECIES	RECOGNIZED HOSTS	SIZE (μm)	TYPICAL MORPHOLOGY[a]	RECOGNIZED TICK VECTORS	GEOGRAPHIC DISTRIBUTION
B. canis	Domestic dog, wolf, striped jackal, black-backed jackal, fox[b]	2.4 × 5.0	Paired piriform bodies	*Rhipicephalus sanguineus, Dermacentor* spp., *Haemaphysalis leachi, Hyalomma plumbeum*	Worldwide: Africa, Asia, Australia, Europe, Central and South America, Japan, United States
B. gibsoni	Domestic dog, jackal, wolf, fox, mongoose, ferret, badger	1.0 × 3.2	Single, annular bodies	*Haemaphysalis bispinosa, R. sanguineus*	India, Sri Lanka, Malaysia, Korea, Egypt, Japan, United States
B. vogeli	Domestic dog	4.0 × 5.0	Paired piriform bodies	*R. sanguineus*	Asia, Africa
B. cati	Domestic cat, Indian wildcat	1.0 × 2.5		Unknown	India
B. felis	Domestic cat, Sudanese wildcat, puma, leopard	1.0 × 2.3	Single or paired annular bodies	Unknown	South Africa, Sudan
B. herpailuri	Jaguarundi, domestic cat[b]	1.3 × 3.4	Single or paired piriform bodies	Unknown	South America, Africa
B. pantherae	Leopard, domestic cat[b]	1.2 × 2.2		Unknown	Kenya

[a]Extreme variation in morphology may be encountered with a given species of *Babesia*.
[b]Experimentally infected only.

dictable patent periods alternating with dormant periods. The intensity of the parasitemia is variable from one patent period to another.

Intraerythrocytic parasitemia causes both intravascular and extravascular hemolysis. In the acute disease, babesiosis is characterized predominantly by intravascular hemolysis resulting in a regenerative anemia

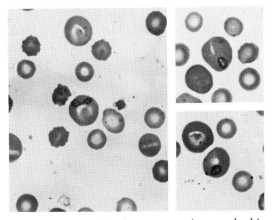

Figure 83–1. Anisocytosis, macrocytosis, several echinocytes, and two *B. canis* organisms in a blood smear from a naturally infected dog. (Wright's-Giemsa stain; × 900). Insets—other red cells containing *B. canis* organisms (× 1100). (Courtesy of Peter MacWilliams, DVM, PhD.)

without suppression of erythropoiesis. Hemoglobinemia, hemoglobinuria, and bilirubinuria develop during the early progressive stages of the disease. Pyrexia develops, presumably due to the release of endogenous pyrogens from erythrolysis and from destruction of the parasite and erythrocytes by the mononuclear phagocyte system. The extent to which immunologic mechanisms contribute to anemia and thrombocytopenia in canine babesiosis remains unclear. A positive Coombs' test result is frequently encountered.[4] As the disease process becomes more advanced, bilirubinemia and icterus develop. Splenic and hepatic enlargements occur due to passive congestion and hyperplasia of the mononuclear phagocyte system.

Hemolysis results in a severe anemic anoxia, anaerobic metabolism, lactic acid generation, and metabolic acidosis.[5] Microvascular damage secondary to hypoxia contributes to the development of DIC, which may be responsible for some of the atypical manifestations of the disease.[6]

Variation in pathogenicity among different strains of *B. canis* contributes to the differences in severity of clinical presentations that are observed in field stiuations. The organism may induce a chronic carrier state without apparent symptomatology or follow-

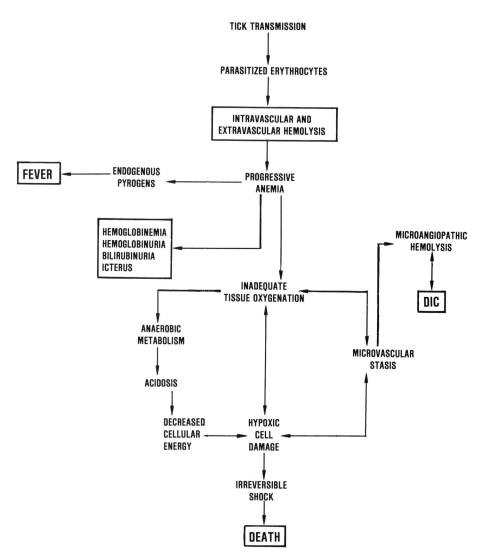

Figure 83–2. Proposed pathogenesis of canine babesiosis.

ing survival of an acute infection. Premunition, characterized by a delicate balance between the parasite and host defenses, develops in chronically infected dogs. This balance may be disturbed by environmental stresses, intercurrent disease, immunodeficiency, splenectomy, or immunosuppressive treatment. Premunition is considered advantageous in endemic areas. Following experimental infection with B. gibsoni, lymphocyte transformation in response to mitogens is depressed during periods of parasitemia.[7]

Pups are more susceptible to certain strains of B. canis and frequently acquire a more severe infection than do adult dogs.[8,9] Concurrent infection with Ehrlichia canis may increase mortality or induce a nonre-

generative anemia (see Clinical Findings, Chapter 37).[10]

Cat

The pathogenesis of feline babesiosis, although less clearly delineated, is in many respects similar to that of canine babesiosis. The severity of hemolytic anemia seen in cats equals that of dogs and may be accompanied by sudden death.[11] Unlike canine babesiosis, fever, acidosis, severe hepatic damage, severe renal damage, and coagulation abnormalities are less severe and less frequently encountered in both clinical and experimental cases.[12]

CLINICAL FINDINGS

Dog

Canine babesiosis can be subclinical, peracute, acute, or chronic. Clinical findings consistent with the typical presentation of canine babesiosis include depression, weakness, anorexia, pale mucous membranes, icterus, pyrexia, and splenomegaly. Often, infected dogs become ill only after being subjected to severe stress, hard work, concurrent infection, or splenectomy. The peracute form of the disease usually occurs in young dogs that are heavily parasitized and in a state of shock despite a short history of illness. Petechial and ecchymotic hemorrhages are observed in severely affected dogs with thrombocytopenia or DIC. Chronic infections can be characterized by intermittent fever, capricious appetite, and a marked loss of body condition. Atypical forms of the disease may cause such unusual manifestations as ascites, asymmetric peripheral edema, ulcerative stomatitis, GI disturbances, CNS signs, muscular aberrations, respiratory symptoms, and circulatory disturbances.[6]

Cat

Feline babesiosis is a disease that primarily affects cats less than 2 years of age and is characterized clinically by inappetance, lethargy, weakness, rough haircoats, and pale mucous membranes. Unlike the disease in dogs, fever and icterus are rarely seen in cats. Yellow- to orange-colored diarrhea has been observed in both natural and experimental cases.[11] Tachycardia, tachypnea, and dyspnea with exertion have been observed in severely anemic cats. Care must be taken when examining these animals to prevent iatrogenic death.

DIAGNOSIS

Dog

Alterations in laboratory parameters will vary with the severity of the clinical presentation. Early laboratory abnormalities include hemolytic anemia, bilirubinemia, bilirubinuria, and hemoglobinuria. Hemato-

logic examination of a Wright's- or Giemsa-stained peripheral blood film usually reveals anisocytosis, poikilocytosis, polychromasia, and nucleated erythrocytes consistent with a regenerative anemia (see Fig. 83–1). Spherocytes are found occasionally. Presence of reticulocytosis confirms a regenerative anemia. The majority of dogs with naturally occurring babesiosis caused by B. canis or B. gibsoni have a positive Coombs' test result.[4] Babesiosis should be included among the differential diagnoses of anemic puppies with suspected ancylostomiasis.

Thrombocytopenia occurs in both mild and severe B. canis infections but is generally more marked in severely affected dogs.[6, 10] The mechanisms responsible for thrombocytopenia have not been clearly established; however, thrombocytopenia may occur independently of DIC, which is a complication of severe canine babesiosis.

Granular and cellular casts and renal tubular epithelium have been observed in urine specimens from dogs with B. canis infections. Increased urinary concentrations of hemoglobin, bilirubin, and protein have been found in severely affected dogs. In contrast to B. canis infections, icterus and hemoglobinuria are rare in dogs infected with B. gibsoni. Azotemia and metabolic acidosis appear to contribute to the morbidity and mortality of severely affected dogs.

The above laboratory findings are consistent with, but not diagnostic of, canine babesiosis. Antemortem confirmation requires microscopic demonstration and species identification of the causative organism. B. canis or B. gibsoni organisms are found more readily in peripheral blood films obtained from a microcapillary system such as the ventral surface of the ear or the toenail. Giemsa-stained blood films are superior to Wright's-stained films for demonstrating organisms.[4]

Despite appropriate staining technique and intensive blood film examination, organisms frequently cannot be found. Blood from a suspect animal can be injected into a splenectomized dog, after which daily blood films are examined for organisms. The IFA test is currently recommended because it appears to represent a reliable means of detecting patent or occult parasitemia in dogs.[13, 14] Titers greater than 1:40 are considered positive for either B. canis or B. gibsoni. Cross-reactivity between B. gibsoni and B. canis necessitates the eventual demonstration of the organism in a blood film for specific identification. Species differentiation is important for selection of an effective chemotherapeutic agent. False-negative results can occur in immature dogs infected with *B. canis* because they are often incapable of mounting a detectable IFA titer.[4, 8] Serology is also useful for characterizing the prevalence of infection within a specified region.[3,15]

Cat

The hematologic findings in experimentally and naturally infected cases of feline babesiosis include a rapid drop in hematocrit. Anemia is most severe approximately 3 weeks following experimental infection. A macrocytic hypochromic anemia is often found in feline babesiosis and is most probably related to a more chronic hemolytic anemia.[16]

Biochemical changes in cats with babesiosis are generally of minimal significance. Renal function is unaffected and venous blood pH remains normal. Occasional alterations in liver enzymes and mild to moderate bilirubinemia have been observed in some cats.

PATHOLOGIC FINDINGS

Gross lesions associated with canine babesiosis include a dark reddish-blue enlarged spleen, enlarged lymph nodes, yellowish discoloration of tissues in icteric animals, pericardial effusion, subcutaneous edema, hemorrhagic lesions, pneumonia, and hepatomegaly. The urinary bladder frequently contains red urine. Varying degrees of congestion, hemorrhage, and necrosis can be seen in the lymph nodes, the proximal GI tract, kidneys, liver, heart, brain, pleura, mesentery, and other tissues.[6] Splenomegaly appears to be the most consistent finding in chronic cases. An impression smear of the spleen can be utilized to substantiate the diagnosis of babesiosis at necropsy (Fig. 83–3).

Pallor, thin watery blood, and hepatomegaly are indicative of feline babesiosis. Urine is usually golden yellow and rarely red. Feces are yellow to orange in color.

In general, histologic lesions are related to inadequate tissue oxygenation causing vas-

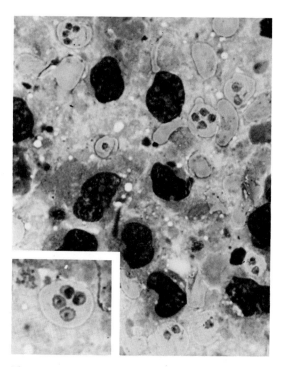

Figure 83–3. Impression smear of the spleen obtained at necropsy from a naturally infected dog. Numerous erythrocytes contain one or more *B. canis* organisms. (Wright's-Giemsa stain; × 1100). (Courtesy of Peter MacWilliams, DVM, PhD, and Charles W Qualls Jr, DVM, PhD.)

cular endothelial damage. In the brain, fibrin thrombi containing aggregates of parasitized erythrocytes and monocytes can be seen in meningeal vessels. Congestion, edema, hemorrhage, and necrosis are seen in tissues that have high metabolic activity, such as the brain, heart, kidney, and intestines. The renal tubules may contain dense eosinophilic, hyaline droplets and hemoglobin droplets or crystals. Tubular epithelial cells may be swollen. In severe cases, renal tubular necrosis and centrilobular hepatic necrosis are prominent findings. *Babesia* organisms may be found in erythrocytes in the vasculature of most tissues in variable numbers.

Erythroid hyperplasia has been seen in the bone marrow. Mononuclear phagocyte system hyperplasia and foci of extramedullary hematopoiesis may be observed in the spleen, lymph nodes, and liver. A mononuclear cell infiltrate can be found in numerous tissues in the late acute to chronic forms of the disease.

Centrilobular necrosis, bile stasis, and extramedullary hematopoiesis are the most consistent histologic lesions in cats. No specific uniform histologic pattern is observed.[12]

THERAPY

Dog

Management of canine babesiosis involves the use of parasiticidal drugs and supportive treatment. When considering a therapeutic regimen, an arbitrary division of clinical cases into two categories that roughly reflect the progression of disease is recommended. The stable uncomplicated case may require only treatment with an antibabesial drug, whereas the complicated case requires intensive medical management. Numerous drugs have been utilized for treatment of canine babesiosis.[17, 18] Properties of antibabesial drugs are compared in Table 83–2. Drug efficacy varies significantly between species of *Babesia* infecting the same host. Some drugs will eliminate the parasitemia without eliminating the infection. Diminazene aceturate, phenamidine isethionate, and imidocarb dipropionate are effective therapeutic agents for *B. canis* (see Aromatic Diamidines, Chapter 77). Imidocarb is a useful agent for treatment of concurrent canine ehrlichiosis and babesiosis.[19] No drug has been completely effective in clearing *B. gibsoni* parasites from erythrocytes.[20]

Transfusion of packed erythrocytes or fresh whole blood from a canine erythrocyte antigen 1.1-, 1.2-, and 7-negative donor is indicated if the hematocrit falls below 15%.

Packed erythrocytes are preferable since little or no plasma loss occurs. Blood for transfusion should be collected in such a manner as to prevent platelet inactivation. The formula

$$\text{ml blood in anticoagulant} = \text{kg} \times K \times \left(\frac{\text{desired hematocrit} - \text{patient hematocrit}}{\text{donor blood hematocrit}} \right)$$

where $K = 60$ (cat), 80 (dog) and (kg) = patient's body weight

can be used to determine the volume of blood for transfusion. Following transfusion, the recipient's hematocrit ideally should be 30%. Exchange transfusion has been utilized to treat human babesiosis. Administration of iron, B complex vitamins, and anabolic steroids can be utilized to assist erythrocyte production.

Studies involving severely complicated canine babesiosis[5, 21] emphasize the importance of sodium bicarbonate for treatment of metabolic acidosis. Severe acidosis appears to represent an important factor that determines survival in severely affected dogs. The formula

$$\text{mEq of sodium bicarbonate} = 0.6 \times \text{kg} \times (25 - \text{patient's serum } HCO_3^-)$$

where kg = patient's body weight

will estimate the total body fluid HCO_3^- deficit. However, the rate of sodium bicar-

Table 83–2. Selected Chemotherapeutic Agents Utilized for Treatment of Canine and Feline Babesiosis[a]

DRUG (PROPRIETARY NAME)	BABESIA			SIDE EFFECTS	DOSE[b] (mg/kg)	ROUTE	INTERVAL (hours)	DURATION (days)
	canis	*gibsoni*	*felis*					
Diminazene aceturate (Berenil, Ganaseg)	+ +	+	±	Polyneuritis, CNS hemorrhage with overdose, encephalomalacia	3.5 (10% solution)	IM	Once	1
Phenamidine isethionate (Lomadine, Phenamidine)	+ +	+	−	Nausea, vomiting, abscess formation at injection site, CNS hemorrhage with overdose	15 (5% solution)	SC	Twice	c
Trypan blue (Trypan blue)	±	−	−	Perivascular sloughing, stains tissue blue	4 (1–2% solution)	IV	Once	1
Imidocarb dipropionate (Imizol)	+ +	ID	−	Transient salivation, serous nasal discharge, diarrhea, dyspnea	2–6	SC, IM	Once	1
Primaquine phosphate (Primaquine)	ID	−	+ + +	Single dose >1 mg/kg is lethal in cats	0.5	PO, IM	Once	1

[a] − = poor, ± = poor to fair, + = good, + + = very good, + + + = excellent, ID = insufficient data, IM = intramuscular, SC = subcutaneous, IV = intravenous, PO = oral.
[b] Dose per administration at specified interval, expressed as mg/kg unless otherwise stated.
[c] Given on two consecutive days.

bonate administration in canine babesiosis has not been clearly established. Replacement of 50% of the HCO_3^- deficit in the first 24 hours is generally recommended for treatment of metabolic acidosis; however, rapid IV administration of 1.0 mEq/kg has been utilized successfully in dogs with anemic shock secondary to *B. canis*.[21] Overzealous administration of sodium bicarbonate can cause severe complications, such as paradoxic CSF acidosis and coma.

Azotemia generally responds readily to blood transfusion and fluid administration such as would be indicated for acute renal failure. Fluid diuresis with normal saline should be initiated in azotemic dogs. Response to therapy can be determined by daily monitoring of BUN and electrolyte values.

The extent to which anticoagulant therapy is beneficial for treatment of DIC secondary to canine babesiosis remains to be determined. Removal of the inciting stimulus with an antibabesial drug may be effective in halting the progression of consumptive coagulopathy.

Cat

Primaquine phosphate, compared with nine other drugs for treatment of *B. felis*, has been found to be highly effective.[22] Dosage and side effects are given in Table 83–2. Unlike *B. felis*, *B. herpailuri* is reported to be susceptible to diminazene treatment.[23] Stress should be minimized to prevent iatrogenic death in cats with severe anemia. In addition to antibabesial drugs, fresh blood should be transfused to anemic cats, in the same manner as for dogs.

PREVENTION IN THE DOG

The primary means of prevention of canine babesiosis is control of the tick vector, which involves a routine dipping program for dogs and spraying of the premises. Animals from an endemic area should be dipped and quarantined for 3 weeks prior to admission to the kennel. In endemic areas total elimination of the parasitemia with the use of babesicidal therapy is not recommended because the animal cleared of the organism is susceptible to reinfection.

A vaccine produced from soluble antigen present in culture supernatant (Pitodoq, Institute Merieux, Lyon, France) is currently marketed in France for prevention of canine babesiosis.[24] Efficacy studies are under way to determine the vaccine's utility in an endemic region. Serologic testing in nonendemic areas may help to identify asymptomatic carriers that can be eliminated or treated so as to remove a source of infection for tick transmission. Blood donors should be screened serologically so that infected, asymptomatic dogs will not be used as donors. Splenectomy is recommended for canine blood donors in endemic regions so that parasitemia develops if a donor becomes infected. A severe outbreak of babesiosis in a kennel of research dogs emphasized the ease with which the disease can be introduced into the environment.[25] The spread of canine babesiosis by transporting asymptomatic animals from an endemic to nonendemic regions is a danger.

PUBLIC HEALTH CONSIDERATIONS

Only in the last decade has *Babesia* been recognized as pathogenic to humans. Human babesiosis has been reported from the United States, Mexico, Europe, and the Soviet Union.[26,27] Thus far, cases of human babesiosis have been caused by *Babesia* that infects rodents or ruminants.

References

1. Roher DP, Anderson JF, Neilsen SW: Experimental babesiosis in coyotes and coy dogs. *Am J Vet Res* 46:256–262, 1985.
2. Futter GJ, Belonje PC: Studies on feline babesiosis: 1. Historical review. *J S Afr Vet Assoc* 50:105–106, 1980.
3. Martinod S, Laurent N, Moreau Y: Resistance and immunity of dogs against *Babesia canis* in an endemic area. *Vet Parasitol* 19:245–254, 1986.
4. Farwell GE, LeGrand EK, Cobb CC: Clinical observations on *Babesia gibsoni* and *Babesia canis* infections in dogs. *J Am Vet Med Assoc* 180:507–511, 1982.
5. Button C: Metabolic and electrolyte disturbances in acute canine babesiosis. *J Am Vet Med Assoc* 175:475–479, 1979.
6. Moore DJ, Williams MC: Disseminated intravascular coagulation: a complication of *Babesia canis* infection in the dog. *J S Afr Vet Assoc* 50:265–275, 1979.
7. Kawamura M, Maede Y, Namioka S: Mitogenic responsibilities of lymphocytes in canine babe-

siosis and the effects of splenectomy on it. *Jpn J Vet Res* 35:1–10, 1987.

8. Breitschwerdt EB, Malone JB, MacWilliams P, et al: Babesiosis in the greyhound. *J Am Vet Med Assoc* 182:978–982, 1983.

9. Harvey JW, Toboada J, Lewis JC: Babesiosis in a litter of pups. *J Am Vet Med Assoc* 192:1751–1752, 1988.

10. Van Heerden J, Reyers F, Stewart CG: Treatment and thrombocyte levels in experimentally induced canine ehrlichiosis and canine babesiosis. *Onderstepoort J Vet Res* 50:267–270, 1983.

11. Futter GJ, Belonje PC: Studies on feline babesiosis 2. Clinical observations. *J S Afr Vet Assoc* 51:143–146, 1980.

12. Futter GJ, Belonje PC, Van Der Berg A, et al: Studies on feline babesiosis 4. Chemical pathology; macroscopic and microscopic postmortem findings. *J S Afr Vet Assoc* 52:5–14, 1981.

13. Ristic J, Lykin JD, Smith AR, et al: *Babesia canis* and *Babesia gibsoni*: soluble and corpuscular antigens isolated from blood of dogs. *Exp Parasitol* 30:385–392, 1971.

14. Anderson JF, Magnarelli LA, Sulzer AJ: Canine babesiosis: indirect fluorescent antibody test for a North American isolate of *Babesia gibsoni*. *Am J Vet Res* 41:2102–2105, 1980.

15. Levy MG, Breitschwerdt EB, Moncol DJ: Antibody activity to *Babesia canis* in dogs in North Carolina. *Am J Vet Res* 48:339–341, 1987.

16. Futter GJ, Belonje PC, Van Der Berg A: Studies of feline babesiosis 3. Hematological findings. *J S Afr Vet Assoc* 51:271–280, 1980.

17. Roberson EL: Antiprotozoan drugs. In Booth NH, McDonald LE (ed): *Veterinary Pharmacology and Therapeutics*, ed 5. Ames, Iowa State University Press, 1982, pp 874–891.

18. Stewart CG: A comparison of the efficacy of isometamidium, amicarbalide and diminazene against *Babesia canis* in dogs and the effect on subsequent immunity. *J S Afr Vet Assoc* 54:47–51, 1983.

19. Price JE, Dolan TT: A comparison of the efficacy of imidocarb dipropionate and tetracycline hydrochloride in the treatment of canine ehrlichiosis. *Vet Rec* 107:275–277, 1980.

20. Ruff MD, Fowler JL, Fernan RC, et al: Action of certain antiprotozoal compounds against *Babesia gibsoni* in dogs. *Am J Vet Res* 34:641–645, 1973.

21. Malherbe WD, Immelman A, Haupt WH, et al: The diagnosis and treatment of acid base deranged dogs infected with *Babesia canis*. *J S Afr Vet Assoc* 47:29–33, 1976.

22. Potgieter FT: Chemotherapy of *Babesia felis* infection: efficacy of certain drugs. *J S Afr Vet Assoc* 52:289–293, 1981.

23. Stewart CG, Hackett KJW, Collett MG: An unidentified *Babesia* of the domestic cat (*Felis domesticus*). *J S Afr Vet Assoc* 51:219–221, 1980.

24. Levy MG: Personal communication. North Carolina State University, Raleigh, NC, 1987.

25. Hirsch D, Hickman PL, Buckholder CR, et al: An epizootic of babesiosis in dogs used for medical research. *Lab Anim Care* 19:204–208, 1969.

26. Brocklesby DW: Human babesiosis. *J S Afr Vet Assoc* 50:302–307, 1979.

27. Healy GR: Babesia infections in man. *Hosp Pract* June:107–116, 1979.

84 ENTERIC PROTOZOAL INFECTIONS

Carl E. Kirkpatrick

The enteric protozoa covered in this chapter are limited to four protozoan genera: *Giardia*, *Pentatrichomonas*, and *Entamoeba* in the phylum Sarcomastigophora and *Balantidium* in the phylum Ciliophora. Salient characteristics of these organisms and the diseases they may cause are presented in Table 84–1. Enteric protozoa of the phylum Apicomplexa are discussed in Chapters 86 (Toxoplasmosis and Neosporosis), 87 (Enteric Coccidiosis), and 88 (Cryptosporidiosis). Detailed coverage of laboratory methods for diagnosis of enteric protozoan infections is presented in Chapter 76 and Appendix 12.

GIARDIASIS

Etiology and Epidemiology

Within the mammalian small intestine, *Giardia* exists as fragile, anaerobic, lumen-dwelling, motile trophozoites. Environmental survival of *Giardia* between hosts is accomplished within resistant, dormant, nonmotile cysts. No intermediate host is required to complete its life cycle (Fig. 84–1).[1]

The piriform, bilaterally symmetric trophozoites divide asexually in the upper small intestine of dogs and in the lower

Table 84–1. Comparison of Some Enteric Protozoa in Dogs and Cats[a]

ORGANISM	STAGE	AVERAGE SIZE (μm)	NATURAL HOSTS	ORGAN PARASITIZED	PATHOGENIC MECHANISMS	CLINICAL SIGNS
Giardia[b]	Tr Cy	15 × 10 × 3 10 × 8	D, C, H, other mammals	Small intestine	Damage to glycocalyx and microvilli on intestinal epithelium; inhibition of some digestive enzymes; host inflammatory response	None to chronic diarrhea, continuous or intermittent; malabsorption
Pentatrichomonas hominis	Tr	8 × 5	D, C, H, other mammals	Large intestine	Probably none; considered harmless commensal but may be opportunistic pathogen	None to diarrhea
Entamoeba histolytica	Tr Cy	25 (diam.) 12 (diam.)	D, C, H, NHP	Large intestine	Invades colonic wall, producing ulcers; may metastasize to extraintestinal sites	None to diarrhea; dysentery
Balantidium coli	Tr Cy	60 × 35 50 (diam.)	D, P, H, NHP	Large intestine	Invades colonic wall, producing ulcers (metastases rare)	None to diarrhea; dysentery

[a]Tr = trophozoite, Cy = cyst, D = dog, C = cat, H = human being, NHP = nonhuman primate, P = pig.
[b]Some *Giardia* spp. may be identical.

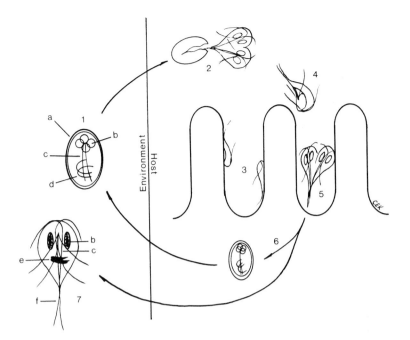

Figure 84–1. Diagram of *Giardia* life cycle, indicating organelles of cyst and trophozoite visible by light microscopy. After cyst (1) is ingested by the host, excystation (2) occurs in the small intestine. Trophozoites (3–5) attach to the mucosa or swim freely in the lumen, where they divide asexually. Following encystment, cysts are excreted (6) in the feces, completing the cycle. Excreted trophozoites (7) do not survive. Key to structural features: a, cyst wall; b, nuclei; c, axonemes (recurrent flagella); d, adhesive disk fragments; e, median bodies; f, flagella. (From Kirkpatrick CE: *Vet Clin North Am [Small Anim Pract]* 17:1377–1387, 1987. Reprinted with permission.)

small intestine of cats (Fig. 84–2). Trophozoite adherence to the brush border of the intestinal mucosa is accomplished by a ventral adhesive disc. Eight flagella propel the trophozoite from one attachment site to another. In dogs, transformation to the relatively resistant cyst form is thought to occur mainly in the cecum.[2] Encystation of trophozoites is stimulated by bile salts and fatty acids at slightly akaline pH.[3] Although tro-

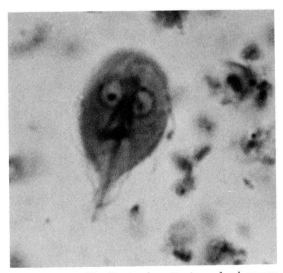

Figure 84–2. *Giardia* trophozoite in a fecal smear stained to enhance the characteristic organelles (compare with Fig. 84–1) (iron hematoxylin; × 2000).

phozoites may be passed in diarrheic stools, cysts are more routinely shed. Whereas cysts may survive for days to weeks in cool, moist conditions, trophozoites do not persist outside the host. On excretion, the relatively resistant, ellipsoidal cysts are immediately infective to another host. Following exposure of ingested cysts to gastric and duodenal fluids, the trophozoites are triggered to emerge and to colonize the small intestinal mucosa.

The prepatent period of *Giardia* infection ranges from 5 to 12 days (mean, about 8 days) in dogs and from 5 to 16 days (mean, about 10 days) in cats. The onset of disease, when it occurs, may precede cyst shedding by 1 to 2 days.

Giardia is worldwide in distribution and infects many species of mammals and birds. Immature animals and immunodeficient adults are most likely to be found infected and clinically ill.[4] For example, adult, IgA-deficient dogs were found to be four times more likely to shed *Giardia* cysts than were dogs with normal serum IgA concentrations.[5] In immunocompetent animals, it is likely that previous exposures confer some degree of immunity to reinfection and disease. Congregations of animals, such as in breeding kennels, catteries, and laboratory animal colonies, have a high prevalence of *Giardia* infection.[6]

Pathogenesis

Putative differences in virulence of *Giardia* strains, as well as host genetics and immune status, probably determine the outcome of an infection.[7] Parasite-related pathogenic factors that have been identified include inhibition of some host intestinal enzymes active in lipid and carbohydrate digestion.[8] Reduction in host enzyme activity apparently results from both mechanical damage to the microvillar glycocalyx and uncharacterized substances made by the parasites. Abnormally rapid sloughing of intestinal epithelial cells leads to failure of new epithelial cells, arising in the crypts, to differentiate fully into columnar cells with microvilli. Blunting of intestinal villi and microvilli results in decreased absorptive surface area. Malabsorption of nutrients, including fat, disaccharides, certain vitamins, and iron, may occur.[1,9] Protein-losing enteropathy has been reported in some human patients. Invasion of the intestinal mucosa or physical occlusion of the mucosa by trophozoites is not generally thought to be significant in the pathogenesis of giardiasis.[8] In the absence of *Giardia* organisms, microscopic changes in the intestine are nonspecific and resemble changes produced by other infections and toxicities.

Clinical Findings

Manifestations of giardiasis are variable.[10,11] Infection may be present without signs of illness. Acute diarrhea may be the owner's complaint for very young puppies or kittens presented early in the course of illness. On the other hand, chronic diarrhea, which may be continuous or sporadic, may persist indefinitely if untreated. Although clinical signs, like pathologic findings, are not specific to giardiasis, an animal with chronic diarrhea and poor response to symptomatic therapy should be suspected as infected. In uncomplicated cases, pale, semiformed, sometimes greasy stools may be passed for weeks or even months. Therapy directed at signs of enteritis (e.g., antimotility drugs, antimicrobials, kaolin or bismuth compounds) may alleviate giardiasis, but diarrhea often returns after withdrawal of treatment. Chronic malabsorption results in weight loss or, in immature animals, poor weight gain, sometimes despite a normal

appetite. Watery or hemorrhagic diarrheas are unlikely to be due solely to *Giardia* infection. Similarly, *Giardia* infection does not in itself produce fever or emesis.

Diagnosis

Since causes of malabsorption and maldigestion other than giardiasis must be considered (e.g., pancreatic exocrine insufficiency), arriving at a definitive diagnosis of giardiasis necessitates finding the organisms (Figs. 84–2 and 84–3). While the favorable response of a patient to anti-*Giardia* drugs may suggest a post hoc diagnosis of giardiasis, these drugs are also effective against some other enteric microorganisms.

Although *Giardia* is among the most prevalent of the intestinal parasites of dogs and cats,[4,6] giardiasis often goes undetected.[12] Reasons for this may include failure to consider it in the differential diagnosis, failure to recognize the organisms, use of inappropriate methods for fecal analysis, and intermittent excretion of organisms in feces of infected individuals.

Relative to most other intestinal parasites of dogs and cats, *Giardia* cysts and trophozoites are small (see Table 84–1). In terms of organism structure, *Giardia* trophozoites may be mistaken for those of *Pentatricho-*

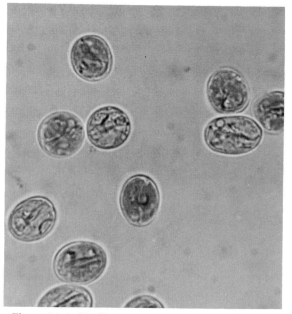

Figure 84–3. *Giardia* cysts concentrated from the feces of a cat by the zinc sulfate centrifugal flotation technique. Cyst wall, nuclei, axonemes, and median bodies are apparent in several of the cysts (iodine; × 1100).

monas hominis, and Giardia cysts may be confused with small coccidian oocysts, Sarcocystis spp. sporocysts, or yeasts.

Giardia trophozoites may be observed in freshly collected, unformed feces of dogs and cats or in duodenal mucus obtained by endoscopy in the dog[13] or by peroral string sampling (EnteroTest, HDC Corp, Mountain View, CA).[14] Endoscopy is less helpful in cats because trophozoites tend to localize in the middle to distal small intestine. To observe living trophozoites, a small amount of sample should be mixed with an isotonic solution and scanned under a minimum of 200 × magnification with reduced light (Chapter 76). Trophozoites are transparent, so overly bright illumination of the specimen may inhibit detection. Either phase-contrast or darkfield illumination is preferable to bright-field illumination. Giardia trophozoites have a characteristically erratic, tumbling motion. Some of them may temporarily adhere to the slide or to the underside of the coverslip, with their ventral flagella still beating in a wavelike manner. In contrast, P. hominis trophozoites have a smoother motion, and, given optimal illumination and contrast, an undulating membrane may be discerned. Adding a drop of iodine solution to the specimen will kill Giardia and P. hominis trophozoites, but iodine will also stain them, thereby facilitating differentiation on the basis of structure (compare Figs. 84–2 and 84–4).[15]

For the detection of Giardia cysts by fecal flotation, the zinc sulfate centrifugal flotation method is preferred (see Appendix 12). Aqueous zinc sulfate solution is prepared to a specific gravity of 1.18 to 1.20. Flotation media more commonly used in veterinary practice, such as sucrose, sodium chloride, and sodium nitrate solutions, are too hypertonic for Giardia cysts. In these solutions, cysts will crumple to the point that they are unrecognizable. Cysts may be distinguished from coccidian oocysts and sporocysts by internal structure and by observing that Giardia cysts will take up iodine, whereas the latter organisms will not. Yeasts also will stain with iodine; however, yeasts are oval, not ellipsoidal, and they are about half the size of Giardia cysts. Furthermore, close observation of yeast cells may reveal budding. In cases of steatorrhea, the high fat content of feces may frustrate attempts at flotation. In such cases, the use of the formalin-ethyl acetate sedimentation method to

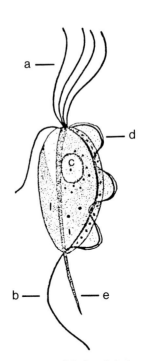

Figure 84–4. Drawing of P. hominis trophozoite indicating some of the characteristic organelles. Key: a, anterior flagella; b, posterior flagellum; c, nucleus; d, undulating membrane; e, axostyle. (Modified from Wenrich SH: J Parasitol 33:177–188, 1947. Reprinted with permission.)

concentrate Giardia cysts from a fecal specimen would be suitable.

The excretion of cysts and trophozoites in host feces is often sporadic (Fig 84–5).[16] Also, the presence of Giardia organisms in feces does not necessarily parallel the severity of clinical signs. Therefore, examination of more than one fecal specimen from a suspected case of giardiasis may be necessary. Likewise, a single negative fecal examination should not be taken as proof of successful therapy. Although not always adequate, analysis of at least three fecal specimens, collected every other day, will enable the detection of Giardia in the majority of cases.

Methods for detecting parasite-specific antigens using ELISA techniques may be more sensitive than microscopy in determining the presence of human Giardia infection.[16a,16b] Such methods (Giardia Direct Detection System, Trend Scientific, St. Paul, MN; ProSpect/Giardia, Alexon Biomedical, Mountain View, CA) offer the ability to screen large numbers of fecal samples. Because of the possibility of false-positive results, microscopic examination is still considered to be the reference standard.

Therapy

In the United States, none of the drugs used to treat giardiasis in small animals is officially approved for that purpose. However, these drugs have been used commonly in human patients. Some of the reportedly effective treatment regimens in dogs and cats are shown in Table 84–2.[17–21] The nitroimidazole compounds (e.g., metronidazole, ipronidazole, tinidazole) and furazolidone are suspected mutagens and carcinogens. However, the results of a controlled epidemiologic study of women indicated no increased risk of cancer due to metronidazole therapy.[22] Little is known of the effect of these drugs in pregnancy. However, since giardiasis is not a life-threatening disease, it seems prudent not to treat pregnant animals. In vitro susceptibility studies have indicated that tinidazole is the most effective drug (in terms of the minimum concentration necessary to kill *Giardia* trophozoites), followed by furazolidone, metronidazole, and quinacrine.[23–26] Quinacrine, at recommended dosages, may cause transient GI upset. Furazolidone may be preferred for use in cats, owing to its palatability and suspension formulation. However, this drug may need to be given for a longer duration than metronidazole to be completely effective. Ipronidazole, a water-soluble nitroimidazole compound, may be preferred in treating large groups of kenneled dogs, as the drug is relatively inexpensive and may be administered in drinking water.[27] The ipronidazole-treated water should be changed daily and offered in nonmetallic containers away from direct sunlight. In dogs, tinidazole has the advantage of efficacy with just one dose per day,[20] but this drug is not widely available.

Treatment failures may occur. As for many infectious diseases, the possibility of reinfection must be considered along with inadequate treatment efficacy. Retreatment with the same or alternative drug should be attempted. There is some recent evidence for the existence of drug-resistant *Giardia* strains.[24,25] In especially stubborn cases of canine giardiasis, concurrent administration of quinacrine and metronidazole at the dosages given in Table 84–2 may be effective.[28]

The question of whether otherwise healthy animals found to be passing *Giardia* cysts warrant treatment is sometimes a subject for debate among clinicians. Points in favor of treating such patients are that signs of giardiasis may recur, the cyst-passing animal serves as a reservoir of infection for other animals, and giardiasis may be a zoonosis.

Public Health Considerations

Giardia is the most common intestinal parasite of people in North America. Many infections are acquired by drinking unfiltered municipal drinking water originating from *Giardia*-contaminated streams, rivers, or lakes. Infants and children in day care facilities appear to have a particularly high risk of infection.[29–31] The results of some biochemical and cross-transmission experi-

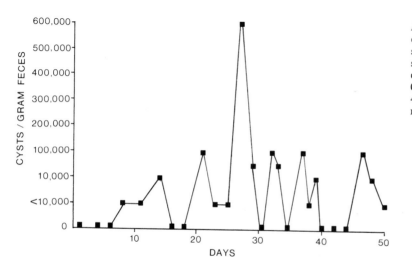

Figure 84–5. The concentration of *Giardia* cysts in feces changes significantly from day to day, as shown in this naturally infected cat. (Modified from Kirkpatrick CE, Farrell JP: *Am J Vet Res* 45:2182–2188, 1984, with permission.)

Table 84–2. Drugs Used to Treat Canine and Feline Giardiasis[a]

DRUG	SPECIES	DOSE[b] (mg/kg)	ROUTE	INTERVAL (hours)	DURATION (days)
Metronidazole	D	15–30[c]	PO	12–24	5–7
	C	10–25	PO	12–24	5–7
Tinidazole	D	44	PO	24	3
Quinacrine	D	9	PO	24	6
	D	6.6	PO	12	5
Ipronidazole	D	126 mg/L[d]	PO	Ad libitum	7
Furazolidone	C	4[e]	PO	12	7–10

[a]D = dog, C = cat, PO = oral.

[b]Dose per administration at specified interval, expressed as mg/kg unless otherwise stated.

[c]Neurotoxicity has been noted with higher doses previously recommended, see Nitroimidazoles, Chapter 77. To facilitate the dosage to smaller animals, the 250 or 500 mg tablets may be ground, or smaller tablet size (50 or 100 mg) may be used.

[d] In drinking water.

[e] In suspension, 200 mg/day maximum.

ments have suggested that *Giardia* spp. are not as highly host-specific as was once thought.[32,32a,32b,33] However, more studies are required to determine conclusively whether cysts of *Giardia* spp. shed by cats and dogs are infective for people.[34,34a] Attempts to induce giardiasis in dogs and cats by administering *Giardia* organisms obtained from people have yielded equivocal results.[35] Epidemiologic studies have not indicated that pet ownership is a significant risk factor for giardiasis in people.[29–31] Nevertheless, it would seem prudent to treat *Giardia*-infected pets as long as uncertainty remains.

Disinfection of cysts on premises can best be accomplished by use of quaternary ammonium compounds.[36] At manufacturers' recommended dilutions, various preparations (Roccal, Winthrop Labs, New York, NY; Totil, Calgon Corp, St. Louis, MO) have inactivated >99% of *G. muris* within 1 minute at 4° to 10°C and 20° to 25°C.

Chlorine disinfection of public drinking water is not effective in controlling giardial contamination, and filtration must be used. Organic chlorine compounds such as N-halamines are stable in water and have shown marked efficacy in inactivating *Giardia* cysts within 2 minutes at 22°C.[36a]

TRICHOMONIASIS

Etiology and Epidemiology

P. hominis is a piriform flagellate inhabiting the large intestines (particularly the cecum) of people, dogs, cats, and some other mammals. Transmission is direct via the fecal-oral route. The organisms exist only in the trophozoite stage. Trophozoites bear five anteriorly directed flagella and a single, posteriorly directed flagellum that arises at the anterior end and courses along the body of the trophozoite attached to the undulating membrane, a characteristic feature of trichomonads. A rigid, rod-shaped organelle, the axostyle, runs through the trophozoite and protrudes from the posterior end (see Fig. 84–4).[15]

Clinical Findings

It is widely thought that *P. hominis* does not cause disease in dogs and cats, although it is possible that it is an opportunistic pathogen. There is no doubt that large numbers of trophozoites may be seen in diarrheic feces of dogs, yet an unambiguous, causal relationship remains to be established.

Diagnosis and Therapy

Microscopic examination of fecal smears, as described previously for *Giardia* trophozoites, will reveal the tiny, motile trophozoites (see Table 84–1). The trophozoites of *P. hominis* must be distinguished from those of *Giardia*. Intercurrent *P. hominis* and *Giardia* infections can occur. If desired, trichomoniasis may be eliminated with metronidazole at the dosages given for *Giardia* (see Table 84–2).

AMEBIASIS

Etiology and Epidemiology

Entamoeba histolytica is a facultatively parasitic ameba that predominantly infects people and nonhuman primates, although dogs and cats also may be infected. Although the prevalence of amebiasis in the United States has declined considerably over the last several decades, *E. histolytica* remains an important parasite in many tropical areas around the world.[37]

Trophozoites either inhabit the colonic lumen as commensals or invade the colonic wall, sometimes metastasizing to liver, lungs, brain, or perianal skin (Figs. 84–6 and 84–7).[38] Various strains of *E. histolytica* differ in virulence. Cysts, passed in human feces, are the infective stages. Because encystment of trophozoites rarely occurs in dogs and cats, amebiasis is among those unusual diseases that are transmissible from humans to pets but seldom vice versa.

Pathogenesis and Pathologic Findings

E. histolytica trophozoites damage the intestine by attaching to and lysing host cells and secrete enzymes that disrupt intercellular connections.[39] The presence of certain bacteria and a host with deficient protein intake contribute to parasite virulence. The host's own cellular immune response to tissue-invading amebas can exacerbate the damage. Secretory diarrhea may be induced by serotonin and other factors secreted by the trophozoites.

In invasive amebiasis, erosion or ulceration of the colonic mucosa results. Microscopic examination of infected colonic tissue may reveal the classical "flask-shaped" ulcer of amebiasis, the result of mucosal undermining by trophozoites in the submucosa. Trophozoites may be seen in sections

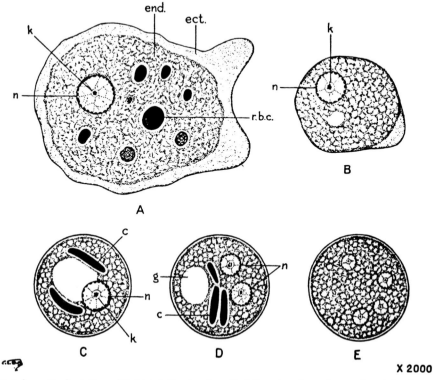

Figure 84–6. Schematic depiction of *E. histolytica* trophozoite (*A*) and various stages of cyst development (*B* to *E*); c, chromatoid bodies; g, glycogen vacuole; k, karyosome; n, nucleus; r.b.c., red blood cell; end., endoplasm; ect., ectoplasm. (From Brown HW, Neva FA: *Basic Clinical Parasitology*, ed 5. Copyright Appleton & Lange, 1983. Reprinted with permission.)

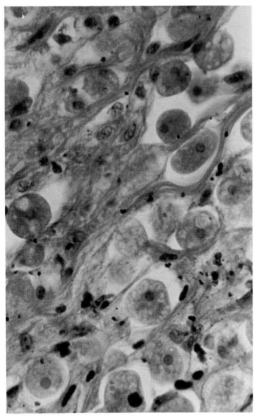

Figure 84–7. Numerous *E. histolytica* trophozoites in a section from the wall of a human colon. Each organism contains a single darkly stained nucleus; in some of the trophozoites, pale vacuoles are apparent (H and E; × 540).

stained with H and E, iron hematoxylin, or PAS reaction (Fig. 84–7).

Clinical Findings

E. histolytica infections may be inapparent or lead to signs of severe ulcerative colitis, including dysentery. Fulminant, untreated amebiasis may prove fatal. Extraintestinal amebiasis, a serious complication, is rare in dogs and unknown in cats. In such cases, signs would be referable to the tissue parasitized (e.g., lung). A case of canine amebiasis was reported in a bitch with vulvar swelling and bloody vaginal discharge. Trophozoites were found in uterine lumen and within ulcers and abscesses in the cervix and vagina.[40]

Diagnosis and Therapy

Definitive diagnosis of amebiasis in dogs and cats requires finding *E. histolytica* tro-

phozoites in feces or in the tissues (see Table 84–1). Trophozoites are difficult to detect in fecal specimens. Direct smears of fresh feces reveal the sluggish, ameboid motility of the trophozoites. In invasive amebiasis, trophozoites may contain erythrocytes. Macrophages in feces may be confused with trophozoites. Methylene blue staining of a wet mount may be helpful in revealing amebas. Trichrome- or iron hematoxylin-stained fecal smears are ideal for diagnosis, but these techniques are best left to a reference laboratory (see Appendix 8). Fecal concentration methods (i.e., flotation or sedimentation) are unsuitable for *E. histolytica* trophozoites. In clinically affected animals, a more reliable means of detecting the trophozoites is the microscopic examination of a sectioned biopsy specimen of colonic mucosa (Fig. 84–7).

Few recent reports on treatment of *E. histolytica*-infected dogs and cats are available. But, based on studies of human patients, metronidazole, at dosages recommended for treatment of giardiasis (see Table 84–2), should be effective against amebiasis.

Public Health Considerations

Although amebiasis is a potentially serious human disease, it is unlikely that dogs and cats are significant reservoirs of these parasites for people. It is more likely that dogs and cats acquire their infections from human feces or from food or water contaminated by human feces. Therefore, although amebiasis is not a zoonosis, the finding of *E. histolytica* in a pet should prompt the veterinarian to suggest that the owners seek medical advice. The owners could have infected the pet or been exposed to a common source of *E. histolytica* cysts.

BALANTIDIASIS

Etiology and Epidemiology

Balantidium coli is a relatively large (see Table 84–1), ciliated protozoan found throughout the world. Although the pig is the most frequently infected animal, dogs and people sometimes become infected with *B. coli*. Infection in the cat has not been reported. Like *E. histolytica*, *B. coli* trophozoites inhabit the colon, either as commen-

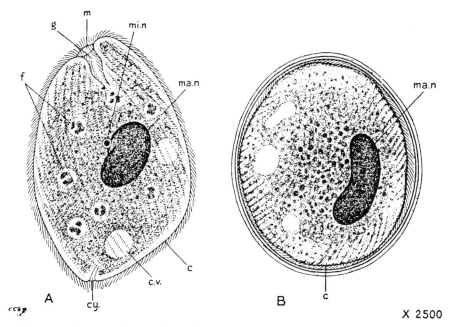

Figure 84–8. Schematic diagram of a *B. coli* trophozoite (A) and cyst (B); c, cilia; c.v., contractile vacuole; cy., cytopyge; f, food vacuole; g, gullet; m, mouth; ma.n, macronucleus; mi.n, micronucleus. (From Brown HW, Neva FA: *Basic Clinical Parasitology*, ed 5. Copyright Appleton & Lange, 1983. Reprinted with permission.)

sals or invasive parasites, and cysts are passed in the feces. Cysts are infective when ingested by a susceptible host.

Pathogenesis and Pathologic Findings

Why normally commensal *B. coli* trophozoites may become virulent in some instances remains a largely unanswered question. Certain colonic bacteria and concurrent *Trichuris vulpis* (whipworm) infection may contribute to *B. coli* invasiveness.

The gross and microscopic features of balantidiasis closely resemble those of amebiasis in the colon. Unlike amebiasis, extraintestinal metastases of *B. coli* trophozoites rarely occur. Routinely processed sections of affected colonic tissue will reveal the trophozoites with their characteristic cilia and bean-shaped macronucleus (Figs. 84–8 and 84–9).

Clinical Findings

Balantidiasis is clinically indistinguishable from some other causes of hemorrhagic colitis, including amebiasis and trichuriasis. There may be a history of contact with

swine. Swine themselves show no signs of disease due to *B. coli* infection.

Diagnosis and Therapy

B. coli cysts and, occasionally, trophozoites may be detected on fecal flotation, using the zinc sulfate centrifugal flotation method. Fresh fecal smears in an isotonic solution are preferred to demonstrate the

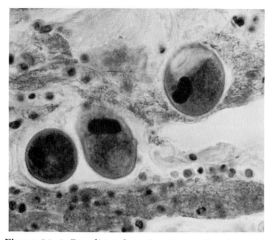

Figure 84–9. *B. coli* trophozoites in a section from the wall of a human colon. Note the prominent parasite macronuclei and the surrounding inflammatory response (H and E; × 250).

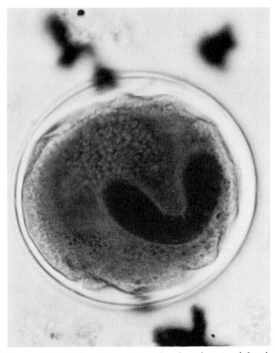

Figure 84–10. B. coli cyst in a fixed and stained fecal smear. The hyaline cyst wall and macronucleus are conspicuous. (Giemsa stain; × 1200).

motile trophozoites. The distinctive macronucleus of both cyst and trophozoite (Figs. 84–8, 84–9, and 84–10) is invisible unless stained. A drop of acidic methyl green solution (1 g methyl green, 1 ml glacial acetic acid, 100 ml water) added to the preparation will reveal the macronucleus in most of the organisms after a few minutes of contact.

Recent reports of therapy of canine balantidiasis are lacking. However, based on human clinical studies, oral metronidazole (see Table 84–2) or tetracyclines should prove effective in the dog.

Public Health Considerations

Since *B. coli*-infected dogs may excrete cysts in their feces, the potential for transmission of the parasite from dog to people exists. Compared with swine, however, dogs are so uncommonly infected that they cannot be considered significant reservoirs of *B. coli* for people.

References

1. Kirkpatrick CE: Giardiasis. *Vet Clin North Am [Small Anim Pract]* 17:1377–1387, 1987.

2. Sogayas MIL, Cur PR, daSilva EF: *Giardia canis* Hegner, 1922. I. Localizacao no tubo digestivo de caes naturalmente infectados. *Arq Bras Med Vet Zoot* 39:265–272, 1987.

3. Gillin FD, Reiner DS, Doncher SE: Small intestinal factors promote incystation of *Giardia lamblia* in vitro. *Infect Immun* 56:705–707, 1988.

4. Kirkpatrick CE: Epizootiology of endoparasitic infections in pet dogs and cats presented to a veterinary teaching hospital. *Vet Parasitol* 30:113–124, 1988.

5. Felsburg PF, Glickman LT, Shofer F, et al: Clinical, immunologic and epidemiologic characteristics of canine selective IgA deficiency. In *Recent Advances in Mucosal Immunity*, Part B. New York, Plenum, 1987, pp 1461–1470.

6. Swan JM, Thompson RCA: The prevalence of *Giardia* in dogs and cats in Perth, Western Australia. *Aust Vet J* 63:110–112, 1986.

7. Nash TE, Herrington DA, Losonsky GA, et al: Experimental human infections with *Giardia lamblia*. *J Infect Dis* 156:974–984, 1987.

8. Smith PD: Pathophysiology and immunology of giardiasis. *Annu Rev Med* 36:295–307, 1985.

9. De Vizia B, Poggi V, Vajro P, et al: Iron malabsorption in giardiasis. *J Pediatr* 107:75–78, 1985.

10. Hahn NE, Glaser CA, Hird DW et al: Prevalence of *Giardia* in the feces of pups. *J Am Vet Med Assoc* 192:1428–1438, 1988.

11. Collins GH, Pope SE, Griffin DL: Diagnosis and prevalence of *Giardia* spp. in dogs and cats. *Aust Vet J* 64:89–90, 1987.

12. Baker DG, Strombeck DR, Gershwin LJ: Laboratory diagnosis of *Giardia duodenalis* infection in dogs. *J Am Vet Med Assoc* 190:53–56, 1987.

13. Roudebush P, Delivorias MH: Duodenal aspiration via flexible endoscope for diagnosis of giardiasis in a dog. *J Am Vet Med Assoc* 187:162–163, 1985.

14. Hall EJ, Rutgers HC, Batt EM: Evaluation of the peroral string test in the diagnosis of canine giardiasis. *J Small Anim Pract* 29:177–183, 1988.

15. Wenrich SH: The species of *Trichomonas* in man. *J Parasitol* 33:177–188, 1947.

16. Kirkpatrick CE, Farrell JP: Feline giardiasis: observations on natural and induced infections. *Am J Vet Res* 45:2182–2188, 1984.

16a. Janoff EN, Craft JC, Pickering LK, et al: Diagnosis of *Giardia lamblia* infections by detection of parasite-specific antigen. *J Clin Microbiol* 27:431–435, 1989.

16b. Stibbs HH, Samadpour M, Manning JF: Enzyme immunoassay for detection of *Giardia lamblia* cyst antigens in formalin-fixed and unfixed human stool. *J Clin Microbiol* 26:1665–1669, 1988.

17. Belosevic M, Faubert GM, Guy R, et al: Observations on natural and experimental infections with *Giardia* isolated from cats. *Can J Comp Med* 48:241–244, 1984.

18. Kirkpatrick CE, Laczak JP: Giardiasis in a cattery. *J Am Vet Med Assoc* 187:161–162, 1985.

19. Kirkpatrick CE: Feline giardiasis: a review. *J Small Anim Pract* 27:69–80, 1986.

20. Zimmer JF, Burrington DB: Comparison of four protocols for the treatment of canine giardiasis. *J Am Anim Hosp Assoc* 22:168–172, 1986.

21. Zimmer JF: Treatment of feline giardiasis with metronidazole. *Cornell Vet* 77:383–388, 1987.

22. Beard CM, Noller KL, O'Fallon WM, et al: Cancer

after exposure to metronidazole. *Mayo Clin Proc* 63:147–153, 1988.

23. Boreham PFL, Phillips RE, Shepherd RW: The sensitivity of *Giardia intestinalis* to drugs in vitro. *J Antimicrob Chemother* 14:449–461, 1984.

24. McIntyre P, Boreham PFL, Phillips RE, et al: Chemotherapy in giardiasis: clinical responses and in vitro drug sensitivity of human isolates in axenic culture. *J Pediatr* 108:1005–1010, 1986.

25. Gordts B, De Jonckheere J, Kasprzak W, et al: In vitro activity of antiprotozoal drugs against *Giardia intestinalis* of human origin. *Antimicrob Agents Chemother* 31:672–673, 1987.

26. Gordts B, DeJonckheere J, Kasprzak W, et al: In vitro activity of antiprotozoal drugs against *Giardia*. *Antimicrob Agents Chemother* 31:672–673, 1987.

27. Abbitt B, Huey RL, Eugster AK: Treatment of giardiasis in adult greyhounds, using ipronidazole-medicated water. *J Am Vet Med Assoc* 188:67–69, 1986.

28. Taylor GD, Wehman WM, Tyrell DJL: Combined metronidazole and quinacrine hydrochloride therapy for chronic giardiasis. *Can Med Assoc J* 136:1179–1180, 1987.

29. Keystone JS, Yang J, Grisdale D, et al: Intestinal parasites in metropolitan Toronto day-care centres. *Can Med Assoc J* 131:733–735, 1984.

30. Woo PTK, Paterson WB: *Giardia lamblia* in children in day-care centres in southern Ontario, Canada, and susceptibility of animals to *G. lamblia*. *Trans R Soc Trop Med Hyg* 80:56–59,1986.

30a. Steketee RW, Reid S, Cheng T, et al: Recurrent outbreaks of giardiasis in a child day care center, Wisconsin. *Am J Public Health* 79:485–490, 1989.

31. Boreham PFL, Phillips RE: Giardiasis in Mount Isa, Northwest Queensland. *Med J Aust* 144:524–528, 1986.

32. Nash TE, Keister DB: Differences in excretory-secretory products and surface antigens among 19 isolates of *Giardia*. *J Infect Dis* 152:1166–1171, 1985.

32a. Erlandsen SL, Sherlock LA, Januschuka M, et al: Cross-species transmission of *Giardia* spp.: inoculation of beavers and muskrats with cysts of human, beaver, mouse, and muskrat origin. *Appl Environ Microbiol* 54:2777–2785, 1988.

32b. Meloni BP, Lymbery AJ, Thompson RC: Isoenzyme electrophoresis of 30 isolates of *Giardia* from humans and felines. *Am J Trop Med Hyg* 38:65–73, 1988.

33. Faubert GM: Evidence that giardiasis is a zoonosis. *Parasitol Today* 4:66–68, 1988.

34. Bemrick WJ, Erlandsen SL: Giardiasis—is it really a zoonosis? *Parasitol Today* 4:69–71, 1988.

34a. Giardiasis—zoonosis or not. *J Am Vet Med Assoc* 194:447–451, 1989.

35. Kirkpatrick CE, Green GA: Susceptibility of domestic cats to infections with *Giardia lamblia* cysts and trophozoites from human sources. *J Clin Microbiol* 21:678–680, 1985.

36. Zimmer JF, Miller JJ, Lindmark DG: Evaluation of the efficacy of selected commercial disinfectants in inactivating *Giardia muris*. *J Am Anim Hosp Assoc* 24:379–385, 1988.

36a. Kong LI, Swango LJ, Blagvurn BL, et al: Inactivation of *Giardia lamblia* and *Giardia canis* cysts by combined and free chlorine. *Appl Environ Microbiol* 54:2580–2582, 1988.

37. Walsh JA: Problems in recognition and diagnosis of amebiasis: estimation of the global magnitude of morbidity and mortality. *Rev Infect Dis* 8:228–238, 1986.

38. Brown HW, Neva FA: *Basic Clinical Parasitology*, ed 5. Norwalk, CT, Appleton-Century-Croft, 1983.

39. Ravdin JI: Pathogenesis of disease caused by *Entamoeba histolytica*: studies of adherence, secreted toxins, and contact-dependent cytolysis. *Rev Infect Dis* 8:247–260, 1986.

40. Yasuda A, Midoro K, Makayama H, et al: Pathology of genital amoebiasis in a female dog. *Jpn J Vet Sci* 50:549–551, 1988.

85 ACANTHAMEBIASIS

Lenn R. Harrison
Rudy W. Bauer

ETIOLOGY

Acanthamoeba is a genus of ubiquitous free-living amebas found in fresh and salt water, soil, and sewage.[1,2] Organisms of this genus cause pneumonia and encephalitis in animals[1,3–6] and humans[1,2,7] and a chronic keratitis in humans.[8,9] Acanthamebiasis has rarely been reported in dogs except possibly in greyhounds.[1,5] *Acanthamoeba* infection has not been described in cats. *Acanthamoeba* has a relatively simple life cycle with two stages: (1) a vegetative trophozoite that feeds mostly on bacteria in nature and (2) a cyst phase that is often able to resist adverse environmental conditions including desiccation.[1] Several *Acanthamoeba* species are pathogenic for animals and people. *A. castellani* and *A. culbertsoni* have been found in canine infections.[5,6]

EPIDEMIOLOGY

In critically ill or debilitated people, *Acanthamoeba* sp. typically causes a chronic granulomatous encephalitis, which may last for more than a week to months before death occurs.[2] Amebic keratitis has been seen in otherwise healthy people who wear contact lenses or who have minor corneal trauma.[8,9] The organism has been shown to persist in ophthalmic solutions for up to 90 days.[9a] Immunosuppressed persons such as organ transplant and acquired immunodeficiency syndrome (AIDS) patients, alcoholics, diabetics, or otherwise debilitated individuals are at high risk and are particularly susceptibile to acanthamebiasis.[2,10]

In dogs, epizootics of acanthamebiasis have been observed in greyhounds,[1,5] while singular cases have been described in a German shepherd[3] and an immunosuppressed Akita.[6] Young dogs appear to be most susceptible. Affected greyhounds varied from 4 to 13 months of age.

The incubation period for canine acanthamebiasis is unknown, nor has the source(s) of the *Acanthamoeba* infection in affected greyhound kennels been found. The route by which dogs acquire the disease has not been determined. The disease appears to occur on farms with good management.

CLINICAL FINDINGS

The clinical signs of canine acanthamebiasis and canine distemper are remarkably similar.[5,6] Initial signs include mild oculonasal discharge, anorexia, and lethargy. Rectal temperature varies from normal to as high as 40.5°C (105°F). Respiratory distress and neurologic signs follow, and most dogs eventually show neurologic dysfunction. Coughing and forced respiratory movements may be observed after a few days. Neurologic signs that develop include incoordination, head tilt, stumbling, dysmetria, walking sideways, and seizures. Severely affected dogs in lateral recumbency are unable to right themselves. Less severely affected greyhound dogs fail to recover sufficiently for performance racing.

DIAGNOSIS

The clinical laboratory abnormalities in acanthamebiasis are nonspecific. Leukopenia is due to marked lymphopenia in greyhounds[5] and a reduction in all types of blood leukocytes in nongreyhound cases.[3,6] The cause of the leukopenia is unknown, but it may be due to concurrent infectious

815

disease, stress, or specific factor(s) produced by the *Acanthamoeba*.

Premortem diagnosis of acanthamebiasis in dogs has been rare. Culture or biopsy of affected tissues would be the most specific means of confirmation. Although lung and CNS tissues are not readily accessible, the possibility of finding organisms in CSF and tracheal washings has not been evaluated. Organisms have been found in corneal scrapings of people with amebic keratitis when the smears were stained with calcofluor-White method.[6a] The organism can be cultured from lesions by special methods that are not done in most laboratories.[7]

PATHOLOGIC FINDINGS

Lung and brain lesions have been observed in all cases. Lung lesions vary from light tan to deep red, raised, semisolid nodules distributed uniformly throughout all lobes.[3,5,6] The nodules show a tendency to coalesce, and intralesional cavitations have been noted. Brain lesions may be large, multifocal, and visible on the meningeal surfaces of the cerebrum and cerebellum and vary from red to tannish-brown as the result of recent hemorrhage or of necrosis.

Microscopically, lung and brain lesions are generally circumscribed to coalescing areas of granulomatous inflammation; however, focally diffuse meningeal inflammatory infiltrates have been seen. Trophozoites and occasional cyst forms of *Acanthamoeba* are seen within alveolar spaces and terminal bronchioles (Fig. 85–1). In brain lesions the amebas are best visualized in perivascular and subarachnoid spaces, and the organisms are generally present in necrotic areas of the neuropil but often are masked by the presence of infiltrating inflammatory cells. Lesions in other tissues are not consistent, but granulomatous foci in glomeruli of some dogs have been observed associated with trophozoites.[5]

Histologic methods and IFA tests are used to demonstrate and identify the organism in tissues.[7] Free-living pathogenic amebas are difficult to differentiate microscopically from certain mammalian cells, especially macrophages.[11] The diagnostic feature of *Acanthamoeba* in histologic sections is the centrally located nucleolus.[1,7] No histochemical stain has been found to be specific for *Acanthamoeba*. PAS and Gomori's methe-

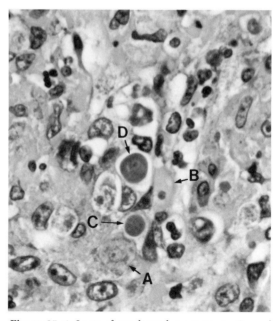

Figure 85–1. Lung of greyhound, pneumonia. Several *Acanthamoeba* are clustered together. Note the morphologic progression from trophozoite to cyst form (*arrows* A–D) (H and E; × 400).

namine silver methods stain only the cyst wall (Fig. 85–2). The IFA test is specific and reliable on deparaffinized sections of formalin-fixed tissue and, when properly done,

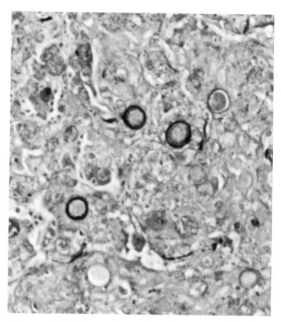

Figure 85–2. Lung of greyhound, pneumonia. Same case as Figure 85–1. Only the cell wall of the cyst form is stained. The body of the *Acanthamoeba* apart from the cell wall takes up the background stain (Gomori's methenamine silver stain; × 320).

allows identification of species of *Acanth-amoeba*.

THERAPY AND PREVENTION

There is no known effective therapeutic regimen for systemic acanthamebiasis. However, sulfadiazine has been effective in treating experimental infection in mice.[11] Other drugs are being tested for efficacy.[7] In vitro studies have shown the organism to be susceptible to natamycin, neomycin, paromomycin, ciclopiroxolamine, and ketoconazole.[7a]

Dogs may be exposed to low numbers of *Acanthamoeba* throughout their lifetimes. Since these are free-living amebas, prevention is accomplished by avoiding access to contaminated water. Pathogenic free-living amebas are found more frequently in thermally enriched water collections or thermally polluted discharge water from industrial plants, or in lakes or swimming pools.[2] Non-thermally enriched water contains fewer amebas. A 0.5% solution of sodium hypochlorite is a satisfactory disinfectant. Since *Acanthamoeba* feed on bacteria, water sources should be initially screened for amebas by testing for coliforms.

PUBLIC HEALTH CONSIDERATIONS

There is no known transmission of infection between hosts, and infections are thought to originate solely from environmental sources.[12] The dog, however, may serve as a sentinel for human infections due to a common environmental exposure.

References

1. Griffin JL: Pathogenic free-living amoeba. *In* Krier JP (ed): *Parasitic Protozoa*, Vol II. New York, Academic Press, 1978, pp 507–549.
2. Martinez AJ: *Free-living Amebas: Natural History, Prevention, Diagnosis, Pathology, and Treatment of Disease.* Boca Raton, FL, CRC Press, 1985.
3. Ayers KH, Billups LH, Garner FM: Acanthamoebiasis in a dog. *Vet Pathol* 9:221–226, 1972.
4. Culbertson CG, Smith JW, Minner JR: *Acanthamoeba*: observations on animal pathogenicity. *Science* 127:1506, 1958.
5. Harrison LR, Liggett AD, Chandler FW, et al: *Acanthameba* infection of greyhounds. *J Am Vet Med Assoc.* Submitted, 1989.
6. Pearce JR, Powell HS, Chandler FW, et al: Amebic meningoencephalitis caused by *Acanthamoeba castellani* in a dog. *J Am Vet Med Assoc* 187:951–952, 1985.
6a. Osato M, Robinson N, Wilhelmus K, et al: The laboratory diagnosis of *Acanthamoeba* keratitis, 29th Intersci Conf Antimicrob Agents Chemother, Houston, Sept 1989, p 187. (Abstr).
7. Visvesvara GS: Free-living pathogenic amoebae. *In* Lennette EH (ed): *Manual of Clinical Microbiology,* ed 4. Washington, DC, American Society for Microbiology, 1985, pp 626–628.
7a. Osato M, Robinson N, Wilhelmus K, et al: Standardization of in vitro antimicrobial susceptibility tests for *Acanthamoeba.* 29th Intersci Conf Antimicrob Agents Chemother, Houston, Sept 1989, p 187. (Abstr).
8. Moore MB, McCulley JP, Luckenback M, et al: *Acanthamoeba* keratitis associated with soft contact lenses. *Am J Ophthalmol* 100:396–403, 1985.
9. Newton C, Driebe WT, Gordon LR, et al: *Acanthamoeba* keratitis associated with contact lenses—United States. *MMWR* 35:405–408, 1986.
9a. Brandt FH, Ware DA, Visvesvara GS: Viability of *Acanthamoeba* cysts in ophthalmic solutions. *Appl Environ Microbiol* 55:1144–1146, 1989.
10. Wiley CA, Safrin RE, Davis CE, et al: *Acanthamoeba* meningoencephalitis in a patient with AIDS. *J Infect Dis* 155:130–133, 1987.
11. Culbertson CG: The pathogenicity of soil amebas. *Annu Rev Microbiol* 25:231–254, 1971.
12. Visvesvara GS: The public health importance and disease potential of small free-living amebae. *2nd International Conference on the Biology and Pathogenicity of Small Free-living Amoebae*, 1980.

86

TOXOPLASMOSIS AND NEOSPOROSIS

J. P. Dubey
Craig E. Greene
Michael R. Lappin

Toxoplasmosis

ETIOLOGY

Toxoplasma gondii is an obligate intracellular coccidian parasite that infects virtually all species of warm-blooded animals, including people. Domestic cats and other Felidae are the definitive hosts and all nonfeline hosts are intermediate hosts. There are three infectious stages: sporozoites in oocysts, invasive tachyzoites (actively multiplying stage), and encysted bradyzoites (slowly multiplying stage). Oocysts are excreted in feces, whereas tachyzoites and bradyzoites are found in tissues.

Three major ways of transmission are congenital infection, ingestion of infected tissues, and ingestion of oocyst-contaminated food or water (Fig. 86–1). Other minor modes of transmission include infected milk and transfusion of fluids or transplantation of organs.

Enteroepithelial Life Cycle

This cycle is found only in the definitive feline host. Most cats become infected by ingesting intermediate hosts infected with tissue cysts. Bradyzoites are released from the tissue cysts in the stomach and intestine when the cyst wall is dissolved by digestive enzymes. Bradyzoites penetrate the epithelial cells of small intestine and initiate the five types (A to E) of predetermined asexual stages (Fig. 86–2). These types, A to E, are equivalent to schizonts of other intestinal coccidia. After an undetermined number of

generations, merozoites released from type D or E form male (micro) or female (macro) gamonts. The microgamont divides and forms several biflagellate microgametes, which are released and swim to and penetrate macrogamonts. A wall is formed around the fertilized macrogamont to form an oocyst. Oocysts are round to oval, 12 × 10 μm, and are unsporulated (uninfective) when passed in feces. After exposure to air and moisture, oocysts sporulate and contain two sporocysts, each with four sporozoites. Sporozoites are banana-shaped, approximately 8 × 2 μm, and can survive in the oocyst for many months even under harsh environmental conditions.

The entire enteroepithelial (coccidian) cycle of *T. gondii* can be completed within 3 days after ingestion of tissue cysts. However, following ingestion of oocysts or tachyzoites, the formation of oocysts is delayed until 3 weeks or more, but differences in the life cycle that account for this delay are uncertain.

Extraintestinal Life Cycle

The extraintestinal development of *T. gondii* is the same for all hosts, including dogs, cats, and people, and is not dependent upon whether tissue cysts or oocysts are ingested. After the ingestion of oocysts, sporozoites excyst in the lumen of the small intestine and penetrate intestinal cells including the cells in the lamina propria. Sporozoites divide into two by an asexual process known

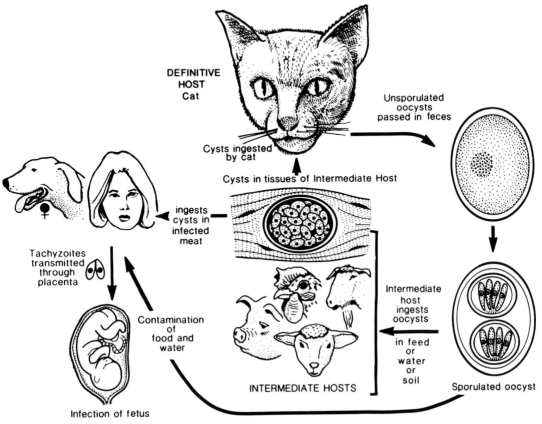

Figure 86–1. Life cycle of T. gondii.

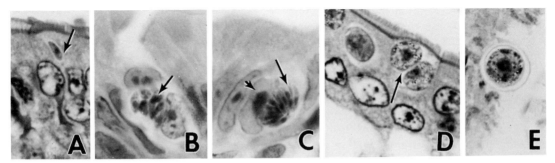

Figure 86–2. Enteroepithelial stages of T. gondii in the small intestine of cats (H and E; × 1000). A, Merozoite (arrow) above the epithelial cell nucleus. B, Type B meront (arrow). C, Type C meront (arrow) in banana-shaped merozoites. The epithelial cell nucleus (arrowhead) is hypertrophied. D, Two female gamonts on right (arrow), each with one nucleus, and a male gamont on left. E, Unsporulated oocyst in intestinal lumen.

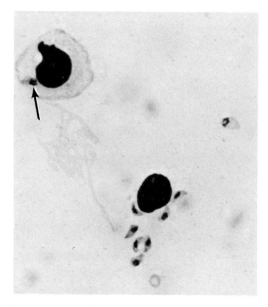

Figure 86–3. Tachyzoites of *T. gondii* in impression smear from lung. One tachyzoite is within a macrophage (*arrow*), and others are being liberated from the host cell (Giemsa; × 1250). (Courtesy of Dr. J. P. Dubey, Zoonotic Diseases Laboratory, US Department of Agriculture, Beltsville, MD.)

as endodyogeny and become tachyzoites. Tachyzoites are lunate in shape, approximately 6 × 2 μm (Figs. 86–3 and 86–4),[1] and multiply in almost any cell of the body. If the cell ruptures, they infect new cells. Otherwise, they multiply intracellularly for an undetermined period and eventually encyst. Tissue cysts grow intracellularly and contain numerous bradyzoites (Figs. 86–5 and 86–6). Bradyzoites resemble tachyzoites in structure except that they are thinner and the nucleus is located at the posterior end of the parasite. Biologically, bradyzoites differ from tachyzoites in that they can survive the digestive process in stomach, whereas tachyzoites cannot. Tissue cysts vary in size from 10 to 50 μm and usually conform to the shape of the parasitized cell. Cysts are separated from the host cell by a thin (0.5 μm) elastic wall (Fig. 86–5). Tissue cysts are formed in the CNS, muscles, and visceral organs and probably persist for the life of the host. Tissue cysts in muscles are longer than those in the brain.

Congenital Transmission

Parasitemia during pregnancy can cause placentitis followed by spread of tachyzoites to the fetus. In people or sheep, congenital transmission occurs only when the woman or ewe becomes infected during pregnancy. Little is known of transplacental toxoplasmosis in cats or dogs, although its prevalence is thought to be less common than that occurring in sheep and goats.

PATHOGENESIS

The type and severity of clinical illness with *T. gondii* infections are dependent on the degree and localization of tissue injury. Cell necrosis is due to the intracellular growth of *Toxoplasma*; *T. gondii* does not produce a toxin. In infections acquired after the ingestion of tissue cysts or oocysts, initial clinical signs are due to the necrosis of intestine and associated lymphoid organs by tachyzoites. *T. gondii* then spreads to extraintestinal organs via blood or lymph and focal necrosis may develop in many organs (Fig. 86–7). The clinical outcome is determined by the extent of injury to these organs, especially vital organs such as the heart, eye, and adrenal glands. Although acute disseminated infections can be fatal, the host often recovers.

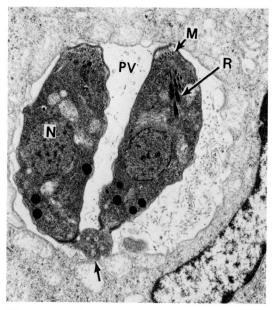

Figure 86–4. Transmission electron micrograph of tachyzoites of *T. gondii*. Tachyzoites are separated from the host cell cytoplasm by a parasitophorous vacuole (PV). One tachyzoite has divided into two progeny that are still attached at the posterior end. Note central nucleus (N), rhoptries (R), and micronemes (M) anterior to the nucleus (× 10,000). (Courtesy of Dr. C. A. Speer, Montana State University, Bozeman, MT.)

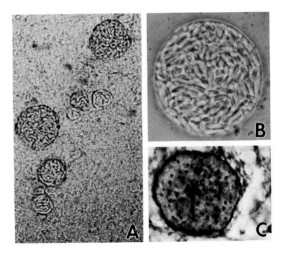

Figure 86–5. T. gondii tissue cysts from brain of experimentally infected mice. A, Different-size tissue cysts (unstained smear; × 300). B, High magnification to show a thin cyst wall and banana-shape bradyzoites (unstained smear, × 1000). C, Tissue cyst in section. The cyst wall is argyrophilic (silver stain; × 1000). (Courtesy of Dr. J. P. Dubey, Zoonotic Diseases Laboratory, US Department of Agriculture, Beltsville, MD.)

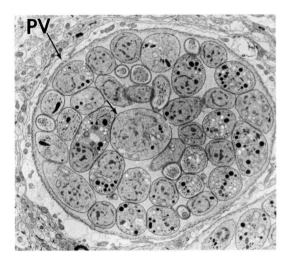

Figure 86–6. Transmission electron micrograph of a young tissue cyst of T. gondii in the brain of a mouse, 21 days PI. The tissue cyst is separated from the cytoplasm of the neuron by a parasitophorous vacuole (PV). One tachyzoite (arrow) is dividing (× 6500). (Courtesy of Dr. D. J. P. Ferguson, Oxford University, England.)

Figure 86–7. Liver of a kitten congenitally infected with T. gondii. Numerous white-yellowish areas of discoloration are due to necrosis produced by tachyzoites. (Courtesy of Dr. J. P. Dubey, Zoonotic Diseases Laboratory, US Department of Agriculture, Beltsville, MD.)

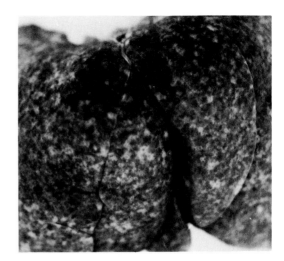

By about the third week after infection, tachyzoites begin to disappear from visceral tissues and may localize as tissue cysts, perhaps in response to host immune mechanisms. Tissue cysts may rupture and released bradyzoites may initiate a clinical relapse during immunosuppression, such as with antitumor or glucocorticoid therapy (Fig. 86–8).[2, 3] The mechanism of reactivation is not known.

Why some infected dogs or cats develop clinical toxoplasmosis whereas others remain well is not fully understood. Age, sex, host species, strain of *T. gondii*, and the number of organisms and stage of the parasite ingested may account for some of these differences. Postnatally acquired toxoplasmosis is generally less serious than prenatally acquired infection. Stress may also aggravate *T. gondii* infection. Concomitant illnesses or immunosuppression may make a host more susceptible because *T. gondii* proliferates as an opportunistic pathogen. Clinical toxoplasmosis in dogs is often associated with canine distemper or other infections or glucocorticoid therapy, but in some cases predisposing disorders cannot be found.[4] Similarly, some cases of clinical feline toxoplasmosis have been observed concomitantly with haemobartonellosis, feline

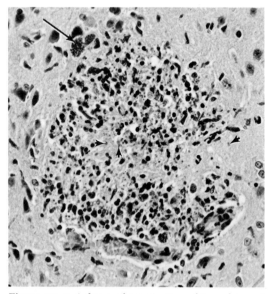

Figure 86–8. A focus of reactivation of toxoplasmosis in the cerebrum of a chronically infected cat medicated with corticosteroids. Tissue cysts (*arrow*) are present at the periphery of the lesion. Numerous tachyzoites (*arrowheads*) are present in the necrotic area but are not visible at this magnification (H and E; × 400). (From Dubey JP, Frenkel JK. *Vet Pathol* 11:350–379, 1974, with permission.)

leukemia and immunodeficiency virus infections, and feline infectious peritonitis.[5, 5a]

CLINICAL FINDINGS

Cats

Clinical toxoplasmosis is most severe in transplacentally infected kittens.[6, 7] Affected kittens may be stillborn or die before weaning. Kittens may continue to suckle until death. Clinical signs reflect inflammation of the liver, lungs, and CNS. Affected kittens may have an enlarged abdomen because of enlarged liver and ascites. Encephalitic kittens may sleep most of the time or cry continuously.

Anorexia, lethargy, and dyspnea owing to pneumonia have been commonly recognized features of postnatal toxoplasmosis. Other clinical signs now have been recognized.[5] These signs, which may not be present in all cases, include persistent or intermittent fever, anorexia, weight loss, icterus owing to hepatitis or cholangiohepatitis, vomiting, diarrhea, abdominal effusion, hyperesthesia on muscle palpation, stiffness of gait, shifting leg lameness, and neurologic deficits. Ocular signs include uveitis involving both anterior and posterior chambers, iritis, iridocyclitis, keratic precipitates, and detachment of retina. Retinitis may occur in both eyes and in both tapetal and nontapetal areas (see Toxoplasmosis, Chapter 13).[5, 6] Clinical signs may be sudden or have a slow onset. The disease may be rapidly fatal in some cats with severe respiratory or CNS signs.

Dogs

Clinical signs may be localized in respiratory, neuromuscular, or gastrointestinal systems or may be caused by generalized infection. The neurologic form of toxoplasmosis may last for several weeks without involvement of other systems, whereas severe disease involving the lungs and liver may kill dogs within a week. Generalized toxoplasmosis is seen mostly in dogs less than 1 year of age and is characterized by fever, tonsillitis, dyspnea, diarrhea, and vomiting. Icterus usually results from extensive hepatic necrosis. Myocardial involvement is usually subclinical, although arrhythmias and heart failure may develop as predominant findings in some older dogs.

The most dramatic clinical signs in older dogs have been associated with neural and muscular systems. Neurologic signs depend on the site of lesion in the cerebrum, cerebellum, or spinal cord.[8, 8a] Seizures, cranial nerve deficits, tremors, ataxia, or paresis or paralysis may be seen. Dogs with myositis may initially have an abnormal gait, muscle wasting, or stiffness.[9, 10] Paraparesis and tetraparesis may rapidly progress to profound tetraplegia with lower motor neuron dysfunction. These animals are depressed, have marked muscle atrophy and hyperesthesia, are unable to move, and have loss of cranial and spinal reflexes. Canine toxoplasmosis is clinically similar to *Neospora caninum* infection, which was previously confused with toxoplasmosis (see Neosporosis, this chapter).

There are only a few reports of ocular lesions associated with toxoplasmosis in dogs.[11] Retinitis, anterior uveitis, iridocyclitis, hyperplasia of ciliary epithelium, and optic nerve neuritis have been noted (see Toxoplasmosis, Chapter 13).

DIAGNOSIS

Clinical Laboratory Findings

Routine hematologic and biochemical parameters may be abnormal in cats and dogs with acute systemic toxoplasmosis. Leukopenia seen in severely affected cats may persist until death and is usually characterized by an absolute lymphopenia and neutropenia with an inappropriate left shift, eosinopenia, and monocytopenia. Leukocytosis may be seen in the recovery phase of illness.

Biochemical abnormalities during the acute phase of illness include hypoproteinemia and hypoalbuminemia. Marked increases in serum ALT (formerly SGPT) and AST (formerly SGOT) activities have been noted in animals with acute hepatic and muscle necrosis. Dogs generally have increased serum ALP activity with hepatic necrosis. Serum creatine phosphokinase (CPK) activity is also increased in cases of muscle necrosis. Serum bilirubin level has been increased in animals with acute hepatic necrosis and especially in cats that develop cholangiohepatitis or hepatic lipidosis. Cats that develop cholangiohepatitis also may show increased serum ALP activity.[12, 13]

Cerebrospinal Fluid

In encephalomyelitic dogs and cats, both protein and leukocytes may be increased in CSF. Cells in CSF are usually a mixed population of large and small mononuclear cells and neutrophils.

Cytology

Tachyzoites may be detected in various body fluids during the acute illness (Fig. 86–3). They are rarely found in blood, CSF, or transtracheal washings but are more common in the peritoneal and thoracic fluids of animals developing thoracic effusions or ascites.

Radiology

Thoracic radiographic findings, especially in cats with acute disease, consist of a diffuse interstitial to alveolar pattern with a mottled lobar distribution. Diffuse symmetric homogeneous increased density due to alveolar coalescence has been noted in severely affected animals. Mild pleural effusion can be present. Abdominal radiographic findings may consist of masses in the intestines or mesenteric lymph nodes or homogeneous increased density as a result of effusion.

Fecal Examination

Despite the high prevalence of serum antibodies in cats worldwide, the prevalence of *T. gondii* oocysts in feces is low. In the United States, less than 1% of cats shed oocysts on any given day.[14] Because cats usually shed *T. gondii* oocysts for only 1 to 2 weeks following their first exposure, oocysts are rarely found in routine fecal examination. Moreover, cats usually are not clinically ill during the period of oocyst shedding.

T. gondii oocysts in feline feces are morphometrically indistinguishable from oocysts of *Hammondia hammondi* and *Besnoitia darlingi*, which also occur in cats.

Oocysts of these coccidians can be differentiated only by sporulation and subsequent animal inoculation. If 10-μm-sized oocysts are found, they should be considered to be T. gondii until proved otherwise. Further inoculations should be attempted only by a competent diagnostic laboratory because of the infectious nature of the organism.

Because of their small size, oocysts of T. gondii are best demonstrated by centrifugation using Sheather's sugar solution (see Appendix 12). Five to ten grams of feces is mixed with water to a liquid consistency and the mixture is strained with gauze. Two parts Sheather's sugar solution (500 g sugar, 300 ml water, and 6.5 g melted phenol crystals) is added to one part fecal suspension and centrifuged in a capped centrifuge tube. Care should be taken not to fill the tube to the top to prevent spillage or aerosols. Following centrifugation at 1000 × g for 10 minutes, remove 1 to 2 drops from the meniscus by a dropper, place on a microscope slide, cover with a coverslip, and examine at low-power (100 ×) magnification. T. gondii oocysts are about one-fourth the size of Isospora felis and one-eighth the size of Toxocara cati, the common roundworm of the cat (Fig. 86–9).[15]

Serologic Testing

Once infected, animals harbor toxoplasmic tissue cysts for their life. Serologic surveys indicate that T. gondii infections are prevalent worldwide. Approximately 30% of cats and dogs in the United States have T.

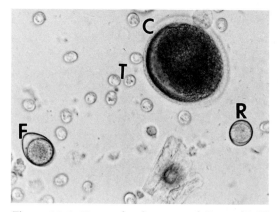

Figure 86–9. Unsporulated oocysts of T. gondii (T), Isospora felis (F), and I. rivolta (R) and an egg of the roundworm Toxocara cati (C) in a flotation of feline feces (unstained; × 410). (Dubey JP. J Am Vet Med Assoc 169:1061–1078, 1976, with permission.)

gondii antibodies.[14, 16, 16a, 17, 18] The prevalence of seropositivity increases with age of the cat or dog because of chance of exposure rather than susceptibility.

Until recently, serologic testing of cats and dogs has involved the measurement of IgG antibodies. Some cats may not develop IgG titers to T. gondii for 4 to 6 weeks. Therefore, tests for IgG antibodies are not an indicator of oocyst shedding. In fact, increased IgG titers to T. gondii indicate only prior infection.[18a] However, serologic testing using IgM-based assays in dogs and cats may be of value in diagnosing clinical toxoplasmosis. For proper interpretation, precautions must be taken concerning the timing and number of samples collected, the type of serologic test performed, and whether IgM or IgG antibodies are being measured.

Five main types of serologic tests have been used in the diagnosis of toxoplasmosis. The methylene blue dye binding (MBD or Sabin-Feldman) method is highly sensitive and specific for human toxoplasmosis but not necessarily for cats. Moreover, the test is too technical to perform in diagnostic laboratories and uses live T. gondii.[19] The indirect immunofluorescent antibody (IFA) technique is comparable to the dye test but does not require the use of live antigen. Some false-positive polar-staining, which can occur with the IFA test, has been attributed to Fc receptors on the surface of T. gondii trophozoites that nonspecifically bind immunoglobulin.[16a] The indirect hemagglutination (IHA) test similarly does not require the use of live antigen and has been adapted for use in a commercially available kit form. It is less sensitive than the MBD and IFA tests. Its main drawback is that it primarily measures IgG and is usually not positive during acute infections. Latex agglutination tests have been adapted to commercially available kits. Although this is an adequate procedure for serologic screening, it cannot be used to distinguish immunoglobulin classes, and primarily detects IgG. The modified agglutination test detects only IgG antibodies but is extremely sensitive. A modification of this test is useful for detecting recently acquired infections in cats.[19] It is also available in a kit form. See Appendix 8 for a listing of available kits for the above procedures. The agglutination test has been improved in its sensitivity and specificity in distinguishing acute or chronic Toxoplasma infections in people by using formalin-fixed or acetone-fixed tachyzoites.[18a] The ELISA methods have been shown to be as sensitive as those of IFA.[20] Immunoblot procedures improve the specificity and sensitivity of the IFA and ELISA assays.[21] The major advantage of these two assay methods is that they may be modified such that IgM titers can be evaluated, making them useful in detecting recent infection in animals.

The IgM-ELISA has been adapted to detect antibodies in cats. Most experimentally infected cats developed IgM antibodies by 2 weeks postinoculation (PI) but became negative by 16 weeks PI (Fig. 86–10).[22, 23] In contrast, IgG antibodies increased beginning 3 to 4 weeks PI and remained so for at least 1 year. Because circulating *T. gondii* antigen has been detected intermittently for at least 1 year, it is unsuitable in separating acute from chronic infections in cats.[23] Results of urine antigen measurements have been positive in rodents with acute experimental toxoplasmosis,[23a] but the specificity of such assays for active infection is uncertain.

In humans, an IgG titer of 1:1024 or more usually indicates acute infection, and a fourfold rise in antibody titer confirms the diagnosis of acute toxoplasmosis. However, IgG titers of 1:1024 or greater in dogs and cats *do not* necessarily indicate acute infections. Furthermore, elevated IgG titers in a single serum sample cannot be equated with clinically active toxoplasmosis in a suspect animal. Chronic persistence of high IgG titers merely reflects continued presence of the *Toxoplasma* antigen. Increases in IgG and IgM titers also may occur during reactivation of chronic infection. A serial fourfold rise in serum titer in blood samples taken 2 to 3 weeks apart is required to confirm active infection using a test that measures IgG. However, both samples must be compared on one test run because of day-to-day variability in measuring antibody titers. Simultaneous measurement of IgG and IgM antibodies offers the most reliable means of determining the presence and duration of feline and canine toxoplasmosis with a single sample. Severe immunosuppressive disorders, such as feline immunodeficiency viral infections, have been associated with impaired increases in antibody titer or lack of class shift from IgM to IgG antibody responses.

Protozoal Isolation

The presence of *T. gondii* can be confirmed by animal or cell culture inoculation. Laboratory mice are the most susceptible animals. Homogenized suspensions of tissues or body fluids obtained at necropsy or by biopsy may be used to infect laboratory mice or tissue culture.[24] Cleaned, sporulated oocysts obtained from feces similarly may be used to infect mice. Generally mice are inoculated SC or intraperitoneally. Beginning 4 to 6 days PI, peritoneal exudates of mice are examined for tachyzoites of *T. gondii* in intraperitoneally inoculated mice. Tissue cysts are present 4 to 6 weeks PI, mostly

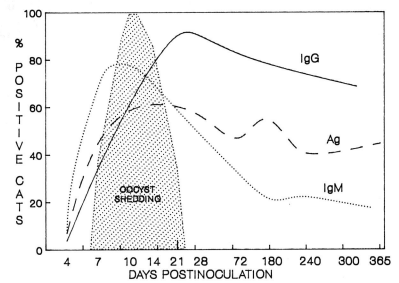

Figure 86–10. Stylized graph showing the relative time periods for oocyst shedding and increases in serum IgG, IgM, and *Toxoplasma* antigen in feline sera based on a number of cats showing a positive test result during the course of experimental toxoplasmosis. (Data from Lappin MR, et al: *Am J Vet Res.* In press.)

in neural tissue. *Toxoplasma* antibodies in mice have developed by 3 weeks PI and can be demonstrated by any one of the serologic tests mentioned above. Lack of parasite demonstration does not mean that the mice are not infected with *T. gondii*, and serologic verification is necessary.

PATHOLOGIC FINDINGS

Dogs

Grossly, necrosis is the predominant lesion, particularly in the brain, lung, liver, and mesenteric lymph nodes. The pulmonic lesion consists of gray-white nodular foci up to 5 mm in diameter and is found subpleurally and in the parenchyma. The bronchial lymph nodes are often enlarged and necrotic. Grossly visible necrotic foci are also seen in pancreas, liver, kidneys, and spleen. Multiple ulcers up to 10 mm in diameter can be seen in the stomach and small intestines. In the CNS, areas of discoloration and necrosis up to 12 mm in diameter and cerebellar atrophy have been observed.[25]

Myositis involving the muscles of the limbs has been observed in dogs with *T. gondii* infections.[9, 10] The affected muscles are pale, flaccid, and reduced in mass and in severe chronic cases are grossly replaced by connective tissue.

Microscopically, pulmonic lesions consist of fibrinous exudation and necrosis involving alveolar walls, blood vessels, and bronchioles. The alveolar lumina are filled with fibrin and occasionally with lymphocytes, neutrophils, and eosinophils. The alveolar lining and terminal epithelial cells are hypoplastic and infiltrated with lymphocytes, plasma cells, and multinucleated giant cells. Necrosis, the predominant muscular lesion, involves myofibers, small blood vessels, and surrounding connective tissue. Necrosed myofibers are replaced by fibrosis. Neural lesions consist of necrosis, gliosis, and vasculitis and are characteristic of a multifocal nonsuppurative meningoencephalomyelitis.[10, 25] Early lesions seen in blood vessels consist of endothelial cell proliferation, necrosis, and perivascular cuffing. Neuronal necrosis, mild malacia, and some astrocytosis may be seen. Multifocal leptomeningeal infiltrates of macrophages, plasma cells, and some lymphocytes and neutrophils are found. In dogs with *T. gondii* polymyositis,

noninflammatory degenerative changes are seen in peripheral nerves and nerve roots.[10] Immunoperoxidase staining can be used to demonstrate *T. gondii* definitively in tissues.[26]

Cats

The gross and microscopic findings may be similar to those seen in dogs; however, in feline toxoplasmosis, necrosis is predominantly seen in the liver (Fig. 86–7), mesenteric lymph nodes, pancreas, and lungs. CNS lesions are similar to those found in dogs. Granulomas may be present in intestines and mesenteric lymph nodes. Cholangiohepatitis, found in cats infected with *Toxoplasma*,[12, 13] has not been reported in any other host. The bile ducts are hyperplastic and plugged with desquamated bile duct epithelium and exudate. *T. gondii* schizonts (not tachyzoites) were seen in the biliary epithelium in both naturally occurring and experimentally induced disease.[1, 27]

THERAPY

Available drugs usually suppress replication of *T. gondii* and are not completely effective in killing the parasite. Dosages for these drugs are summarized in Table 86–1.

Clindamycin is the drug of choice for treating clinical toxoplasmosis in dogs and cats.[3, 5, 9, 28] Because of its good intestinal absorption, oral and parenteral dosages are similar. Clindamycin dosages for treating toxoplasmosis are greater than those used to treat anaerobic infections for which the drug is marketed.

Clinical signs of systemic illness usually begin to resolve within 24 to 48 hours following institution of therapy. Appetite improves, hyperesthesia disappears, and fever usually subsides. Lower motor neuron deficits and muscle atrophy may take 1 to 2 weeks to resolve in animals with polymyositis. Clindamycin has been effective in crossing the blood-brain and blood-vascular barriers in *Toxoplasma*-infected animals and people.[29, 29a] Neurologic deficits improve but some signs persist because of permanent damage caused by CNS inflammation. Anterior uveitis usually improves and active chorioretinitis subsides within 1 week. Complete resolution of inflammation may require

Table 86–1. Therapy for Toxoplasmosis[a]

DRUG	SPECIES	DOSAGE[b] (mg/kg)	ROUTE	INTERVAL (hours)	DURATION (weeks)
Extraintestinal Cycle (Systemic Infection)					
Clindamycin	D	3–13[c]	PO, IM	8	2
	D	10–20	PO, IM	12	2
	C	8–17	PO, IM	8	2
	C	12.5–25	PO, IM	12	2
Sulfonamides[d]	B	30	PO	12	2
and					
Pyrimethamine[e]		0.25–0.5	PO	12	2
Enteroepithelial Cycle (Oocyst Shedding by Cats)					
Clindamycin	C	50	PO, IM	24	1–2
	C	12.5–25	PO, IM	12	1–2
Sulfonamides[d]	C	100	PO	24	1–2
and					
Pyrimethamine		2.0	PO	24	1–2
Monensin	C	[f]	PO	24	1–2
Toltrazuril	C	5–10	PO	24	2

[a]D = dog, C = cat, PO = oral, IM = intramuscular.
[b]Dose per administration at specified interval, expressed as mg/kg unless otherwise stated.
[c]Use proportionally higher dosages/kg/ in small (<5 kg) dogs.
[d]Twice this dosage is used if sulfonamides are used alone.
[e]Available only in 25-mg tablets. For proper dosing of cats, must be divided.
[f]Mixed as 0.02% (w/w) concentration in dry weight of food.

additional treatment with 1% prednisone drops in each eye every 6 to 8 hours for 2 weeks.[5] Cats with concurrent feline immunodeficiency virus (FIV) infections do not respond as well to therapy.

Oral clindamycin causes anorexia, vomiting, or diarrhea in dogs and cats, especially at higher dosages.[9, 30] This appears to be related to local GI irritation, since parenteral therapy at similar dosages does not cause these signs in the same animals. The side effects stop soon after the dosage is reduced or therapy is discontinued. *Clostridium difficile* overgrowth has not been documented in dogs and cats as it has been in people treated with clindamycin (see Lincomycin and Clindamycin, Chapter 43).

Although less suitable than clindamycin, the combination of rapid-acting sulfonamides, such as sulfadiazine or triple sulfas, with pyrimethamine is synergistic in the therapy of systemic toxoplasmosis. Because mental depression, anemia, leukopenia, and thrombocytopenia from bone marrow suppression develop rapidly in cats, frequent hematologic monitoring is required during treatment, especially if therapy lasts longer than 2 weeks. Although trimethoprim-sulfonamide crosses the blood-brain barrier well,[31, 32] it has been reported to be ineffective in treating a dog with severe uveitis and optic neuritis.[11]

Bone marrow suppression can often be corrected with the addition of folinic acid (5.0 mg/day) or by adding brewer's yeast (100 mg/kg/day) to the animal's diet. Brewer's yeast, which contains folic acid, is inexpensive and as effective as folinic acid. The parasite utilizes preformed folic acid better than folinic acid. Nevertheless, pyrimethamine and sulfonamides inhibit folic-folinic acid metabolism in the parasite to a greater extent than in the mammalian cell, so that supplementation with folic acid does not completely reverse therapeutic efficacy when pyrimethamine and sulfonamides are used *in combination*.

Several new drugs, such as trimetrexate and piritrexin, which are antifolates; roxithromycin and azithromycin, both macrolides; and arprinocid, a purine analog and an anticoccidial drug, have been effective in treating experimental toxoplasmosis in mice,[31, 33–37] but they are not available for clinical use in cats or dogs. Doxocycline alone and in combination with sulfonamides has shown efficacy against acute disseminated toxoplasmosis in mice.[37a] Trioxane derivatives have been shown to be effective against *T. gondii* in vitro.[38] Spiramycin, used in Europe for prevention of transplacental transmission of *Toxoplasma*, has not been as effective in treating postnatally infected people.[24, 35]

Oocyst Shedding in Cats

This has been partially controlled only when high dosages of pyrimethamine and sulfonamide have been used (see Table 86–1). Oocyst excretion also has been reduced by the dosages of clindamycin recommended for systemic chemotherapy.

Monensin, an anticoccidial drug used in poultry and cattle feeds, is effective in suppressing oocyst shedding when placed in dry cat food within 1 to 2 days PI.[39] Its use did not prevent infected cats from developing immunity against shedding of oocysts in subsequent exposure to *Toxoplasma*. Toxicity was not noted when the drug was fed for extended periods, despite its known tendency to produce a myopathy in dogs and horses.[40] Toltrazuril has been highly effective when given on a daily basis in preventing oocyst shedding following infection or reshedding after glucocorticoid-induced immunosuppression.[40a] Use of these drugs may be beneficial in treating cats owned by pregnant women, to reduce the risk of potential exposure of the fetus to oocysts.

PREVENTION

Preventing toxoplasmosis in dogs and cats involves measures intended to reduce the incidence of feline infections and subsequent shedding of oocysts into the environment. Cats preferably should be fed only dry or canned, commercially processed cat foods. The prevalence of canine and feline toxoplasmosis has been higher in countries where raw meat products are fed to pets. Household pets should be restricted from hunting and eating potential intermediate hosts or mechanical vectors, such as cockroaches, earthworms, and rodents. If meat is fed, it should always be thoroughly cooked, even if frozen prior to feeding. Cats should be prevented from entering buildings where food-producing animals are housed or feed storage areas.

PUBLIC HEALTH CONSIDERATIONS

Worldwide, nearly 500 million people have *T. gondii* antibodies. The seroprevalence of *T. gondii* is highest (approaching 100%) in warm, moist, or tropical climates and lowest in arid and frigid regions of the world.[17] The rate of congenital infection varies among countries, being higher in continental Europe and South America than in North America.[17] In the United States, prevalence is highest in the East and in the Appalachian mountain regions and is lowest in the arid Southwest and northwestern mountain regions. Approximately 25% to 50% of people tested in the United States have antibodies to *Toxoplasma*.[17]

Clinical disease in people is similar to that seen in infected intermediate hosts, such as dogs. Retinochoroiditis is the primary clinical disease in congenitally infected children. Prenatal detection of fetal infection and treatment of the pregnant mother has greatly reduced the morbidity of disease in newborn infants.[24]

Postnatally acquired infections are generally asymptomatic and self-limiting, usually persisting for 1 to 12 weeks. Such infections with persistent or recurrent lymphadenopathy may resemble infectious mononucleosis or Hodgkin's disease and usually are not fatal unless the host is severely immunosuppressed and the infection becomes disseminated. Reactivation of chronic latent (encysted) infection also is possible and has been seen in AIDS patients when *Toxoplasma* encephalitis is the predominant illness.[17, 41]

Oocyst survival is an important determinant of the distribution and maintenance of the disease in nature. Oocysts, which are shed by cats, contaminate the environment and are ingested by herbivorous animals, who subsequently infect carnivorous animals higher in the food chain, such as humans. People become infected by ingesting infected meat (usually pork, goat, or lamb). Ingestion of raw goat's milk may be an additional source of human toxoplasmosis.

Although oocysts are key in the epidemiology of toxoplasmosis, there is no correlation between toxoplasmosis and cat ownership. Most cats become infected from carnivorism soon after weaning and shed

Table 86–2. Effects of Temperature on Toxoplasma *Oocyst Sporulation*

TEMPERATURE	DAYS
23.8°C (75°F)	1–3
15°C (59°F)	5–8
11°C (51.8°F)	21

oocysts for only short periods thereafter.[14] Cats found to be shedding *T. gondii* oocysts should be hospitalized and treated to eliminate shedding, particularly when a pregnant woman is present in the household. Therefore, to prevent inadvertent environmental contamination, cat owners should practice proper hygienic measures on a routine basis. Since infected cats rarely have diarrhea and since they groom themselves regularly, direct fecal contact when handling infected cats is unlikely.[14]

Litter boxes should be changed daily, since at least 24 hours usually are necessary for oocysts to reach the infective stage. Oocyst sporulation depends on environmental temperature (Table 86–2). Unsporulated oocysts are more susceptible to disinfection and environmental destruction; therefore control efforts should be directed at this stage. Litter pans should be disinfected with scalding water. Cat feces should be disposed of in the septic system, incinerated, or sealed tightly in a plastic bag before placing in a sanitary landfill. Only organic litters that are biodegradable should be placed in the septic system. High-temperature composting to kill oocysts remains to be proved. Under no circumstances should litter boxes be dumped into the environment.

Oocysts survive best in warm, moist soil, factors that help to explain the high prevalence of disease in temperate and tropical climates. Exposure to constant freezing temperatures, drying, and high environmental temperatures is lethal to oocysts (see Table 86–3). Sporulated oocysts may survive in soil for 18 months or more, especially if they are covered and out of direct sunlight. A cat's natural instinct to bury or hide its feces provides the protected environment for oocyst survival. Children's sandboxes should be covered to prevent cats from defecating in them. Mechanical vectors, such as sowbugs, earthworms, and houseflies, have been shown to contain oocysts, and cockroaches and snails are additional mechanical vectors.[42] Control of these invertebrates will help reduce the spread of infection.

Sporulated oocysts resist most disinfectants, and only ammonia is effective when it is in contact with contaminated surfaces for extended periods (see Table 86–3). Because of the time required for chemical disinfection and the fumes produced by ammonia, immersing litter pans in boiling or scalding water usually is the easiest means of disinfection. Steam cleaning can be used to decontaminate hard impervious surfaces.

Outbreaks of human infection have been reported when oocyst-contaminated dust particles were inhaled or ingested.[43] Dispersion of oocysts can also occur by earthmoving or cultivating equipment, shoes, animal feet, wind, rain, and fomites. Streams can become contaminated via water runoff. Stray and wild cats have been known to contaminate streams. A report of military recruits infected by drinking oocyst-contaminated stream water in a jungle has been made.[44] Water from streams or ponds should always be boiled prior to drinking.

Prevention of human toxoplasmosis involves avoiding exposure of susceptible hosts, which includes the unborn fetus and immunosuppressed adults. Risk of exposure by contact with infected meat can be avoided by cooking all meat to greater than 66°C (see Table 86–3)[44a].

Although freezing of meat in home freezers will help reduce the prevalence of infection, it is not a consistently reliable method for killing organisms. Good personal hygiene dictates that hands be washed well after handling raw meat. Animal care technicians cleaning cat cages should wear masks and protective clothing.[14]

Table 86–3. Survival of Toxoplasma

CONDITIONS	MAXIMAL SURVIVAL TIME
Bradyzoites	
−6°C (21.2°F)	1 day
50°C (122°F)	20 min
64°C (147.2°F)	1 min
Oocysts	
Unsporulated	
−21°C (−5.8°F)	1 day
37°C (98.6°F)	1 day
Sporulated	
−20°C (−4°F)	28 days
50°C (122°F)	30 min
5% Ammonia	60 min

Neosporosis

ETIOLOGY

Neospora caninum is a newly described protozoan that has been previously confused with *T. gondii*.[45] Its tachyzoites and tissue cysts resemble those of *T. gondii* under the light microscope. The complete life cycle of this organism is unknown. Tachyzoites are 5 to 7 μm by 1 to 5 μm, depending on the stage of division (Fig. 86–11). They divide into two zoites by endodyogeny. In infected carnivores tachyzoites are found within macrophages, polymorphonuclear cells, spinal fluid, and neural and other cells of the body. Individual organisms are ovoid, lunate, or globular. They contain one or two nuclei and are arranged either singly, in pairs, or in groups of four or more.

Nonseptate tissue cysts (up to 100 μm in diameter) are found in neural cells (Fig. 86–12). They may be round or elongated. The cyst wall is 1 to 4 μm thick and encloses slender PAS-positive bradyzoites.

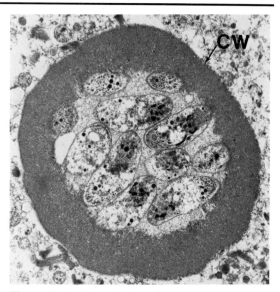

Figure 86–12. Transmission electron micrograph of a tissue cyst of *N. caninum* in the brain of a dog. Note the thick cyst wall (CW) and slender bradyzoites (× 9939). (Courtesy of Dr. J. P. Dubey, Zoonotic Diseases Laboratory, US Department of Agriculture, Beltsville, MD.)

CLINICAL FINDINGS

Naturally occurring infections were reported only in dogs and calves but, experimentally, domestic cats are also susceptible.[45–47, 47a] In general, clinical findings are similar to those of toxoplasmosis, but neurologic deficits and muscular abnormalities

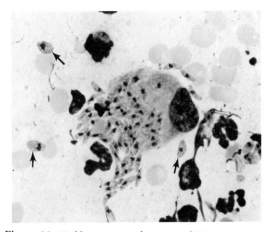

Figure 86–11. Numerous tachyzoites of *N. caninum* in a smear of an ulcer in the skin of a dog. Dividing tachyzoites (*arrows*) are thicker than nondividing tachyzoites (Giemsa; × 750). (Courtesy of Dr. J. P. Dubey, Zoonotic Diseases Laboratory, US Department of Agriculture, Beltsville, MD.)

predominate. Both pups and older dogs are affected and the infection can be transmitted congenitally.[48] Older dogs have had signs of multifocal CNS involvement, polymyositis, myocarditis, dermatitis, or multifocal dissemination.[45] The most severe infections have been seen in young (<6-month-old) dogs presented with ascending paralysis of limbs. Features that distinguish neosporosis from other forms of paralysis are gradual muscle atrophy and stiffness, usually as an ascending paralysis with the pelvic limbs being more severely affected than the thoracic limbs. It progresses to rigid contracture of the muscles of the affected limb (Fig. 86–13). Cervical weakness, dysphagia, and death develop with time. This syndrome of progressive polyradiculomyositis of young dogs has been recognized previously.[49–54] Explanation for the musculoskeletal rigidity are that lower motor neuron injury occurs to the developing neuromuscular system of young animals and that nerve root and muscle involvement is extensive. It is likely that many cases diagnosed as toxoplasmosis were due to *N. caninum* infection. Ultrastructural and immunochemical methods have confirmed this organism to be distinct from *T. gondii*.[45, 55–59]

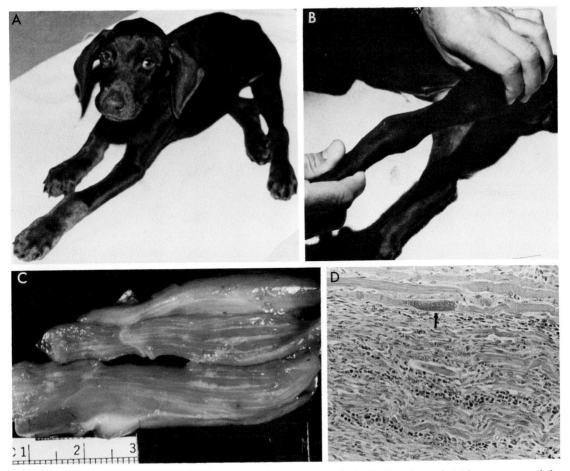

Figure 86–13. A, Three-month-old Doberman pinscher with tetraplegia. B, Atrophy and rigid contracture of the puppy's limbs are apparent. C, Gross and D, microscopic appearances of muscle fibers in chronic myositis. A group of organisms (*arrow*) is shown in D (H and E; × 40).

DIAGNOSIS

Hematologic and biochemical findings have been variable, depending on the organ system of involvement. With muscle disease, CPK and AST activities have been increased. CSF abnormalities have included mild increases in protein (>20 but <50 mg/dl) and nucleated cell (>10 but <50 cells/dl) concentrations. Differential leukocyte counts included monocytes, lymphocytes, neutrophils, and eosinophils in decreasing numbers, respectively. Electromyographic abnormalities have consisted of reduced insertion potentials and fibrillation potentials. Antisera used to detect *T. gondii* antibodies do not cross-react with N. *caninum*, so that serum or CSF antibody titers to *T. gondii* are negative.

N. *caninum* may be found in CSF and biopsy tissues and may be detected with any stain used to stain blood films. N. *caninum* can be differentiated from *T. gondii* by its location in the host cell cytoplasm. N. *caninum* tachyzoites are usually located in the host cell cytoplasm (Fig. 86–14), whereas *T. gondii* is always separated from the cytoplasm by a parasitophorous vacuole. Tissue cysts of N. *caninum* have thicker walls than those of *T. gondii* (Fig. 86–15). N. *caninum* can be grown in cell culture and in rodents. A fluorescent antibody test using cell-cultured N. *caninum* can detect N. *caninum*-specific antibodies, and N. *caninum* can be distinguished from *T. gondii* in sections by an immunochemical stain.[46,59]

PATHOLOGIC FINDINGS

Nonsuppurative encephalomyelitis, polyradiculoneuritis, myositis, and myofibrosis

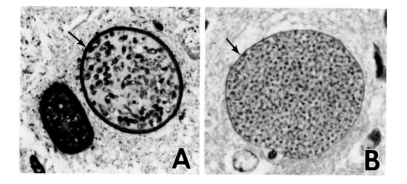

Figure 86–15. Comparison of tissue cysts of *N. caninum* (A) and *T. gondii* (B) in the brain (H and E, × 750). The cyst wall (*arrows*) of *N. caninum* is thicker than that of *T. gondii*. (Courtesy of Dr. J. P. Dubey, Zoonotic Diseases Laboratory, US Department of Agriculture, Beltsville, MD.)

are the predominant findings (see Fig. 86–13). Necrosis of other tissues also occurs.[45] *N. caninum* appears to induce more inflammation than *T. gondii* and has been found to cause severe phlebitis and dermatitis.

THERAPY

Information on effective therapy for this disease is limited. However, drugs used for therapy of toxoplasmosis should be tried early in the course of illness. In one instance, clindamycin given at a daily dosage of 40

mg/kg, divided into three doses, did not reverse the signs of paralysis in an affected dog.[60] The degree of muscle contracture was so marked at the time of therapy that clinical improvement was not expected. Progression of the disease might be arrested by treatment. In experimental infections in mice, treatment with sulfadiazine was effective in reducing clinical severity of neosporosis.[61]

References

1. Dubey JP: *Toxoplasma, Hammondia, Besnoitia, Sarcocystis,* and other tissue cyst-forming coccidia of man and animals. In Kreier JP (ed): *Parasitic Protozoa,* Vol 3. New York, Academic Press, 1977, pp 101–237.
2. Dubey JP, Frenkel JK: Immunity to feline toxoplasmosis: modification by administration of corticosteroids. *Vet Pathol* 11:350–379, 1974.
3. Lappin MR, Greene CE, Dawe DW: Methyl prednisolone acetate effect on serology and oocyst shedding in cats with chronic toxoplasmosis. *Am J Vet Res.* In press, 1990.
4. Dubey JP, Carpenter JL, Topper MJ, et al: Fatal toxoplasmosis in dogs. *J Am Anim Hosp Assoc.* In press, 1989.
5. Lappin MR, Greene CE, Winston S, et al: Clinical feline toxoplasmosis: serologic diagnosis and therapeutic management of 15 cases. *J Vet Intern Med.* In press, 1989.
5a. Witt CJ, Moench TR, Gittelsohn AM, et al: Epidemiologic observations on feline immunodeficiency virus and *Toxoplasma gondii* coinfection in cats in Baltimore, Md. *J Am Vet Med Assoc* 194:229–232, 1989.
6. Dubey JP, Johnstone I: Fatal neonatal toxoplasmosis in cats. *J Am Anim Hosp Assoc* 18:461–467, 1982.
7. Dubey JP: Unpublished observations, Agricultural Research Service, U.S. Dept. of Agriculture, Beltsville, MD, 1988.
8. Averill DR, de Lahunta A: Toxoplasmosis of the canine nervous system: clinicopathologic findings in four cases. *J Am Vet Med Assoc* 159:1134–1141, 1971.
8a. Hass JA, Shell L, Saunders G: Neurological manifestations of toxoplasmosis: a literature review and case summary. *J Am Anim Hosp Assoc* 25:253–260, 1989.

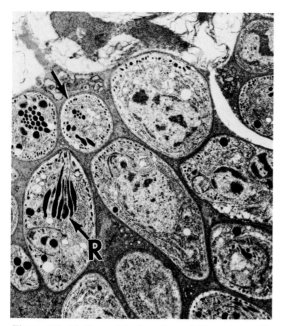

Figure 86–14. Several tachyzoites of *N. caninum* directly in the cytoplasm of a myelinated cell (*arrow*) in the spinal cord of a dog. Several tachyzoites are dividing into two by endodyogeny. Numerous rhoptries (R) in tachyzoites distinguish *N. caninum* from *T. gondii* (× 10,425). (Courtesy of Dr. J. P. Dubey, Zoonotic Diseases Laboratory, US Department of Agriculture, Beltsville, MD.)

9. Greene CE, Cook JP, Mahaffey EA: Clindamycin for treatment of *Toxoplasma gondii* polymyositis in a dog. *J Am Vet Med Assoc* 187:631–634, 1985.

10. Braund KG, Blagburn BL, Toivio-Kinnucan M, et al: *Toxoplasma* polymyositis/polyneuropathy—a new clinical variant in two mature dogs. *J Am Anim Hosp Assoc* 24:93–97, 1988.

11. Bussanich MN, Rootman J: Implicating toxoplasmosis as the cause of ocular lesions. *Vet Med* 80:43–51, 1985.

12. Smart ME, Downey RS, Stockdale PHG: Toxoplasmosis in a cat associated with cholangitis and progressive pancreatitis. *Can Vet J* 14:313–316, 1973.

13. Neufeld JL, Brandt RW: Cholangiohepatitis in a cat associated with a coccidia-like organism. *Can Vet J* 15:156–159, 1974.

14. Dubey JP: Toxoplasmosis in cats. *Feline Pract* 16:12–45, 1986.

15. Dubey JP: A review of *Sarcocystis* of domestic animals and of other coccidia of cats and dogs. *J Am Vet Med Assoc* 169:1061–1078, 1976.

16. Dubey JP: Toxoplasmosis in dogs. *Canine Pract* 12:7–28, 1985.

16a. Budzko DB, Tyler L, Armstrong D: Fc receptors on the surface of *Toxoplasma gondii* trophozoites: a confounding factor in testing for anti-*Toxoplasma* antibodies by indirect immunofluorescence. *J Clin Microbiol* 27:959–961, 1989.

17. Dubey JP, Beattie CP: *Toxoplasmosis of Animals and Man*. Boca Raton, FL, CRC Press, 1988, pp 1–220.

18. Lappin MR, Greene CE, Prestwood AK, et al: *Toxoplasma gondii* serologic prevalence of infection as determined by enzyme-linked immunosorbent assays for detection of immunoglobulin M, immunoglobulin G, and circulating antigens in healthy and clinically ill cats in Georgia. *Vet Parasitol*. In press.

18a. Suzuke Y, Israelski DM, Danneman BR, et al: Diagnosis of toxoplasmic encephalitis in patients with acquired immunodeficiency syndrome by using a new serologic method. *J Clin Microbiol* 26:2542–2543, 1988.

19. Dubey JP, Thulliez PH: Serologic diagnosis of toxoplasmosis in cats fed *Toxoplasma gondii* tissue cysts. *J Am Vet Med Assoc* 194:1297–1299, 1989.

20. Pappas MG, Lunde MN, Hajkowski R, et al: Determination of IgM and IgG antibodies to *Toxoplasma* using the IFA test, ELISA, and dot-ELISA procedures. *Vet Parasitol* 20:31–42, 1986.

21. Partenen P, Turunen HJ, Paasivuo RTA, et al: Immunoblot analysis of *Toxoplasma gondii* antigens by human immunoglobulins G, M, and A antibodies at different stages of infection. *J Clin Microbiol* 20:133–135, 1984.

22. Lappin MR, Greene CE, Prestwood AK, et al: Diagnosis of recent *Toxoplasma gondii* infection in cats utilizing an enzyme-linked immunosorbent assay for immunoglobulin M. *Am J Vet Res* 50:1580–1585, 1989.

23. Lappin MR, Greene CE, Prestwood AK, et al: Enzyme-linked immunosorbent assay for the detection of circulating antigens of *Toxoplasma gondii* in the serum of cats. *Am J Vet Res* 50:1586–1589, 1989.

23a. Huskinson J, Stepick-Biek P, Remington JS: Detection of antigens in urine during acute toxoplasmosis. *J Clin Microbiol* 27:1099–1101, 1989.

24. Daffas F, Forestier F, Capella-Pavlovsky M, et al: Prenatal management of 746 pregnancies at risk for congenital toxoplasmosis. *N Engl J Med* 318:271–275, 1988.

25. Koestner A, Cole CR: Neuropathology of canine toxoplasmosis. *Am J Vet Res* 21:831–844, 1960.

26. Conley FK, Jenkins KA, Remington JS: *Toxoplasma gondii* infection of the central nervous system. Use of the peroxidase-antiperoxidase method to demonstrate *Toxoplasma* in formalin-fixed, paraffin embedded tissue sections. *Human Pathol* 12:690–698, 1981.

27. Dubey JP, Frenkel JK: Cyst-induced toxoplasmosis in cats. *J Protozool* 19:155–177, 1972.

28. Dubey JP, Yeary RA: Anticoccidial activity of 2-sulfamoyl-4,4-diaminodiphenylsulfone, sulfadiazine, pyrimethamine and clindamycin in cats infected with *Toxoplasma gondii*. *Can Vet J* 18:51–57, 1977.

29. Rolston KVI, Hoy J: Role of clindamycin in the treatment of central nervous system toxoplasmosis. *Am J Med* 83:551–554, 1987.

29a. Danneman BR, Israelski DM, Remington JS: Treatment of toxoplasmic encephalitis with intravenous clindamycin. *Ann Intern Med* 148:2477–2482, 1988.

30. Greene CE, Lappin MR, Marks M: Clinical and biochemical changes in healthy cats given clindamycin. Unpublished information. University of Georgia, Athens, GA, 1989.

31. Luft BJ, Remington JS: Toxplasmic encephalitis. *J Infect Dis* 157:1–6, 1988.

32. Weiss LM, Harris C, Berger M, et al: Pyrimethamine concentrations in serum and cerebrospinal fluid during treatment of acute *Toxoplasma* encephalitis in patients with AIDS. *J Infect Dis* 157:580–583, 1988.

33. Luft BJ: Potent in vivo activity of arprinocid, a purine analogue, against murine toxoplasmosis. *J Infect Dis* 154:692–694, 1986.

34. Araujo FG, Guptill DR, Remington JS: In vivo activity of piritrexin against *Toxoplasma gondii*. *J Infect Dis* 156:828–830, 1987.

35. Araujo FG, Guptill DR, Remington JS: Azithromycin, a macrolide antibiotic with potent activity against *Toxoplasma gondii*. *Antimicrob Agents Chemother* 32:755–757, 1988.

36. Chang HR, Pechere J-CF: Effect of roxithromycin on acute toxoplasmosis in mice. *Antimicrob Agents Chemother* 31:1147–1149, 1987.

37. Kovacs JA, Allegra CJ, Chabner BA, et al: Potent effect of trimetrexate, a lipid-soluble antifolate, on *Toxoplasma gondii*. *J Infect Dis* 155:1027–1032, 1987.

37a. Chang HR, Conte R, Pechere JC: In vitro and in vivo activity of doxycycline against *Toxoplasma gondii*. 29th Intersci Conf Antimicrob Agents Chemother, Houston, September 1989, p 141. (Abstr).

38. Chang HR, Jefford CW, Pechere J-CF: Potent activity of new 1,2,4-trioxanes against *Toxoplasma gondii*. Abstr, 28th Annu Intersci Conf Antimicrob Agents, Los Angeles, October 1988, p 291.

39. Frenkel JK, Smith DD: Inhibitory effects of monensin on shedding of *Toxoplasma* oocysts by cats. *J Parasitol* 68:851–855, 1982.

40. Wilson JS: Toxic myopathy in a dog associated with the presence of monensin in dry food. *Can Vet J* 21:30–31, 1980.

40a. Rommel M, Schnieder T, Krause HD, et al: Trials to suppress the formation of oocysts and cysts of

Toxoplasma gondii in cats by medication of the feed with toltrazuril. Vet Med Rev 2:141–153, 1987.

41. Luft BJ, Brooks RG, Conley FK, et al: Toxoplasmic encephalitis in patients with acquired immune deficiency syndrome. JAMA 252:913–917, 1984.

42. Frenkel JK, Ruiz A, Chinchilla M: Soil survival of Toxoplasma oocysts in Kansas and Costa Rica. Am J Trop Med Hyg 24:439–443, 1975.

43. Teutsch SM, Juranek DD, Sulzer A, et al: Epidemic toxoplasmosis associated with infected cats. N Engl J Med 300:695–699, 1979.

44. Benenson MW, Takbujl ET, Lemon SM, et al: Oocyst-transmitted toxoplasmosis associated with ingestion of contaminated water. N Engl J Med 307:666–669, 1982.

44a. Dubey, JP, Kotula AW, Sharar A, et al: Effect of high temperature on infectivity of Toxoplasma gondii "tissue cysts." J Parasitol. In press, 1990.

45. Dubey JP, Carpenter JL, Speer CA, et al: Newly recognized fatal protozoan disease of dogs. J Am Vet Med Assoc 192:1269–1285, 1988.

46. Dubey JP, Hattel AL, Lindsay DS, et al: Neonatal Neospora caninum infection in dogs: isolation of causative agent and experimental transmission. J Am Vet Med Assoc 193:1259–1263, 1988.

47. Dubey JP, Lindsay DS: Fatal Neospora caninum infection in kittens. J Parasitol 75:148–151, 1989.

47a. Dubey JP, Leathers CW, Lindsay DS: Neospora caninum-like protozoon associated with fatal myelitis in newborn calves. J Parasitol 75:146–148, 1989.

48. Dubey JP, Lindsay DS: Transplacental transmission of Neospora caninum infection in dogs. Am J Vet Res 50:1578–1579, 1989.

49. Holliday TA, Olander HJ, Wind AP: Skeletal muscle atrophy associated with canine toxoplasmosis: a case report. Cornell Vet 53:288–301, 1963.

50. Drake JC, Hime JM: Two syndromes in young dogs caused by Toxoplasma gondii. J Small Anim Pract 8:621–626, 1967.

51. Nesbit JW, Lourens DC, Williams MC: Spastic paresis in two littermate pups caused by Toxoplasma gondii. J S Afr Vet Assoc 52:243–246, 1981.

52. Core DM, Hoff EJ, Milton JL: Hindlimb hyperextension as a result of Toxoplasma gondii polyradiculitis. J Am Anim Hosp Assoc 19:713–716, 1983.

53. Greene CE, Prestwood AK: Coccidial infections. In Greene CE (ed): Clinical Microbiology and Infectious Diseases of the Dog and Cat. Philadelphia, WB Saunders Co, 1984, pp 824–858.

54. Suter MM, Hauser B, Palmer DG: Polymyositis-polyradiculitis due to toxoplasmosis in the dog: serology and tissue biopsy as diagnostic aids. Zentrabl Vet Med [A] 31:792–798, 1984.

55. Bjerkäs I, Mohn SF, Presthus J: Unidentified cyst-forming sporozoon causing encephalomyelitis and myositis in dogs. Z Parasitenkd 70:271–274, 1984.

56. Bjerkäs I, Landsverk T: Identification of Toxoplasma gondii and Encephalitozoon cuniculi by immunoperoxidase techniques and electron microscopy, in stored, formalin-fixed, paraffin-embedded tissue. Acta Vet Scand 27:11–22, 1986.

57. Hilali M, Lindberg R, Waller T, et al: Enigmatic cyst-forming sporozoon in the spinal cord of a dog. Acta Vet Scand 27:623–625, 1986.

58. Cummings JF, de Lahunta A, Suter MM, et al: Canine protozoan polyradiculoneuritis. Acta Neuropathol 76:46–54, 2988.

59. Lindsay DS, Dubey JP: Immunohistochemical diagnosis of Neospora caninum in tissue sections. Am J Vet Res. In press, 1989.

60. Hay WH, Shell LG, Lindsay DS, et al: Diagnosis and treatment of Neospora caninum in a dog. J Am Vet Med Assoc. In press, 1990.

61. Lindsay DS, Dubey JP: Unpublished data. USDA, Beltsville, MD, 1989.

87 ENTERIC COCCIDIOSIS

J. P. Dubey
Craig E. Greene

Coccidia are obligate intracellular parasites normally found in the intestinal tract. They belong to phylum Apicomplexa, class Sporozoasida, order Eucoccidiorida, family Eimeriidae, Cryptosporidiidae, or Sarcocystidae. Coccidian genera that infect cats and dogs are *Isospora* (also called *Cystoisospora*), *Hammondia*, *Besnoitia*, *Sarcocystis*, *Toxoplasma*, and *Cryptosporidium*. The last two genera are discussed in Chapters 86 and 88, respectively. An undefined *Caryospora*-like infection is discussed in this section. Another coccidian genus, *Eimeria*, found commonly in herbivores and rodents, is found in feces of dogs and cats only after they ingest intestinal contents or feces from herbivores or rodents; the oocysts pass unchanged through the feline or canine intestine. Some coccidians of dogs remain unclassified.

Intestinal Coccidiosis

All coccidians have an asexual and a sexual cycle. In some genera, such as *Sarcocystis*, the asexual and sexual cycles occur in different hosts, whereas in *Isospora* both the cycles may be found in the same host (Table 87–1 and Fig. 87–1). The oocyst is the environmentally resistant stage in the life cycle of all coccidia and is excreted in feces of the definitive host.

A typical coccidian life cycle is best represented by the description that follows. Oocysts are passed unsporulated in feces and contain a single nucleated mass called sporont, which almost fills the oocyst (Fig. 87–2).[1] After exposure to air, warm (20° to 37°C) temperatures, and moisture, oocysts sporulate, and two sporocysts are formed. Within each sporocyst are four sporozoites

Table 87–1. Comparison of Some Coccidial Genera that Infect Dogs and Cats[a]

	SEXUAL CYCLE: INTESTINAL REPLICATION		MEANS OF TRANSMISSION	ASEXUAL CYCLE: EXTRAINTESTINAL REPLICATION	
	Definitive Hosts	Form of Oocyst Passed	Direct Transmission Possible	Intermediate or Paratenic Hosts	Location of Tissue Cysts
Isospora	B	U	Yes	Dog, cat, many other mammals	Extraintestinal or lymphoid tissues (monozoic)
Besnoitia	C	U	No	Many vertebrates	Fibroblasts
Hammondia	B	U	No	Herbivores, rodents	Skeletal muscle
Sarcocystis	B	S[b]	No	Many vertebrates	Cardiac and skeletal muscle
Cryptosporidium	B	S[c]	Yes	None	None
Toxoplasma	C	U	Yes	Many vertebrates	Many tissues

[a]B = both dog and cat, C = cat, U = unsporulated, S = sporulated.
[b]Free sporocysts.
[c]Naked sporozoites.

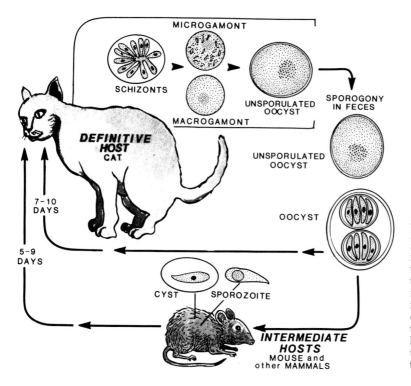

Figure 87–1. Life cycle of *Isospora felis*, which is typical of the *Isospora* spp. The mode of transmission may be direct, via ingestion of sporulated oocysts from the environment, or indirect, via ingestion of cysts in prey animals. Sexual and asexual reproduction of the parasite occur in the intestines of the definitive host (in this case, a cat), and unsporulated oocysts are shed in the feces of definitive hosts.

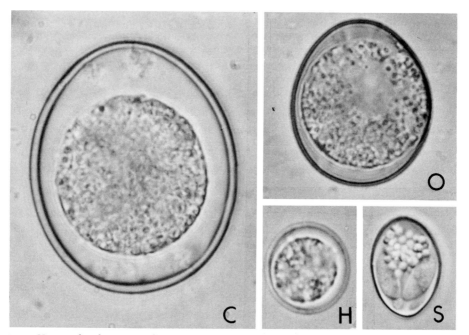

Figure 87–2. Unsporulated oocysts of *Isospora canis* (C), *I. ohioensis* (O), and *Hammondia heydorni* (H) and sporulated sporocyst of *Sarcocystis* sp. (S) from canine feces (unstained; × 1700). (From Dubey JP. *J Am Vet Med Assoc* 169:1061–1078, 1976, with permission.)

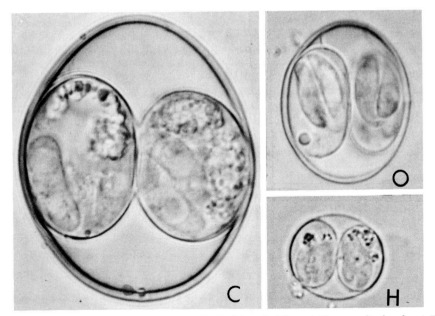

Figure 87–3. Sporulated oocysts of *Isospora canis* (C), *I. ohioensis* (O), and *Hammondia heydorni* (H). Compare with Fig. 87–2 (unstained; × 1700). (From Dubey JP. *J Am Vet Med Assoc* 169:1061–1078, 1976, with permission.)

(Fig. 87–3). The sporozoites are banana-shaped and are the infective stage (Fig. 87–4).[2] They can survive environmental exposure inside the oocysts for many months. After the ingestion of sporulated oocysts by cats or dogs, sporozoites excyst in the intestinal lumen, and the sporozoites initiate the formation of schizonts or meronts. During schizogony or merogony, the sporozoite nucleus divides into two, three, or more nuclei, depending upon the parasite and the stage of the cycle. After nuclear division, each nucleus is surrounded by cytoplasm, forming a merozoite. The number of merozoites within a schizont varies from two to several hundred, depending upon the stage of the cycle and the species of coccidia. Merozoites are released from a schizont when the host cell ruptures. The number of schizogonic cycles vary with the parasite. First genera-

Figure 87–4. *Isospora canis* sporulated oocyst treated with 5.25% sodium hypochlorite solution to dissolve part of the oocyst wall (OW). Two sporocysts occupy most of the oocyst. Each sporocyst has a thin sporocyst wall (SW), four banana-shaped sporozoites (S), and a sporocystic residual body (SR). The SR may be compact or dispersed (unstained; × 1600). (From Kirkpatrick CE, Dubey JP. *Vet Clin North Am [Small Anim Pract]* 17:1405–1420, 1987, with permission.)

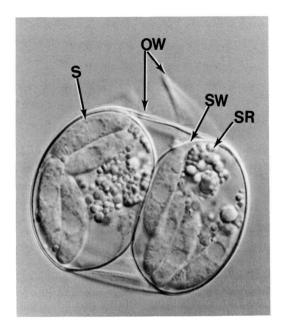

tion merozoites either repeat the asexual cycle and form second generation schizonts or may transform into male (micro) and female (macro) gamonts. The microgamont divides into many tiny microgametes. A microgamete fertilizes a macrogamete, and an oocyst wall is formed around the zygote. The life cycle is completed when unsporulated oocysts are excreted in feces.

ISOSPORA (CYSTOISOSPORA)

Members of the genus Isospora, the most commonly recognized coccidians infecting dogs or cats, are species-specific for the definitive host. At least four species, I. canis, I. ohioensis, I. burrowsi, and I. neorivolta, infect dogs; two species, I. felis and I. rivolta, infect cats.

The life cycle of Isospora infecting dogs and cats is similar to the basic coccidian intestinal cycle, except an asexual cycle can also occur in the definitive or intermediate host.[3] Upon ingestion by definitive or suitable paratenic (intermediate) hosts, oocysts excyst in the presence of bile, and free sporozoites invade the intestine. Some sporozoites penetrate the intestinal wall and enter mesenteric lymph nodes or other extraintestinal tissues, where they form enlarging unicellular cysts (Fig. 87–5). Since no replication occurs, the term paratenic, rather than intermediate, host is used. Monozoic cysts of Isospora may remain in extraintestinal tissues of definitive and paratenic hosts for the life of the host.[4] In dogs and cats, these "cysts" may serve as a source of intestinal reinfection and relapse of enteric coccidiosis. Ingestion of monozoic cysts in paratenic hosts leads to intestinal infection in the definitive dog and cat host. The life cycle after the ingestion of paratenic host is the same as after the ingestion of sporulated oocysts from feces.

Clinical Findings

Diarrhea with coccidiosis in immunocompetent animals probably represents incidental or concurrent infections with coccidia and other infectious agents, since coccidial infection can be present in the absence of clinical illness. Enzootic infections are frequently found in catteries or kennels where animals are congregated, with clinical signs being most apparent in neonates. Experimental studies have shown that clinical signs of intestinal disease are uncommon unless large numbers of oocysts are fed to very young (<1 month old) or immunosuppressed animals.[3] Clinically, severe diarrhea has been associated with naturally occurring coccidiosis in immunosuppressed dogs and cats.[5,6] Diarrhea with weight loss and dehydration and, rarely, hemorrhage is the primary sign attributed to coccidiosis in dogs and cats. Anorexia, vomiting, mental depression, and death may be seen in severely affected animals. Severely immunosuppressed dogs and cats may have extraintestinal stages in macrophages of their lymphocyte-depleted mesenteric lymph nodes or extraintestinal tissues.

Intestinal coccidiosis may be manifested clinically when dogs or cats are shipped or weaned or when there is a change in ownership. Diarrhea might result from the extraintestinal stages of Isospora returning to the intestines. Monozoic cysts do not cause clinical disease in paratenic hosts.

Diagnosis

Diagnosis of intestinal coccidial infection in dogs and cats is made by identification of the oocysts by any of the fecal flotation methods commonly used to diagnose parasitic infections (see Fecal Examination, Chapter 86 and Appendix 12). In dogs, only I. canis can be identified with certainty by oocyst size and shape (see Fig. 87–2). The two species of Isospora occurring in cats can be readily distinguished by oocyst size (see Fig. 86–9). Oocysts of I. felis in cats and I. canis in dogs are large and easily distinguished from small oocysts, whereas it is almost impossible to distinguish I. rivolta, I. burrowsi, and I. ohioensis morphologically (Fig. 87–6; see also Fig. 86–9). Although I. felis-, I. rivolta-, I. canis-, and I. ohioensis-like oocysts are passed unsporulated in freshly excreted feces, they sporulate partially by the time fecal examination is made. Partially sporulated oocysts contain two sporocysts without sporozoites. Isospora spp. may sporulate within 8 hours of excretion, and these Isospora are highly infectious.

Therapy

The presence of underlying disease or host immunosuppression should be suspected

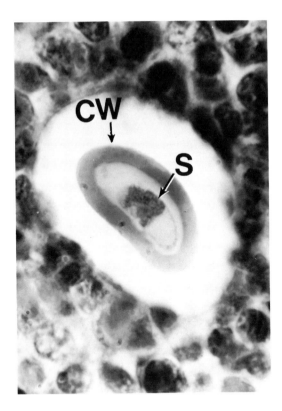

Figure 87–5. Tissue cyst of *Isospora felis* in smear of mesenteric lymph node of an experimentally-infected mouse. The sporozoite (S) is surrounded by a thick cyst wall (CW). The vacuole around the cyst wall is a fixation artifact (PAS; × 1250).

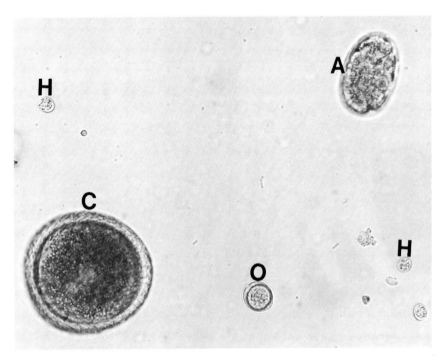

Figure 87–6. Unsporulated oocysts of *Isospora ohioensis* (O) and *Hammondia heydorni* (H) compared with eggs of the nematodes *Toxocara canis* (C) and *Ancylostoma caninum* (A) in a flotation of canine feces (unstained; × 385). (From Dubey JP. *J Am Vet Med Assoc* 169:1061–1078, 1976, with permission.)

whenever coccidial infections persist for extended periods in older animals or seem to be associated with chronic diarrhea. Treatment is often indicated in bitches and their newborn puppies because of the severity of clinical signs at this age. If diarrhea or dehydration is severe, parenteral fluid therapy must be considered as a supportive measure. Blood transfusions may be required when severe intestinal hemorrhage results in anemia.

Specific therapy involves the use of drugs that are coccidiostatic rather than curative (Table 87–2). However, as with many protozoal diseases, the presence of low-level infection may lead to premmunity.

Sulfonamides have long been the drugs of choice for the treatment of coccidiosis. Rapid-acting sulfonamides, such as sulfadimethoxine or sulfaguanidine, can be used alone or in combination with other antifolate drugs such as trimethoprim. Trimethoprim-sulfonamide offers the advantage of being readily available and is of lower toxicity compared with other drugs. It should be considered a drug of first choice. Nitrofurazone can be used alone or in combination with sulfonamides. Nitrofurazone is also available as a 4.59% soluble powder that can be added to drinking water (up to 1 g/2 L) for 7 days.

Amprolium is considered effective preventive and treatment procedure for coccidiosis in kenneled puppies. Although it is not presently approved for use in dogs, it can be administered as an undiluted liquid or paste, but it is unpalatable in these forms. Use of gelatin capsules is recommended when puppies object to the drug in food or water. One gelatin capsule containing 100 mg of 20% amprolium in soluble powder can be given daily for 7 to 12 days to 6-week old puppies of small breed (<10 kg in adult weight) dogs. Puppies of larger breeds should receive 200 mg as a total daily dosage for the same interval. Anorexia may develop in puppies that eat more than 300 mg of amprolium on a daily basis.[11] Amprolium also can be used in drinking water in which 29.6 ml (1 ounce) of 9.6% solution is added to 4 liters (1 gallon) of water for 7 to 10 days; no other source of water is provided.

Toxic side effects of amprolium include anorexia, diarrhea, depression, and CNS signs related to thiamine deficiency. Signs of toxicity may be reversed if parenteral thiamine therapy (1 to 10 mg/day IM or IV) is instituted early.

Quinacrine, spiramycin, toltrazuril, and roxithromycin are drugs that have been used on a limited basis to treat canine and feline coccidiosis. Their use might be considered if more established treatment regimens fail or protozoal resistance develops.

Table 87–2. Anticoccidial Drugs for Dogs and Cats[a]

DRUG	SPECIES	DOSE[b] (mg/kg)	ROUTE	INTERVAL (hours)	DURATION (days)
Sulfamethoxine[c, 7]	B	50–60	PO	24	5–20
Sulfaquanidine[7, 8]	B	100–200	PO	8	5
Trimethoprim-sulfonamide[9]	D	30–60[d]	PO, SC	24	5
	B	15–30[e]	PO, SC	12–24	5
Ormetoprim-sulfadimethoxine[6]	D	66[f]	PO	24	7–23
Furazolidone[g, 10]	B	8–20	PO	12–24	5
Amprolium[11, 12]	D	300–400[h] (total)	PO	24	5
	D	110–200[i] (total)	PO	24	7–12
	C	60–100 (total)	PO	24	7
Quinacrine[13]	B	10	PO	24	5
Spiramycin[7, 14]	H	50–100[j] (total)	PO	24	5
Toltrazuril[15]	D	10	PO	Medicated feed	2–6
Roxithromycin[16]	H	2.5	PO	12	15

[a]B = dog and cat, D = dog, C = cat, H = human, PO = oral.

[b]Dose per administration at specified interval, expressed as mg/kg unless otherwise stated.

[c]Other sulfonamides, such as sulfadimidine and sulfaquanadine can be used, but sulfaquinoxaline should be avoided owing to its interference with vitamin K synthesis with potential hemorrhagic complications.[16a]

[d]Greater than 4 kg body weight.

[e]Less than 4 kg body weight.

[f]Consists of 11 mg ormetoprim and 55 mg of sulfadimethoxine.

[g]When furazolidone is combined with sulfonamides, 50% of this dose is used.

[h]Total dose/day. Lower dosage recommended for puppies and maximum of 300 mg total/day (see text).

[i]Total dose/day. Combine 150 mg amprolium and 25 mg sulfadimethoxine/kg/day for 14 days.[17]

[j]Total dose/day. Dose on a mg/kg basis is listed in Table 77–2.

Prevention

Coccidiosis tends to be a disease problem in areas of poor sanitation. The fecal shedding of large numbers of environmentally resistant oocysts makes infection likely under such conditions. Animals should be housed so as to prevent contamination of food and water bowls by contaminated soil or infected feces. Feces should be removed daily and incinerated. Oocysts survive freezing temperatures. Runs, cages, food utensils, and other implements should be disinfected by steam cleaning or immersion in boiling water or with 5% ammonia solutions (see Table 86–3). Animals should have limited access to intermediate hosts and should not be fed uncooked meat. Insect control is essential in animal quarters and food storage areas, since cockroaches and flies may serve as mechanical vectors of oocysts. Coccidiostatic drugs can be given to infected bitches prior to or soon after whelping to control the spread of infection in puppies.

HAMMONDIA

There are two species of *Hammondia* in domestic animals: *H. hammondi*, with cats as definitive host, and *H. heydorni* with dogs and coyotes as definitive hosts. Unlike *Isospora* spp., *H. hammondi* and *H. heydorni* have obligatory two-host life cycles similar to *Toxoplasma* (see Chapter 86 and Table 87–1). For *H. hammondi*, goats and rats are natural intermediate hosts, and the domestic cat (*Felis catus*) and the European wild cat (*Felis sylvestris*) are the definitive hosts. *H. hammondi* does not invade extraintestinal tissues of the cat, and cats are only infected by eating tissue cysts. Experimentally, many warm-blooded animals, including monkeys, cattle, sheep, goats, pigs, rabbits, guinea pigs, and mice can serve as intermediate hosts. Intermediate hosts become infected by ingesting sporulated oocysts that resemble those of *T. gondii*. Sporozoites excyst in the intestinal lumen, invade the intestinal wall, and multiply as tachyzoites in the intestines, mesenteric lymph nodes, and other tissues. The parasite eventually encysts principally in muscles (Fig. 87–7).

H. heydorni's life cycle is similar to that of *H. hammondi* except that dogs and coyotes are definitive hosts. Cattle, sheep, goats, buffaloes, camels, moose, and deer are its intermediate hosts. The structure of the parasite in the intermediate hosts is not known. Both *H. hammondi* and *H. heydorni* are nonpathogenic. Therefore, no treatment is necessary.

BESNOITIA

Cats, but not dogs, are definitive hosts for two species of *Besnoitia* in the United States:

Figure 87–7. *Hammondia hammondi* tissue cyst in section of abdominal muscle of an experimentally infected mouse. Note the thin cyst wall enclosing hundreds of PAS-positive bradyzoites (PAS; × 750).

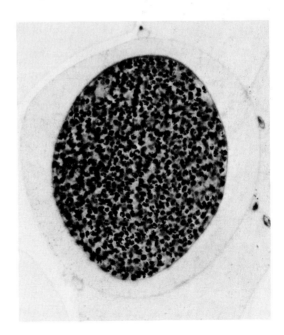

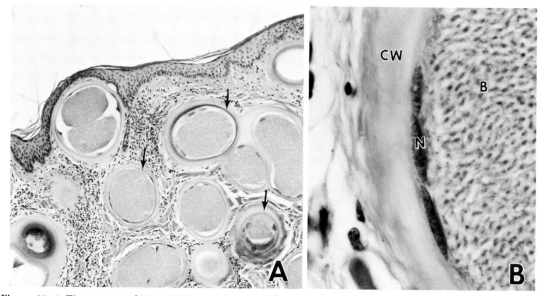

Figure 87–8. Tissue cysts of *Besnoitia besnoiti* in skin of a naturally infected cow (H and E). *A,* Arrows point to thick cyst walls (× 150). *B,* Note thick cyst wall (CW) incorporating host cell nuclei (N) and numerous bradyzoites (B) (× 750).

B. wallacei of rats and mice and *B. darlingi* of opossums and, possibly, of lizards.

The life cycle of *Besnoitia* is similar to those of *H. hammondi* and *T. gondii* (Table 87–1). Cats become infected by ingesting tissue cysts (Fig. 87–8), and schizonts and gamonts are formed in intestinal goblet cells. Unsporulated oocysts are shed in feces, and they are difficult to distinguish from those of *H. hammondi.* Intermediate hosts become infected by ingesting sporulated oocysts. The parasite develops in connective tissue,

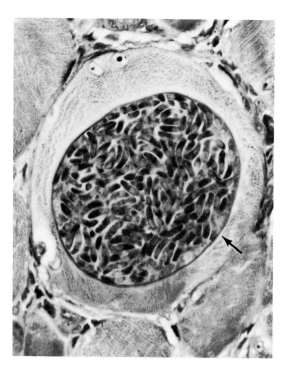

Figure 87–9. Cross section of sarcocyst of *Sarcocystis muris* in a myocyte. The sarcocyst wall (*arrow*) is thin and encloses numerous banana-shaped bradyzoites. There is no host reaction around the sarcocyst (Giemsa stain, × 750).

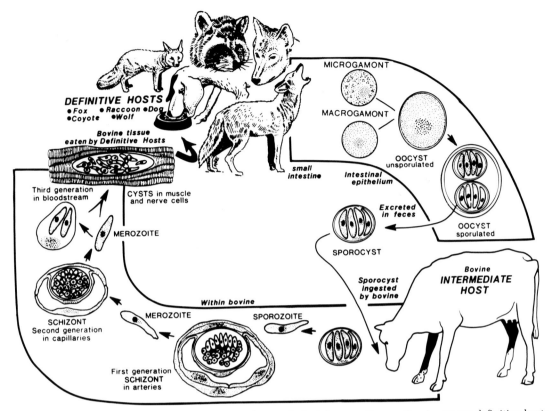

Figure 87–10. Life cycle of *Sarcocystis cruzi*, which is typical of *Sarcocystis* spp. Carnivores are definitive hosts, supporting the sexually replicating stages of the parasite, and herbivores are intermediate hosts, supporting the asexually replicating stages of the parasite. Sporulated oocysts or, more commonly, sporocysts are excreted in the feces of carnivores (Modified from Dubey JP, Fayer R. *Br Vet J* 139:371–377, 1983, with permission.)

Figure 87–11. Sporocysts (*arrows*) in the lamina propria of small intestine of dog fed S. *cruzi*-infected beef (H and E; × 1250).

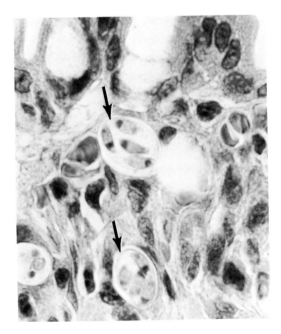

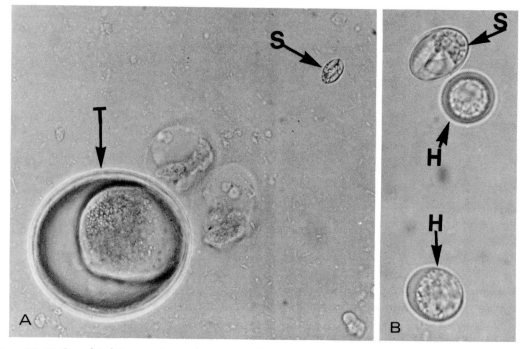

Figure 87–12. Sporulated *Sarcocystis cruzi* sporocysts (S), unsporulated *Hammondia hammondi* (H), and *Toxascaris leonina* egg (T) in fecal flotation of canine feces (unstained; *A*, × 430; *B*, ×1250). (From Dubey JP. *J Am Vet Med Assoc* 169:1061–1078, 1976, with permission.)

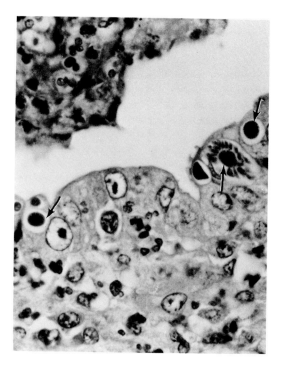

Figure 87–13. Bile duct from a dog with severe obstructive jaundice reported by Lipscomb and colleagues, 1989.[26] Parasites (*arrows*) are present in epithelial cells of bile duct. One schizont has merozoites radiating from a residual body. Inflammatory cells are present in bile duct lumen (H and E; × 750). (Courtesy of Dr. J. P. Dubey, Zoonotic Laboratory, US Department of Agriculture, Beltsville, MD.)

and cysts may become macroscopic. *Besnoitia* is considered nonpathogenic for cats, and no treatment is necessary.

SARCOCYSTIS

Infections due to *Sarcocystis* are ubiquitous in reptiles, birds, and warm-blooded animals. Virtually all cattle and sheep are infected with this parasite. There are over 90 species of *Sarcocystis*.[18,19] *Sarcocystis* spp. have an obligatory two-host life cycle (see Table 87–1). Carnivores (predators) are definitive hosts, and herbivores (prey) are intermediate hosts. As the name implies, the parasite forms tissue cysts (called sarcocysts) in muscles and neural tissues. Sarcocysts are thin or thick walled, and the zoites are usually separated from each other by septa (Fig. 87–9). Cats and dogs become infected by ingesting sarcocysts. The life cycle of *Sarcocystis* is distinct from other coccidians of domestic animals in that oocysts sporulate within the definitive host and are excreted in the feces in an infective form (Fig. 87–10). The intermediate hosts become infected by ingesting sporocysts or oocysts. One to three generations of schizogony occur in blood vessels or in hepatocytes (depending on the species of intermediate hosts), and merozoites then invade skeletal muscles and nerve cells, where they form sarcocysts (Figs. 87–10 and 87–11). Certain species of *Sarcocystis*, transmissible via dogs, are pathogenic in cattle, sheep, goats, pigs, and mule deer, whereas species transmissible via cats are generally nonpathogenic.

There are over 20 species of *Sarcocystis* for both cats and dogs. It is not possible to differentiate species based on measurements of sporocysts. *Sarcocystis* is excreted in feces fully sporulated, often as free sporocysts when examined microscopically (Fig. 87–12). They are small and because of low density, lie at a different plane of focus than other parasites.

Sarcocystis species are not pathogenic for dogs or cats, and no treatment is necessary. Infections can be prevented by feeding only cooked meat. Occasionally, sarcocysts are found in skeletal muscles of immunosuppressed cats and dogs, but their life cycle is unknown.[21,21a]

Cutaneous Coccidiosis: Suspected Caryosporiosis

An unidentified coccidium has been reported from cutaneous nodules in two dogs from Italy,[22] a dog from Columbia, Missouri,[23] and a dog from Tifton, Georgia.[24] All four dogs were 4 to 6 months old, and at least the two dogs from the United States had concurrent distemper virus–like illness.

The skin nodules were up to 2 cm in diameter, and some had a central ulcerated area through which serohemorrhagic exudate could be expressed. Microscopically, the dermatitis was characterized by edema and infiltrations by polymorphonuclear cells, eosinophils, and macrophages. Schizonts and male and female gamonts were seen in macrophages.

In the absence of further structural details, it is impossible to identify the organisms in the infected dogs described. The location of the organism in dermis and within macrophage-like cells indicates that the organism might be a species of coccidium of the genus *Caryospora*.

Members of the genus *Caryospora* have an oocyst with one sporocyst that contains eight sporozoites, and they typically parasitize mostly reptiles and raptors. At least two species, *C. bigenetica* and *C. simplex* are parasitic in rodents and snakes. *Caryospora* spp. have a complicated life cycle involving asexual and sexual multiplication both in the prey (rodent) and the predator (snake).[25] In addition to usual schizonts and gamonts, sporulated oocysts and monozoic cysts (called caryocysts) are formed in connective tissue cells of the prey; these sporulated oocysts and caryocysts have not been found in the tissues of dogs.

Intrahepatic Biliary Coccidiosis in Dogs

Intrahepatic biliary coccidiosis is a rare condition in dogs. Clinical signs are those associated with hepatic disease: icterus, weight loss, and vomiting.[26] Small and large bile ducts are enlarged because of inflammation and desquamation of epithelial cells. Lesions may extend into hepatic parenchyma. Asexual stages (schizonts) of an unidentified coccidium are found in biliary epithelial cells (Fig. 87–13). This coccidium is different from *Toxoplasma*, *Sarcocystis*, *Hammondia*, *Cryptosporidium*, or any other known coccidium of the dog.

References

1. Dubey JP: A review of `Sarcocystis of domestic animals and other coccidia of cats and dogs. J Am Vet Med Assoc 169:1061–1078, 1976.
2. Kirkpatrick CE, Dubey JP: Enteric coccidial infections. Isospora, Sarcocystis, Cryptosporidium, Besnoitia, and Hammondia. Vet Clin North Am Small Anim Pract 17:1405–1420, 1987.
3. Dubey JP: Life cycle of Isospora rivolta (Grassi, 1879) in cats and mice. J Protozool 26:433–443, 1979.
4. Frenkel JK, Dubey JP: Rodents as vectors for feline coccidia Isospora felis and Isospora rivolta. J Infect Dis 125:69–72, 1972.
5. Dubey JP, Weisbrode SE, Rogers WA: Canine coccidiosis attributed to an Isospora ohioensis-like organism: a case report. J Am Vet Med Assoc 173:185–191, 1978.
6. Dunbar MR, Foreyt WJ: Prevention of coccidiosis in domestic dogs and captive coyotes (Canis latrans) with sulfadimethoxine-ormetoprim combination. Am J Vet Res 46:1899–1902, 1985.
7. Böch J, Gobel E, Heine J, et al: Isospora-Infektionen bei Hund und Katze. Berl Munch Tierarztl Wochenschr 94:384–391, 1981.
8. Correa WM, Correa CNM, Langoni H, et al: Canine isosporosis. Canine Pract 10:44–46, 1983.
9. Dürr UM: Klinische Erfahrungen mit Trimethoprim-Sulfadiazin (Tribrissen^R) bei der Kokzidiose bei Hund und Katze. Tierarztl Umschau 31:177–178, 1976.
10. Greene CE: Antimicrobial chemotherapy. In Greene CE: Clinical Microbiology and Infectious Diseases of the Dog and Cat. Philadelphia, WB Saunders Co, 1984, pp 144–188.
11. Smart J: Amprolium for canine coccidiosis. Mod Vet Pract 52:41, 1971.
12. Boch J: Die Kokzidiose der Katze. Tierarztl Prax 12:383–390, 1984.
13. Euzebey J: Les coccidies parasites du chien et du chat: incidences pathogéniques et épidémiologiques. Rev Med Vet 131:43–61, 1980.
14. Böch J, Mannl A, Weiland G, et al: Die Sarkosporidiose des Hundes—Diagnose und Therapie. Prax Tierarztl 8:637–644, 1980.
15. Rommel M, Schneider T, Westerhoff J, et al: The use of toltrazuril-medicated food to prevent the development of Isospora and Toxoplasma oocysts. Symp Biol Hung 33:445–449, 1986.
16. Musey KL, Chidiac C, Beaucaire G, et al: Effectiveness of roxithromycin for treating Isospora belli infection. J Infect Dis 158:646, 1988.
16a. Patterson JM, Grenn HH: Hemorrhage and death in dogs following administration of sulfaquinoxaline. Can Vet J 16:265–268, 1975.
17. Olsen ME: Coccidiosis caused by Isospora ohioensis-like organisms in three dogs. Can Vet J 26:112–114, 1985.
18. Levine ND: The taxonomy of Sarcocystis (Protozoa, Apicomplexa) species. J Parasitol 72:372–382, 1986.
19. Dubey JP, Speer CA, Fayer R: Sarcocystosis of Animals and Man. Boca Raton, FL, CRC Press, 1989, pp 1–215.
20. Dubey JP, Fayer R: Sarcocystosis. Br Vet J 139: 371–377, 1983.
21. Edwards JF, Ficken MD, Lutgen PJ, et al: Dissseminated sarcocytosis in a cat with lymphosarcoma. J Am Vet Med Assoc 193:831–832, 1988.
21a. Hill JE, Chapman WL, Prestwood AK: Intramuscular Sarcocystis sp. in two cats and a dog. J Parasitol 74:724–727, 1988.
22. Marcone G: Sporozoen-Dermatosen des Hundes. Zeit Infekt Parasitenk Hyg Haust 4:5–32, 1908.
23. Shelton GC, Kintner LD, MacKintosh DO: A coccidia-like organism associated with subcutaneous granulomata in a dog. J Am Vet Med Assoc 152:263–267, 1968.
24. Sangster LT, Styer EL, Hall GA: Coccidia associated with cutaneous nodules in a dog. Vet Pathol 22:186–188, 1985.
25. Upton SJ, Current WL, Barnard SM: A review of the genus Caryospora Leger, 1904 (Apicomplexa: Eimeriidae). Syst Parasitol 6: 3–21, 1986.
26. Lipscomb TP, Pletcher JM, Dubey JP, et al: Intrahepatic biliary coccidiosis in a dog. Vet Pathol. 26:343–345, 1989.

88 CRYPTOSPORIDIOSIS

Annie K. Prestwood

ETIOLOGY AND EPIDEMIOLOGY

Cryptosporidium is a ubiquitous coccidian genus in the suborder Eimeriina, family Cryptosporidiidae of the phylum Apicocomplexa that inhabits the epithelium of the respiratory and digestive systems of reptiles, birds, and mammals. Infections of the ileum are most common, but gastric, respiratory, and conjunctival infections have been seen in many hosts. Its oocyst is extremely small, measuring either 4 to 5 μm or 6 to 8 μm in diameter and often is difficult to demonstrate in the feces without special techniques. Although numerous species have been described, only two are recognized in mammals based on oocyst sizes, namely *C. parvum* and *Cryptosporidium* sp., respectively. The biology of *Cryptosporidium* sp. is not well known and will not be considered further. In contrast, *C. parvum* is by far the most commonly occurring species in mammals and, similar to *Toxoplasma*, has a wide mammalian host range.[1] It has been reported from rodents, domestic livestock, cats, dogs, people, and numerous wild mammals. Ruminants, especially calves, are considered reservoir hosts. Cross-infection between various mammalian hosts occurs. Cryptosporidia found in reptiles and birds apparently do not infect mammals, and some species may be relatively host-specific. A high prevalence of serum antibodies to cryptosporidia in most species tested suggests that exposure to the parasite is common.[2]

The life cycle of cryptosporidia differs from that of most other coccidians (Fig. 88–1). They are located in parasitophorous vacuoles at the cell's microvillous surface rather than within the host cell cytoplasm (Fig. 88–2).[2a] Furthermore, the oocyst contains four naked sporozoites and sporulates within the body of the host so that oocysts are directly infective when shed. Upon ingestion by a susceptible host, sporozoites excyst and invade the microvillous border of the intestine. Two stages (types I and II) of meronts, which reproduce asexually, have been identified. Within 24 hours, trophozoites and type I meronts, containing six to eight merozoites, are present. The number of asexual multiplications by this type I meront is unknown but is more than one, as evidenced by the persistence of this stage. By 48 hours there are numerous type II meronts, each containing four merozoites. By days 3 to 8, all developmental stages are present—i.e., meronts differentiate into microgametocytes and macrogametes that, following fertilization, form oocysts. Some oocysts that are produced are thick walled, whereas others are thin walled. Sporulation occurs endogenously, and thick-walled oocysts are shed with the feces. Thin-walled oocysts excyst within the lumen of the gut and invade other cells, thus providing a means for the maintenance and progression of bowel infection in the absence of reinfection.

Oocysts of cryptosporidia are spread via the fecal-oral route, and fecal contamination of food or drinking water is a common source of infection. Apparently, relatively few oocysts are necessary to precipitate disease in people, as evidenced by waterborne transmission through municipal water supplies and accidental infection of laboratory personnel.

PATHOGENESIS

Cryptosporidia are either primary pathogens or secondary invaders in a variety of immunosuppressive diseases of animals and people. Crowding and unsanitary practices increase the risk of exposure. Cryptosporidial diarrhea is common among calves in "calf nurseries," where it can be a primary pathogen. Similarly, this parasite is an important

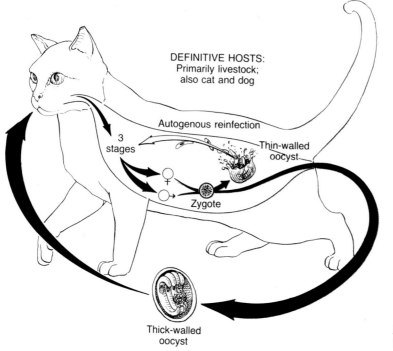

DEFINITIVE HOSTS:
Primarily livestock;
also cat and dog

Autogenous reinfection

3 stages

Thin-walled oocyst

Zygote

Thick-walled oocyst

Figure 88–1. Life cycle of *Cryptosporidium*.

cause of diarrhea among children in day-care centers.

It is uncertain as to what host immunologic factors are involved in defense against these parasites. Immunocompetence is involved in the degree and duration of illness. Some individuals develop few or no signs of disease, whereas others develop a severe diarrheal disease that is self-limiting (hours or days). Other individuals, when severely stressed or immunosuppressed owing to viral or other agents, may develop a diarrheal disease of several weeks' to months' duration. Concomitant infection with other agents, e.g. numerous enteric viruses such as rotavirus, bacteria such as *Campylobacter* or *Salmonella*, and protozoa such as other coccidia and *Giardia* serve to complicate and exacerbate the diarrheal syndrome. In dogs and cats, severe cryptosporidiosis most often is secondary to immunosuppressive agents such as canine distemper and feline leukemia viruses and concurrent infection with other intestinal pathogens.

Healthy neonatal pups and kittens have been experimentally infected with cryptosporidia, but clinical signs of disease have not been observed. Neonates shed oocysts for 5 to 12 days postinfection (PI).

Decreased intestinal microvillar disac-

charidases have been found in the distal small intestine. Blunting and fusion of intestinal villi may decrease the absorptive surface area of the bowel. Whether these pathologic processes are due to parasite metabolites or host immune responses is uncertain.

CLINICAL FINDINGS

Cats

The potential to cause diarrhea has been questioned since infection of healthy adult cats[3] or healthy 6-week-old kittens[4] resulted in nonsymptomatic infection. Diarrhea can be self-limiting or absent in naturally infected immunocompetent cats.[5] Pathogenicity undoubtedly is greater in immunodeficient cats. Intestinal cryptosporidiosis in other feline leukemia virus–negative[6] or –positive cats[7, 8] has also been associated with chronic anorexia, weight loss, and persistent diarrhea. The diarrhea may be of small bowel nature, characterized by high-volume, low-frequency stools with significant weight loss. Tenesmus, fresh blood, swelling, and discomfort may be seen with chronicity.

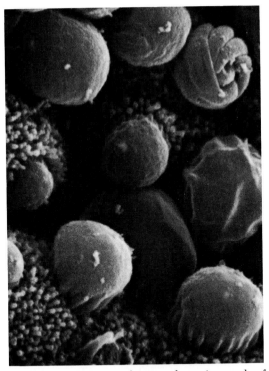

Figure 88–2. Scanning electron photomicrograph of various stages of *Cryptosporidium* on the epithelial cell microvillous surface of the cloaca of a young chicken (× 5000). (Courtesy of Sandy L. White, Lilly Research Labs, Greenfield, IN. From Current WL: *ASM News* 54:605–612, 1988, with permission.)

Dogs

Experimental infection of healthy pups resulted in oocyst shedding without accompanying disease.[4] Naturally occurring cryptosporidiosis has been reported in a 1-week-old pup that died after an episode of diarrhea and dyspnea,[9] whereas other pups, infected with cryptosporidia, did not show clinical signs suggestive of infection.[10] Cryptosporidiosis has been described in two immunosuppressed pups with distemper.[11,12] Cryptosporidial infection has been diagnosed in an adult dog with persistent diarrhea, lymphoplasmacytic enteritis, and malabsorption syndrome and no obvious cause for immunosuppression.[13]

Calves and Other Animals

Cryptosporidial infection is an important cause of fulminating diarrhea among young calves. Cryptosporidial diarrhea also is an important disease among young ruminants found in zoos. Less severe infections have been reported in young swine, lambs, and foals. The coccidian is fairly common in birds, infecting the digestive and respiratory tracts and the bursa of Fabricius, and may be a primary pathogen. In captive snakes, *Cryptosporidium* causes gastritis and subsequent vomiting, since it parasitizes the stomachs of these reptiles.

People

People of all ages may become infected with cryptosporidia, and severity of disease depends upon the immunocompetence of the host. Fulminating, rapidly fatal disease occurs in people with AIDS. Individuals with congenital immunodeficiency disease may survive for years with persistent cryptosporidiosis. Immunocompetent persons may be infected readily with *Cryptosporidium*, and outbreaks of epizootic proportions have occurred because of contamination of municipal water supplies. Most people develop transient clinical signs and recover. Infection among veterinary students is common after contact with infected calves. Severe stress or concurrent infection by viruses or bacteria serve to exacerbate the diarrheal syndrome.

In people, there has been a causal connection between oocysts being shed in the stool and GI signs.[14] The typical prepatent period is 5 to 7 days. Clinical signs that may last from 2 to 26 days in immunocompetent people may include nausea, abdominal cramps, low-grade fever, and anorexia. Occasionally, episodes last longer.[15] Diarrhea may be profuse, and dehydration is a common sequela. Nonsymptomatic infections do occur, especially in recovery phases of the illness.[16] Conversely, symptomatic patients can have intermittently negative stools.[14]

DIAGNOSIS

Fecal Examination

Since cryptosporidial oocysts are directly infective when shed in the feces, caution must be used to avoid accidental infection. To destroy the oocyst, 1 part 100% formalin (38% formaldehyde) should be mixed with 9 parts fluid feces before performing fecal examination procedures. Samples should also be formalinized prior to shipment to a diagnostic laboratory and should be placed in a nonbreakable container. The outside of the container should be disinfected to avoid infection of laboratory personnel. Oocysts rarely passed in formed stools may be seen microscopically on direct smears of feces, but concentration techniques, such as Sheather's sugar solution, can be used (see Appendix 12). Because oocysts are the same size as or smaller than erythrocytes and because of their transparency, unstained preparations using conventional light microscopy do not permit accurate identification.

Oocysts are small, either 4 to 5 μm or 6 to 8 μm in diameter, and refractile. On Sheather's flotation, they cling to the coverslip; therefore, one must focus immediately beneath the coverslip. Oocysts appear as circular, sometimes concave, discs that are refractile and pink with bright-field microscopy. Dark shadows of sporozoites may be seen within the oocysts.

Other procedures used to demonstrate cryptosporidial oocysts in fluid stools include formalin–ethyl acetate sedimentation technique or examination of direct smears of feces or intestinal contents by using negative stains such as Kinyoun's modified carbolfuchsin or crystal violet (Table 88–1). A modification of the acid-fast staining technique using dimethyl sulfoxide (DMSO) has simplified the procedure and has stained the internal structure of the organism.[17] For a description of these sedimentation and staining techniques, see Appendix 12. Staining methods allow for easier detection of the oocysts and their differentiation from yeasts. Yeasts stain darker and are slightly smaller than cryptosporidia, are oval, appear in clumps, and may show budding. When searching for cryptosporidial oocysts on unstained preparations, phase-contrast microscopy is often recommended; however, bright-field microscopy can be used (Fig. 88–3). A wet preparation with crystal violet is used on fluid stools, and oocysts can readily be seen since they do not stain (Fig. 88–4). An indirect fluorescent antibody (IFA) procedure for staining cryptosporidial oocysts in feces is commercially available (Merifluor, Meridian Diagnostics, Cincinnati, OH; see also Appendix 8).[17a] An accurate ELISA procedure to detect cryptosporidial antigen in feces has also been developed.[17b]

Animal Inoculation

Oocysts for animal inoculation may be harvested by sugar centrifugation and stored in a refrigerator in 2.5% potassium dichromate for up to 6 months without appreciable loss of viability. Neonatal mice are inoculated per os, and their intestinal tissues are examined microscopically 1 week later. Chick embryos also have been infected successfully with *Cryptosporidium*.[18] It should be emphasized that people may be infected with cryptosporidia of animal origin, and precautions should be taken to minimize exposure of personnel and animals and to prevent environmental contamination.

Intestinal Biopsy

Gross lesions consist of enlarged, congested mesenteric lymph nodes, and changes are most severe in the distal ileum. The mucosa is hyperemic and may contain watery, yellow contents. Biopsy specimens can be taken from the intestine and processed routinely and stained with H and E (Fig. 88–5). Organisms may be missed unless multiple surgical samples are taken. A procedure

Table 88–1. Appearance of Stained Cryptosporidial Oocysts

	APPEARANCE	
STAIN	Oocyst	Yeast
None (bright-field)	Semitranslucent, nonrefractile, difficult to visualize	Same as oocyst
None (phase-contrast)	Dull blue with highly refractile residual body	Not refractile, indeterminate content
Giemsa	Pale blue, red granule	Same as oocyst
Kinyoun's carbolfuschin	Unstained, refractile (negative stain)	Stain darkly
Modified Ziehl-Nielson	Deep red, blue granules, some remain unstained	Unstained
DMSO-Ziehl-Nielson	Pink to red, internal vacuoles, some remain unstained	Blue-green

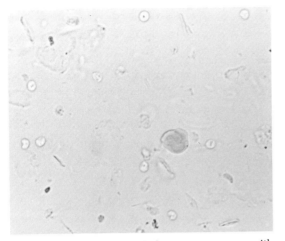

Figure 88–3. Cryptosporidial oocyst as seen with bright-field microscopy using Sheather's sugar flotation (× 160).

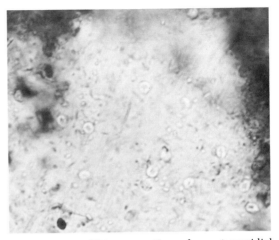

Figure 88–4. Wet preparation of cryptosporidial oocysts. Their appearance is accentuated by lack of internal staining (crystal violet; × 125).

has been described whereby tissue impressions were stained with stains used for blood cells.[19] Excellent results were obtained.

Specimens may be fixed in Bouin's or formalin solutions (see Appendix 12). Samples must be fixed within hours of death or biopsy because autolysis causes rapid loss of the intestinal surface containing the organisms. Microscopic lesions consist of varying degrees of villous atrophy, reactive lymphoid tissue, and inflammatory infiltrates in the lamina propria, consisting of neutrophils, macrophages, and lymphocytes. Parasites may be found throughout the intestines but are usually most numerous in the distal small intestine.

THERAPY

To date, there have been few drugs used successfully for treating cryptosporidiosis.[20] Infections in immunocompetent animals or persons are self-limiting, and full recovery soon ensues. Fluid replacement may be necessary to combat the severe dehydration that accompanies the disease. Parenteral fluids usually are more effective than oral fluids, since in some cases, addition of fluid to the GI tract may stimulate more diarrhea. Antibiotic therapy for eliminating secondary bacterial invaders may be necessary.

Spiramycin, a macrolide antibiotic (see Spiramycin, Chapter 77), has been somewhat effective in treating, but not curing, chronic cryptosporidiosis in people with AIDS.[21,22] Results of treating infected infants have been less encouraging.[22a] The recommended dose for people is 30 mg/kg, given orally every 12 hours for 1 to 6 weeks. It is not currently licensed for use in the United States; use in animals is limited, and established doses are not available. Clindamycin was not effective in reducing oocyst numbers excreted in the feces of an infected dog.[13]

PUBLIC HEALTH CONSIDERATIONS

Cryptosporidial infection in people was not recognized until 1976. Since that time,

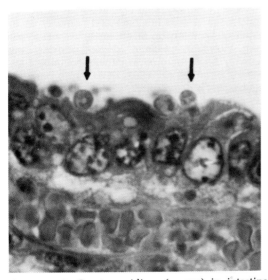

Figure 88–5. Cryptosporidium (arrows) in intestine from an infected calf is characteristically located at the microvillous border (H and E; × 250).

it has been diagnosed with increasing frequency. Animal handlers, medical personnel, people living or traveling in developing countries, and children in day-care facilities have the highest risk of exposure.[23] Between 4% to 7% of human patients admitted to hospitals for gastroenteritis had cryptosporidiosis.[24,25] In both reports, infections were more common during the warm, humid months. Waterborne outbreaks of epizootic proportions have been described in Texas and Georgia.[25a] There are numerous reports, published and unpublished, of cryptosporidiosis among veterinary students who have had contact with calves with diarrhea. Calves with diarrhea must be considered a potential source of cryptosporidia for human infection. Intestinal cryptosporidiosis and diarrhea developed in a child receiving chemotherapy for leukemia.[5,26] The child's kitten was found to be nonsymptomatically infected and shedding oocysts in its stool. An infected dog was the presumed source of infection for a veterinary student.[13] Most serious cryptosporidiosis occurs in patients with AIDS, and in these persons the prognosis usually is grave.

Cryptosporidial agents are resistant to commercial bleach (5.25% sodium hypochlorite), and routine chlorination of drinking water probably has no effect on their viability. Of the commonly used disinfectants, only formol saline (10% solution) and ammonia (5% solution) were effective in destroying the viability of cryptosporidial oocysts. However, oocysts had to be in contact with the disinfectants for 18 hours. More concentrated (50%) ammonia solutions have been effective after 30 minutes.[27] Moist heat (steam or pasteurization [$>55°C$]), freezing and thawing, or thorough drying are more practical means of disinfection.[23,28] Excellent sanitation and liberal use of boiling water for scalding food and water bowls should minimize contamination in a clinical environment.

References

1. Fayer R, Ungar BLP: Cryptosporidium and cryptosporidiosis. Microbiol Rev 50:458–483, 1986.
2. Kirkpatrick CE, Farrell JP: Cryptosporidiosis. Compend Cont Educ Pract Vet 6:5154–5165, 1984.
2a. Current WL: The biology of Cryptosporidium. ASM News 54:605–612, 1988.
3. Iseki M: Cryptosporidium felis sp n (Protozoa: Eimeriina) from the domestic cat. Jpn J Parasitol 28:285–307, 1986.
4. Current WL, Reese NC, Ernst JV, et al: Human cryptosporidiosis in immunocompetent and immunodeficient persons. N Engl J Med 308:1252–1257, 1983.
5. Bennett M, Baxby D, Blundell N, et al: Cryptosporidiosis in the domestic cat. Vet Rec 116:73–74, 1985.
6. Poonacha KB, Pippin C: Intestinal cryptosporidiosis in a cat. Vet Pathol 19:708–710, 1982.
7. Greene CE, Prestwood AK: Coccidial infections. In Greene CE (ed): Clinical Microbiology and Infectious Diseases of the Dog and Cat. Philadelphia, WB Saunders Co, 1984, pp 824–858.
8. Monticello TM, Levy MG, Bunch SE, et al: Cryptosporidiosis in a feline leukemia virus–positive cat. J Am Vet Med Assoc 191:705–706, 1987.
9. Wilson RB, Holscher MA, Lyles SJ: Cryptosporidiosis in a pup. J Am Vet Med Assoc 183:1005–1006, 1983.
10. Sisk DB, Gosser HS, Styer EL: Intestinal cryptosporidiosis in two pups. J Am Vet Med Assoc 184:835–836, 1984.
11. Kukushima K, Helman RG: Cryptosporidiosis in a pup with distemper. Vet Pathol 21:247–248, 1984.
12. Turnwald GH, Barta O, Taylor HW, et al: Cryptosporidiosis associated with immunosuppression attributable to distemper in a pup. J Am Vet Med Assoc 192:79–81, 1988.
13. Greene CE, Jacobs GJ, Prickett D: Intestinal malabsorption and cryptosporidiosis in an adult dog. J Am Vet Med Assoc. In press, 1990.
14. Jokipii L, Jokipii A: Timing of symptoms and oocyst excretion in human cryptosporidiosis. N Engl J Med 315:1643–1647, 1986.
15. Wolfson JS, Richter JM, Waldron MA, et al: Cryptosporidiosis in immunocompetent patients. N Engl J Med 312:1278–1282, 1985.
16. Zar F, Geiseler PJ, Brown VA: Asymptomatic carriage of Cryptosporidium in the stool of a patient with acquired immunodeficiency syndrome. J Infect Dis 151:195, 1985.
17. Pohjola S, Jokipii L, Jokipii A: Dimethylsulphoxide-Ziehl-Nielsen staining technique for detection of cryptosporidial oocysts. Vet Rec 115:442–443, 1984.
17a. Rusnak J, Hadfield TL, Rhodes MM, et al: Detection of Cryptosporidium oocysts in human fecal specimens by an indirect immunofluorescence assay with monoclonal antibodies. J Clin Microbiol 27:1135–1136, 1989.
17b. Ungar B, Quinn C: Enzyme immunoassay for the detection of Cryptosporidium in fecal specimens. 29th Intersci Conf Antimicrob Agents Chemother, Houston, September, 1989, p 262. (Abstr).
18. Current WL, Long PL: Development of human and calf Cryptosporidium in chicken embryos. J Infect Dis 148:1108–1113, 1983.
19. Latimer KS, Goodwin M: Rapid cytologic diagnosis of respiratory cryptosporidiosis in chickens. Avian Dis 32:826–830, 1988.
20. Moore JA, Blagburn BL, Lindsay DS: Cryptosporidiosis in animals, including humans. Compend Cont Educ Pract Vet 10:275–287, 1988.
21. Portnoy D, Whiteside ME, Buckley E, et al: Treatment of intestinal cryptosporidiosis with spiramycin. Ann Intern Med 101:202–204, 1984.
22. Centers for Disease Control: Update: treatment of cryptosporidiosis in patients with acquired immunodeficiency syndrome (AIDS). MMWR 33:117–119, 1984.

22a. Wittenberg DF, Smith EG, vanden Ende J, et al: Spiramycin is not effective in treating *Cryptosporidium* diarrhea in infants: results of a double blind randomized trial. *J Infect Dis* 159:131–132, 1989.

23. Moon HW, Woodnansee DB: Cryptosporidiosis. *J Am Vet Med Assoc* 189:643–646, 1986.

24. Tzipori S, Smith M, Birch C, et al: Cryptosporidiosis in hospital patients with gastroenteritis. *Am J Trop Med Hyg* 32:931–934, 1983.

25. Mata L, Bolanos H, Pizarro D, et al: Cryptosporidiosis in children from some highland Costa Rican rural and urban areas. *Am J Trop Med Hyg* 33:24–29, 1984.

25a. Hayes EB, Matte TD, O'Brien TR, et al: Large community outbreak of cryptosporidiosis due to contamination of a filtered public water supply. *N Engl J Med* 320:1372–1376, 1989.

26. Lewis IS, Hart CA, Baxby D: Diarrhea due to *Cryptosporidium* in acute lymphoblastic leukemia. *Arch Dis Child* 60:60–62, 1985.

27. Sundermann CA, Lindsay DS, Blagburn BL: Evaluation of disinfectants for ability to kill avian *Cryptosporidium* oocysts. *Companion Anim Pract* 1:36–39, 1987.

28. Anderson BC: Moist inactivation of *Cryptosporidium* sp. *Am J Public Health* 75:1433–1434, 1985.

89

PNEUMOCYSTOSIS

Craig E. Greene
Francis W. Chandler

ETIOLOGY

Pneumocystis carinii, the etiologic agent of pneumocystosis, occurs worldwide and infects several animal species, including people. A saprophyte of low virulence, it exists in temperate and tropical climates at altitudes of up to 5,000 feet. Its primary habitat is the mammalian respiratory tract, and estimates of latent human infection range from 1% to 10% of the population. Subclinical or latent infections also are common in rats, mice, guinea pigs, rabbits, cats, sheep, and wild animals.[1,2] Clinical pneumonia has been reported to occur spontaneously in dogs, pigs, horses, goats, nonhuman primates, and people. Most reports of clinical pneumonia are linked with documented or suspected immunodeficiency in the host.[3] Increased prevalence of the disease in recent years is due not only to greater awareness of it but also to the increased use of immunosuppressive therapy.

The taxonomy of *P. carinii* is uncertain. It has been classified by use of freeze-fracture techniques as a unicellular protozoan belonging to the phylum Sarcomastigophora, subphylum Sarcodina. Ultrastructurally, however, its reproductive behavior is similar to the ascospore formation of yeast cells, and its organelles resemble those of some pathogenic fungi. Ribosomal RNA sequencing demonstrates it to be a member of the fungi.[4, 4a] Biologically, it behaves like a protozoan and is sensitive to drugs used to treat sporozoan infections. The morphology of the organism and the histopathology of lesions produced by human and animal isolates throughout the world are similar. Only a single species name has been assigned to the genus *Pneumocystis*, but antigenic differences suggest that several strains may exist.[4] Biologic differences between isolates from different hosts are suggested by the relative difficulty of experimental interspecies transmission.

EPIDEMIOLOGY

P. carinii appears to be maintained in nature by transmission from infected to susceptible animals within a species. Organisms found in the soil do not appear to be a likely source of infection.[5] The primary mode of spread is thought to be airborne droplet transmission between hosts. The contagious nature of pneumocystosis is suggested by the epidemic spread that has occurred in institutionalized humans. Sporadic case reports may represent an activation of infection by stress, crowding, and immunosuppressive therapy during hospitalization of latent carriers. Clinical disease has also been experimentally activated after glucocorticoid therapy, cytotoxic therapy, and irradiation of laboratory rodents.[6]

The parasite's entire life cycle is completed within the alveolar spaces, where organisms adhere in clusters to the lining cells. Ultrastructural studies have contributed a large body of information concerning the life cycle of *P. carinii* organisms (Fig. 89–1). *Pneumocystis* infections are usually limited to the lung; however, organisms have occasionally been reported in extrapulmonary sites in humans, and in one instance were reported in a dog.[7] Severe immunodeficiency states in people, such as AIDS, can be associated with lymphatic or hematogenous dissemination of the organisms from the lungs to other tissues.[8,9]

PATHOGENESIS

Pneumocystis organisms rarely multiply to large numbers in the lungs of subclinically

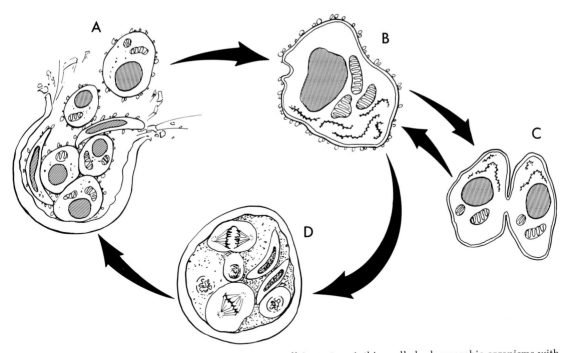

Figure 89–1. Life cycle of *P. carinii*. Trophozoites are small (2- to 5-μm), thin-walled, pleomorphic organisms with reticular cytoplasm and eccentric nuclei (A). They increase in size to form larger (4- to 7-μm) trophozoites (B), which reproduce either by binary fission, dividing into two identical but smaller trophozoites (C) or by forming a thick-walled cyst (D). The cyst undergoes a process similar to ascospore formation in yeasts whereby nuclear division results in separate chromatin masses in the cytoplasm. Cytoplasmic and nuclear membranes form multiple thin-walled ovoid or crescent-shaped intracystic sporozoites, which are released after rupture of the cyst wall (A).

infected hosts. Instead, impaired host resistance or preexisting lung pathology allows them to proliferate. The overgrowth and clustering of *P. carinii* within alveolar spaces may lead to alveolar-capillary blockage and decreased gaseous exchange. Intra-alveolar organisms are often accompanied by thickening of alveolar septa, but they seldom invade the pulmonary parenchyma and are rarely found in alveolar macrophages. With an adequate immune response, the body may eliminate the infection, although the removal of large amounts of alveolar exudate and cellular debris may take up to 8 weeks.

CLINICAL FINDINGS

In general, *Pneumocystis* infections of cats and dogs are latent or subclinical, as they are in people. The organism has been found in the lungs of cats, but no clinical disease was reported.[1] Lung specimens examined from cats suffering from feline leukemia virus infection, interstitial pneumonia, or both have not had evidence of pneumocystosis.[10]

Most canine cases have been in dachshunds less than 6 months old with suspected congenital immunodeficiency,[11–14] although one case of disseminated pneumocystosis in a Shetland sheepdog has also been reported.[7]

The clinical features of *Pneumocystis* pneumonia are similar to those caused by other infectious agents except for dry lung sounds, a nonproductive cough, and lack of fever. The typical clinical history in dogs is that of gradual weight loss and respiratory difficulty, progressing over 1 to 4 weeks. The weight loss, which occurs in spite of a good appetite in most dogs, may be associated with diarrhea and occasional vomiting. Coughing is not always reported, but reduced exercise tolerance is uniformly seen. Infected animals have responded minimally or temporarily to antibiotic or glucocorticoid therapy.

Abnormalities seen on physical examination include dyspnea, tachycardia, and increased dry respiratory sounds on thoracic auscultation. Animals are usually in poor condition and cachectic. Although the mucous membranes are generally normal in color, they may be cyanotic in severely affected animals. Affected dogs remain relatively alert and afebrile, although slight (1° to 2°C [1.8° to 3.6°F]) elevations of rectal temperature have been reported. Fluid may be present in the thoracic and peritoneal cavities of some dogs. Ocular fundic lesions known as "cotton wool spots" rarely occur in human patients with pneumocystosis, and they represent infarction of the nerve fiber layer. They have not been reported in animal infections.

DIAGNOSIS

Hematologic abnormalities are usually nonspecific, and a neutrophilic leukocytosis with a shift suggesting inflammation is seen most consistently. Less frequently, eosinophilia and monocytosis are found. Polycythemia may occur secondarily to arterial hypoxemia from impaired gaseous exchange. Thrombocytopenia, which can be significant enough to cause bleeding, has been a complication in humans. Biochemical alterations are usually nonspecific. Arterial hypoxemia ($PO_2 \leq 80$), hypocapnia ($PCO_2 \leq 35$), and increased arterial blood pH indicate an uncompensated respiratory alkalosis.

Findings on thoracic radiography include diffuse, bilaterally symmetric, alveolar to interstitial lung disease, with compensatory emphysema in severely infected animals. A solitary lesion, unilateral involvement, a cavitary lesion, spontaneous pneumothorax, or a lobar infiltrate may occasionally be present. Tracheal elevation, right-sided heart enlargement, and pulmonary arterial enlargement reflect cor pulmonale secondary to diffuse pulmonary disease.

Serologic tests have been developed for use in people with pneumocystosis, but their diagnostic value is uncertain. Unfortunately, many immunodeficient patients who develop pneumocystosis fail to produce antibody titers, and healthy contacts of pneumocystosis patients frequently have higher titers than the patients themselves. Increased antibody titers to P. carinii persist for long periods, offering a valuable index of exposure in epidemiologic studies. However, they are of limited use for an immediate diagnosis. An increase in titer over 2 to 3 weeks is needed to confirm active infection. Circulating Pneumocystis antigen has been detected in human serum by counterimmu-

noelectrophoresis and ELISA methods.[14a] However, antigenemia is also found in up to 15% of clinically normal humans who have been tested.

P. carinii has been successfully propagated on cell culture media but not on a continuous basis. Methods have been developed using density gradient centrifugation or antibody-facilitated sedimentation of leukocytes to isolate and concentrate cyst forms from fluids or tissue specimens for cultivation and diagnostic purposes.[15,15a]

Owing to the uncertainties of serologic testing, a diagnosis of pneumocystosis usually is confirmed by demonstrating the organism in biopsy specimens or respiratory fluids. Sputum, transtracheal washings, gastric contents, and oropharyngeal secretions may contain organisms. Percutaneous needle aspiration is a rapid and simple diagnostic procedure. A 1-inch, 22-gauge needle is inserted through the right thoracic wall into the pulmonary parenchyma, and tissue is rapidly aspirated into 0.2 ml of sterile saline. Samples for cytology may be obtained by endobronchial brushing or transbronchoscopic biopsy, but these procedures require special endoscopic equipment and involve the risk of general anesthesia. Transtracheal or transbronchial lavage is more available to practitioners, and studies have shown good correlation between these procedures and transbronchoscopic biopsy in confirming a diagnosis.[16] None of the cytologic techniques are as reliable or as definitive as lung biopsy for documenting active pneumocystosis. Unfortunately, lung biopsy has the greatest risk of complications. Hemorrhage, secondary infection, pneumothorax, and deaths from anesthesia have been reported in dogs. Antimicrobial therapy can begin 24 to 48 hours before specimen collection in patients suspected of having pneumocystosis without masking the presence of organisms in the biopsy sample.

Impression smears for cytologic study should be made from all tissues before fixation for histologic evaluation in order to facilitate early diagnosis and treatment, because smears can be prepared and stained more rapidly than tissue sections. The cytologic material is placed on a glass microscope slide to dry, after which it is selectively stained with methenamine silver for cysts or with Giemsa stain for intracystic sporozoites and trophozoites (Fig. 89–2).[17]

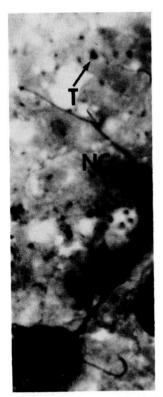

Figure 89–2. Impression smear of lung tissue from a rat infected with *P. carinii*. Nucleated cysts (NC) and trophozoites (T) are readily demonstrated with Giemsa stain (× 1500).

Direct fluorescent antibody (FA) testing or enzyme immunoassay (ELISA) has been used effectively to detect antigen in sputum and tracheal aspirates.[18,18a] An FA test kit is available (see Appendix 8). An immunoperoxidase technique also has been developed for staining *P. carinii* in lung sections or impression smears.

PATHOLOGIC FINDINGS

Pathologic findings in pneumocystosis are primarily confined to the lungs, although dissemination to regional lymph nodes and other organs has been reported. On gross examination, the lungs are firm, consolidated, and pale brown or gray (Fig. 89–3). They do not collapse when the chest cavity is opened. Fluid is not expressed from cut surfaces of the lung, as occurs in many pneumonic processes. The pulmonary and mediastinal lymph nodes are often enlarged. Despite the apparent lack of pleural inflammation, small amounts of fluid may be found in the pleural cavity. Cardiac enlargement,

when present, has been right-sided in all cases.

Appropriate histologic staining is essential to ensure detection of *P. carinii* organisms (Table 89–1). The routine H and E stain does not readily demonstrate the organism, which may explain why the disease is not found more frequently. With this stain, only the nuclei of the intracystic sporozoites are demonstrated. Various modifications of methenamine silver staining can be used to stain the cyst walls brownish-black, but trophozoites will not be detected (Fig. 89–4). Overstaining with methenamine silver may cause erythrocytes in alveolar spaces to be mistaken for the organisms. Polychrome stains, such as Wright's, Gram, Giemsa, and methylene blue, will show the trophozoites and nucleated sporozoites within cysts in cytologic specimens, but the thick walls of cyst forms will not be apparent (see Fig. 89–2).

On histologic examination, alveolar spaces are found to be filled with amorphous, foamy, eosinophilic material that has a honeycombed pattern. A few macrophages and desquamated alveolar lining cells may also be present, but polymorphonuclear leukocytes are absent. There is little or no phagocytosis of intact *Pneumocystis* organisms. However, nonviable organisms, such as those seen after treatment, are often phagocytosed, and macrophages may contain Gomori's methenamine silver–positive granular material that represents the residuum of cyst wall degradation. In some in-

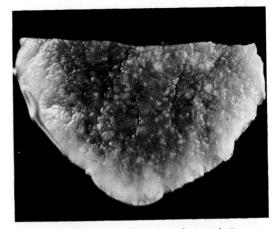

Figure 89–3. Lung of a rhesus monkey with *Pneumocystis* pneumonia in an early stage. The surface of the lung is covered with scattered, pinpoint, grayish-white lesions. These lesions were found throughout the lung when it was sectioned (× 3).

Table 89–1. Comparison of Staining Methods for Demonstrating Pneumocystis
in Clinical Specimens

	REACTION OF		
STAIN	**Trophozoite**	**Cyst Wall**	**Internal Structures**
H and E	Unstained	Unstained	Weakly basophilic
Methenamine silver	Unstained	Brownish-black	Unstained
Toluidine blue	Unstained	Purplish-violet	Unstained
PAS	Unstained	Red	Unstained
Giemsa	Unstained	Unstained	Magenta
Gram	Unstained	Positive	Positive

stances, alveolar septa are markedly thickened by dense accumulations of plasma cells, lymphocytes, and macrophages, and septa may be widened by fibrosis in chronic infections. With methenamine silver stain, cyst forms appear as spherical, ovoid, or crescent-shaped structures that range from 4 to 7 μm in diameter and have dot-like focal cyst wall thickenings (Fig. 89–5; see also Fig. 89–4).[19] Cyst walls also can be demonstrated with other stains (see Table 89–1) and will fluoresce when stained with orange G of a Papanicolaou stain.[20,21] Trophozoites in tissue sections are best demonstrated with Giemsa stain, especially using Wolbach's procedure. On ultrastructural examination, intact alveoli appear crowded with trophozoite and cyst stages that totally fill the existing air spaces. Trophozoites commonly line alveoli.

THERAPY

Supportive care is essential for any patient with *Pneumocystis* pneumonia because of disturbed alveolar gaseous exchange. Oxygen therapy administered by cage, mask, or intubation is needed, and ventilatory assistance also may be required. Aerosol therapy with mucolytics has been recommended to assist in the dissolution of alveolar debris. Anti-inflammatory dosages of glucocorticoids have been beneficial in reducing the pulmonary inflammation associated with infection.[21a] Immunosuppressive agents should be temporarily discontinued whenever pneumocystosis is diagnosed in an animal receiving such therapy.

Specific chemotherapy is most beneficial in cases in which the disease is suspected

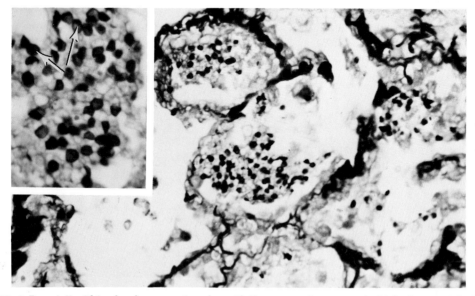

Figure 89–4. P. *carinii* within alveolar spaces in a dog with *Pneumocystis* pneumonia. Light, honeycombed matrix contains trophozoites and cellular debris. Darker ovoid, irregular, and crescent-shaped structures are cysts (× 300). *Inset,* Details of cysts that commonly show darker oval focus of cyst wall (*arrows*) (Gomori's methenamine silver stain; × 600).

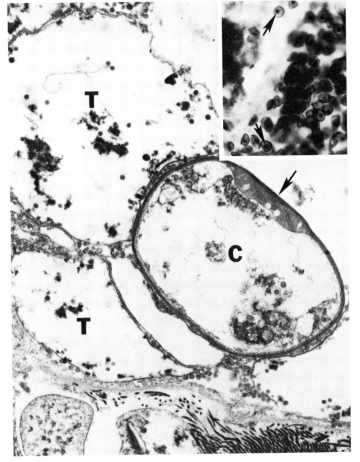

Figure 89–5. Pulmonary pneumocystosis. Alveolar space contains thin-walled trophozoites (T) and a cyst form (C) of *P. carinii*. Segmental, lamellated thickening of cyst wall (*arrow*) corresponds to darkly stained "intracystic" foci seen by light microscopy (uranyl acetate and lead citrate stain; × 22,000). *Inset, P. carinii* cysts in touch imprint contain spherical to oval foci of enhanced staining (*arrows*) that in profile are contiguous with cyst wall (Gomori's methenamine silver stain; × 560).

or diagnosed during its early stages (Table 89–2). Two major chemotherapeutic agents have been used to treat pneumocystosis successfully. Pentamidine isethionate is an aromatic diamidine that has been used to reduce fatalities from the disease in humans. Its major side effects include impaired renal function, hepatic dysfunction, hypoglycemia, hypotension, hypocalcemia, urticaria, and hematologic disorders. BUN and glucose are monitored daily during treatment, and the drug is discontinued or dosage is reduced if complications or azotemia occur.

This drug has been used successfully to treat a dog with pneumocystosis, with the only side effect localized pain at the site of injection.[11] Pentamidine has also been used successfully at a reduced dosage in combination with sulfonamides to lower its toxic side effects. Pentamidine, administered by aerosol on a periodic basis for prophylaxis against pneumocystosis in human AIDS patients, has had less toxicity than parenteral use (see Aromatic Diamidines, Chapter 77).

The combination of trimethoprim and sulfamethoxazole has been found more effec-

Table 89–2. Therapy for Pneumocystosis[a]

GENERIC NAME (Trade Name)	DOSE[b] (mg/kg)	ROUTE	INTERVAL (hours)	DURATION (weeks)
Trimethoprim-sulfonamide (Tribrissen, Bactrim, Septra)	15	PO	6	2[c]
Pentamidine isethionate (Pentam, Lomidine)	4	IM	24	2
Carbutamide[d]	50	IM	12	3

[a]PO = oral, IM = intramuscular.
[b]Dose per administration at specified interval, expressed as mg/kg unless otherwise stated.
[c]Suggested canine dosage is half the human dosage.
[d]Not commercially available.

tive and less toxic than pentamidine in treating and preventing *Pneumocystis* pneumonia in immunosuppressed humans. A relatively high oral dosage of 30 mg/kg, given every 6 hours for 2 weeks, has been recommended in humans so that the drug reaches therapeutically effective serum concentrations. Long-term (up to 2 years) prophylactic therapy for pneumocystosis at this dosage has caused no bone marrow toxicity in children, although changes in oral and fecal microflora have been noted. An increased incidence of mucocutaneous candidiasis was found. Half this dose might be used to treat dogs. IV trimethoprim-sulfonamide therapy has been shown to be as effective or more so than oral therapy and has the advantage of ease of administration in severely depressed or comatose patients. Folic acid supplementation should be used if side effects such as leukopenia or anemia are observed or if long-term therapy is required.

Carbutamide, a sulfonylurea compound, has been shown to be effective in treating and preventing *P. carinii* pneumonia in glucocorticoid-treated rodents.[22] It may offer an alternative to treatment when toxicity to the other available drugs develops. Combination therapy using clindamycin and primaquine has been effective in both in vivo and in vitro studies, whereas neither drug is effective alone.[23] Further investigation on the naturally occurring disease will be needed. Other aromatic diamidines, such as diminazene, imidocarb, and amicarbalide, have been more effective than pentamidine in treating experimental *P. carinii* pneumonia (see also Chapter 77).[24] Dapsone and trimethoprim, used in combination, have been effective in experimental animals and clinical trials in immunosuppressed people with pneumocystosis.[25,26] Trimetrexate, a lipid-soluble antifoliate, has been given concomitantly with leucovorin to people with *Pneumocystis carinii* pneumonia and AIDS.[27] As with most of the other drugs, neutropenia with or without thrombocytopenia has been the main side effect.

Pneumocystosis in humans and animals is prima facie evidence of immunodeficiency. For this reason, prophylactic treatment with trimethoprim-sulfonamide drugs has been used in hospitalized humans who are receiving irradiation or immunosuppressive agents or who have immunodeficiencies and debilitating diseases. Similar precautions are not warranted in pets because pneumocystosis has not been recognized with similar frequency in such instances.

References

1. Settnes OP, Hasselager E: Occurrence of *Pneumocystis carinii* Delanoë & Delanoë, 1912, in dogs and cats in Denmark. *Nord Vet Med* 36:179–181, 1984.
2. Shimizu A, Kimura F, Kimura S: Occurrence of *Pneumocystis carinii* in animals in Japan. *Jpn J Vet Sci* 47:309–311, 1985.
3. Chandler RW, McClure HM, Campbell WG, et al: Pulmonary pneumocystosis in nonhuman primates. *Arch Pathol Lab Med* 100:163–167, 1976.
4. Huges WT, Gigliotti F: Nomenclature for *Pneumocystis carinii*. *J Infect Dis* 157:432–433, 1988.
4a. Markus MB: Nomenclature of *Pneumocystis carinii*. *J Infect Dis* 159:366, 1989.
5. Hughes WT, Bartley DL, Smith BM: A natural source of infection due to *Pneumocystis carinii*. *J Infect Dis* 147:595, 1983.
6. Chandler FW, Frenkel JK, Campbell WG: Animal model: *Pneumocystis carinii* pneumonia in the immunosuppressed rat. *Am J Pathol* 95:571–574, 1979.
7. Tvedten HW, Langham RF, Beneke ES: Systemic *Pneumocystis carinii* infection in a dog. *J Am Anim Hosp Assoc* 10:592–594, 1974.
8. Eng RHK, Bishburg E, Smith SM: Evidence for destruction of lung tissues during *Pneumocystis carinii* infection. *Arch Intern Med* 147:746–749, 1987.
9. Pilon VA, Echols RM, Celo JA, et al: Disseminated *Pneumocystis carinii* infection in AIDS. *N Engl J Med* 316:1410–1411, 1987.
10. Hagler DN, Kim CK, Walzer PD: Feline leukemia virus and *Pneumocystis carinii* infection. *J Parasitol* 73:1284–1286, 1987.
11. Farrow BRH, Watson ADJ, Hartley WJ, et al: Pneumocystis pneumonia in the dog. *J Comp Pathol* 82:447–453, 1972.
12. Copland JW: Canine pneumonia caused by *Pneumocystis carinii*. *Aust Vet J* 50:515–518, 1974.
13. Botha WS, Van Rensburg IBJ: Pneumocystosis: a chronic respiratory distress syndrome in the dog. *J S Afr Vet Assoc* 50:173–179, 1979.
14. McCully RM, Lloyd J, Kuys D, et al: Canine pneumocystis pneumonia. *J S Afr Vet Assoc* 50:207–213, 1979.
14a. Pifer LW, Wolf BL, Weems JJ, et al: *Pneumocystis carinii* antigenemia in acquired immunodeficiency syndrome. *J Clin Microbiol* 26:1357–1361, 1988.
15. Settnes OP: Isolation and buoyant density of *Pneumocystis carinii* in percoll gradients. *Nord Vet Med* 37:306–311, 1985.
15a. Pesanti EL, McCarron BA: Rapid separation of *Pneumocystis carinii* from lung lavage fluids. *J Clin Microbiol* 26:1598–1599, 1988.
16. Rorat E, Garcia RL, Skolom J: Diagnosis of *Pneumocystis carinii* pneumonia by cytologic examination of bronchial washings. *JAMA* 254:1950–1951, 1985.
17. Shimono LH, Hartman B: A simple and reliable rapid methenamine silver stain for *Pneumocystis carinii* and fungi. *Arch Pathol Lab Med* 110:855–856, 1986.

18. Kovacs JA, Ng VL, Masur H, et al: Diagnosis of Pneumocystis carinii pneumonia: improved detection in sputum with use of monoclonal antibodies. N Engl J Med 318:589–593, 1988.

18a. McNabb SJ, Graves DC, Kosanke SD, et al: Pneumocystis carinii antigen detection in rat serum and lung lavage. J Clin Microbiol 26:1763–1771, 1988.

19. Watts JC, Chandler FW: Pneumocystis carinii pneumonitis. The nature and diagnostic significance of the methenamine silver–positive "intracystic bodies." Am J Surg Pathol 9:744–751, 1985.

20. Ghalli VS, Garcia RL, Skolom J: Fluorescence of Pneumocystis carinii in Papanicolaou smears. Hum Pathol 15:907–909, 1984.

21. Flint A, Beckwith AL, Naylor B: Pneumocystis carinii pneumonia. Cytologic manifestations and rapid diagnosis in routinely prepared Papanicolaou-stained preparation. Am J Med 81:1009–1010, 1986.

21a. Lambertus MW, Goetz MB: Treatment of Pneumocystis pneumonia in AIDS. N Engl J Med 318:988–989, 1988.

22. Hughes WT, Smith-McCain BL: Effects of sulfonyl-urea compounds on Pneumocystis carinii. J Infect Dis 153:944–947,1986.

23. Queener SF, Bartlett MS, Richardson JD: Activity of clindamycin with primaquine against Pneumocystis carinii in vitro and in vivo. Antimicrob Agents Chemother 32:807–813, 1988.

24. Walzer PD, Kim CK, Foy J, et al: Cationic antitrypanosomal and other antimicrobial agents in the therapy of experimental Pneumocystis carinii pneumonia. Antimicrob Agents Chemother 32:896–905, 1988.

25. Mills J, Leong G, Medina I, et al: Dapsone treatment of Pneumocystis carinii pneumonia in the acquired immunodeficiency syndrome. Antimicrob Agents Chemother 32:1057–1060, 1988.

26. Walzer PD, Kim CK, Foy JM: Inhibitors of folic acid synthesis in the treatment of Pneumocystis carinii pneumonia. Antimicrob Agents Chemother 32:96–103, 1988.

27. Allegra CJ, Chabner BA, Tuazon CU, et al: Trimetrexate for the treatment of Pneumocystis carinii pneumonia in patients with the acquired immunodeficiency syndrome. N Engl J Med 317:978–985, 1987.

90 NEUROLOGIC DISEASES OF SUSPECTED INFECTIOUS ORIGIN

Marc Vandevelde

Granulomatous Meningoencephalitis Versus Primary Reticulosis

Granulomatous meningoencephalitis (GME) has been reported to occur in dogs in the United States,[1-3] Australia,[4] New Zealand,[5] and several European countries[6] and is characterized by disseminated inflammatory lesions in the CNS with perivascular granuloma formation.

The term *primary reticulosis* of the CNS encompasses a range of morphologically different lesions that are thought to be essentially proliferative reactions of the reticulo-histiocytic elements originating from the adventitia of the blood vessels, the lepto-meninges, and the so-called microglia.[7] With the exception of the very rare diffusely growing microgliomatosis, reticulosis is characterized by perivascular mononuclear cuffs containing many histiocytic elements. Adjacent cuffs may merge, leading to the formation of tumor-like lesions. Based on cytologic criteria, some lesions have been classified as inflammatory and others as neoplastic reticuloses in addition to transitional forms.[7]

In the late 1970s, GME was recognized as a disease entity based on clinical and pathologic studies.[1] Retrospective morphologic and immunocytochemical studies demonstrating lymphocytic and histiocytic cell markers have shown that many cases previously classified as reticulosis, especially those with multifocal lesions, have been GME.[8,9] In fact, GME can be associated with the formation of tumor-like mass lesions that usually coexist with characteristic disseminated lesions in other areas of the brain.[3] When such typical disseminated lesions are lacking, other diseases have to be considered. Immunocytochemistry demonstrating various immunoglobulin classes reveals that some of these focal mass lesions are in fact primary lymphosarcomas.[10] In conclusion, GME accounts for the vast majority of lesions previously called reticulosis. The remaining cases are mostly lymphosarcomas, and in a few mass lesions, some suspicion remains that they are true histiocytic tumors.[9]

ETIOLOGY

There is little doubt that GME is an infectious disease. However, experimental studies to transmit the infectious agent in dogs using GME-brain tissue have been unsuccessful.[11] Bacteria and fungi can cause granulomatous lesions in the CNS of small animals, but it is unlikely that such agents would have escaped detection on light microscopic examination of GME. It is possible the the PAS-positive and acidophilic inclusions in macrophages in lesions in some cases may be an unidentified infectious agent.[2] Other investigators have searched unsuccessfully for an infectious organism by electron microscopic examination of the tissues.[12] Serologic tests for toxoplasmosis have been carried out in a few cases, but the results have been negative.[1] The possibility of rickettsial infection as an underlying cause should also be considered. Certain viral infections such as equine infectious anemia, feline infectious peritonitis, and visna are also associated with granulomatous lesions of the CNS. The author believes that the most likely cause of GME is a virus. Canine distemper virus (CDV), which is responsible for a variety of CNS lesions, can be excluded as a cause of GME, since systematic immunocytochemical studies in a large number of GME cases failed to find CDV antigen in the lesions.[13] The presence of anti-CDV antibody titers in the CSF of seven dogs with GME[14] is difficult to explain in view of the negative immunocytochemical findings. Sophisticated culturing techniques will be necessary to identify the agent. Simultaneous onset of the clinical signs in two related Afghan hounds suggests that the disease may be associated with common exposure or genetic predisposition.[14a]

CLINICAL FINDINGS

The disease occurs in young to middle-aged dogs. Females are more often affected than males, and there is a higher prevalence for smaller breeds, especially poodles.[3] In dogs with disseminated lesions, there is usually an acute onset, and the disease is always progressive, with death generally occurring within 1 to 8 weeks. Definitive neurologic signs cannot be expected because the lesions are disseminated in the CNS. Signs are associated with the site of most extensive damage and may involve disturbances in gait and postural reactions, with ataxia, dysmetria, paresis, and paralysis; changes in mental status (confusion, lethargy, and coma); and deficits in cranial nerve function. In the acute stage of the disease more than half of the animals have fever, and many animals exhibit paraspinal discomfort[14] or cervical pain.[2] Chronic disease (several months) is possible in the focal form of GME. Large tumor-like masses may develop into focal GME, with clinical signs suggestive of a space-occupying mass. Presenting signs refer to a single site of involvement, most frequently to the posterior fossa, with brain stem and cerebellar signs, and sometimes to the cerebrum. A particular localization of GME, previously called ocular reticulosis,

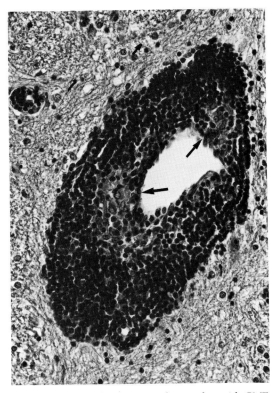

Figure 90–1. Histologic section from a dog with GME, showing perivascular mononuclear cuffing with eccentrically situated nodular foci of macrophages (*arrows*) (H and E; × 250).

occurs with acute unilateral or bilateral blindness and ophthalmoscopic evidence of optic neuritis.[3]

DIAGNOSIS

Typical hematologic and biochemical findings are lacking. Neutrophilia may be present in the acute disease.[14] The CSF is abnormal, with a marked pleocytosis; cell counts of 100 to more than 1000 WBCs/μl are usual. Mononuclear cells predominate, but some neutrophils also are present in most cases.[15] Cytologic examination of the CSF may reveal large anaplastic mononuclear cells with abundant lacy cytoplasm.[3] Electrophoretic examination of the CSF may suggest blood-brain barrier disruption and intrathecal immunoglobulin synthesis.[14] Such changes are not specific for GME. In focal GME, the tumor-like lesions can be detected with computerized axial tomography.[3] Electroencephalographic patterns studied in some dogs with GME were found to be abnormal.[1]

PATHOLOGIC FINDINGS

Lesions are found in the meninges, brain, and spinal cord, especially in the cervical segments. White matter is generally more severely affected than gray matter. Although the lesions are disseminated, the cerebral hemispheres, the midbrain, and regions around the fourth ventricle are most frequently involved. The lesions, which are strictly associated with the vasculature, consist of perivascular cuffing of monocytes, lymphocytes, plasma cells, and sometimes a few neutrophils. The formation of eccentrically situated nodular foci of macrophages within these cuffs is a characteristic finding in GME (Fig. 90–1). The cuffs can become very large and merge with adjacent cuffs, leading to the formation of tumor-like granulomas.

THERAPY

There is no specific therapy for GME, although improvement frequently has been observed after glucocorticoid administration. However, all known cases have eventually died of the disease despite steroid treatment.

Pug Dog Encephalitis

This disease, which occurs only in the pug dog breed, has been known for several years in the United States and has been recorded not only in California and the Northeastern states[16] but also in the Southeast.[17] The prevalence of this disease outside the United States is uncertain. This breed is relatively uncommon in Europe. Three histologically confirmed cases have been observed in Switzerland, and one clinically suspected case has been seen in southern Italy.[6]

ETIOLOGY

The etiology of pug dog encephalitis is unknown. The distribution and morphology of the lesions are unique for this disease and totally different from the histologic findings in other known CNS infections in small animals. The pathologic findings are, nevertheless, strongly suggestive of an infectious process. Bacteria, fungi, and protozoal organisms may probably be ruled out as potential causes because they would have been detected on histologic examination. The predominantly mononuclear inflammation suggests a viral etiology. Viral isolation attempts in two cases however were unsuccessful.[16] The restriction of this disease to a single breed is highly unusual for infections of small animals and strongly suggests predisposing genetic factors. It could be speculated that pug dogs may have a breed-specific tissue antigen that could act as a receptor for a hitherto unknown virus or may have a breed-specific composition of the immune response genes leading to an atypical immunologic reaction toward a known pathogen. The predilection of the cerebral hemispheres for involvement with a necrotic inflammatory process is similar to the features seen with α-herpesvirus encephalitides of other species.[15a]

CLINICAL FINDINGS

The disease may occur at any age and affects both sexes. The course of the disease is usually 1 to 6 months, but occasionally pug dogs may die a few days after the onset of signs. The most consistent sign is the occurrence of partial or generalized seizures. Other cerebral signs include decreased consciousness, abnormal behavior, compulsive circling, blindness, generalized ataxia and paresis, and deficient postural reactions. A few animals may exhibit brain stem signs. The disease is always progressive, and many animals die as a result of severe seizures.[16]

DIAGNOSIS

There are no typical hematologic and biochemical findings. CSF analysis is abnormal in most dogs, with a predominantly mononuclear pleocytosis (usually 90 to 600 cells/μl) and increased protein concentration; (usually 50 to 200 mg/dl);[15a,18] however, these are not specific, since other encephalitides are associated with similar CSF changes. The massive necrotizing lesions in the cerebrum could be detected with computerized axial tomography.

PATHOLOGIC FINDINGS

Necrotizing lesions in the cerebrum may be visible on macroscopic examination. The histologic findings are unusual and highly typical for this disease, a disseminated meningitis, chorioiditis, and encephalitis with greatest involvement of the cerebrum. The perivascular and meningeal inflammatory infiltrates consisting of lymphocytes, plasma cells, histiocytes, and macrophages have a strong tendency to invade the parenchyma.

There are extensive compact subpial and subventricular lesions that may extend deep into the underlying brain tissue, with unusually intense microglial proliferation and total destruction of the original tissue elements. In some areas, there is frank cerebrocortical necrosis. The cerebral white matter also is severely affected, with intense perivascular cuffing and gliosis, and in some areas there is leukomalacia with liquefaction and cavitation of the tissue (Fig. 90–2).

THERAPY

There is no treatment for this disease. Glucocorticoids do not alter the course of pug dog encephalitis, and antiepileptic drugs are often ineffective to control the seizures.[16]

Hydrocephalus with Periventricular Encephalitis in Dogs

Hydrocephalus is probably the most common developmental abnormality of the CNS in dogs and may be the result of congenital or acquired stenosis of the mesencephalic aqueduct.[19] Acquired hydrocephalus usually is a result of infectious or neoplastic diseases that lead to obstruction of the CSF drainage pathways. A particular form of acquired hydrocephalus in young dogs is associated with severe periventricular inflammation. It probably has existed for a long time but was first described as an entity in the United States in 1977.[20] A series of cases from western Europe was reported in 1981.[21]

ETIOLOGY

Because of the severe inflammatory changes seen with hydrocephalus, an infectious cause has been suspected. On bacteriologic examination of brain tissue and CSF in two dogs with this disease, three different bacteria were isolated; however, these were thought to be contaminants. It is possible that the disease is caused by a virus, although no infectious agent was found on

electron-microscopic study of the periventricular tissues of two dogs.[21] Canine parainfluenza virus has caused hydrocephalus in dogs after experimental inoculation (see Chapter 20).[22,23] However, the clinical and pathologic findings in experimental parainfluenza–induced hydrocephalus are totally different from the condition described herein. Serum neutralizing antibodies against canine parvovirus were absent in the sera of two dogs in the previously mentioned study.[21]

CLINICAL FINDINGS

This disease occurs in puppies between 2 and 6 months of age. There is no predilection for miniature breeds as occurs with congenital hydrocephalus. The animals are normal at birth and exhibit normal development for the first 2 months of life. At 2 or 3 months of age, acute neurologic signs occur, together with rapidly progressing skull enlargement. Neurologic signs include behavioral changes such as depression, dullness, and hyperactivity. There is progressive incoordination

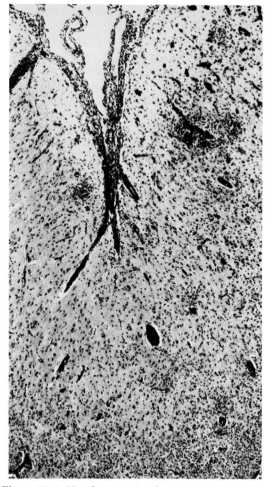

Figure 90–2. Histologic section from a case of pug dog encephalitis. Severe perivascular and meningeal inflammation as well as necrosis of large areas of the cerebral cortex (H and E; × 100).

in all limbs, and most animals develop neurologic blindness. Less consistent findings are cranial nerve deficits, which may include deafness, abnormal eye motility, head tilt, and dysphagia. The course of the disease is usually progressive over several days to a few weeks. In some animals, the clinical condition may stabilize.

DIAGNOSIS

There are no consistent hematologic or biochemical findings associated with this form of hydrocephalus. CSF abnormalities consist of xanthochromia, increased protein concentration, and pleocytosis consisting of erythrocytes, mononuclear cells, and macrophages containing erythrocytes. Radiographic examination of the skull reveals abnormalities such as thinning of the cranial vault and homogeneous appearance of the intracranial contents. However, these findings are indicative of hydrocephalus, regardless of its cause.[19] The same can be said for the EEG findings typical of hydrocephalus.[19]

PATHOLOGIC FINDINGS

There is massive enlargement of the cerebral ventricles, which are filled with cloudy, hemorrhagic CSF. The internal surface of the ventricles is focally roughened, with a brownish discoloration. A typical finding is the presence of large dissecting cavities also called false diverticula in the cerebral mantle (Fig. 90–3A). These communicate with the lateral ventricles. Histologically, there is a severe inflammation with necrosis of the ependymal and subependymal tissues. The lesions are always hemorrhagic. Hemosiderin-laden macrophages are found in old lesions. There is perivascular cuffing with inflammatory cells and in acute lesions, diffuse infiltration with neutrophils and macrophages (see Fig. 90–2B and 2C). Glial mesenchymal repair tissue is formed later in the course of the disease.

THERAPY

By the time the condition becomes evident to the owner, severe damage has already taken place. In most cases, the disease is rapidly progressive, leading to severe neurologic impairment. However, in those cases in which the condition stabilizes, conservative therapy with glucocorticoids or surgical treatment may be considered.[19]

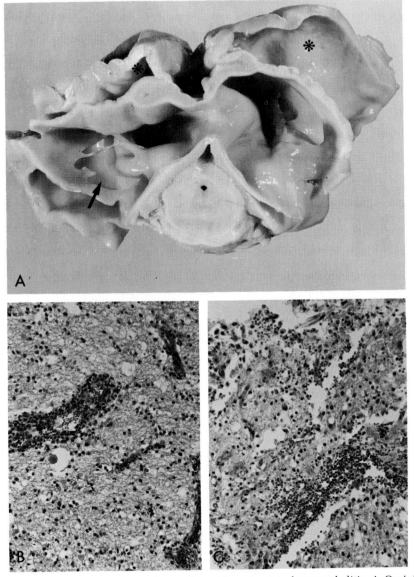

Figure 90–3. Gross and histologic specimens from a dog with periventricular encephalitis. *A*, Occipital area at the level of the midbrain showing greatly enlarged ventricles. False diverticulum (*asterisk*) communicates with the lateral ventricle through a defect (*arrow*) in the ventricular wall. *B*, Inflammatory changes (cuffing) in the periventricular tissue (H and E; × 100). *C*, Hemorrhage and malacia in periventricular tissue (H and E; × 100). (*A* from Wouda W et al: *Zentralbl Veterinärmed [A]* 28:481–493, 1981, with permission.)

Feline Poliomyelitis

Poliomyelitis in domestic cats was first reported in North Africa and Ceylon in the 1950s. In recent years additional cases have been described in North America and Europe.[24-26] A clinically and pathologically similar condition occurs in large Felidae (lions and tigers) held in captivity.[27,28]

ETIOLOGY

Pathologic findings indicate that poliomyelitis in cats is almost certainly caused by a virus. However, ultrastructural studies to demonstrate a specific causal virus in domestic cats have not yet been performed, and the considerable efforts to identify such a virus in lions and tigers, including tissue culture studies, animal inoculation, and serologic studies for known viruses,[28] have all been unsuccessful. Comparative pathologic studies suggest that several known spontaneously occurring or experimentally induced viral infections of cats are unlikely to cause poliomyelitis; however, the role of togaviruses should be investigated further.[26] The role, if any, of feline immunodeficiency virus has not been investigated.

CLINICAL FINDINGS

Feline poliomyelitis is an insidious disease; its onset is slow and progresses over weeks to months. In many instances, the neurologic signs may stabilize, and some animals may recover. Immature, as well as adult, cats appear to be susceptible. In cats, the disease is sporadic; to the author's knowledge, no outbreaks have been recorded in catteries. However, outbreaks in which several lions and tigers were simultaneously affected have occurred in zoologic gardens.[27,28] The predominant signs are problems in locomotion, including paresis, ataxia, and depressed postural reactions in the pelvic and thoracic limbs. Lower motor neuron involvement is characterized by muscle atrophy and decreased tendon reflexes. Hyperesthesia in the thoracic and lumbar areas is apparent is some cases. Additional neurologic signs, which occur rarely, include epilepsy, cerebellar signs, and pupillary abnormalities.

PATHOLOGIC FINDINGS

Disseminated inflammatory lesions are found in the brain and spinal cord (Fig. 90–4). The spinal cord and medulla oblongata

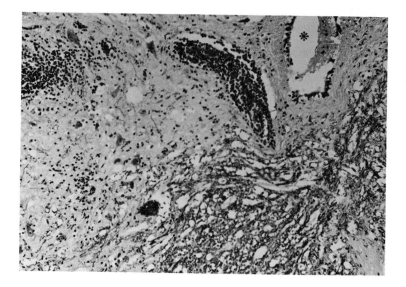

Figure 90–4. Histologic section from the spinal cord of a cat with poliomyelitis, showing perivascular cuffing and nodular gliosis in the gray matter. Asterisk indicates central canal (H and E; × 250).

are most severely affected. The lesions consist of perivascular mononuclear cuffing, gliosis, and neuronal degeneration, the last being most obvious in the ventral horns of the spinal cord. In chronic cases very little inflammation may be seen, but neuronal loss and intense astrogliosis in the cord are striking. As a result of neuronal damage, there also is marked diffuse Wallerian degeneration of the lateral and ventral columns, resembling a primary degenerative disorder. There are no consistent lesions in other organ systems.

THERAPY

There is no curative treatment for the suspected viral infection. Contact between unaffected cats and those suspected to have the disease should be avoided. The prognosis is not always unfavorable, as large Felidae suspected of having the infection have been known to recover.[27]

Conclusions

It is to be expected that additional CNS diseases of suspected infectious origin will be recognized in dogs and cats. The ability to characterize infectious agents in these diseases is limited when formalin-fixed tissues are used. Fresh material for culture should be collected when clinical findings are compatible with one of these disorders. In addition to brain tissue taken for isolation procedures, serum and CSF should be collected and screened for antibody activity against a wide variety of known infectious agents. It also is possible that more systematic ultrastructural studies of appropriately fixed tissues taken from lesions and sites indicated by the clinical examination may be useful in detecting infectious agents. For a discussion of meningitis of suspected infectious or immune-mediated causes, see Bacterial Infections of the Central Nervous System, Chapter 12.

References

1. Braund KG, Vandevelde M, Walker TL, et al: Granulomatous meningoencephalomyelitis in six dogs. *J Am Vet Med Assoc* 172:1195–1200, 1978.
2. Cordy DR: Canine granulomatous meningoencephalomyelitis. *Vet Pathol* 16:325–333, 1979.
3. Braund KG: Granulomatous meningoencephalomyelitis. *J Am Vet Med Assoc* 186:138–141, 1985.
4. Glastonbury JRW, Frauenfelder AR: Granulomatous meningoencephalitis in a dog. *Aust Vet J* 57:186–189, 1981.
5. Alley MR, Jones BR, Johnstone AC: Granulomatous meningoencephalitis of dogs in New Zealand. *NZ Vet J* 31:117–119, 1983.
6. Vandevelde M: Unpublished observation, University of Bern, Bern, Switzerland, 1987.
7. Fankhauser R, Fatzer R, Luginbühl H et al: Reticulosis of the central nervous system in dogs. *Adv Vet Sci* 16:35–71, 1972.
8. Higgins JR: Morphologic and histochemical characteristics of GME and reticulosis: one disease or two? The California perspective. *Proceedings ACVIM Forum*, Washington, DC, 1986.
9. Vandevelde M: Morphologic and histochemical characteristics of GME and reticulosis: one disease or two? The Bern perspective. *Proceedings ACVIM Forum*, Washington, DC, 1986.
10. Vandevelde M, Fatzer R, Fankhauser R: Immunohistologic studies on primary reticulosis of the canine brain. *Vet Pathol* 18:577–588, 1981.
11. Luttgen P: Personal communication, University of Texas A and M, College Station, TX, 1986.
12. Cork L: Personal communication, University of Georgia, Athens, GA, 1974.
13. Higgins RJ: Personal communication, University of California, Davis, CA, 1986.
14. Sorjonen DC: Granulomatous meningoencephalomyelitis: clinical and histopathologic correlations. *Proceedings ACVIM Forum*, San Diego, 848–850, 1987.
14a. Harris CW, Didier PJ, Parker AJ: Simultaneous central nervous system reticulosis in two related Afghan hounds. *Compend Cont Educ Pract Vet* 10:304–310, 1988.
15. Bailey CS, Higgins RJ: Characteristics of cerebrospinal fluid associated with canine granulomatous meningoencephalomyelitis: a retrospective study. *J Am Vet Med Assoc* 188:418–421, 1986.
15a. Cordy DR, Holliday TA: A necrotizing meningoencephalitis of pug dogs. *Vet Pathol* 26:191–194, 1989.
16. De Lahunta A: *Veterinary Neuroanatomy and Clinical Neurology*. Philadelphia, WB Saunders Co, 1983.
17. Greene CE: Personal communication, University of Georgia, Athens, GA, 1987.
18. Holliday TA: Personal communication, University of California, Davis, CA, 1986.
19. Hoerlein BF: *Canine Neurology*. Philadelphia, WB Saunders Co, 1978.
20. Higgins RJ, Vandevelde M, Braund KG: Internal hydrocephalus and associated periventricular encephalitis in young dogs. *Vet Pathol* 14:236–246, 1977.

21. Wouda W, Vandevelde M, Kihm U: Internal hydro-cephalus of suspected infectious origin in young dogs. *Zentralbl Veterinärmed [A]* 28:481–493, 1981.

22. Baumgärtner WK, Krakowka S, Koestner A, et al: Acute encephalitis and hydrocephalus in dogs caused by canine parainfluenza virus. *Vet Pathol* 19:79–92, 1982.

23. Baumgärtner WK, Krakowka S, Koestner A, et al: Ultrastructural evaluation of acute encephalitis and hydrocephalus in dogs caused by canine parainflu-enza virus. *Vet Pathol* 19:305–314, 1982.

24. Kronevi T, Nordström M, Moreno W, et al: Feline ataxia due to nonsuppurative meningoencephalo-myelitis of unknown etiology. *Nord Vet Med* 26:720–725, 1974.

25. Vandevelde M, Braund KG: Polioencephalomyelitis in cats. *Vet Pathol* 16:420–427, 1979.

26. Hoff EJ, Vandevelde M: Non-suppurative encepha-lomyelitis in cats suggestive of a viral origin. *Vet Pathol* 18:170–180, 1981.

27. Flir K: Encephalomyelitis in the big cats. *Dtsch Tierarztl Wochenschr* 80:401–404, 1973.

28. Melchior G: Meningoencephalitis in lions and ti-gers. *In* Ippen R, Schröder H (eds): *Diseases of Zoo Animals*. Proceedings of the XV International Sym-posium on Zoo Animal Diseases (Kolmarden). Ber-lin, Akademie-Verlag, 1973, pp 245–254.

APPENDICES

APPENDIX 1. Canine Immunization Recommendations[a]

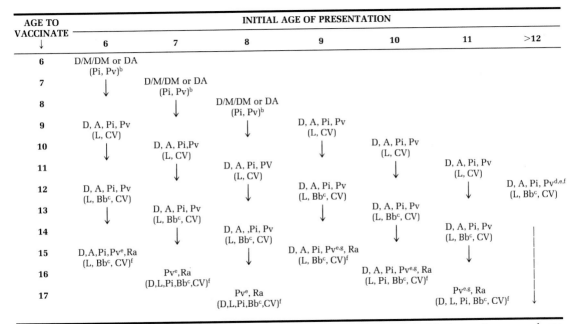

AGE TO VACCINATE ↓	INITIAL AGE OF PRESENTATION						
	6	7	8	9	10	11	>12
6	D/M/DM or DA (Pi, Pv)[b]						
7	↓	D/M/DM or DA (Pi, Pv)[b]					
8	↓	↓	D/M/DM or DA (Pi, Pv)[b]				
9	D, A, Pi, Pv (L, CV)	↓	↓	D, A, Pi, Pv (L, CV)			
10	↓	D, A, Pi,Pv (L, CV)	↓	↓	D, A, Pi, Pv (L, CV)		
11	↓	↓	D, A, Pi, PV (L, CV)	↓	↓	D, A, Pi, Pv (L, CV)	
12	D, A, Pi, Pv (L, Bb[c], CV)	↓	↓	D, A, Pi, Pv (L, Bb[c], CV)	↓	↓	D, A, Pi, Pv[d,e,f] (L, Bb[c], CV)
13	↓	D, A, Pi, Pv (L, Bb[c], CV)	↓	↓	D, A, Pi, Pv (L, Bb[c], CV)	↓	
14	↓	↓	D, A, ,Pi, Pv (L, Bb[c], CV)	↓	↓	D, A, Pi, Pv (L, Bb[c], CV)		(line)
15	D,A,Pi,Pv[e],Ra (L, Bb[c], CV)[f]	↓	↓	D, A, Pi, Pv[e,g], Ra (L, Bb[c], CV)[f]	↓	↓	
16		Pv[e],Ra (D,L,Pi,Bb[c],CV)[f]	↓		D, A, Pi, Pv[e,g], Ra (L, Pi, Bb[c], CV)[f]	↓	
17			Pv[e], Ra (D,L,Pi,Bb[c],CV)[f]			Pv[e,g], Ra (D, L, Pi, Bb[c], CV)[f]	↓

[a]Ages are listed in weeks. Suggested optional antigens are in parentheses. Colostric immunity assumed; see Colostric-Deprived Neonates, below, for that circumstance. For accompanying text, see Vaccination Recommendations for Canine Diseases, Chapter 2, and sections on prevention in respective disease chapters. Evidence indicates that IM vaccination with measles and rabies gives better protection as compared to SC inoculation. However, the latter route is associated with more discomfort and potential allergic reactions.

Continued on following page

[b]Pv is recommended and is not optional in high prevalence areas. Some feel that Pv vaccine in puppies less than 9 weeks of age should precede or be given alternately with D vaccine; however, this is not necessary. Coronaviral vaccination is delayed until 9 weeks to minimize potential allergic reactions; however, it may be given earlier if outbreaks are noted in young puppies.

[c]If *Bordetella* and parainfluenza antigens are given as an MLV-intranasal preparation, then only one inoculation with those antigens is needed, given at either time, instead of the two listed in the series.

[d]Give a second vaccination 2 to 3 weeks later with same antigen and also give Ra antigen.

[e]Additional optional Pv vaccination may be given 2 to 3 weeks later when experience dictates that vaccine breaks will occur due to maternal antibody interference with the recommended protocol. A small percentage of puppies may show this blockade up to 18 weeks of age using any of the presently available vaccines. Certain breeds should be vaccinated up to 18 weeks of age (see Vaccination Recommendations for Canine Parvoviral Infection, Chapter 2).

[f]For coronaviral vaccination, at least two vaccinations are recommended, given 2 to 3 weeks apart. Pups completing this series prior to 12 weeks of age should be given an additional dose between 12 and 16 weeks of age.

[g]Administration of at least four parvoviral vaccines in the neonatal vaccination series has been associated with more consistent seroconversion. An additional Pv vaccine may be given 2 to 3 weeks after this inoculation when outbreaks in previously vaccinated dogs have been noted.

BOOSTERS: D, A, Pi (L, Bb, CV) yearly. I-FeO-Pv every 3 to 6 months; MLV-FeO-Pv or I-CaO-Pv every 6 to 12 months; or MLV-CaO-Pv yearly. Ra every 1 or 3 years, depending on product used, dog's age, and local public health laws.

PREGNANT FEMALES: Do not use any MLV vaccines. Only effective I products are A, L, Pv, Ra, and Bb.

COLOSTRUM-DEPRIVED NEONATES: Start D, A, at 2 to 3 weeks of age and repeat every 3 weeks until the animal is 12 weeks old. Add L (Pi optional) between 9 to 12 weeks of age and Ra on the last visit. Use inactivated Pv until dog is >5 weeks old and a live product thereafter along with the other antigens. Vaccination of certain breeds or those in high prevalence areas should continue until 18 weeks of age for Pv protection.

OUTBREAK:

Distemper—vaccinate within 4 days of initial exposure.

Respiratory disease—booster with Pi or Bb (IN preferred).

Leptospirosis—two doses 2 to 3 weeks apart every 3 to 6 months.

Parvoviral enteritis—use MLV-CaO in exposed dogs.

ABBREVIATIONS: D = distemper (MLV); M = measles (MLV); A = adenovirus-1 (hepatitis) or adenovirus-2 (respiratory virus) (MLV or I); L = *Leptospira* (I); Pi = parainfluenza (MLV): Pv = parvovirus (FeO = feline origin; CaO = canine origin); CV = coronavirus (I); Ra = rabies (MLV or I); Bb = *Bordetella*; I = inactivated (noninfectious); MLV = modified live virus; IN = intranasal.

APPENDIX 2. *Feline Immunization Recommendations*[a]

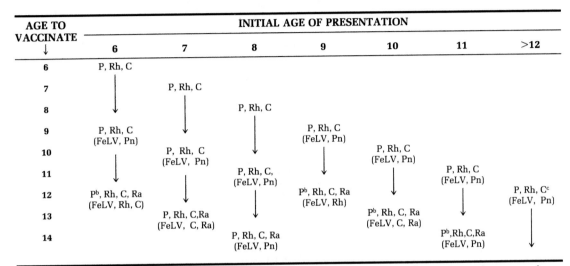

AGE TO VACCINATE ↓	INITIAL AGE OF PRESENTATION						
	6	7	8	9	10	11	>12
6	P, Rh, C						
7		P, Rh, C					
8			P, Rh, C				
9	P, Rh, C (FeLV, Pn)			P, Rh, C (FeLV, Pn)			
10		P, Rh, C (FeLV, Pn)			P, Rh, C (FeLV, Pn)		
11			P, Rh, C, (FeLV, Pn)			P, Rh, C (FeLV, Pn)	
12	P[b], Rh, C, Ra (FeLV, Rh, C)			P[b], Rh, C, Ra (FeLV, Rh)			P, Rh, C[c] (FeLV, Pn)
13		P, Rh, C,Ra (FeLV, C, Ra)			P[b], Rh, C, Ra (FeLV, C, Ra)		
14			P, Rh, C, Ra (FeLV, Pn)			P[b],Rh,C,Ra (FeLV, Pn)	

[a]Ages are listed in weeks. Suggested optional antigens are in parentheses. Colostric immunity assumed; see Colostric-Deprived Neonates below for that circumstance. For accompanying text, see Vaccination Recommendations for Feline Diseases, Chapter 2, and sections on prevention in respective disease chapters. A feline infectious peritonitis vaccine (Primucell FIP) is under development by Norden Laboratories, Lincoln, NE. The vaccine is administered intranasally as two doses given at a 3-week interval beginning at 9 weeks of age. Evidence indicates that IM vaccination with feline respiratory and FeLV vaccines gives better protection as compared to SC inoculation. However, the latter route is associated with more discomfort and potential allergic reactions.

[b]If I product is used, then repeat 2 to 3 weeks later.

[c]Give a second vaccination 2 to 3 weeks later with same antigen and also give rabies antigen. Only one P is essential if MLV is used; only one Rh and C if IN is used.

BOOSTERS: P and Ra yearly; Rh, C, FeLV, and FIP are optional, depending on prevalence of disease in area.

PREGNANT FEMALES: Two I-P, Rh, and C should be given 3 weeks apart with I-Ra on last visit. (DO NOT USE MLV VACCINES).

COLOSTRUM-DEPRIVED NEONATES: Presented <4 weeks old: two I-P, Rh, C 3 weeks apart, then complete series as listed above. Presented 4 to 6 weeks old: MLV-P, C immediately and 3 weeks later, then complete series as listed above. Presented >6 weeks old: follow series as listed above.

OUTBREAK:
Panleukopenia
No colostral immunity or previous vaccination—<6 weeks old: 2 to 4 ml/kg feline serum SC or IM, then 2 weeks later start series above; >6 weeks old: MLV-P immediately.
Vaccinated 1 year previously—MLV-P immediately.
Respiratory disease: MLV-IN-Rh, C; MLV-Pn (optional).

ABBREVIATIONS: P = panleukopenia (MLV, I); Rh = rhinotracheitis (MLV, I); C = calicivirus (MLV, I); Ra = rabies (MLV, I); Pn = pneumonitis (Chlamydia, MLV); FeLV = feline leukemia virus (I); FIP = feline infectious peritonitis virus (MLV): I = inactivated; MLV = modified live virus; SC = subcutaneous; IM = intramuscular; IN = intranasal.

APPENDIX 3. Immunization Guidelines and Available Biologics for

VACCINE ANTIGENS AND RECOMMENDATIONS[a]	RAB-I	RAB-L	CORONA	PARV-FL	PARV-CI
Type of antigen[b]	I	L	I	L	I
Route[c]	IM, SC	IM	SC	SC	SC
Earliest neonatal vaccination (weeks)[d]	12	12	6	6	6
Latest neonatal vaccination (weeks)[d]	N	N	12–16	16–18	16–18
Booster interval[e]	A, T	A, T	A	A	A

MANUFACTURERS AND AVAILABLE COMBINATIONS[f]

	RAB-I	RAB-L	CORONA	PARV-FL	PARV-CI
112, 189, C112, C189	—	—	×	—	—
189, C189	—	—	—	—	—
272	—	—	—	—	×
112, 189, C189	—	—	×	—	—
112, 189, B8, C189, C112	—	—	×	—	—
195, 264, B1, B3, B7, C29	—	—	—	—	—
112, 189, 195, 264, A1, A2, A3, B1, B3, B7, B8, B9, C29, C189	—	—	—	—	—
272	—	—	—	—	×
189, C189	—	—	—	—	—
107, 112, 189, 195, 264, C29	—	—	—	—	—
112, 189, 195, 264, A1, A2, C29, C107, C112, C189, C264, N1	—	—	—	—	—
107, 189, 195, B8, C29, C189	—	—	—	—	×
112, 124, 188, 195, 225, 264, 272, B2	—	—	—	—	—
112, 124, 225, 264, 272, B2	—	—	—	—	—
112, 225, 264	—	—	—	—	—
189	—	—	—	—	—
189	—	—	—	—	—
189, 264	—	—	—	—	—
124, 165	—	—	—	—	—
165, 189, 195, 225, 264, 272, C189	—	—	—	—	—
189	—	—	—	—	—
B1	—	—	—	—	—
124, B3	—	—	—	—	—
B5, B6	—	—	—	—	—
B1, B3, B5	—	—	—	—	×
B2	—	—	—	×	—
B2, B8	—	—	—	—	—
B9	—	—	—	—	—
A3, B1, B7, B8, B9, C29, C189	—	—	—	—	—
B5	—	—	—	—	×
B3, B5	—	—	—	—	—
A3, B1, B3, B5, B6, C10, C29, C107, C112, C189, N1	—	—	—	—	×
B8	—	—	—	—	—
C29, C107, C112, C189, C264	—	—	—	—	—
B1, B3	—	—	—	—	×
B1, B7	—	—	—	—	—
C10	—	—	—	—	×
C10	—	—	—	—	×
189, C189	—	—	—	—	—
112, 189, C189	—	—	×	—	—
C29, C189	—	—	—	—	—
107, 112, 124, 188, 189, 195, 225, 264, 272, 298 B1, B2, B3, B7, B8, B9 }	—	—	—	—	—
107, 112, 165, 189, 195, 225, 298, 302 B2, B7, B9, C10, C29, C107, C112, C189, C298 }	×	—	—	—	—
189, C189	—	×	—	—	—
B4	—	—	—	—	—

[a]Rab-I = inactivated rabies virus; Rab-L = attenuated rabies virus; Corona = inactivated coronavirus; Parvo-FL = attenuated feline-origin parvovirus; Parvo-CI = inactivated canine-origin parvovirus; Parvo-CL = attenuated canine-origin parvovirus; Bord-LN = attenuated intranasal *Bordetella*; Bord-IP = inactivated parenteral *Bordetella*; Para-LN = attenuated intranasal parainfluenza virus; Para-IP = inactivated parenteral parainfluenza virus; Lepto = inactivated *Leptospira canicola* and *L. icterohemorrhagiae* antigens; Adeno2 = attenuated adenovirus-2; Adeno1I = inactivated adenovirus-1; Adeno1L = attenuated adenovirus-1; Measles = measles virus; Dist = attenuated distemper virus.

[b]L = attenuated live; I = noninfectious or inactivated

[c]IM = intramuscular; SC = subcutaneous; IN = intranasal

[d]Ages are assuming that neonate received colostrum. If neonate did not receive colostrum, see Table 2–2 and Appendix 1. N = not applicable.

[e]A = annual; T = triennial; B = biannual

[f]See Appendix 5 for a list of manufacturers designated by alphanumeric code based on license numbers. No letter prefix = United States; B = Great Britain; C = Canada; A = Australia, N = New Zealand.

Specific Canine Infectious Diseases

PARV-CL	BORD-LN	BORD-IP	PARA-LN	PARA-IP	LEPTO	ADENO2	ADENO1I	ADENO1L	MEASLES	DIST
L	L	I	L	L	I	L	I	L	L	L
SC	IN	SC	IN	SC	SC	SC	SC	SC	IM, SC	SC
6	4	6	4	6	6	6	6	6	6	6
16–18	12	12–16	12	12–16	12–16	12–16	12–16	12–16	12	12–16
A	A,B	A,B	A,B	A,B	A	A	A	A	N	A
—	—	—	—	—	—	—	—	—	×	×
—	—	—	—	—	—	×	—	—	—	—
×	—	—	—	—	—	—	—	—	—	—
×	—	—	—	×	—	×	—	—	—	×
—	—	—	—	—	—	×	—	—	—	×
—	—	—	—	×	g	×	—	×	—	×
—	—	—	—	×	g	×	—	—	×	×
—	—	—	—	×	g	×	—	—	—	×
×	—	—	—	×	g	×	—	—	—	×
—	—	—	—	×	g	×	—	—	—	×
—	—	—	—	—	—	—	—	×	—	×
—	—	—	—	×	g	—	—	×	—	×
×	—	—	—	×	g	—	—	×	—	×
—	—	—	—	—	—	—	—	×	—	×
—	—	—	—	×	—	—	—	—	—	—
—	—	—	—	×	—	—	—	—	—	—
—	×	—	×	—	—	—	—	—	—	—
—	—	×	—	—	—	—	—	—	—	—
—	—	×	—	—	×	—	—	—	—	—
—	—	—	—	—	×	—	×	—	—	—
—	—	—	—	—	—	—	—	—	×	—
—	—	—	—	—	×	—	×	—	—	×
—	—	—	—	—	×	—	×	—	—	—
—	—	—	—	—	×	—	—	—	—	—
×	—	—	—	—	—	—	×	—	—	×
×	—	—	—	—	—	—	—	—	—	—
×	—	—	—	—	×	—	×	—	—	×
—	—	—	—	—	×	—	×	—	—	—
—	—	—	—	×	×	—	—	—	×	×
×	—	—	—	×	×	×	—	—	—	×
—	—	—	—	×	×	—	—	—	—	—
×	—	—	—	—	—	×	—	—	—	×
—	—	—	—	×	—	—	×	—	—	×
—	—	—	—	×	×	—	×	—	—	×
—	—	×	—	×	—	×	—	—	—	×
×	—	—	—	×	×	×	—	—	—	×
—	—	—	—	×	×	×	—	—	—	×
—	—	—	—	—	×ʰ	—	—	—	—	—
—	—	—	—	—	—	—	—	—	—	—
—	—	—	—	—	—	—	—	—	—	—
—	—	—	—	—	—	—	—	—	—	—
—	×	—	—	—	—	—	—	—	—	—

ᵍIn the United States, these combined products may have Lepto added in lieu of diluent. British, Canadian, Australian, and New Zealand products containing Lepto are designated by an × in this column.

ʰListed companies in the United States that market Lepto alone and, as indicated in footnote g, as a diluent in combined vaccines.

APPENDIX 4. Immunization Guidelines and Available Biologics for Specific Feline Infectious Diseases

VACCINE ANTIGENS AND RECOMMENDATIONS[a]	RAB-I	RAB-L	FeLV	CHLA	CAL-IP	CAL-LP	CAL-LN	RHIN-IP	RHIN-LP	RHIN-LN	PAN-IP	PAN-LP	PAN-LN
Type of antigen[b]	I	L	I	L	I	L	L	I	L	L	I	L	L
Route[c]	IM, SC	IM	IM, SC	IM, SC	IM, SC	IM, SC	IN	IM, SC	IM, SC	IN	IM, SC	IM, SC	IN
Earliest neonatal vaccination (weeks)[d]	12	12	9–10	6	6	6	3–4	6	6	3–4	6	6	3–4
Latest neonatal vaccination (weeks)[d]	N	N	12–14	12–14	12–14	12–14	12	12–14	12–14	12	12–14	12–14	12
Booster interval[e]	A, T	A, T	A	A	A	A	A	A	A	A	A	A	A

MANUFACTURERS AND AVAILABLE COMBINATIONS[f]

	RAB-I	RAB-L	FeLV	CHLA	CAL-IP	CAL-LP	CAL-LN	RHIN-IP	RHIN-LP	RHIN-LN	PAN-IP	PAN-LP	PAN-LN
112, 189, 213, 264, 312, C189	—	—	×	—	—	—	—	—	—	—	—	—	—
213, C29, C264, C189	—	—	×	—	—	×	—	—	×	—	—	×	—
124, 189, 195, 225, 264, 272, A1, A2, A3, B1, B2, B3, B7, B8, C29, N1	—	—	—	—	—	—	—	—	—	—	—	×	—
107, 112, 189, 195, 225, 264, 272, A3, B1, B2, B3, B5, B6, B8, C189, N1	—	—	—	—	—	—	—	—	—	—	×	—	—
107	×	—	—	—	—	—	—	—	—	—	×	—	—
264	—	—	—	—	—	—	—	—	×	—	—	—	—
107, 124, 189, 195, 225, 264, 272, B2, B3, B5, C189	—	—	—	—	—	×	—	—	×	—	—	—	—
124, 189, 195, 225, 272, A1, A2, A3, B2, B7, B8, N1	—	—	—	—	—	×	—	—	×	—	—	×	—
112, 195, 213, C10, C112	—	—	—	—	×	—	—	×	—	—	×	—	—
107, 225, 264, 272, B2, B3, B5, C29, C107, C264	—	—	—	—	—	×	—	—	×	—	×	—	—
185, 195, C29, C189	—	—	—	×	—	×	—	—	×	—	—	×	—
195, C29	—	—	—	×	—	×	—	—	×	—	×	—	—
195	×	—	—	×	—	×	—	—	×	—	—	×	—
112, C10, C112	×	—	—	—	×	—	—	×	—	—	×	—	—
107, 195, C29, C10, C107	×	—	—	—	—	×	—	—	×	—	×	—	—
264	—	—	—	—	—	—	—	—	×	—	×	—	—
195, C29	—	—	—	×	—	—	—	—	—	—	—	—	—
189	—	×	—	—	—	—	—	—	—	—	—	—	—
107, 112, 165, 189, 195, 225, 298, 302, C107	×	—	—	—	—	—	—	—	—	—	—	—	—
124	—	—	—	—	—	—	×	—	—	×	—	—	×
189, B3	—	—	—	—	—	—	×	—	—	×	—	—	—
C29	×	—	—	×	—	×	—	—	×	—	×	—	—

[a]Rab-I = inactivated rabies virus; Rab-L = attenuated rabies virus; FeLV = inactivated feline leukemia virus; Chla = attenuated Chlamydia; Cal-IP = inactivated parenteral calicivirus; Cal-LP = attenuated parenteral calicivirus; Cal-LN = attenuated intranasal calicivirus; Rhin-IP = inactivated parenteral rhinotracheitis virus (feline herpesvirus-1); Rhin-LP = attenuated parenteral rhinotracheitis virus; Rhin-LN = attenuated intranasal rhinotracheitis virus; Pan-IP = inactivated parenteral panleukopenia virus; Pan-LP = attenuated parenteral panleukopenia virus; Pan-LN = attenuated intranasal panleukopenia virus.

[b]L = attenuated live; I = noninfectious or inactivated.

[c]IM = intramuscular; SC = subcutaneous; IN = intranasal.

[d]Ages are assuming that neonate received colostrum. If neonate did not receive colostrum, see Table 2–2 and Appendix 2.

[e]A = annual; T = triennial.

[f]See Appendix 5 for a list of manufacturers designated by alphanumeric code based on license numbers. No letter prefix = United States; B = Great Britain; C = Canada.

876

APPENDIX 5. Manufacturers of Canine and Feline Biologics in the United States, Australia and New Zealand, Great Britain, and Canada[a]

COUNTRY	LICENSE CODE[b]	MANUFACTURER	ADDRESS	PRODUCT
United States	107	COOPERS ANIMAL HEALTH INC.[c]	2000 South 11th Street Kansas City KS 66103 800-255-4456 913-321-1070	D: Epivaxine C: Premune, Epifel, Cytorab R: Cytorab, Trirab, Epirab
	112	FORT DODGE LABORATORIES INC.	Fort Dodge IA 50501 800-247-1776 515-955-4600	D: Duramune C: Fel-O-Vax R: Annumune, Trimune
	124	BIO-CEUTIC LABORATORIES Boehringer Ingelheim	2621 North Belt Highway St. Joseph MO 64502 816-233-2804	D: D-Vac, Narammune C: Rhinolin
	165	SCHERING CORPORATION	P.O. Box 3113 Omaha NE 68103 800-228-9663 201-558-4000	D: Intra-trac R: Biorab
	188	COLORADO SERUM COMPANY	4950 York Street Denver CO 80216 303-295-7527	D: Canine Dist-Hep-Lepto
	189	NORDEN LABORATORIES[d]	P.O. Box 80809 Lincoln NE 68501 800-366-5201 800-742-7588	D: Vanguard, Firstdose, Coughguard C: Felocell, Felocine, Felomune, Leukocell R: Endurall, Rabguard
	195	SOLVAY VETERINARY INC. Fromm Laboratories	703 Lake Shore Road Grafton WI 53024 800-524-1645 609-987-2600	D: Parvoid, Galaxy, Leptobac C: Eclipse, Psittacoid R: Rabvac
	213	DIAMOND SCIENTIFIC	P.O. Box 328 Des Moines IA 50302 800-333-9341 515-262-9341	C: Covenant, Confirm
	225	BEECHAM LABORATORIES[d]	P.O. Box 221 White Hall IL 62092 800-251-7040 800-821-0279	D: Sentryvac C: Panvac, Panacine R: Rabcine (distributor)
	243	CEVA LABORATORIES	7101 College Boulevard Overland Park KS 66210 800-255-6444 800-538-2382	D: DHP-LCI Parvo
	264	PITMAN-MOORE INC.[c]	P.O. Box 344 Washington Crossing NJ 08560 800-525-9840	D: Quantum, Tissuvax C: FVR-C-P R: Imrab (distributor)
	272	TECHAMERICA GROUP INC. Fermenta Animal Health	7410 NW Tiffany Springs Pk Kansas City MO 64190-1350 816-891-5500	D: Paramune, Bronchicine, Adenomune, Parvocine C: Rhinopan, Respomune R: Biorab
	298	RHONE MERIEUX	115 Transtech Drive Athens GA 30601 404-548-9292	R: Imrab (manufacturer)
	302	IMMUNOVET INC.	5910-G Breckenridge Parkway Tampa FL 33610 813-621-9447	R: Dura-Rab, Rabcine (manufacturer)
	312	SYNBIOTICS CORP.	11011 Via Frontera San Diego CA 92127 619-451-3770	C: Vac SYN

Continued on following page

APPENDIX 5. Manufacturers of Canine and Feline Biologics in the United States, Australia and New Zealand, Great Britain, and Canada[a] Continued

COUNTRY	LICENSE CODE[b]	MANUFACTURER	ADDRESS	PRODUCT
Australia and New Zealand	A1	ARTHUR WEBSTER PTY LTD[e]	23 Victoria Avenue Castle Hill NSW 2154 (02) 899–2111	D: Websters C: Websters
	A2	COMMONWEALTH SERUM LABS[e]	45 Poplar Road Parkville Vic 3052 (03) 389–1356	D: CSL C: CSL
	A3	PITMAN-MOORE–COOPERS	P.O. Box 777 North Ryde, NSW 2113 (02) 888–4011	D: Vaxitas C: FVR-C-P, Vaxitas
	N1	PITMAN-MOORE–COOPERS	33 Whakatiki St. Private Bag Upper Hutt NZ FAX (04) 279–144	D: Quantum, Vaxitas C: FVR-C-P, Vaxitas
Great Britain	B1	COOPERS ANIMAL HEALTH LTD[c]	Crewe Hall, Crewe Cheshire CW1 1UB 0270-580131	D: Epivax, Vaxitas, Leptovax C: Fiovax, Vaxicat
	B2	C-VET LTD.	Minster House, Western Way Bury St. Edmunds Suffolk IP33 3SU 0284-61131	D: Boostervac, Delcavac C: Feli-pan, Feliflu, C-Vet
	B3	DUPHAR	Solvay House, Flanders Road Hedge End, Southampton Hants. SO3 4QH 048-92-81711	D: Kavak C: Katavac
	B4	GIST-BROCADES ANIMAL HEALTH	Cut Hedge Farm, London Road Braintree Essex CM7 8QH 0376-21721	D: Intrac
	B5	GLAXOVET	Breakspear Road South Harefield, Uxbridge Middlesex UB9 6LS 0895-630266	D: Canilep C: Purtect
	B6	HOECHST	Walton Manor, Milton Keynes Bucks. MK7 7AJ 0908-665050	D: Maxavac C: Felidovac
	B7	INTERVET	Science Park, Milton Road Cambridge CB4 4FP 0223-311221	D: Nobi-vac C: Nobi-vac R: Nobi-vac
	B8	NORDEN LABORATORIES[d]	Cavendish Road, Stevenage Herts. SG1 2EJ 0438-367881	D: Enduracell, Lepto C: Felocine, Felocell
	B9	RMB ANIMAL HEALTH	Rainham Road South, Dagenham Essex RM10 7XS 01-592-3060	D: Caniffa R: Rabiffa, Rabisin

APPENDIX 5. *Manufacturers of Canine and Feline Biologics in the United States, Australia and New Zealand, Great Britain, and Canada*[a] Continued

COUNTRY	LICENSE CODE[b]	MANUFACTURER	ADDRESS	PRODUCT
Canada	C10	LANGFORD INC.	400 Michener Road Guelph ON N1K 1E4 519-837-2040	D: Canlan, Pavlan C: Felan R: Immunorab
	C107	COOPERS AGROPHARM INC.[c]	695 Westney Road South P.O. Box 430 Ajax ON L1S 3C5 416-427-0455	D; Epivaxine, Bovax C: Cytorab, Epifel R: Epirab
	C112	AYERST LABORATORIES	1025 Blvd Laurentien Saint Laurent PQ H4R 1J6 514-744-6771	D: Duramune C: Fel-O-Vax R: Trimune
	C189	NORDEN LABORATORIES[d]	6581 Kitmat Road, Unit 8 Mississauga ON L5N 3T5	D: Vanguard, Firstdose, Coughguard C: Felocell, Felocine, Leukocell R: Endurall, Rabguard
	C264	PITMAN-MOORE[c]	421 East Hawley Street Mundelein IL 60060 312-949-3198	D: Quantum C: FVR-C-P
	C29	SOLVAY VETERINARY	209 Maintou Drive Kitchener ON N2C 1L4 519-748-5473	D: Galaxy, Fromm, Parvac, Parvoid C: Eclipse, Psittacoid R: Rabvac
	C298	RHONE POULENC AGRICULTURE DIV.	2000 Argentia Road Plaza 3, Suite 400 Mississauga ON L5N 1V9 416-821-4450	R: Imrab

[a]Composition of products from manufacturers is described in Appendices 3 and 4. D = products for dogs; C = products for cats; R = products for rabies.
[b]License code is a real designation in the United States and Canada and an arbitrary number for other countries.
[c]Coopers Animal Health, Inc. and Pitman-Moore have merged.
[d]Norden Laboratories and Beecham Laboratories have merged.
[e]Export to New Zealand, which also imports Nobi-Vac from Europe.
Information on biologics from Australia was provided by Dr. David Watson, University of Sydney, NSW, Australia; from New Zealand, by Dr. Elizabeth Lee, Massey University, Palmerston North, New Zealand; those from Great Britain are from Evans J(ed): *The Henston Veterinary Vade Mecum: Small Animals*, ed 7. Surrey, Update—Siebert Publications Ltd, 1988; and those from Canada, from *Canadian Compendium of Veterinary Pharmaceuticals, Biologicals and Specialties*, ed 1. Hensall, ON, 774569 Ontario Ltd, 1989.

APPENDIX 6. *Compendium of Animal Rabies Control, 1990**

National Association of State Public Health Veterinarians, Inc.

The purpose of these recommendations is to provide information on rabies vaccines to practicing veterinarians, public health officials, and others concerned with rabies control. This document serves as the basis for animal rabies vaccination programs throughout the United States. Its adoption will result in standardization of procedures among jurisdictions which is necessary for an effective national rabies control program. These recommendations are reviewed and revised as necessary before each calendar year. All animal rabies vaccines licensed by the United States Department of Agriculture (USDA) and marketed in the United States are listed in Part II of this Compendium; Part III describes the principles of rabies control.

Part I: Recommendations for Immunization Procedures

A. VACCINE ADMINISTRATION: All animal rabies vaccines should be restricted to use by or under the supervision of a veterinarian.

B. VACCINE SELECTION: In comprehensive rabies control programs, only vaccines with a 3-year duration of immunity should be used. This eliminates the need for annual vaccination and constitutes the most effective method of increasing the proportion of immunized dogs and cats. (See Part II.)

C. ROUTE OF INOCULATION: Unless otherwise specified by the product label or package insert, all vaccines must be administered intramuscularly at one site in the thigh.

D. WILDLIFE VACCINATION: Vaccination of wildlife is not recommended since no rabies vaccine is licensed for use in wild animals. Neither wild nor exotic animals susceptible to rabies should be kept as pets. Offspring of wild animals bred with domestic dogs or cats are considered wild animals.

E. ACCIDENTAL HUMAN EXPOSURE TO VACCINE: Accidental inoculation may occur during administration of animal rabies vaccine. Such exposure to inactivated vaccines constitutes no rabies hazard. No rabies in humans has resulted from needle or other exposure to a licensed modified-live virus vaccine in the United States.

F. IDENTIFICATION OF VACCINATED DOGS: All agencies and veterinarians should adopt the standard tag system. This practice will aid the administration of local, state, national and international procedures. Dog license tags should be distinguishable in shape and color from rabies tags. Anodized aluminum rabies tags should be no less than 0.064 inches in thickness.

1. RABIES TAGS

CALENDAR YEAR	COLOR	SHAPE
1990	Orange	Fireplug
1991	Green	Bell
1992	Red	Heart
1993	Blue	Rosette

2. RABIES CERTIFICATE: All agencies and veterinarians should use the NASPHV Form #50 "Rabies Vaccination Certificate" which can be obtained from vaccine manufacturers. Computer generated forms containing the same information are acceptable.

THE NASPHV COMPENDIUM COMMITTEE
Suzanne R. Jenkins, VMD, MPH, Chair
Keith A. Clark, DVM, PhD
Russell W. Currier, DVM, MPH
Russell J. Martin, DVM, MPH
Grayson B. Miller, Jr., MD
F. T. Satalowich, DVM, MSPH
R. Keith Sikes, DVM, MPH

CONSULTANTS TO THE COMMITTEE
Melvin K. Abelseth, DVM, PhD
George M. Baer, DVM, MPH, Centers for
 Disease Control
David W. Dreesen, DVM, MPVM, AVMA Council on
 Public Health and Regulatory Veterinary Medicine
Robert B. Miller, DVM, MPH, APHIS, USDA
Robert H. Miller, PhD, Veterinary Biologics Section,
 Animal Health Institute
William G. Winkler, DVM, MS

ENDORSED BY:
American Veterinary Medical Association (AVMA)
Council of State and Territorial Epidemiologists (CSTE)

* Address all correspondence to: Suzanne R. Jenkins, VMD, MPH
Virginia Department of Health
Office of Epidemiology
109 Governor Street
Richmond, Virginia 23219

Part II: Vaccines Marketed in U.S. and NASPHV Recommendations

Product Name	Produced By	Marketed By	For Use In[1]	Dosage[2]	Age at Primary Vaccination[3]	Booster Recommended
A) MODIFIED LIVE VIRUS ENDURALL-R	Norden License No. 189	Norden	Dogs	1 ml	3 mos. & 1 yr. later	Triennially
			Cats	1 ml	3 months	Annually
B) INACTIVATED TRIMUNE	Fort Dodge License No. 112	Ft. Dodge	Dogs Cats	1 ml 1 ml	3 mos. & 1 yr. later	Triennially Triennially
ANNUMUNE	Fort Dodge License No. 112	Ft. Dodge	Dogs Cats	1 ml 1 ml	3 months 3 months	Annually Annually
BIORAB-1	Schering License No. 165-A	Biologics Corp.	Dogs Cats	1 ml 1 ml	3 months 3 months	Annually Annually
DURA-RAB 1	ImmunoVet License No. 302-A	ImmunoVet & Vedco, Inc. Fermenta Animal Health	Dogs Cats	1 ml 1 ml	3 months 3 months	Annually Annually
DURA-RAB 3	ImmunoVet License No. 302-A	ImmunoVet & Vedco, Inc. Fermenta Animal Health	Dogs Cats	1 ml 1 ml	3 mos. & 1 yr. later 3 mos. & 1 yr. later	Triennially Triennially
RABCINE 3	ImmunoVet License No. 302-A	Beecham	Dogs Cats	1 ml 1 ml	3 mos. & 1 yr. later 3 mos. & 1 yr. later	Triennially Triennially
RABCINE	Beecham License No. 225	Beecham	Dogs Cats	1 ml 1 ml	3 months 3 months	Annually Annually
ENDURALL-K	Norden License No. 189	Norden	Dogs Cats	1 ml 1 ml	3 months 3 months	Annually Annually
RABGUARD-TC	Norden License No. 189	Norden	Dogs Cats Sheep Cattle Horses	1 ml 1 ml 1 ml 1 ml 1 ml	3 mos. & 1 yr. later 3 months 3 months 3 months	Triennially Triennially Annually Annually Annually
CYTORAB	Coopers Animal Health Inc. License No. 107	Coopers	Dogs Cats	1 ml 1 ml	3 months 3 months	Annually Annually
TRIRAB	Coopers Animal Health Inc. License No. 107	Coopers	Dogs Cats	1 ml 1 ml	3 mos. & 1 yr. later 3 months	Triennially Annually
RABVAC 1	Solvay Animal Health, Inc. License No. 195-A	Solvay Animal Health, Inc.	Dogs Cats	1 ml 1 ml	3 months 3 months	Annually Annually
RABVAC 3	Solvay Animal Health, Inc. License No. 195-A	Solvay Animal Health, Inc.	Dogs Cats Horses	1 ml 1 ml 2 ml	3 months 1 year later 3 months	Triennially Triennially Annually
IMRAB	Rhone Merieux, Inc. License No. 298	Pitman-Moore	Dogs Cats Sheep Cattle Horses	1 ml 1 ml 2 ml 2 ml 2 ml	3 months & 1 year later 3 months & 1 year later 3 months & 1 year later 3 months 3 months	Triennially Triennially Triennially Annually Annually
IMRAB-1	Rhone Merieux, Inc. License No. 298	Pitman-Moore	Dogs Cats	1 ml 1 ml	3 months 3 months	Annually Annually
EPIRAB	Coopers Animal Health Inc. License No. 107	Coopers	Dogs Cats	1 ml 1 ml	3 months & 1 year later 3 months & 1 year later	Triennially Triennially
C) COMBINATION ECLIPSE 3 KP-R	Solvay Animal Health, Inc. License No. 195-A	Solvay Animal Health, Inc.	Cats	1 ml	3 months	Annually
ECLIPSE 4 KP-R	Solvay Animal Health, Inc. License No. 195-A	Solvay Animal Health, Inc.	Cats	1 ml	3 months	Annually
CYTORAB RCP	Coopers Animal Health Inc. License No. 107	Coopers	Cats	1 ml	3 months	Annually
FEL-O-VAX PCT-R	Fort Dodge License No. 112	Fort Dodge	Cats	1 ml	3 months & 1 year later	Triennially
ECLIPSE 4-R	Solvay Animal Health, Inc. License No. 195-A	Solvay Animal Health, Inc.	Cats	1 ml	3 months	Annually

[1]Refers only to domestic species of this class of animals.
[2]All vaccines must be administered <u>intramuscularly</u> at one site in the thigh unless otherwise specified by the label.
[3]Three months of age (or older) and revaccinated one year later.

Continued on following page

Compendium of Animal Rabies Control, 1990 Continued

Part III: Rabies Control

A. PRINCIPLES OF RABIES CONTROL

1. HUMAN RABIES PREVENTION: Rabies in humans can be prevented either by eliminating exposures to rabid animals or by providing exposed persons with prompt local treatment of wounds combined with appropriate passive and active immunization. The rationale for recommending preexposure and postexposure rabies prophylaxis and details of their administration can be found in the current recommendations of the Immunization Practices Advisory Committee (ACIP), of the Public Health Service (PHS). These recommendations, along with information concerning the current local and regional status of animal rabies and the availability of human rabies biologics, are available from state health departments.

2. DOMESTIC ANIMALS: Local governments should initiate and maintain effective programs to remove strays and unwanted animals and to ensure vaccination of all dogs and cats. Such procedures in the United States have reduced laboratory confirmed rabies cases in dogs from 6,949 in 1947 to 128 in 1988. Since more rabies cases are reported annually among cats than among dogs, immunization of cats should be required. The recommended vaccination procedures and the licensed animal vaccines are specified in Parts I and II of this NASPHV Compendium.

3. RABIES IN WILDLIFE: The control of rabies among foxes, skunks, raccoons, and other terrestrial animals is difficult. Selective reduction of these populations may be useful when indicated, but the success of this procedure depends heavily on the circumstances surrounding each rabies outbreak. (See C. Control Methods in Wild Animals.)

B. CONTROL METHODS IN DOMESTIC AND CONFINED ANIMALS

1. PREEXPOSURE VACCINATION AND MANAGEMENT
Animal rabies vaccines should be administered only by or under the direct supervision of a veterinarian. This is the only way to assure the public that the animal has been properly immunized. Within 1 month after primary vaccination, a peak rabies antibody titer is reached and the animal can be considered to be immunized. (See Parts I and II for recommended vaccines and procedures.)

(a) DOGS AND CATS
All dogs and cats should be vaccinated against rabies at 3 months of age and revaccinated in accordance with Part II of this Compendium.

(b) LIVESTOCK
It is neither economically feasible nor justified from a public health standpoint to vaccinate all livestock against rabies. However, consideration should be given to the vaccination of livestock located in areas where wildlife rabies is epizootic, especially animals which are valuable and/or may have frequent contact with humans. (See Part II for recommended vaccines.)

(c) OTHER ANIMALS
(1) ANIMALS MAINTAINED IN EXHIBITS AND IN ZOOLOGICAL PARKS
There is no rabies vaccine licensed for use in wild animals. Captive animals not completely excluded from all contact with local rabies vectors can become infected. Moreover, such animals may be incubating rabies when captured. Exhibit animals susceptible to rabies should be quarantined for a minimum of 180 days. Animal workers at such facilities should receive preexposure rabies immunization. This practice may reduce the need for euthanasia of valuable animals for rabies testing after they have bitten a handler.

(2) WILD OR EXOTIC ANIMALS
Because of the risk of rabies in wild animals (especially raccoons, skunks and foxes), the AVMA, the NASPHV, and the CSTE strongly recommend the enactment of state laws prohibiting the importation, distribution, relocation, or keeping of wild animals and wild animals crossbred to domestic dogs and cats as pets. Because the period of rabies virus shedding in infected wild or exotic animals (including ferrets) is unknown, confinement and observation of those animals that bite humans are not appropriate.

2. STRAY ANIMALS
Stray dogs or cats should be removed from the community, especially in areas where rabies is epizootic. Local health departments and animal control officials can enforce the pick up of strays more efficiently if owned animals are confined or kept on leash. Strays should be impounded for at least 3 days to give owners sufficient time to reclaim animals and to determine if human exposure has occured.

3. QUARANTINE
(a) INTERNATIONAL. Present PHS regulations (42 CFR No. 71.51) governing the importation of dogs and cats are insufficient to prevent the introduction of rabid animals into the United States. All dogs and cats imported from countries with enzootic rabies should be vaccinated against rabies at least 30 days prior to entry into the United States. CDC regulates the importation of these animals into the United States. The public health official of the state of destination should be notified within 72 hours of any animal conditionally admitted into his jurisdiction. The conditional admission into the United States of such animals is subject to state and local laws governing rabies. Failure to comply with these requirements should be promptly reported to the director of the respective quarantine center.

(b) INTERSTATE. Dogs and cats should be vaccinated against rabies according to the Compendium's recommendations at least 30 days prior to interstate movement. While in transit they should be accompanied by a currently valid NASPHV Form #50, Rabies Vaccination Certificate.

4. ADJUNCT PROCEDURES
Methods or procedures which enhance rabies control include:

(a) LICENSURE. Registration or licensure of all dogs and cats may be used to control rabies by reducing the stray animal population. A fee is frequently charged for such licensure and revenues collected are used to maintain rabies or animal control programs. Vaccination is an essential prerequisite to licensure.

(b) CANVASSING OF AREA. House-to-house canvassing by animal control personnel enforces vaccination and licensure requirements.

(c) CITATIONS. Citations are legal summonses issued to owners for violations, including the failure to vaccinate or license their animals. The authority for officers to issue citations should be an integral part of each animal control program.

(d) LEASH LAWS. All communities should adopt leash laws that can be incorporated in their animal control ordinances.

5. POSTEXPOSURE MANAGEMENT
ANY ANIMAL BITTEN OR SCRATCHED BY A WILD, CARNIVOROUS MAMMAL (OR A BAT) NOT AVAILABLE FOR TESTING SHOULD BE REGARDED AS HAVING BEEN EXPOSED TO RABIES.

(a) DOGS AND CATS. Unvaccinated dogs and cats bitten by a rabid animal should be euthanized immediately. If the owner is unwilling to have this done, the animal should be placed in strict isolation for 6 months and vaccinated 1 month before being released. Dogs and cats that are currently vaccinated should be revaccinated immediately and confined and observed for 90 days.

(b) LIVESTOCK. All species of livestock are susceptible to rabies; cattle and horses are among the most susceptible of all domestic animals. Livestock bitten by a rabid animal and currently vaccinated with a vaccine approved by USDA for that species should be revaccinated immediately and observed for 90 days. Unvaccinated livestock should be destroyed (slaughtered) immediately. If the owner is unwilling to have this done, the animal should be kept under very close observation for 6 months.

The following are recommendations for owners of unvaccinated livestock exposed to rabid animals:

(1) If the animal is slaughtered within 7 days of being bitten, its tissues may be eaten without risk of infection, provided liberal portions of the exposed area are discarded. Federal meat inspectors will reject for slaughter any animal known to have been exposed to rabies within 8 months.

(2) Neither tissues nor milk from a rabid animal should be used for human or animal consumption. However, since pasteurization temperatures will inactivate rabies virus, drinking pasteurized milk or eating cooked meat does not constitute a rabies exposure.

(c) WILD OR EXOTIC ANIMALS. Wild or exotic animals bitten by a rabid animal should be euthanized immediately. Such animals currently vaccinated with a vaccine approved by USDA for that species may be revaccinated immediately and placed in strict isolation for at least 90 days.

6. MANAGEMENT OF ANIMALS THAT BITE HUMANS
A healthy dog or cat that bites a person should be confined and observed for 10 days and evaluated by a veterinarian at the first sign of illness during confinement. Any illness in the animal should be reported immediately to the local health department. If signs suggestive of rabies develop, the animal should be humanely killed, and its head removed and shipped under refrigeration for examination by a qualified laboratory designated by the local or state health department. Any stray or unwanted dog or cat that bites a person may be killed immediately and the head submitted as described above for rabies examination.

C. CONTROL METHODS IN WILD ANIMALS

The public should be warned not to handle wild animals. Wild carnivorous mammals and bats (as well as the offspring of wild animals crossbred with domestic dogs and cats) that bite people should be killed and the brain submitted to the laboratory for rabies examination. A person bitten by any wild animal should immediately report the incident to a physician who can evaluate the need for antirabies treatment. (See current rabies prophylaxis recommendations of the ACIP)

1. TERRESTRIAL MAMMALS
Continuous and persistent government-funded programs for trapping or poisoning wildlife are not cost effective in reducing wildlife rabies reservoirs on a statewide basis. However, limited control in high-contact areas (picnic grounds, camps, suburban areas) may be indicated for the removal of selected high-risk species of wild animals. The state wildlife agency should be consulted early to manage any elimination programs in coordination with the state health department.

2. BATS
(a) Rabid bats have been reported from every state except Alaska and Hawaii, and have caused rabies in humans in the United States. It is neither feasible nor desirable, however, to control rabies in bats by areawide programs to reduce bat populations.

(b) Bats should be excluded from houses and surrounding structures to prevent direct association with humans. Such structures should then be made bat proof by sealing entrances.

APPENDIX 7. Health and Vaccination Requirements for Interstate and International Shipment of Dogs and Cats

STATE OR COUNTRY	HEALTH CERTIFICATE		RABIES VACCINATION		MINIMUM AGE (Months)	VACCINATION	
	Canine	Feline	Canine	Feline		Type	Timing
Alabama	+	+	+	+	>3	AL	Less than 1 year prior to entry
Alaska	+	+	+	+		AL	As per the Compendium of Animal Rabies Vaccines[b]
Arizona	−	−	+	−	4	AL	Vaccination is current
Arkansas	+	+	+	+	>3	AL	Less than 1 year prior to entry
California	c	c	+	−	>4	AL	
Colorado	+[d]	+[d]	+	+	>3	AL	Less than 1 year prior to entry
Connecticut	+	−	+	−		AL	Between 21 days and 6 months prior to entry
Delaware	+	+	+	−	>4	AL	
Florida	+	−	+	−		AL	Less than 6 months prior to entry
Georgia	−	−	+	−		AL	As per the Compendium of Animal Rabies Vaccines[b]
Guam[e]	−	−	−	−			
Hawaii[f]	+	+	+	+		MLV	Within 4 months of entry
Idaho	+	+	+	+	≥3	AL	As per the Compendium of Animal Rabies Vaccines[b]
Illinois	+	−	+	−	>4	AL	As per the Compendium of Animal Rabies Vaccines[b]
Indiana	?	?	+	+	>3	AL	Within 1 year of entry
Iowa	+	+	+	+	>4	AL	Within 1 year of entry
Kansas	+	+	+	+	≥3	AL	
Kentucky	+	+	+	+	>4	I, MLV	I within 1 year, MLV within 2 years, Cat: within 1 year
Louisiana	+	−	+	−	>2	CE, NT	Dog: CE within 2 years, NT within 1 year
Maine[g]	+	+	+	+	≥6	AL	Within 10 days of entry
Maryland	+	−	+	−	>4	AL	Within 1 year of entry
Massachusetts	+	−	+	−		AL	Within 1 year of entry
Michigan	−	−	+	−	>6	AL	
Minnesota	+	−	+	−	>3	AL	Within 1 year of entry
Mississippi	+	−	+	+	>3	AL	Within 6 months of entry
Missouri	+	−	+	−	>4	AL	As per the Compendium of Animal Rabies Vaccines[b]
Montana	+	+	+	+	>3	AL	As per the Compendium of Animal Rabies Vaccines[b]
Nebraska	+	+	+	+		AL	Within 1 month of entry
Nevada	+	+	+	+	>3	AL	As per the Compendium of Animal Rabies Vaccines[b]

APPENDIX 7. Health and Vaccination Requirements for Interstate and International Shipment of Dogs and Cats Continued

STATE OR COUNTRY	HEALTH CERTIFICATE		RABIES VACCINATION		MINIMUM AGE (Months)	VACCINATION	
	Canine	Feline	Canine	Feline		Type	Timing*
New Hampshire[h]	+	+	+	+	>3	AL	Between 7 days and 1 year of entry, pups <3 months of age should be vaccinated within 30 days of entry
New Jersey	+	−	−	−			
New Mexico	+	+	+	+	≥3	AL	Within 1 year of entry
New York	+						
North Carolina[i]							
North Dakota	+	+	+	+	>3	AL	
Ohio	+	−	+	−	>6	AL	Dependent on the type
Oklahoma	+	−	+	−		AL	Within 1 year of entry
Oregon	+	+	+	+	>4	AL	
Pennsylvania	+	−	+	−	>3	AL	Dependent on the type
Puerto Rico	−	−	+	+	>2	AL	
Rhode Island	+	−	+		>4	I, MLV	I between 1 and 6 months, MLV within 2 or 3 years
South Carolina	+	+	+	+		AL	Within 1 year of entry
South Dakota	+	+	+	+	>3	AL	Within 1 year of entry
Tennessee	+	+	+	+	>3 (D), >6 (C)	AL	Within 1 year of entry
Texas[j]							
Utah	+	+	+	+	>4	I, MLV	I within 1 year, MLV within 2 years
Vermont	+	+	+	+	>6	Tri	Within 1 year of entry
Virgin Islands	+	+	+	+	>2	AL	Within 6 months of entry
Virginia	+	+	+	+	>4	I, MLV	I within 1 year, MLV within 3 years
Washington	+	+	+	+		AL	Dependent on type
West Virginia	+	+	+	+	>5	AL	Within 1 year of entry
Wisconsin	+	−	+	−	6	AL	Dependent on type
Wyoming	+	+	+	+	≥3	AL	As per the Compendium of Animal Rabies Vaccines[b]
Afghanistan	+	+	+	+			Within 30 days prior to entry
Albania	+	+					
Algeria	+	+	+	+			Within 3 months prior to entry
Angola	+	+	+	+			Within 4 months prior to entry
Argentina[k,l]	+	+	+	+			Within 10 days prior to departure
Aruba[m]	+	+	+	+			
Australia[n]							
Austria[o]	+	+	+	+			Within 1 month to 1 year prior to entry
Bahamas[p]	+	+	+	+	>6		Within 10 days to 9 months prior to entry
Bahrain[q]	+	+	+	+			
Bangladesh	+	+					
Barbados[q,r]	+	+					
Belgium	+	+	+	+			Within 1 month prior to entry

*For countries for which no type or timing of vaccine is indicated, check with the embassy or consulate of the country of destination.

Continued on following page

STATE OR COUNTRY	HEALTH CERTIFICATE		RABIES VACCINATION		MINIMUM AGE (Months)	VACCINATION	
	Canine	Feline	Canine	Feline		Type	Timing*
Belize	+	+	+	+			Within 30 days prior to entry
Benin	+	+	+	+			Within 30 days prior to entry
Bermuda[s,t]	+	+	+	+	>4		Within 1 month to 1 year prior to entry
Bolivia[k]	+	+	+	+			
Botswana[u]							
Brazil[k]	+	+	+	+			
Brunei[m]	+	+	+	+			
Bulgaria	+	+	+	+			Dog: within 1 month to 1 year prior to entry
							Cats: within 1 to 6 months prior to entry
Burkina Faso[v]	+	+	+	+			Within 3 weeks to 6 months prior to entry
Burma (Myanmar)	+	+					
Burundi[w,x]	+	+	+	+			Depending on type
Cameroon	+	+	+	+			Within 48 hours of departure
Canada[y]	+	+	+	+			
Canary Islands (see Spain)							
Cape Verde	+	+	+	+			
Cayman Islands[k,z,aa]	+	+	+	+	2		
Central African Republic[v]	+	+	+	+			Within 2 weeks to 6 months of entry
Chad	+	+	+	+			
Chile[k]	+	+	+	−			More than 1 month prior to arrival
China	+	+	+	+	2		Within 4 months prior to entry
Colombia[k,bb]	+	+	+	+			Within 15 days to 3 years prior to entry
Congo	+	+	+	+			Within 3 weeks to 6 months prior to entry
Cook Island[cc]							
Corsica (see France)							
Costa Rica[k,m,bb,dd]	+	+	+	+			
Cuba[k]	+	+	+	−			
Cyprus	+	+	+	+			
Czechoslovakia[v,ee]	+	+	+	+			
Denmark[t,v]	+	+	+	+	>3		Within 1 month to 1 year prior to entry
Djibouti	+	+	+	+	>6		Within 1 month to 1 year prior to entry
Ecuador[k]	+	+	+	−			Within 2 weeks prior to entry
Egypt[z]	+	+					
El Salvador[k]	+	+	+	+			Within 3 months prior to entry
Equatorial Guinea			+	+			
Ethiopia	+	+					
Faeroe Islands[ff]							
Fiji[gg]							
Finland[hh]	+	+					
France[ii]	+	+	+	+	>3		Within 1 month to 1 year prior to entry

*For countries for which no type or timing of vaccine is indicated, check with the embassy or consulate of the country of destination.

APPENDIX 7. Health and Vaccination Requirements for Interstate and International Shipment of Dogs and Cats Continued

STATE OR COUNTRY	HEALTH CERTIFICATE		RABIES VACCINATION		MINIMUM AGE (Months)	VACCINATION	
	Canine	Feline	Canine	Feline		Type	Timing*
French Guinea (see France)							
French Polynesia[ff]							
French West Indies (see France)							
Gabon	+	+	+	+	>3		Within 3 days prior to departure
Gambia	+	+					
Democratic[jj] Republic of Germany (East)	+	+	+	+			Within 1 to 12 months prior to entry
Federal Republic[v] of Germany (West)	+	+					
Ghana	+	+	+	+			Within 1 month prior to entry
Gibraltar[kk]	+	+	+	+			Within 28 days of entry
Greece	+	+	+	+			Dog: within 6 days to 1 year prior to entry Cat: within 6 days to 6 months prior to entry
Greenland[ll]							
Grenada	+	+					
Guadeloupe (see French West Indies)							
Guatemala[k]	+	+					
Republic of Guinea	+	+	+	+			
Guinea-Bissau	+	+	+	+			Within 1 month of entry
Guyana[m]							
Haiti	+	+	+	+			Within 60 days of entry
Honduras[k,mm]	+	+	+	−			Within 60 days of entry
Hong Kong[z]	+	+					
Hungary[z,nn]	+	+	+	+			
Iceland[oo]							
India[pp]	+	+	+	+		NT CE	NT: 1 month to 1 year prior to entry CE: 1 month to 3 years prior to entry
Indonesia[ii]	+	+	+	+			
Iran[qq]							
Iraq	+	+	+	+			
Ireland[v]							
Israel	+	+	+	+			Within 1 month to 1 year prior to entry
Italy[rr]	+	+	+	+			Within 20 days to 11 months prior to entry
Ivory Coast	+	+	+	+			Within 3 days of departure
Jamaica[ss]							
Japan[s]	+	−	+	−			Within 1 month to 1 year prior to entry
Jordan	+	+	+	+			Within 1 month prior to entry
Kenya	+	+	+	+			Within 5 days of departure
Kiribati[tt]							
Korea (South)[m]	+	+	+	+			
Kuwait[uu]	+	+	+	+			Within 1 month to 1 year prior to entry
Laos	+	+	+	+			Within 1 month prior to entry

*For countries for which no type or timing of vaccine is indicated, check with the embassy or consulate of the country of destination.

Continued on following page

APPENDIX 7. Health and Vaccination Requirements for Interstate and International Shipment of Dogs and Cats Continued

STATE OR COUNTRY	HEALTH CERTIFICATE		RABIES VACCINATION		MINIMUM AGE (Months)	VACCINATION	
	Canine	Feline	Canine	Feline		Type	Timing*
Lebanon	+	+					
Leeward Islands	+	+	+	+			
Lesotho[vv]							
Liberia[k]	+	+	+	+			
Libya	+	+	+	+			
Luxembourg (See Belgium)							
Macao[nn]	+	+	+	+			
Madagascar[x]	+	+	+	+	D: >3 C: >6		Within 1 month to 1 year prior to entry
Malawi[m]	+	+	+	+			
Malaysia[mm]	+	+					
Maldive Islands[ww]							
Malta[ff]							
Martinique (see French West Indies)							
Mauritania[xx]	+	+	+	+	>3		
Mauritius[yy]	+	+	+	+			
Mexico[k,l]	+	+	+	+			
Monaco[zz]	+	+	+	+			Within 1 to 6 months prior to entry
Morocco[k,l]	+	+	+	+			
Mozambique	+	+	+	+	>6		Within 6 months prior to entry
Nauru[Al]							
Nepal	+	+	+	+			
Netherlands (see Belgium)							
Netherlands Antilles[s]	+	+	+	−			Within 30 days prior to entry
New Zealand[B1]							
Nicaragua[k]	+	+	+	+			Within 60 days prior to entry
Niger[ee]	+	+					
Nigeria[C1]	+	+	+	+			
Norway[D1]	+	+					
Oman[E1]	+	+		+			Within 1 month prior to entry
Pakistan	+	+	+	+			
Panama[nn]	+	+	+	+			Within 1 to 16 months prior to entry
Papua New Guinea[F1]							
Paraguay	+	+					
Peru[k]	+	+					
Philippines[k]	+	+	+	+			
Poland[G1]	+	+					
Portugal[k]	+	+	+	+			D: within 1 year prior to entry C: within 6 months prior to entry
Qatar	+	+					
Reunion (see France)							
Romania	+	+	+	+			D: within 1 month to 1 year prior to entry C: within 1 to 6 months prior to entry
Rwanda[H1]	+	+	+	+			Within 15 days prior to entry
Santa Lucia[v]							
Saint Martin (see Netherlands Antilles)							
Samoa (American)[ff]							
Sao Tome and Principe	+	+	+	+			

*For countries for which no type or timing of vaccine is indicated, check with the embassy or consulate of the country of destination.

STATE OR COUNTRY	HEALTH CERTIFICATE		RABIES VACCINATION		MINIMUM AGE (Months)	VACCINATION	
	Canine	Feline	Canine	Feline		Type	Timing*
Saudi Arabia[l1]		+		+			Within 1 month to 1 year prior to entry
Senegal[j1]	+	+	+	+			Within 1 to 6 months prior to entry
Seychelles[m]							
Sierra Leone[K1]	+	+	+	+			
Singapore[r]	+	+					
Somalia	+	+					
South Africa	+	+	+	+			Within 2 months to 1 year prior to entry
Spain[k]	+	+	+	+			
Sri Lanka	+	+					
Sudan	+	+	+	+			
Surinam	+	+	+	+			Within 1 month prior to entry
Swaziland[L1]							
Sweden[M1]							
Switzerland	+	+	+	+			Within 20 days prior to entry
Syria	+	+					
Taiwan[m]	+	+	+	−			
Tanzania[N1]	+	+	+	−			
Thailand	+	+	+	+			
Tonga[ff]							
Trinidad and Tobago[N1]	+	+	+	+			Within 30 days prior to entry
Tunisia	+	+	+	+			Within 1 to 6 months prior to entry
Turkey[k,l]	+	+	+	+			
Tuvalu	+	+	+	+			
Uganda[O1]	+	+					
United Arab Emirates	+	+					
United Kingdom[m]							
United States (Also see state listing above)			+	+		NT	NT: within 1 to 12 months prior to entry
						CE	CE: within 1 month to 3 years prior to entry
Uruguay[l]	+	+	+	+			Within 1 month to 1 year prior to entry
USSR[s]	+	+					
Vanuatu[P1]							
Venezuela[l]	+	+	+	+			
Western Samoa[Q1]							
Yemen	+	+					
Yugoslavia[x]	+	+					
Zaire[x]	+	+	+	+		Kelev	Within 1 month to 1 year prior to entry
						Flury	Within 1 month to 3 years prior to entry
Zambia	+	+	+	+			
Zimbabwe[R1]							

[a]+ = required, − = not required, D = dog, C = cat, AL = any licensed vaccine type, I = inactivated vaccine, MLV = modified live virus vaccine, CE = chicken embryo, NT = inactivated nerve tissue, Tri = triennial, ? = Check with state health department, embassy, or consulate of the specific state or country. Data compiled from APHIS: State and Federal Health Requirements and Regulations Governing the Interstate and International Movement of Livestock and Poultry, Washington, DC, US Department of Agriculture, Animal and Plant Health Inspection Service, on-line computer listing 1989; Canadian Travel Information, 1982/1983, Canadian Government Office of Tourism, Ottawa, Ontario, under authority of Minister of Industry, Trade, and Commerce; and "Traveling with Your Pet," American Society for the Prevention of Cruelty to Animals, New York, NY 10128. These requirements should be used as guidelines. Because regulations are subject to change without notice, for any additional vaccinations or requirements that may be needed, the reader is advised to contact the state health department, embassy, or consulate of the destination well in advance of planned travel. Accredited veterinarians within the United States can call The Voice Response Service, US Dept of Agriculture at (800) 234–8732 for additional information.

[b]See Appendix 6.

[c]Health certificate recommended.

[d]Certificate stating that animal is free from exposure to rabies and if over 3 months of age that the animal has been immunized for rabies within the previous 12 months.

*For countries for which no type or timing of vaccine is indicated, check with the embassy or consulate of the country of destination.

Footnotes continued on following page

^e*Importation* requires only 120-day quarantine.

^f*Importation* requires only 120-day quarantine if animal from rabies-endemic area. If animal is from certified rabies-free area, health certificate and current rabies vaccination is all that is required.

^gAll animals must be vaccinated for distemper between 7 and 30 days of entry into the state.

^hAll animals must be vaccinated for the common viral diseases between 7 days and 1 year of entry into the state.

ⁱContact: North Carolina Department of Health, P.O. Box 209, Raleigh, NC 27611, (919) 733-3410.

^jContact: Texas Department of Health, 1100 West 49th Street, Austin, TX 78756, (512) 458-7111.

^kHealth certificate must be legalized (fee) by that country's Consulate.

^lHealth certificate must be validated by USDA veterinarian.

^mAnimals subject to quarantine period.

ⁿContact Australian Quarantine Service, c/o Dept. of Primary Industry, Canberra, A.C. T 2600, Australia.

^oDocumentation must be translated in German.

^pHealth certificates must be issued within 24 hours prior to departure.

^qDogs and cats from the United Kingdom require certificates from the Ministry of Agriculture and Fisheries that animal is rabies free.

^rHealth certificate must be issued within 7 days of departure.

^sHealth certificate must be issued within 10 days of departure.

^tAnimals from United Kingdom and other rabies-free areas need no health certificate.

^uContact Director of Veterinary Services, Private Bag 003, Gaborone, Botswana.

^vHealth certificate must state that animal is from a rabies-free area.

^wHealth certificate must state that animal is free from ticks.

^xHealth certificate must be issued within 15 days of departure.

^yAnimals from United States must be vaccinated within 3 years of entry. Animals from rabies-free countries are not required to have rabies inoculation. Animals from other countries must have rabies inoculation within 1 month to 1 year prior to entry.

^zHealth certificate must be issued within 2 weeks prior to entry.

^{aa}Animals must also be vaccinated against distemper, hepatitis, leptospirosis, and parvovirus infection.

^{bb}Animals must also be vaccinated against distemper and hepatitis.

^{cc}For more information, contact Ministry of Agriculture, PO Box 96, Rarotunga, Cook Island.

^{dd}Dogs and cats must also have *Taenia echinococcus* vaccination certification.

^{ee}Health certificate must be issued within 3 days prior to departure and state that other contagious diseases have not occurred in the area of origin.

^{ff}Import of pets is prohibited.

^{gg}Dogs and cats from New Zealand and Australia only.

^{hh}Dogs and cats must be vaccinated against distemper and be free from worms.

ⁱⁱHealth certificate must be issued within 5 days prior to entry.

^{jj}Visits limited to 28 days.

^{kk}Restricted to residents of Europe.

^{ll}Contact the Danish Embassy or Consulate.

^{mm}Health certificates must be dated within 10 days of departure. Animals from rabies-free areas need notarized statement that they were residents of that area for at least 120 days prior to departure.

ⁿⁿDogs must also be vaccinated against hepatitis.

^{oo}Animals must also be inoculated against distemper.

^{pp}Dogs are prohibited. For permission to import cats, contact Chief Veterinarian, Yfirdralaeknir, Reykjavik, Iceland.

^{qq}Dogs must be certified free from distemper, Aujesky's disease, leishmaniasis, and leptospirosis. Cats must be certified free from panleukopenia.

^{rr}For information, contact Algerian Embassy.

^{ss}Health certificates are valid for 30 days.

^{tt}Dogs (other than Seeing Eye dogs) and cats are subject to a 3- to 6-month quarantine. Seeing Eye dogs must have a health certificate and must have been inoculated against rabies at least 6 months prior to departure.

^{uu}Health certificates must be issued within 10 days of departure.

^{vv}For information contact Chief Agricultural Officer, PO Box 267, Bikenibeau, Tarawa.

^{ww}Health certificate must be obtained within 1 month of departure.

^{xx}Contact the Lesotho Embassy.

^{yy}Contact the Ministry of External Affairs for information.

^{zz}Cats must be vaccinated against typhus.

^{A1}Health certificate must be issued within 3 weeks prior to arrival. Animals must be vaccinated against distemper, hard pad, infectious hepatitis, and leptospirosis.

^{B1}Health certificates must be issued within 3 days of departure.

^{C1}Contact the Republic of Nauru.

^{D1}Health certificates must be issued at least 10 days prior to departure.

^{E1}Contact Director General, Ministry of Agriculture and Fisheries, Animal Health Division, PO Box 2298, Wellington, New Zealand.

^{F1}Contact embassy prior to departure, since regulations are subject to change.

^{G1}Health certificate must document that animal is free from leptospirosis. Animals are subject to a 4-month quarantine at the owner's expense.

^{H1}Dogs must also be vaccinated against distemper, leptospirosis, hepatitis, and typhus. Cats must also be vaccinated against feline enteritis, panleukopenia, and hepatitis.

^{I1}Contact Chief Quarantine Officer (Animals), Dept. of Agriculture, Stock and Fisheries, Port Moresby, Papua New Guinea.

^{J1}Health certificates for dogs must be obtained 1 month to 1 year prior to entry and those for cats must be obtained 1 to 6 months prior to entry.

^{K1}Dogs must be vaccinated with Flury Low Egg Passage rabies vaccines and cats must be vaccinated with Flury High Egg Passage rabies vaccines.

^{L1}Only watch, hunting, Seeing Eye, and Hearing Ear dogs are permitted and must have health certificates.

^{M1}Health certificates must be issued within 48 hours of departure.

^{N1}Dogs must also be vaccinated against distemper, hard pad, infectious canine hepatitis, and leptospirosis. Cats must also be vaccinated against feline panleukopenia.

^{O1}Contact Secretary, Ministry of Agriculture and Cooperatives, PO Box 162, Mbabane, Swaziland.

^{P1}Contact National Board of Agriculture, Director of Contagious Animal Diseases, S-551 83 Jonkoping.

^{Q1}Dogs must also be vaccinated against distemper, hepatitis, and parvoviral enteritis.

^{R1}Health certificate must be issued within 6 days prior to departure.

^{S1}Contact Chef d'Elevage at Por Vila.

^{T1}Contact Director of Agriculture, Apia, Western Samoa.

^{U1}Contact Director of Veterinary Services, PO Box 8012, Causeway, Zimbabwe.

APPENDIX 8. Laboratory Testing
for Confirmation of Infectious Diseases[a]

INFECTIOUS DISEASE	SAMPLE (AMOUNT OR HANDLING)	TYPE OF TEST (LABORATORY[b] OR TEST KIT[c])	INTERPRETATION
	Viral and Rickettsial Infections (see Chapter 14)		

Canine Distemper (see Chapter 16)

INFECTIOUS DISEASE	SAMPLE (AMOUNT OR HANDLING)	TYPE OF TEST (LABORATORY[b] OR TEST KIT[c])	INTERPRETATION
Antemortem	Blood or buffy coat smear, conjunctival scraping, CSF, transtracheal wash (cytologic smears are air dried and refrigerated, alcohol- or acetone-fixed)	Ag: DFA (many) Ag: ELISA (research)	Positive result confirms infection with proper technique; false-negatives possible in chronic (CNS) infections; false-positives due to lab technique
	Serum: paired sample taken 10–14 days apart (2–3 ml, refrigerated)	Ab: VN (many) Ab: IFA (many) Ab: ELISA (research, 25)	Paired samples: rising (4-fold) titer confirms active infection; > 1:100 single VN titer indicates relative immune protection against disease
	CSF (1–3 ml, refrigerated)	Ab: VN (25, 39) Ab: IFA (research) Ab: ELISA (research, 25)	Positive titer confirms CNS infection if serum contamination is excluded or if CSF titer is high relative to serum titer; some inconsistencies have been noted
Postmortem	Lung, bladder, cerebellum (refrigerated)	Ag: DFA (many) Ag: VI (many)	Positive result confirms infection
	Lung, bladder, brain, liver, stomach (formalin-fixed)	Histol (many)	Inclusion body detection with compatible histologic changes indicates infection; some false-positive and false-negative results

Infectious Canine Hepatitis (see Chapter 17)

INFECTIOUS DISEASE	SAMPLE (AMOUNT OR HANDLING)	TYPE OF TEST (LABORATORY[b] OR TEST KIT[c])	INTERPRETATION
Antemortem	Oropharyngeal swabs, urine, feces (refrigerated)	Ag: VI (many) Ag: EM (6)	Positive result confirms infection
	Serum: paired samples taken 10–14 days apart (2–3 ml, refrigerated)	Ab: VN (many)	Paired samples: rising (4-fold) titer confirms active infection
Postmortem	Liver (fresh impression smear)	Cytol (many)	Presence of intranuclear inclusions supportive of diagnosis
	Spleen, liver, brain (refrigerated)	Ag: DFA (9, 21)	Positive result confirms infection
	Liver, gallbladder, kidney, lung, stomach, brain (formalin-fixed)	Histol (many)	Compatible histologic changes indicate infection

Canine Herpesvirus Infection (see Chapter 18)

INFECTIOUS DISEASE	SAMPLE (AMOUNT OR HANDLING)	TYPE OF TEST (LABORATORY[b] OR TEST KIT[c])	INTERPRETATION
Antemortem	Nasal swab, vaginal swab (refrigerated)	Ag: VI, DFA (many) Ag: EM (16)	Positive result confirms infection
	Serum: paired samples taken 10–14 days apart (2–3 ml, refrigerated)	Ab: VN (35, 39) Ab: IFA (29)	Paired samples: rising (4-fold) titer confirms active infection; single titer interpretation only determines prior exposure
Postmortem	Neonates—lung, liver, kidney, CNS (refrigerated)	Ag: VI (many) Ag: FA (9)	Positive result confirms infection

Canine Parainfluenza Infection (see Chapters 19 and 20)

INFECTIOUS DISEASE	SAMPLE (AMOUNT OR HANDLING)	TYPE OF TEST (LABORATORY[b] OR TEST KIT[c])	INTERPRETATION
	Transtracheal washing, oropharyngeal swab, CSF (refrigerated)	Ag: VI (many)	Positive result confirms infection
	Serum or CSF (2–3 ml, refrigerated)	Ab: VN (34, 39) Ag: IFA (34)	Paired serum samples: rising (4-fold) titer confirms active infection; CSF-positive titer confirms infection

Continued on following page

APPENDIX 8. *Laboratory Testing*
for Confirmation of Infectious Diseases[a] Continued

INFECTIOUS DISEASE	SAMPLE (AMOUNT OR HANDLING)	TYPE OF TEST (LABORATORY[b] OR TEST KIT[c])	INTERPRETATION
Canine Viral Enteritis (see Chapter 21)			
PARVOVIRUS			
Antemortem	Serum: paired samples taken 10–14 days apart (2–3 ml, refrigerated)	Ab: HA-I (many) Ab: VN (many) Ab: IFA (many) Ab: ELISA (Kit 1)	Positive titers (level varies with lab) indicate protection; paired samples: rising (4-fold) titer confirms active infection; IgG titer usually increased by the time clinical signs are observed, so high serum IgM titer or fecal Ag examination is more diagnostic of active infection
	Feces (refrigerated)	Ag: HA (many) Ag: EM (many) Ag: DFA (many) Ag: ELISA (Kit 2)	Positive result confirms infection; clinical disease associated with shedding of *large* quantities of virus; some shedders are nonsymptomatic; false-negatives after 4–7 days of clinical illness
Postmortem	Small intestine, heart—neonate (refrigerated)	Ag: DFA (many) Ag: VI (many)	Positive result confirms infection
	Intestine (formalin-fixed)	Histol	Postive result indicates infection
CORONAVIRUS			
Antemortem	Serum: paired samples taken 10–14 days apart (2–3 ml, refrigerated)	Ab: IFA (many, Kit 2a)	Single high IgG titer indicates exposure only; serum titer does not reflect degree of protection against infection. Paired samples: rising (4-fold) IgG titer confirms infection
	Feces (refrigerated)	Ag: VI (9) Ag: EM (6, 21, 35)	Positive result showing high particle numbers confirms infection; some shedders are nonsymptomatic carriers
Postmortem	Intestine (refrigerated)	Ag: DFA (many, 20, 21)	Positive result confirms infection
	Intestine (formalin-fixed)	Histol	Positive result suggests infection
ROTAVIRUS (see also Chapter 21)			
Antemortem	Serum (2–3 ml, refrigerated)	Ab: ELISA (38) Ab: IFA (38)	Paired samples: rising (4-fold) titer confirms active infection
	Feces (fresh, refrigerated)	Ag: EM (35) Ag: ELISA (39, Kit 3) Ag: LAAD (many, Kit 4)	Positive result confirms infection; some shedders may be nonsymptomatic carriers
Postmortem	Tissue (intestine, refrigerated)	Ag: DFA (24)	Positive result confirms infection
Canine Papillomatosis (see Chapter 22)			
	Oral tissue (formalin-fixed)	Histol (many)	Positive result suggests infection
Feline Panleukopenia (see Chapter 23)			
Antemortem	Serum: paired samples taken 10–14 days apart (2–3 ml, refrigerated)	Ab: IFA, VN (many, 34, 39) Ab: HA-I (25)	Paired samples: rising (4-fold) IgG titer confirms active infection
	Feces (fresh, refrigerated)	Ag: VI (6) Ag: EM (6, 35)	Positive result confirms infection; some shedders are nonsymptomatic carriers
Postmortem	Intestine, mesenteric lymph nodes, lung, pharyngeal swab (fresh or refrigerated)	Ag: DFA (many) Ag: VI (9, 13, 39)	Positive result confirms infection

APPENDIX 8. Laboratory Testing
for Confirmation of Infectious Diseases[a] Continued

INFECTIOUS DISEASE	SAMPLE (AMOUNT OR HANDLING)	TYPE OF TEST (LABORATORY[b] OR TEST KIT[c])	INTERPRETATION
Feline Infectious Peritonitis (see Chapter 24)			
Antemortem	Serum, fluid effusion (1–2 ml, refrigerated)	Ag: IFA (many) Ab: VN (many) Ab: ELISA (many, Kit 5) Ag: PE (many)	Positive serum titer suggests exposure to FIPV; however, titers can also be due to cross-reactions with enteric coronaviruses
Postmortem	Liver, small intestine (refrigerated)	Ag: DFA (many) Ag: VI (research)	Positive result confirms infection
	Liver, small intestine, kidney (formalin-fixed)	Histol (many)	Compatible histologic changes indicate infection
Feline Leukemia Virus Infection (see Chapter 26 and Table 26–3)			
Antemortem	Blood film or buffy coat or bone marrow smear (air dried)	Ag: IFA (many)	Positive result confirms infection; more specific for bone marrow infections than ELISA
	Serum or anticoagulated whole blood (1–2 ml)	Ag: ELISA (many, Kits 6 & 7)	Positive result confirms infection; more sensitive than IFA
	Serum (2–3 ml, refrigerated)	Ab: FOCMA (2, 35)	Positive result confirms current antitumor protection; may change with time
Postmortem	Blood (heparinized) or tissue (refrigerated, fresh)	Ag: VI (25)	Positive result confirms infection
Feline Immunodeficiency Virus Infection (see Chapter 26)			
	Serum, whole blood (1–2 ml, refrigerated)	Ab: ELISA (many, Kits 7 & 8)	Positive result confirms exposure and probable infection with virus; few animals may test seropositive but be nonsymptomatic carriers
Feline Respiratory Disease (see Chapter 27)			
RHINOTRACHEITIS VIRUS			
Antemortem	Serum: paired samples taken 10–14 days apart (2–3 ml, refrigerated)	Ab: IFA (34, 34a) Ab: VN (many)	Paired samples: rising (4-fold) titer confirms active infection
	Nasal swab (refrigerated)	Ag: VI (many)	Positive result indicates infection
Postmortem	Lung, liver, kidney (frozen or refrigerated)	Ag: DFA (many) Ag: VI (many)	Positive result confirms infection
CALICIVIRUS			
Antemortem	Serum: paired samples taken 10–14 days apart (2–3 ml, refrigerated)	Ab: IFA (34, 34a) Ab: VN (many)	Paired samples: rising (4-fold) titer confirms active infection
	Oropharyngeal swabs, intestinal and fecal swabs (refrigerated)	Ag: VI (many) Ag: EM (6)	Positive result confirms infection
Postmortem	Trachea, lung, kidney, intestine (refrigerated)	Ag: VI (many) Ag: DFA (9) Ag: IFA (9)	Positive result confirms infection
FELINE COWPOX INFECTION (see Chapter 30)			
Antemortem	Scabs (dry, sterile vial)	Ag: EM (many)	Positive result confirms infection with poxvirus
	Serum (2–3 ml, refrigerated)	Ab: VN (55)	Positive titer confirms exposure but not necessarily active infection

Continued on following page

APPENDIX 8. Laboratory Testing
for Confirmation of Infectious Diseases[a] Continued

INFECTIOUS DISEASE	SAMPLE (AMOUNT OR HANDLING)	TYPE OF TEST (LABORATORY[b] OR TEST KIT[c])	INTERPRETATION
Rabies (see Chapter 31)			
Antemortem	Vibrissae biopsy (refrigerated, in dry sterile vial)	Ag: DFA (6, 15)	Positive result confirms infection
	CSF (2–3 ml, refrigerated)	Ab: VN (many)[d]	High titer means CNS is infected (vaccine or virulent virus); takes 1–2 weeks to develop a titer and must compare to serum value
Postmortem	Brain (refrigerated)	Ag: DFA (many)[d]	Positive result confirms infection; more sensitive than Negri body detection
	Brain (formalin-fixed)	Histol (many)[d]	Negri bodies not present in all cases; false-positive and false-negative results can occur
Pseudorabies (see Chapter 32)			
Antemortem	Serum: paired samples taken 10–14 days apart (2–3 ml, refrigerated)	Ab: VN (many)	Positive result indicates exposure; paired samples; rising (4-fold) titer confirms active infection
Postmortem	Brain, tonsils, lung, cervical lymph nodes, salivary glands, spleen (refrigerated)	Ag: DFA (many) Ag: VI (many)	Positive result confirms infection
	Brain (formalin-fixed)	Histol (many)	Compatible histologic changes indicate infection
Ehrlichiosis (see Chapter 37)			
Antemortem	Blood films, bone marrow smears (refrigerated or alcohol-fixed)	Cytol (many)	Positive result confirms infection; many false-negatives due to low numbers of organisms
	Serum (2–3 ml, refrigerated)	PE (many)	Nonspecific hyperglobulinemia seen with other disorders
	Serum: single sample (2–3 ml, refrigerated)	Ab: IFA (E. canis: 13, 16a, 27, 28, 35) (E. platys: 16a) (E. ristici: 13) (E. equi: 13)	Positive titer confirms active infection unless animal was recently treated with appropriate drugs, must be infected for at least 30 days to have positive titer
Rocky Mountain Spotted Fever (see Chapter 38)			
Antemortem or Postmortem	Skin biopsy or other tissues (formalin-fixed)	Ag: DFA (12)	Positive result confirms infection; many false-negatives; no need for species specificity
	Serum: paired samples taken 10–14 days apart (1–2 ml, refrigerated)	Ab: IFA-IgG (11, 12, 17)	Paired samples: rising (4-fold) IgG titer confirms active infection; species-specific testing required
	Serum: single sample (1–2 ml, refrigerated)	Ab: IFA-IgM (11)	Single positive IgM titer indicates active infection; a second titer may be needed to clarify some low titers.
		Ab: LAB (many, Kit 9)	Single positive latex titer indicates active infection since measures IgM; false-negative results occur
Q Fever (see Chapter 38)			
	Serum (2–3 ml, refrigerated)	Ab: IFA (24, 35) Ab: ELISA (18)	Acute: high phase II antibodies. Convalescent: intermediate to high phase I and II antibodies. Chronic: phase I lipopolysaccharide antibodies high

APPENDIX 8. Laboratory Testing
for Confirmation of Infectious Diseases[a] Continued

INFECTIOUS DISEASE	SAMPLE (AMOUNT OR HANDLING)	TYPE OF TEST (LABORATORY[b] OR TEST KIT[c])	INTERPRETATION
Haemobartonellosis (see Chapter 39)	Blood films (unstained and unfixed)	Cytol (many)	Positive result confirms infection; stained artifacts must be viewed cautiously
Chlamydial Infection (see Chapter 40)	Serum (2–3 ml, refrigerated)	Ab: CF (30, 35)	Paired samples: rising (4-fold) titer confirms active infection
	Nasal and ocular swabs, lung (refrigerated)	Cult (25, 30, 35) Ag: ELISA (many, Kit 10)	Positive result confirms infection; large numbers of organisms more indicative of active infection
	Conjunctival smear (refrigerated)	Ag: FA (34a, Kit 10a)	Positive result confirms infection; large numbers of organisms more indicative of active infection
Mycoplasmal Infection (see Chapter 41)	Nasal swab, trachea (refrigerated)	Cult (many)	Positive result confirms infection; many infections are nonsymptomatic since part of resident microflora

Bacterial Infections
(see Chapter 42)

Leptospirosis (see Chapter 45)			
Antemortem	Serum: paired samples taken 10–14 days apart (2–3 ml, refrigerated)	Ab: MA (many) Ab: SAT (many)	Paired samples: rising (4-fold) titer confirms active infection; single positive titer 1:300 confirms recent exposure in nonvaccinate; lower titers associated with vaccination; titer $\geq$1:800 by itself suggests recent infection
	Urine (1–2 ml, refrigerated)	DF (many)	Positive result suggests infection; nonpathogenic spirochetes and artifacts make unreliable
	Urine, blood (2–3 ml, refrigerated)	Cult (25, 37, 41, 42)	Positive result confirms infection
Postmortem	Urine, blood, kidney (in transport media)	Ag: DFA (9, 25) Cult (25) DF (25, 41, 42)	Positive result confirms infection Positive result suggests infection; nonpathogenic spirochetes and artifacts make unreliable
Canine Lyme Borreliosis (see Chapter 46)	Serum: paired samples taken 10–14 days apart (2–3 ml, refrigerated)	Ab: IFA (many) Ab: ELISA-IgG (many) Ab: ELISA-IgM (11)	Paired samples: rising (4-fold) IgG titer confirms active infection with *Borrelia* spp. Single high IgM titer confirms recent or active infection with *Borrelia* spp.
	Ticks (moistened container, refrigerated or at room temperature)	Cult (17)[d] Ag: IFA (research)	Positive result confirms tick infection
Botulism (see Chapter 47)	Feces, blood, serum, intestinal contents (refrigerated)	MI (35)	Test performed with and without specific antisera for confirmation of type involved

Continued on following page

APPENDIX 8. Laboratory Testing
for Confirmation of Infectious Diseases[a] Continued

INFECTIOUS DISEASE	SAMPLE (AMOUNT OR HANDLING)	TYPE OF TEST (LABORATORY[b] OR TEST KIT[c])	INTERPRETATION
Anaerobic Infections (see Chapter 49)			
	Lesion exudate (refrigerated in airtight or anaerobic transport system)	Cult (many)	Positive result confirms infection but may be contaminants to wound exudates
Enteric Bacterial Infections (see Chapter 50)			
SALMONELLOSIS			
Antemortem	Serum: paired samples taken 10–14 days apart (2–3 ml, refrigerated)	Ab: HA-I (16)	Paired samples: rising (4-fold) titer confirms active infection; single positive titer is nonspecific
	Feces or fecal swab (3 g fresh or refrigerated)	Cult (many)	Positive result confirms active infection; may be subclinical carrier
	Blood (1–2 ml, sterilely collected in blood culture broth media)	Cult (many)	Positive result confirms clinically significant bacteremic infection
Postmortem	Intestinal lymph nodes, spleen, many internal organs other than intestine (refrigerated)	Cult (many)	Positive result confirms active septicemic infection
CAMPYLOBACTERIOSIS			
	Feces (2–3 g fresh, in sterile airtight container; add Thioglycollate transport medium)[e]	Cult (many)	Positive result confirms infection; may be subclinical carrier
	Intestine, colon, lymph node, lung, spleen (formalin-fixed)	Histol (many)	Compatible histologic changes indicate infection
Mycobacteriosis (see Chapter 51)			
	Tissue specimen or exudate (fresh or frozen)	Cult (many)	Positive result confirms infection
	Tissue (formalin-fixed)	Histol (many)	Finding acid fast bacteria must be combined with bacterial culture for determining organism involved
Brucellosis (see Chapter 52)			
Antemortem	Serum: single sample (2–3 ml, refrigerated until sent)	Ab: SAT (many, Kit 11)	Positive result confirms infection, but many false-positives; do 2ME modification and TAT next to determine titer or ID for increased specificity
		Ab: TAT (many)	>1:50 suspicious; >1:100 positive; >1:200 usually bacteremic; some false-negatives and false-positives; do ID next
		Ab: ID (25)	May detect rare seronegatives, more specific test; use to check TAT positives
Nocardiosis (see Chapter 53)			
	Peritoneal, pleural, and pericardial fluid	Cult (many)	Positive result confirms infection
Plague (see Chapter 59)			
	Serum (2–3 ml, refrigerated)	Ab: (7, 24)	Positive result confirms exposure; rising (4-fold) titer confirms active infection
	Exudates (2–3 ml, refrigerated)	Ab: FA (7, 24)[f]	Positive result confirms infection
	Exudates (swabs)	Cult (7, 34)[f]	Positive result confirms infection

APPENDIX 8. Laboratory Testing
for Confirmation of Infectious Diseases[a] Continued

INFECTIOUS DISEASE	SAMPLE (AMOUNT OR HANDLING)	TYPE OF TEST (LABORATORY[b] OR TEST KIT[c])	INTERPRETATION
Tularemia (see Chapter 60)			
	Serum (2–3 ml, refrigerated)	Ab: (24)[f]	Positive result confirms exposure; rising (4-fold) titer confirms active infection
	Swab or exudate on ice	Cult (24)[f]	Positive result confirms infection

Fungal Infection
(see Chapter 62)

INFECTIOUS DISEASE	SAMPLE (AMOUNT OR HANDLING)	TYPE OF TEST (LABORATORY[b] OR TEST KIT[c])	INTERPRETATION
Dermatophytosis (see Chapter 64)			
	Lesion (scabs or plucked hairs in sterile dry tubes)	Cult (many, Kit 12)	Positive result confirms infection; some cats may be non-symptomatic carriers
Blastomycosis or Histoplasmosis (see Chapters 65 and 66, respectively)			
Antemortem or Postmortem	Serum: single sample (2–3 ml, refrigerated)	Ab: CF (many) Ab: (many, 21)	Positive result confirms exposure but not necessarily active infection
	Tissue or fluid aspirates (1–2 ml in sterile container)	Cult (6)[g] Cytol (many, can be done in practice)	Positive result confirms infection
	Tissue biopsy (formalin-fixed)	Histol (many)	Positive result confirms infection
Cryptococcosis (see Chapter 67)			
	Serum or CSF: single sample (1–2 ml in sterile container, refrigerated)	Ag: LAAD (6, 11, Kit 13)	Positive result confirms active infection
	Serum (2–3 ml, refrigerated)	Ab: ID (34)	Positive titer confirms exposure but not necessarily active infection
	Tissue or fluid aspirate (in sterile container, refrigerated)	Cult (many, 6)	Positive result confirms infection
		Cytol (many, can be done in practice)	Positive result confirms infection
	Tissue (in sterile container, refrigerated)	Ag: DFA (12a)	Positive result confirms infection
Coccidioidomycosis (see Chapter 68)			
	Serum: single or paired samples (2–3 ml, refrigerated)	Ab: ID (many) Ab: CF (2, 9)	See Table 68–1 for interpretation
	Tissue or fluid aspirate (1–2 ml, refrigerated)	Cult (6)[g]	Positive result confirms infection
	Tissue (refrigerated)	Cytol (many, can be done in practice)	Positive result confirms infection
Sporotrichosis (see Chapter 69)			
	Exudate from lymphatics (1–2 ml, refrigerated)	Cytol (many, can be done in practice)	Positive result confirms infection
	Tissue (refrigerated)	Ag: DFA (12a) Cult (41, 42)	Positive result confirms infection
	Serum (2–3 ml, refrigerated)	Ab: SAT (30)	Positive result confirms exposure but not necessarily active infection
Aspergillosis (see Chapter 71)			
	Serum: single sample (2–3 ml, refrigerated)	Ab: ELISA (13, 32a) Ab: ID (many) Ab: CF (many)	Positive result confirms exposure but not necessarily active infection
	Tissue or exudate (refrigerated)	Cult (many)	Positive result confirms infection; can be a contaminant
Prototheosis (see Chapter 75)			
	Tissue (refrigerated)	Ag: DFA (12a) Cult (41, 42)	Positive result confirms infection

Continued on following page

APPENDIX 8. Laboratory Testing
for Confirmation of Infectious Diseases[a] Continued

INFECTIOUS DISEASE	SAMPLE (AMOUNT OR HANDLING)	TYPE OF TEST (LABORATORY[b] OR TEST KIT[c])	INTERPRETATION
Protozoal Infections (see Chapter 76)			
Trypanosomiasis (see Chapter 78)			
	Serum: single sample (2–3 ml, refrigerated)	Ab: IFA (35)	Positive result confirms recent or previous infection
	Blood film (thick and thin)	Cytol (many)[h]	Positive result confirms infection
Leishmaniasis (see Chapter 79)			
	Serum or dried blood spots on filter paper	Ab: IFA (65)[h]	Positive result confirms infection; infection usually persists
Hepatozoonosis (see Chapter 80)			
	Blood film	Cytol (35)	Positive result confirms infection
Encephalitozoonosis (see Chapter 81)			
	Serum: single sample (2–3 ml, refrigerated)	Ab: IFA (18b)	Positive result confirms previous exposure but not necessarily active infection
Cytauxzoonosis (see Chapter 82)			
	Blood films, bone marrow	Cytol (many, 21)	Positive result confirms infection; may be uncommon in peripheral blood films
Babesiosis (see Chapter 83)			
	Blood film	Cytol (many, 2, 9)	Positive result confirms infection, may be uncommon in peripheral blood films
	Serum: single sample (2–3 ml, refrigerated)	Ab: IFA (13, 27, 35)	Positive titer >1:40 indicates active or very recent infection
Enteric Protozoal Infections (see Chapter 84)			
	Feces (refrigerated)	Flot, Sed (many) Ag: ELISA (Kit 13a)	Positive result indicates infection; some animals may be nonsymptomatic carriers
Toxoplasmosis (see Chapter 86)			
	Serum: paired samples taken 10–14 days apart (2–3 ml, refrigerated)	Ab: HA-I (many, Kit 14) Ab: IFA-IgG (many, 35) Ab: CF (certain) Ab: ELISA-IgG (many, 6, 11) Ab: LAB (Kit 14a)	Paired samples: rising (4-fold) IgG titer confirms active infection; single positive titer is nonspecific
		Ab: ELISA-IgM (6, 11)	A single high IgM titer indicates active or recent infection; evaluation of IgG and IgM simultaneously is not informative
	Feces (cat only, refrigerated)	Flot (many)	Oocyst identification is positive, although inoculation into intermediate host is often needed to confirm exact species
	Tissue biopsy (formalin-fixed)	Histol (many)	Positive for infection; if detected, clinical significance must be determined
Neosporosis (see Chapter 86)			
	Serum: paired samples taken 10–14 days apart (2–3 ml, refrigerated)	Ab: IFA (18a)[f]	Paired samples: rising (4-fold) IgG titer confirms active infection; single positive titer indicates previous exposure
	Tissue biopsy (formalin-fixed or refrigerated)	Ag: DFA (18a)[f]	Positive result confirms infection

APPENDIX 8. *Laboratory Testing for Confirmation of Infectious Diseases*[a] Continued

INFECTIOUS DISEASE	SAMPLE (AMOUNT OR HANDLING)	TYPE OF TEST (LABORATORY[b] OR TEST KIT[c])	INTERPRETATION
Coccidiosis (see Chapter 87)			
	Feces (refrigerated)	Flot (many)	Oocyst identification is positive
Cryptosporidiosis (Chapter 88)			
	Feces (refrigerated)	Flot (many)	Oocyst identification is positive
		Ag: FA (20, Kit 15)	Positive result confirms infection
		Ag: ELISA (research)	
Pneumocystosis (see Chapter 89)			
	Sputum, lung aspirates (refrigerated)	Cytol (many)	Positive result suggests infection, difficult to find and numerous artifacts make visualization difficult
		Ag: FA (many, Kit 16)	Positive result confirms infection

[a]Ab = antibody
Ag = antigen
Biop = biopsy
CF = complement fixation
Cult = culture
Cytol = cytology
DF = darkfield microscopy
DFA = direct immunofluorescence (IFA substituted in some cases)
ELISA = enzyme-linked immunosorbent assay
EM = electron microscopy
Flot = fecal flotation
FOCMA = feline oncornavirus cell membrane antibody
HA = hemagglutination
HA-I = hemagglutination-inhibition
Histol = histology
ID = immunodiffusion
IFA = indirect immunofluorescence
LAAD = latex agglutination antigen determination
LAB = latex agglutination antibody determination
MA = microscopic agglutination
2ME = 2-mercaptoethanol modification of TAT
MI = mouse inoculation
PE = protein electrophoresis
SAT = slide agglutination test
TAT = tube agglutination test
VI = virus isolation
VN = virus neutralization

[b]Designated laboratories responded to a survey sent to laboratories that process veterinary samples. Any comments or additions concerning laboratories to be listed in future editions should be sent to the editor. Laboratories referred to by number in this column are listed at the end of this appendix, on pages 900–903. Information on laboratories in Great Britain compiled from Evans J (ed): *The Henston Veterinary Vade Mecum*, ed 7. Surrey, Update—Siebert Publications Ltd, 1988.

[c]Commercially available test kits for infectious disease are referred to in this column as a numbered kit, and a list of the respective products follows the list of laboratories, on pages 903–904.

[d]Many public health laboratories test animals only in cases of human exposure.

[e]Campy-BAP (for culture) and Thioglycollate medium (transport), BBL Microbiological Systems, Cockeysville, MD 21030

[f]Contact laboratory before submitting specimen.

[g]Culture has public health risk.

[h]Specimens have public health risk.

Continued on following page

Laboratories Listed by Number

UNITED STATES

Alabama

1. The Charles S. Roberts Veterinary Diagnostic
   Laboratory
   PO Box 2209
   Auburn, AL 36831–2209
   (205) 844–4987

Arizona

2. Southwest Veterinary Diagnostics, Inc.
   13633 North Cave Creek Road
   Phoenix, AR 85022
   (602) 971–4110
   (602) 275–7460

California

3. San Diego County Veterinary Laboratory
   5555 Overland Avenue, Building 4
   San Diego, CA 92123–1274
   (619) 694–2838
4. California Veterinary Diagnostics Inc.
   P.O. Box V
   3911 West Capitol Avenue
   West Sacramento, CA 95691
   (916) 372–4200
5. Veterinary Reference Laboratory
   National Office: Dallas, TX
   Natl: (800) 527–7673;
   CA: (800) 422–7328
   Northern CA: (800) 772–3287
   Metro: 352–7960
   Southern CA: (800) 432–7305
   Metro: 937-0161

Colorado

6. Veterinary Diagnostic Laboratory
   Colorado State University
   Fort Collins, CO 80523
   (303) 491–1281
7. Plague Branch, VBDD
   The Centers for Disease Control
   PO Box 2087
   Fort Collins, CO 80522
   (303) 221–6465

Delaware

8. State of Delaware
   Department of Agriculture
   2320 South DuPont Highway
   Dover, DE 19901
   (302) 736–4811

Florida

8a. Bureau of Diagnostic Laboratories
   Florida Department of Agriculture
   PO Box 460
   Kissimmee, FL 32742
   (407) 847–3185

Georgia

9. Diagnostic Assistance Laboratory
   College of Veterinary Medicine
   University of Georgia
   Athens, GA 30602
   (404) 542–5568

10. Tifton Veterinary Diagnostic
    and Investigational Laboratory
    University of Georgia
    Tifton, GA 31793
    (912) 386-3340
11. Infectious Diseases Laboratory
    Department of Small Animal Medicine
    College of Veterinary Medicine
    University of Georgia
    Athens, GA 30602
    (404) 542–9384
12. Smith Kline Veterinary Laboratory
    1777 Montreal Circle
    Tucker, GA 30084
    Natl: (800) 631–3974; GA: (800) 533–3950
12a. Centers for Disease Control
    Mycology Unit or Bacteriology Unit
    US Department of Health and Human Services
    Atlanta, GA 30333

Illinois

13. Department of Veterinary Pathobiology
    2001 South Lincoln Avenue
    University of Illinois
    Urbana, IL 61801
    (217) 333-2671

Indiana

14. Indiana State Board of Health
    1330 West Michigan Street
    PO Box 1964
    Indianapolis, IN 46206
    (317) 633–0376

Kansas

15. Veterinary Diagnostic Laboratory
    College of Veterinary Medicine
    Veterinary Medical Center
    Mahattan, KS 66506
    (913) 532-5660

Kentucky

16. Veterinary Diagnostic and Research Center
    Murray State University
    PO Box 2000 North Drive
    Hopkinsville, KY 42240
    (502) 886–3959

Louisiana

16a. Louisiana Veterinary Medical
    Diagnostic Laboratory
    School of Veterinary Medicine
    Louisiana State University
    Baton Rouge, LA 70803
    (504) 346–3193

Maryland

17. State of Maryland
    Department of Health and Mental Hygiene
    Laboratories Administration
    Howard and Biddle Streets
    PO Box 2355
    Baltimore, MD 21203
    (301) 383–2883

APPENDIX 8. Laboratory Testing
for Confirmation of Infectious Diseases Continued

18. Maryland Medical Laboratory Inc.
    1901 Sulfur Spring Road
    Baltimore, MD 21227
    (301) 247–9100
18a. J. P. Dubey
    Zoonotic Diseases Laboratory
    Livestock & Poultry Sciences Institute
    USDA, BARC-East, Bldg. 1040
    Beltsville, MD 20705
    (301) 344–2128
18b. AnMed/Biosafe Inc.
    7642 Standish Pl.
    Rockville, MD 20855
    (301) 762–0366

Massachusetts
19. Tufts University
    School of Veterinary Medicine
    Division of Diagnostic Laboratories
    305 South Street
    Jamaica Plain, MA 02130
    (617) 522-2125

Mississippi
20. Mississippi Board of Animal Health & Veterinary
        Diagnostic Laboratory
    2531 North West Street
    PO Box 4389
    Jackson, MS 39216
    (601) 354–6091

Missouri
21. Veterinary Medical Diagnostic Laboratory
    University of Missouri—Columbia
    Columbia, MO 65211
    (314) 882–6695

Nebraska
22. University of Nebraska
    Department of Veterinary Science
    Veterinary Diagnostic Center
    Lincoln, NE 68583–0907
    (402) 472–1434
23. Institute of Agriculture and Natural Resources
    West Central Research and Extension Center
    Route 4, Box 46A
    North Platte, NE 69101
    (308) 532–3611

New Mexico
24. New Mexico Department of Agriculture
    Veterinary Diagnostic Services
    700 Camino de Salud, NE
    Albuquerque, NM 87106
    Natl: (800) 432-9110

New York
25. Diagnostic Laboratory
    New York State College of Veterinary Medicine
    Box 786
    Cornell University
    Ithaca, NY 14850
    (607) 256–6541
26. Veterinary Research Associates
    333 West Merrick Road
    Valley Stream, NY 11580
    Natl: (800) 872–7828; NY: (800) 872–1001

North Carolina
27. North Carolina State University
    School of Veterinary Medicine
    4700 Hillsborough Street
    Raleigh, NC 27606
    (919) 829–4347
28. Roche Biovet
    Division of Roche Biomedical Labs
    PO Box 2230
    Burlington, NC 27215
    Natl: (800) 334–5161; NC: (800) 672–3646

North Dakota
29. North Dakota State University of Agriculture and
        Applied Science
    Veterinary Science
    Fargo, ND 58105
    (701) 237–7511

Oklahoma
30. Oklahoma Animal Disease Diagnostic Laboratory
    Oklahoma State University
    Stillwater, OK 74078
    (405) 744–6623

Oregon
31. Veterinary Diagnostic Laboratory
    Oregon State University
    PO Box 429
    Corvallis, OR 97339–0429
    (503) 754–3261
32. Veterinary Reference Laboratory
    National Office: Dallas, TX
    Natl: (800) 527–7673; Western
    States: (800) 854–7133
    Portland 252–0444

Pennsylvania
32a. Laboratory of Pathology
    School of Veterinary Medicine
    University of Pennsylvania
    Philadelphia, PA 19104
    (215) 898–8859

South Carolina
33. College of Agricultural Science
    Division of Livestock Poultry
    Clemson University
    PO Box 218
    Elgin, SC 29045–0218
    (605) 688–5171

Tennessee
34. Specialized Assays
    PO Box 25110
    1808 Hayes Street
    Nashville, TN 37202
    Natl: (800) 443–3648; TN: (800) 541–9061
34a. C. E. Kord Animal Disease Laboratory
    PO Box 40627, Melrose Station
    Nashville, TN 37204
    (615) 360–0125

Texas
35. Texas Veterinary Medical Diagnostic Laboratory
    Drawer 3040
    College Station, TX 77840
    (409) 845–3414

Continued on following page

APPENDIX 8. Laboratory Testing
for Confirmation of Infectious Diseases Continued

36. Veterinary Reference Laboratory
    3191 Commonwealth Road
    Dallas, TX 75247
    Natl: (800) 527–7673; TX: (800) 442–1661
    Western States (800) 854–7133
    Offices in California and Oregon

Virginia

37. State of Virginia
    Department of Agriculture and Consumer Services
    Division of Animal Health
    Bureau of Laboratory Services
    1 North 14th Street, Room 162
    Richmond, VA 23219
38. Riverside Veterinary Laboratories
    8132 Forest Hill Avenue
    PO Box 3889
    Richmond, VA 23235
    Natl: (800) LAB–0100; VA: (800) 828–5228

Washington

39. Washington Animal Disease Diagnostic
       Laboratory
    College of Veterinary Medicine
    Washington State University
    PO Box 2037
    Pullman, WA 99164
    (509) 335–9696

West Virginia

40. State of West Virginia
    Department of Health
    Office of Laboratory Services
    167 11th Street
    South Charleston, WV 25303
    (304) 348–3530

Wisconsin

41. Wisconsin Department of Agriculture, Trade and
       Consumer Protection
    Animal Health Division (Central Lab)
    6101 Mineral Point Road
    Madison, WI 53705
    (608) 266–2465
42. Wisconsin Department of Agriculture, Trade and
       Consumer Protection
    Animal Health Division (Regional Lab)
    1418 East LaSalle Avenue
    Barron, WI 54812
    (715) 537–3151

Wyoming

43. Wyoming State Veterinary Laboratory
    1190 Jackson Street
    Laramie, WY 82070
    (307) 742–6638

GREAT BRITAIN

44. Animal Health Trust
    PO Box No. 5
    Balaton Lodge, Snailwell Road
    Newmarket
    Suffolk CB8 7DW
    (0638) 661111

45. Barnard and Partner
    424 Victoria Avenue
    Southend-on-Sea
    Essex SS2 6NB
    (0702) 432020
46. Bloxham Laboratories
    George Street
    Teignmouth
    Devon TQ14 8AH
    (06267) 7884415
47. Bristol University
    Clinical Pathology Diagnostic Services
    Department of Veterinary Medicine
    University of Bristol
    Langford House
    Bristol BS18 7DU
    (0934) 852581
48. Cambridge University
    Clinical Pathology Laboratories
    Department of Clinical Veterinary Medicine
    Madingly Road
    Cambridge CB3 0ES
49. Canine Infectious Diseases Research Unit
    University of Glasgow Veterinary School
    Bearsden, Glasgow
    G61 1QH
    041–330–5776
50. Feline Infectious Diseases Research Unit
    University of Glasgow Veterinary School
    Bearsden, Glasgow
    G61 1QH
    041–330–5777
51. Glasgow University
    Department of Veterinary Pathology
    University of Glasgow Veterinary School
    Bearsden, Glasgow
    G61 1QH
    041–330–5773
52. Grange Laboratories
    PO Box 4
    Wetheby Yorks
    LS22 5JU
    (0937) 61649
53. LabPak Limited
    661 Foleshill Road
    Coventry
    CV6 5JQ
    (0203) 666123
54. Leeds Veterinary Laboratories Limited
    Unit 3, Westfield Mills
    Kirk Lane, Yeadon
    Leeds LS19 7LX
    (0532) 507556
55. Liverpool University
    Department of Clinical Pathology
    PO Box 147
    Liverpool L68 3BX
    051–709–6022
56. Mansi Laboratories Limited
    Herons Way
    Wey Road, Weybridge
    Surrey KT13 8HS
    (0932) 45354/42855

APPENDIX 8. Laboratory Testing
for Confirmation of Infectious Diseases Continued

57. The Microbiology Laboratories
56 Northumberland Road
North Harrow
Middx HA2 7RE
01–868–4050

58. North Western Laboratories
    Limited
Addon Road
Poulton le Fylde
Lancs FY6 8JL
(0253) 899215

59. Royal Veterinary College
    Field Station
Department of Pathology
Hawkshead House
Hawkshead Lane
North Mymms
Hatfield, Herts
AL9 7TA
(0707) 55486

60. St. David's Laboratory
43 St. David's Hill
Exeter
Devon EX4 4DJ
(0392) 56719

61. Salvet Laboratories Limited
Avon Lodge
21 Stratford Road
Salisbury, Wilts
SP1 3JN
(0722) 29663

62. Vetdiagnostics
Shamrock Farms (Great Britain) Ltd
Victoria House
Small Dale, Henfield
Sussex BN5 9XE
(0273) 493933

63. Vetlab Services
Unit 11 Station Road
Southwater, Harsham
West Sussex RH13 7QH
(0403) 730176

64. Wickham Laboratories Limited
Winchester Road
Wickham, Fareham
Hants PO17 5EU
(0329) 832511

65. Diagnostic Laboratory
London School of Hygiene
London, England

NAME OF KIT		TYPE OF TEST		MANUFACTURER*
Canine Enteric Viral Infections				
Kit 1	DiaSystems Canine Parvovirus Antibody Test Kit	Ab: ELISA	U:	TechAmerica Diagnostics, Ellwood, KS 66024, Natl: (800) 891-5550 (Fermenta Animal Health Co., Kansas City, MO 64190)
	CITE Parvovirus	Ab: ELISA	U:	IDEXX Corp., Portland, ME 04101, Natl: (800) 548–6733
	Ocetia Canine Parvovirus	Ab: ELISA	B:	IDS Ltd, Washington, Tyne & Wear NE37 3HS, 091-417-6530
Kit 2	DiaSystems Canine Parvo Antigen Kit	Ag: ELISA	U:	TechAmerica Diagnostics, Ellwood, KS 66024, Natl: (800) 891–5550 (Fermenta Animal Health Co., Kansas City, MO 64190)
Kit 2a	Ocetia Canine Coronavirus	Ab: ELISA	B:	IDS Ltd, Washington, Tyne & Wear NE37 3HS, 091-417-6530
Kit 3	Rotazyme	Ag: ELISA	U:	Abbott Laboratories, Diagnostics Division, North Chicago, IL 60064, Natl: (800) 323–9100
	Rotaclone	Ag: ELISA	U:	Cambridge Bioscience, Worcester, MA 01605, (508) 797–5777
Kit 4	MERITEC-Rotavirus	Ag: LAAD	U:	Meridian Diagnostics, Inc., Cincinnati, OH 45244, Natl: (800) 543-1980; OH: (513) 271–3700
Feline Infectious Peritonitis				
Kit 5	DiaSystems FIP Test Kit	Ab: ELISA	U:	TechAmerica Diagnostics, Ellwood, KS 66024, Natl: (800) 891–5550 (Fermenta Animal Health Co., Kansas City, MO 64190)
	Ocetia Feline Infectious Peritonitis	Ab: ELISA	B:	IDS Ltd, Washington, Tyne & Wear NE37 3HS, 091–417–6530
Feline Retroviral Infections				
Kit 6	DiaSystems FeLV Test Kit	Ab: ELISA	U:	TechAmerica Diagnostics, Ellwood, KS 66024, Natl: (800) 891-5550 (Fermenta Animal Health Co., Kansas City, MO 64190)
	Leukassay FII	Ab: ELISA	U:	Pitman-Moore, Washington Crossing, NJ 08560, Eastern US: (800) 241-3166; Western US: (800) 525–9480
	Leukassay	Ab: ELISA	B:	C-Vet, Ltd, Suffolk IP33 3SU, (0284) 61131

Continued on following page

APPENDIX 8. Laboratory Testing
for Confirmation of Infectious Diseases Continued

NAME OF KIT	TYPE OF TEST		MANUFACTURER*
Kit 6 *Continued*			
CITE FeLV	Ab: ELISA	U:	IDEXX Corp., Portland, ME 04104, Natl: (800) 548–6733
		B:	Glaxovet Ltd, Middlesex UB9 6LS (0895) 630266
ViroCheck/FeLV Test Kit	Ab: ELISA	U:	Synbiotics Corp, San Diego, CA 92127, Natl: (800) 228–4305; CA; (800) 992–6868
Kit 7 CITE FeLV and FIV	Ab: ELISA	U:	IDEXX Corp., Portland, ME 04101, Natl: (800) 548–6733
Kit 8 CITE FIV	Ab: ELISA	U:	IDEXX Corp., Portland, ME 04101, Natl: (800) 548–6733
		B:	Glaxovet Ltd, Middlesex UB9 6LS, (0895) 630266
Rickettsial and Chlamydial Infections			
Kit 9 Latex-*Rickettsia rickettsii* Kit	Ab: LAB	U:	Integrated Diagnostics Inc., Baltimore, MD 21227, Natl: (800) TEC-INDX; MD: (301) 247–2570
Kit 10 Chlamydia Antigen Test	Ag: ELISA	U:	Orthodiagnostics Systems Inc., Raritan, NJ 88869
Chlamydiazyme	Ag: ELISA	U:	Abbott Laboratories, Diagnostics Division, North Chicago, IL 60064, Natl: (800) 323–9100
Kit 10a Chlamydia Detection Kit	Ag: FA	U:	Whittaker Bioproducts Inc., Walkersville, MD 21793, Natl: (800) 538–3961; MD: (301) 898–7025
Bacterial Infections			
Kit 11 D-TEC-CB	Ab: SAT	U:	Pitman-Moore, Washington Crossing, NJ 08560, Eastern US: (800) 241–3166; Western US: (800) 525–9480
Fungal Infections			
Kit 12 Fungassay	Culture	U:	Pitman-Moore, Washington Crossing, NJ 08560, Eastern US: (800) 241–3166; Western US: (800) 525–9480
		B:	C-Vet, Ltd, Suffolk IP33 3SU, (0284) 61131
Kit 13 Cryptococcal latex antigen kit	Ag: LAAD	U:	Meridian Diagnostics Inc, Cincinnati, OH 45244, Natl: (800) 543–1980; OH: (513) 271–3700
		U:	American Scientific Products, McGaw Park, IL
Protozoal Infections			
Kit 13a Giardia Direct Detection System	Ag: ELISA	U:	Trend Scientific Inc, St. Paul, MN, (612) 633–0925
ProSpecT/Giardia	Ag: ELISA	U:	Alexon Biomedical, Mountain View, CA 94043, (415) 961–3436
Kit 14 Toxo HA-I	Ab: HA-I	U:	Wampole Laboratories, Division of Carter Wallace, Inc., Cranbury, NJ 08512, (609) 655–6000
Ket 14a Toxotest-MT (Eiken)	Ab: LAB	U:	Tanabe USA Inc, 7930 Convoy Court, San Diego, CA 92111, (619) 571–8410
Kit 15 Meriflour-Cryptosporidium	Ag: IFA	U:	Meridian Diagnostics Inc., Cincinnati, OH 45244, Natl: (800) 543–1980; OH: (513) 271–3700
Kit 16 Meriflour-Pneumocystis	Ag: IFA	U:	Meridian Diagnostics Inc., Cincinnati, OH 45244, Natl: (800) 543–1980; OH: (513) 271–3700

*U = United States; B = Great Britain.

APPENDIX 9: *Environmental Survival of Certain Microorganisms and Some Effective Biocidal Agents*[a]

TYPE OF MICROORGANISM	Temperature (°C)	Time	Type	Concentration (%)	Time (min)	Temperature (°C)	Reference[b]
Enveloped Viruses							
HERPESVIRUSES							
Feline rhino-	4	154 days	Heat		4–5	56	1–3
tracheitis virus	25	33 days	Alc	70	10	25	
(see Chapter 27)	37	3 hr	HC	3.12	10	25	
			HI	100	10	25	
			Phen	3.12	10	25	
			QUAT	0.5	10	25	
			AF	4	10	25	
			AG	2	10	25	
			Big	0.78	10	25	
Canine	4	48 hr	Heat		4	56	4, 5
herpesvirus (see	37	48 hr	LS	10	15		
Chapter 18)							
PARAMYXOVIRUS							
Canine distemper	4	7–8 wk	Heat		30	60	2, 6
virus (see	25	7–8 wk	LS	0.3	10		
Chapter 16)			AF	0.1	120		
			Phen	1	Hours		
			QUAT	0.2	30		
RHABDOVIRUS							
Rabies virus (see			Heat		15	70	2, 6
Chapter 31)	4	Weeks	UV		Rapid		
	25	Days	Phen	3	15		
TOGAVIRUS							
Louping-ill virus	4–8	2 wk	Heat		10	58	6
(see Chapter 35)					2–5	60	
Unenveloped Viruses							
PARVOVIRUSES							
Canine parvovirus	Very stable		Heat		15	56	7
(see Chapter 21)	in the						
	environ-						
	ment						
	25	3 mo					
Feline	Very stable		Phen	0.05	Rapid		2, 3
panleukopenia	in the		HC	3.12	10	25	
virus (see	environ-		AF	4	10	25	
Chapter 23)	ment		AG	2	10	25	
			Big	0.78	10	25	
PAPOVAVIRUS							
Canine papilloma	4–8	63 days	Heat		60	45–80	6, 8
virus (see	37	6 hr					
Chapter 22)							
ADENOVIRUS							
Infectious canine	4	2 mo	Heat		3–5	60	5, 8, 9
hepatitis virus	25	14 days	UV		120		
(see Chapter 17)	37	6 hr	AF	0.2	24 hr		
PICORNAVIRUS							
Feline calicivirus	7–20	10 days	Heat		30	50	1, 2, 10
(see Chapter 27)			Phen	3.12	10	50	
			HC	3.12	10	25	
			AF	4	10	25	
			AG	2	10	25	

Continued on following page

APPENDIX 9: *Environmental Survival of Certain Microorganisms and Some Effective Biocidal Agents*[a] Continued

TYPE OF MICROORGANISM	ENVIRONMENTAL SURVIVAL		BIOCIDAL AGENT				
	Temperature (°C)	Time	Type	Concentration (%)	Time (min)	Temperature (°C)	Reference[b]
REOVIRUSES Canine reovirus and rotavirus Feline reovirus	24 37	2 days 19 hr	Heat Alc AF	70 3	30 60 30	60 25 56	2, 11
Rickettsiae **CHLAMYDIA** (see Chapter 40)	0 25	24 hr 7 days	Heat LS QUAT	0.5	15 30 Effective	60	1, 2, 5
MYCOPLASMAS (see Chapter 41)	28	21 days	Heat Phen AF	1 0.5	15 Minutes Minutes	55	2, 12
Bacteria **GRAM-POSITIVE STAPHYL-OCOCCI** (see Chapter 57)	4	Several months	Heat Phen	1	30 15	60	13
BRUCELLA (see Chapter 52)	25	3 mo	Heat Phen	1	15 15	60	12, 14, 15
SALMONELLA (see Chapter 50)	25	12–14 wk (in pasture)	Heat		20	60	2, 16
MYCOBACTERIUM TUBER-CULOSIS (see Chapter 51)	25	Weeks (in dried sputum)	Heat UV Phen HC	15 5 5	60 Several hours Minutes 15	25	2, 17
CLOSTRIDIUM SPORES (see Chapters 47 and 48)	Very resis-tant in environment		Heat Phen	5	10 10–12 hrs	120	5, 18
ACTINOMYCETES (see Chapter 53)			Heat		20	60	2
LEPTOSPIRA (see Chapter 45)			Heat		10	50	2
Protozoa **TOXOPLASMA CYSTS** (see Chapter 86)	4	68 days	Heat Freeze drying		10–15	56	19
ISOSPORA (CYSTOISOSPORA) (see Chapter 87)	25	24 hr	Heat		4 hr	50	20

APPENDIX 9: *Environmental Survival of Certain Microorganisms and Some Effective Biocidal Agents*[a] Continued

| TYPE OF MICROORGANISM | ENVIRONMENTAL SURVIVAL | | BIOCIDAL AGENT | | | | |
	Temperature (°C)	Time	Type	Concentration (%)	Time (min)	Temperature (°C)	Reference[b]
ENTAMOEBA HISTOLYTICA (see Chapter 84)							
Trophozoite	25	2–5 days	Heat		60–90	45	21
Cyst			Heat		5		22

[a]Alc = alcohol (methyl or ethyl); HC = Sodium hypochlorite (bleach); HI = iodophor; Phen = phenolic; QUAT = quaternary ammonium compound; AF = formaldehyde; AG = glutaraldehyde; Big = biguanide (chlorhexidine); LS = lipid solvent (ether or chloroform); UV = ultraviolet light (2537 Å.) (See Chapter 1 for a discussion of these disinfecting agents.)

[b]References refer to the following list:

1. Ott RL: Viral diseases. *In* Catcott EJ (ed): *Feline Medicine and Surgery*, ed 2. Santa Barbara, American Veterinary Publications, 1975, pp 17–62.
2. Buxton A, Fraser G: *Animal Microbiology*. Oxford, Blackwell Scientific Publications, 1977.
3. Scott FW: Virucidal disinfectants and feline viruses. *Am J Vet Res* 41:410–414, 1980.
4. Hirai K, Mihoshi A, Yagami K, et al: Isolation of a herpesvirus from a naturally occurring case with hemorrhagic and necrotizing lesions of puppies. *Res Bull Fac Agr Gifu Univ* 41:139–153, 1978.
5. Gillespie JH, Timoney JF: *Hagan and Bruner's Infectious Diseases of Domestic Animals*, ed 7. Ithaca, Cornell University Press, 1981.
6. Merchant IA, Packer RA: *Veterinary Bacteriology and Virology*, ed 7. Ames, Iowa State University Press, 1967.
7. Pollack RVH, Carmichael LE: Newer knowledge about canine parvovirus. *In Proceedings*. 30th Gaines Symposium, 36–40, 1981.
8. Joklik WK: The inactivation of viruses. *In* Joklik WK, Willett HP, Amos DB (eds): *Zinsser Microbiology*. ed 17. New York, Appleton-Century-Crofts, 1980, pp 1026–1029.
9. Larain NM: The mechanisms of immunity in canine virus hepatitis. *Br Vet J* 115:35–45, 1959.
10. Povey RC, Johnson RH: Observations on the epidemiology and control of viral respiratory disease in cats. *J Small Anim Pract* 11:485–494, 1970.
11. Rosen L: Reovirus group. *In* Horsfall FL, Lamm I (ed): *Viral and Rickettsial Diseases of Man*, ed 4. Philadelphia, JB Lippincott Co, 1965, pp 569–579.
12. Tan RJS, Miles JAR: Characterization of mycoplasmas isolated from cats with conjunctivitis. *NZ Vet J* 21:27–32, 1973.
13. Pelczar MJ, Reid RD: *Microbiology*, ed 2. New York, McGraw-Hill Book Co, 1965.
14. Smith IM: *Brucella* species (brucellosis). *In* Mandell GL, Douglas RG, Bennett JE (eds): *Principles and Practice of Infectious Diseases*. New York, John Wiley & Sons, 1979, pp 1772.
15. Wilfert CM: *Brucella*. *In* Joklik WK, Willett HP, Amos DB (eds): *Zinsser Microbiology*, ed 17. New York, Appleton-Century-Crofts, 1980, pp 796–803.
16. Joseland SW: Survival of *Salmonella typhi murium* in various substances under natural conditions. *Aust Vet J* 27:264–266, 1951.
17. Farer LS: *Mycobacterium tuberculosis*: bacteriology, epidemiology and treatment. *In* Mandell GL, Douglas RG, Bennett JE (eds): *Principles and Practice of Infectious Diseases*. New York, John Wiley & Sons, 1979, pp 1905–1925.
18. Osterhaut S, Willett HP: *Clostridium botulinum*. *In* Joklik WK, Willett HP, Amos DB (eds): *Zinsser Microbiology*, ed 17. New York, Appleton-Century-Crofts, 1980, pp 854–863.
19. Jacobs L, Remington JS, Melton ML: The resistance of the encysted form of *Toxoplasma gondii*. *J Parasitol* 46:11–21, 1960.
20. Mahrt JL: Sporogony of *Isospora rivolta* oocysts from the dog. *J Protozool* 15:35–45, 1968.
21. Jones MJ, Newton WI: The survival of cysts of *Entamoeba histolytica* in water at room temperatures between 45°C and 55°C. *Am J Trop Med* 30:53, 1950.
22. Caberra HA, Porter RJ: Survival time and critical temperatures of various strains of *Entamoeba histolytica*. *Exp Parasitol* 7:285–291, 1958.

APPENDIX 10.   Commercially Available Environmental Disinfectants and Their Uses

ACTIVE INGREDIENT	BRAND NAME	MANUFACTURER	DILUTION FOR KENNEL[a]	SUSCEPTIBLE ORGANISMS[b]
Halogens				
Sodium hypochlorite	Clorox	Clorox Co.	1:32	coronaviruses, parvoviruses, feline respiratory viruses, canine infectious tracheobronchitis viruses, *Coxiella burnetii*
Sodium chlorite	Alcide LD, ABQ	Alcide Corp.	undiluted	
Organic iodine	Betadine	Purdue Frederick	1:20 to 1:150	Canine adenoviruses
Aldehydes				
Glutaraldehyde	Sonacide, Cidex	Ayerst Labs	undiluted	*Coxiella burnetii, Clostridium*
Glutaraldehyde-phenate	Sporocidin	Sporocidin Int.	1:16	
Phenolics				
Ortho-benzyl-para-chlorophenol	O-syl Calgo-San	National Labs Calgon Corp.	1:128 1:128	*Salmonella*, canine adenoviruses
Quaternary Ammonium Compounds				
Octyl decyl dimethyl ammonium chloride Alkyl dimethyl benzyl ammonium chloride	Quatsyl 256 Totil-Plus Roccal-D Quintricide	National Labs Calgon Corp. Winthrop Vet Shorline Mfg.	1:256 1:128 1:200 1:128	*Brucella canis, Giardia* cysts
Biguanides				
Chlorhexidine diacetate	Nolvasan	Fort Dodge Labs	3:128	Canine infectious tracheobronchitis virus, feline respiratory viruses

[a]1:128 dilution approximates 1 ounce per gallon of water.

[b]All disinfectant categories listed are effective against canine distemper virus, feline leukemia and immunodeficiency viruses, rabies virus, herpesviruses, chlamydia, *Rickettsia, Leptospira*, and *Borrelia*.

APPENDIX 11. Infectious Disease Rule-Outs for Medical Problems[a]

INTEGUMENTAL PROBLEMS
Ulcerative, Fistulous, or Nodular Lesions

Canine viral papilloma (22)
Feline lymphosarcoma (26)
Feline immunodeficiency virus infection (26)
Feline cowpox virus infection (30)
Melioidosis (50)
Glanders (50)
L-form infections (50)
Mycobacterial infections (51)
Canine brucellosis (52)
Actinomycosis (53)
Nocardiosis (53)
Dermatophilosis (54)
Feline abscesses (55)
Streptococcal infections (56)
Staphylococcal infections (57)
Bite infections (58)
Plague (59)

Tularemia (60)
Blastomycosis (65)
Histoplasmosis (66)
Cryptococcosis (67)
Coccidioidomycosis (68)
Sporotrichosis (71)
Aspergillosis, disseminated (71)
Candidiasis, disseminated (72)
Trichosporosis (73)
Pythiosis (74)
Zygomycosis (74)
Pseudallescheriosis (74)
Phaeohyphomycosis (74)
Eumycotic mycetoma (74)
Prototothecosis (75)
Leishmaniasis (79)
Caryosporiosis, cutaneous coccidiosis (87)

Pruritus
Pseudorabies (32)

Pustular or Vesicular Lesions
Bacterial skin infections (5)
Canine distemper (16)
Canine herpesvirus infection, neonatal and adult (18)
Feline immunodeficiency virus infection (26)

Feline herpesvirus infection (27)
Streptococcal infections (56)
Staphylococcal infections (57)
Dermatophytosis (64)

Extremity Edema
Bacterial endocarditis (7)
Infectious canine hepatitis (17)
Canine ehrlichiosis (37)

Rocky Mountain spotted fever (38)
Aspergillosis, disseminated (71)
Babesiosis (83)

MUSCULOSKELETAL PROBLEMS

Muscle Inflammation
Anaerobic bacterial infections (6, 49)
Feline abscesses (55)
Trypanosomiasis (78)

Hepatozoonosis (80)
Toxoplasmosis (86)
Neosporosis (86)

Joint Inflammation
(Infectious or Immune-Mediated)
Bacterial skin infection (5)
Feline calicivirus infection (27)
Feline syncytial virus infection (28)
Canine ehrlichiosis (37)
Rocky Mountain spotted fever (38)
Mycoplasmal infections (41)
Endotoxemia (44)
Canine Lyme borreliosis (46)

L-form infections (50)
Actinomycosis (53)
Feline abscesses (55)
Streptococcal infections (56)
Coccidioidomycosis (68)
Aspergillosis, disseminated (71)
Leishmaniasis (79)

Bone Inflammation
(Osteomyelitis, Periostitis)
Bacterial or fungal discospondylitis (6)
Anaerobic bacterial infections (49)
Mycobacterial infections (51)
Actinomycosis (53)
Nocardiosis (53)
Feline abscesses (55)
Staphylococcal infections (57)

Blastomycosis (65)
Histoplasmosis (66)
Coccidioidomycosis (68)
Aspergillosis, disseminated (71)
Candidiasis, disseminated (72)
Phaeohyphomycosis (74)
Leishmaniasis (79)
Hepatozoonosis (80)

Continued on following page

APPENDIX 11.   Infectious Disease Rule-Outs
for Medical Problems[a] Continued

CARDIOVASCULAR PROBLEMS

Heart Muscle
(Cardiomyopthy, Myocarditis)

Bacterial endocarditis (7)
Canine distemper, neonatal (16)
Canine parvovirus infection, neonatal or prenatal (21)
Pseudorabies (32)
Rocky Mountain spotted fever (38)
Canine Lyme borreliosis (46)

Streptococcal infection, neonatal (56)
Coccidioidomycosis (68)
Trypanosomiasis (78)
Hepatozoonosis (80)
Toxoplasmosis (86)

RESPIRATORY PROBLEMS

Upper Respiratory
(Rhinitis, Sinusitis, Tracheobronchitis)

Bacterial respiratory infections (8)
Canine distemper (16)
Canine adenovirus-2 infection, also adenovirus-1 (17)
Canine herpesvirus infection (18)
Canine tracheobronchitis (19)
Bordetella infection (19)
Canine parainfluenza (20)
Feline immunodeficiency virus infection (26)
Feline rhinotracheitis (27)
Feline calicivirus infection (27)

Salmon poisoning disease (36)
Canine ehrlichiosis (37)
Rocky Mountain spotted fever (38)
Chlamydial infection (40)
Mycoplasmal infection (41)
Staphylococcal infection (56)
Cryptococcosis (67)
Rhinosporidiosis (70)
Aspergillosis, nasal (71)
Trichosporosis (73)

Radiographic/Pulmonary Pattern
(Alveolar-Interstitial)

Bacterial pneumonia (8)
Streptococcal pneumonia (8, 56)
EF-4 infection (8)
Canine distemper (16)
Infectious canine hepatitis (17)
Feline calicivirus infection (27)

Endotoxemia (44)
Mycobacterial infections (51)
Plague (59)
Toxoplasmosis (86)
Pneumocystosis (89)

(Interstitial)

Canine adenovirus-2 infection (17)
Canine herpesvirus infection (18)
Canine parainfluenza (19)
Feline calicivirus infection (27)

Canine ehrlichiosis (37)
Rocky Mountain spotted fever (38)
Leishmaniasis (79)

(Interstitial-Nodular)

Melioidosis (50)
Glanders (50)
Mycobacterial infections (51)
Blastomycosis (65)

Histoplasmosis (66)
Cryptococcosis (67)
Coccidioidomycosis (68)
Acanthamebiasis (85)

Pleural Effusion

Bacterial pyothorax (8)
Feline infectious peritonitis (24)
Feline viral neoplasia (26)
Anaerobic bacterial infections (49)

Actinomycosis (53)
Nocardiosis (53)
Feline abscesses (55)
Toxoplasmosis (86)

GASTROINTESTINAL PROBLEMS

Oral Ulcerative or Vesicular Lesions

Chronic ulcerative stomatitis (9)
Canine herpesvirus infection (18)
Canine parvovirus infection (21)
Feline leukemia virus infection (26)
Feline immunodeficiency virus infection (26)

Feline rhinotracheitis (27)
Feline calicivirus infection (27)
Rocky Mountain spotted fever (38)
Leptospirosis (45)
Candidiasis (72)

Dental Enamel Hypoplasia

Canine distemper (16)

Feline panleukopenia (23)

APPENDIX 11. *Infectious Disease Rule-Outs for Medical Problems*[a] Continued

GASTROINTESTINAL PROBLEMS Continued

Icterus, Hepatomegaly, Hepatic Failure

Hepatic abscesses (10)
Cholangitis/cholangiohepatitis (10)
Infectious canine hepatitis (17)
Canine herpesvirus infection, neonatal (18)
Feline infectious peritonitis (24)
Feline viral neoplasia (26)
Feline herpesvirus infection, neonatal (27)
Haemobartonellosis (39)

Leptospirosis (45)
Tyzzer's disease (50)
Mycobacterial infections (51)
Streptococcal infections, neonatal (56)
Histoplasmosis (66)
Encephalitozoonosis (81)
Cytauxzoonosis (82)
Babesiosis (83)
Toxoplasmosis (86)

Vomiting

Intra-abdominal infections (9)
Cholangitis/cholangiohepatitis (10)
Canine distemper (16)
Infectious canine hepatitis (17)
Canine herpesvirus infection, neonatal (18)
Canine parvovirus infection (21)
Feline panleukopenia (23)
Feline infectious peritonitis (24)
Feline lymphosarcoma (26)

Salmon poisoning disease (36)
Rocky Mountain spotted fever (38)
Leptospirosis (45)
Salmonellosis (50)
Shigellosis (50)
Campylobacteriosis (50)
Tyzzer's disease (50)
Mycobacterial infections (51)
Listeriosis (56)
Pythiosis (74)

Diarrhea

Enteric infections (9)
Bacterial overgrowth (9)
Canine distemper (16)
Paramyxoviral infection (20)
Canine viral enteritis (21)
Feline panleukopenia (23)
Astroviral infection (25)
Rotaviral infection (25)
Feline lymphosarcoma (26)
Feline immunodeficiency virus infection (26)
Enterovirus infections (33)
Salmon poisoning disease (36)
Endotoxemia (44)
Leptospirosis (45)

Salmonellosis (50)
Shigellosis (50)
Campylobacteriosis (50)
Tyzzer's disease (50)
Yersiniosis, intestinal (50)
Listeriosis (56)
Histoplasmosis (66)
Protothecosis (75)
Giardiasis (84)
Balantidiasis (84)
Amebiasis (84)
Trichomoniasis (84)
Toxoplasmosis (86)
Coccidiosis (87)
Cryptosporidiosis (88)

Acute Abdominal Pain

Intra-abdominal infections (9)
Infectious canine hepatitis, acute (17)
Canine herpesvirus infection, neonatal (18)
Feline panleukopenia (23)

Feline infectious peritonitis (24)
Rocky Mountain spotted fever (38)
Leptospirosis (45)
Salmonellosis (50)

Abdominal Effusion

Intra-abdominal infections (9)
Infectious canine hepatitis (17)
Feline infectious peritonitis (24)
Feline lymphosarcoma (26)
Anaerobic bacterial infections (49)
Actinomycosis (53)

Nocardiosis (53)
Streptococcal infections, neonatal (56)
Histoplasmosis (66)
Trypanosomiasis (78)
Toxoplasmosis (86)

Abdominal Mass

Intra-abdominal infections (9)
Hepatic abscesses (10)
Feline infectious peritonitis (24)
Feline viral neoplasia (26)
Mycobacterial infections (51)
Actinomycosis (53)

Nocardiosis (53)
Histoplasmosis (66)
Coccidioidomycosis (68)
Pythiosis (74)
Zygomycosis (74)
Toxoplasmosis (86)

Continued on following page

APPENDIX 11.   *Infectious Disease Rule-Outs*
for Medical Problems[a] Continued

URINARY PROBLEMS
Renal Failure

Pyelonephritis (11)
Feline lymphosarcoma (26)
Canine ehrlichiosis (37)
Rocky Mountain spotted fever (38)
Leptospirosis (45)

Canine Lyme borreliosis (46)
Coccidioidomycosis (68)
Leishmaniasis (79)
Encephalitozoonosis (81)
Babesiosis (83)

GENITAL PROBLEMS
Scrotal Enlargement or Drainage

Orchitis, epididymitis (11)
Feline infectious peritonitis (24)
Canine ehrlichiosis (37)

Rocky Mountain spotted fever (38)
Canine brucellosis (52)
Blastomycosis (65)

Reproductive Failure, Infertility, Abortion, Birth of Ill (Fading) Neonates

Pyometra, endometritis (11)
Canine distemper (16)
Canine herpesvirus infection (18)
Canine parvovirus-1 infection (21)
Feline panleukopenia (23)
Feline infectious peritonitis (24)
Feline leukemia virus infection (26)

Feline herpesvirus infection (17)
Q fever (38)
Salmonellosis (50)
Canine brucellosis (42)
Streptococcal infection, neonatal (56)
Toxoplasmosis (86)

HEMOLYMPHATIC PROBLEMS
Lymphadenopathy

Bacteremia, any type (7)
Canine distemper (16)
Infectious canine hepatitis, acute (17)
Canine viral papillomatosus (22)
Feline infectious peritonitis, mesenteric (24)
Feline leukemia virus infection (26)
Feline immunodeficiency virus infection (26)
Mumps virus infection (34)
Salmon-poisoning disease (36)
Canine ehrlichiosis (37)
Rocky Mountain spotted fever (38)
Q fever (38)
Salmonellosis (50)
Melioidosis (50)
Glanders (50)
L-form infections (50)
Mycobacterial infections (51)
Canine brucellosis (52)
Actinomycosis (53)
Nocardiosis (53)

Streptococcal infections (56)
Plague (59)
Tularemia (60)
Cat scratch disease (61)
Blastomycosis (65)
Histoplasmosis (66)
Cryptococcosis (67)
Coccidioidomycosis (68)
Sporotrichosis (69)
Aspergillosis, disseminated (71)
Candidiasis (72)
Trichosporosis (73)
Pythiosis (74)
Zygomycosis (74)
Phaeohyphomycosis (74)
Prototothecosis (75)
Trypanosomiasis (78)
Leishmaniasis (79)
Encephalitozoonosis (81)
Cytauxzoonosis (82)
Babesiosis (83)
Toxoplasmosis (86)

Splenomegaly

Bacteremia, any type (7)
Feline leukemia virus infection (26)
Feline immunodeficiency virus infection (26)
Canine ehrlichiosis (37)
Rocky Mountain spotted fever (38)
Q fever (38)
Haemobartonellosis (39)

Endotoxemia (44)
Mycobacterial infections (51)
Plague (59)
Tularemia (60)
Trypanosomiasis (78)
Leishmaniasis (79)
Cytauxzoonosis (82)
Babesiosis (83)

APPENDIX 11. Infectious Disease Rule-Outs for Medical Problems[a] Continued

HEMOLYMPHATIC PROBLEMS Continued

Immunodeficiency
See Table 3–3

Anemia

Regenerative
Feline leukemia virus infection (26)
Feline immunodeficiency virus infection (26)
Haemobartonellosis (39)
Hepatozoonosis (80)
Cytauxzoonosis (82)
Babesiosis (83)

Nonregenerative
Feline infectious peritonitis (24)
Feline leukemia virus infection (26)
Feline immunodeficiency virus infection (26)
Canine ehrlichiosis (37)
Histoplasmosis (66)
Leishmaniasis (79)

Circulating Cellular Inclusions

Bacteremia (7)
Canine distemper, lymphocytes, polychromatophilic erythrocytes (16)
Feline infectious peritonitis, neutrophils (24)
Canine ehrlichiosis, neutrophils, lymphocytes or platelets (37)
Haemobartonellosis, erythrocytes (39)
Histoplasmosis, monocytes or neutrophils (66)

Trypanosomiasis, monocytes (78)
Leishmaniasis, monocytes (79)
Hepatozoonosis, neutrophils and monocytes (80)
Cytauxzoonosis, erythrocytes (82)
Babesiosis, erythrocytes (83)
Toxoplasmosis, leukocytes (86)

Persistent Lymphopenia

Bacteremia (7)
Canine distemper, acute (16)
Canine parvovirus infection (21)
Feline leukemia virus infection (26)

Feline immunodeficiency virus infection (26)
Canine ehrlichiosis (37)

Leukocytosis

Bacteremia (7)
Canine herpesvirus infection, neonatal (18)
Feline infectious peritonitis (24)
Feline viral neoplasia (26)
Feline leukemia virus infection (26)
Salmon poisoning disease (36)
Rocky Mountain spotted fever (38)
Leptospirosis (45)
Anaerobic bacterial infections (49)
Salmonellosis (50)
Actinomycosis (53)
Nocardiosis (53)

Feline abscesses (55)
Streptococcal infections, neonatal (56)
Staphylococcal infections (57)
Plague (59)
Blastomycosis (65)
Histoplasmosis (66)
Coccidioidomycosis (68)
Aspergillosis (71)
Candidiasis, disseminated (72)
Hepatozoonosis (80)
Acanthamebiasis (85)

Neutropenia

Bacteremia (7)
Canine parvovirus infection (21)
Feline panleukopenia (23)
Feline leukemia virus infection (26)
Feline immunodeficiency virus infection (26)

Salmon poisoning disease (36)
Canine ehrlichiosis (37)
Endotoxemia (44)
Salmonellosis, acute (50)

Thrombocytopenia (Petechial Hemorrhages)

Primary
Feline leukemia virus infection (26)
Canine ehrlichiosis, chronic (37)

Associated with DIC-Increased Consumption
Bacteremia (7)
Infectious canine hepatitis (17)
Canine herpesvirus infection, neonatal (18)
Canine parvovirus infection (21)
Feline panleukopenia (23)
Feline infectious peritonitis (24)
Feline leukemia virus infection (26)
Canine ehrlichiosis, acute or chronic (37)
Ehrlichia platys infection (37)
Rocky Mountain spotted fever (38)
Endotoxemia (44)
Leptospirosis (45)
Salmonellosis (50)
Histoplasmosis (66)
Babesiosis (83)

Continued on following page

APPENDIX 11. Infectious Disease Rule-Outs
for Medical Problems[a] Continued

MISCELLANEOUS LABORATORY PROBLEMS

Increased Liver Enzymes

Cholangiohepatitis (10)
Hepatic abscesses (10)
Infectious canine hepatitis (17)
Canine herpesvirus infection, neonatal (18)
Feline panleukopenia (23)
Feline infectious peritonitis (24)
Feline lymphosarcoma (26)
Feline myeloproliferative disease (26)
Canine ehrlichiosis (37)

Rocky Mountain spotted fever (38)
Endotoxemia (44)
Leptospirosis (45)
Tyzzer's disease (50)
Histoplasmosis (66)
Aspergillosis, disseminated (71)
Trypanosomiasis (78)
Hepatozoonosis (80)
Babesiosis (83)
Toxoplasmosis (86)

Feline leukemia virus infection (26)
Canine ehrlichiosis (37)

Positive Coombs' Testing

Haemobartonellosis (39)
Babesiosis (83)

Azotemia

Pyelonephritis (11)
Canine herpesvirus infection, neonatal (18)
Feline leukemia virus infection (26)
Canine ehrlichiosis, chronic (37)
Rocky Mountain spotted fever (38)

Endotoxemia (44)
Leptospirosis (45)
Canine Lyme borreliosis (46)
Coccidioidomycosis (68)
Encephalitozoonosis (81)
Babesiosis (83)

Icterus

Cholangiohepatitis (10)
Infectious canine hepatitis (17)
Feline infectious peritonitis (24)
Feline leukemia virus infection (26)
Endotoxemia (44)
Leptospirosis (45)

Tyzzer's disease (50)
Histoplasmosis (66)
Cytauxzoonosis (82)
Babesiosis (83)
Toxoplasmosis (86)

Hyperfibrinogenemia

Feline infectious peritonitis (24)

Bacterial endocarditis (7)

Proteinuria

Rocky Mountain spotted fever (38)
Leptospirosis (45)
Canine Lyme borreliosis (46)
Coccidioidomycosis (68)
Leishmaniasis (79)

Bacteremia (7)
Urinary tract infections (11)
Infectious canine hepatitis (17)
Feline infectious peritonitis (24)
Feline leukemia virus infection (26)
Canine ehrlichiosis (37)

Hypoalbuminemia

Rocky Mountain spotted fever (38)
Endotoxemia (44)
Salmonellosis (45)
Blastomycosis (65)
Histoplasmosis (66)

Bacteremia (7)
Canine parvovirus infection (21)
Feline infectious peritonitis (24)
Feline viral neoplasia (26)
Salmon poisoning disease (36)
Canine ehrlichiosis (37)

Hypoglobulinemia

Canine distemper, neonatal or prenatal (16)

Hyperglobulinemia

Bacteremia (7)
Chronic ulcerative stomatitis (9)
Cholangiohepatitis (10)
Feline infectious peritonitis (24)
Feline viral neoplasia (26)
Feline immunodeficiency virus infection (26)
Canine ehrlichiosis (37)

Canine brucellosis (52)
Blastomycosis (65)
Histoplasmosis (66)
Cryptococcosis (67)
Coccidioidomycosis (68)
Leishmaniasis (79)
Encephalitozoonosis (81)

Hypoglycemia

Hepatozoonosis (80)

Bacteremia (7)
Actinomycosis (53)

APPENDIX 11. *Infectious Disease Rule-Outs for Medical Problems*[a] Continued

CNS PROBLEMS

Primary Meningitis/Secondary Encephalitis

Bacterial meningitis (12)
Brain abscesses (12)
Feline infectious peritonitis (24)
Canine ehrlichiosis (37)
Rocky Mountain spotted fever (38)
Anaerobic bacterial infections (49)
Canine brucellosis (52)
Actinomycosis (53)
Feline abscesses (55)
Listeriosis (56)
Blastomycosis (65)

Histoplasmosis (66)
Cryptococcosis (67)
Coccidioidomycosis (68)
Zygomycosis (74)
Phaeohyphomycosis (74)
Protothecosis (75)
Encephalitozoonosis (81)
Babesiosis (83)
Acanthamebiasis (85)
Granulomatous meningoencephalitis (90)
Pug encephalitis (90)

Primary Encephalitis/Secondary Meningitis

Canine distemper (16)
Infectious canine hepatitis (17)
Canine herpesvirus infection,
  neonatal and prenatal (18)
Canine paramyxovirus encephalitis (20)
Feline panleukopenia, neonatal and prenatal (23)
Feline paramyxovirus infection (29)

Rabies (31)
Pseudorabies (32)
Arbovirus infections (35)
Louping ill (35)
Babesiosis (83)
Toxoplasmosis (86)
Neosporosis (86)
Feline poliomyelitis (90)

CSF Results

CSF Protein and Mononuclear Cells

Canine distemper (16)
Paramyxoviral encephalitis (20, 29)
Rabies (31)
Pseudorabies (32)
Arboviral infections (35)
Canine ehrlichiosis (37)
Granulomatous meningoencephalitis (90)
Feline polioencephalomyelitis (90)
Pug encephalitis (90)
Hydrocephalus with periventricular encephalitis (90)

CSF Protein and Neutrophils

Feline infectious peritonitis (24)
Rocky Mountain spotted fever (38)
Canine brucellosis (52)
Listeriosis (56)
Blastomycosis (65)
Cryptococcosis (67)
Phaeohyphomycosis (74)
Protothecosis (75)
Encephalitozoonosis (81)
Toxoplasmosis (86)
Neosporosis (86)

Epidural or Extradural Compression of Spinal Cord/Discospondylitis

Feline lymphosarcoma (26)
Canine brucellosis (52)
Actinomycosis (53)
Feline abscesses (55)

Staphylococcal infections (57)
Aspergillosis (71)
Paecilomycosis (74)

Hydrocephalus

Canine paramyxovirus encephalitis (20)
Feline infectious peritonitis (24)

Periventricular encephalitis (90)

Ocular Problems
See Table 13–5

[a]For further discussion, refer to chapters designated in parentheses.

Some Preservation, Staining, and Microscopy Techniques for Infectious Disease Agents

STAINING PROCEDURES

Gram Stain

Uses: Bacterial classification

Reagents

1. Crystal (gentian) violet solution
Crystal violet, 99% dye content	10 g
Methanol, absolute	500 ml
2. Iodine solution
Iodine crystals	6 g
Potassium iodide	12 g
Distilled water	1800 ml
3. Decolorizer
   Ethanol, 95%
4. Counterstain
Safranin, 99% dye content	10 g
Distilled water	1000 ml

Procedure

1. Air-dry smears on clean microscope slides, and heat fix by passing over a flame.
2. Flood slides with crystal violet solution for 1 minute, and rinse slides with tap water.
3. Flood slides with iodine solution for 10 seconds, and rinse with tap water.
4. Decolorize until no more color comes off thin areas, and rinse with tap water.
5. Flood slides with counterstain for 10 seconds, rinse slides with tap water, drain, and blot dry.

Interpretation: Gram-positive organisms stain blue; gram-negative organisms stain red.

Acid-Fast Stain (Kinyoun Carbol Fuchsin)

Uses: Mycobacterial and actinomycetes,[a] demonstration of cryptosporidial oocysts

Reagents

1. Carbol fuchsin
Basic fuchsin	4 g
Phenol, melted	8 ml
Ethanol, 95%	20 ml
Distilled water	68 ml

   Mix phenol, ethanol, and 50 ml of water in a bottle with a stopper. Add dye and shake. Allow to stand overnight at room temperature. Add the remaining water and filter through coarse paper. Store in stoppered bottle.
2. Decolorizer
Hydrochloric acid, concentrated	12 ml
Ethanol, 95%	388 ml
3. Counterstain
Methylene blue	4 g[a]
Water	400 ml

Procedure

1. Air-dry smears on clean microscope slides, and heat fix by passing over a flame.
2. Cover slides with strips of coarse filter paper, and flood with carbol fuchsin for 5 minutes.
3. Remove the filter paper, and rinse slides with tap water.
4. Decolorize until thick areas of the smear are clear.
5. Rinse the slides with tap water.
6. Flood the slides with counterstain for 1 minute.
7. Rinse with tap water, drain, and blot dry.

Interpretation: Acid-fast organisms stain red. The background and other organisms stain blue.

New Methylene Blue Stain

Uses: Rapid cytologic staining. Poor for bacterial or protozoal staining. Some fungal elements can be identified with this procedure.

Reagents
New methylene blue (powdered)	0.5 g
Physiologic saline (0.85%)	100 ml
Formalin, concentrated	1 ml

Filter and store the stain in a dark bottle. It can be used immediately and has a long shelf-life if evaporation is prevented.

Procedure

1. Prepare blood film or impression smear on a clean glass microscope slide and allow to air dry.
2. Add a drop of stain to a clean coverglass, and place the coverglass on the slide. Avoid air bubble formation.

The wet-mount is ready for immediate microscopic examination. The stain is not permanent but can be preserved for a few hours if the coverglass is ringed with nail polish.

Lactophenol Cotton Blue Stain

Uses: To aid in the microscopic detection of fungal elements in culture

Reagents
Phenol, crystals	20 g
Lactic acid	20 g
Glycerin	40 g
Distilled water	20 ml
Cotton blue dye	0.05 g

Mix lactic acid, glycerin, and water; then add phenol and dissolve, gently heating over a water bath. Add the dye when ingredients are completely dissolved.

Procedure

1. Place a drop of lactophenol cotton blue stain on a clean microscope slide.
2. Place a small piece of the specimen in the stain and gently tease apart with clean teasing needles.
3. Gently lower a coverslip; do not push down, but allow the stain to flow to the edges of the coverslip.
4. Wipe the excess stain from the edges of the coverslip, and seal the coverslip with nail polish. If properly prepared, this preparation will keep for months.

KOH Solution

Uses: For clearing of tissue preparations to visualize fungal arthrospores

Reagents
Potassium hydroxide	10–20 g
Distilled water	100 ml

---

[a]For actinomycetes, use 2.5% methylene blue in 95% ethyl alcohol as counterstain. *Nocardia* stain acid-fast.

916

APPENDIX 12. Some Preservation, Staining, and Microscopy Techniques for Infectious Disease Agents Continued

STAINING PROCEDURES Continued

Procedure

1. Mix the specimen (tissue or exudate) with a drop of the solution on a clean slide. Cover with a coverglass and press to make a thin mount. Slight warming with a flame may help clearing. Ten minutes to 24 hours may be required for clearing, depending on the viscosity of the specimen. Keep the slide in a moist chamber for prolonged incubation.
2. Scan under low power with reduced lighting. Switch to high power to check for fungal elements.

Lugol's Solution

Uses: For staining direct fecal smear for *Giardia*. Used as a component in the merthiolate-iodine-formalin solution below.

Reagents

Iodine, crystals	5 g
Potassium iodide	10 g
Distilled water	100 ml

Add iodine crystals after potassium iodide has dissolved in water, filter, and store in a brown bottle. *Dilute 2 to 4 times with water immediately before use for direct smears.* Overstaining may obscure internal structures. (See Merthiolate-Iodine-Formalin Preservative for additional use.)

Methylene Blue in Acetate Buffer

Uses: Protozoal identification (does not stain other organisms well)

Reagents

Methylene blue	0.06 g
Acetate buffer is mixture of two stock solutions:	
1. 0.02 M acetic acid	
Glacial acetic acid	11.55 ml
Distilled water	1000 ml
2. 0.2 M sodium acetate	
Sodium acetate	
$NaC_2H_3O_2$	16.0 g
or	
$NaC_2H_3O_2 \cdot 3H_2O$	27.2 g
Distilled water	1000 ml

Mix 46.3 ml of acetate buffer solution 1 and 3.7 ml of acetate buffer solution 2, add 50 ml of distilled water, and then add dye.

Procedure

Allow 5 to 10 minutes for stain to penetrate the organism. The cytoplasm stains light blue and the nucleus stains darker blue. Examine within 30 minutes of staining.

Acid Methyl Green

Uses: Identification of *Balantidium coli*

Reagents

Methyl green	4 g
Glacial acetic acid	1 ml
Distilled water	100 ml

Interpretation: Protozoal nuclei stain bright green, whereas the cytoplasm is colorless to bluish gray.

Giemsa Stain and Buffer Solutions

Uses: For cytologic demonstration of viral, mycoplasmal, chlamydial, and ehrlichial inclusions and *Leishmania* and *Trypanosoma* in blood films

Reagents

Giemsa stain is commercially available as a ready-to-use stain or can be made using the following formula:

Giemsa powder	3.41 g
Glycerin	222 ml
Methanol, absolute	225 ml

Add Giemsa powder to glycerin a little at a time. Allow to stand overnight in a water bath at 55° C. Add methanol. The stain must age for 2 months before it can be used. Filter before use.

The working buffer is composed of 2 stock solutions:

1. Monobasic phosphate buffer	
Potassium phosphate, monobasic	9.07 g
Distilled water	1000 ml
2. Disodium phosphate buffer	
Disodium phosphate	9.59 g
Distilled water	1000 ml

Mix 3.5 ml of solution 1 and 9 ml of solution 2 immediately before use.

Working stain:	
Giemsa stain	1 ml
Working buffer	5 ml
Distilled water	45 ml

Giemsa-Staining Thin Blood Films

1. Fix blood films that are completely dry in absolute methanol for 3 minutes.
2. Place slides in working stain for 25 to 30 minutes.
3. Place container under running tap water until all stain is removed. This will prevent stain precipitates from adhering to the films.

Giemsa-Staining Thick Blood Films

1. Omit step 1 in previous procedure.
2. Continue as for thin blood films.

Wright's Stain and Buffer

Uses: For staining blood films and cytologic specimens for cellular morphology and presence of viral inclusions, rickettsia *(Ehrlichia)*, bacteria, fungi, or protozoa

Reagents

Wright's stain is commercially available as a ready-to-use stain or can be made using the following formula:

Wright's stain powder	0.3 g
Glycerin	3 ml
Methanol, absolute	100 ml

Mix Wright's powder with glycerin in a mortar and pestle and grind thoroughly. Rinse mortar with small amounts of methanol and pour into a dark container. Mix with a magnetic stirrer for about 1 week, but do not heat. Filter before use.

Continued on following page

APPENDIX 12.   Some Preservation, Staining, and Microscopy Techniques for Infectious Disease Agents Continued

STAINING PROCEDURES Continued

Phosphate buffer:

Monobasic potassium phosphate	5.47 g
Dibasic sodium phosphate	3.80 g

Distilled water to bring to a total volume of 1000 ml in a volumetric flask.

Wright's-Staining Thin Blood Films
1. Allow film to dry completely before staining.
2. Place slide on a level rack in a horizontal position, and cover the film completely with stain. Do not allow adjacent slides to touch each other or slides to dry during the procedure. Stain for 1 to 3 minutes.
2. Add an equal amount of buffer and blow on the slide to ensure thorough mixing. A metallic green sheen should form. Allow to stand for 3 to 5 minutes.
4. Flood the slide with water to rinse metallic scum from surface. Do not pour the buffer off, as this will leave staining precipitates on the film.

Wright's-Staining Thick Blood Films
The staining procedure is the same as described above; however, thick films must be laked in water prior to staining in Wright's stain. In addition, the staining time may need to be increased. Care should be taken to prevent excess precipitate formation during the water rinse.

Gimenez Stain for Rickettsiae
Uses: Staining of Chlamydiae and rickettsiae

Reagents

Stock carbol fuchsin contains

10% (wt/vol) fuchsin		100 ml
Fuchsin	10 g	
Ethanol, 95%	100 ml	
4% (vol/vol) aqueous phenol		250 ml
Phenol	4 ml	
Distilled water	100 ml	
Distilled water		650 ml

This stock solution should be held at 37°C for 48 hours before use.

Phosphate buffer (pH 7.45)

0.2 M NaH$_2$PO$_4$	3.5 ml
0.2 M Na$_2$HPO$_4$	15.5 ml
Distilled water	19 ml

Working stain solution is composed of the stock solution diluted 1:2.5 with the phosphate buffer. The working solution is immediately filtered and is filtered again before every stain. It is usable for 3 to 4 days.

Counterstain

Malachite green	0.8 g
Distilled water	100 ml

Procedure
1. Heat-fix the smear.
2. Stain with fuchsin for 1 to 2 minutes.
3. Wash with tap water.
4. Stain with malachite green for 6 to 9 seconds.
5. Wash with tap water.
6. Restain with malachite green for 6 to 9 seconds.
7. Wash with tap water and blot dry.

Interpretation: Most elementary bodies will stain red against a greenish background.

DMSO-Modified Acid-Fast Stain for Cryptosporidia

Uses: Demonstration of cryptosporidial oocysts in feces

Reagents

Stain 1: primary stain

Fuchsin crystals	4 g
Ethanol, 95%–99%	25 ml
Phenol crystals	12 g
Glycerin	25 ml
DMSO	25 ml

Mix fuchsin, alcohol, and phenol, then glycerin, DMSO, and add water to volume of 160 ml. Mix well and let stand 30 minutes, then filter. Store in brown screw-capped bottle at room temperature.

Stain 2: decolorizer, counterstain

Light or malachite green	4.4 g
Glacial acetic acid	30 ml
Glycerin	50 ml
Distilled water	220 ml

Mix green dye and water, then add acetic acid and glycerin. No need to filter. Store in capped bottle at room temperature.

Procedure
1. Mix feces with 10% formalin solution.
2. Concentrate oocysts by sedimentation or flotation.
3. Apply fecal extract to slide.
4. Fix 9 to 10 seconds in absolute methanol.
5. Place in stain 1 for 5 minutes.
6. Rinse with tap water, and drain excess water.

Interpretation: Oocysts stain pink to red. They are 4 to 6 μm and may be round or oval with internal vacuole or residual bodies that clump to the side. Sporozoites may be seen internally. Ghosts (empty cysts) may stain partially. Yeasts and WBC stain blue-green.

FIXATION PROCEDURES

Michel's Medium
Uses: Preservation of tissue specimens for immunofluorescent detection of antibodies

Reagents

Buffer is a mixture of three stock solutions:
1. 1 M potassium citrate buffer (pH 7.0)

Potassium citrate	3.240 g
Distilled water	10 ml

2. 0.1 M magnesiun sulfate

Magnesium sulfate	0.120 g
Distilled water	10 ml

3. 0.1 M N-ethylmaleimide

N-ethylmaleimide	0.125 g
Distilled water	10 ml

APPENDIX 12.   Some Preservation, Staining, and Microscopy Techniques for Infectious Disease Agents Continued

FIXATION PROCEDURES

Make up each of the above solutions in a separate flask, then mix 2.5 ml of solution 1, 5.0 ml of solution 2, and 5.0 ml of solution 3 with 87.5 ml of distilled water. Adjust the final pH to 7.0 with 1 M KOH or HCl.

Fixative	
$(NH_4)_2SO_4$	55 g
Buffer	100 ml

Fixative must be between pH 7.0 and 7.2; adjust with 1M KOH or HCl. It has a long shelf-life. For use for skin biopsy specimens for immunofluorescent testing.

Bouin's Fixative

Uses: For optimal fixation of ocular tissue

Reagents

Picric acid, saturated aqueous solution	75 ml
Formalin, concentrated	25 ml
Acetic acid, glacial	5 ml

Extreme caution should be used when handling picric acid since it is highly explosive—it MUST be handled as a saturated solution.

The fixative is rapid acting, but it is advisable to leave the tissues in the solution for several hours. It is best not to leave the specimen in the fixative for longer than 4 to 5 days. Transfer the specimen from Bouin's fixative to 50% alcohol and then to 70% alcohol. Wash repeatedly with changes of 70% alcohol, not water.

Polyvinyl Alcohol Preservative

Uses: Preservation of feces
Reagents

Polyvinyl alcohol (PVA, Elvanol 71-24)	10 g
Ethanol, 95%	62.5 ml
Mercuric chloride, saturated aqueous	125 ml
Glacial acetic acid	10 ml
Glycerin	3 ml

Mix liquid ingredients, then add PVA, but do not stir. Cover the container and allow to stand undisturbed overnight. Slowly heat the solution to 75° to 80°C. Remove from heat and swirl the container for 30 seconds or until the solution becomes homogeneous and milky.

Procedure
1. For bulk fixation of feces mix 1 part feces with 9 parts PVA preservative and store in brown bottles.
2. For fecal smears
   a. Place a small amount of feces on a clean microscope slide.
   b. Add 3 drops of PVA preservative and mix with feces using an applicator stick.
   c. Spread the material over one third of the slide and dry in an incubator at 37°C overnight. Slides must be completely dry before staining.
   d. Stain slides immediately or store for subsequent staining.

Merthiolate-Iodine-Formalin Preservative

Uses: Preservation of feces and staining of parasitic eggs and oocysts
This fixative is composed of two stock solutions that are mixed immediately before use.

Reagents
1. Merthiolate-formalin solution

Distilled water	50 ml
Formaldehyde (USP)	5 ml
Tincture or merthiolate, 1:1000	40 ml
Glycerin	1 ml

2. Lugol's solution (formula appears earlier in this appendix)

Mix 9.4 ml of solution 1 with 0.6 ml of solution 2 just before use.

Procedure
1. Add 1 g of feces to preservative and mix with an applicator stick.
2. Allow to stand undisturbed overnight. Three distinct layers will form. The top layer is a mixture of water and formaldehyde. The second layer (the interface) may contain some parasites; however, most protozoa will be found throughout the bottom layer.
3. Using a pipet, withdraw samples from the middle and bottom layers and examine systematically.

FECAL CONCENTRATION PROCEDURES

Sheather's Sugar Flotation Solution

Uses: Flotation of protozoal oocysts

Reagents

Sugar	2268 g (5 lb)
Distilled water	1452 ml
Phenol, crystals melted in hot water bath	29.5 g

Procedure
1. Soften feces with water and strain through a tea strainer or 2 layers of cheesecloth.

2. Thoroughly mix the aqueous fecal suspension with twice the volume of sugar solution.
3. Pour into a centrifuge tube, add enough sugar solution to form a meniscus on the top of the tube, and place a coverslip on the top of the tube.
4. Balance the tubes in the centrifuge and centrifuge at 300 × g for 10 minutes.
5. Remove the coverslip and place it on a clean slide.

Focus on the air bubbles; organisms and air bubbles adhere to the coverslip. Slides sealed with nail polish

Continued on following page

APPENDIX 12. Some Preservation, Staining, and Microscopy Techniques for Infectious Disease Agents Continued

FECAL CONCENTRATION PROCEDURES Continued

will keep for weeks, although some resistant nematode eggs will embryonate (e.g., *Toxocara canis*).

Zinc Sulfate Solution (Specific gravity = 1.18)

Uses: Flotation of *Giardia* cysts

Reagents

Zinc sulfate	300 g
Distilled water	670 ml

This formula approximates the proper specific gravity.

Procedure

1. Thoroughly mix 1 g of feces with 2 ml of water and pour into a centrifuge tube, filling the tube to within 2 mm of the top with water.
2. Balance the tubes in the centrifuge and centrifuge at 300 × g for 1 minute.
3. Pour off supernatant, and add 2 ml of zinc sulfate solution. Mix thoroughly, and fill the tube with zinc sulfate solution to within 2 mm of the top.
4. Strain the suspension through a tea strainer or two layers of cheesecloth.
5. Return the strained suspension to the centrifuge tube. A few drops of Lugol's iodine may be added at this time. Formula for Lugol's iodine appears earlier in this appendix.
6. Balance the tubes and centrifuge at 300 × g for 1 minute. Allow the centrifuge to come to a complete stop without disturbance.
7. If iodine was added previously, add saline to a clean microscope slide. If iodine was not added previously, add a drop of iodine to a clean slide.

8. Without removing the centrifuge tube, remove 1 or 2 drops from the surface of the suspension with a freshly flamed and cooled bacteriologic loop (5 to 7 mm in diameter) and add to the prepared slide.
9. Coverslip and systematically examine for parasites.

Formalin Ether or Ethyl Acetate Sedimentation Technique

Uses: Flotation of *Giardia* cysts

Procedure

1. Thoroughly mix feces in physiologic saline to obtain a volume of 12 ml.
2. Strain suspension through a tea strainer or 2 layers of cheesecloth to remove debris and pour into a 15-ml glass centrifuge tube.
3. Centrifuge at 300 × g for 2 minutes, then decant supernatant (about 1 to 2 ml of sediment should remain).
4. Add 10 ml of 10% formalin to the sediment and mix thoroughly.
5. Add 3 ml of reagent-grade ether or ethyl acetate, stopper the tube, and shake vigorously.
6. Centrifuge at 300 × g for 2 minutes.
7. Loosen the debris plug that forms at the top of the tube with an applicator stick and discard.
8. Decant supernatant.
9. Remove a drop or 2 of sediment (there should be adequate fluid to make a wet mount), place on a clean microscope slide, coverslip, and examine systematically for parasites.

A drop of iodine may be added to the slide to help visualize internal morphology.

APPENDIX 13. *Choice of Appropriate Antimicrobial Therapy*[a]

COMMON INFECTING ORGANISMS	FIRST CHOICE(S)	SECOND CHOICE(S)
Integumentary (see Chapter 5; for dosages, see Table 5–3 and Appendix 14)		
Superficial pyoderma		
Staphylococci	ery, meth, TS, clox, oxo	ceph, amp, mac, linc, chlor, clind
Dermatophilus	pen	amp
Deep pyoderma		
Gram-positive organisms		
Staphylococci	ery, TS, oxa, meth, clav, BRP	linc, chlor, clind, gent
Streptococci	amp, pen	ceph, ery, chlor, clav
Actinomyces	pen	dox, min, ceph, rif
Gram-negative organisms		
Proteus	amp, gent, chlor	ceph, quin, amg
Pseudomonas	carb, gent, tet	tob, poly, chlor, quin, carb + gent, 3ceph
Escherichia coli	clav, chlor, tet, gent	ceph, quin, TS
Other organisms		
Nocardia	sulf, amp	TS, dox, min, ery
Musculoskeletal (see Chapter 6; for dosages, see Table 6–2 and Appendix 14)		
Appendicular osteomyelitis		
Gram-positive organisms		
Staphylococci	ceph, meth, clox, clind, oxa, clav	pen + amg, clind, vanc
Streptococci	amp	pen, ery, ceph
Gram-negative organisms		
E. coli	amp	ceph, tob, quin, gent
Pasteurella	pen	ery, tet
Proteus	amp	ceph, quin, gent
Pseudomonas	carb, quin	gent, tob
Other organisms		
Anaerobes	clind, met	chlor
Vertebral osteomyelitis		
Gram-positive organisms		
Staphylococci	ceph, clind, meth, clox, BRP	pen, clav, gent
Streptococci	amp, clox, BRP	pen, clav, chlor
Corynebacteria	ery	pen
Actinomyces	pen, clind, amp, ery	tet, min, rif, chlor
Gram-negative organisms		
E. coli	amp	ceph, quin, tob, gent
Proteus	amp	ceph, quin, amg
Pseudomonas	quin	ticar, amg
Pasteurella	pen, amp	ery, tet
Brucella	min + gent	tet + strep
Other organisms		
Nocardia	TRS	TS, min, ami, 3ceph, amp, ery, imi
Anaerobes	clind, met	chlor
Otitis media-externa		
Gram-positive organisms		
Staphylococci	clav, clind, clox	ceph
Streptococci	amp, amox, clav	pen
Gram-negative organisms		
Proteus	amp	ceph, quin
Pseudomonas	carb	gent, tob, quin
Joint infections		
Staphylococci	clox, meth, quin	pen, ceph, 2ceph
Streptococci	amp	pen, clav
Mycoplasma	ery, tyl	tet, quin
Erysipelothrix	pen	
L-forms	tet	
Rickettsiae	tet	chlor, quin
Ehrlichia	tet	dox, min, chlor

Continued on following page

APPENDIX 13. *Choice of Appropriate Antimicrobial Therapy*[a] Continued

COMMON INFECTING ORGANISMS	FIRST CHOICE(S)	SECOND CHOICE(S)
Musculoskeletal		
Muscle Infections		
Staphylococci	meth, clox	pen, ceph
Clostridia	pen, clind	ceph, ery, tet
Toxoplasma	clind	PS
Cardiovascular		
(see Chapter 7; for dosages see Table 7–7 and Appendix 14)		
Sepsis		
Gram-positive organisms		
Staphylococci	BRP, ceph, dox	amg, vanc, 3ceph
Streptococci	pen	amox, amp, ceph, ery, chlor
Gram-negative organisms		
E. coli	pen or 3ceph + gent or tob, quin, TS	amg, carb, ticar, pip, imi, 3ceph
Pseudomonas	carb + gent or tob, quin, pip	amp, carb, ticar, 3ceph, imi
Other organisms		
Anaerobes	clind, pen	chlor, met
Respiratory		
(see Chapter 8; for dosages see Appendix 14)		
Upper tract: rhinitis		
Gram-positive organisms		
Streptococci	amp, pen	ceph, ery
Staphylococci	meth, clox	ceph, clind
Gram-negative organisms		
E. coli	amp	ceph, gent, tob, quin, TS
Pasteurella	pen	ery, tet
Bacteroides	met, chlor, clind	ceph, tet
Other organisms		
Mycoplasma	ery, tet	tyl
Chlamydia	tet	chlor, ery, quin
Tonsillitis-pharyngitis		
Gram-positive organisms		
Staphylococci	meth, clox	ceph
Streptococci	pen, amp	ceph, ery
Gram-negative organisms		
E. coli	amp	ceph, gent, tob
Klebsiella	ceph	gent, tob, TS, chlor
Pseudomonas	carb, gent, tob, quin	ceph, ticar, poly
Pasteurella	pen	ery, tet
Bordetella	tet, chlor	ery, amp, amg, TS
Other organisms		
Mycoplasma	ery	tet
Lower tract: pneumonia		
Gram-positive organisms		
Staphylococci	meth, clox	ceph, clind
Streptococci	pen, amp	ceph, ery
Corynebacteria	ery	pen
Gram-negative organisms		
Pseudomonas	carb, gent, ticar, quin, pip	carb + gent, imi
E. coli	amp, TS	ceph, gent, tob, quin, pip, imi
Klebsiella	amg, TS	ceph, chlor, quin, pip, imi
Bordetella	tet, ery	chlor
Pasteurella	amp	ery, tet
Enterobacter	amg	carb

APPENDIX 13. *Choice of Appropriate Antimicrobial Therapy*[a] Continued

COMMON INFECTING ORGANISMS	FIRST CHOICE(S)	SECOND CHOICE(S)

Respiratory

Pleural Infections
  Gram-negative organisms

Pasteurella	pen, amp	ery, tet
E. coli	amp	ceph, gent, tob
Pseudomonas	carb, quin	gent, tob, ticar
Proteus	amp	ceph
Klebsiella	ceph	gent, tob, chlor
Enterobacter	amg	carb
Bacteroides	met, clind, ery	ceph, tet
Fusobacterium	pen	met, chlor

  Other organisms

Actinomyces	pen	ery, tet
Nocardia	TS, sulf, dox	chlor, ery, min
Anaerobes	met, clind, pen	chlor, ticar, carb, clav, 3ceph

Gastrointestinal
(see Chapter 9; for dosages see Tables 9–2 and 9–5 and Appendix 14)

Oral cavity
  Gram-positive organisms

Staphylococci	meth, clox, BRP	ceph, clind
Streptococci	pen	ceph, ery
Corynebacteria	ery	pen, amp, amox

  Gram-negative organisms

Fusobacteria	pen	met, tet, ery, clind
Proteus	amp, chlor, carb	ceph, amg
Pseudomonas	gent, carb, quin	poly, tob, carb + gent
E. coli	amp, chlor	tet, amg, poly, ceph, quin
Pasteurella	pen	ery, tet, amp

  Other organisms

Anaerobes	met, clind	chlor, clav, pen

Small and large intestine
  Gram-positive organisms

Staphylococci	meth, clox, mac, clind, vanc	ceph, chlor, linc
Clostridia	pen	ery, ceph, tet

  Gram-negative organisms

Salmonella	chlor, quin	TS, poly, amox
E. coli	amp, gent, cef, TS	pen, ceph, amg, quin
Campylobacter	ery, tyl	amg, chlor, quin
Shigella	amp	amg, chlor, quin
Klebsiella	ceph, amg	

Intra-abdominal sepsis[b]
  Gram-positive organisms

Streptococci	amp	pen, ceph, ery, dox
Clostridia	pen, spect	ceph, carb, clind, tet

  Gram-negative organisms

Salmonella	chlor, quin	TS, poly, amox
E. coli	amp, gent, cef, TS	pen, ceph, amg, quin
Campylobacter	ery, tyl	amg, chlor, quin
Shigella	amp	chlor, quin
Klebsiella	ceph, amg	chlor, quin
Proteus	amp, chlor	ceph, amg
Pseudomonas	carb, gent, quin	poly, tob, carb + gent
Bacteroides	clind, met	chlor, tet

Hepatobiliary[c]
(see Chapter 10; for dosages see Table 10–1 and Appendix 14)

  Gram-positive organisms

Staphylococci	amp, amox, clind	ceph, tet
Clostridia	pen	met, chlor

Continued on following page

APPENDIX 13. *Choice of Appropriate Antimicrobial Therapy*[a] Continued

COMMON INFECTING ORGANISMS	FIRST CHOICE(S)	SECOND CHOICE(S)
Hepatobiliary[c]		
Gram-negative organisms		
E. coli	kan, gent, amp	ceph, chlor, quin
Klebsiella	ceph	gent, tob
Salmonella	kan, gent, quin	amp, amox, 3ceph
Pasteurella	amp, BRP	ery, tet
Enterobacter	kan, gent, tob	carb, ami
Bacteroides	pen, clind, met	ceph
Genitourinary		
(see Chapter 11; for dosages see Table 11–6 and Appendix 14)		
Cystitis and pyelonephritis		
Gram-positive organisms		
Staphylococci	amp, amox, TS, pen	ceph, chlor, BRP, nit
Streptococci	pen, amp, amox, TS	ceph, chlor, tet, ery, nit
Gram-negative organisms		
E. coli	sulf, TS, amp, amox, clav, nit	ceph, 3ceph, quin, BRP, carb, chlor, tet, gent, kan
Pseudomonas	tet, TS, carb, gent	poly, ceph, 3ceph, quin, carb + gent
Proteus	amp, TS, amox, pen, chlor	ceph, clav, 3ceph amg
Klebsiella	ceph, TS, amg	chlor, clav, 3ceph
Enterobacter	amg, nit, TS	carb, ceph, chlor
Prostatitis (acute)[d]		
Gram-positive organisms		
Staphylococci	meth, clox, mac	ceph, chlor, clind, olean, TS, linc
Streptococci	pen, amp	ceph, TS, ery
Gram-negative organisms		
E. coli	amp, TS	olean, ceph, chlor, tet, carb, quin, amg
Proteus	amp, chlor	ceph, carb, quin, sulf
Pseudomonas	quin, carb, amg	poly, carb + gent, chlor
Female reproductive system (metritis, vaginitis)		
Gram-positive organisms		
Streptococci	pen, amp	ceph, ery
Staphylococci	clav, TS, ceph	
Gram-negative organisms		
Brucella canis	min + gent, dox + gent	tet + strep
Proteus	amp, chlor, clav	ceph, amg
E. coli	tet, chlor, amp, TS, clav	amg, quin, ceph, poly
Male reproductive system (orchitis, epididymitis)		
Gram-positive organisms		
Streptococci	amp, amox, chlor, TS	
Staphylococci	meth, clox, clav, TS, mac	ceph, chlor, linc
Gram-negative organisms		
B. canis	min + gent	tet + strep
E. coli	amp, chlor, tet, TS	amg, ceph, poly
Proteus	amp, chlor	ceph, TS, quin, amg
Klebsiella or Enterobacter	ceph, amg	chlor, quin
Pseudomonas	tet, carb, amg	quin, carb + gent, chlor
Central Nervous System		
(see Chapter 12; for dosages see Table 12–4 and Appendix 14)		
Meningoencephalitis		
Gram-positive organisms		
Staphylococci		
Coagulase negative	amp, TS	pen, ceph
Coagulase positive	meth, clox, clav, TS	ceph, 3ceph, vanc, chlor
Streptococci	amp	pen, ceph, ery
Actinomyces	amp	min

APPENDIX 13. *Choice of Appropriate Antimicrobial Therapy*[a] Continued

COMMON INFECTING ORGANISMS	FIRST CHOICE(S)	SECOND CHOICE(S)
Central Nervous System		
Gram-negative organisms		
E. coli	amp	TS, chlor, mox
Pseudomonas	carb, quin	chlor, gent,[e] 3ceph, pip
Pasteurella	amp, pen	tet, ery, TS
Salmonella	chlor, TS	amp, mox, quin
B. canis	min + gent	tet + strep
Other organisms		
Anaerobes	pen, amp, met	clind, chlor, carb
Leptospira	pen	ery, tet
Ehrlichia	tet	min, dox
Rickettsia	tet	min, chlor
Ocular		
(see Chapter 13; for dosages see Table 13–4 and Appendix 14)		
Conjunctivitis/keratitis[f]		
Gram-positive organisms		
Staphylococci	amp, chlor	NBP, ery
Streptococci	pen	ceph, ery
Gram-negative organisms		
E. coli	chlor	ceph, gent, NBP
Proteus	chlor	gent, ceph, amp
Pseudomonas	gent, tet	
Salmonella	chlor	gent
Intraocular		
Gram-positive organisms		
Staphylococci	meth, clox	ceph, clav, clind
Streptococci	pen	ceph, ery
Gram-negative organisms		
B. canis	min + gent	tet + strep
Salmonella	chlor, TS	amp, quin
E. coli	amp, chlor	ceph, quin, TS, tob, gent
Other organisms		
Leptospira	pen, ery, tet	

[a]First choices are based on lower cost and attempt to reserve more potent antimicrobials for resistant strains of bacteria. Because drug resistance may develop, antimicrobial susceptibility testing should be performed when possible.

amg = aminoglycoside
ami = amikacin
amox = amoxicillin
amp = ampicillin
BRP = β-lactamase-resistant penicillin
carb = carbenicillin
cef = cefamandole
ceph = 1st generation cephalosporins
2ceph = 2nd generation cephalosporins
3ceph = 3rd generation cephalosporins
chlor = chloramphenicol
clav = clavulanate-amoxicillin
clind = clindamycin
clox = cloxacillin
dox = doxycycline
ery = erythromycin
gent = gentamicin
imi = imipenem-cilastatin
kan = kanamycin
linc = lincomycin
mac = macrolide
met = metronidazole

meth = methicillin
min = minocycline
mox = moxalactam
NBP = neomycin-bacitracin-polymyxin
nit = nitrofurantoin
olean = oleandomycin
oxa = oxacillin
pen = penicillin
pip = piperacillin
PS = pyrimethamine-sulfonamide
quin = quinolone
rif = rifampin
spect = spectinomycin
strep = streptomycin
sulf = sulfonamide
tet = tetracycline
ticar = ticarcillin
tob = tobramycin
TRS = trisulfapyrimidines
TS = trimethoprim-sulfonamide
tyl = tylosin
vanc = vancomycin

[b]Combination antimicrobials against anaerobic and aerobic organisms are desirable.
[c]The presence of icterus contraindicates use of biliary-excreted drugs such as tet, linc, ery, TS, chlor, dox, rif, clind.
[d]For use in chronic cases: ery, chlor, dox, TS, olean.
[e]Intrathecal administration of gent is needed to achieve high concentrations in CSF.
[f]Topical administration.

APPENDIX 14. Dosages of Antimicrobial Drugs*[,a]

GENERIC DRUG	SPECIES	DOSE LEVEL	DOSE[b] (mg/kg)	ROUTE	INTERVAL[c] (hrs)	FOOTNOTES AND TABLES
AMIKACIN	D	L	5.0	SC	8–12	[d,e]11–6, 43–4
AMIKACIN	B	I	5.0–7.5	IV, IM, SC	8	[d]
AMIKACIN	C	H	5.0–10.0	IV, IM, SC	8–12	[d,f]51–5, 53–2
AMOXICILLIN	B	L	15.0–20.0	PO	8–12	[e]9–2, 11–6, 43–1, 45–2, 50–1, 54–1
AMOXICILLIN	D	L	11.0	PO	8	[e]10–1, 11–6
AMOXICILLIN	B	I	20.0–25.0	IV, IM, SC, PO	8	49–5
AMOXICILLIN	B	H	30.0–50.0	IV, IM, SC, PO	8	[f]
AMOXICILLIN-CLAVULANATE	B	I	11.0–22.0	PO	8	[g]5–3, 43–1
AMPHOTERICIN B	D	M	0.4–0.5	IV	30 days	[h,i]68–2
AMPHOTERICIN B	D	L	0.2–0.4	IV	48	[d,i]65–1, 66–1, 67–3, 75–1
AMPHOTERICIN B	D	H	0.4–0.5	IV	48–72	[d,i,j]63–2, 68–2
AMPHOTERICIN B	C	L	0.2–0.3	IV	48	[d,i,k]63–2, 65–1, 66–1, 75–1
AMPHOTERICIN B	C	H	0.3–0.5	IV	48	[d,i]12–4, 67–3
AMPICILLIN	B	L	10.0–20.0	IV, IM, SC	8	[e]10–1, 43–1, 45–2
AMPICILLIN	B	I	20.0–50.0	IV, IM, SC, PO	8	6–2, 11–6, 12–4, 46–1, 53–1, 53–2, 55–2
AMPICILLIN	B	H	20.0–40.0	IV	6	[f]7–7, 44–1, 53–1
AMPICILLIN-SULBACTAM	P	I	20.0	IV, IM	6–8	[g]
AMPROLIUM	D	L	110.0–200.0 mg total	PO	24	[l]87–2
AMPROLIUM	D	H	300.0–400.0 mg total	PO	24	[l,m]87–2
AMPROLIUM	C	L	60.0–100 mg total	PO	24	[l]87–2
AZLOCILLIN	P	I	75.0	IV	6–8	[n]
BACAMPICILLIN	P	I	50.0	PO	12	[o]
BENZNIDAZOLE	D	I	5.0	PO	24	78–1
CARBENICILLIN	B	L	10.0–30.0	IV, IM	4–8	[p]12–4, 43–1
CARBENICILLIN	B	I	20.0–30.0	PO	8	[e]
CARBENICILLIN	B	H	30.0–100.0	IV, IM	6–8	[f]
CARBUTAMIDE	H	I	50.0	IM	12	89–2
CEFACLOR	P	L	6.6	PO	8	43–3
CEFACLOR	P	H	13.3	PO	8	[f,m]
CEFADROXIL	B	I	22.0	PO	12	[e]5–3, 43–3
CEFAMANDOLE	P	L	20.0	IV	6	[i]43–3
CEFAMANDOLE	P	I	15.0–30.0	IM	8	[i]
CEFAMANDOLE	P	H	10.0–15.0	IV	4	[i]
CEFAZOLIN	P	L	8.3	IV, IM	8	43–3
CEFAZOLIN	P	I	15.0	IV, IM	8–12	
CEFAZOLIN	P	H	33.3	IV, IM	8	
CEFOPERAZONE	P	L	30.0	IM	6	43–3
CEFOPERAZONE	P	H	30.0	IV	4	[f]
CEFOTAXIME	D	I	20.0–80.0	IV, IM, SC	8	43–4, 53–2
CEFOTAXIME	P	I	6.0–40.0	IV, IM	4–6	[f,p]12–4
CEFOXITIN	P	L	25.0	IV, IM	6–8	49–5
CEFOXITIN	P	H	30.0–40.0	IV, IM	6	
CEFTAZIDIME	B	I	25.0	IM, SC	8–12	43–3
CEFTIOFUR	B	L	1.0	IM, SC	12–24	[e]
CEFTRIAXONE	P	I	20.0	IV, SC	12	46–1
CEPHALEXIN	B	L	20.0–40.0	PO	8–12	5–3, 43–3, 49–5, 50–1, 56–2
CEPHALEXIN	B	H	40.0–60.0	PO	8	[f,p]12–4
CEPHALOTHIN	B	L	15.0–25.0	IV, IM, SC	8	7–7
CEPHALOTHIN	B	H	25.0–40.0	IV, IM, SC	6–8	[f]7–7, 44–1
CEPHAPIRIN	B	L	20.0–30.0	IV, IM, SC	8	

---

*For additional information, also see: ophthalmic drugs: Table 13–4; antiviral drugs: Table 15–1; antifungal drugs: Table 63–2; antiprotozoal drugs: Table 77–2.

926

GENERIC DRUG	SPECIES	DOSE LEVEL	DOSE[b] (mg/kg)	ROUTE	INTERVAL[c] (hrs)	FOOTNOTES AND TABLES
CEPHAPIRIN	B	H	30.0–40.0	IV, IM, SC	6–8	[f,p,q]9–2, 12–4
CEPHRADINE	B	L	12.0	PO	6	43–3
CEPHRADINE	B	I	20.0–40.0	IV, IM, PO	8	6–2
CEPHRADINE	B	H	6.0–25.0	IV, IM	6–8	[f]
CHLORAMPHENICOL	D	L	33.0	PO	8	[e]11–6
CHLORAMPHENICOL	B	I	15.0–25.0	IV, IM, SC, PO	6–8	[q]7–7, 9–2, 37–2, 38–3, 39–1, 49–5, 50–1
CHLORAMPHENICOL	D	H	25.0–50.0	IV, IM, SC, PO	6–8	[f,p,r]5–3, 6–2, 12–4, 44–1, 53–1, 56–2, 59–1
CHLORAMPHENICOL	C	H	50.0	IV, IM, SC	12	
CHLORTETRACYCLINE	B	I	20.0	PO	8	
CIPROFLOXACIN	B	L	5.0–11.0	PO	12	[s]43–10
CIPROFLOXACIN	D	H	10.0–15.0	PO	12	[t]7–7, 43–10
CLINDAMYCIN	B	L	5.0–10.0	IV, IM, PO	12	6–2, 9–2, 48–2, 49–5, 53–1, 55–2
CLINDAMYCIN	B	L	5.0–11.0	IV, IM, PO	8	[u]48–2
CLINDAMYCIN	D	H	10.0–20.0	IM, SC, PO	12	[v]77–2, 86–1
CLINDAMYCIN	D	H	3.0–13.0	IV, IM, PO	8	[f,v]86–1
CLINDAMYCIN	C	I	8.0–17.0	IV, IM, PO	8	[f,v]86–1
CLINDAMYCIN	C	H	50.0	PO	24	[w]86–1
CLINDAMYCIN	C	H	12.5–25.0	PO, IM, IV	12	[f,v]86–1
CLOFAZAMINE	C	I	2.0–8.0	PO	24	51–5
CLOXICILLIN	B	I	10.0–15.0	IV, IM, PO	6	6–2, 43–1
COLISTIMETHATE SODIUM	P	I	1.0–1.5	IV, IM	8	[d]
DAPSONE	D	L	0.3–0.6	PO	8–12	[h]51–5
DAPSONE	B	I	1.1	PO	6–8	[x]51–5
DAPSONE	C	H	12.5–25.0 mg total	PO	12–24	[y]51–5
DEMECLOCYCLINE	P	I	6.0–12.0	PO	6–12	43–6
DICLOXICILLIN	B	L	10.0–20.0	PO	8	43–1
DICLOXICILLIN	B	H	50.0	PO	8	[f]
DIHYDROSTREPTOMYCIN	B	L	5.0–10.0	IM, SC	12	[d]43–4, 51–4, 52–2
DIHYDROSTREPTOMYCIN	B	I	7.5	IM, SC	8–12	[d]
DIHYDROSTREPTOMYCIN	B	H	12.5	IM, SC	8–12	[d]45–2
DIHYDROSTREPTOMYCIN	D		10.0–20.0	PO	6	[z]
DIIODOHYDROXYQUIN	P	I	10.0	PO	8	[aa]
DIMINAZENE ACETURATE	B	I	2.0–3.5	IM	once	77–2, 80–1, 83–1
DOXYCYCLINE	B	L	5.0–10.0	IV, PO	12	45–2, 51–5, 55–2
DOXYCYCLINE	B	H	15.0–20.0	PO	12	37–3, 38–3, 43–6, 52–2
ENILCONAZOLE	D	I	20.0	topical	12	71–2
ENROFLOXACIN	B	L	2.5–5.0	PO	12	[s]43–10
ENROFLOXACIN	B	H	5.0–15.0	PO	12	[t]7–7, 43–10
ERYTHROMYCIN	D	L	2.0–4.0	IM, SC	12–24	
ERYTHROMYCIN	B	I	8.0–20.0	PO	8–12	46–1, 50–1, 53–2, 56–2
ERYTHROMYCIN	B	H	10.0–20.0	PO	8	5–3, 56–5
ETHAMBUTOL	P	I	15.0	PO	24	51–4
FLUCONAZOLE	B	I	2.5–5.0	PO	12	63–2, 66–1, 71–2
FLUCYTOSINE	B	I	30.0–50.0	PO	6–8	12–4, 63–2, 67–3
FLUCYTOSINE	B	H	50.0–75.0	PO	8	63–2, 67–3
FLUCYTOSINE	C	L	75.0	PO	12	67–3
FRAMYCETIN	P	I	20.0	PO	6	[z]
FURAZOLIDONE	B	I	2.2	PO	8	[r]43–8
FURAZOLIDONE	B	I	8.0–10.0	PO	12–24	77–2, 87–2
FURAZOLIDONE	C	I	4.0	PO	12	[bb]84–2
GENTAMICIN	B	L	2.0	IM, SC	12	[d,r,s]6–2, 10–1, 43–4, 50–1, 51–5, 59–1
GENTAMICIN	B	I	2.0	IV, IM, SC	6–8	[d,f,r,t]4–2, 11–6, 44–1, 52–2, 54–1
GENTAMICIN	B	H	3.0–4.0	IV, IM, SC	8	[d,r,f]7–7, 44–1
GRISEOFULVIN (microsized)	B	I	25.0–60.0	PO	12	[cc]63–2, 64–6
GRISEOFULVIN (ultramicrosized)	B	I	5.0–15.0	PO	12–24	[dd]63–2, 64–6
HETACILLIN	B	L	10.0–20.0	PO	8–12	[e]43–1
HETACILLIN	B	H	20.0–40.0	PO	8	[f]11–6
HETACILLIN	C	L	50.0 mg total	PO	8–12	
IMIDOCARB DIPROPIONATE	D	I	2.0–6.0	IM	once	37–2, 77–2, 83–1
IMIPENEM-CILASTATIN	B	I	2.0–5.0	IV	8	53–2

Continued on following page

APPENDIX 14. Dosages of Antimicrobial Drugs*,a Continued

GENERIC DRUG	SPECIES	DOSE LEVEL	DOSE[b] (mg/kg)	ROUTE	INTERVAL[c] (hrs)	FOOTNOTES AND TABLES
IPRONIDAZOLE	D	I	126.0 mg/l water	PO	ad lib	bb84–2
ISONIAZID	P	I	10.0–20.0	PO	24	ee51–4
ITRACONAZOLE	B	L	5.0	PO	12–24	63–2, 65–1, 66–1
ITRACONAZOLE	B	I	5.0–10.0	PO	12	63–2, 65–1, 67–3, 71–2, 72–1, 75–1
ITRACONAZOLE	C	H	20.0	PO	24	67–3
KANAMYCIN	D	I	4.0	SC	12	d,e11–6, 43–4
KANAMYCIN	B	L	4.0	IV, IM, SC	8	d,e
KANAMYCIN	B	I	5.0–7.5	IM, SC	12	d51–5, 59–1
KANAMYCIN	B	H	4.0–6.0	IM, SC	6	d,f
KANAMYCIN	B	I	10.0–12.0	PO	6	d,z
KETOCONAZOLE	B	I	10.0–30.0	PO	24	63–2, 64–6, 67–3
KETOCONAZOLE	B	H	5.0–15.0	PO	12	9–2, 63–2, 65–1, 67–3, 71–2, 72–1, 75–1
KETOCONAZOLE	D	M	2.0–5.0	PO	24	h68–2
KETOCONAZOLE	D	L	5.0–10.0	PO	8–12	68–2
KETOCONAZOLE	D	I	5.0–30.0	PO	12–24	69–1, 71–2
KETOCONAZOLE	D	H	15.0–20.0	PO	12	p65–1
KETOCONAZOLE	C	L	5.0–10.0	PO	12–24	65–1, 66–1, 69–1
KETOCONAZOLE	C	I	10.0–15.0	PO	24–48	63–2
KETOCONAZOLE	C	H	50.0–100.0 mg total	PO	12–48	66–1, 68–2, 72–1
LINCOMYCIN	D	L	20.0	PO	12	5–3, 56–5
LINCOMYCIN	D	L	10.0	IV, IM	12	
LINCOMYCIN	D	H	15.0	PO	8	
MEGLUMINE ANTIMONIATE	D	I	50.0–100.0	IV, IM, SC	24	ff77–2, 79–4
METHENAMINE MANDELATE	B	I	10.0	PO	6–12	
METHICILLIN	D	L	25.0–40.0	IM	6	
METRONIDAZOLE	B	I	22.0–50.0	PO	24	bb,gg9–5
METRONIDAZOLE	B	I	8.0–25.0	PO	12	bb,gg9–2, 9–5, 77–2
METRONIDAZOLE	B	I	7.5–15.0	PO	8	r,gg7–7, 9–2, 9–5, 48–2, 49–5, 50–1
METRONIDAZOLE	B	I	10.0–15.0	IV, PO	8–12	r,gg7–7, 9–2, 10–1, 12–4, 47–1, 49–5, 55–2
MEZLOCILLIN	P	I	75.0	IV, IM	8	hh
MINOCYCLINE	B	I	5.0–15.0	PO	12	6–2, 37–3, 38–3, 53–1, 53–2
MINOCYCLINE	D	H	12.5	PO	12	ii52–2
MINOCYCLINE	D	H	25.0	PO	24	ii52–2
MONENSIN	C	L	0.02 (%)	by wt, in food	24	86–1
MOXALACTAM	P	I	50.0	IV, IM	6–8	43–3
NAFCILLIN	P	I	10.0–25.0	IV, IM, PO	6	hh43–1
NAFCILLIN	P	H	25.0–50.0	IV	4–6	hh
NALIDIXIC ACID	D	I	18.0	PO	6	jj
NEOMYCIN	B	I	2.5–10.0	PO	6–12	z43–4
NETILMICIN	P	I	1.0–2.0	IM, SC	8	
NIFURTIMOX	P	I	8.0–10.0	PO	24	77–2
NIFURTIMOX	D	I	2.0–7.0	PO	6–12	78–1
NITROFURANTOIN	D	I	4.4	PO	8	e11–6, 43–8
NORFLOXACIN	D	I	5.0–11.0	PO	12	s43–10
NORFLOXACIN	D	H	22.0	PO	12	t43–10
NOVOBIOCIN	D	I	10.0	PO	8	
ORMETOPRIM-SULFONAMIDE	D	I	66.0	PO	24	87–2
OXACILLIN	B	I	15.0–25.0	PO	6–8	5–3, 43–1
OXACILLIN	B	H	8.8–20.0	IV, IM	4–6	p12–4
OXYTETRACYCLINE	B	I	22.0	PO	8	43–6
OXYTETRACYCLINE	B	I	7.0–12.0	IV, IM	12	kk36–1
OXYTETRACYCLINE (REPOSITOL)	D	I	20.0	IM	1 week	kk52–2
PAROMOMYCIN	B	I	10.0	PO	8	n,z77–2
PARVAQUONE	C	I	10.0–30.0	IM	24	82–1
PENICILLIN G (AQUEOUS)	B	I	20.0–40.0 × 1000 units	IV, IM	4–6	f,q,p,hh7–7, 9–2, 12–4, 46–1, 47–1, 48–2
PENICILLIN G (AQUEOUS)	B	I	40.0–100.0 × 1000 units	IV, IM	6	hh43–1, 48–2, 49–5, 53–1

APPENDIX 14. *Dosages of Antimicrobial Drugs**,a Continued

GENERIC DRUG	SPECIES	DOSE LEVEL	DOSE[b] (mg/kg)	ROUTE	INTERVAL[c] (hrs)	FOOTNOTES AND TABLES
PENICILLIN G (BENZATHINE)	B	I	40.0 × 1000 units	IM	120	43–1
PENICILLIN G (PROC. + BENZ.)	B	I	13.0–30.0 × 1000 units	IM, SC	48	
PENICILLIN G (PROCAINE)	B	I	10.0–30.0 × 1000 units	IM, SC	12	47–1, 49–5, 56–2
PENICILLIN G (PROCAINE)	B	H	30.0–50.0 × 1000 U/kg	IM, SC	12	45–2, 48–2, 53–1, 55–2
PENICILLIN G (TABLETS)	D	H	37.0 × 1000 U/kg	PO	8	[e]11–6
PENICILLIN G (TABLETS)	B	H	50.0–165.0 × 1000 units	PO	6–8	[f]43–1, 53–1
PENICILLIN V	B	I	20.0–30.0	PO	8	11–6, 55–2, 56–2
PENICILLIN V	B	H	30.0–50.0	PO	6–8	[f]6–2, 53–1
PENTAMIDINE ISETHIONATE	P	I	4.0	IV, IM	24	[d,hh,kk]89–2
PHENAMIDINE ISETHIONATE	B	I	15.0	SC	24	77–2, 83–1
PHTHALYSULFATHIAZOLE	B	I	100.0	PO	12	[z]43–9
PIPERACILLIN	B	I	50.0–70.0	IV, IM	6–8	[f]43–1
PIPERACILLIN	B	H	50.0	IV, IM	4	f
POLYMYXIN E (COLISTIN)	B	I	1.5–5.0	PO	8	d,z
POTASSIUM IODIDE	C	I	20.0	PO	12	69–1
POTASSIUM IODIDE	D	I	40.0	PO	8	69–1
PRIMAQUINE PHOSPHATE	B	I	8.0–15.0 mg base tot	IM	24	n
PYRAZINAMIDE	B	I	15.0–40.0	PO	24	[jj]51–4
PYRIMETHAMINE (+SULFONAMIDE)	B	I	0.5–1.0	PO	24	[r,ll]77–2
PYRIMETHAMINE (+SULFONAMIDE)	C	L	0.3–0.5	PO	12	[mm]86–1
PYRIMETHAMINE (+SULFONAMIDE)	C	I	2.0	PO	24	[nn]86–1
QUINACRINE HYDROCHLORIDE	D	I	50.0–100.0 mg total	PO	8–12	[r]84–2
QUINACRINE HYDROCHLORIDE	D	L	6.0–11.0	PO	12–24	[bb]77–2, 84–2, 87–2
RIFAMPIN	B	I	10.0–20.0	PO	12	[jj]51–4, 51–5, 53–1
SISOMICIN	P	L	1.0	IM, SC	8	43–4
SISOMICIN	P	H	2.0	IM, SC	8	
SODIUM IODIDE	D	I	20.0–40.0	PO	8–12	63–2
SODIUM IODIDE	C	I	20.0	PO	24	63–2
SODIUM STIBOGLUCONATE	D	I	30.0–50.0	IV, SC	24	[ff]77–2, 79–4
SODIUM STIBOGLUCONATE	D	H	50.0–100.0	IV, IM	24	[ff]79–4
SPECTINOMYCIN	B	I	20.0	PO	12	f,z
SPECTINOMYCIN	B	I	5.0–12.0	IM	12	f
SPIRAMYCIN	B	I	8.0–10.0	PO	12	77–2
SPIRAMYCIN	P	I	50.0–100.0	PO	24	77–2, 87–2, 88–1
STREPTOMYCIN	B	I	20.0	PO	6	[d,z]43–4
STREPTOMYCIN	B	L	7.5	IM, SC	12	d,hh
STREPTOMYCIN	B	I	10.0–20.0	IM, SC	12	[d]6–2
STREPTOMYCIN	B	H	11.0	IM, SC	8	f,d
STREPTOMYCIN	C	I	5.0	IM, SC	12	[d]59–1
SULFADIAZINE	B	L	50.0–66.0	IV, PO	12	[oo]43–9, 53–2
SULFADIAZINE	D	I	30.0	IV, PO	6	oo
SULFADIAZINE	D	H	110.0	PO	12	oo
SULFADIMETHOXINE	B	I	25.0	IV, IM, SC, PO	12–24	[bb]43–9, 87–2
SULFADIMETHOXINE	B	I	50.0–60.0	PO	24	[bb]87–2
SULFAGUANIDINE	B	I	100.0–200.0	PO	8	[bb]43–9, 87–2
SULFAMETHAZINE	B	I	50.0–55.0	IV, PO	8–12	
SULFAMETHOXAZOLE	B	I	30.0	PO	12	[oo]43–9
SULFASALAZINE	D	I	12.5	PO	6	[z]9–5, 43–9
SULFASALAZINE	D	H	10.0–25.0	PO	8	[z]9–5
SULFASALAZINE	C	L	5.0–10.0	PO	8	[z]9–5
SULFASALAZINE	C	H	25.0	PO	24	[z]9–5
SULFISOXAZOLE	B	I	40.0–50.0	PO	8–12	[e]11–6, 43–9
SULFISOXAZOLE	D	H	22.0	PO	8	[e]11–6, 43–6, 53–2
TETRACYCLINE	B	I	22.0	PO	8	6–2, 37–3, 38–3, 39–1, 45–2, 46–1, 59–1, 75–1

Continued on following page

APPENDIX 14. *Dosages of Antimicrobial Drugs**,a Continued

GENERIC DRUG	SPECIES	DOSE LEVEL	DOSE[b] (mg/kg)	ROUTE	INTERVAL[c] (hrs)	FOOTNOTES AND TABLES
TETRACYCLINE	B	H	25.0–50.0	PO	6–8	[f]48–2, 50–1
TETRACYCLINE	D	H	20.0–40.0	PO	12–24	9–2
TETRACYCLINE	D	H	18.0	PO	8	[e]11–6
THIABENDAZOLE	D	I	20.0	PO	12	9–5, 71–2
THIACETARSAMIDE SODIUM	B	I	2.2	IV	24	39–1
THIACETARSAMIDE SODIUM	C	I	2.2	IV	12	82–1
TICARCILLIN	B	I	40.0–75.0	IV, IM	6–8	[f]43–1
TICARCILLIN-CLAVULANATE	B	L	30.0–50.0	IV	6–8	f,g
TINIDAZOLE	D	I	44.0	PO	24	[bb]84–2
TOBRAMYCIN	D	I	1.0	SC	8	[e]11–6, 43–4
TOBRAMYCIN	P	I	1.0–2.0	IV, IM, SC	8	e
TOLTRAZURIL	B	I	10.0	PO	24	[l,bb]77–2, 87–2
TRIMETHOPRIM- SULFONAMIDE	D	I	13.0	PO	12	[e,pp]5–3, 11–6, 43–9, 50–1, 51–5
TRIMETHOPRIM- SULFONAMIDE	B	L	15.0–30.0	PO	24	[d,pp]77–2, 87–2
TRIMETHOPRIM- SULFONAMIDE	B	I	15.0–30.0	PO, SC, IV	12	[f,n,pp]7–7, 12–4, 59–1
TRIMETHOPRIM- SULFONAMIDE	D	H	30.0–60.0	PO	24	[pp,qq]77–2, 87–2
TRIMETHOPRIM- SULFONAMIDE	P	H	15.0	PO	6–8	[pp,qq]7–7, 12–4, 89–2
TRISULFAPYRAMIDINE (TRI.SULF.)	B	I	50.0	IV, PO	12	[f]43–9, 53–2
TRYPAN BLUE	B	I	4.0	IV	once	[rr]77–2, 83–1
TYLOSIN	B	L	5.0–10.0	PO	8–12	50–1
TYLOSIN	B	I	5.0–15.0	IV, IM	6–8	f
TYLOSIN	D	H	10.0–25.0	PO	8	9–5
VANCOMYCIN	B	I	5.0–12.0	PO	6	
VANCOMYCIN	B	I	20.0	IV	12	

[a]Abbreviations

    Species: D = dog, B = dog and cat, C = cat, P = people; dose level: L = low, I = intermediate, H = high, M = maintenance
    Route: SC = subcutaneous, IV = intravenous, IM = intramuscular, PO = oral

[b]Dose per administration at specified interval, expressed as mg/kg unless otherwise stated.

[c]Interval of administration expressed in hours unless otherwise stated.

[d]Nephrotoxic potential; monitor renal function periodically with serum urea nitrogen and complete urinalysis.

[e]Low dose primarily effective for urinary tract infections.

[f]High dose effective for severe multisystemic or hard-to-reach infections.

[g]Dosage based on penicillin derivative fraction of the drug.

[h]Maintenance dose restricted for long-term therapy once infection has been controlled.

[i]Reduce dose or avoid use of drug in animals with renal insufficiency.

[j]Canine maximum total dose of 8 to 11 mg/kg as needed to achieve remission. See also cited antifungal tables. Dose can be reduced in combination with azole derivatives.

[k]Feline maximum total dose of 4 mg/kg as needed to achieve remission. See also cited antifungal tables. Dose can be reduced in combination with azole derivatives.

[l]Treat for 7 to 10 days, administering medication in food.

[m]Dosage for particularly resistant infections.

[n]Do not give longer than 2 weeks without reevaluation of patient.

[o]Better absorbed than ampicillin after oral administration.

[p]High dose for CNS infections.

[q]Only one dose of the prescribed regimen is given just before or during anesthesia for dental prophylaxis. See also Table 9–2.

[r]Do not give longer than 1 week without reevaluation of patient.

[s]Lower dosage for urinary tract and some soft tissue infections.

[t]Higher dosage for multisystemic or resistant skin or soft tissue infections.

[u]Dosage for anaerobic infections.

[v]Dosage for treatment of toxoplasmosis.

[w]Dosage for maintenance to control oocyst shedding by cats.

[x]Loading or induction dose for initial therapy.

[y]Do not give dose longer than 2 weeks. Cat dose is typically 50 mg total per administration. Maximum daily dose per cat is 200 mg.

[z]Not absorbed with intact intestinal mucosa. Use this dose and route for enteric infections only.

[aa]Maximum daily dose is 2 g.

[bb]Dose for treatment of intestinal protozoa.

[cc]Treat for a minimum of 4 to 6 weeks. Dose is lower than that because of microsize.

[dd]Treat for a minimum of 4 to 6 weeks. Dose is very low because of ultramicrosize.

[ee]Maximum dose is 300 mg/day.

[ff]Dose must be calculated on the basis of antimony in compound. Supplied preparations usually contain 30% antimony by weight.

APPENDIX 14.   Dosages of Antimicrobial Drugs*,ª Continued

ggNeurotoxicity is possible at higher dosages (>30 mg/kg/day). See discussion under metronidazole, Chapter 43.

hhInfuse drug given IV slowly over 10 to 15 minutes minimum.

iiDose for treatment of brucellosis. See cited table. A tetracycline is combined with an aminoglycoside.

jjHepatotoxicity may develop.

kkIM administration is painful and irritating. Use deep IM injection.

llDose expressed as pyrimethamine alone. Add sulfonamide per administration of 60 mg/kg. Watch for signs of CNS depression or bone marrow toxicity. See Chapters 43, 77, and 86 for further information on these drugs.

mmDose expressed as pyrimethamine alone. Add sulfonamide per administration of 30 mg/kg. Watch for signs of CNS depression or bone marrow toxicity. See Chapters 43, 77, and 86 for further information on these drugs.

nnDose for prevention of oocyst shedding. Add sulfonamide per administration of 100 mg/kg.

ooSulfonamide dose only: see trimethoprim-sulfonamide for combined dosage formulation.

ppDose expressed as total trimethoprim and sulfonamide in a 1:5 ratio.

qqHigh dosages may be associated with sulfonamide urolithiasis in dogs and nephrotoxicity in cats. See trimethoprim-sulfonamide, Chapters 5 and 43.

rrUsually made as a 1% to 2% sterile solution filtered for IV inoculation.

*For additional information, also see: ophthalmic drugs: Table 13–4; antiviral drugs: Table 15–1; antifungal drugs: Table 63–2; antiprotozoal drugs: Table 77–2.

INDEX

Note: Page numbers in *italics* refer to illustrations; page numbers followed by (t) refer to tables.